Pediatric Interventional Radiology

Pediatric Interventional Radiology

Edited by

Richard Towbin MD
Professor and Radiologist-in-Chief, Department of Radiology, Phoenix Children's Hospital, Phoenix;
Professor of Radiology, Mayo Clinic College of Medicine; and
Professor, Department of Child Health, University of Arizona, Phoenix College of Medicine, Phoenix, AZ, USA.

Kevin M. Baskin MD
Former Assistant Professor, Department of Radiology, University of Pittsburgh Medical Center, and former Chief of Pediatric Interventional Radiology, Children's Hospital of Pittsburgh, Pittsburgh, PA, USA

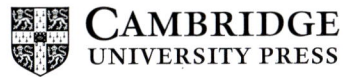

CAMBRIDGE
UNIVERSITY PRESS

University Printing House, Cambridge CB2 8BS, United Kingdom

Cambridge University Press is part of the University of Cambridge.

It furthers the University's mission by disseminating knowledge in the pursuit of education, learning and research at the highest international levels of excellence.

www.cambridge.org
Information on this title: www.cambridge.org/9781107042629

© Cambridge University Press 2015

This publication is in copyright. Subject to statutory exception and to the provisions of relevant collective licensing agreements, no reproduction of any part may take place without the written permission of Cambridge University Press.

First published 2015

Printed in the United Kingdom by Bell and Bain Ltd

A catalog record for this publication is available from the British Library

Library of Congress Cataloging in Publication data
Pediatric interventional radiology (Towbin)
Pediatric interventional radiology / edited by Richard Towbin, Kevin M. Baskin.
   p.; cm.
Includes index.
ISBN 978-1-107-04262-9 (Hardback)
I. Towbin, Richard B., editor. II. Baskin, Kevin, M., editor. III. Title.
[DNLM: 1. Radiography, Interventional–methods. 2. Adolescent.
3. Child. 4. Infant. WN 200]
RC78
616.07′572–dc23   2014037662

ISBN 978-1-107-04262-9 Hardback

Cambridge University Press has no responsibility for the persistence or accuracy of URLs for external or third-party internet websites referred to in this publication, and does not guarantee that any content on such websites is, or will remain, accurate or appropriate.

. . . .

Every effort has been made in preparing this book to provide accurate and up-to-date information which is in accord with accepted standards and practice at the time of publication. Although case histories are drawn from actual cases, every effort has been made to disguise the identities of the individuals involved.

Nevertheless, the authors, editors and publishers can make no warranties that the information contained herein is totally free from error, not least because clinical standards are constantly changing through research and regulation. The authors, editors and publishers therefore disclaim all liability for direct or consequential damages resulting from the use of material contained in this book. Readers are strongly advised to pay careful attention to information provided by the manufacturer of any drugs or equipment that they plan to use.

Contents

List of contributors vi
Acknowledgements vii

1 **Introduction** 1
Richard Towbin, Kevin M. Baskin, David Aria and Robin Kaye

2 **Central venous access** 22
Kevin M. Baskin and Richard Towbin

3 **Thoracic interventions** 97
Richard Towbin, Kevin M. Baskin, David Aria and Carrie Schaefer

4 **Abdominopelvic interventions** 151
Kevin M. Baskin and Richard Towbin

5 **Hepatobiliary interventions** 250
Kevin M. Baskin, Richard Towbin, David Aria and Robin Kaye

6 **Genitourinary interventions** 297
Richard Towbin, Kevin M. Baskin and David Aria

7 **Musculoskeletal and soft tissue interventions** 356
Kevin M. Baskin, Richard Towbin, David Aria and Carrie Schaefer

8 **Vascular interventions** 404
Richard Towbin, Kevin M. Baskin, David Aria and Carrie Schaefer

Index 477

Contributors

David Aria MD
Department of Radiology, Phoenix Children's Hospital, Phoenix, AZ, USA

Kevin M. Baskin MD
Former Assistant Professor, Department of Radiology, University of Pittsburgh Medical Center, and former Chief of Pediatric Interventional Radiology, Children's Hospital of Pittsburgh, Pittsburgh, PA, USA

Robin Kaye MD
Department of Radiology, Phoenix Children's Hospital
Associate Professor, Department of Child Health, University of Arizona, Phoenix College of Medicine
Assistant Professor, Department of Radiology, Mayo Clinic College of Medicine, Phoenix, AZ, USA

Carrie Schaefer MD
Department of Radiology, Phoenix Children's Hospital
Assistant Professor, Department of Child Health, University of Arizona, Phoenix College of Medicine
Instructor, Department of Radiology, Mayo Clinic College of Medicine, Phoenix, AZ, USA

Richard Towbin MD
Professor and Radiologist-in-Chief, Department of Radiology, Phoenix Children's Hospital
Professor of Radiology, Mayo Clinic College of Medicine
Professor, Department of Child Health, University of Arizona, Phoenix College of Medicine, Phoenix, AZ, USA

Acknowledgements

This book, like life, has had many ups and downs and has taken more time than it should have to come to this point. In many ways it is akin to one of my loves, cycling. In order to be successful you have to work hard to learn the basics, be ready to work through the tough times when your energy and creativity are low and, no matter what, never stop pedaling until you reach the top of the mountain. Cycling also teaches that the riders will always do their best when they work with a committed and effective team. Once at the top of a mountain it is important to stop for a short time to enjoy the achievement and incredible view, enjoy the thrill of the ride down and get ready for the next climb.

In my journey I have been very fortunate to work with incredibly dedicated and talented people in all facets of Radiology. All have taught me a lot and left an imprint on me. While it is difficult to thank each person individually everyone who has been part of this adventure should feel the same pride that I do for helping to develop the field of Pediatric Intervention. This journey began at Cincinnati Children's Hospital with the prescience and continuous support of J. Scott Dunbar, M.D. and Corning Benton, M.D. to help a young radiologist develop an idea and the daily and lifelong support of Robert Kaufman, M.D. to keep it real and moving forward. The development continued at Children's Hospital of Michigan with the help of Tom Slovis, M.D. but took its full form at Children's Hospital of Pittsburgh. After a brief stop in Philadelphia the interventional program is now thriving in the capable hands of Anne Marie Cahill, M.D. Now, my personal odyssey is likely in its last phase at Phoenix Children's Hospital. I am a very lucky man to be able to work with Drs. Robin Kaye, Carrie Schaefer and David Aria who make it fun and educational to come to work every day. I do not know what I would do without their friendship. During this incredible journey there have been numerous talented fellows, all of whom I owe a debt of gratitude to for their commitment and tireless work and willingness to teach me. Over the past several decades there has been one individual, Robin Kaye, M.D., who has been there for almost the entire time. Robin's contributions to Pediatric Interventional Radiology and our practices have been so significant that it is impossible to remember where the ideas came from and how it all happened. Wonderfully, it just did.

A special thanks to Kevin Baskin who rejuvenated the project. Without Kevin's energy and input I doubt this book would have been finished. Thanks to Birck Cox (bcillustration.com) for the wonderful illustrations. Thanks to Laurie Johnson, RN for assistance assembling the manuscript.

Naturally, none of these accomplishments could have happened without my wife, Janet. She is the foundation that everything is built on and provides the everlasting, no questions asked, support that any successful person needs and boy-o-boy do I have.

The book is dedicated to the memory of my mother, Sue, my father Gene and my terrific children Alex and Emily and their respective spouses Meredith and Michael and my grandchildren Ross, Philip, and Anna.

Richard Towbin, M.D.

This book has been, for both Rich and myself, a labor of love and friendship. Rich conceived the need for this text early on, recognizing that the care of children who require image-guided interventions constitutes its own domain within the continuum of medical practice, and that achieving best practices requires thoughtful application of foundational principles that differ from other disciplines within pediatric care and from similar practices in the care of adult patients. I joined him in this quest more than 15 years ago, and have been inspired by him continually over the ensuing time to give all within our power to deliver a message that is accessible, correct, and useful. I am pleased that we release this work to a community that is growing and shares our passion for the care of children, and look forward to the achievements of coming generations as they build on the foundation of the experiences expressed here and echoed elsewhere among our respected colleagues.

No work of this scope emerges without support and sacrifice. I wish to acknowledge here the love and encouragement offered by my uncle, Luis, my mother, Ina, and my son, Lukas. I would be remiss if I did not also recognize the inspiration of the late Jack O'Connor, MD, who I first encountered as a pediatric resident as he was giving lactation advice to a new mother. He taught me that a radiologist is first and foremost a physician, a lesson I have never forgotten and one to which I hope Rich and I have given our own expression of respect through this book.

Kevin M. Baskin, M.D.

Chapter 1

Introduction

Richard Towbin, Kevin M. Baskin, David Aria and Robin Kaye

History 1
Overview 2
A modular approach to interventional radiology 4
Core module 4
Transitional module 5
Completion modules 5
Ultrasound-guided access 5
Clinical practice development 7
Approach 7
The interventional radiology team 8
Facilities, equipment, and supplies 9
Angiography suite 9
Ultrasound 10
Miscellaneous equipment 10
Catheters, wires, and things 10
Patient preparation and safety 10
General principles 10
Patient preparation 10
Informed consent 10

NPO status 11
Preprocedure medications 12
Laboratory studies 12
Prophylactic antibiotics 12
Patient safety 12
Contrast reactions and premedication 12
Emergency premedication 13
Radiation dose management 13
Positioning and padding 15
Sedation for interventional procedures 15
Sedation formulary 16
Topical, local, tumescent, and regional anesthesia 17
Anxiolytics 17
Hypnotic sedatives 18
Opioid analgesics 19
Treatment of sedation complications 19
Emergence delirium (paradoxical reaction) 19
Reversal agents 19
Postprocedure pain management 21

History

The subspecialty of interventional radiology has its roots in the late 1950s and early 1960s with the development of catheterization techniques for cardiovascular angiography. The following two decades resulted in a remarkable growth and development of both diagnostic radiologic techniques and biologically compatible materials. This evolution of equipment and methodology has played a major role in the development, acceptance, and utilization of interventional radiology.

Cross-sectional imaging with ultrasound (US), computed tomography (CT), and magnetic resonance imaging (MRI) has, in most instances, allowed the radiologist to accurately localize and describe a pathologic process anywhere in the body. More recently, the addition of positron emission tomography (PET) has allowed radiologists to observe the regional physiology of a lesion and help plan interventional procedures accordingly. Using these powerful imaging techniques, the interventionalist can plan the safest approach to the lesion and target the most active region while avoiding uninvolved structures.

The development of new devices, especially in small sizes, has led to an ever-increasing number of non-vascular and vascular interventional procedures in the pediatric population. The advances in materials were generally targeted for use in the adult population. However, it was not long until children were also benefiting as a result of the creativity of interventionalists working with all ages and sizes of pediatric patients. Over the last several years there has been a substantial increase in the number of interventionalists specifically trained to treat children as well as a rapid growth in the number of interventional procedures being performed.

Pediatric Interventional Radiology, ed. Richard Towbin and Kevin M. Baskin. Published by Cambridge University Press. © Cambridge University Press 2015.

An overview of our practice growth over the last three decades defines the changes that have occurred in the field. In the late 1970s we began to make the transition in the name of the specialty from special procedures to interventional radiology. In the early years the practice consisted mainly of the "ographies" – diagnostic angiography, myelography, arthrography, etc. In this period a busy service might do 50 to 75 cases per year. The introduction of cross-sectional imaging with CT and US significantly propelled the field of pediatric interventional radiology forward.

The 1980s were a time of innovation and experimentation that resulted in a markedly expanded procedural menu. Many new image-guided procedures were introduced including aspiration and drainage of fluid collections, percutaneous biopsy, percutaneous feeding (nasojejunal tube insertion, percutaneous gastrostomy, percutaneous gastrojejunostomy), esophageal dilation, nephrostomy tube insertion, ureteral stent placement, Whitaker perfusion testing, and endopyelotomy, to name a few. Toward the end of the 1980s, procedural volumes had increased by more than five- to ten-fold, with the busiest services reaching a milestone of 1,000 procedures per year and rivaling the pediatric surgical services in both complexity and volume of procedures.

The period of the 1990s continued the trend of rapid growth but in a more sophisticated manner. The most substantial group of new procedures of this decade were in the area of venous access. During this period we learned and perfected the approaches to insertion of tunneled central lines, ports, and peripherally inserted central catheters (PICCs). New procedures of this era also centered around the biliary tree with a substantial volume of percutaneous transhepatic cholangiograms, biliary drainages and dilations, liver biopsies in patients with liver transplants, transjugular liver biopsy, hepatic chemoembolization, and an occasional pediatric transjugular intrahepatic portosystemic shunt (TIPS) or experimental liver cell transplant. Also, new vascular procedures such as arterial and venous thrombolysis and IVC filter placement were added to the emerging procedural menu. The interventional treatment of children with hemangiomas and vascular malformations began in earnest and quickly became a unique area of subspecialization for pediatric interventional radiologists. Additionally, musculoskeletal procedures such as bone and soft tissue biopsy, joint injections, and percutaneous excision of osteoid osteoma were becoming more frequent. By the end of this decade procedural volumes had again more than doubled.

This led into the new millennium. For the past 14 years the menu of new procedures has been growing; as the maturing caseload has increased so has the complexity and acuity of the patients. There are now a number of practices in North America with high (>70%) utilization rates in two, three, or more interventional suites. There has been a parallel shift toward greater clinical involvement in the patient's care and management both before and after procedures, with a greater interventional radiology presence at the bedside, in clinical conferences, and in specialty and multidisciplinary clinics. Perhaps one of the most encouraging elements of current pediatric interventional radiology practice is that it has achieved a seamless position alongside other procedure-based medical specialties. In reviewing the history of our specialty to date, we have come a long way from the days when we were defined by the "special procedures" we performed. It has been both a difficult and an immensely rewarding journey so far; fraught with political, clinical, and philosophical challenges, as well as the fulfillment of seeing so many children enjoy beneficial outcomes, especially those referred as poor medical and surgical risks. Today, our value exists in the body of technique, experience, judgment, and clinical acumen that defines the interventional practitioner, leading often to more frequent success and significantly fewer complications for the same procedure when performed by the interventional service than by any other. The future is certainly exciting and bright. New frontiers such as molecular medicine, cell- and gene-based therapies, and nanotechnology will change the nature of interventions and of medical care for the better and whatever happens, we are certain that pediatric interventional radiology will be in the center of it.

Overview

This text is designed to fulfill three overarching functions: guidance, advisory, and reference, and to integrate these three functions across the scope of practice of the pediatric interventional radiologist organized under the theme of a modular approach to procedure development. In terms of clinical and procedural guidance, each procedure is introduced with some context regarding its history and its differentiation over time from procedural alternatives. Since in the majority of cases an interventional procedure has been developed as an alternative to an open surgical procedure, relevant comparisons are presented that highlight both advantages and challenges relative to the surgical alternative. Next, clinical indications and contraindications are identified that will assist the reader in achieving the correct response at the right time in the right patient, as well as understanding conditions under which a given procedure should be altered, deferred, or avoided in order to optimize both safety and effectiveness. Although this text is focused on the practical rather than the academic, the authors have extensively reviewed the literature on each topic to assure that the advice we offer from our own experience is in line with best practices and peer-reviewed evidence where it is available and applicable to pediatric conditions.

Next, the technical aspects of each procedure are given. We have adopted a "cookbook" approach, listing the equipment and supplies we have found to be of practical value in daily use over an extensive and comprehensive experience. The intent is not to be prescriptive, exhaustive, or encyclopedic, but to provide a basic compendium that works. Individual practitioners will likely find local solutions that add value in their practice for their patients; this is characteristic of the inherent tendency to innovate that is a hallmark of interventional radiology in general and of pediatric interventions in particular. It has been our goal to provide a foundation with a proven record of success; a reliable starting place that can also serve as a point of departure as practitioners gain individual experience. Likewise, issues of patient preparation are reviewed for each procedure that focus the reader's attention especially on items that should be incorporated into effective planning. Such issues will include preprocedure imaging, laboratory analysis, prophylactic medications, necessary preparation of the operative site, positioning, comfort, protection (i.e., from cardiorespiratory compromise, hypothermia, nerve compression or stretching, hyper- or hypovolemia, etc.), and preprocedure consultation and discussion that will all contribute to a safer, more orderly, and more satisfying procedural event.

The heart of each section is the description of the "standard procedure." Again, this is meant to be practical but not prescriptive. The idea is that a practitioner with appropriate training in the fundamental techniques of interventional radiology and associated clinical care, and with suitable experience in the diagnosis, care, and treatment of pediatric disorders should be able to safely and effectively reproduce each of the procedures described in the "ordinary" case. We have attempted to apply the Pareto Principle (also known as the "80–20" rule) to help the reader focus attention on those elements of a procedure that really make a difference to the outcome.

Where we have used or have knowledge of common or particularly helpful alternative approaches to the standard procedure, these are presented as "technical variations." In some cases, these alternatives are simply another common approach to accomplish the same end (for example, transgluteal versus transrectal drainage of a pelvic abscess). One alternative may fit better with the practitioner's "comfort zone" than the other, or may provide a workable option when there is some impediment to the standard procedure. In other cases, the alternatives presented may allow the practitioner to select from a menu of relative advantages – where selection of a modality, use of ionizing radiation, patient position, or other factors may make one choice safer, better, faster, or less expensive than the other for a given patient on a given day. In some cases, such as aspiration and drainage procedures in the abdomen and pelvis, there are regional considerations that represent variations on a general theme, so that after a general description of the drainage procedure, only those elements that differentiate one variation from the other are necessary (e.g., drainage of a deep pelvic abscess versus drainage of a pancreatic pseudocyst, etc.).

The reader is then directed to "postprocedure and follow-up care" for issues in longitudinal care of the interventional patient. A number of procedures have an associated "technical problems and pitfalls" section intended to help prepare the reader to anticipate and recognize issues that can lead to a failed procedure or an adverse outcome, to prevent these where possible, and to respond to them systematically and effectively when they do occur. A "complications" section outlines those adverse events that may be expected over time when a volume of these procedures are performed, both from our own experience and a review of the literature. In many cases, there is insufficient data available regarding complication rates in pediatric patients. Here, we have tried to extrapolate reasonably from the literature in adult patients and from the limited information available in children in order to help pediatric practitioners communicate more realistically with patients, families, and colleagues, as well as offering general guidelines for the purposes of quality assurance and continuous process improvement.

In constructing each chapter, we have grouped procedures by anatomic location or organ system. Where overlaps occur, procedures had to be delegated to a single chapter to avoid redundancy, but these instances are noted in other related chapters to assist readers in finding information efficiently. Chapters build on the unifying modular procedure development theme (see next section), from procedures based primarily on target visualization and access to those that develop the access tract to those that modify completion elements. Numerous transitional elements (e.g., guide wire stabilization, simultaneous biplane techniques, non-linear and curvilinear pathway development, percutaneous reduction and internal fixation, methods of parent artery protection) are offered to the reader to illustrate solutions integral to the procedures with which they are associated, but also to provide an intellectual framework that encourages the reader to think in broad and abstract ways when trying to solve more complex clinical problems. These elements should support practitioners' own innovation as they seek solutions to problems beyond the scope of this text as well as those not yet imagined.

In this spirit, Chapter 2 focuses on venous access and acquired disorders of the central venous system. The emphasis is on optimizing both decision-making and technique to minimize opportunity for complication, and to develop high-value options for the management of common challenges. Chapter 3 provides a comprehensive view of thoracic procedures from the management of parapneumonic effusions, mediastinal collections, and pulmonary abscesses through intrathoracic biopsies to tracheobronchial stenting. Chapter 4 offers a tour de force of interventional diversity in the abdomen and pelvis. The gastrointestinal procedures, which, with central venous access, form the backbone of most pediatric interventional practices, are surveyed in detail, followed by application of drainage and biopsy procedures across the spectrum of abdominopelvic places and spaces. The chapter concludes with treatments of strictures and retrieval of foreign bodies in the hollow viscera. In contrast, Chapter 5 delves into the more high-end, high-risk procedures in the liver, gallbladder, and spleen that characterize treatment of liver transplant patients. Throughout this text, the reader familiar with adult interventional radiology will recognize that despite the different disease profile in children, the procedural armamentarium of the pediatric interventional radiologist is every bit as demanding and sophisticated and, perhaps, even more complex. Chapter 6 presents procedures in the genitourinary system, which are emblematic of the modular procedural development concept, from target visualization and access (e.g., renal biopsy, Whitaker perfusion test) to tract development (e.g., nephrostomy, percutaneous nephrolithotomy) to modification of completion elements (e.g., treatment of ureteral strictures, percutaneous endopyelotomy). Chapter 7 highlights interventional applications in the musculoskeletal system and soft tissues, an area where pediatric interventional radiologists have led their adult colleagues in innovation and integration of techniques from across other procedural specialties, largely owing to the historic nature of pediatric interventional radiology as a multimodality, multisystem specialty and to its early adoption of ultrasound as an especially potent and versatile guidance modality. The text concludes in Chapter 8, where classic angiography and endovascular procedures meet the pediatric subspecialty treatment of vascular malformations.

A modular approach to interventional radiology

Historically, interventional radiology (IR), like other subspecialties of radiology and other procedure-based specialties, developed episodically and empirically. New procedures, imaging technologies, and techniques originated and evolved based on a variety of needs and opportunities. For example, in the past a child with an osteoid osteoma was conventionally treated by open surgical resection of the tumor, using inexact image guidance with portable fluoroscopy or nuclear imaging. Disadvantages of this approach included frequent persistence or recurrence of the tumor, a high rate of postoperative morbidity, prolonged hospitalization, and high cost. Now, increasing use of percutaneous removal or ablation with CT guidance has improved outcomes and shortened treatment time while reducing morbidity and cost.

Over the past few years we have tried to think more systematically about how and why our interventional radiology practice has grown and developed new and more complex procedures. We have struggled to find a logical basis for our approach. Like Neo in *The Matrix*, who received this guidance from the boy bending spoons with his mind, *"Do not try to bend the spoon. That's impossible. Instead only try to realize the truth..."* we were struck by the need to simplify our approach to problem-solving but not to be confined to conventional approaches. As a result of this introspection we have come to better understand the underlying unifying and organizing process that initially was subliminal but now has become conscious.

We have come to recognize two central themes. First, new procedure development must be driven not by the tools and procedures with which we are familiar but by the problems that our patients need to have solved. This applies in practice what many experts have been advocating in theory; a learner-centered, problem-based approach to learning. The second, and perhaps more evolutionary, theme is that there is no simple continuum of expertise. Rather, we must be willing to use whatever tools are available to us regardless of the practice area in which they reside, or to create new tools when our current practice is insufficient to solve a problem. Sometimes we are forced to laboriously reason forward in step-by-step fashion, as novices often do, linking known facts in a line from problem to solution. This is an inherently laborious process because of the numerous possibilities that branch from each step, and the therefore relatively high likelihood of less effective choices that may crowd out or obscure the "best" choice or that may lead to a procedural dead-end.

When our deeper expertise permits, we may be able to more expeditiously create a solution in fewer steps using existing procedural elements through *backward reasoning*, working from the intended goal back along a chain of modular procedural elements that logically connect the end objective of the procedure to an achievable beginning. When gaps remain they may require innovation or invention to create a continuous linkage between elements and so achieve an effective solution. The smaller that the gaps can be made, the more easily they may be overcome. Recognizing the "modularity" of new procedure development frees us to attack new procedures by breaking them down into a series of smaller tasks that are less daunting, because most of the modular tasks are already familiar to us (although perhaps in other locations or applications).

The concept of a modular approach to pediatric IR is intended to present a "thought template" to be considered when trying to solve technical or intellectual problems. It is in no way intended to suggest that this is the best or only way to modify existing approaches or to create novel solutions. On the contrary, it is our hope that this will be used as a springboard to open up thinking and enhance creativity so that we may be able to consider unexplored opportunities and to merge what on the surface may seem to be disparate or contradictory methods, materials, techniques, and technology into new, minimally invasive diagnostic techniques and interventional therapies for the patients that we treat.

Core module

The core module can be defined in several ways. We can look at an individual technique such as image-guided needle placement or a whole procedure such as nephrostomy tube insertion as a basic unit. The core module should, however, be the most fundamental building block of the procedure being performed. For example, the retrograde gastrostomy procedure can be considered the core module for cecostomy insertion (Chapter 4). Some procedures may involve linkage of two or more core procedures, such as hemangioma (interstitial/venocapillary) sclerotherapy (Chapter 8), lymphocele (cystic) sclerotherapy (Chapter 4), and abscess drainage (Chapter 4), which when linked together provide the conceptual basis for sclerotherapy and partial gland ablation of ranula (Chapter 7).

Transitional module

A transitional module is one that facilitates completion of the procedure or development of a new procedure, but on its own does not complete the task. One of the most common modular techniques that fits this definition is insertion of a guide wire. The guide wire enables the use of dilators or the placement of sheaths and catheters, but on its own does not bring the procedure to an endpoint. Any device that fulfills the same function can be used in the same modular context, from the introducer catheter of an Amplatz® serial dilator (Figure 4.20) in the dilation of a nephrostomy tract for percutaneous nephrolithotomy (Chapter 6) to the Steinman pin (Figure 7.23b) for delivery of a compression screw for internal fixation of a fracture (Chapter 7). Another common transition module is tract development. Tract dilation with or without placement of a sheath is frequently done to develop and maintain a connection between the skin surface and target site. This subset of modular techniques and procedures is very important as it enables the development of more complex or layered procedures and unlocks the door to creative solutions to clinical problems.

Completion modules

Completion modules are the evolutionary components of the procedural groups. It is by combining and adding new modular subunits that new solutions and novel procedures are born. These modules may already be in your toolbox, reside in the toolbox of another subspecialty, or may need to be developed anew. When considering a new approach to a problem, the addition of a creative completion module is a perfect place to "think outside of the box." Novel combinations of materials, methods, and technologies are the raw materials that can lead to new and exciting outcomes.

Consider a few examples of successful new procedures using completion modules, which at the time might have seemed to be unusual or to merge discordant techniques and technologies, such as the use of a radio frequency probe through a guide needle to ablate tumors, or using endoscopes in collaboration with urologists to incise a stenotic ureteropelvic junction or to remove a stone. In the future the only limitation to replacing open surgery with minimally invasive techniques may be our imagination and ingenuity. There are certainly many resources and combinations that remain untried and in time many new materials and possibilities will be made available. However, the exciting prospect is that we all have the opportunity to discover new solutions.

Ultrasound-guided access

Image-guided needle placement is a fundamental core module, as it forms the basis for the majority of percutaneous image-guided procedures in pediatric IR. With the advent of cross-sectional imaging and improvements in instrumentation, many procedures previously performed under surgical control are now done more safely, effectively, and economically with minimally invasive techniques using image guidance. Real-time two-dimensional US has played a major role in this transition. Sonographic guidance of needle placement serves as a prototypical modular procedure, as it is useful for such a broad variety of applications in many organ systems. For this reason, its general elements are discussed here, rather than repeating the discussion in the majority of chapter sections that follow throughout this text.

Since US is portable and radiation free, it can be used at the bedside, in the emergency room, in the operating room, or in the interventional suite. In experienced hands, US guidance facilitates precision needle placement and is a useful initial modality in multimodality procedures; for example, in conjunction with fluoroscopy or CT when necessary. In inexperienced hands, US may increase the risk of adverse events over conventional non-image-guided alternatives when a poor understanding of the image volume leads the operator to violate vital structures and treat non-target tissues. The authors have borne witness to numerous examples over the years of iatrogenic injuries and catastrophic complications resulting from misuse of US guidance. Several are recounted within the remaining chapters of this text.

A preliminary scan should be performed to thoroughly evaluate the target lesion and plan the route. When choosing the needle entry site it is important to know the technique that will be used. In other words, the skin entry site will be different depending on whether a biopsy guide or freehand technique is being used. (A brief word here on the use of biopsy guides: many experienced interventionalists do not use them, others do. They should be considered a part of the armamentarium, with this caution: a needle guide will not keep the needle in plane and on-target in all circumstances, and the "needle guides" on the monitor are only a suggestion of where the needle is likely to go if it is not deflected.) The skin entry site will also be influenced by a choice to scan in the long or short axis. Once the entry site has been determined the skin is marked. The skin is then sterilely prepared and draped with the skin mark positioned appropriately in the field.

Before beginning the procedure it is helpful to position the US machine so that the monitor is as close as possible, and directly in the operator's line of sight (Figure 2.9). This will maximize hand–eye coordination and comfort. Always perform the procedure in the most physically comfortable position possible. Physical discomfort is both fatiguing and distracting and can significantly impair performance. We find that it is usually best to grasp the transducer in the non-dominant hand (when feasible), keeping the ulnar surface of this hand in contact with the patient when the transducer contacts the skin (Figure 1.1). This position will improve stability and reduce fatigue of the scanning hand.

Ideally, when scanning in long axis, the entire course of the needle, including its tip, and the target lesion should be seen in the imaging field throughout the procedure. A common source of difficulty in accomplishing this objective arises when the

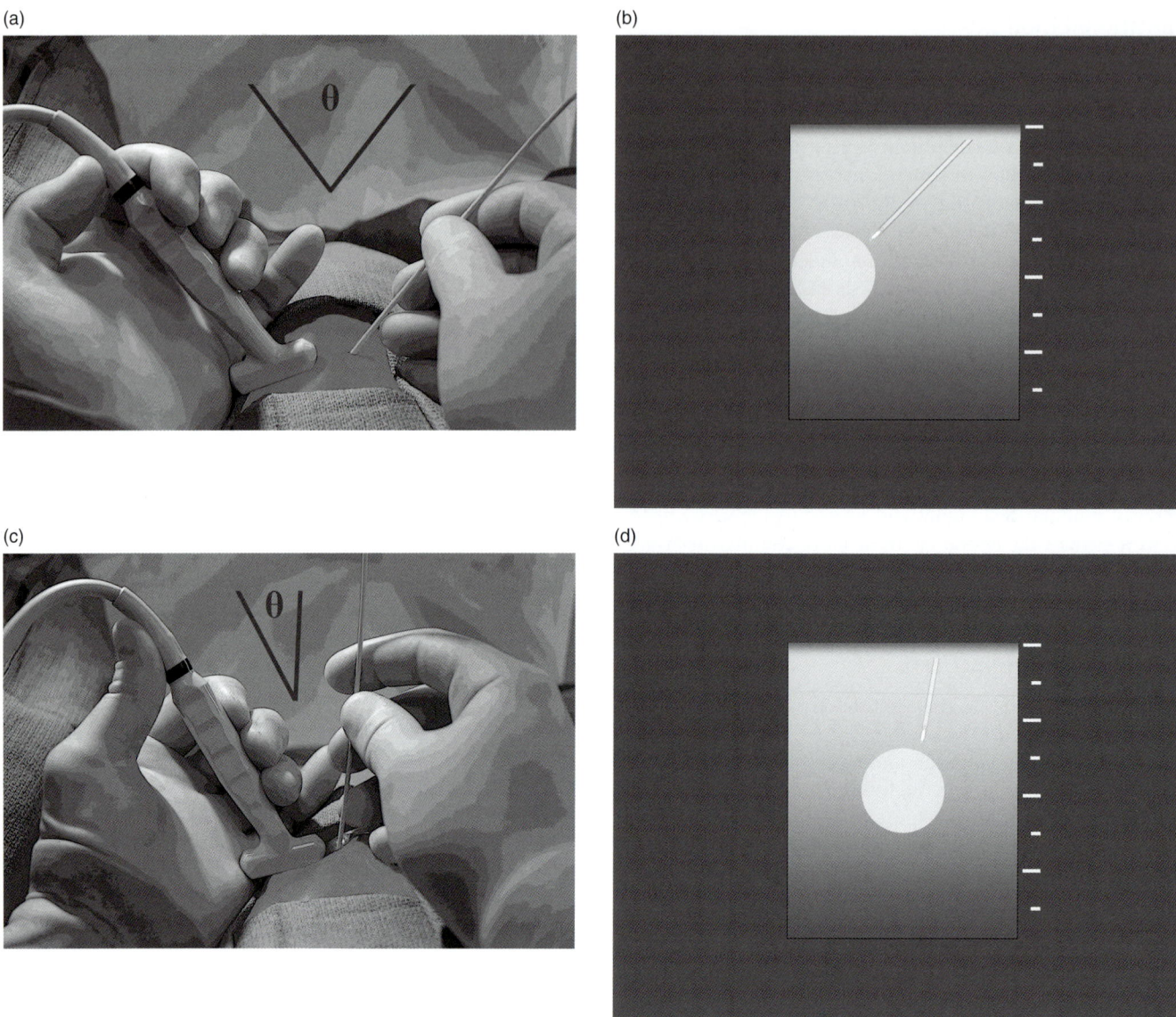

Figure 1.1 (a) Resting some part of each hand against the body surface reduces fatigue and unwanted motion during ultrasound-guided needle access. Obtaining a wide angle (Θ) between the ultrasound transducer and the needle, by entering the skin some distance apart from the transducer, will significantly improve conspicuity of the needle. (b) The wide angle between the needle and the transducer and eccentric location of the lesion within the imaging field allows earlier and more conspicuous visualization of the needle shaft and tip in plane with the target lesion, increasing the opportunity for a successful outcome. (c) A narrow angle (Θ) between the needle and transducer, often created by moving the needle too close to the transducer, may severely impair visualization. (d) With an acute angle between the needle and the transducer, and with the target centered in the imaging field, the needle is visualized poorly and over only a short part of its path. Partial visualization of the needle shaft, motion artifact, and less careful management of the tip location contribute to a higher likelihood of adverse outcomes. (e) When operating at a curved body surface, a needle entry point well away from the transducer allows an optimal (parallel) relationship between the needle and the transducer face. (f) Achieving the ideal parallel relationship between the transducer face and the needle shaft optimizes conspicuity of the needle, including the tip (due to "comet-tail" or "ring-down" artifact) and the entire length of the shaft (with "reverberation artifact"). Again, locating the target eccentrically in the imaging field allows visualization of the greatest possible length of the needle, including tip and shaft, in plane with the target lesion.

needle is located too close to the transducer, and at too acute an angle. Desirable specular reflections from the needle are maximized when the needle is parallel to the face of the transducer and perpendicular to the sound beam. This optimal geometry is difficult to accomplish in practice. Deviation of only 10 degrees from parallel with respect to the transducer face may be enough to impair visualization of the needle. This may require that the needle enter the skin 1–3 cm or more away from the edge of the transducer. Locate the target eccentrically or peripherally in the scanning field, so that the needle can be tracked throughout its entire course.

Although one may wish to scan periodically with color Doppler to identify and avoid vessels, it is best to turn color off or to narrow the color box to just show the relevant vascular structure at risk while advancing the needle in order to keep the screen refresh rate high enough to detect needle tip

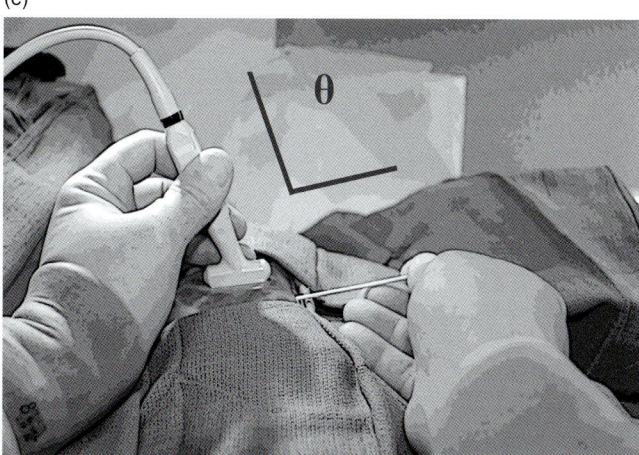
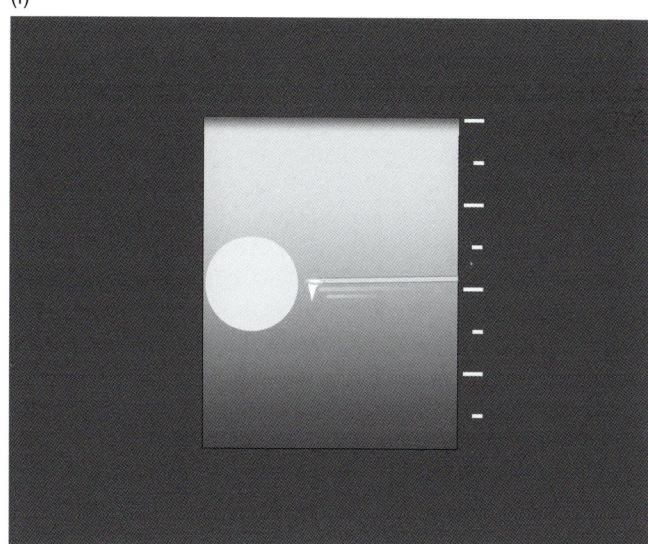

Figure 1.1 (cont.)

motion in a timely fashion (Figure 3.23f). Raise the focal zone toward the surface to visualize the needle entering the field. Advance slowly until the tip enters the target, moving the focal zone as necessary.

As much as possible, one should be able to visualize the needle shaft and tip in plane with the target. If at any time this is not what you see, stop. **Look at your hands!** (Unlike diagnostic US, the key to interventional US is relating physical space with the imaging space. Staring at the monitor while moving both the needle and the transducer is unlikely to accomplish this goal, while holding the transducer on target and *looking at* the relationship of the needle to the transducer may be the most efficient way to bring the needle tip and the target into simultaneous view.) With the transducer properly positioned adjust the angle of the needle until it is in plane with the sound beam (parallel to the long axis of the transducer face at its midpoint). If uncertainty persists after repeatedly trying to locate the needle tip, it may be better to withdraw and begin again.

If a lesion is located near a curved body surface (e.g., a focal renal lesion), it can be helpful to scan in long axis and position the long axis of the transducer and the needle entry site perpendicular to each other, ideally arranging the needle path as perpendicular to the sound beam as possible, even if this means that the needle enters the skin several centimeters from the transducer (Figure 1.1e,f). Such an arrangement can increase the conspicuity of the needle significantly.

Clinical practice development
Approach

There is no single right way to approach practice development. However, in over 30 years of being a pediatric interventionalist, my colleagues and I have found that certain approaches work better than others. Here are some of the lessons we have learned. There are three main keys to success: focusing on customer service, being willing to help without reservation, and being an expert.

If we look at critical aspects of the patient/family encounter we find it is important to develop a trusting relationship at the initial meeting. This is made easier when the practitioner presents a professional and positive attitude. Simple gestures that recognize the patient as a person are easy to overlook but have a profound effect on rapport. For example, we try to always introduce ourselves to the patient and the family. If the patient is old enough to understand what is going on, it is often good to talk first with the patient and address their concerns and questions and then talk with the parents. In all cases we give a sufficiently detailed outline of the procedure with a reasonable account of the alternatives, benefits, and risks so the patient and family can understand the implications and choices involved, and give an estimate of how long it will take so they can have realistic expectations about the scope and nature of the encounter. We let the patient and parents know what to expect after the procedure in terms of pain and any limitations that might be imposed, and when the patient will be able to eat again and return to baseline activities.

If there are delays before the procedure (for example, if prior cases are running longer than expected), our staff give a face-to-face explanation and update to help dissipate the heightened stress and frustration that can be magnified by uncertainty and a feeling of being "neglected." During the procedure, especially if it is taking longer than predicted, it is very helpful to give the family updates. Finally, when the procedure is over it is important to give the family an overview of how the procedure went and to discuss any issues or problems. It is vital to developing an effective trust relationship that the patient and family are given ample time and encouragement to express concerns and to ask questions, from the initial consultation and consent discussion through to the recovery period and any follow-up visits. The referral service also needs to be informed, ideally personally via a phone call, of the outcome of the procedure and any issues or complications that may have arisen. The clinical team also needs to know what postprocedural needs the patient may have and what the plan for future follow-up or intervention may be.

The impact and importance of providing quality customer service is probably obvious to all of us, but somehow it is often difficult to accomplish. You certainly know good service when you see it! The essence of good customer service is to treat everyone – clinicians, patients, and families – as you would like to be treated. However, something crazy often happens when people become the service *provider* – they become less flexible, need to follow both real and imaginary rules, and come up with lots of excuses for not doing something. As one might guess, this approach does not usually get the customer response and positive feeling that is desired. Yet this is the "black hole" into which a service will inevitably be drawn without positive effort and energy. Avoiding this unfortunate state and making customer service a strong point of a practice are complex issues about which many books have been written.

In our experience, a simple and successful solution to this complex problem begins with the most effective, but at times painful, answer to the question, "Will you/can you do…?". Say: "Yes." When the conversation begins with "No" it is *very* difficult to walk away with a satisfied customer. Ironically, we have all had these experiences on call when prolonged contentious discussions ultimately result in the requested case being performed anyway, but with both parties feeling very stressed and dissatisfied. As someone who has been in that situation more than once (or even one thousand times), "No" is seldom the *right* answer even when it seems to be the *correct* answer.

Saying "Yes" instantly changes the tenor of the discussion and makes you an ally of the person seeking your help. Saying "Yes" does not mean that you will do anything and everything asked of you but it does indicate your willingness to meet the other party halfway and to enter into an open discussion that hopefully ends with a mutually satisfying plan to care for the *patient*, which obviously is the real priority. When a requester hears "No" they tend to feel polarized and threatened with an inability to find a solution to their problem; they may escalate rhetoric and tension in a bid to avoid being abandoned. When the requester hears "Yes" they can relax and better hear recommendations about alternative solutions. Thus, saying "Yes" even to a request for help with a hopeless problem or a clearly contraindicated procedure can provide the support and shared responsibility the requester may need to accept and act appropriately on a difficult or challenging reality.

The medical expert engenders confidence in others and is able to solve a wide range of problems. Other professionals will seek out the expert to get their opinions on subjects within the expert's scope of practice and will be open to the expert's advice. In order to gain expert status it is essential for the interventional radiologist to be current in the field, attend and, if possible, participate in local, regional, and national meetings, maintain high professional standards, and expect and strive for excellent outcomes.

Seek out mentors and advisors. Very few who perform pediatric interventional procedures have the luxury of multiple colleagues within the same practice, and every pediatric interventionalist, from the most experienced to the most recently trained, benefits from sharing ideas, concerns, and outcomes with others who have overlapping interest, experience, and scope of practice. Early in your career this is essential in order to form foundational technical skills and problem-solving approaches to a variety of cases. It is also important to maintain relationships with mentors and colleagues with whom you can discuss challenging cases and problems throughout your career because all of us are continually learning. When we exchange ideas we challenge what we think we know. The excellent practitioner can learn from everyone, including practitioners outside of our field.

The interventional radiology team

One of the major keys to developing a successful pediatric interventional practice is building a strong interventional team. A typical pediatric interventional team consists of interventionalists, interventional radiology technologists, and pediatric radiology nurses. Each member brings a skill set that is additive and helps provide the highest level of care. Substitution for or omission of any one of these individuals can significantly impair the team's effectiveness. The number of persons in each subgroup depends on many factors including the number of interventional suites that are in use per day, the number and type of cases performed, and the availability of adjunctive staff such as schedulers, aides, or others to answer phones and assist with other functions. With increasing volume, efficiencies improve significantly with at least two full-time equivalent pediatric interventionalists, nurses, and technologists.

The leader of the team is an interventional radiologist who is committed to the concept and ideal of pediatric interventional radiology. The team leader must have knowledge of pediatric conditions, diseases, and special needs, the technical training to deal with this diverse patient population, and the commitment to focus on the care of children. The pediatric interventional radiologist must also be able to develop a rapport with the pediatricians, pediatric surgeons, and pediatric subspecialists who will be referring patients to the interventional service. They must demonstrate a willingness to participate in a child's care regardless of the type of procedure or level of difficulty that is required. A willingness to live in the pediatric world, to be responsive to pediatric problems and an investment in the "art of the possible" characterizes the practice leader likely to achieve success. The practitioner who works at the end of an "umbilical cord" from another practice environment, who is willing to do only what must be done, and who conceives of pediatric interventions as an imposition on other priority commitments, is not likely to inspire the interventional team or potential referring clinicians.

The interventional technologist also has a complex and challenging job. Their skills and enthusiasm make them an indispensable member of the team. In many practices, the lead technologist is responsible for workflow management, as well as purchasing and inventory control. The technologists are responsible for setting up instrument and supply trays, anticipating the technical needs of the case, and safely and effectively setting up the equipment. On many occasions, a technologist will be the first assistant during a procedure. We always have a technologist, together with a nurse, circulate in the room to supply equipment and technical support as needed. Compared to technologists in the adult interventional environment, the pediatric interventional technologist is often significantly more integrally involved in the performance of the procedure, rather than simply managing the related imaging and documentation. At the completion of the procedure the technologist will complete paperwork and label and submit images to the picture archiving and communication system (PACS) for review and interpretation.

Pediatric interventional nurses are the third vital part of an effective IR team. The interventional nurse must have advanced skills in pediatric patient care, usually with critical care experience such as in the intensive care unit, transport team, or emergency department, with skills and experience in the evaluation, assessment, and care of children with a wide variety of illnesses, acuities, and developmental levels. Unfortunately, in some places this type of pediatric nurse is left off the team or substituted for with a nurse trained in other areas of pediatrics, which can leave a significant deficit in team composition.

When familiar with the procedures, the IR nurse adds to the breadth and complexity of procedures that may be performed on a sedated or anesthetized child. The nurse working in the IR suites will meet the family, ready the child for the procedure, and discuss nursing issues relating to the forthcoming procedure to be performed. If a procedure is performed with the patient under sedation the nurse is responsible for administering the medication and monitoring the child's vital signs. At the completion of the procedure, the nurse is responsible for coordinating the patient's recovery, either until discharge to home or until transfer to a recovery facility (i.e., pediatric anesthesia care unit or intensive care unit) or to an acute care unit. If the child is to be discharged home, written instructions are given to the family and questions are answered by the nurse. The day after the procedure nurses make follow-up phone calls to check on the patient and make sure all questions are answered. In addition to these duties, the interventional nurse is often involved with the team making hospital rounds and seeing children in IR clinic. And finally, in our practice, in addition to nursing duties during cases, the nurse is responsible for same-day patient scheduling and daily case management. On its best day and in all but the quietest practices, interventional radiology is a study in controlled chaos. With all these responsibilities it is important that the interventional nurse be well trained, flexible, friendly, and fast.

Some practices also incorporate mid-level providers (i.e., nurse practitioners or physician assistants) who act as physician extenders and work within the scope of practice of the supervising physician to perform procedures, provide patient histories and physical examinations, participate in clinic visits, consultations, ward rounds, and patient and provider education. They can become the face of the practice to the patient and provider community, tying loose ends, improving communication and accessibility, and freeing the interventional radiologist to focus on "big picture" elements essential to the long-term success of the practice.

Facilities, equipment, and supplies

Another key to having an effective pediatric IR service is having the correct equipment and supplies to do a wide variety of cases. In pediatric IR this means making sure that you have wires, catheters, drains, etc., to use on patients of all sizes. Especially in infants and small children you just cannot "make do" with adult-sized materials. This section is included for someone interested in building a pediatric IR lab from the ground up. It is not intended to be a fully comprehensive list of every single item or piece of equipment you will ultimately use, but rather it is a basic list of materials and equipment that will allow you to start a program and be able to perform a wide variety of basic cases as well as a few of the more complex cases you will be asked to perform.

Angiography suite

Because the conventional access point for many angiographically guided interventions is the adult groin, the location of central and auxiliary components of these angiographic units is oriented to serving the needs of the operator at this location. Pediatric interventions tend to differ in a major way – they are far more often conducted at a location closer to the X-ray generator and detector, the more so the smaller the patient. The head of an adult patient may be under the detector during a neurologic intervention while the operator stands comfortably at the groin, 2 to 3 feet (0.6 to 0.9 meters) away from the detector, looking directly at the monitor, hands easily at the controls. The whole body of a pediatric patient may be under the detector while the operator stands as close to the patient as the pedestal and foot controls will allow, struggling to see the patient in the dark shadows under the detector while craning around the C-arm to see monitors that may not orient easily for viewing from this position, and out of immediate reach of controls. The images generated under such conditions may not reflect these challenges, but the ease and speed of the procedure, the safety of the patient and staff, and the fatigue of the operator may well reflect them. These are all items that should be considered when evaluating potential equipment (and when preparing for a given procedure).

There are different philosophies regarding what the minimal needs of an IR section are. In our view, in order to be able to do the broadest menu of cases it is best to begin with a biplane angiography suite. On the other hand, having only a high-quality single plane suite takes very few procedures off the table. The equipment should have all the modern technology to be able to perform digital subtraction angiography at low dose and do suitable postprocessing of images. A small focal spot (≤0.4 mm) and pediatric-specific presets are central to achieving optimal image quality while conserving total delivered dose of radiation (see "Radiation dose management" below). Rotational angiography is great if affordable and the service is substantial enough in size and complexity to justify the expense. If a second room is needed single plane suites will usually suffice.

Ultrasound

The majority of cases will involve a combination of US for guidance of needle placement followed by fluoroscopic monitoring of the remainder of the procedure. We have found it preferable to have a dedicated diagnostic quality US machine equipped with a full range of transducer sizes, types, and frequencies. An absolute must is a linear high-frequency transducer with a small footprint, which in our practice is our workhorse probe, especially for venous access. More portable notebooks and limited, miniature US machines may have a limited role and can be adequate for less demanding applications but do not have the penetrating power that high-quality machines possess. Although the features of a high-end machine are only intermittently required, it is impossible to predict which cases will *not* require them, so the lower quality machines have not proved adequate for a full service IR department in our experience.

Miscellaneous equipment

The suite must have a high-quality power injector that can accurately inject small volumes of contrast. Ideally the injector is linked digitally to filming.

Safety devices such as Velcro® straps (or "seat belts" in pediatric parlance) that can be cut to desired lengths are a must in order to secure the patient on the table. Also, we often use an Octostop® cradle to secure small infants (<10 kg) and facilitate positioning. This can sometimes reduce the need for sedation and can shorten procedure time, especially for feeding tube insertion and other minor procedures. Other safety devices for positioning patients include arm boards, sponges, gel rolls, and bolsters all in a variety of shapes and sizes.

Warming devices are a must to keep small children warm and dry in order to maintain their body temperature. These can include warming lights, warming blankets, and chemical warming pads. We prefer warm blown air. We use a Bair Hugger® that comes with a variety of sizes and shapes of air blankets, which can be placed under or over the patient depending on the needs of the case. We also find having a blanket warmer in the suite indispensible for patient comfort at both the beginning and end of cases.

Pulse Doppler is a sensor that we place over the dorsalis pedis or posterior tibialis pulse so that we can monitor the distal pulse while compressing the arterial puncture site after catheter/sheath removal.

Catheters, wires, and things

A basic, limited set of catheters will accommodate the vast majority of intravascular procedures (Table 1.1). To the extent possible all catheters should be in 3, 4, and 5 French sizes. Specialty catheters may be in selected sizes for specific uses. The core guide wires are 0.018-inch and 0.035-inch although 0.038-inch can be substituted. The length of the wire is also relevant. The 0.018-inch wires are maintained in 65, 100, and 150 cm when available. Table 1.1 reflects a core stock that we have found covers most situations. Additional equipment and supplies will depend upon the local mix of cases and operator preferences. Procedure-specific equipment and supplies accompany each procedure set throughout the text.

Patient preparation and safety

General principles

Most cases are performed with US guidance with confirmatory fluoroscopy and less frequently with CT guidance. Ultrasound generally allows for shorter and safer procedures. The ability to have continuous needle visualization almost certainly results in greater accuracy in needle tip positioning and a lower incidence of untoward effects. Computed tomography guidance, because of its large radiation dose, is reserved for only those cases in which US guidance is not possible. The result of the improvement in techniques, image guidance for procedures and new and improved materials is an increasing total number of minimally invasive procedures, many of which are being performed safely and effectively on an outpatient basis, e.g., feeding procedures, biopsy, vascular access, angiography, sclerotherapy, arthrography, and lumbar punctures.

It is important that the IR suite is treated like an operating room and strict sterile technique and adherence to universal precautions is maintained. In our practice IR suite entry is restricted. All personnel entering the IR suite must wear hospital scrubs, surgical hats, and masks. Those performing the procedure, including the interventionalist and any assistants, must wear sterile gowns and gloves.

Patient preparation

Informed consent

For interventional procedures, informed consent is necessary prior to elective and urgent cases, and where possible for emergency cases as well. Policies regarding emergency procedures when consent cannot be obtained vary from hospital to

Table 1.1 Equipment: core set

- Catheters: Pigtail, JB-1, Harwood Nash or Weinberger (WNBG), C-1, Cobra, microcatheters (depending upon case types, from 3 French to 1.2 French tips)
- Guide wires: Bentson, mandril, angled Glidewire®, Roadrunner®, Amplatz Stiff® and Superstiff®, Rosen, Newton
- Specialty guide wires are not stocked in all sizes and lengths. These wires are primarily for microcatheters and are usually 0.014-inch although smaller gauge wires are stocked to match the microcatheters
- Vascular (single-wall) puncture needles, micropuncture needles, angiocatheters from 24 to 18 gauge, Seldinger
- Abscess drainage and large collection needle: Yueh 5 French sheathed needle
- Drainage catheters: Towbin Duan 5 French pigtail, 6.3 French to 24 French locking pigtails
- Biopsy needles:
  - Fine needle aspiration (FNA): 22-gauge or 18-gauge Chiba needles
  - Soft tissue core biopsy needles (18 gauge, 16 gauge): end-cutting automated, side-cutting semi-automated; with coaxial sets
  - Transjugular liver biopsy kit
  - Bone biopsy needles: Ackerman, Craig (can be used with a power drill), T-Lok, Jamshidi
- Embolic materials:
  - Liquid agents: dehydrated alcohol, sodium tetradecyl sulfate, doxycycline, bleomycin, thrombin
  - Temporary particulate agents including Gelfoam® and Avitene®
  - Permanent agents: tissue adhesives and liquid embolics, e.g., Histoacryl® and Onyx®
  - Embospheres or PVA particles: 100 to 300, 300 to 500, 500 to 700, 700 to 900, and 900 to 1,200 micron particles
  - Coils:
    - 0.018-inch: Hilal 0.5 cm, 1.0 cm straight plus complex shapes with 1 to 2 cm diameters
    - A wide range of 0.035-inch coils in diameters from 3 mm to 12 mm and lengths to 15 cm
  - Vascular plugs
- Feeding catheters:
  - Frederick–Miller nasogastric tube (8 French)
  - Primary gastrostomy tube for antegrade insertion
  - Button (low profile) gastrostomy and button gastrojejunostomy (balloon-tipped)
  - Balloon-tipped replacement gastrostomy (14 to 24 French) that can be converted to a gastrojejunostomy with the coaxial addition of a Frederick–Miller tube
- Venous access:
  - PICC: 3 French single lumen, 4, 5 French single and double lumen, standard and antibiotic-impregnated
  - Cuffed central lines: 3 French single lumen, 4, 5 French single and double lumen, standard and antibiotic-impregnated
  - Temporary and apheresis catheters: 6 to 12 French
  - Hemodialysis catheters: 8 to 14.5 French; 15 to 27 cm
  - Ports: petite and standard up to 5 to 7 French

hospital, and usually involve attestation in the medical record from clinicians not performing the procedure that the procedure is critical to the welfare of the patient and that delay to obtain consent would pose an unacceptable risk.

The basic elements of informed consent include a description of the planned procedure, expected benefits, known significant risks, and available alternatives, ideally presented in a language and form that the consenter can adequately understand. It is useful to record these elements in the medical record. Consent is obtained from the patient when they are 18 years of age (or of majority) or are an emancipated minor. However, for the majority of pediatric patients informed consent is obtained from the parent or legal guardian, who must be present or at least available by phone. When appropriate, assent is obtained from the minor patient. If the child is a ward of the state consent issues should be addressed early since it can take hours to days to get consent from the appropriate state-appointed official.

NPO status

Patients scheduled for an interventional procedure are fasted according to hospital policies regarding sedation and anesthesia. In our practice, patients are kept NPO for six to eight hours for formula or solids, four hours for breast milk, and two hours for clear liquids. Emergency cases may require deviations from these guidelines, which must be considered on a case-by-case basis. If proper fasting cannot be assured, procedural sedation may not be appropriate. All patients that require sedation or anesthesia should have adequate intravenous access. In order that patients fasting for a procedure do not become dehydrated, especially neonates, infants, and young children, orders for maintenance intravenous fluids should be part of routine preprocedure orders. This is especially important for patients who will be receiving intravascular contrast during the procedure. Good communication with the referring service will help identify those patients with specific fluid restrictions or requirements.

Preprocedure medications

Children who are on anticoagulation have these medications held. Typically we withhold enoxaparin (Lovenox®) for 24 hours, which usually amounts to the doses the night before and the morning of the procedure. Heparin needs to be withheld for two to four hours. Warfarin may need to be withheld for one to several days depending upon the specific regimen. If non-steroidal anti-inflammatory agents are to be withheld (usually only for high-risk elective procedures), at least a week is required to replace affected platelets. There are certain patients in whom cessation of anticoagulation may not be safe, and in those cases a decision about whether to move forward with the procedure is made after consultation with the referring service. Non-steroidal anti-inflammatory agents, reversible platelet inhibitors, may need to be withheld for only 24 hours.

All *necessary* medications (usually anti-seizure medications) that cannot be given intravenously (IV) should be taken the morning of the procedure with small sips of water, at least two hours before the procedure. The insulin dose in diabetic patients may be cut in half on the morning of a procedure for the fasting patient, although appropriate endocrinologic consultation will provide more specific guidance.

Laboratory studies

Routine laboratory tests are seldom required prior to most procedures unless there is a known or suspected bleeding diathesis, a significant possibility of postprocedural bleeding related to the type of procedure being performed (e.g., pancreatic biopsy), or there is a pertinent medical condition. In such cases, a CBC, platelet count, PT, PTT, and INR are the baseline studies usually obtained. There is generally a poor correlation between abnormalities in the coagulation profile or platelet counts and procedure-related bleeding complications. Not all laboratory abnormalities of coagulation are associated with increased risk of a significant bleeding complication. However, there have been no prospective studies on the predictive value of coagulation parameters in pediatric patients undergoing image-guided procedures. Medical history appears to be the most important factor in predicting the risk of bleeding complications in patients undergoing percutaneous procedures. For example, patients with a history of malignancy or bone marrow transplantation are at a five-fold greater risk of hemorrhagic complications following liver biopsy, regardless of preprocedure coagulation parameters, number of passes, needle size, or operator experience. No matter what the numbers, a sick child or one with a history of bleeding problems should be treated with great caution.

Platelet dysfunction can be congenital or acquired, qualitative or quantitative. Acquired conditions such as liver disease, renal failure (uremia), and aspirin administration cause a qualitative defect whereas a consumptive coagulopathy results in a quantitative defect. For qualitative platelet dysfunction, alternatives include desmopressin (DDAVP), platelet transfusion, or cryoprecipitate administration. Extrinsic pathway abnormalities, signaled by a prolonged PT or an elevated INR, are seen most often with warfarin administration, nutritional (vitamin K) deficiency, and disseminated intravascular coagulopathy. In the face of an elevated INR, in addition to holding warfarin (or replacing with heparin), vitamin K or fresh frozen plasma may be indicated. Intrinsic pathway abnormalities, with prolonged PTT, most often result from treatment with heparin or enoxaparin. In addition to holding heparin, fresh frozen plasma may be helpful. Specific circumstances may require factor replacement or other specialized interventions to correct the abnormal value. In all cases, agents such as platelets and fresh frozen plasma that achieve peak blood levels at the time they are infused should be administered as close to the time of the procedure as possible for maximum effect. Close consultation with the referring clinical service and with a hematologist in such situations is essential.

Policies regarding pregnancy testing before imaging and interventional procedures vary from hospital to hospital. In general, every female patient capable of conception should have affirmative evaluation (β-HCG testing) before exposure to ionizing radiation or to an invasive procedure.

Prophylactic antibiotics

Prophylactic antibiotics are not routinely given except for children with congenital heart disease. Antibiotic prophylaxis is recommended in the following high-risk cardiac conditions: prosthetic cardiac valve, history of infective endocarditis, congenital heart disease (CHD) including unrepaired cyanotic CHD with or without palliative shunts and conduits, completely repaired congenital heart defect with prosthetic material or device during the first six months after the procedure, repaired CHD with residual defects at the site or adjacent to the site of a prosthetic patch or prosthetic device, and cardiac transplantation recipients with cardiac valvular disease. Antibiotic prophylaxis is no longer recommended for any other congenital cardiac defect than those listed above. Those children with high-risk CHD who require prophylaxis receive PO amoxicillin (50 mg/kg, not to exceed 2 grams/dose) or IV ampicillin (50 mg/kg IV/IM, not to exceed 2 grams/dose) administered 30 to 60 minutes before the procedure. Patients who are allergic to penicillin and cephalosporins receive vancomycin (20 mg/kg over an hour).

Patients with a congenital or acquired immune deficiency, such as patients with HIV, SCIDS, SSA, DM, or autoimmune disease, cancer patients on chemotherapy, patients with bone marrow or solid organ transplant, or patients on chronic steroid therapy, may be at high risk for infectious complications. Antibiotic prophylaxis for interventional procedures on these patients is decided on a case-by-case basis.

Patient safety

Contrast reactions and premedication

The incidence of reactions to non-ionic contrast media is quite low in the pediatric population and ranges from about 0.2% to

3.5%. When an adverse event occurs it may be classified as minor or major depending upon its severity. Minor reactions may be dose dependent and include sensations of warmth and pain, nausea and vomiting, a metallic taste, bradycardia, hypotension, and vasovagal reactions. Other minor events that can occur can be classified as thromboembolic, vascular injury, tissue injury, volume overload, and allergic events.

Major reactions to iodinated contrast may also occur but are far less common. These events are usually dose independent and the child may have predisposing factors such as renal insufficiency, a history of a reaction to contrast injection, a strong allergic history including asthma, food or drug allergies, or complex medical issues. It is important to identify these patients so that a pretreatment protocol can be initiated if indicated.

Several *premedication regimens* have been proposed to reduce the frequency or severity of reactions to contrast media, although only two are most frequently used. In the first regimen the patient receives prednisone (50 mg PO) thirteen hours, seven hours, and one hour before receiving contrast. In addition the patient receives diphenhydramine (Benadryl®) (50 mg PO, IV, or IM) one hour before receiving contrast. In the second regimen the patient receives methylprednisolone (Medrol®) (32 mg PO) twelve hours and two hours before receiving contrast. As in the first option, an antihistamine can also be added to this regimen.

If the patient is unable to take oral medication, 200 mg of hydrocortisone IV may be substituted for oral prednisone.

Emergency premedication

In case of the emergent need to perform a study that requires IV contrast in a patient with suspected or known sensitivity then there are three main premedication regimens, given in decreasing order of preference. In the first regimen methylprednisolone sodium succinate (Solu-Medrol®) 40 mg IV or hydrocortisone sodium succinate (Solu-Cortef®) 200 mg IV is given every four hours until the contrast study is performed. In addition diphenhydramine 50 mg IV is given one hour prior to contrast injection. In the second regimen dexamethasone sodium sulfate (Decadron®) 7.5 mg IV or betamethasone 6 mg IV is given every four hours until the contrast study is performed. In addition diphenhydramine 50 mg IV is given one hour prior to contrast injection. In the last regimen, in cases where the study must be done immediately, steroids are omitted entirely and diphenhydramine 50 mg IV is given just prior to contrast injection. Note: IV steroids have not been shown to be effective when administered less than four to six hours prior to contrast injection.

Radiation dose management

As interventional radiologists, we must be sensitive to both stochastic and tissue reaction effects of the ionizing radiation we use to diagnose disease, guide procedures, and evaluate outcomes. As pediatric interventionalists, the urgency of this responsibility is significantly increased, as the time that our patients have to experience adverse effects is greater in general than for adult patients. In fact, the attributable lifetime risk of a radiation-induced cancer from one Sievert of dose is believed to be about 3% for middle-aged adults, but rises to about 12 to 15% for a child in the first decade of life.

Because the impact of stochastic effects is so uncertain, we must evaluate the basis for each potential exposure. However, it would be a mistake to view each exposure as an independent event, or to promote the idea that reducing instantaneous dose is a valid objective. If images are not adequate to discern target structures or to guide the procedure, not only may the operator attempt to compensate with prolonged exposure, but the substandard images also introduce risk of catastrophic complications in their own right.

The overarching concept is to reduce total cumulative dose to the degree possible while facilitating safe completion of the intended procedure. Sometimes, perhaps counterintuitively, increasing the instantaneous dose will result in a lower total cumulative dose. For example, doubling the dose per frame may substantially increase conspicuity of target structures. However, because the large number of photons required to achieve optimal images in larger adults is not needed in smaller children, the pulse width can be decreased by several times, yielding better imaging with a much smaller total dose.

The risk of tissue reactions, or dose-dependent radiation injury (formerly known as deterministic effects), should also influence our decision-making during interventional procedures. Certainly, we should be aware of and limit acute dose to vulnerable tissues and organs, including the lens of the eye, gonads, red marrow, breast, intestinal mucosa, skin, etc. We should also be aware that tissue effects of acute dose are not limited to cell killing, but are also subject to an orchestrated biological response to cell injury, including fibrosis, cytokine activation, and other non-lethal signaling responses that can influence the extent of tissue injury and that can have both acute and delayed effects.

In the effort to reduce unnecessary exposure of patients to medical radiation there is no substitute for properly trained staff operating properly configured equipment in the delivery of thoughtfully planned care. A full consideration of these objectives is beyond the scope of this text. Nevertheless, there are a number of guidelines that can help reduce both acute and cumulative dose exposure for patients undergoing interventional procedures, as well as for the IR personnel and others in the room during procedures.

Avoid use of ionizing radiation where possible:

Use radiation effectively. Do not perform studies that will not influence management, and do not perform interventions that will not influence outcome.

Use alternative modalities when possible. A large proportion of interventions performed in children can make substantial use of US as an alternative to CT or fluoroscopy.

Limit the number of recorded images. If high temporal resolution is not necessary to adequate visualization or diagnosis, lower the pulse rate. If higher spatial resolution is not required, lower the dose and use last-image-hold, fluoroscopic-image-grab, or fluoro-loop-store/playback to evaluate progress and to document events rather than radiographic/angiographic acquisitions. The patient dose associated with a single fluoroscopic frame is approximately one-tenth the dose of a single standard recorded radiographic image.

Limit redundant imaging. Use last image hold rather than continuous fluoroscopy to evaluate relationships. Road mapping and three-dimensional road mapping can save dose, contrast, and procedure time. Three-dimensional road mapping in complex vascular procedures can reduce the dose at a given location and orientation by allowing re-orientation of the C-arm without acquiring a new road map, provided the patient is not moved relative to the original road map acquisition. When the operator expects to toggle between two or more fixed C-arm and table positions, as often occurs during musculoskeletal interventions, saving the positions as assignable presets allows safe and rapid transition between positions without active imaging.

Optimize imaging moment by moment:

Optimize hardware and standard imaging configurations for use in children. Imaging devices "out of the box" are usually optimized for adult patients. The vendor and medical physicist must work together to provide configurations adapted to the enormous dynamic range demanded by the spectrum of path lengths and tissue characteristics found in pediatric patients. Then, interventional staff must become properly trained to use the correct features and options for each specific situation.

"Stand down" promptly after prior events if they required elevated dose parameters. A given task event (e.g., bypassing a staghorn calculus with a fine guide wire during placement of a percutaneous nephroureterostomy, or manipulation of a catheter during intravascular procedures in a small child) may require imaging parameters that deliver a higher dose, such as increased frame rate or electronic magnification. During this period, dose may accumulate much more quickly than usual. At the end of this period, the motivation to return to lower quality imaging parameters may be impeded by the relief experienced by the operator enjoying continuation of the higher than necessary image quality. It is important to adjust these parameters for each task as it arises, and to measure and monitor dose as it is delivered.

Consider biplane imaging for select studies. Small vessel caliber in children requires a higher contrast concentration to achieve adequate subject contrast. Since total contrast dose is limited, use of biplane imaging may allow timely acquisition of images necessary for diagnosis within contrast constraints.

Use the appropriate X-ray tube focal spot. The kW rating of the focal spot should be matched to the imaging task to generate the best available geometric image sharpness for the intended imaging path length (usually, but not always, related to the size of the patient). If available, small (e.g., 0.3 mm) focal spots should be used for small children up to the early teen years.

Know when to use a grid. The grid on most angiographic units is removable, and should be removed when the imaging path length is less than 8 to 12 cm. (A grid with reduced lead content should be used when the patient size/imaging path length is 12 to 20 cm.) When imaging a small pediatric patient, removing the grid, increasing the source-to-image-receptor (SID) distance (e.g., from 85 cm to 125 cm), and increasing the field-of-view (e.g., to 23 cm to 37 cm) can reduce dose by 30 to 60% while *improving* image quality and convenience to the operator (i.e., more room to work under the detector)!

Use appropriate filtration. As patient (or body part) size decreases, adding spectral (e.g., copper) filtration to the standard aluminum filtration, decreasing pulse width, and reducing tube voltage to maintain adequate subject contrast, allows significant dose reduction. For neonates, up to 0.9 mm of copper filtration can be added. Radiographic technique factors, X-ray tube voltage (kV), tube current (mA), pulse width (msec), and added filter thickness are the fundamental controls used to manage patient dose and image quality.

Collimate appropriately. Position of the collimator blades should be represented on a static image so that irradiation during adjustment is not required. On the angiographic unit, the collimator should be an adjustable (wedge) equalization filter. Used properly, collimators improve image quality and reduce dose to the patient. If collimators (or shielding or radio-opaque gloves on the operator or internal hardware in the patient) shade the automated exposure control (AEC) sensors, they may cause dose to increase substantially in an attempt to maintain brightness in the displayed image!

Use appropriate shielding. Non-target radiosensitive tissues should be shielded when they are potentially exposed to significant radiation dose. However, as noted above, shielding should not be allowed to shade the AEC sensors or to impair the operator's visualization of important target structures.

It is also important to consider radiation risk to non-patients during interventional procedures. Non-essential personnel and those with recognized vulnerability (e.g., pregnant women) should be excused from the interventional suite during periods when ionizing radiation is in use. In addition to normal protective (shielded) clothing and eyewear, during radiographic acquisitions ideally all personnel should leave the room, but essential personnel that cannot leave should be provided additional shielding and should stand as far as possible from the X-ray generator.

Personnel should be aware at all times of their relationship to the X-ray beam, and should take precautions to minimize dose. The reality is that for some procedures it is not possible to keep hands out of the beam (e.g., transgastric gastrojejunostomy tube replacement), but supination of the hand close to the beam and judicious collimation can greatly reduce personnel exposure. Operators should avoid electively introducing hard attenuators (e.g., radio-opaque gloves, spinal hardware, etc.) within the scope of automatic exposure control (AEC) detectors where this would tend to elevate patient entry dose without significant benefit to the operator or to the exam.

Pediatric interventional radiologists benefit from the minimal scatter radiation generated by small pediatric bodies and body parts. However, the "pediatric" spectrum also includes patients who exceed common stated weight restrictions and are sometimes referred for interventional radiologic procedures as a last resort. Other patients may require non-orthogonal path lengths that may exceed even the typical lateral path length for a large adult. These patients may include adolescents to elderly adults, and they can challenge practitioners' ability to generate clinically useful fluoroscopic, angiographic, or computed tomographic images despite very high doses and prolonged attempts. The extraordinary path lengths may also subject medical staff to much higher levels of scatter radiation than are normally encountered.

Management of radiation exposure and reduction of associated risk is a core competency of radiologists. Interventional radiologists are in the best position to provide guidance and oversight on these issues within a health care institution. While radiologists are optimally involved in all medical imaging, especially when ionizing radiation is involved, the reality is that other providers, including surgeons, cardiologists, anesthesiologists, emergency medicine physicians, intensivists, nephrologists, nurse practitioners, and physician assistants may also be using this equipment. Appropriate requirements and thresholds for privileging and credentialing practitioners who are allowed to use this equipment should be addressed within each institution. Just as anesthesiologists are often the gatekeepers regarding use of anesthetic and sedative agents, so should radiologists be the gatekeepers for use of ionizing radiation, and interventional radiologists be the gatekeepers for use of medical imaging for guidance of invasive procedures.

Positioning and padding

The first objective of positioning the patient in the interventional suite is to provide optimal access for the interventional team to comfortably and efficiently visualize target structures and structures at risk, and to manipulate equipment and instruments so as to achieve the desired outcome safely and effectively. While specific issues of positioning are addressed as necessary with each procedure in the text, patients may be positioned in almost every conceivable orientation, from supine to prone to lateral decubitus, and even in a lithotomy position or seated or tilted one way or another, as the needs of each case dictate. At the same time, heavy equipment may be moving around the patient, sometimes at relatively high speeds, including the CT gantry (which may be tilted as well) and the angiographic C-arm, which may spin rapidly (e.g., during rotational imaging). These positional issues have implications for potential physiologic responses, position-related complications, and mechanical injury hazards. Most related injuries or physiologic compromise can be anticipated and avoided if staff take the time to evaluate the patient in light of these positional issues before and during each case.

In general, these risks can be grouped into three major classes: nerve injury (including stretch, compression, ischemia, and metabolic injury), ocular injury (including corneal drying) and soft-tissue trauma, and pressure sores. For example, the brachial plexus is especially at risk when the upper extremity is abducted and externally rotated, and the head is turned to the contralateral side. The nose and eyes may be compressed during prone procedures. Respirations, ventilation, and systemic venous return may be compromised by shifting abdominal contents in prone or supine positions, while differential ventilation of the two sides can be expected in a lateral position. For long cases, and for any case performed under regional anesthesia, deep sedation or general anesthesia, padding of pressure points (e.g., egg crate foam, gel pads, diapers or other cloth) to avoid neuropathy or other injury is essential. Prior to the beginning of a procedure, at frequent intervals throughout, and at any time heavy equipment will be moved or apparatus near limbs and digits will be assembled or disassembled, the patient should be carefully inspected to avoid position-related injuries.

Sedation for interventional procedures

Historically, provision of sedation for pediatric procedures, especially the ability to develop and maintain a deep plane of sedation safely and reliably in children of all ages and sizes, was a signature element of the most successful pediatric interventional radiology practices. In the past five years there has been a significant shift in the approach to the sedation of patients in the IR suite. Today, an increasing number of cases are done under general anesthesia or, at some institutions, under sedation managed by a non-radiologist, usually from a hospital-wide sedation service. Although the pendulum is swinging, the end of this story has probably not yet been told. One telling (and ironic) development: adult interventional practices are developing an increasing interest in IR-managed sedation! No matter what unfolds, it is certain that a deeper understanding of the management of patient comfort and consciousness will strengthen any interventionalist's practice.

Both sedation and general anesthesia have compelling strengths and complex challenges. Sedation allows more flexibility in case scheduling and case flow with more efficient use of the IR suite, and is significantly less costly than general anesthesia. The main absolute disadvantage is the limitation in patient selection: at least 20 to 30% of interventional patients will not be suitable candidates for sedation, due to cardiorespiratory vulnerabilities, need for paralysis, other contraindications to sedation medications, or prior sedation failure. Additionally, interventional sedation is a sophisticated art form that requires an experienced team and, ideally, a supervising clinician who is not performing the interventional procedure. The advantages of general anesthesia are that even very ill or unstable patients can undergo procedures, patients are motionless and pain free, respirations can be controlled, and frankly, it takes away the added pressure of directing sedation from the interventionalist while performing the case. These advantages assure that general anesthesia will have an essential role in any serious interventional practice. Its disadvantages are primarily logistic and economic: transitions between cases take much longer, scheduling is not as easy, and it is much more expensive. Additionally, although obscured by the methodology of complication reporting, the rates of anesthesia failure and minor complications are non-trivial.

The fact of the matter is that there is no single optimal solution for management of comfort, consciousness, and safety for pediatric interventional radiology procedures. For most practices, the best solution will involve an amalgam of modalities. As many procedures as can be safely done with sedation will improve utilization and cost efficiency while giving the interventional service maximum control over workflow. The most seriously ill patients, those with risky airway issues, and those who must be paralyzed will require anesthesia, either from the anesthesiology service or, for patients already in the ICU, under the supervision of the intensivists. Anesthesia with a managed airway will also be useful for patients who have complex medical or surgical conditions and for procedures that are expected to be long (over two hours) or are known to be associated with a significant amount of pain or discomfort.

The authorship group has a combined experience approaching 150,000 pediatric sedations. We have learned to value experience over theory, and to understand that while every sedation encounter needs to be individualized to the patient and procedure, the principal guardian of safety is consistency. In this context, consistency of sedation practice begins with a sedation protocol and formulary. This ensures an organized, consistent approach for every sedation. The IR staff must be fully trained in airway management and sedation pharmacology and be certified in basic life support (BLS) and pediatric advanced life support (PALS). The suite must be calm, quiet, and at times dimly lit to provide an environment that is conducive for sedation. Monitoring equipment, including pulse oximetry, EKG, BP, respirations, and end tidal CO_2, must be present. Additionally, suction, O_2, N_2O, and the full range of age- and size-appropriate accessory equipment to facilitate sedation, such as nasal cannula, masks, valve bags, oral airways, nasal trumpets, etc., should be available. Finally, there must be a readily accessible resuscitation cart that includes medications and equipment such as laryngoscopes, ET tubes, and a defibrillator to perform resuscitation if needed.

Table 1.2 Risk index classification of the American Society of Anesthesiology (ASA)

Classification	Patient condition
1	Normal, healthy patient without organic, physiologic, or psychiatric disturbance
2	Patient with controlled medical conditions without systemic effects
3	Patient with medical conditions with significant systemic effects intermittently associated with significant functional impairment
4	Patient with poorly controlled medical condition that is associated with significant dysfunction and is a potential threat to life
5	Patient with a critical medical condition that is associated with little chance of survival, with or without a surgical procedure

When considering children for sedation, those who are American Society of Anesthesiology (ASA) Class 1 or 2 are the best candidates. ASA classifications are provided in Table 1.2. For patients in ASA Class 3 and 4, anesthesiology consultation is advised prior to sedation. Anesthesiology back-up should be considered, and there should be a low threshold for transfer of the case to the supervision of a pediatric anesthesiologist. Given these limitations, we have provided sedation in numerous selected cases in these classes without incident. ASA Class 5 represents an absolute contraindication to sedation under the supervision of the interventional radiologist. These cases are universally performed by the anesthesiology service in virtually all institutions. In general it is also recommended that patients with congenital heart disease or severe cardiorespiratory compromise who are to undergo an IR procedure be anesthetized by a pediatric anesthesiologist who is specially trained or experienced in cardiac anesthesia.

Sedation formulary

A sedation formulary is not an encyclopedic compendium of sedation medications, but a practical selection of medications that are familiar to the practitioners and supportive of the goals of the practice. There are numerous medications from a variety of drug classes that may be used. The drugs mentioned in this section reflect our current practice and are a very *basic* list.[‡] We believe choosing a limited number of drugs, which are effective at sedation, analgesia, and anxiolysis, and with which the practice group are very familiar and confident, is the best approach. The sedation drugs available to a given

---

[‡] Every effort has been made to ensure the accuracy of drug doses; however readers must confirm and follow the doses and schedules set out by manufacturers. This material is not intended as a substitute for consulting qualified health care professionals. Patient circumstances will vary and some information may have become outdated as a result of more recent medical developments.

Table 1.3 Common local anesthetics

Drug	Routes for use	Dose	Side effects/comments
Buffered lidocaine	Infiltration	Add 1 ml sodium bicarbonate to 9 ml lidocaine Dose: 3–5 mg/kg	Less painful on injection than lidocaine alone
EMLA® – eutectic mixture of local anesthetics (prilocaine 2.5% & lidocaine 2.5%)	Topical use on intact skin	preemies >30 gestational weeks: 0.5 g for 60 min/day Full-term neonates: 1 g Infants & children: 2–3 g (area: <10 kg 100 cm^2, 10–20 kg 600cm^2, >20 kg 2,000 cm^2) for 60–90 min prior to procedure	Use on intact skin Used for neonatal circumcision, IV placement, chest tube removal, spinal taps, portacath access Watch for s/s of methemoglobinemia
Elamax-4 – topical anesthetic cream (lidocaine 4%)	Topical – may be used on minor cuts, abrasions, or minor burns	Thick layer to skin, may be covered with Tegaderm® (skin area: <10 kg 100 cm^2, 10–20 kg 200 cm^2) for 30–60 min	Contraindicated in patients with a known history of sensitivity to local anesthetics

Courtesy of Janet Semenova PNP, John S. Jones MD, Analgesic Reference Resource, Pain Management Services, Phoenix Children's Hospital.

practice are regulated by institutional policies, usually set by a hospital-wide anesthesia/sedation committee that includes anesthesiologists, intensivists, hospitalists, interventionalists, and others, and the rules for use of these sedation drugs are bounded by hospital guidelines as well as national guidelines. Two precautionary notes: first, the institution must be committed to providing the facilities, equipment, and support necessary to run a successful sedation program. Second, the sedation team must recognize its own limitations in experience and expertise, and know when to say no. If the experience, expertise, and support are not sufficient to provide a safe sedation for a given case, then the case should be scheduled with anesthesia.

The ideal sedative would have the fastest time to action, the fewest adverse effects, the greatest difference between effective dose and toxic dose, and the shortest half-life, which would allow the patient to return to baseline as fast as possible. That being said – there is no perfect sedation drug! We use three main classes of agents for sedation: anxiolytics, hypnotic sedatives, and opioid analgesics alone or, more commonly, in combination. Sedative doses should be calculated on a weight (i.e., mg/kg) basis. The selected agents should be titrated to effect, and sufficient time allowed to elapse between doses to achieve peak drug effect before administration of additional drugs. The doses of any pertinent reversal agents should be known before the case starts, although the drugs do not necessarily need to be drawn up.

Topical, local, tumescent, and regional anesthesia

All children who are not receiving general anesthesia benefit from effective local anesthesia (Table 1.3: Common local anesthetics). When done properly, local anesthesia can decrease the amount of analgesia required for a case. Currently we begin skin (topical) anesthesia with a J-Tip®. The J-Tip® uses CO_2 to propel 1% lidocaine into the dermis via the pores, which instantly results in quite rapid and effective local topical anesthesia. The J-Tip® can be applied at the site of an IV start as well as at the expected needle insertion site for an intervention. Then, once the skin of the site has been sterilely prepared and draped, using a 30-gauge needle and buffered 1% lidocaine the remainder of the access tract is anesthetized. We recommend infusing the local anesthetic very slowly. In our practice the J-Tip® has replaced topical agents (e.g., EMLA® or ELA-Max® cream) for most applications since the latter requires at least 30 to 60 minutes for skin anesthesia to be accomplished plus prior selection of the entry site for the procedure. For some specific applications, tumescent or regional anesthesia are useful. For example, endovenous ablation is improved if a tumescent mixture of dilute (i.e., 0.1%) buffered lidocaine in normal saline is injected under US guidance within the connective tissue sheath surrounding the target vessel, compressing the vessel around the treatment catheter and protecting surrounding non-target tissues from thermal injury. Regional anesthesia (nerve block) can provide a pain-free field within the distribution of the target nerve(s), such as multilevel intercostal blockade prior to subcutaneous port pocket formation.

Anxiolytics

Benzodiazepines, including diazepam (Valium®), lorazepam (Ativan®), and midazolam (Versed®), form the most common class of drugs used for anxiolysis (Table 1.4: Drug formulary for sedation). We almost exclusively use midazolam given IV at 0.05 to 0.1 mg/kg for this purpose because it is short acting and can be easily titrated to effect. Onset of action after IV injection is usually <60 seconds with a duration of 15 to 30 minutes. Doses can be repeated, allowing two to five minutes between doses, until the desired effect is achieved. For prolonged cases, doses can be repeated every hour, beginning at 25% of the dose originally required to achieve sedation. When used in combination with an opioid analgesic, the two medications are often alternated to effect, although the medication choice at each time-point should be responsive to the dominant need of the child at that point

Table 1.4 Drug formulary for sedation

Drug	Dose	Route	Maximum dose
Midazolam HCl (Versed®)	0.05 to 0.10 mg/kg 0.30 to 0.75 mg/kg	IV, IM PO	0.3 mg/kg 15 mg
Chloral hydrate (Notec®)	50 to 75 mg/kg	PO, PR	100 mg/kg or 1 g
Pentobarbital sodium (Nembutal®)	2 to 4 mg/kg	IV, IM, PO	6 mg/kg
Fentanyl citrate (Sublimaze®)	1 µg/kg	IV, IM	50 µg

(i.e., sedative to affect level of consciousness, analgesic to affect response to painful stimulus).

Beside the well-known CNS depressant effects, midazolam also can cause short-term retrograde amnesia, which means that children often do not remember the events surrounding their procedure, although not all children experience this effect. Potential complications include respiratory depression, apnea, respiratory and cardiac arrest. Paradoxical agitation and combativeness have been reported. The respiratory depressant effects may be increased when used in conjunction with barbiturates or opioid analgesics. Midazolam is metabolized by the liver and excreted in the urine.

The drug can also be administered orally (PO) at 0.3 to 0.7 mg/kg, intranasally (IN) at 0.2 to 0.4 mg/kg, or intramuscularly (IM) at 0.08 to 0.1 mg/kg. Oral or intranasal Versed® has become a useful strategy for calming and sedating children who do not have intravenous access, especially those less than five or six years of age. It is especially useful for calming an anxious or agitated child prior to starting an IV or as an adjunct to another sedative. Onset of action with oral or intranasal administration is about 15 minutes with a duration of 30 minutes. The oral form of the drug has a very bitter taste that many children will not tolerate. Mixing it with cherry or other fruit-flavored syrup is one way to make it more palatable. The intranasal form really stings when it comes in contact with the nasal mucosa. Also, the drug is absorbed by the nasal mucosa and is inactivated by gastric acid, so the maximum volume that can be given intranasally is usually less than 1 ml per side. It should be given slowly so that it stays in contact with the nasal mucosa and is not just swallowed.

Hypnotic sedatives

Chloral hydrate (Notec®) is a non-barbiturate hypnotic sedative and is the oldest member of the hypnotic group (Table 1.4: Drug formulary for sedation). We use this drug only in patients under one year of age who do not have venous access. Due to its unpredictable nature and frequent failure, we have found very few remaining applications for its use in the interventional practice. Doses administered range from 75 to 100 mg/kg, with a usual initial dose of 50 mg/kg in preemies and neonates, and 75 mg/kg in older infants. The maximum single dose is one gram. If the desired sedation level is not achieved with the first dose additional doses may be given up to a maximum of 100 mg/kg. Time to action is relatively slow, 20 to 30 minutes, and duration of action is about 60 to 90 minutes. Like the barbiturates, chloral hydrate has no analgesic activity. It may be combined with fentanyl for procedures that have painful components. Potential complications include respiratory depression, hypotension, skin rash, and gastritis. Chloral hydrate is metabolized in the liver and kidney and is excreted in the urine.

Pentobarbital sodium (Nembutal®) is a barbiturate hypnotic sedative that has non-selective CNS depression and is capable of producing all levels of CNS mood alterations from excitation to deep coma. We usually administer the drug IV with an initial dose of 2 to 3 mg/kg. Maximum single dose is 100 to 200 mg, depending on the size of the patient. It is important to give the dose with a rapid push as the maximum sedative effect depends on as high a concentration in the blood as possible. Onset of action is about one to two minutes with a duration in the range of 45 to 60 minutes. Like midazolam this drug can be titrated to effect. Additional doses at 1 to 2 mg/kg may be given every five to ten minutes up to a maximum of 7 mg/kg. Pentobarbital can also be given IM, but its onset and duration of action are unpredictable when given by this route, so we avoid it if at all possible.

Barbiturates have almost no analgesic effect in sedative doses and indeed can actually make children hypersensitive to environmental or physical stimulation. Therefore it is imperative to have the IR suite calm, quiet, and if possible, dimly lit, and to not physically stimulate the patient by rubbing or patting them. This means that for procedures we must give a separate analgesic drug. Pentobarbital is a respiratory depressant in a dose-dependent manner. When given in standard sedative doses the respiratory depression noted is similar to sleep with a slight decrease in heart rate and blood pressure. The respiratory depressant effect is synergistic and additive with opioids and midazolam. Potential complications include respiratory depression, apnea, laryngospasm, vasodilation with fall in blood pressure, and paradoxical excitement (about 6%).

In our experience, paradoxical excitement most often occurs when children are confused and disoriented during sedation induction, due to either inadequate dosing or prolonged dose delivery (slow push). Pentobarbital is metabolized in the liver and excreted in the urine and less often in the feces.

Opioid analgesics

Fentanyl citrate (Sublimaze®) is a short-acting narcotic analgesic 100 times more potent than morphine sulfate and 750 times more potent than meperidine (Demerol®). However, its duration of action is about 30 to 60 minutes compared to three to four hours for morphine sulfate. Fentanyl is an excellent adjunct to barbiturates in that it effectively desensitizes the patient to painful stimuli and is additive to the hypnotic effect. In general, it tends to decrease the total dose of pentobarbital needed to complete the diagnostic test or intervention. The drug is given slow IV push in 1 μg/kg doses with an onset of action of two to three minutes. The maximum single dose we use is 50 μg. This drug, like midazolam and pentobarbital, can also be titrated to effect and repeat doses of 1 μg/kg can be given every five to ten minutes up to a maximum of 5 to 7 μg/kg.

The potential complications of fentanyl include facial itching, respiratory depression, apnea, and chest muscle rigidity (the dreaded "wooden chest" syndrome). Wooden chest syndrome is most likely to occur if the drug is given in rapid bolus form or in high doses. The best treatment for this complication is avoidance. It is our practice to never inject fentanyl directly into an IV. Instead, it is administered slowly through the side port of infusion tubing with fluids running. If, in spite of this precaution, wooden chest syndrome occurs, immediately give Narcan®, an opioid reversal agent, and call for the emergent help of an anesthesiologist. A neuromuscular blocking agent is usually the treatment of choice, along with intubation and mechanical ventilation. Fentanyl is metabolized by the liver and cleared mostly in the urine and to a lesser extent in the feces.

Treatment of sedation complications

We have been utilizing this drug formulary for over 30 years and have found it to be extremely safe and effective. Major complications of sedation are rare and occur in much less than 0.1% of cases. Respiratory depression, apnea, and rarely respiratory arrest are the most common adverse effects. Fortunately, these respiratory difficulties are generally easy to recognize and treat provided they are promptly diagnosed. In our practice whenever a child's oxygen saturation goes below 92%, supplemental oxygen is given (usually at 2 to 3 L/min), by mask, nasal cannula, or blow by, to maintain O_2 saturation above 95%. If necessary, the child is stimulated, and the head is repositioned with the neck mildly extended and the jaw thrust forward to straighten the airway. If necessary, the nose and mouth are suctioned, and an oral airway inserted. This type of respiratory depression is usually seen shortly after a drug bolus and is short-lived. If the respiratory depression is persistent, reversal of narcotics or benzodiazepines is considered. If these maneuvers fail, the resuscitation team should be called.

Although minor complications such as emergence delirium, (also known as paradoxical hyperactivity), skin rash, respiratory depression, facial itching, and bronchospasm can be seen in 7 to 10% of cases, in no instance has these problems led to permanent injury or death.

Extreme caution should be exercised in children who are very ill, especially those with hepatic or renal failure. These children are more prone to acute drug toxicity because of their inability to metabolize and excrete drugs and are poor candidates for intravenous sedation.

Emergence delirium (paradoxical reaction)

Children who experience paradoxical excitement are very difficult to manage due to their extreme agitation and inability to be consoled. It is very important to protect the patient and to emotionally support the parents. The patient is awake but "out of it" and can be extremely hyperactive. This effect may last hours and is very distressing for parents and caretakers to watch, even though it has no lasting effect on the patient. In the past we tried to treat this with little success by attempting to keep the child immobilized. More recently, intranasal or intravenous midazolam was tried with only slightly better results. However, we have found that caffeine can have a calming effect on most children with this reaction. Intravenous caffeine citrate can be administered IV at 20 mg/kg with a maximum dose of 200 mg.

Reversal agents

Naloxone hydrochloride (Narcan®), an opioid antagonist, prevents or reverses the effects of opioids including respiratory depression, sedation, and hypotension (Table 1.5: Reversal agents). Narcan® is most effectively given IV. While the American Academy of Pediatrics does not endorse subcutaneous or intramuscular administration in opiate intoxication since absorption may be erratic or delayed, if an IV route of administration is not available, Narcan® may be administered intramuscularly or subcutaneously. The usual initial dose in children is 0.01 mg/kg. If this dose does not result in the desired degree of clinical improvement, a subsequent dose of 0.1 mg/kg may be administered every two minutes to a maximum dose of 2 mg. When Narcan® is administered intravenously, the onset of action is generally apparent within two minutes. The half-life of Narcan® is about one hour but may be up to three hours in neonates. Since the duration of action of Narcan® may be shorter than that of some opiates, the effects of the opiate may return as the effects of Narcan® dissipate. Therefore, although the opiate-intoxicated child responds dramatically to Narcan®, they must be continuously monitored with EKG, SpO_2, and blood pressure checked frequently, and repeat doses of Narcan® may be required. The adverse effects of Narcan®

Table 1.5 Reversal agents

Drug	Usual adult dose >50 kg	Usual pediatric dose <50 kg	Comments, side effects, contraindications
Naloxone (Narcan®)	**Opioid-induced respiratory depression:** 0.1–0.2 mg IV q 2–3 min until reversal of symptoms. **Rapid titration method for opioid-induced respiratory depression:** Remove 0.4 mg (1 ml) from vial. Add to 9 ml NS = 0.04 mg/ml. Give 0.5 ml IV q 2–3 min until reversal of symptoms. **Opioid-related side effects (e.g., pruritus, N/V, urinary retention):** 0.01–0.02 mg IV q 2–3 min to max three doses in one hour. **Emergency situations (e.g., unknown ingestion) IV/IM:** 0.4–2 mg IV q 2–3 min.	**Opioid-induced respiratory depression:** 0.01 mg/kg IV q 2–3 min until reversal of symptoms. **Rapid titration method for opioid-induced respiratory depression:** Remove 0.1 mg (0.25 ml) from ampule of 0.4 mg/ml. Add to 9.75 ml NS = 0.01 mg/ml. Give 0.25–0.5 ml q 2–3 min until reversal of symptoms. **Opioid-related side effects (e.g., pruritus, N/V, urinary retention):** 0.001–0.002 mg/kg IV q 2–3 min to max three doses in one hour. **Emergency situations (e.g., unknown ingestion) IV/IM:** 0.1 mg/kg IV q 2–3 min to max of 2 mg or until reversal of symptoms.	Use cautiously in opioid-dependent or postoperative patients to avoid large cardiovascular changes (e.g., hypertension), pulmonary edema, and seizures.
Flumazenil (Romazicon®)	**Benzodiazepine sedation/respiratory depression:** 0.2 mg IV q 1 min may repeat as needed × 4 doses. **Max dose: 1–3 mg**	**Benzodiazepine sedation/respiratory depression:** 0.01 mg/kg to max of 0.2 mg/dose IV q 2–3 min until symptoms resolve. **Max dose: 1 mg**	Onset: 1–3 min. Duration of action: 45–60 min. Associated with seizures in benzodiazepine-dependent patients or suspected TCA overdose.

Courtesy of Janet Semenova PNP, John S. Jones MD, Analgesic Reference Resource, Pain Management Services, Phoenix Children's Hospital.

Table 1.6 An approach to mild/moderate postprocedural pain: dosing data for NSAIDs

Drug	Usual adult dose >50 kg	Usual pediatric dose <50 kg	Comments
Acetaminophen	**PO:** 650–1,000 mg q 4 h (max 4 g/day)	**PO:** 10–20 mg/kg q4 h **PR:** 40 mg/kg initially, then 20 mg/kg q 6 h (max 90–120 mg/kg/day)	Lacks the peripheral anti-inflammatory activity of other NSAIDs
Aspirin	**PO:** 650–975 mg q 4 h	**PO:** 10–15 mg/kg q 4 h	The standard against which other NSAIDs are compared. Inhibits platelet aggregation; may cause postoperative bleeding. *Contraindicated with fever or viral illness*
Ibuprofen (Motrin®, others) * elixir concentration = 100 mg/5ml	**PO:** 400 mg q 4–6 h 3.2 g/day max	**PO:** 10 mg/kg q 6–8 h 70 mg/kg/day max	Available as several brand names and as generic; also available as oral suspension; gastritis/platelet dysfunction
Ketorolac tromethamine (Toradol®)	30 or 60 mg IV/IM initial dose followed by 15 or 30 mg q 6 h	0.5 mg/kg q 6 h IV/IM	Duration of therapy not to exceed three days or 12 doses; gastritis/platelet dysfunction

Courtesy of Janet Semenova PNP, John S. Jones MD, Analgesic Reference Resource, Pain Management Services, Phoenix Children's Hospital.

include seizures, drowsiness, nervousness, ventricular tachycardia or fibrillation, tachycardia, hypertension, and asystole. Gastrointestinal problems such as nausea and vomiting may occur as can respiratory depression, hyperpnea, and pulmonary edema. Administering Narcan® to newborns of addicted mothers or to drug addicts may cause seizures and other withdrawal symptoms. The drug is metabolized in the liver and excreted in the urine.

Romazicon® (flumazenil) competitively inhibits the activity at the benzodiazepine recognition site on the GABA/

Table 1.7 An approach to moderate/severe postprocedural pain

Drug	Usual adult dose >50 kg	Usual pediatric dose <50 kg	Comments, side effects, contraindications
Morphine (oral **immediate release IR** – Roxanol®, MSIR®, oral **controlled release CR** – MS Contin®)	**IV:** 5–10 mg q 2–4 h **Continuous IV:** 0.8–1 mg/h **PO IR:** 30 mg q 3–4 h Not PRN **or** 60 mg q 3–4 h PRN **PO CR:** 15–30 mg q 8–12 h	**IV:** 0.05–0.1 mg/kg/dose q 2–4 h; *Neonates:* ½ of pediatric dosing **Continuous IV:** 0.01–0.04 mg/kg/h **POIR:** 0.3–0.6 mg/kg q 3–4 h **PO CR:** 0.3–1 mg/kg per dose q 8–12 h	Histamine release – pruritus Nausea/vomiting, miosis, sedation, urinary retention, respiratory depression, constipation, seizures in newborns. *Metabolized hepatically to M6G. M6G is renally excreted. May accumulate and cause respiratory depression in renal failure.*
Hydromorphone (Dilaudid®)	**IV:** 1.5 mg q 3–4 h **PO:** 6 mg q 3–4 h **PR:** 3 mg q 6–8 h	**IV:** 0.015 mg/kg/dose q 3–4 h **PO:** 0.03–0.08 mg/kg/dose q 3–4 h	Side effects may be less prominent than with morphine. *No active metabolite.*
Fentanyl (IV – Sublimaze®; Patch – Duragesic®)	**IV:** 25–100 mcg **Continuous IV:** 50–100 µg/h **Transdermal:** 25 µg/h or convert from current opioid to equipotent dose	**IV:** 1–5 µg/kg/dose q 30–60 min **Continuous IV:** 1–5 µg/kg/h **Transdermal:** 8–15 µg/kg/h	Rapid infusion may cause chest wall rigidity. Tolerance develops rapidly. Rapid onset, short duration of action. Transdermal – Should not be used in opioid naïve patients; 15–17 h to reach steady state. Absorption accelerated in response to fever or heat.
Oxycodone **IR** with **acetaminophen*** (Percocet®) **CR**: (OxyContin®)	**Recommended starting doses:** **PO IR:** 5–15 mg oxycodone q 3–4 h **PO CR:** 10 mg oxycodone q 12 h	**PO IR:** 0.1–0.2 mg/kg/dose oxycodone q 3–4 h **PO CR:** 0.6–0.8 mg/kg/dose oxycodone q 12 h	N/V, pruritus, constipation, sedation.
Hydrocodone plus acetaminophen* (Lortab®, Vicodin®)	**PO:** 5–10 mg hydrocodone q 3–4 h	**PO:** 0.1–0.2 mg/kg/dose hydrocodone q 3–4 h	Same as oxycodone
Methadone (Dolophine®)	**IV:** 10 mg q 6–8 h **PO:** 20 mg q 6–8 h	**IV:** 0.1 mg/kg q 6–8 h **PO:** 0.2 mg/kg q 6–8 h – acute dosing; for ongoing chronic use, dose may be smaller	Drug may accumulate with repeated dosing due to prolonged half-life, peak CNS and respiratory depression may not be reached for several days following institution of or increase in dose. The effects on respiration appear to last longer than analgesia. Same side effects as morphine.

* Caution: when combining opioid products that contain acetaminophen with prn acetaminophen (90 mg/kg/day max acetaminophen dose) in children and >50 kg max of 4 g/day.
Courtesy of Janet Semenova PNP, John S. Jones MD, Analgesic Reference Resource, Pain Management Services, Phoenix Children's Hospital.

benzodiazepine receptor complex. For the reversal of the sedative effects of benzodiazepines administered for conscious sedation in pediatric patients the recommended initial dose is 0.01 mg/kg (up to a maximum of 0.2 mg) administered intravenously over 15 seconds. If the desired level of consciousness is not obtained after waiting an additional 45 seconds, further injections of 0.01 mg/kg (up to a maximum of 0.2 mg) can be administered and repeated at 60-second intervals up to a maximum total dose of 0.05 mg/kg or 1 mg. Complications of Romazicon® include seizures, weak or shallow breathing, continued drowsiness for longer than two hours, confusion, fear, panic attack, or a fast or uneven heart rate.

Postprocedure pain management

Children commonly experience pain after a majority of procedures. However, the tolerance to pain varies widely between individuals of all age groups. We have found it helpful to anticipate this postprocedural discomfort and give families prescriptions when they go home or speak with house staff of inpatients so that each child is given the necessary drugs to control their discomfort (Table 1.6: An approach to mild/moderate postprocedural pain; Table 1.7: An approach to moderate/severe postprocedural pain). This approach seems to lead to greater patient and family satisfaction.

Chapter 2

Central venous access

Kevin M. Baskin and Richard Towbin

History 23
Interventional radiology and CVC insertion 23
Team approach 23
Route of access 25
Peripherally inserted central catheter (PICC) insertion 27
Introduction 27
Indications 27
Technique 29
Equipment 29
Patient preparation 30
Standard technique 33
Technical variations 36
Catheter measurement 36
Postprocedure and follow-up care 36
PICC removal 36
Technical problems and pitfalls 37
Complications 38
Catheter-related thrombophlebitis 38
Catheter dysfunction 38
Central venous catheter (CVC) insertion 39
Introduction 39
Indications 41
Technique: internal jugular CVC insertion 42
Equipment 42
Patient preparation 43
Standard technique 44
Creation of a subcutaneous tunnel 49
Postprocedure and follow-up care 50
Technical problems and pitfalls 50
Technique: subclavian CVC 51
Equipment and patient preparation 51
Standard technique 51
Technical variations 52

Postprocedure and follow-up care 52
Technique: femoral CVC 52
Equipment and patient preparation 52
Standard technique 52
Technical variations 53
Postprocedure and follow-up care 53
Technique: difficult access 53
Equipment and patient preparation 54
Standard technique: transbrachiocephalic access 54
Standard technique: transhepatic access 58
Postprocedure and follow-up care 59
Standard technique: translumbar access 59
Technical variations 60
Stabilizing the guide wire 60
Postprocedure and follow-up care 61
Technique: venous recanalization 61
Equipment 61
Patient preparation 61
Standard technique 61
Postprocedure and follow-up care 62
CVC removal 62
Complications 65
Infection 65
Malposition 68
Tip occlusion 69
Thrombolysis 70
Thrombosis 73
Mechanical malfunction 74
Intravascular foreign body 75
Indwelling infusaport (port) insertion 76
Introduction 76
Indications 76
Technique 77
Equipment 77
Patient preparation 77

Pediatric Interventional Radiology, ed. Richard Towbin and Kevin M. Baskin. Published by Cambridge University Press. © Cambridge University Press 2015.

Creation of a subcutaneous pocket 77
Technical variations 79
Arm port insertion 79
Postprocedure and follow-up care 81
Technical problems and pitfalls 81
Port removal 81
Conversion of port to CVC 84
Complications 84
Future advances 85
Controversies/issues 86
Conclusions 87

Appendices
Appendix 2.A Blood drawing from a PICC or CVC 88
Appendix 2.B Central venous catheter repair 89
Appendix 2.C Procedure for CVC occlusion: complete or partial 90
Appendix 2.D Heparin locking 92
Appendix 2.E Dressing change 93
Appendix 2.F Accessing an implantable venous access device (IVAD port) 94
Appendix 2.G Critical management for implantable venous access devices (port) 96

History

The history of venous cannulation extends over 250 years. Intravenous therapy was first performed in children in the 1940s. In 1973, Broviac and associates introduced the tunneled silicone central venous catheter (CVC) for prolonged hyperalimentation. Six years later, Hickman and colleagues presented an alternative to the Broviac right atrial catheter with a larger lumen. The Hickman catheter has subsequently gained popularity for a broader range of indications. Initially, tunneled right atrial catheters were inserted by surgical cut-down of the proximal cephalic vein and subcutaneous tunneling to the anterior chest wall. However, this approach was not always successful because of the small caliber of the cephalic vein. Thus, cut-down of the larger and more central internal or external jugular veins was introduced in the early 1980s, and soon after methods were described for percutaneous insertion of subclavian venous catheters. Over the years, surgical techniques have been adapted so that central lines could be inserted percutaneously without and with imaging guidance.

Interventional radiology and CVC insertion

In the past, interventionalists were primarily consulted to evaluate and treat catheter dysfunction or catheter-related complications, through diagnostic venography as well as image-guided redirection of malpositioned catheters and retrieval of intravascular catheter fragments. Advances in imaging, especially sonography, and in interventional techniques allowed interventionalists to gain venous access even in patients whose major venous pathways (jugular, subclavian, and femoral) had become occluded. In the late 1980s, surgical techniques for placement of central lines were adapted to allow for primary percutaneous insertion. Since that time, successful placement of CVCs in angiography suites has become the norm in virtually all facilities worldwide where interventional services are available. The percutaneous technique is equally adaptable for both children and adults. Over the last few years, referrals for insertion of CVCs have increased dramatically. In many large pediatric centers, pediatric interventionalists provide leadership of the multispecialty coalition responsible for the many diverse aspects of care of the complex population of patients who require central venous access. Image-guided percutaneous insertion of central and peripheral catheters for venous access is now the fastest growing segment of pediatric interventional practice. Venous access insertion and salvage procedures performed by interventional radiologists have proven to be safer, more cost effective, and more durable than alternative options, especially for patients at highest risk for catheter-related complications.

Team approach

Vascular access is one of the most ubiquitous interventions within tertiary health care centers. For some patients (e.g., with cystic fibrosis) central access is a predictable feature of their admission. It is helpful to plan the procedure prior to the patient's arrival in hospital. For others (e.g., hemophiliacs and children with intestinal failure) long-term access is an essential component of their lives, and thorough coordination of their home care should be planned, when possible, in advance of their discharge.

Although in the past central venous access had been accomplished primarily by the surgical service, it is now clear that the entire spectrum of access catheters and ports can be accurately and safely placed in the interventional suite with a comparable or improved rate of successful insertion, reduced complication rates, and prompt (often same-day) service. The success rate, complication rate, and accuracy of catheter positioning in the interventional suite compares favorably to CVC insertion in the operating room. In our practice successful insertion of a CVC is accomplished in over 99% of cases. The complication rate is about 2% with presumptive perioperative infection being most common. In general, placement using interventional techniques is now considered the approach of choice in many institutions. Minimally invasive, image-guided placement has the advantage of being less costly since it usually is accomplished using intravenous sedation outside of the operating room and does not require same-day surgery, recovery room, or anesthesiology services. Perhaps the most important consideration is that image-guided CVC insertion avoids using the subclavian vein. This is relevant because the subclavian vein is the final common pathway from the ipsilateral extremity and neck to the heart and its use for central access is associated with the highest

Table 2.1 Procedure and outcome measures

Guidelines are available in the literature for (1) quality improvement, (2) prevention of catheter-related infections, and (3) reporting standards for CVC placement. To improve outcome and quality assurance analysis, it may be helpful to record the following information for each central venous access device referral or deployment:

- Demographic information (patient name, unique identification number, date and time of procedure, age, sex, weight, date of birth, etc.)
- Underlying disease, patient acuity, comorbid illness, ASA class, competence of patient or primary caregiver
- Any contraindicating or complicating factors
  - coagulopathy
  - fever, sepsis, known infection, immunodeficiency, nutritional status
  - venous stenosis
  - acute thrombosis
  - local skin infection
- Referring service and provider; inpatient or outpatient status
- Provider or patient preference for CVC device or position
- Indication(s) for venous access placement or replacement; intended function (e.g., dialysis, plasmapheresis, phlebotomy, simultaneous delivery of medications that cannot be mixed)
- Anticipated endpoint for venous access
- Provider responsible for access (interventionalist, surgeon, nurse, etc.)
- Procedure location (interventional suite, operating room, bedside, etc.)
- Provider responsible for anesthesia/sedation (anesthesiologist, nurse, etc.)
- Preprocedural interventions (e.g., antibiotics, blood products, imaging)
- Initial access
  - entry side and site (e.g., basilic vein, internal jugular vein, common femoral vein)
  - method (e.g., visual, fluoroscopic venography, ultrasound)
  - device (e.g., angiocatheter, single wall needle)
  - number and location of unsuccessful and successful attempts
  - complications (e.g., arterial puncture, pneumothorax)
  - reason for deferral, discontinuation or failure, if insertion not completed
- Access device and position
- Catheter manufacturer, description, lumen number and diameter, final length, composition, coating or impregnation, etc.
- Implanted, tunneled or direct? (If tunneled, length and exit site)
- Cuffed or uncuffed? (If cuffed, material and position)
- Tip position and catheter function (Satisfactory position? How were position and function confirmed?)
- Method of catheter fixation, wound closure and dressing
- Equipment and supplies used; cost
- Procedure time, fluoroscopy time or estimated radiation dose
- Type, duration, and adequacy of anesthesia/sedation/analgesia
- Procedural complications (e.g., venospasm, extravasation) and management
- Adjunctive therapies required (e.g., papaverine, nitroglycerine, tissue plasminogen activator (tPA), hot packs)
- Complications, including:
- Catheter-related infection (include dates)
  - type (phlebitis; catheter-related sepsis; bacteremia; colonization; exit site, tunnel or pocket infection, etc.)
  - suspected (basis) or proven (method and results)
  - management (e.g., antibiotics, catheter removal, repeat cultures)
  - result of catheter-tip and blood cultures
  - outcome
- Catheter dysfunction (include dates)
  - type (e.g., phlegmasia, extravasation or infiltration, fracture, fragment embolization, etc.)
  - management
  - outcome
- Occlusion, fibrin sheath formation or thrombosis (include dates)
  - method of diagnosis or documentation
  - location and extent
  - management
  - outcome
- Dislodgment, migration or malposition (include dates)
  - method of diagnosis or documentation
  - management
  - outcome
- Other catheter-related complications or interventions
- Complications, additional details:
  - Major
    - admission to hospital for therapy
    - unplanned increase in level of care
    - prolonged hospitalization
    - permanent adverse sequelae
    - death
  - Minor
    - no sequelae
    - nominal therapy
    - short hospital stay (for observation)
  - Procedurally related (within 24 hours of insertion)
  - Early (within 30 days of placement)
  - Late
- Removal or replacement (reason and date; endpoint achieved?)

rate of complications. Even asymptomatic thrombotic occlusion is important in that it significantly reduces the number of potential access sites.

While most central access in large pediatric centers today can be managed by the interventional and nursing services, there is frequent need for expert support from services across the spectrum of specialization, including radiology, surgery, nursing, anesthesiology, intensive care, oncology, hematology, nephrology, emergency services, infectious diseases, epidemiology, hemodialysis and apheresis services, discharge planning, and home health care. Such coordination of care, in some cases under the auspices of a central venous access service, is essential for optimal management of this large and diverse patient population.

A substantial proportion of costs and complications related to central venous access may be reduced through improved allocation of resources, aggressive education of patients, families and health care practitioners who become involved with central access devices, improved communication between health care providers, preventive care and early intervention for expected complications, and careful quality control through outcomes information management and dissemination (Table 2.1).

Route of access

Although there is less reported experience with image-guided placement of CVCs in children than in adults, many of the stated indications pertinent to the older age groups are also relevant in childhood. Today, when central venous access is considered, a variety of possibilities exist. For both CVCs and peripherally inserted central catheters (PICCs) one can select from non-tunneled catheters, tunneled catheters, or ports. The most frequent referrals to the interventional service for venous access are children who need total parenteral nutrition, medium- to long-term antibiotics or chemotherapy, frequent blood drawing, fluid replacement, and severely ill children in the intensive care unit. However, in general, any child requiring one or more weeks of intravenous therapy or those who require venous access for recurrent blood drawing have become candidates for insertion of either a PICC or CVC (Appendix 2.A). With the large number of choices currently available the type of catheter used for central venous access can now be tailored to children of all ages and sizes.

Currently, there are no specific criteria for deciding whether to place a CVC or PICC. In our practice, the choice of a CVC or PICC is based on physician preference, patient size and age, vessel patency, predicted length of time that central access is needed, family or patient preference, and underlying illness. In general, we prefer to insert PICCs for children older than one year who need venous access for a short period of time (two to four weeks), older children with larger peripheral veins, and children with pulmonary disease or abnormal pulmonary function. The latter group of children (e.g., cystic fibrosis, positive pressure ventilation) could have their life threatened by a pneumothorax complicating central venous access. In most of the situations described above, a 3 French (for children less than 10 kg) or 4 French (for children greater than 10 kg) single lumen non-tunneled PICC is inserted. With newer materials and catheter treatments (e.g., antibiotic-impregnated catheters), we are evolving toward longer term use of PICCs in select situations.

In our patient population a peripheral port is not commonly inserted because of its expense and the short time that lines are needed in general. Ports for central or peripheral lines are used for individuals who need long-term, intermittent venous access. Ports are now available in single and double lumen designs in a variety of sizes. In the pediatric population children requiring chemotherapy or long-term blood component replacement are the primary recipients. A CVC (usually 5 to 7 French) is preferred in a wide variety of circumstances, especially for children receiving chemotherapy, children with organ transplants, severely ill patients in the ICU, those requiring dialysis, apheresis, or frequent blood draws, hyperalimentation, or drug infusion therapy.

Once the appropriate access device has been selected, a pathway for placement must be planned. This includes determination of the insertion site, the intravascular course, and the tip position of the intended access. Preferred pathways are well established, although particular variations are seen from institution to institution, and reflect local experience and preferences. In general, a PICC line proceeds from a vein in the upper extremity through the basilic, brachial, or cephalic vein. Whenever possible the basilic or brachial veins are selected since they are the largest, most accessible, and have the straightest course. Whether initial puncture is via the superficial system (e.g., basilic vein) or deep system (e.g., brachial vein) appears to have no measurable impact on outcomes.

The cephalic vein is an interesting and challenging alternative. In young children the terminal arch appears to mature at a different rate than the rest of the veins of the extremity and is often 1 to 2 French smaller than the proximal cephalic vein. As a result the "infantile" form of the terminal segment may challenge the interventionalist to navigate its terminal "C" or "Z" shape. We have found that in order to be able to go from the cephalic vein into the subclavian vein one may need to use advanced techniques including fluoroscopic road mapping, a directional catheter, preferably a 3 French directional catheter, and an angled glide wire, that significantly increase the complexity, duration, and cost of the procedure. In some instances it is wise to simply stop and puncture another vein.

Ports and jugular lines are tunneled from the chest wall through a central vein. Whenever possible, the internal jugular vein is the preferred route of access. Subclavian lines are avoided whenever possible but can also be tunneled from a similar position on the chest wall. For each of these, the tip is positioned at the entrance to the right atrium (see below). Femoral lines proceed from the common femoral vein to one of two preferred positions: short lines that end in the infrarenal IVC, and long lines that end between the diaphragm and the inferior third of the right atrium, preferably below the seventh thoracic interspace.

The anatomy of the cavoatrial junction is seldom detailed in discussions of catheter tip placement, and improved understanding of this region may assist those who insert central venous access devices to position the catheter with greater confidence and fewer complications. The *entrance to the right atrium* (true cavoatrial junction) is that portion of the cavoatrial junction adjacent to the embryologic true atrium. The cavoatrial junction (Figure 2.1a) is formed developmentally by absorption of the right horn of the sinus venosus, bounded at its inferior margin by the crista terminalis anterolaterally, and the remnant of septum secundum (crista dividens or superior limbic band) posteromedially.

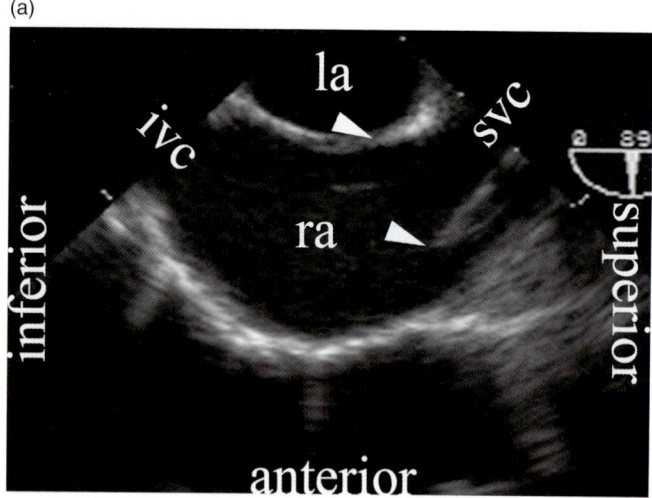
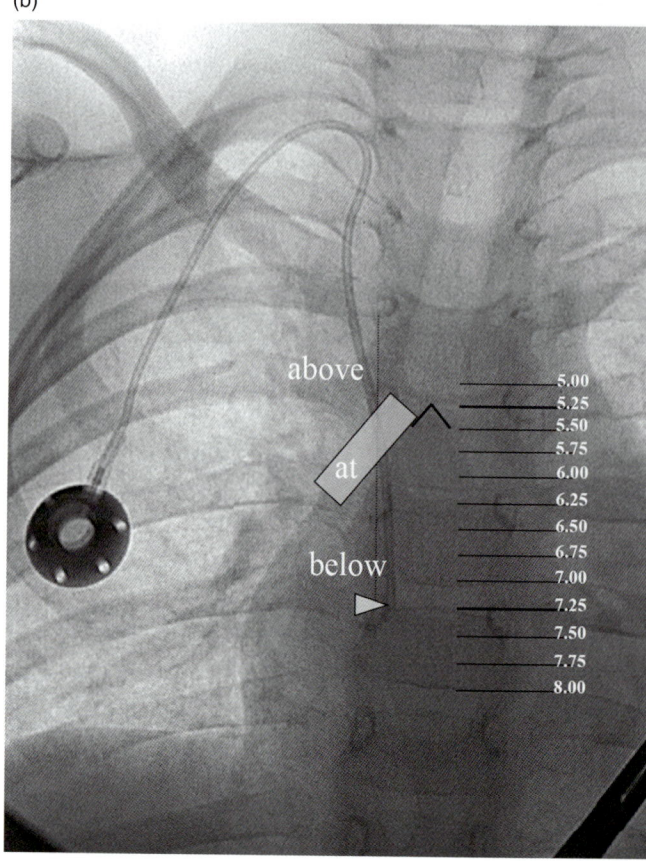

Figure 2.1 Four-year-old male with murmur. (a) This transesophageal echocardiogram demonstrates the structures that form the inferior margin of the superior vena cava (*svc*) in the right atrium (*ra*), including the crista dividens (remnant of the septum secundum) in the intra-atrial septum (*posterior arrowhead*), and the crista terminalis (*anterior arrowhead*). Image courtesy of Meryl Cohen, MD. (b) A right internal jugular indwelling venous port catheter tip is positioned with its tip (*arrowhead*) two vertebral bodies below the carina, below the right mainstem bronchus. Three-dimensional analysis of the chest CT obtained at the same time as this topogram confirmed this point to be precisely at the cavoatrial junction in this patient.

This region corresponds to a point two vertebral bodies below the carina on a posterior–anterior (PA) chest radiograph (Figure 2.1b), and *not* to the upper margin of the right cardiac silhouette. In fact, CVCs that seem to be located high in the right atrium by chest radiograph are often actually in the superior vena cava (SVC) and pose little risk of cardiac perforation. Catheter tip position in the region of the entrance to the right atrium helps assure that the catheter tip will float freely and more centrally within the vascular lumen, less prone to malposition through respiratory and other patient motion, fixation or occlusion against the lateral wall of the SVC, or vascular injury and perforation, especially for catheters entering from the left side.

Challenges may arise when preferred pathways are not accessible, due to venospasm, venous thrombosis or fibrosis, overlying scar, inflammation, burns, infection, or other factors. Prolonged attempts at a difficult site often show rapidly diminishing returns. In patients without a history of prior access, simply moving to the contralateral side or to an alternate preferred site is usually sufficient for success. This may require changing access devices as well, perhaps selecting jugular CVC insertion when venospasm prevents passage of a PICC, for example. Anticipation of such changes in plan is reflected in preprocedural discussions with referring physicians, patients, and parents, so the child leaves the interventional suite with adequate access despite unforeseen obstacles. In patients with a history of difficult access, more careful pathway planning becomes important.

Magnetic resonance angiography has been suggested for mapping potential pathways for central venous access in patients with a history of chronic deep venous thrombosis (DVT). However, it is in just those most challenging patients with extensive collateralization that MR angiography is least accurate. Ultrasonography (US) performed just prior to access frequently displays patent veins as well as obstacles to access such as intravascular thrombosis and anatomic variation. However, the limited field of view compared to CT or fluoroscopy makes it less useful for demonstrating collateral pathways. Once collaterals are identified, US can be used to guide needle insertion. In patients with a history of difficult access, it is sensible to perform contrast venography at the time vascular access is first obtained, even if initial access is achieved under US control. Even if a direct pathway (i.e., via named vessels) to the right atrium is not available, alternate pathways are often visualized.

These pathways may be quite complex (e.g., jugular → paravertebral → hemizygos → azygos → right atrium; Figure 2.2),

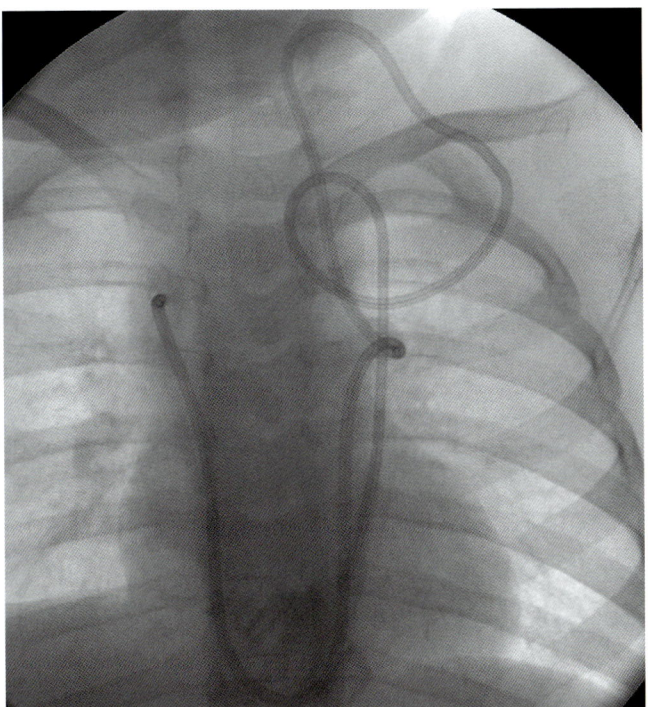

Figure 2.2 This child with chronic intestinal failure, dependent on parenteral nutrition, presented for central venous access insertion after therapy for a prior central line associated bloodstream infection. All conventional venous pathways above the diaphragm were occluded. This double lumen catheter was advanced over a wire that had been manipulated through a complex route from left jugular vein through the paravertebral vein, hemizygos vein, and azygos vein to the right atrium, where it was snared from a right transfemoral approach and exteriorized for stability. The central venous catheter could not be advanced beyond the azygos arch due to the tortuosity of the pathway, but provided adequate access until liver transplantation was performed.

and may require unusual methods to navigate as variously described in "Technical variations," below. Procedures for access via some alternative pathways (e.g., translumbar (Figure 2.3) and transhepatic (Figure 2.4)) have been well described. Other alternate pathways, such as retroclavicular brachiocephalic access (Figure 2.5), are not well known and require advanced ultrasound guidance skills but offer very safe and durable access in patients with extensive central venous occlusions. In the end, one must weigh the needs of the patient against the time and cost of pursuing difficult access. For a relatively short course of antibiotics, serial peripheral angiocatheters might provide adequate access. For a line-dependent child, more novel, complex, and higher risk procedures may be warranted.

Peripherally inserted central catheter (PICC) insertion

Introduction

Silicone catheters were first introduced in 1961 by Stewart and Stanislow and have subsequently gained favor. Development of the silastic catheter and insertion techniques has helped make long-term indwelling catheter insertion one of the most commonly performed procedures in both the pediatric and adult populations. Peripherally inserted central catheters (PICCs), introduced for parenteral nutrition in neonates by Shaw, have been in use since the 1970s. These small-gauge silastic or polyurethane catheters are advanced through peripheral veins, usually of the upper arm or forearm, with the tip positioned centrally. Initially, these were passed through a short peel-away sheath preloaded over a single wall access needle, and passed blindly without a guide wire a predetermined distance calculated to place the tip in the mid- to distal-portion of the SVC. This method is still in use for bedside placement on the ward and in intensive care units. It is associated with a high rate of complication, including failed insertions and frequent malposition or non-central position.

Various methods have been used since to assure proper positioning, including radiographic and US guidance, and use of adjuncts such as intra-atrial EKG monitoring. Many institutions now find it cost-effective to stratify candidates for PICC insertion, assigning straightforward insertions to specially trained nurses, and reserving complicated patients for image-guided placement by an interventional radiologist. This again emphasizes the importance of coordination of vascular access services across the institution.

Indications

There is a general perception that nearly all patients will require a peripheral intravenous angiocatheter on admission to the hospital. This perception may delay consideration of PICC or CVC insertion in the substantial proportion of patients for whom prolonged therapy (greater than one to two weeks) can be anticipated on or prior to admission. For this reason, many children are subjected to the discomfort and increased complications associated with frequent replacement of peripheral angiocatheters, and end up with a PICC anyway. Since their introduction, their scope of use has been broadened considerably (Table 2.2).

Originally, PICCs were used predominantly as an alternative to serial peripheral angiocatheters, allowing safer administration of sclerosing medications, avoiding the need for frequent catheter replacement, and permitting substantial improvements in nutrient delivery and weight gain. PICCs are now also used as an effective alternative to tunneled central venous catheters in many applications. They are most commonly used in children to deliver long-term parenteral nutrition, but are also helpful for intermediate- to long-term access for delivery of chemotherapy, antibiotics, blood products, and fluids and electrolytes, as well as for patients who require frequent blood sampling.

Because children can receive care at home with a PICC in place, central venous access via a PICC line can allow them to be discharged earlier from tertiary care institutions to receive care closer to home, lowering the cost of care as well as the impact on the patient and family. PICC insertion with imaging guidance is safe and effective for patients of all ages and sizes,

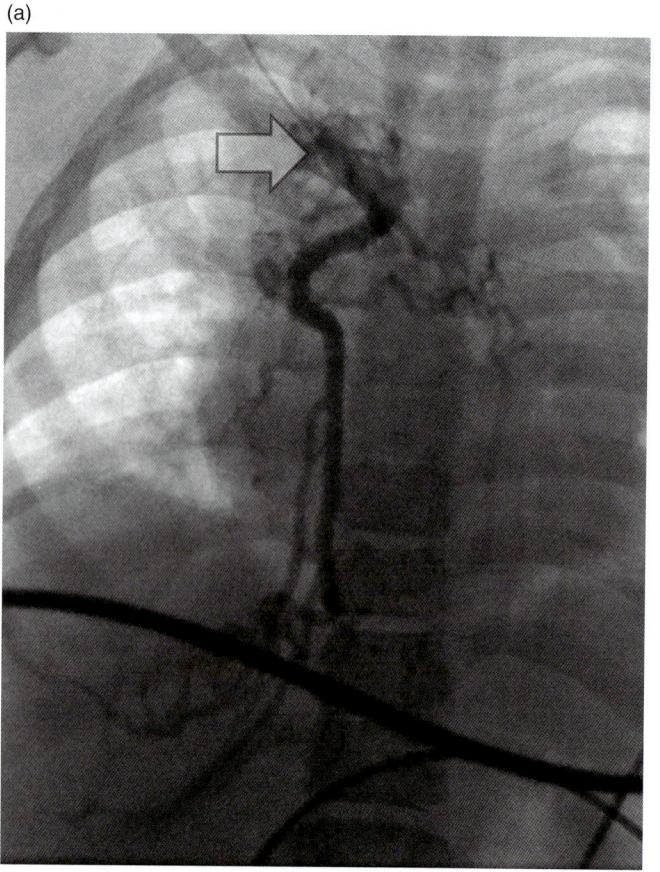
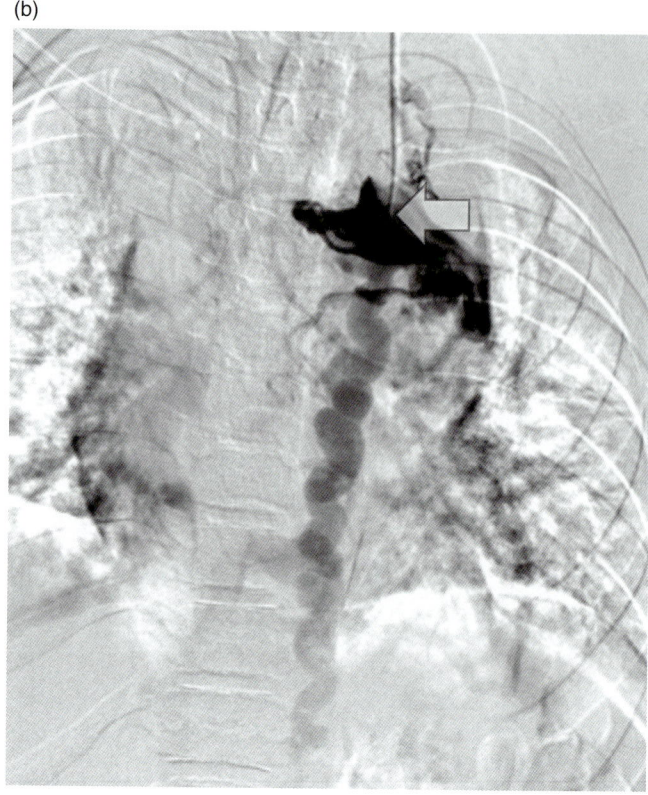
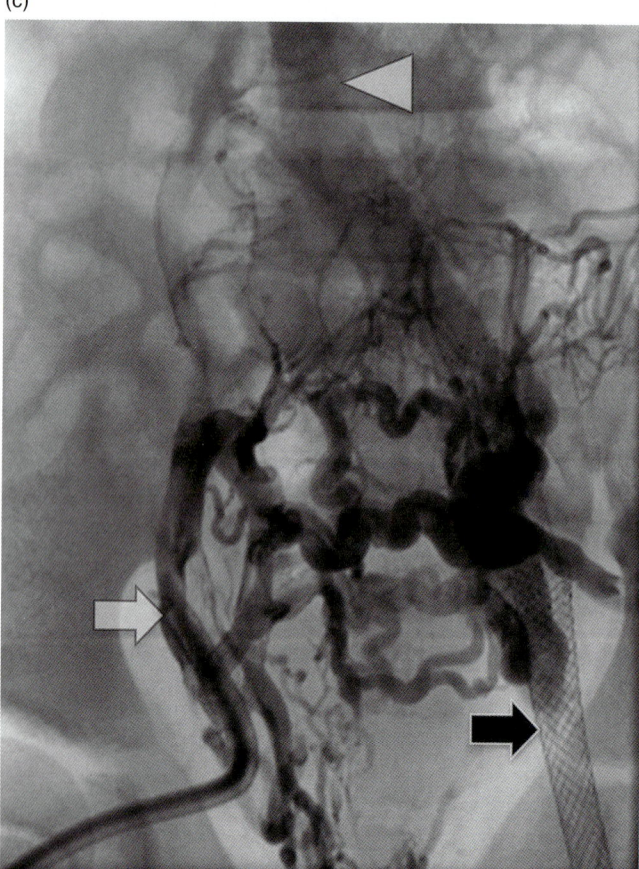
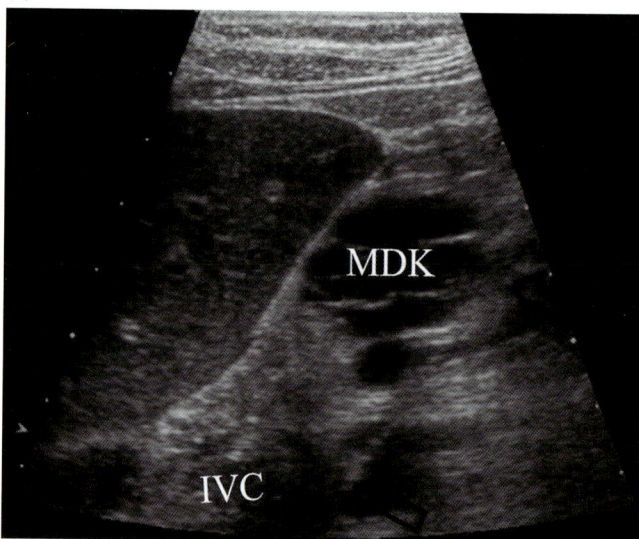

Figure 2.3 A nine-year-old boy with multicystic dysplastic kidneys, after numerous venous procedures, had complete occlusion of all six conventional central venous pathways despite vigorous recanalization efforts. (a) Venography from the junction (*arrow*) of the right internal jugular and subclavian veins demonstrates complete occlusion of the systemic veins and azygos arch with drainage below the diaphragm through azygos and hemizygos collaterals. (b) Venography from the contralateral side (*arrow*) shows complete occlusion of the left internal jugular, subclavian, and brachiocephalic veins with drainage below the diaphragm via hemizygos collaterals. (c) Contrast injection through the existing right external iliac hemodialysis catheter (*white arrow*) shows complete occlusion of the pelvic veins with reconstitution of the IVC (*arrowhead*) via somatic collaterals. A left femoral vein stent (*black arrow*), placed several years

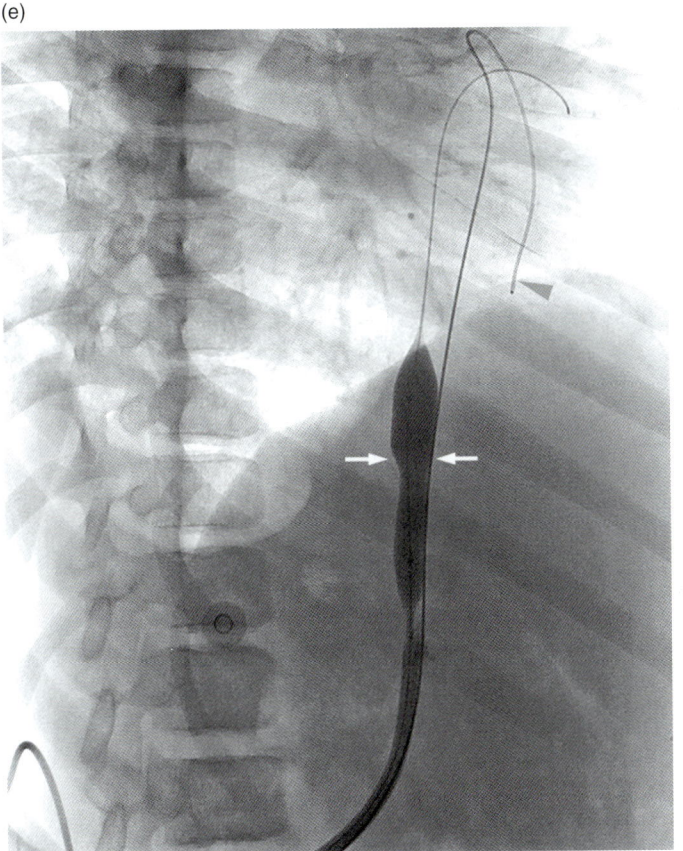 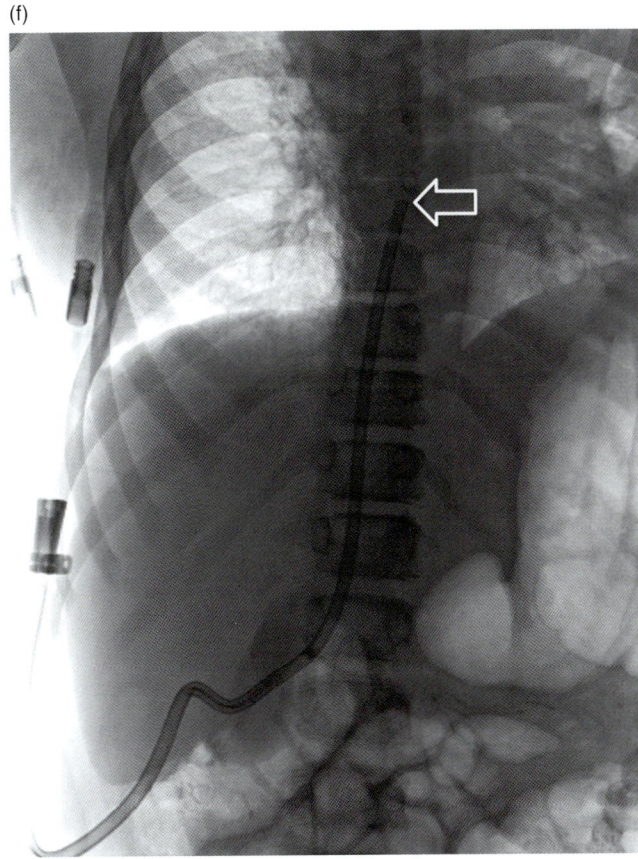

Figure 2.3 (cont.) previously by interventional cardiology, is also completely occluded. (d) After pathway planning with three-dimensional rotational venographic reconstruction, the infrarenal inferior vena cava (*IVC*) was accessed under US guidance with a 15-cm 22-gauge Chiba needle (*arrows*), passing inferior to the kidney (*MDK*). (e) Secondary patency was retained after balloon disruption of a fibrin sheath (*arrows*) and catheter replacement over a superstiff guide wire. A second guide wire (*arrowhead*) was placed outside the sheath as a safety wire. (f) The tip (*arrow*) of the dialysis catheter is within the right atrium per Kidney Disease Outcomes Quality Initiative (KDOQI) guidelines. This pathway remained in use for hemodialysis over two years later.

and is associated with a high rate of success and a low rate of infections and other complications.

Technique

Equipment

The selection of needles, catheters, guide wires, and other equipment varies considerably depending on the experience and preference of the interventionalist and the size, age, and condition of the patient (Table 2.3). In the pediatric age group a range of access needle sizes, catheter diameters, and lengths of single and double lumen catheters are needed (Figure 2.6).

The needle size selected for venipuncture depends on the child's weight and size. A sheathed needle (angiocatheter) or a single wall needle is usually preferred. A Potts–Cournand or Seldinger single wall needle attached to a slip-tip saline syringe is occasionally helpful during fluoroscopically guided access to keep the operator's hand out of the beam. We recommend an access needle thin enough to decrease risk of vasospasm but with a bore large enough to pass at least a 0.018-inch guide wire. For very small infants it is occasionally necessary to begin with a smaller needle and wire, exchanging for a larger dilator or peel-away sheath once access is achieved. Children weighing 10 to 20 kg are usually accessed with 20- or 22-gauge needle. Occasionally, in larger children, 19- or 18-gauge needles are used.

PICCs are available in a range of sizes (2 to 7 French as single lumen catheters, 3.5 to 7 French as double lumen catheters) constructed of polyurethane in fixed lengths or of silicone/silastic, tailored to the desired length during the procedure. Most clinical indications for PICC insertion in children may be satisfied with a 3 or 4 French single lumen catheter. If desired, the silicone PICC lines are made with cuffs and can be tunneled or connected to a port. They are non-tapered and have a high friction coefficient. Thus, they are best inserted through a peel-away sheath and are more difficult to insert over a guide wire than catheters constructed of other materials. In contrast, the polyurethane catheters are firmer, have larger lumens and greater flow rates relative to French size, and are easier to insert. Since they have tapered ends they do not require a peel-away sheath and travel over a guide wire with considerably less effort. Their stiffness may increase the risk of vascular perforation in certain applications.

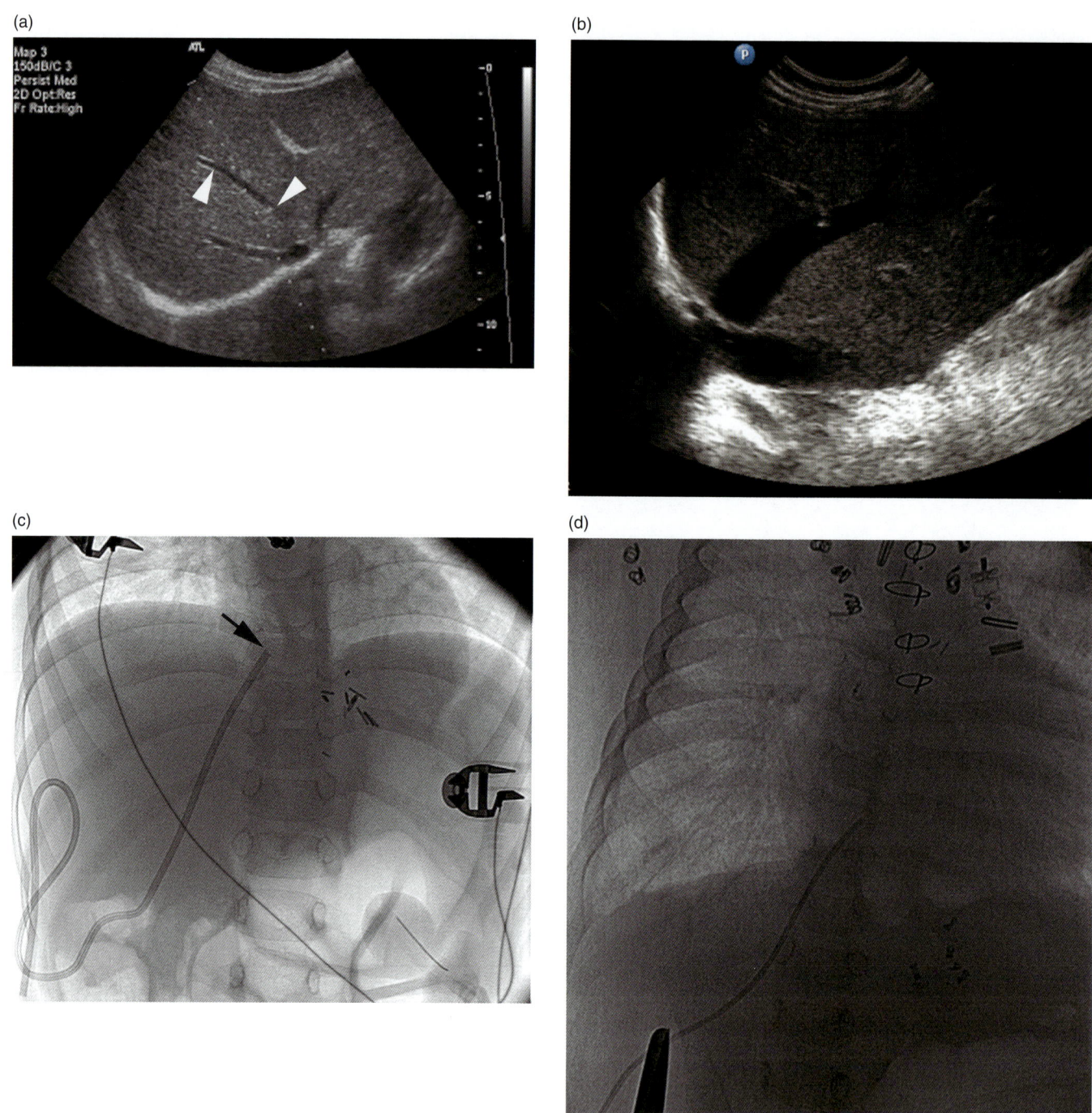

Figure 2.4 Nine-month-old female with congenital heart disease and occluded peripheral and central access. (a,b) Ultrasound-guided placement of needle within hepatic vein. (c,d) 4 French cuffed, tunneled central line placed with tip in the base of the right atrium.

Patient preparation

Informed consent for PICC insertion generally includes discussion of the technical aspects of line insertion, the differences between a CVC and PICC, the procedural risks, benefits and alternatives to PICC insertion. The lower risk of PICC insertion is stressed but the more common, adverse effects including local phlebitis, hematoma formation and infection, are noted. We find it helpful to draw a diagram of the proposed procedure to aid patient and parental understanding and answer questions. Because PICC insertion is never a certain outcome, especially in very sick or small children, we routinely prepare patients, parents, and referring clinicians for the possibility of CVC insertion as an alternative to abandoning or

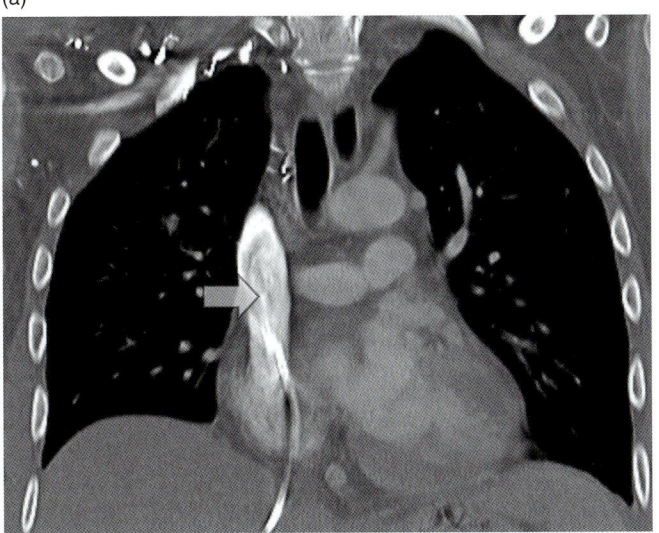
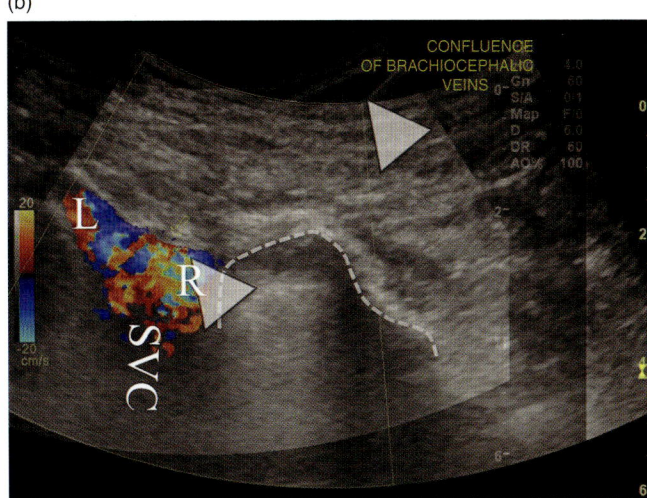
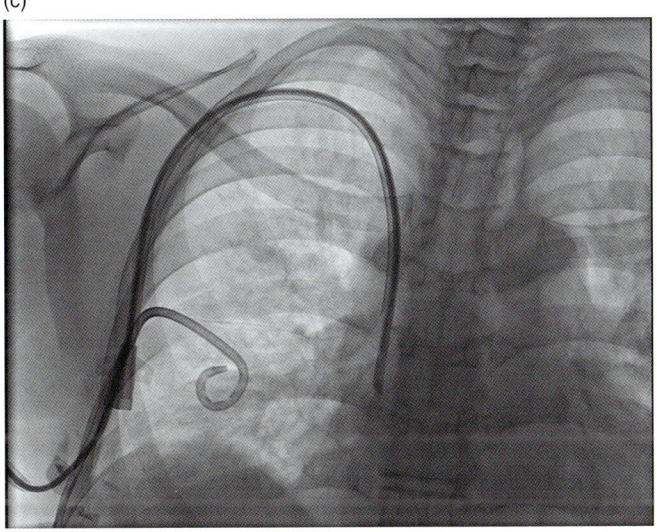

Figure 2.5 A 17-year-old male with long-standing renal failure after liver transplantation requires a hemodialysis catheter. The IVC is occluded at the confluence of common iliac veins. (a) Contrast injection through a preexisting middle hepatic venous catheter shows complete occlusion of the brachiocephalic veins at the confluence, with a patent proximal SVC. (b) An overlay of two right retroclavicular coronal ultrasound images demonstrates color Doppler signal in the SVC, at the confluence of the right (*R*) and left (*L*) brachiocephalic veins. A 21-gauge Chiba needle (*arrowheads*) has been advanced from the base of the neck into the stump of the right brachiocephalic vein, just medial to the superior-medial pleural margin (*dotted line*). (c) Contrast is seen in one lumen of the tunneled right brachiocephalic vein. 14-Fr hemodialysis catheter inserted using the access shown in (b). A preexisting right pleural pigtail thoracostomy drain is also seen, unrelated to this procedure.

unduly protracting a difficult or unfeasible attempt at PICC insertion.

All children are kept NPO for at least six hours so that they can be safely sedated. The occasional child requiring general anesthesia (GA) will be prepared according to the anesthesiology department protocol as if the child were to go to the operating room. When possible, children not receiving GA may benefit from topically applied anesthesia (e.g., eutectic mixture of local anesthetic, or EMLA®, cream or J-tip) placed at likely access sites at least one hour prior to the planned procedure. Laboratory tests are seldom required prior to PICC insertion, unless there is a known or suspected bleeding diathesis, or other pertinent medical condition. In such cases, tests may include a CBC, platelet count, PT, PTT, and rarely a bleeding time. Even so, PICC insertion may be accomplished with due care even in patients with an uncorrectable coagulopathy if the indication warrants, although every effort is made to normalize coagulation. Similarly, with appropriate caution and image guidance PICC lines and perhaps even CVCs may be inserted in patients receiving concurrent anticoagulant therapy. Prophylactic antibiotics are not routinely given, even for children with heart disease, congenital or acquired immune deficiency, sepsis, or high risk for infectious complications, as they do not measurably decrease the catheter-related infection rate in these children, but may increase antibiotic resistance in the at-risk population.

Once in the room, the child is placed on the angiography table and lightly secured with Velcro straps to reduce motion and avoid falling. All children are monitored with pulse oximetry and an automated blood pressure device. A sensor for pulse oximetry is secured to a finger, toe, foot, or an earlobe. Leads are placed for cardiovascular monitoring. Reusable sensors are available for small babies. An intravenous line is started, if possible in the basilic or cephalic vein, or in the hand of the same arm where PICC placement is anticipated. Currently, venographic guidance for entry site selection is rarely used

(Figure 2.7). Instead, US is almost exclusively used for entry site selection and real-time guidance of venipuncture. Although it is sometimes faster and easier to perform a standard venipuncture without imaging guidance at or just below the antecubital fossa with an angiocatheter to gain access into the venous system, the superficial access and location of the catheter at the crease of the elbow may increase the risk of "blown" veins, phlebitis, and mechanical injury to the catheter. We have found it preferable to access under US guidance in nearly all cases, in the upper arm

Table 2.2 Indications for PICC and CVC insertion

Temporary (non-tunneled) CVC (short-term access: <7 days)
- Urgent or emergent access
- Fluid and electrolyte resuscitation
- Antibiotic therapy
- Hemodialysis and apheresis

PICC (short- to long-term access: two weeks to >three months)
- Antibiotic therapy
- Hyperalimentation
- Fluid and electrolyte therapy
- Phlebotomy

Permanent (tunneled) CVC (intermediate- to long-term access: two weeks to >three months)
- Chemotherapy
- Hyperalimentation
- Antibiotics
- Blood product administration
- Fluid and electrolyte therapy
- Phlebotomy
- Chelation therapy
- Hemodialysis and apheresis

Indwelling port (long-term access, intermittent)
- Chemotherapy
- Hyperalimentation
- Blood product administration
- Fluid and electrolyte therapy

Table 2.3 Equipment for PICC and CVC insertion

PICC
- Access needle
  - angiocatheter (22–18 gauge)
  - single wall needle
  - Potts–Cournand needle
  - Seldinger needle
- Peel-away sheath (3–5 French)
- Catheter (3–5 French) (single or double lumen)
- Guide wire (glide wire, Newton wire, mandril wire," J" wire)
- Heparin (<10 kg = 1.5 ml 1:1,000, >10 kg = 3 ml 1:1,000)
- Suture (3–0 silk, 4–0 vicryl)
- Clear occlusive dressing

CVC
- Access needle
  - single wall needle
  - angiocatheter (22 gauge)
- Micropuncture kit
- Tapered vascular dilators
- Peel-away sheath (3.5 to 17 French)
- Tunneling device
- Scalpel
- Central line (single, double, or triple lumen)
  - polyurethane (3 to 7 French) (length: 5, 8, 12, 15 cm)
  - silastic (3 to 9 French) (length: tailored to patient size)
  - apheresis (7 to 12 French; double lumen)
  - dialysis (7 to 14 French; double lumen)
- Guide wire (Newton wire, "J" wire, glide wire, Amplatz Stiff® wire)
- Heparin (<10 kg = 1.5 ml 1:1,000, >10 kg = 3 ml 1:1,000)
- Suture (3–0 silk; 2–0, 3–0, 4–0 vicryl)
- Clear occlusive dressing

(a)

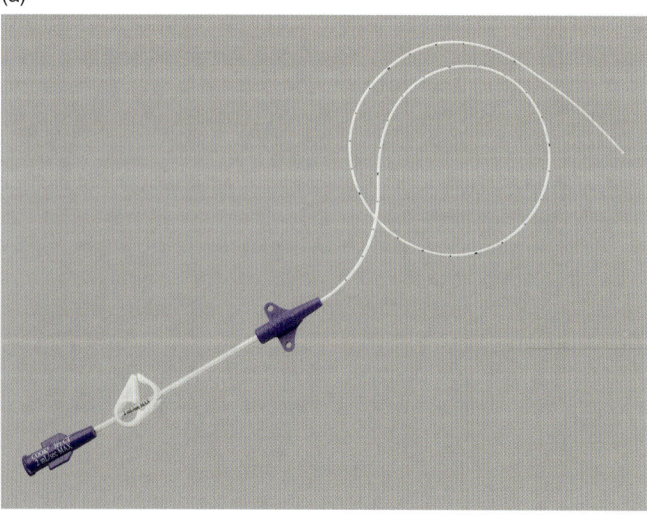

(b)

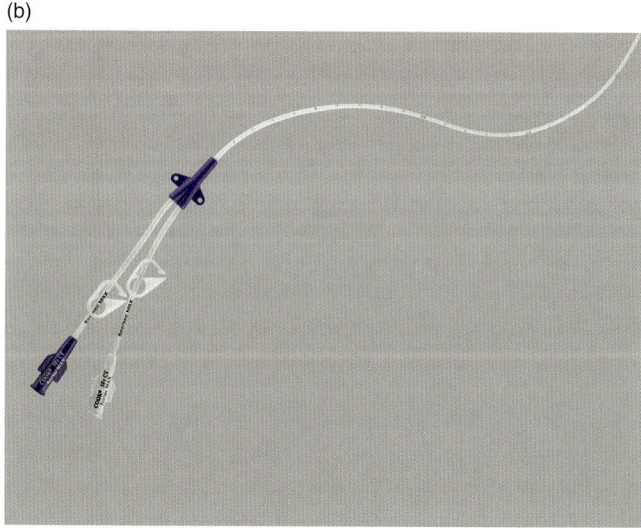

Figure 2.6 (a) 3 French single lumen PICC (Cook Medical). (b) 5 French dual lumen CT compatible PICC (Cook Medical).

Table 2.4 Procedural summary: PICC insertion

- Preprocedural laboratory studies usually not needed.
- Insert IV with ultrasound guidance. If access is uncertain or complicated consider contrast injection with fluoroscopy. If access may be tenuous or difficult, be prepared to insert a guide wire immediately.
- Prepare and drape skin.
- Locally anesthetize entry site.
- Small skin incision at entry site.
- Puncture basilic or brachial vein. Avoid cephalic vein if possible.
- Insert guide wire to or beyond right atrium.
- Dilate tract.
- Exchange dilator for peel-away sheath.
- Measure distance from entry site to upper right atrium or cavoatrial junction.
- Cut PICC to length *(for silicone catheters)*.
- Insert PICC.
- Inject contrast to confirm satisfactory position.
- Secure line in place (e.g., with Stat-loc or suture).
- Cover entry site with a 2 × 2 gauze and occlusive dressing.
- Heparinize PICC.

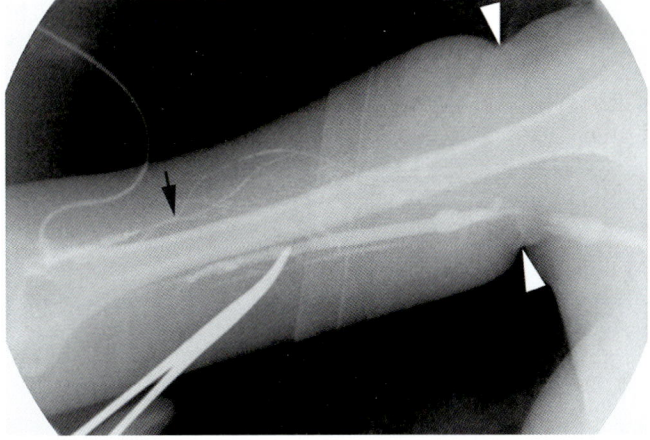

Figure 2.7 After cannulation of a collateral vein (*arrow*) in the arm of an 18-year-old woman with cystic fibrosis, injected contrast refluxes into the basilic vein. A hemostat tip is used to localize the basilic vein prior to venographically guided access. An elastic tourniquet (*arrowheads*) effaces the axillary vein.

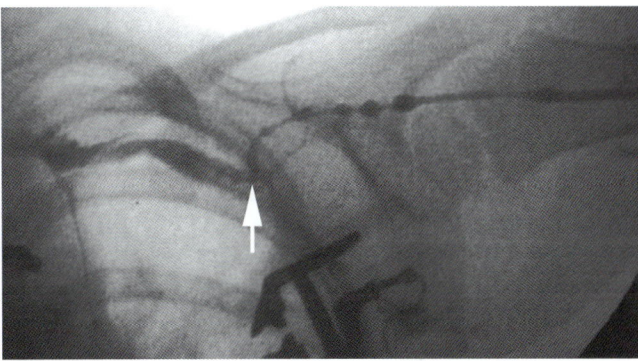

Figure 2.8 Venography performed after injection of intravenous contrast into a hand vein in a six-month-old boy fills the cephalic vein and demonstrates the typical acute angle (*arrow*) at the junction of the cephalic and axillary veins.

above the antecubital fossa, where the deeper veins are more stable.

A diagnostic venogram is not routinely performed prior to PICC insertion. We have found a venogram to be beneficial in the following situations: children who have had cut-downs; children who have had numerous venipunctures; those with a history of difficult or limited venous access; small children; and whenever there is difficulty maneuvering a catheter or guide wire into position. A venogram will show the venous anatomy and demonstrate the presence of collaterals, small, angulated connecting veins, and vasospasm.

Standard technique

There are variations in the order of steps, equipment, and monitoring used to place PICCs in various interventional practices (Table 2.4). In some practices, initial access is accomplished aseptically, with or without image guidance, according to the preference of the interventionalist. Our approach is to sedate or anesthetize the child, select the entry site, locally anesthetize the skin and subcutaneous tissue, and to use image guidance to assist venipuncture. Regardless how initial access is achieved, strict sterile technique and adherence to universal precautions is required for insertion of all central lines. The interventional suite is closed and entry restricted. All personnel entering the IR suite must wear hospital scrubs, surgical hats, and masks. The interventionalists and any ultrasonographer or other interventional assistants also must wear sterile gowns and gloves. The skin of the entry site is sterilely prepared and draped. For small children, we have found a fenestrated transparent cover to be useful. A large sterile field is created with sterile sheets to accommodate equipment, wires, etc., without risk of contamination. In addition, the imaging equipment is covered with sterile plastic covers.

The selection of the entry site is important to the child and should be chosen after an understanding of the individual's handedness and needs has been developed. The skin (and tunnel tract if necessary) is generously anesthetized using a thin (27- or 30-gauge) needle with buffered lidocaine. A small (1–2 mm) skin incision is made at the entry site, either prior to initial access, or alongside the wire once access has been achieved. Once the wire is in place, the prospective tract may be dilated by blunt dissection with the tips of a thin hemostat to ease passage of the dilator or peel-away sheath. Whenever possible, the basilic or brachial vein is punctured at least 2 to 3 cm above the antecubital area. Passage of a catheter from the cephalic vein to the right atrium is often more difficult, especially in small children, due to the small size and angulation (Z shape) of the terminal segment of the cephalic vein (Figure 2.8). Additionally, the risk of PICC-related venous thrombosis appears most highly related to cephalic placement or tip malposition, rather than to age, sex, or catheter size. The brachial vein is approached with caution and always under US control because of the higher risk of arterial puncture and nerve injury. The nerve and artery should be positively identified in each case of brachial vein access to avoid such injuries.

Other sites may be considered when more preferable sites are not available, including the lower forearm and hand, the saphenous vein, and scalp veins. However, if elaborate methods are necessary to pass a PICC, central access (e.g., internal jugular or common femoral vein CVC insertion) should be considered as a more cost- and time-effective alternative. Recently, we have begun to move away from peripheral access as a primary choice in children less than 12 months of age. Also, in small children in whom peripheral access is selected we limit the number of attempted venipunctures and time spent to less than 30 minutes. In these children we prefer to insert a tunneled femoral venous line. In our preliminary experience the procedure is easier, less time consuming and has a similar rate of complications. In some cases a directional wire, and on occasion a directional catheter (e.g., JB-1), are necessary to gain access into the right atrium under fluoroscopic guidance (see "Stabilizing the guide wire" under "CVC insertion," below).

When needed, the choice of imaging modality for initial venous access is multifactorial and ultimately strongly operator dependent. Venographic guidance using fluoroscopy (Figure 2.8) allows the operator to get an excellent idea of the size and position of the vein to be punctured and to visualize it in real time in its long axis as it is punctured. Also, fluoroscopy gives the interventionalist a good feel of when the needle is in contact with the vein as the contrast column becomes effaced and the vein changes position. However, the three-dimensional orientation of the vein is substantially more difficult to appreciate in the planar fluoroscopic image, and may require either angulation of the beam or rotation of the extremity to better define anatomic relationships. Perhaps the most problematic aspect of fluoroscopic guidance is the radiation dose to both the child and interventionalist.

Ultrasound also provides an accurate real time method for guidance of the venipuncture. Ultrasound guidance allows the operator to choose the long or short axis to monitor needle insertion. In addition, because the vein is seen in cross-section, the relationship of the needle to the vein is more precisely visualized. However, for US to be effective, especially in small veins (e.g., premature neonates), quality equipment must be available. The currently available portable US units often do not adequately image peripheral veins in small children.

To use US successfully the operator must commit one hand, at least intermittently, to the US transducer (Figure 2.9) or rely upon the assistance of a technologist. Previous US scanning experience is extremely helpful if this approach is selected, and the learning curve may be steep for interventionalists not already well versed in US-guided interventions (Figure 2.10). Ultrasound equipment and associated personnel may place a burden on already crowded interventional suites.

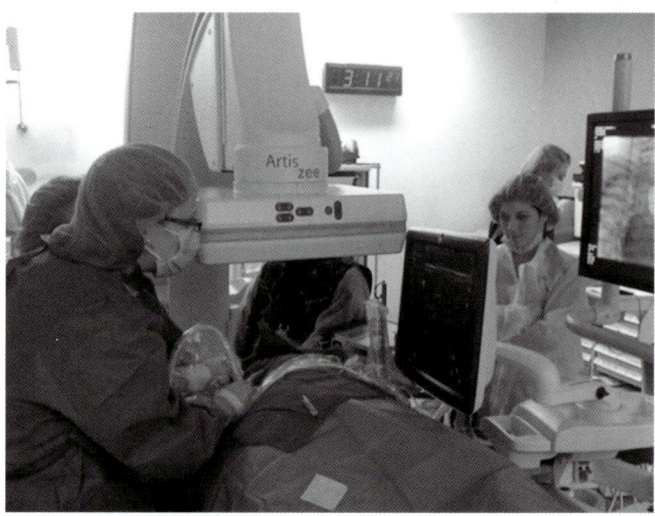

Figure 2.9 Ultrasound guidance for venous access. The transducer is placed in a sterile cover containing gel, and sterile gel is applied to the skin. The access needle, target vein, transducer, and US monitor are organized ergonomically in line to reduce operator fatigue. This may require that a second person operate the US keyboard and controls.

Ultimately, once facility is gained by the operator the frequency of success should be high with both methods, and the complication rate associated with both techniques are indistinguishable. Regardless of the guidance technique used for initial access, once the venous system is entered a guide wire is inserted and positioned in the right atrium or IVC and the catheter is inserted under fluoroscopic control.

If a silastic catheter is chosen, a peel-away sheath is necessary. Although in some cases no tract dilation is necessary, we find that dilating the tract 0.5 to 1.0 French larger than the sheath is helpful and may reduce venospasm. Whether tract dilation is routinely performed, it seems to be extremely important in young infants due to the presence of tough connective tissue about the vein, which catches on the transition zone of the peel-away sheath. This is particularly true when 3 French systems are utilized. Unfortunately, 3 French sheaths have rough transition zones with a rather abrupt change in caliber between the dilator and sheath. In some situations, changing to a longer 3 French dilator (10 cm) in the peel-away sheath helps. If the tip of the peel-away portion becomes deformed it must be replaced or damage to the vein is likely.

Once the peel-away sheath is in place, location of the catheter tip in the preferred final position must be assured. Of the several techniques available to accomplish this, we prefer a modification of the "bent wire" technique, which we have found reliable, quick, and easy to perform. Additional methods are described in "Technical variations," below. To determine the length to which the silastic catheter should be trimmed, the guide wire is passed through the peel-away sheath and its tip positioned at the entrance to the right atrium under fluoroscopic guidance. Anatomic landmarks that may be used to approximate the appropriate tip position include a point two vertebral bodies below the carina, the inferior

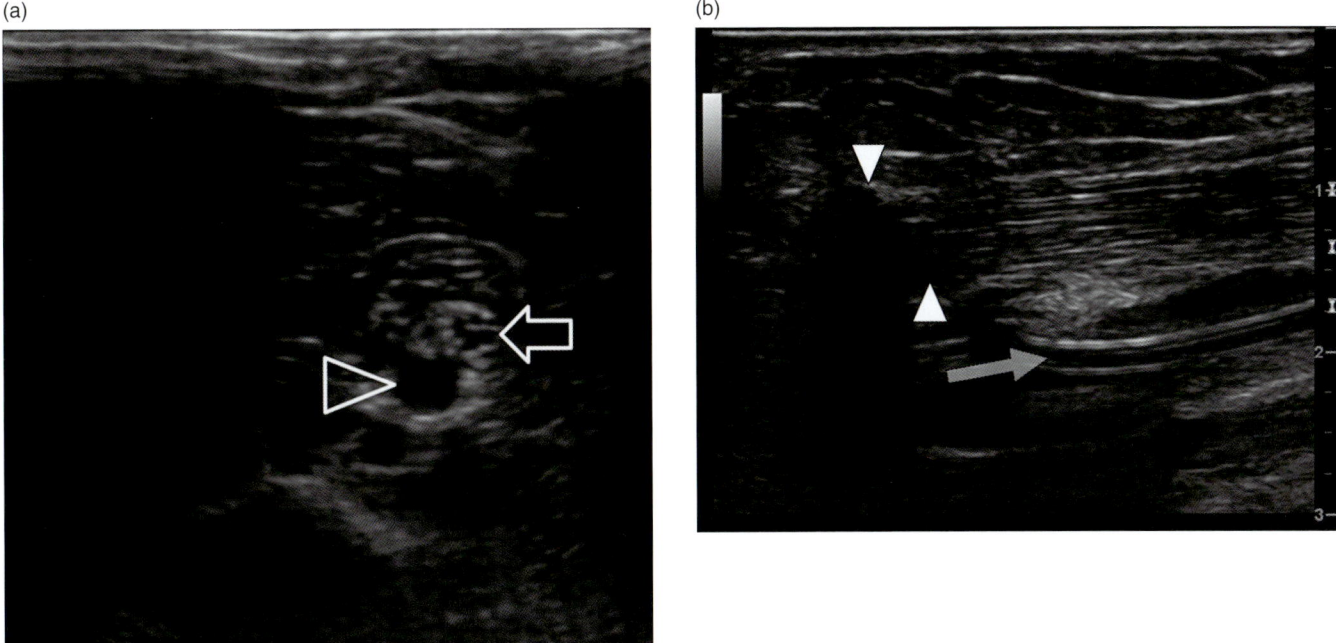

Figure 2.10 (a) Transverse US through the distal arm shows the brachial nerve (*arrow*) anterior to the brachial vein (*arrowhead*). (b) In this long axis view, a PICC placed by an IV nursing team at the bedside passes through the brachial nerve (*arrowheads*) before entering the brachial vein (*arrow*). When the PICC was removed, the patient's pain and paresthesia subsided.

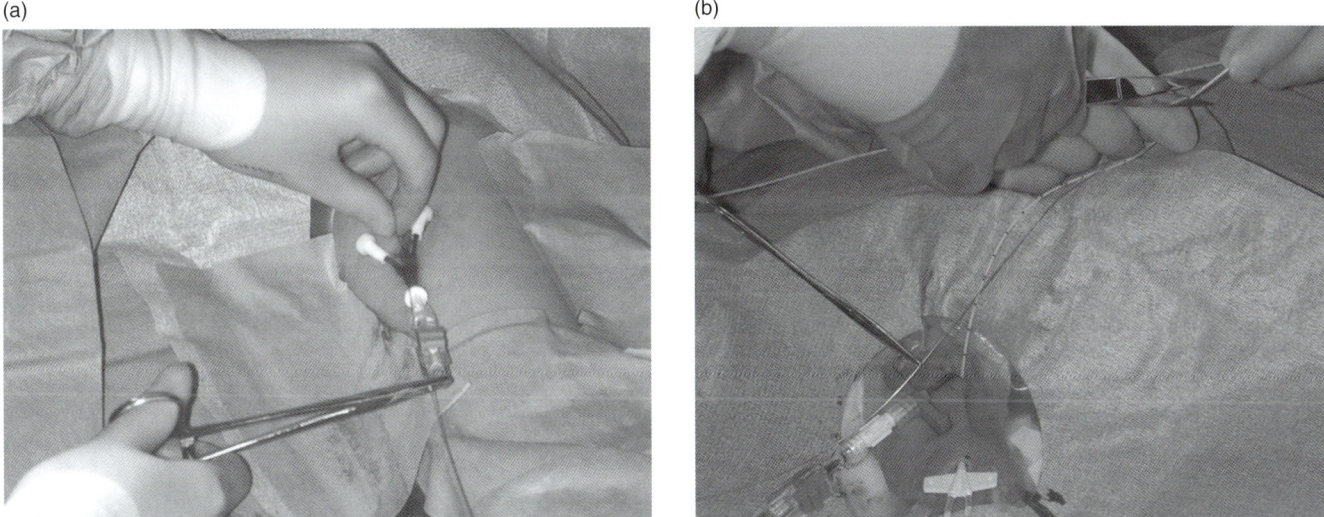

Figure 2.11 Modified "bent guide wire" technique for catheter measurement. (a) The tip of the guide wire is positioned under imaging guidance at the desired location (i.e., entrance to the right atrium), and a hemostat is clamped to the wire as it exits the hub. (b) The guide wire is removed. Once the distance from the hub to the skin entry site has been subtracted, the length of wire remaining is used to mark the point at which the catheter should be cut.

margin of the right mainstem bronchus, or the level of the sixth thoracic vertebra.

A hemostat is clamped to the wire at its exit from the sheath (Figure 2.11a), and the wire is completely withdrawn. The length of the external portion of the sheath is subtracted from the marked length of wire, and the hemostat moved to this shortened length (Figure 2.11b). With the hemostat positioned at the point on the catheter where it will exit the skin, the distal end of the wire now marks the point at which the catheter should be trimmed. Some PICCs have a zone where the catheter has a larger diameter just proximal to its hub. Failure to include this area in the total catheter measurement will leave the catheter too long. The dilator is removed from the peel-away and the PICC, having been cut to the desired length, is inserted.

In some instances, the catheter can be successfully positioned by just advancing it through the peel-away sheath into the venous system, allowing venous flow to carry the tip to its desired intra-atrial position. In our practice a 0.018-inch hydrophilic glide wire is inserted into the PICC and together they are advanced into position. This practice is used in most situations since it reduces procedure time and makes catheter positioning easier. Use of a guide wire is generally required for placement of a PICC via the cephalic vein.

When a guide wire is used, an angled glide wire is usually selected since silastic and silicone catheters do not move easily over non-hydrophilic guide wires. A glide wire must be kept wet to function properly, and wiping the wire frequently with a saline-soaked, lint-free pad (e.g., Telfa) kept in hand facilitates its use. On occasion 3 French catheters will not move easily over a moistened hydrophilic guide wire. One must be careful with a wet or lubricated hydrophilic wire since it can easily slip even through a moderately tight grip and the hard won access can be lost in a moment of inattention.

Once the catheter is positioned at the entrance to the right atrium its location is confirmed fluoroscopically by injection of contrast. Any suspicion of malposition or unexpected catheter deviation should be explored with multiplanar imaging. Any catheter tip that impinges on the vessel wall at greater than a 40-degree angle should be repositioned so that it lies as parallel to the long axis of the vessel as possible to avoid perforation. The catheter hub is then secured to the skin (e.g., with a Stat-Lock® or SorbaView® shield) and covered with a sterile, dry, transparent dressing.

When imaging guidance and interventional techniques are used for central venous access, postprocedure radiographs need not be obtained on a routine basis. Occasionally convenience or other circumstances dictates selection of an alternate location for the catheter tip other than the entrance to the right atrium. Regardless, if available a central location is usually preferred. Catheters that end in tributaries of the vena cava have a much higher frequency of complications. Correct position of the tip, as described in "Route of access," above, is especially important in PICC insertions, as the tip may move up to 3 to 5 cm with changes in arm position and respiration. If the tip is too high in the SVC, it can easily become malpositioned and may require forward flushing or more extensive maneuvers to reposition.

Technical variations
Catheter measurement
Alternatives to the bent guide wire technique include the use of a "single wire" method that allows the operator to leave the initial glide wire in position once access to the right atrium is achieved. This is important when passage from the arm entry site to the right atrium has been difficult due to challenging anatomic factors or venospasm. First, the wire tip is positioned at the projected catheter tip position at the entrance to the right atrium. Subtracting the distance from the back end of the wire (outside of the patient) to the skin entrance site from the total wire length will determine the appropriate length of the PICC to be inserted.

Alternatively, appropriate PICC length can be indirectly measured by anticipating the course of the catheter. The catheter may be placed on top of the child following the course of the wire as monitored by fluoroscopy, from the skin entry site to the desired tip position at the entrance to the right atrium. The PICC is then cut to length and advanced through the peel-away sheath over the glide wire into position. The sheath is peeled open to the skin surface so that the final length of the catheter may be verified before and after the sheath and guide wire are removed.

Postprocedure and follow-up care
At the completion of the procedure catheter course and tip position are documented with fluoroscopy and an image retained.

The catheter is flushed with 1.5 ml of a heparin solution (10 U/ml). The final catheter length and position of the catheter is recorded in the patient's chart along with any other pertinent details of the procedure (see Table 2.1). Prior to discharge, the patient and family receive thorough education in home care of the catheter and dressing from a member of the interventional staff or vascular access service. When PICCs are placed at the bedside without imaging guidance the catheter tip may not be in a satisfactory position in more than 20% of cases. Therefore all of these patients have a postprocedural chest radiograph to document catheter course and tip position. If the catheter is coiled or is not in the distal SVC or upper right atrium the interventional team repositions the PICC. If the catheter is coiled in the proximal venous system but is long enough it is treated using the flush technique. A 3 ml or 5 ml syringe filled with sterile saline is used to forcefully inject the catheter. In most instances the jet effect at the catheter tip pushes the catheter forward into the appropriate position (Figure 2.12). If the catheter is too short or cannot be flushed into position it is replaced in the IR suite. Parenthetically, we believe that catheter tips positioned in the subclavian vein, brachiocephalic vein, or proximal SVC are of concern, especially those above the SVC. It has been our experience that the short or midline catheters are many times more prone to complication than those placed centrally.

PICC removal
At the endpoint of therapy, or when other conditions indicate, someone familiar with the device and the procedure supervises removal of the PICC. A first precaution deserving consideration is that CVCs are easier to remove than to replace. It is sometimes wiser to leave the catheter in place until the endpoint is certain rather than remove it prematurely and subject the patient to a second procedure a short time later.

An uncuffed silicone or polyurethane PICC may simply be pulled out, keeping gentle pressure at the exit site until hemostasis is achieved, then covering the wound with a clean, dry dressing. For every PICC removal, the catheter is inspected for defects, measured, and its length documented and compared

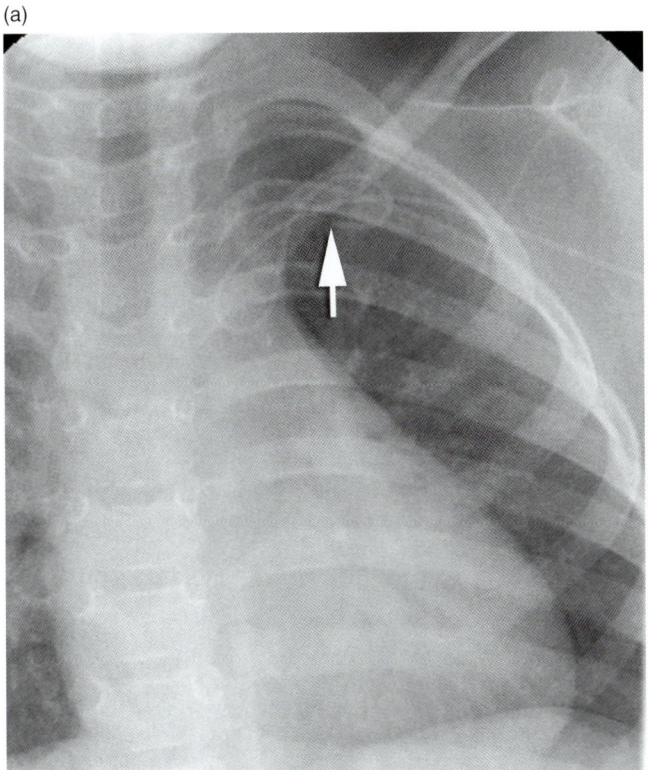 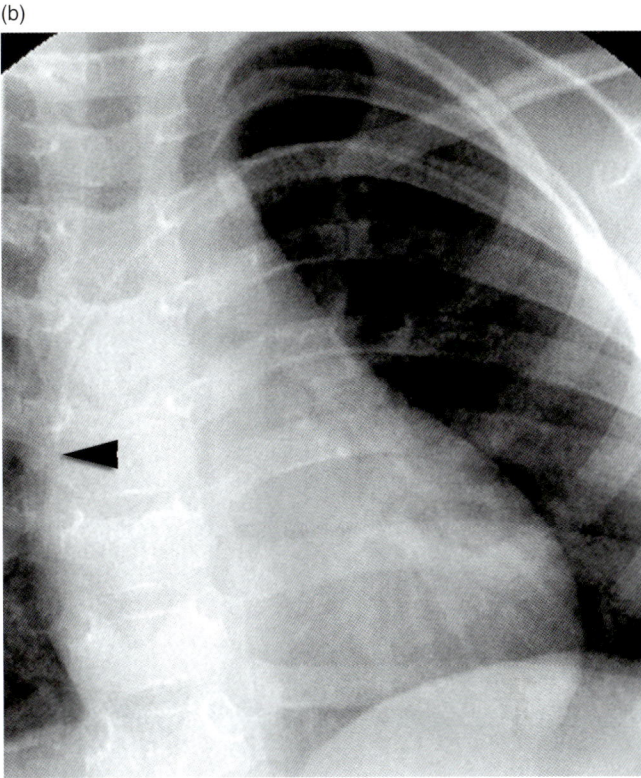

Figure 2.12 Four-year-old girl with septic arthritis for antibiotics. (a) PICC placed by IV team without imaging guidance is coiled in the subclavian vein (*arrow*). (b) After forceful saline flush using a 3-ml syringe, the catheter tip (*arrowhead*) is correctly positioned near the entrance to the right atrium.

with the length recorded at insertion. A significant difference implies fragmentation and possible embolization of the distal fragment. If the PICC is being removed because of suspected catheter infection, the tip is secured under sterile conditions in a suitable container and transported promptly for Gram stain and culture.

A cuffed PICC may sometimes be removed in the same fashion; especially if it is removed before significant tissue ingrowth occurs (ten days to two weeks). However, if there is substantial resistance, or if the patient experiences pain during a brief attempt to extract the catheter, this approach may be abandoned in favor of the following.

If extraction of the cuffed PICC is inhibited by tissue ingrowth, it may be removed using a minor surgical procedure after the distal tract and exit site have been generously infiltrated with local anesthetic. The external component of the catheter and the area around the exit site are prepared and draped in sterile fashion. Using a narrow hemostat, the exit site is dissected, opening the tract to the cuff. With gentle traction on the catheter, the cuff is brought into view. Using care not to damage the catheter itself, the pseudo-capsule of connective tissue is dissected from the circumference of the catheter just proximal to the cuff with blunt dissection and iris scissors. Once free, the catheter will pull out effortlessly. Vigorous traction on the catheter should be avoided due to risk of catheter fracture and embolization. Once hemostasis is achieved, the exit wound is cleaned, bandaged, and left to heal by secondary intention. A suture is not placed, as the wound is considered "dirty".

Technical problems and pitfalls

When venospasm occurs it is difficult to resolve, makes successful placement unlikely, adds a considerable amount of time to the case, and usually adds to the cost since other drugs, catheters, and guide wires may be necessary. When venospasm occurs, a variety of approaches may be tried. Unfortunately, no single approach has been especially helpful. In our experience, most venospasm is due to vessel trauma with a guide wire. Therefore, it is best to avoid pushing a wire tip into the wall even if you feel that it is harmless. Also, one should be careful about spinning a directional guide wire as this "helicopter" action may cause minor intimal injury and venospasm. If the cuff is buried too far above the entry point to safely free it in the manner described above, one may perform a cut-down from a point directly superficial to the cuff, taking care not to damage the catheter. The cuff is then freed and the catheter removed as previously described, except that this wound is closed primarily.

When present, there are several options to treat venospasm. Parenthetically, it may be best to find another site for catheter insertion before embarking on this time consuming and potentially costly journey. Reducing the size of the PICC by 1 French may be helpful and is our first choice if luminal patency, albeit diminished, is noted (i.e., if a wire can be passed beyond the region of spasm). Venospasm may be broached from a physiological, mechanical, or pharmacological basis. First, 5 to 30 minutes of patience may be rewarded with relaxation of the spastic region. If a catheter or dilator is already positioned just proximal to the area of venospasm, a brisk infusion of saline may break the episode long enough to allow passage of the catheter. Should spasm persist, various pharmacologic agents have been used with variable success, including nitroglycerine, papaverine, priscoline, calcium channel blockers, or (if the child is under general anesthesia), halothane.

Attempting to pass a silastic catheter through a spastic or narrow region often causes the catheter body to "accordion" distal to the narrow area. A polyurethane catheter may be stiff enough to pass successfully in these situations. While pulling the wire back to a position proximal to the spasm may allow adequate reduction in the catheter circumference to allow it to pass, this maneuver risks losing access entirely and is not usually recommended.

A similar situation may be encountered when attempting to exchange a silicone PICC over a guide wire. If the PICC becomes accordioned even over a glide wire, we have found it very effective to coat the wire, and even the catheter itself, with a biologically inert lubricant, such as sterile mineral oil or silicone spray. The marked reduction in friction that results is often sufficient to allow passage of the catheter beyond the narrow region.

Complications

Infection, thrombophlebitis, tip occlusion, catheter damage and mechanical malfunction, dislodgment and malposition are the most common complications associated with PICC lines. In general, complications associated with PICC lines and other central venous access devices are similar in nature, differing primarily in frequency. Phlebitis and catheter dysfunction are discussed below. A more complete discussion of catheter-related infections, malposition, tip occlusion, thrombosis, mechanical malfunction, and intravascular foreign body management is provided under "Complications" in the section on "Central venous catheter (CVC) insertion."

Catheter-related thrombophlebitis

Although there have been reports of thrombosis in as many as 23 to 38% of PICC lines, more recently the prevalence of PICC-related thrombosis in children when placed by an experienced interventional radiology team is less than 1%. The incidence of thrombosis was related to the site of access, with the highest incidence in the cephalic vein (57%), followed by the basilic (14%), and the brachial (10%). There is a substantial prevalence of phlebitis (defined as erythema, swelling, pain, or palpable cord overlying the catheter course) associated with PICC insertions. Since this is often a self-limited process, it is important to differentiate phlebitis from catheter-related infection, to prevent unnecessary catheter removal. When phlebitis is suspected, treatment with a warm compress and a tincture of time is often sufficient to resolve symptoms within 24 hours. If necessary, treatment with a non-steroidal anti-inflammatory drug (e.g., intravenous Torudol®) is helpful and may be diagnostic of non-infectious inflammation. Heparin solutions (either 1 U heparin/ml infusion given continuously, or 100 U/ml of intermittent flush each six to eight hours in locked catheters) significantly decreases the risk of phlebitis in peripheral angiocatheters. To our knowledge no prospective trial has proven similar effect in PICC lines. However, this seems a reasonable intervention in situations where phlebitis is suspected, or an increased risk of phlebitis can be anticipated (e.g., difficult insertion, venospasm at insertion, small difference between vessel and catheter diameter).

There has been increased interest in recent years in "midline" or non-central placement of peripherally inserted catheters, especially as a method to salvage difficult PICC insertions complicated by venospasm, venous tortuosity, venous valves, or other factors. It is clear, however, that non-central location of the PICC tip significantly increases the risk of phlebitis, occlusion, leakage, and other complications. In fact, we recommend that if a catheter tip is noted to be outside the ideal "landing zone," that is, between the inferior margin of the right mainstem bronchus and a point two vertebral bodies below the carina, that the tip should be repositioned or the catheter replaced, especially in patients at high risk of catheter-related complications or those with a chronic diagnosis likely to require central access into the foreseeable future.

Catheter dysfunction

Catheter dysfunction usually presents as loss of ability to obtain blood return, total occlusion (catheter does not flush or draw), or pain during flushes or drug administration. These problems can be managed according to a logical protocol that emphasizes a definitive diagnosis and management plan, preserves access safely when possible, and conserves cost.

When pain or edema accompanies infusion, this problem should be evaluated promptly with contrast-enhanced dynamic fluoroscopy. Other studies either delay a definitive diagnosis or increase risk of injury. Pain during injection is usually caused by extravasation of fluid causing increased interstitial pressure in the subcutaneous or perivascular tissues. The principal purpose of the examination is to identify the location and etiology of the extravasation. At times, fluid extravasates through a very subtle pinhole defect in the catheter, often related to rough handling of the catheter during insertion. It is imperative to image the entire course of the catheter prior to contrast injection, and to compare this with the course and position of the catheter at the time of initial insertion. If the position has changed, the tip may no longer be intravascular. One must then carefully observe as the contrast first flows through the catheter.

Extension of a fibrin sheath from the tip to the venous entry site may allow reflux along the distal length of the catheter and into the perivascular tissues. Attempts to resolve a fibrin sheath with instillation of a fibrinolytic agent are occasionally effective, but this is often simply a temporizing intervention. Stripping the catheter with a transfemoral snare is usually successful, but should be reserved for those cases where access is lifesaving or difficult to achieve. The simplest and most definitive therapy is to change the catheter over a wire.

Catheter fractures and tears are among the most common PICC-related complications, occurring in up to one in ten patients. Most of these may be attributed to tearing of the catheter during insertion, overpressuring during injection (e.g., injecting forcefully through a small-caliber syringe), or traction on the catheter hub junction. Such damage to the catheter may range from a pinhole to outright disruption, and may appear on imaging as a subtle line of contrast along the outer wall of the catheter to frank extravasation to an apparent discontinuity in the catheter itself. This common problem has received little attention in most reviews of CVCs and PICCs, especially how to repair leaks and tears in silastic catheters. Although it is technically easy, physicians seldom perform the procedure and it is therefore not widely known (Appendix 2.B). When there is any evidence of damage to the catheter, strict caution should be employed during its removal to avoid catheter fragmentation and embolization of the distal fragment. At least, the catheter should be removed under fluoroscopic control. If embolization appears imminent, the distal component may be guided gently during removal with a transfemoral snare.

Complete occlusion of a CVC (inability to flush or draw) may be due to tip thrombus or fibrin sheath formation, catheter kinking, malposition, or a variety of factors discussed elsewhere in this section. Again, simple causes of dysfunction should be explored before more costly or invasive studies are pursued. For example, it is surprising how often disengaging the clamp, unkinking the external portion of the catheter or unclogging the hub is all that is necessary to restore function. Since it is difficult to perform a contrast study through a catheter that will not flush, it may be worthwhile attempting a forceful injection of contrast or saline prior to removing the catheter. Serial attempts may be made with successively smaller syringes (from 5 ml to 1 ml), remembering that smaller syringes generate greater pressure. Only experienced personnel should use syringes smaller than 10 ml, to avoid damaging the catheter and causing tissue injury.

Inability to obtain blood return when the catheter still flushes often relates to a ball-valve mechanism operating at the catheter tip, due to one of several factors: wedging of the catheter tip against the vessel wall (malposition or fibrinous adherence to the wall), tip thrombus, or fibrin sheath. A contrast-enhanced fluoroscopic study may be required to differentiate these causes in order to direct specific treatment. However, simpler causes may be ruled out first. For example, a change in patient position (elevation of the ipsi- or contralateral arm, rolling from supine to prone, deep inspiration or expiration, etc.) may be enough to free the catheter tip and achieve adequate blood return.

A high calcium phosphate product in the infused solution, or certain acidic or basic drugs may cause precipitation along the catheter anywhere from the hub to the tip. Similarly, a nutrient admixture or piggybacked lipid solution may cause a slow build up of lipid thrombus at the tip. A review of the patient's medical course may reveal such a common cause of occlusion. Treatment depends on the precipitating factor (Appendix 2.C).

If the medication history is unproductive, and tip thrombus is suspected, a trial of thrombolytic therapy is warranted (Appendix 2.C). However, prior to administration of tissue plasminogen activator (tPA) a chest radiograph is obtained to confirm the intravascular course of the catheter in order to avoid tissue injury or bleeding complications. Irregularity of tip position, catheter conformation, or catheter motion may prompt further investigation with contrast-enhanced fluoroscopy. Angulation of the fluoroscope may help resolve real kinks or conformational abnormalities from apparent kinking caused by tortuosity of the catheter course through the imaging plane.

In addition to watching for extravasation and abnormalities of catheter position, the catheter length and motion of the tip is carefully observed. If the catheter is shortened compared to prior studies, this may indicate fragmentation, and the distal (embolized) fragment must be located and, if possible, recovered (Figure 2.13). If the tip moves freely, but the contrast jet streaming from the tip "sprays" diffusely or appears to be deflected (Figure 2.14), this indicates likely tip thrombus or fibrin sheath, as discussed elsewhere. Abnormal tip motion or lack of tip mobility may signify adherence of the tip to the vessel wall, or entrapment of the tip within a deep venous thrombus (Figure 2.15). This finding cannot be adequately evaluated with contrast through the catheter alone, and a focused venogram or US scan may be indicated. If venography is used, it is performed with simultaneous bilateral contrast injection if possible, with gentle compression of the jugular vein, to reduce inflow artifact. For this reason, we routinely request that patients referred for venographic catheter studies are provided with peripheral angiocatheters bilaterally prior to transport to interventional radiology.

Central venous catheter (CVC) insertion

Introduction

Compared to PICC insertion, placement of CVCs is usually technically easier, faster, and more often successful, particularly in small children. The internal jugular vein (IJV) is the preferred venous entry site. If the IJV is not available, a PICC,

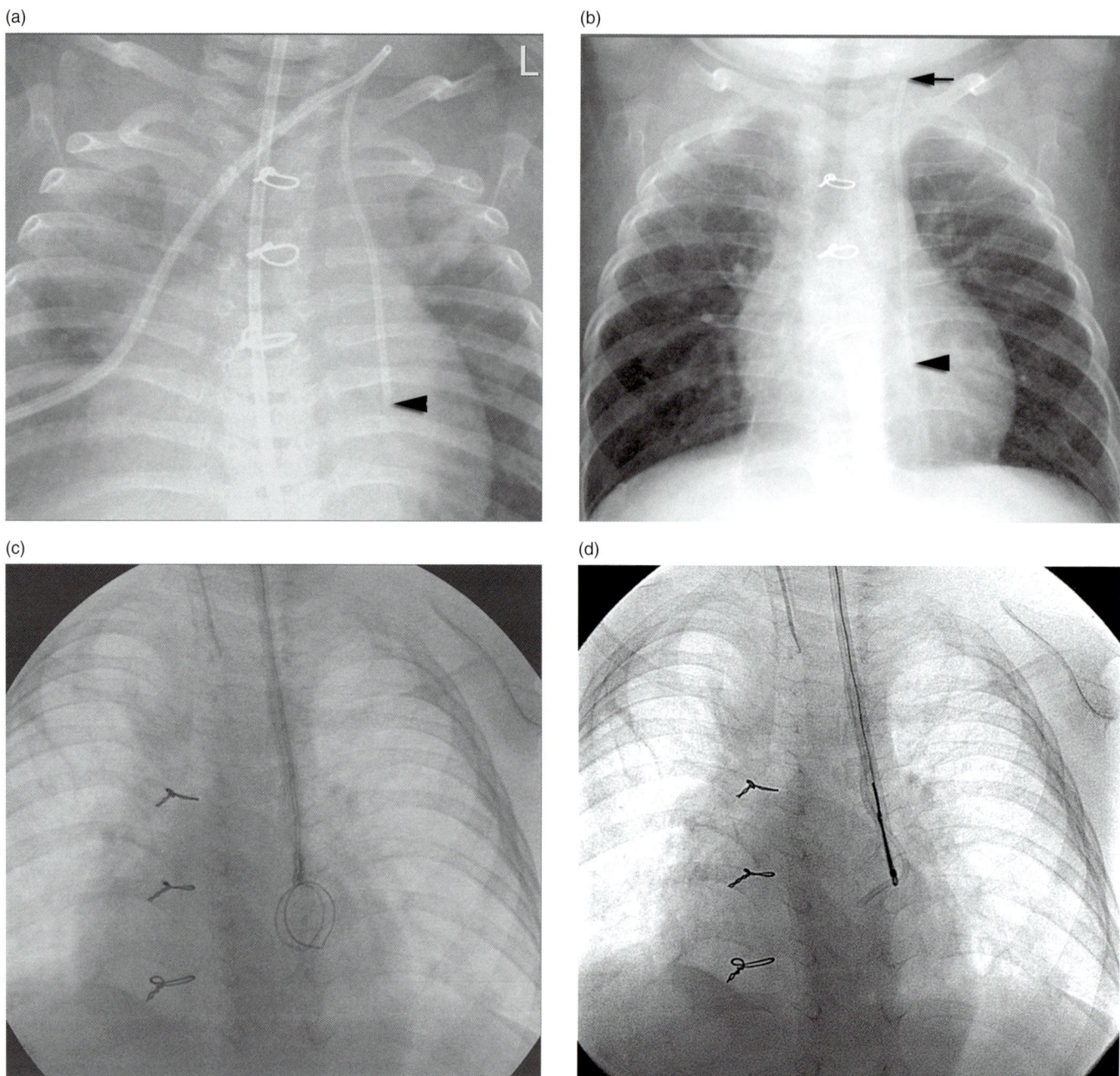

Figure 2.13 A one-year-old girl with trisomy-21, atrioventricular canal repair, and intestinal failure had a left IJ tunneled central venous catheter inserted by the surgical service for nutrition. (a) The catheter tip (*arrowhead*) is positioned within the persistent left SVC. (b) Four months later, the catheter fractured (*arrow*) during attempted removal. (c) A 15-mm snare is deployed through a transjugular sheath passed into the left SVC. (d) The loop snare was closed over the tip of the catheter, and the fragment was recovered through the sheath without further complication.

femoral CVC, or subclavian vein (SCV) can be used. In the past, the use of the femoral vein for CVC insertion has generally been discouraged due to restriction of patient movement and higher likelihood of infection especially in younger children who wear diapers. However, the use of a tunneled, cuffed CVC has made this route useful especially in young children, children with occluded IJVs, those with complex congenital heart disease, and for emergent indications or temporary access (e.g., CVC, apheresis, hemodialysis). Additional considerations regarding femoral location and device selection in older patients may include cosmetic appearance as well as interference with clothing, sport, sexual relations, and seatbelt use, for example. It is generally accepted that subcutaneous tunneling of long-term CVCs significantly reduces the risk of complications, especially catheter-related infection. There is some evidence that tunneling may also reduce the risk of

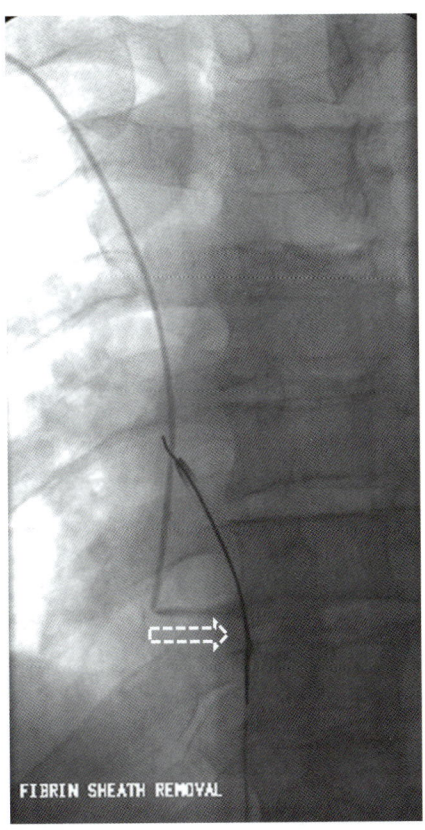

Figure 2.14 A loop snare is gently engaged above the tip of a catheter occluded by a tip clot (note medially deviated contrast "jet" (arrow)). After the snare was pulled down and the clot stripped off, the catheter regained normal function until it was removed at the end of therapy.

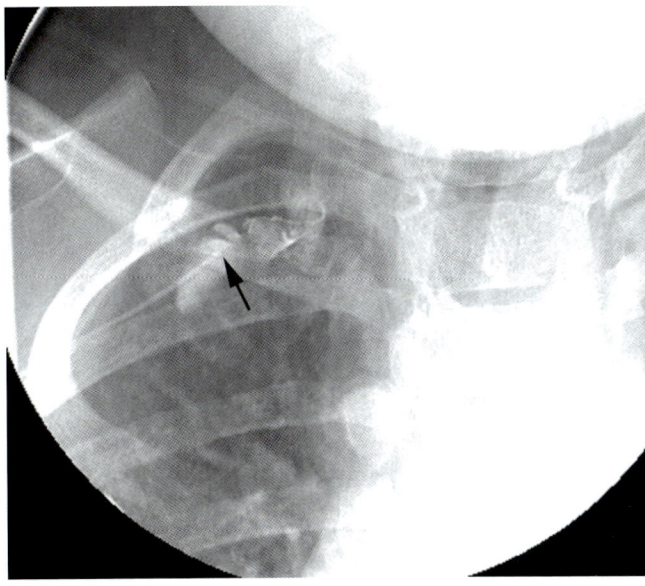

Figure 2.15 PICC inserted with tip (arrow) in mid-subclavian vein. Contrast injection demonstrates occlusive thrombus.

infection in short-term CVCs, especially transjugular CVCs, although prospective evidence in children is not yet available.

In our opinion, use of the subclavian vein as a primary choice for venous access should be discouraged. If the subclavian vein is used it should be only after all other options have been considered. There are several reasons why the subclavian vein should not be considered as a primary choice for venous access including its strategic position as the inflow vessel from the ipsilateral extremity and the neck, and its higher rate of complications when compared to the IJV.

Indications

Central venous catheters are indicated for treatment of both emergent and chronic conditions. Emergent access for volume replacement, blood sampling, or administration of life-saving medications is probably best achieved by the most expedient method available. Usually, this means "blind" percutaneous insertion using anatomic landmarks, or even intraosseous access, by emergency department, intensive care, or surgical personnel. Image-guided placement is normally best reserved for less urgent indications. In the future there will likely be more US-guided bedside insertion of CVCs by interventionalists and other physician and nurse groups (Table 2.2).

Some of the more common indications for CVC placement in the pediatric population are for chemotherapy in oncology patients; for parenteral nutrition; and for dialysis in nephrology patients. Central catheters are also helpful for blood product replacement in hematology patients; prolonged antibiotic therapy (e.g., in cystic fibrosis and osteomyelitis patients); fluids, electrolytes, and medications in intensive care patients and children with metabolic diseases; and a variety of similar applications.

Few contraindications to placement of CVCs exist. An uncorrectable coagulopathy has traditionally been a contraindication for invasive procedures. However, it is precisely these seriously ill children who require central venous access for therapy. Thus, it has been our practice to take all appropriate measures to correct abnormal laboratory data. In cases where correction of low platelets or prolonged PTT has been attempted without success, we perform the procedure with platelets or fresh frozen plasma infusing to maximize safety. Hemophiliac patients with high titers of inhibitors who require central access for factor and blood product replacement are particularly challenging. Although these patients may benefit from immune tolerance treatment and recombinant factor replacement they are usually best approached in close consultation with a pediatric hematologist. Frankly, if uncontrollable bleeding is observed after US-guided access to a neck vessel, one ought first look for mechanical disruption of the catheter (e.g., perforation by a retention suture) before attributing the bleeding to a coagulopathy.

In these situations, an easily accessible peripheral site for PICC or a large central vein well visualized by US is selected. In the latter case the right internal jugular vein (RIJV) is strongly preferred. The RIJV has the advantage of being the largest and easiest central vein to cannulate with the most direct course to the right atrium. It also facilitates accurate measurement of catheter length, and allows for the shortest procedure time.

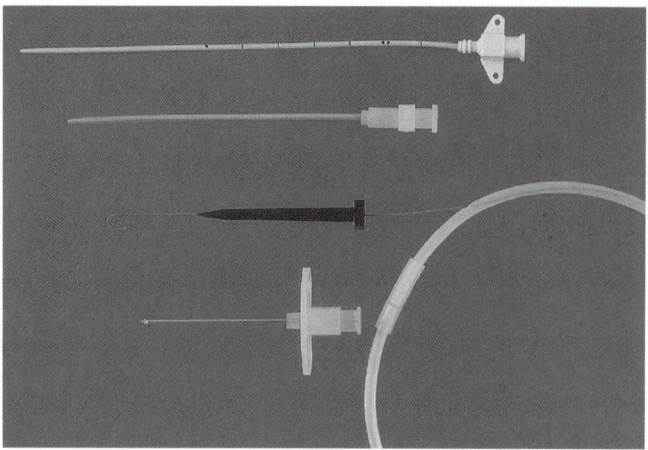

Figure 2.16 3-French tapered non-cuffed polyurethane temporary central venous catheter with access needle, guide wire, and dilator.

In addition, in these instances a temporary CVC (tapered polyurethane CVC) may be inserted (Figure 2.16). Since neither tract dilation nor a peel-away sheath is required procedure time is minimized. Additionally, because the catheter completely fills the tract and venous puncture site, the risk of bleeding is decreased. In both theory and practice cannulation of an IJV has the lowest risk of complications since hemothorax and pneumothorax are less likely to occur. Another significant advantage of the RIJV approach is the ease of achieving postoperative hemostasis and monitoring for delayed bleeding. Placing the patient in a reverse Trendelenburg or semi-upright (sitting) position to lower venous pressure will facilitate hemostasis when the IJV is used.

A word of caution when inserting temporary CVCs! These catheters are stiffer than silastic or silicone CVCs and have a tapered tip (Figure 2.17). Thus, it is important to avoid contact with the cardiac wall, floor, or ceiling. If forward pressure is placed on the cardiac wall perforation and tamponade may occur. The IR or diagnostic radiologist should be mindful of the catheter position and the conformation of its path and tip location. If the tapered catheter abuts the wall and is bowed one should be concerned about the potential for injury and have the catheter repositioned as soon as possible.

Technique: internal jugular CVC insertion
Equipment

The selection of needles, catheters, guide wires, and other equipment varies considerably depending on the experience and preference of the interventionalist and the size, age, and condition of the patient (Table 2.3). In the pediatric age group a range of access needle sizes, catheter diameters, and lengths should be available to the interventionalist. The needle size selected depends on the child's weight and size.

When a CVC is inserted, a single wall needle is preferred since it is more echogenic than an angiocatheter. For very small infants it is occasionally necessary to begin with a smaller

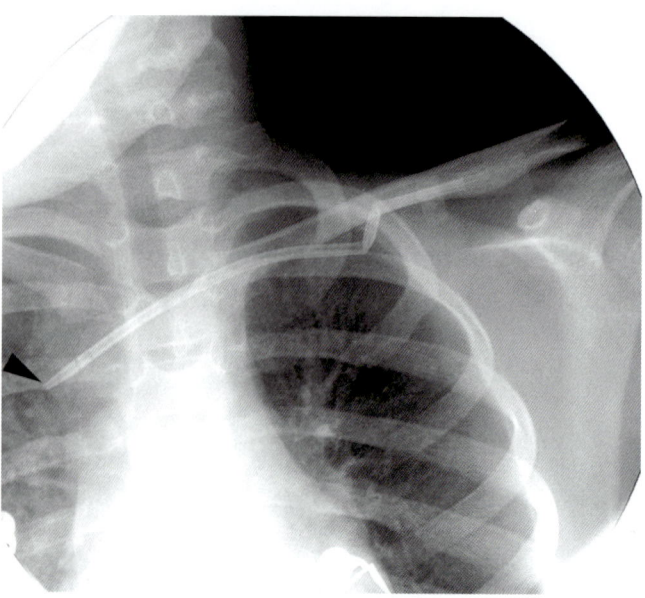

Figure 2.17 Ten-year-old boy with thrombotic thrombocytopenic purpura requiring plasmapheresis was unable to receive therapy due to catheter malfunction. The temporary pheresis catheter is kinked at the venotomy site, a complication similar to catheter "pinch off" previously described. Note the tapered tip (*arrowhead*) of this stiff catheter projecting toward the lateral wall of the SVC. This patient is at increased risk of vessel perforation.

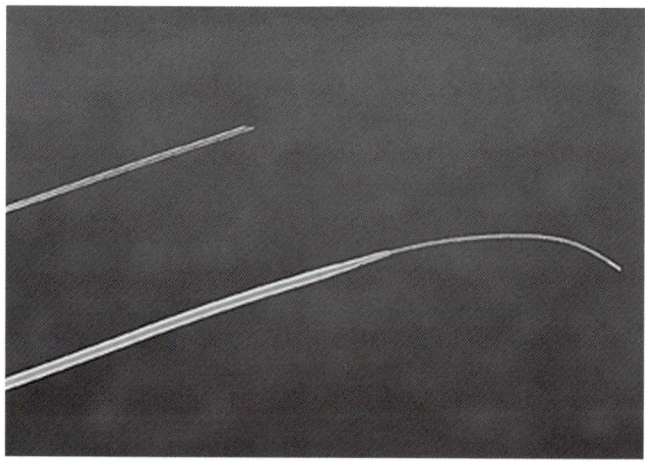

Figure 2.18 Micropuncture introducer sets, such as the one pictured here (Cook, Bloomington, IL) are usually introduced over a 0.018-inch platinum tipped (nitinol) or stainless steel wire, placed through a 21-gauge access needle. Once the coaxial introducer is in position, the inner core is removed, leaving a 4 or 5 French outer catheter in place, which will accept a 0.035- or 0.038-inch guide wire.

needle and wire, such as a micropuncture kit (Figure 2.18), exchanging for a larger dilator or peel-away sheath once access is achieved. Children weighing 10 to 20 kg are usually accessed with 20- or 22-gauge needles. Occasionally, in larger children, 19- or 18-gauge needles are used. Again, the needle selected is often based on operator preference since all types work well.

Regardless of the needle selected, we prefer to place a connecting tube between the needle and the syringe so that gentle suction can be applied. Once "free" blood flows into the tube one can be confident that the needle tip is intraluminal. Also, use of a connecting tube protects against significant movement or accidental dislodgment of the needle tip with unexpected patient or operator motion.

Central venous catheters are available in a wide range of sizes and configurations. In most instances the choice of access device in a given case is made giving consideration to a combination of factors such as the referring physician's preference, the child's illness, and anticipated length of treatment. Our recommendations are included under "Route of access," above. Catheters from 3 French to 9 French are available for use in the pediatric population. Five and 7 French single lumen catheters are the catheters most commonly used. Dialysis or apheresis catheters are generally 7 to 14 French in size. One may choose from a variety of catheter types including PICCs, non-tunneled (temporary) catheters, tunneled catheters, dialysis catheters, and indwelling ports. The final choice depends on the expected catheter use and the dwell time. In addition, one may choose catheters with single, double, or triple lumens. It is important to recognize that for the same outer diameter increasing lumen number decreases cross-sectional area (and therefore, flow) by at least 16 times. Also, blood return is substantially more difficult to obtain in 3 French and smaller catheters making them undesirable for some uses. In general, the catheter with the fewest number of lumens and smallest internal diameter *that will satisfy the clinical need* is selected. This will maximize the diameter of the lumen and flow through it, while minimizing the potential for catheter dysfunction especially in the small French sizes.

Patient preparation

As is the case for all major interventional procedures, informed consent is obtained from the patient when age permits, or from the parent or legal guardian. When appropriate, assent is obtained from the minor patient. For CVC insertion the technical aspects of the procedure and its risks are reviewed with the consenting adult, usually in the presence of the child. The technical factors, most common risks, benefits, and alternatives are carefully explained, including sedation problems, bleeding that could require transfusion or operative intervention, pneumothorax, hemopneumothorax, and infection. Uncommon problems such as catheter fragmentation and distal embolization are rarely discussed in detail.

The evaluation of the individual prior to placement of a CVC varies with the indication and the status of the child. In general, a coagulation profile is obtained for documentation of the PT, PTT, CBC, and platelet count. In rare instances the bleeding time is measured.

For CVC insertion the IJV vein is the preferred entry site, especially when there is an increased risk of bleeding or if the child is severely ill. A decision to tunnel the catheter is made on a case-by-case basis. A tunneled catheter is placed in children who are expected to go home with the central line in place, require access for at least two weeks, or those who will

Table 2.5 Procedural summary: internal jugular CVC insertion

- Obtain preprocedural laboratory studies.
- Select entry site with US.
- Prepare and drape skin.
- Locally anesthetize entry site.
- Small skin incision at entry site.
- Puncture internal jugular vein using real-time US guidance.
- Aspirate until free blood return. Confirm position with venography if necessary.
- Insert guide wire into right atrium, IVC, or hepatic vein.
- Dilate tract (if silastic catheter used).
- Exchange dilator for peel-away sheath.
- Measure distance from entry site to upper right atrium.
- Insert CVC.
- Inject contrast to confirm satisfactory position.
- Suture incision closed.
- Cover entry site with a 2 × 2 gauze and occlusive dressing.
- Heparinize CVC.
- Document procedure in medical record.

need frequent access. In high-risk situations, especially in children with an uncorrected coagulopathy, tunneling is avoided because of the potential for bleeding and subsequent infection. If necessary, tunneling can be performed at a later date when the risk level is appropriate. In a high-risk population, a temporary line may be preferred over a silastic catheter for ease of insertion, shorter procedure time, and avoidance of tract dilation and need for a peel-away sheath. There appears to be a lower incidence of postprocedural bleeding with this approach because of the avoidance of tract dilation and the precise fit of the polyurethane catheter into the vein promotes hemostasis.

Prior to CVC insertion, all children are kept NPO for at least six hours so that they can be safely sedated. The child requiring general anesthesia is prepared according to the anesthesiology department protocol as if the child were to go to the operating room. Standard laboratory tests include a CBC, platelet count, PT, PTT, and (rarely) a bleeding time. Prophylactic antibiotics are not routinely given.

Once in the room, the child is placed on the angiography table and secured with Velcro straps to avoid falling. If the procedure is performed on a tilting angiography table, placing the patient in approximately 10- to 15-degree Trendelenburg fills the jugular vein more prominently, allowing the vein to be punctured with less risk to surrounding structures, and decreasing the risk of air embolism. All children are monitored with pulse oximetry and an automated blood pressure device. A sensor for pulse oximetry is secured to a finger, toe, foot, or rarely an earlobe. Leads are placed for cardiovascular monitoring. Reusable sensors are available for small babies.

Children presenting for primary CVC insertion have a peripheral IV placed if one is not already present. Preprocedural US is performed and the prospective entry site is marked on the skin with an ink marker.

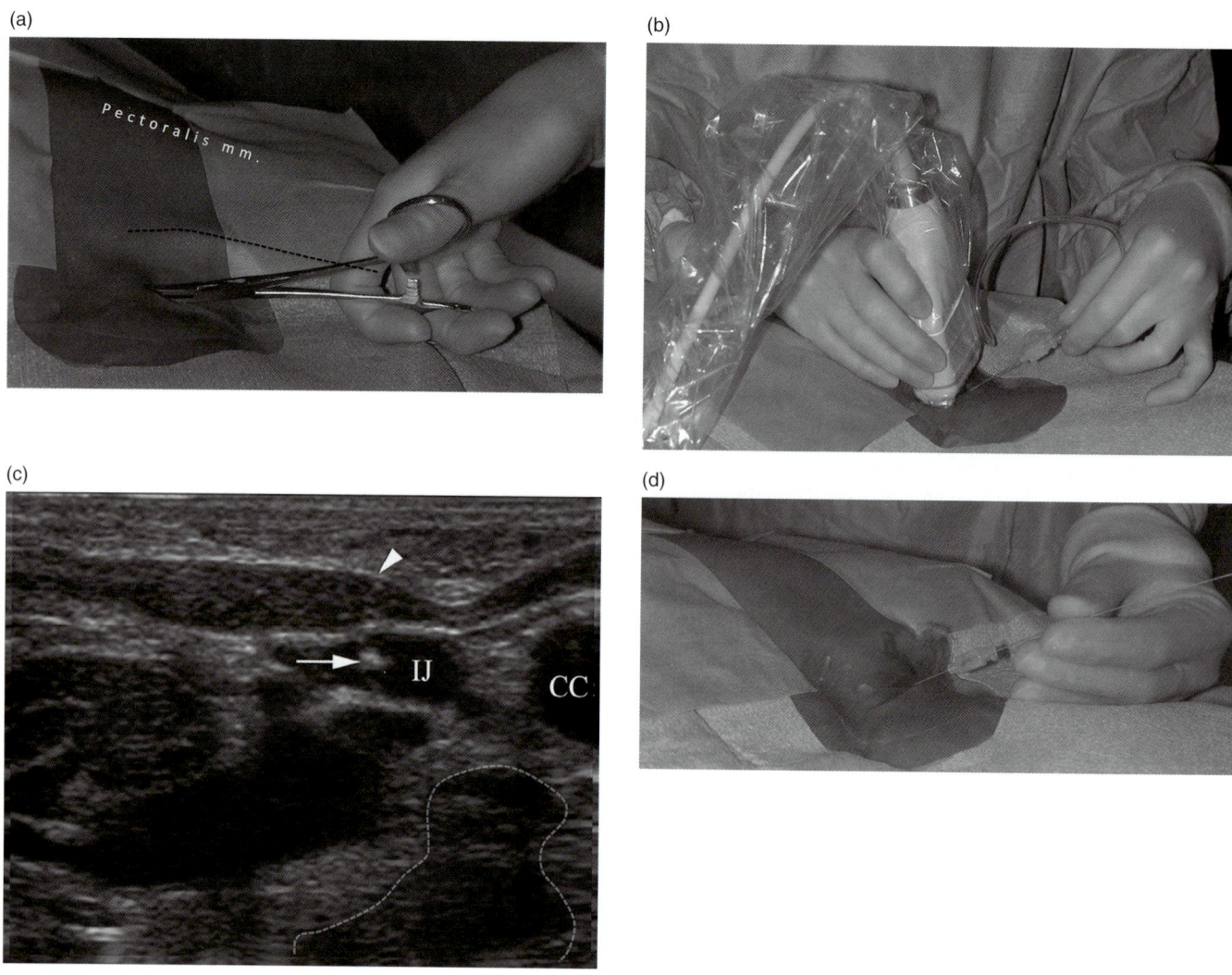

Figure 2.19 Ten-year-old girl with nephrotic syndrome for IJV dialysis catheter insertion. (a) A short skin incision is made at least 2 to 3 cm from the clavicle (*dotted line*), up to halfway between the clavicle and the angle of the jaw. The tract is dilated by blunt dissection with a curved Kelly forceps. (b) Under US guidance the IJV is punctured with an access needle (c) as shown in this linear US image, passing through the sternal head of the sternocleidomastoid muscle (*arrowhead*). The needle tip (*arrow*) is seen within the lumen of the internal jugular (*IJ*). Care must be used to distinguish the vein from the common carotid artery (*CC*), by compression and Doppler flow, and to guard against inadvertent puncture of other vessels, nerves, or the cupola of the lung (*dotted line*). (d) A 0.018-inch mandril guide wire is advanced through the micropuncture needle, and the needle is exchanged for an introducer sheath. (e) After verifying the position of the guide wire tip at the entrance to the right atrium under fluoroscopy, the wire is clamped at the hub and withdrawn. The difference between the clamp and the skin entry site (*arrows*) is subtracted from the initial measurement (*arrowheads*) to determine the length of the catheter from the venotomy site to the proximal lumen tip. (f) This is shown on the catheter as the distance between the *white arrow* and *arrowhead*. The remaining distance (*arrowhead* to *black arrow*) is measured. (g) This becomes the distance from the venotomy site to the skin entry site. The skin entry site and the subcutaneous tract are generously infiltrated with local anesthetic. (h–i) The tunneling device (*arrowhead*) is attached to the catheter (*arrow*) and the subcutaneous tract is formed, keeping the tip of the tunneler (*asterisk*) in the subcutaneous layer but superficial to the clavicle. (j) The catheter is pulled through the tract, until the cuff (*asterisk*) is several centimeters beyond the skin entry site. Both the check-flow valve on the introducer (*arrowheads*) and the clamps on the catheter (*arrow*) should be closed to prevent air embolus. (k) With the catheter (*arrows*) through the subcutaneous tunnel, the mandril wire and inner core of the introducer are removed and a 0.038-inch guide wire is inserted, as deep as the IVC if possible. (l) The tract is prepared with serial dilators up to the diameter of the peel-away sheath. (m) Dilations and sheath insertion are performed under fluoroscopic control, maintaining the dilators (*arrowheads*) parallel to the mediastinum and plenty of wire beyond the tip to prevent inadvertent injury to the heart or great veins. (n) Split dialysis catheters are designed for the proximal tip (*black arrow*) to be positioned at the entrance to the right atrium, in this case approximately two vertebral bodies below the carina (*arrowhead*), with the distal tip (*white arrow*) in the atrium itself, to maximize flow and minimize recirculation. Note that the cuff (*asterisk*) is well beyond the skin entry site (*wavy line*) to assure in-growth and long-term stability.

Standard technique

In most instances the IJV, usually the right, is the largest and easiest central vein to puncture (Table 2.5). This is particularly important in small infants in whom access of the subclavian vein may be challenging and carries a higher risk of malposition, pneumothorax, and other complications.

Caution should be exercised when selecting the site of entry into the internal jugular system. The distance from the jugular bifurcation to its junction with the subclavian vein is short in

Chapter 2 Central venous access

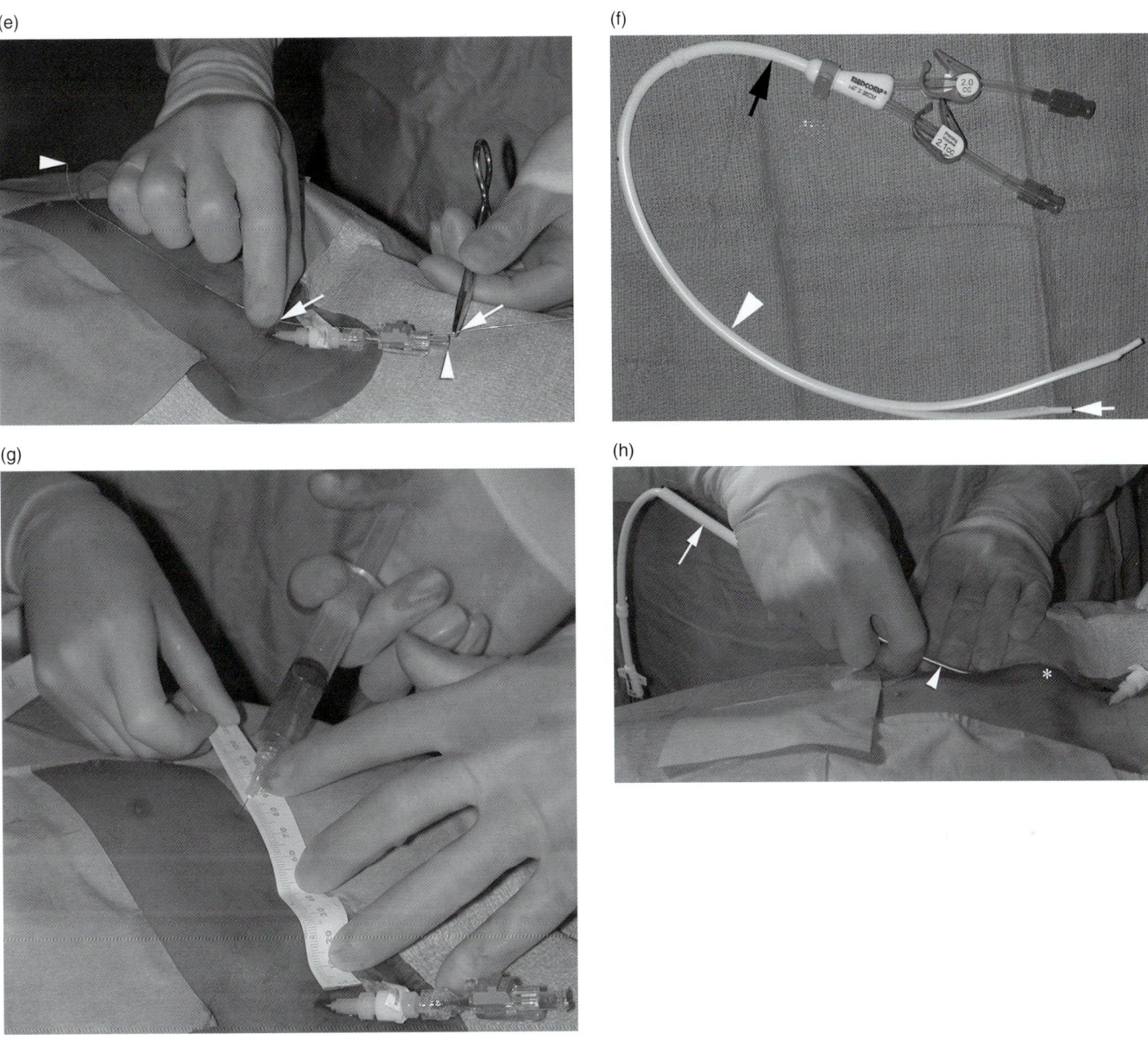

Figure 2.19 (cont.)

small infants and children with short necks. Therefore, it is important to choose an entry site at least 2 to 3 cm superior to the clavicle (Figure 2.19) to minimize the risk of penetrating the posterior wall of the distal jugular or subclavian vein and entering the apical pleural space, or injuring the subclavian artery. If these complications occur, a life-threatening hemothorax may occur. To avoid this problem it is our practice to select an entry site two fingerbreadths superior to the clavicle and to puncture the vessel with the needle at about a 6-degree inclination.

Although venous access may be achieved by non-guided puncture using anatomic landmarks, real-time image guidance to assist venous entry is safer and more efficient in most cases. In our laboratory US is used preferentially. We have found that imaging the vessel in the short axis is best since it nicely demonstrates the relationship of the needle to the middle of the vessel. The long axis can also be successfully used for guidance and some operators prefer this approach. Ultrasound may also identify anatomic reasons for difficult access in some cases. Conversely, use of US without adequate training and experience and without knowledge of the patient's venous history can lead to severe complications (Figure 2.20), including venous or arterial injury, pneumo- or hemothorax, pulmonary hemorrhage, hypovolemic shock, and death.

Selecting the correct catheter length can be challenging, more so when entering from the left IJV. With a longer length of catheter and tunnel for the CVC to recoil into, the degree of shortening tends to be greater. Especially with tunneled

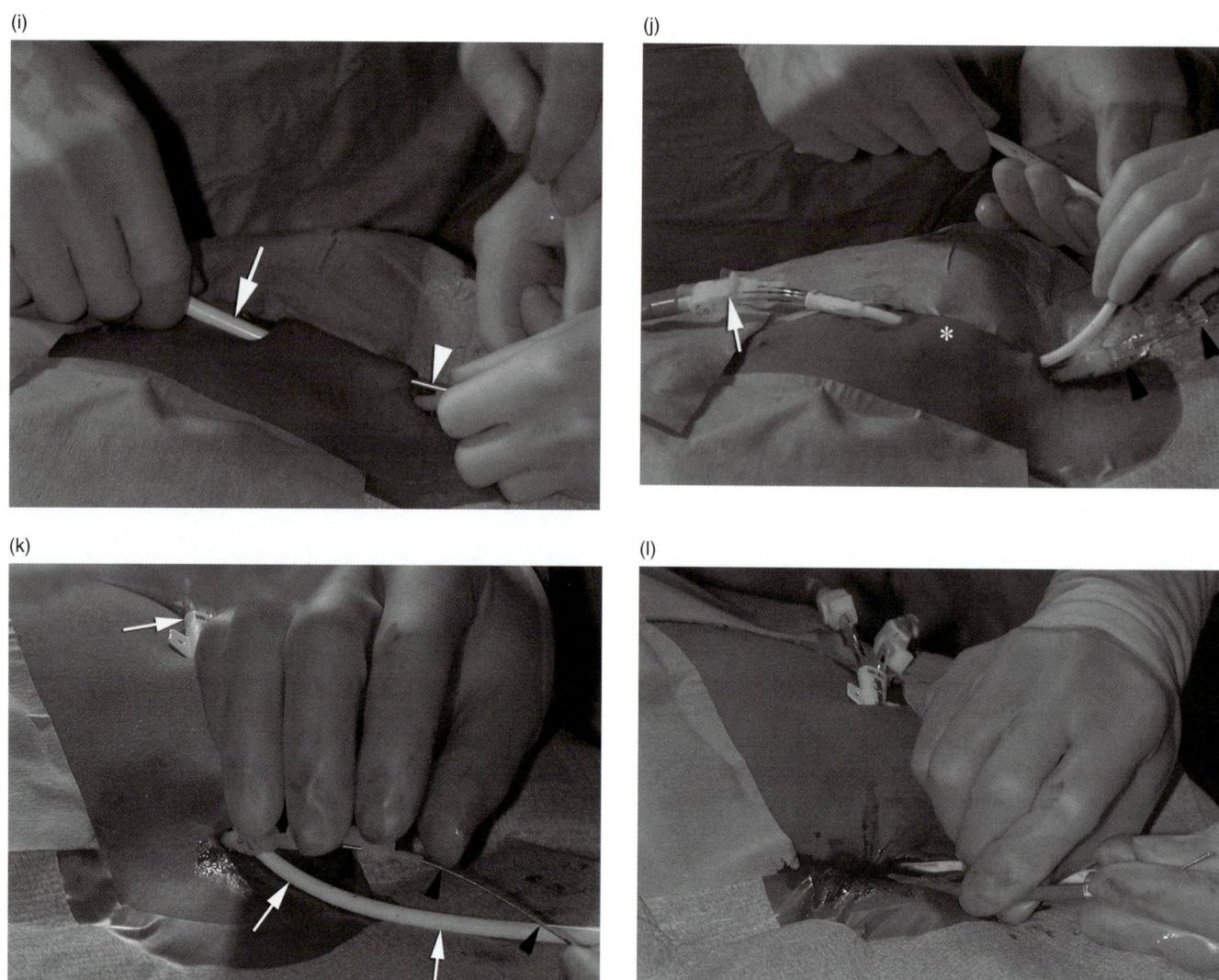

Figure 2.19 (cont.)

catheters, it is easier to pull the catheter back a short distance to achieve appropriate position than to advance it forward the same distance. Therefore, if in doubt it is helpful to measure the catheter a few millimeters longer than otherwise anticipated. When a tunneled catheter or port is placed in an obese or large-breasted patient, care must be taken to account for differences in location of soft tissues between the recumbent and upright positions. The degree of catheter migration may be unexpected and may result in several centimeters of upward movement in the catheter tip (Figure 2.21).

While somewhat complex non-radiographic methods have been described for positioning the catheter tip (such as intra-atrial electrocardiography and transesophageal echocardiography), radiological control is definitive and non-invasive, and obviates postprocedure radiographic confirmation in most cases. The inferior margin of the right mainstem bronchus, the right tracheobronchial angle, the carina, the level of the sixth thoracic vertebra, the level of the third anterior intercostal space, and the lateral deflection of the radiographic "right heart border" have all been suggested as anatomic landmarks that may be used to determine the appropriate catheter length. None of these recommendations arise from prospective study of the relationship between an unequivocal catheter position and the associated rate of mechanical or other complications. Many who respond to rare events such as cardiac perforation and lethal tamponade caution against positioning the catheter tip closer to the atrium than the pericardial reflection. In a particularly erudite editorial, Fletcher and Bodenham note that this latter recommendation is likely to lead to equally serious if less dramatic complications. We agree with their conclusion that "the catheter tip should be placed in as large a vein as possible, ideally (for non-dialysis catheters) outside the heart and parallel with the long axis of the vein such that the tip does not abut the vein or heart wall end-on." Until an appropriate

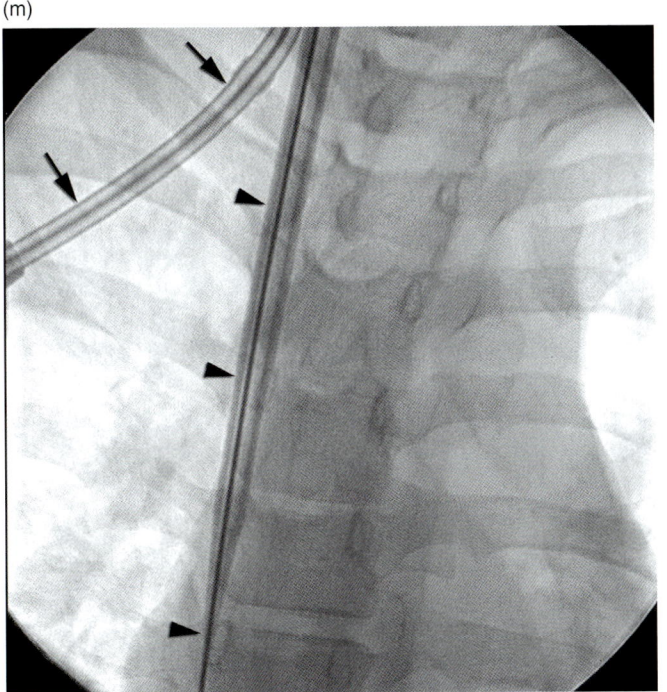
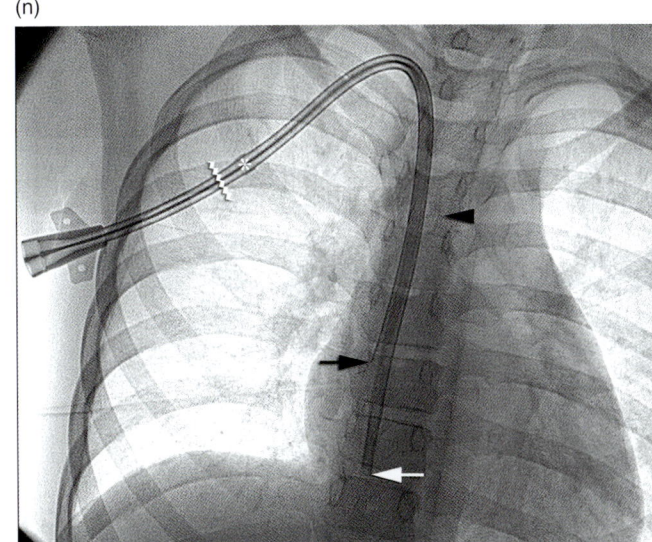

Figure 2.19 (cont.)

study is completed in children, we recommend that (1) the position of each catheter tip be recorded unequivocally, as the number of vertebral bodies (whole and fractional) the tip is located below the carina on a fluoroscopic image or plain chest radiograph, and (2) a position from the intersection of the catheter with the inferior margin of the right mainstem bronchus to a point two vertebral bodies below the carina is the safest "landing zone" overall in our experience.

Once the prospective entry site has been sonographically evaluated and marked, the sterile equipment is uncovered and the entry site (including the chest wall if a tunneled line or port is planned) is prepared and draped in sterile fashion. The skin (and tunnel tract if necessary) is then generously anesthetized using a 30-gauge needle with buffered lidocaine. A small skin incision is made (just large enough to accommodate the diameter of the catheter or cuff to be inserted, Figure 2.19a) and a single wall or sheathed needle, is used to access the vein, according to the operator's preference. If it is consistently difficult to achieve a clean single wall puncture without undue compression of the vein, it may be helpful to use an access needle with a more acutely angled bevel.

In young children the puncture needle is maintained somewhat upright at approximately a 60-degree angle to the skin. The US transducer is kept perpendicular to the skin surface with some cranial angulation (Figure 2.19b) to improve conspicuity of the bevel. The jugular vein must be differentiated from the carotid artery (Figure 2.19c). In general, the jugular vein is larger, non-pulsatile, and enlarges with Valsalva maneuver or a Trendelenburg position. Compression and color Doppler imaging are helpful in verifying the appropriate vessel. If the jugular vein is superficial to the artery, lateral angulation of the US may separate the two vessels and allow a safe window for access.

The puncture needle is directed toward the center of the transducer to its anticipated focal point. An 8 MHz curvilinear to 18 MHz linear transducer, covered with a sterile plastic sleeve, is most commonly used for imaging. The vessel is imaged in the transverse plane so that the relationship of the needle tip to the center of the vessel can be appreciated. Because the jugular vein is highly compliant, care must be taken to achieve a clean puncture of the anterior wall without perforating structures posterior to the vessel lumen. The needle is attached to a connecting tube and 10 ml syringe containing normal saline and suction is applied as the needle is withdrawn. In neonates, the IJV is extremely collapsible. As a result, it is sometimes useful to substitute a smaller syringe in order to avoid collapsing the vessel and interrupting free blood return. When blood return freely flows the tube is disconnected. A guide wire is then inserted and directed into the right atrium or IVC under fluoroscopic control (Figure 2.19d).

If a polyurethane catheter (e.g., temporary central lines) is selected the catheter may be inserted directly without tract dilation or placement of a peel-away sheath. Because they cannot be cut to length, the correct length of temporary, apheresis, and dialysis catheters needs to be selected (Figure 2.19d–f). If a non-tunneled or tunneled silastic or silicone catheter is chosen (see "Creation of a subcutaneous tunnel,"

Chapter 2 Central venous access

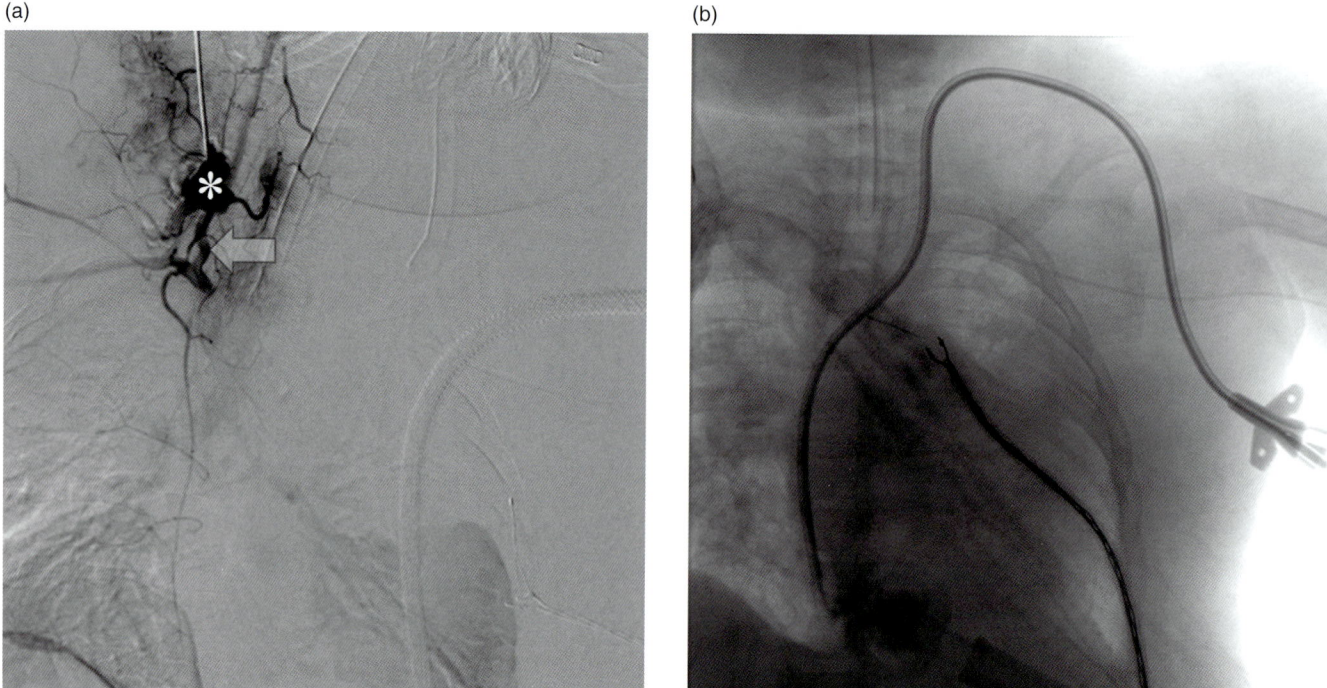

Figure 2.20 Urgent access of the right internal jugular vein was attempted with US guidance by ICU personnel in this one-year-old female in renal failure who had had the right jugular vein ligated with extracorporeal membrane oxygenation (ECMO) as a newborn. (a) Diagnostic angiography after puncture of a vascular mass the following morning demonstrates a pseudoaneurysm (*asterisk*) of the right vertebral artery (*arrow*). (b) A 9.5 Fr double lumen catheter was successfully placed via the left internal jugular vein that provided satisfactory hemodialysis for three months until the patient's death from unrelated sepsis.

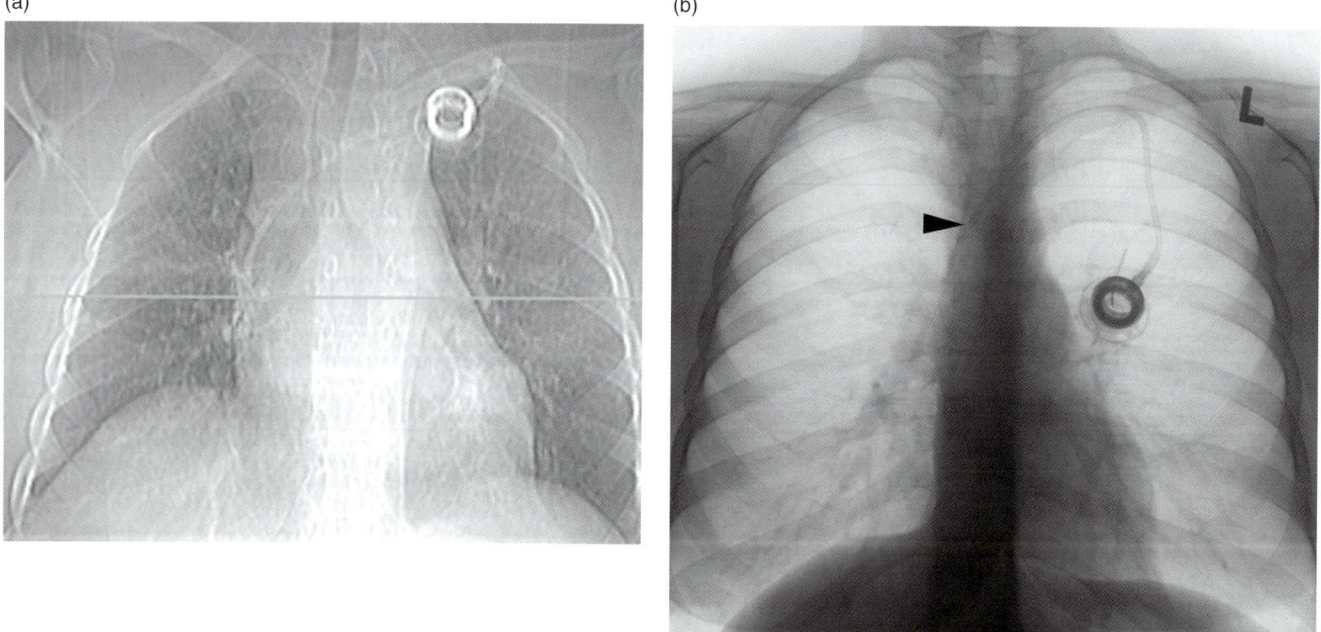

Figure 2.21 Sixteen-year-old girl with acute lymphoblastic leukemia (ALL) and an indwelling port insertion for chemotherapy. (a) With the patient recumbent, the port catheter tip appears to be in a satisfactory position. The horizontal line on this CT topogram indicates the level of the most inferior axial image on which the tip was still visible. (b) In an upright position, movement of breast tissue results in superior migration of the port catheter tip, approximately 1¾ vertebral levels, with the tip (*arrowhead*) now abutting the lateral wall of the SVC. Taping down the breast tissue before catheter insertion may help achieve a more reliable final position.

Table 2.6 Procedural summary: subcutaneous tunnel

Select exit site for the tunnel.

Prepare and drape sterile field.

Apply generous local anesthetic to tract.

Make small incision for catheter exit.

Insert tunneler and create a tract.

Pull a suture through the tract.

Tie the suture to the tip of the CVC and pull through tract until cuff is positioned within distal 1/2 to 1/3 of tract.

Insert CVC into upper right atrium via peel-away sheath.

Remove peel-away sheath.

Inject contrast to confirm satisfactory catheter position.

Close incisions.

Cover with 2 × 2 gauze and occlusive dressing.

Heparinize catheter.

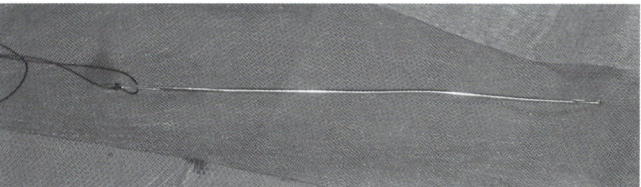

Figure 2.22 A uterine sound or similar blunt-ended malleable device is used to create a subcutaneous tunnel for central venous line insertion.

Regardless what catheter type is used, the CVC length is determined using the bent guide wire technique (Figure 2.19e–g) also described under "Peripherally inserted central catheter (PICC) insertion," above (Figure 2.11). At the completion of the procedure contrast is injected to document catheter position and evaluate for potential adverse events. After contrast injection the CVC is flushed with saline and the line is heparinized. The catheter is then sutured in position and covered with a clear plastic, sterile, occlusive dressing (e.g., Opsite® or Tegaderm®).

Creation of a subcutaneous tunnel

In patients needing medium- to long-term venous access (weeks to months) a tunneled line is indicated (Table 2.6). A subcutaneous tunnel is created after initial venous access has been secured. In appropriate situations (e.g., patients on certain bone marrow transplant protocols) a preexisting indwelling port may be safely exchanged for a tunneled CVC, either using the existing tract or preferably developing a new subcutaneous tunnel.

Once guide wire access to the vessel is secured, the prospective course of the tunnel should be carefully planned. One must avoid sharp turns or angulation that might result in catheter kinking. This is especially important for insertion sites higher in the neck, where the risk of catheter kinking is increased.

The preferred sites for catheter exit are over the lateral chest wall (superolateral to the nipple is preferred) or superomedial to the nipple. It is important not to injure the breast bud, which could result in abnormal breast development. Once the path of the tunnel and the exit site are chosen, the tract is anesthetized (Figure 2.19g) using a long thin-gauge needle (e.g., 22-gauge Chiba). An incision just large enough to receive the tunneling device and retention cuff is made.

A variety of instruments may be used for tunneling including a hemostat or curved Kelly for short tunnels, or one of many rigid or malleable tunnelers for longer tracts. We prefer to use a malleable uterine sound (Figure 2.22), which has a hole in its tip through which a long suture can be tied. The device is inserted in either end of the potential tract and advanced through the subcutaneous tissue until it exits through the other end (Figure 2.19h–j).

Occasionally, especially when inserting lines into the IJV there is too much angulation in the course of the tract at the level of the clavicle for the rigid tunneler to safely and easily get

below), a peel-away sheath must be inserted before the catheter can be introduced. The tract is dilated to the diameter of the peel-away sheath prior to its introduction. For small diameter catheters, this is performed as a single dilation. For large bore catheters, this may require two or three intermediate dilations. For example, in anticipation of a 14 French dialysis catheter (which requires a 17 French peel-away sheath), the tract may be serially dilated with 10, 12, and 16 French dilators (Figure 2.19l). Each dilation is monitored fluoroscopically, taking care to maintain proper alignment with the vessel, and to maintain an adequate length of guide wire beyond the tip of the dilator, to prevent vascular or atrial injury (Figure 2.19m).

Three points may be considered with regard to the peel-away sheath. First, to avoid accidental dislodgment or malposition, it is important that the tip of the outer sheath be positioned deeply enough in the vena cava that secure access will be maintained when the inner dilator is removed. Second, to avoid vascular or atrial perforation the peel-away sheath is best advanced over a guide wire under fluoroscopic control and should not be seated deeply within the right atrium. Third, to assure that the catheter may be introduced easily without undue blood loss, at least 2 to 3 cm of the outer sheath are left outside the skin at the venous entry site.

The wire and dilator are carefully removed, and the sheath is clamped at the skin before the dilator is completely withdrawn (the wire must be pulled back within the tip of the dilator so it is not clamped in the sheath!). This allows unhurried introduction of the first 2 to 3 cm of the catheter tip with very little risk of air embolus or substantial blood loss, as described below. The sheath is unclamped and the rest of the catheter is advanced. The tip position is verified with fluoroscopy before the peel-away sheath is removed.

to the entry site. Thus, a third incision at the level of the clavicle may be required to create an "interrupted" tunnel. The best location for this incision is at the point of maximal angulation. The tunneler can be brought out at this point and reinserted making it easier to complete the tunnel. In this situation it is important to be sure that the new tract starts deeply enough so that the catheter does not come through the skin.

The silastic central line is attached to the tunneler and pulled through the tract making sure that the retention cuff is positioned within the distal half to third of the tunnel. Having measured the length of the catheter from the venous entry point in the neck to the entrance of the right atrium using the bent guide wire technique, the catheter is trimmed to the correct length. If a Groshong type catheter is used, the measuring steps can be omitted since it can be trimmed from its proximal end once the tip is properly positioned.

The catheter is then inserted through the peel-away sheath and its final position confirmed. To accomplish this, a hemostat is positioned transversely across the outer sheath near its entry point at the skin. The inner dilator is slowly removed from the peel-away sheath, clamping the outer sheath closed with the hemostat prior to removing the last couple centimeters of the dilator. In this manner, the first few centimeters of the catheter may be introduced to the level of the clamp without concern for blood loss or air embolus.

With the distal catheter and proximal sheath held firmly, the clamp is carefully removed and the circumference of the sheath restored to allow the catheter to be advanced without difficulty. This step is most easily accomplished with the help of an assistant. Especially with narrow diameter catheters (e.g., 3 or 4 French), there may be resistance to initial passage of the catheter through the sheath. If so, a non-toothed pick-up may be used to assist the catheter's advancement, taking small bites in close proximity to the end of the sheath. Care must be exercised to avoid abrading or perforating the catheter wall during this manipulation.

As the final centimeters of the catheter are inserted, the sheath may be peeled back (*not* advanced) to the level of the skin, and the position of the catheter tip is evaluated prior to complete removal of the sheath. With the tip in a satisfactory position, the sheath is peeled back and removed, taking care not to withdraw or dislodge the catheter during this step. The last bit of catheter is advanced into the neck incision and the skin is closed, usually with a single 4-0 resorbable suture reinforced with two short Steri-Strips® or Dermabond® and Steri-Strips®. If the patient was maintained in the Trendelenburg position during insertion, the table may be restored to a horizontal or even slight anti-Trendelenburg position to facilitate hemostasis.

Postprocedure and follow-up care

All children receiving a CVC have a postoperative chest radiograph or a spot fluoroscopic image to confirm appropriate course and position of the catheter (Figure 2.19n) and to identify a possible pneumothorax, hemopneumothorax, or other complication. Elevating the head of the bed 15 to 45 degrees minimizes postprocedural bleeding. Frequent monitoring of vital signs and close observation for complications are performed. Typically, heart rate and blood pressure are monitored every 15 minutes for a half hour, every 30 minutes for one hour, then every hour until the child is alert and responsive. Children are not allowed to eat or drink and are at bed rest until they have returned to their preprocedure baseline. Once awake and responsive, clear fluids are given and the diet is advanced as tolerated. At this time outpatients may be discharged to home. Prior to discharge or transfer, the procedure and any complications, variations, or noteworthy interventions are recorded in the medical record (see Table 2.1).

Antibiotics are not routinely given. If a complication is observed, treatment is tailored to the extent and severity of the problem. In general, major complications are managed in conjunction with a medical, surgical, or intensive care service, as needed. Complications such as pneumothorax, which can be treated using interventional techniques, are managed in the interventional suite. The interventionalist should remain involved in the management of procedural complications whether or not he or she is the primary treating physician.

Technical problems and pitfalls

If the tunneling device is aimed directly from the exit incision on the chest wall to the venous entry point, the subcutaneous tract so formed is likely to be sharply angulated, and may lead to intermittent kinking and catheter dysfunction. To avoid this complication, the tunneler may be curved and advanced in a "sweeping" motion, creating a gently curved tract. For example, if advancing from the lateral chest to the base of the neck, aim the tunneler first toward the lateral third of the clavicle. As it is advanced, gradually reorient the tip toward the neck wound. It is helpful to guide the tip on its subcutaneous journey with the fingertips of the operator's non-dominant hand, to keep the tunneler superficial to the clavicle, well within the subcutaneous tissues, and away from vulnerable structures in the neck.

In most instances, once the peel-away sheath is in position, a guide wire is not needed to advance the CVC into position. If there is a venous anomaly, tortuous pathway, extensive collateralization, or other problems, a directional guide wire, usually a 0.018-inch glide wire, is utilized. When inserting a left subclavian CVC it is important to make the catheter long enough. For the catheter to be in stable position it is important to have the catheter contact the right SVC wall and have the catheter tip beyond this point dangling free within the proximal SVC or upper right atrium. If it is short or withdraws after removal of the peel-away sheath, the tip will likely be in contact with the right lateral wall of the SVC resulting in intermittent obstruction and difficulty aspirating blood (Figure 2.23). Thus it is likely best to anticipate slight shortening and measure approximately 2 cm longer than one would for a right subclavian CVC. Also, one can create a longer tunnel so the cuff can be pulled back if the catheter is too long.

Technique: subclavian CVC

Equipment and patient preparation

Except as noted, equipment and patient preparation required for subclavian vein catheterization is the same as for other CVCs, as described under "Technique: internal jugular CVC insertion," above.

Standard technique

Although venous access may be achieved by non-guided puncture using anatomic landmarks, real-time imaging guidance is used to assist venous entry in most instances. For US-guided puncture of the subclavian vein, an entry site is planned in its proximal third in the concavity just medial to the shoulder (Table 2.7). This location is more peripheral than the site chosen when using anatomic landmarks alone. This location has the advantage of being away from the pleural cavity making the risk of pneumothorax, hemothorax, catheter pinch off, and intravascular foreign body, less likely. Prior to sedation, an entry site is selected with US and marked on the skin with an ink marker. At this point intravenous sedation is usually given. The table controls and tower are draped in sterile fashion and the skin is sterilized. The site is then covered with a sterile drape. Regardless of the drape selected, a sterile cover sheet is also used to create a wide sterile field. This allows the interventionalist to lay out the syringes, wires, etc., without worrying about contaminating the equipment.

Once the prospective entry site has been sonographically evaluated and marked, the sterile equipment is uncovered and the entry site (including the chest wall if a tunneled line or port is planned) is prepared and draped in sterile fashion. The skin (and tunnel tract if necessary) is then generously anesthetized using a thin needle with buffered lidocaine. A small (2–3 mm) skin incision is made and a single wall or sheathed needle is used. In young children the puncture needle is maintained

Table 2.7 Procedural summary: subclavian CVC insertion

- Obtain preprocedural laboratory studies.
- Select entry site with US or fluoroscopy.
- Prepare and drape skin.
- Locally anesthetize entry site.
- Small skin incision at entry site.
- Puncture subclavian vein using real-time US guidance.
- Aspirate until free blood return. Confirm position with venography if necessary.
- Insert guide wire into right atrium, IVC, or hepatic vein.
- Dilate tract (if silastic catheter used).
- Exchange dilator for peel-away sheath.
- Measure distance from entry site to upper right atrium.
- Insert CVC.
- Inject contrast to confirm satisfactory position.
- Suture incision closed.
- Cover entry site with a 2 × 2 gauze and occlusive dressing.
- Heparinize CVC.

(a)
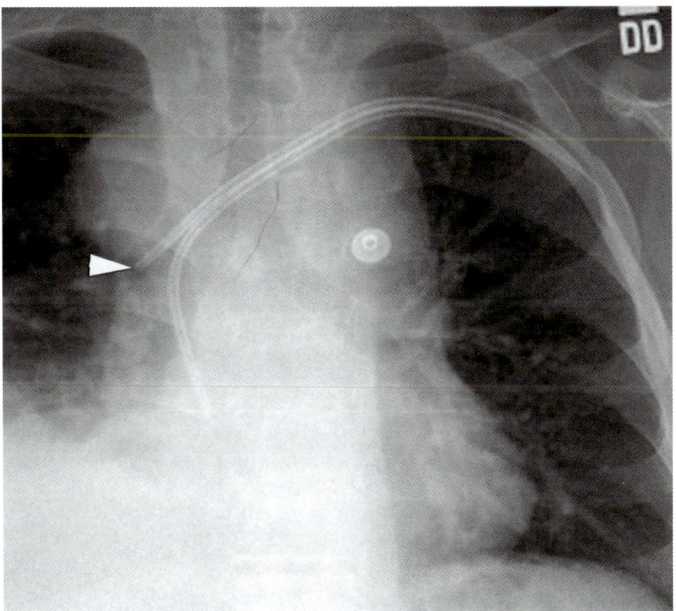

(b)
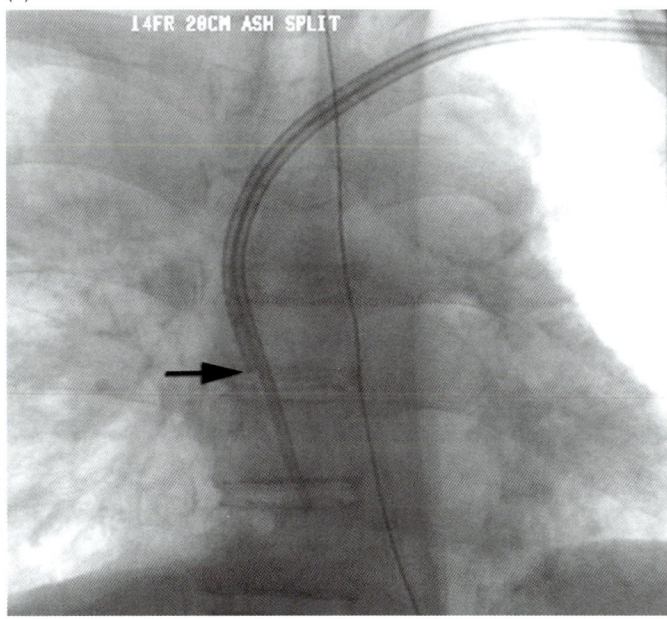

Figure 2.23 Seventeen-year-old girl with end-stage renal disease and pneumonia. (a) Improper insertion of the 14.5 French split lumen dialysis catheter results in the shorter lumen tip (*arrowhead*) projecting against the wall of the SVC. (b) Proper insertion places in the shorter lumen tip (*arrow*) at the entrance to the right atrium, and the long lumen within the true atrium itself. This results in maximal flow and minimal recirculation during dialysis.

somewhat upright at approximately a 60-degree angle to the skin. The US transducer is kept perpendicular to the skin surface carefully avoiding transducer angulation. Slight angulation away from the needle may make the bevel more conspicuous. The puncture needle is then directed toward the center of the transducer to its anticipated focal point. An 8 MHz curvilinear to 18 MHz linear transducer, covered with a sterile plastic sleeve, is used for imaging. The vessel is imaged in the transverse plane so that the relationship of the needle tip to the center of the vessel can be appreciated. The needle is then attached to a connecting tube and 10 ml syringe and suction is applied as the needle is withdrawn. When blood is freely flowing a guide wire is inserted and directed into the right atrium or IVC. If a polyurethane catheter is selected the catheter is inserted directly without tract dilation or placement of a peel-away sheath. If a non-tunneled or tunneled silastic or silicone catheter is chosen, a peel-away sheath must be inserted before a catheter can be placed. In either case the CVC length is determined using the modified bent guide wire method. The choice of catheter length is limited with polyurethane catheters (5 cm, 7 cm, 12 cm, or 15 cm) and in some instances they cannot be utilized. At the completion of the procedure contrast is injected to document catheter position and evaluate for potential adverse events. After contrast injection the CVC is flushed with saline and the line is heparinized. The catheter is then sutured in position and covered with a clear plastic, sterile, occlusive dressing (e.g., Opsite® or Tegaderm®).

Technical variations

If non-guided puncture of the subclavian vein is necessary or elected, venipuncture can safely and successfully be achieved using these simple approaches. Entry of the subclavian vein may be achieved by puncture in the region of the middle third of the clavicle while angling the needle toward the suprasternal notch. While fluoroscopy with injection of contrast via a peripheral vein can be used for subclavian venipuncture, we prefer real-time US guidance.

Postprocedure and follow-up care

Care of the patient receiving a subclavian CVC is identical to that described above for "Technique: internal jugular CVC insertion."

Technique: femoral CVC

The femoral route for central venous catheterization may be useful as a primary or secondary entry site. It is our current practice to consider the femoral route as primary access in a variety of settings including neonates who no longer have umbilical venous access, small children with congenital heart disease, and patients who require emergent access. In addition, in children in whom access to the SVC is relatively contraindicated such as those individuals with venous thrombosis, prior surgical interventions (e.g., Blalock–Tausig shunt), overlying burns, or infection, we have found that the complication rate and longevity of femoral venous CVCs are comparable to other conventional routes of access. In situations where longer term access is required the femoral line is tunneled to the anterolateral thigh, flank, or upper abdomen.

Equipment and patient preparation

Except as noted, the equipment and patient preparation for femoral insertion of a CVC are the same as for other CVC insertions (see "Technique: internal jugular CVC insertion," above). When the patient is positioned on the procedure table, it is helpful to place a roll beneath the hips. This partially reduces the natural anterior angulation of the iliofemoral vessels, and helps to separate the common femoral vein and artery in the coronal plane.

Standard technique

The common femoral vein is easily cannulated without imaging guidance, as described under "Technical variations," below. However, because the vein and artery often overlap in the sagittal plane, especially in younger children, "blind" access does increase the risk of inadvertent arterial puncture, arteriovenous fistula, and prolonged procedure time in those cases where the vein is not easily accessible.

Alternatively, the femoral vein may be readily accessed with a single wall needle under US guidance. For US-guided puncture of the femoral vein, an entry site is planned inferior to the inguinal ligament, preferably superficial to the femoral head. This reduces the risk of retroperitoneal hemorrhage should the artery be inadvertently punctured, and affords a firm platform to apply pressure against if hemostasis is difficult to achieve.

In either case, prior to sedation the entry site is selected and marked on the skin with an ink marker. At this point intravenous sedation is usually given. The table controls and tower are draped in sterile fashion and the skin is sterilized. The site is then covered with a sterile drape. Regardless of the drape selected, a sterile cover sheet is also used to create a wide sterile field. This allows the interventionalist to lay out the syringes, wires, etc., without worrying about contaminating the equipment.

Once the prospective entry site has been evaluated and marked, the sterile equipment is uncovered and the entry site (including the abdomen or thigh if a tunneled line or port is planned) is prepared and draped in sterile fashion (Table 2.8). The skin (and tunnel tract if necessary) is then generously anesthetized using a thin needle with buffered lidocaine.

A small (2–3 mm) skin incision is made and a single wall, or sheathed needle, is used. In young children the puncture needle is maintained somewhat upright at approximately a 60-degree angle to the skin. If US is used, the puncture needle is directed toward the center of the transducer to its anticipated focal point. A 7 to 12 MHz linear transducer, covered with a sterile plastic sleeve, is used for imaging. The vessel is imaged

Table 2.8 Procedural summary: femoral CVC insertion

- Obtain preprocedural laboratory studies.
- Select entry site with US or fluoroscopy.
- Prepare and drape skin.
- Slightly hyperextend hips with roll placed under lower back.
- Locally anesthetize entry site.
- Small skin incision at entry site.
- Puncture common femoral vein using real-time US guidance.
- Aspirate until free blood return. Confirm position with venography if necessary.
- Insert guide wire into right atrium or proximal IVC.
- Dilate tract.
- Exchange dilator for peel-away sheath (if silastic catheter used).
- Measure distance from entry site to lower right atrium or distal IVC, as appropriate.
- Insert CVC.
- Inject contrast to confirm satisfactory position.
- Suture incision closed.
- Cover entry site with a 2 × 2 gauze and occlusive dressing.
- Heparinize CVC.

in the transverse plane so that the relationship of the needle tip to the center of the vessel can be appreciated.

The needle is then attached to a connecting tube and a 10 ml saline-filled syringe and suction is applied as the needle is withdrawn. When blood is freely flowing a guide wire is inserted and directed toward the right atrium. If a polyurethane catheter is selected the catheter is inserted directly without tract dilation or placement of a peel-away sheath. If a non-tunneled or tunneled silastic or silicone catheter is chosen, a peel-away sheath must be inserted before the catheter can be placed. The CVC length is measured using the same methods described for PICC and internal jugular CVC insertion. The catheter tip is either positioned as a long line, between the diaphragm and the inferior third of the right atrium (preferably below the seventh thoracic interspace), or as a short line that ends in the infrarenal IVC.

Just as with other CVCs, femoral lines intended for long-term use may be tunneled and exteriorized, in the fashion of a Hickman or Broviac catheter (Figure 2.24), or internalized as an indwelling port (Figure 2.25), using the approaches described under "Creation of a subcutaneous tunnel," above or "Creation of a subcutaneous pocket," below. Preferred exit sites include the lateral abdomen (between the mid-clavicular and anterior axillary lines, above the waistline, and below the inferior costal margin) and the anteromedial thigh. In either case, the tunnel should be long if possible, to avoid contamination from the diaper or groin region. Again, sharp angulation near the venous entry point must be avoided to prevent catheter kinking and dysfunction.

At the completion of the procedure contrast is injected to document catheter position and evaluate for potential adverse events. After contrast injection the CVC is flushed with saline and the line is heparinized. The catheter is then sutured in position and covered with a clear plastic, sterile, occlusive dressing (e.g., Opsite® or Tegaderm®).

Technical variations

The femoral vein may be accessed "blindly" by aiming the access needle just medial to the palpated femoral pulse, approximately 45 degrees to the skin in the parasagittal plane, and approximately 10 degrees medial to the course of the artery. The single wall needle, attached to a saline-filled syringe, is slowly advanced until it hits bone. Then, gentle suction is applied and the needle is withdrawn until freely flowing blood return is obtained. If no blood return is seen, the process is repeated. After each pass, the needle should be flushed, to prevent occlusion of the needle by a tissue plug or thrombus.

If a temporary femoral line is indicated (e.g., for ICU use or apheresis), the equipment included in commonly available catheter kits is usually sufficient. The catheters are supplied in predetermined lengths, and are intended to be left as a short line. After accessing the vein, a short "J" wire is advanced to the distal IVC, and a small incision is made at the skin entry site. The tract is dilated to the diameter of the catheter, and the catheter is advanced to the hub, which is sutured to the skin and dressed as previously described. These and all *temporary* femoral lines are removed as soon as clinically feasible, preferably within 24 hours, and not more than one week except under extraordinary conditions.

Postprocedure and follow-up care

Care of the patient receiving a femoral CVC is identical to that described above for "Technique: internal jugular CVC insertion."

Infectious complications are more likely in patients with a temporary CVC placed by a femoral route than tunneled femoral CVCs or CVCs inserted via a jugular route, presumably because it is inherently more difficult to maintain a sterile site in the groin than in the neck. This is especially true for patients who are relatively immunocompromised, such as low birthweight neonates, and children with oncologic disease or renal insufficiency. Due to the oblique drainage of lumbar veins into the IVC, especially on the left, care must be taken to avoid malposition of transfemoral catheters into lumbar veins or even the subarachnoid space! Other complications of femoral lines are similar to those found in PICCs and CVCs in general, as discussed elsewhere in this chapter.

Technique: difficult access

In rare instances, especially in children with chronic or severe illnesses (e.g., children with organ transplants or chronic renal failure), all preferred pathways for central venous access including the femoral veins are occluded (Figure 2.26). In these

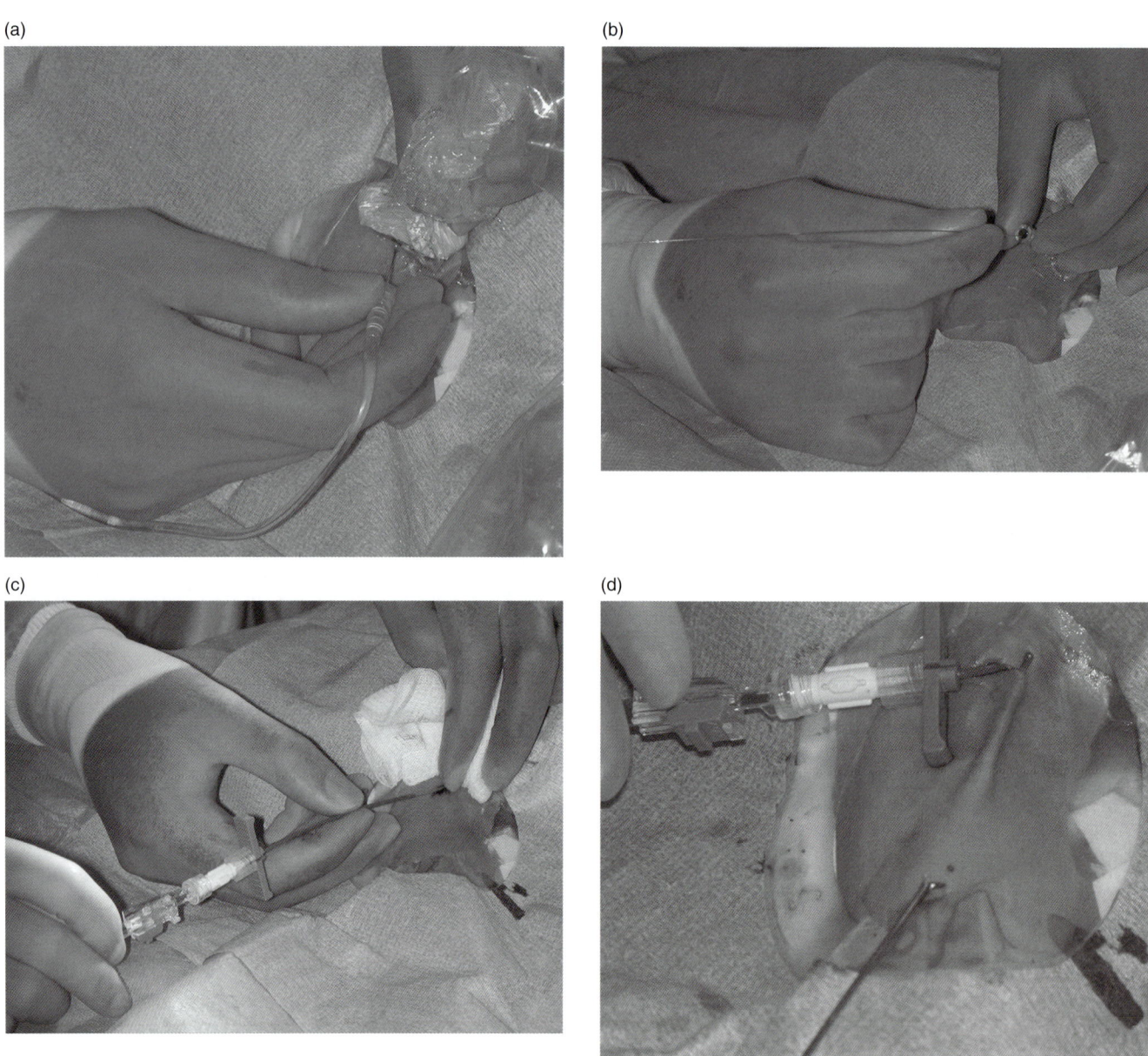

Figure 2.24 Three-month-old girl with hypoglycemia for tunneled femoral central venous line insertion. (a) Using a linear US transducer and a 21-gauge needle the common femoral vein is accessed. (b) A guide wire is advanced through the needle to the right atrium. (c) The needle is exchanged for a dilator, then a peel-away sheath. (d) A tunneling device is used to create a subcutaneous tunnel from the anterolateral thigh to the venotomy site. (e) The central venous catheter is pulled through the tunnel, and cut to length using the modified bent guide wire technique previously described. (f) The trimmed catheter is advanced through the sheath. When proper catheter course and tip position are confirmed with fluoroscopy, the sheath is removed.

cases, a successful search for a safe and useful route for central access may be life-saving. The imagination employed in deriving an alternative pathway for central venous access should be commensurate with need, common sense, and the urgency of the indication.

Equipment and patient preparation

Except as noted, equipment and patient preparation required for catheterization of alternate venous pathways is the same as for other CVCs, as described under "Technique: internal jugular CVC insertion," above.

Standard technique: transbrachiocephalic access

When the major central venous pathways are occluded, one of the brachiocephalic veins is often still patent to the right atrium, although it may not be accessible via a conventional percutaneous route. Conventional venography may not opacify the brachiocephalic vein if the subclavian vein is occluded (e)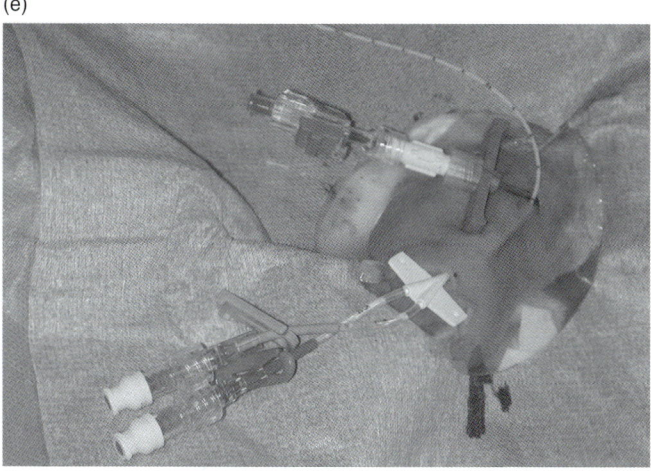

(f)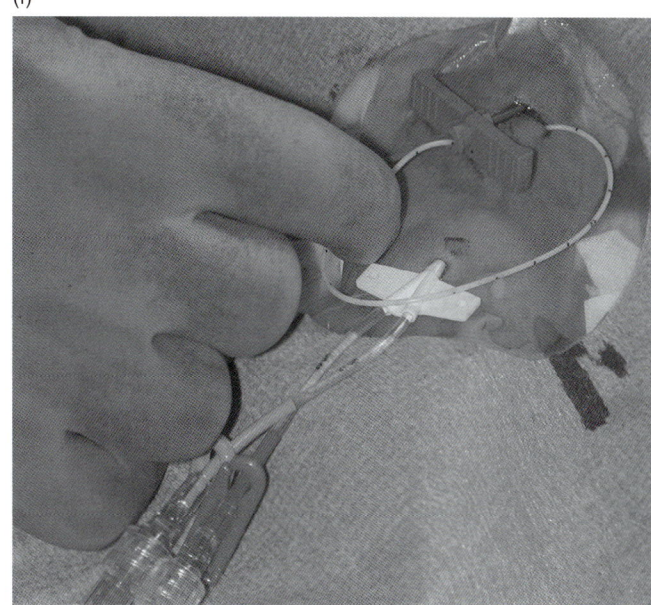

Figure 2.24 (cont.)

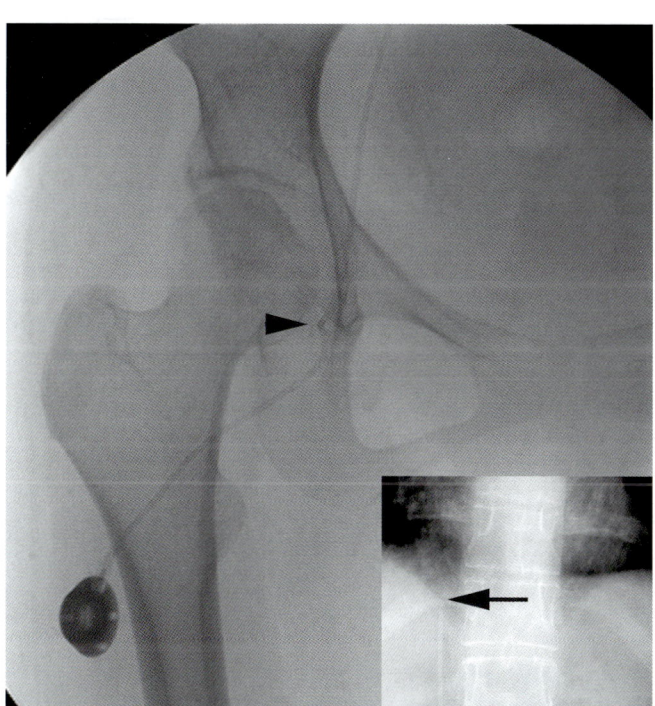

Figure 2.25 Indwelling port placed via a transfemoral route in a 17-year-old girl with cystic fibrosis and a recent history of right atrial thrombosis due to catheter tip malposition. The venotomy site (*arrowhead*) is in the common femoral vein, and the tip (inset, *arrow*) is in the IVC at the level of the diaphragm.

(Figure 2.3). Commonly in this situation, venography shows a network of collateral vessels emptying via the hemizygos and azygos veins to the upper SVC. Gray-scale and color Doppler US imaging in the coronal plane may show a patent brachiocephalic vein, which may be visualized through the confluence into the upper SVC (Figure 2.5). If so, it will often demonstrate a retroclavicular route for access, although the cupola of the lung and the brachiocephalic artery provide a narrow and sometimes complex pathway for access, sometimes directly to the brachiocephalic and sometimes via an enlarged collateral at the base of the neck that drains to the brachiocephalic. Nevertheless, if good technique is employed, this route can usually gain safe access (Table 2.9). Once obtained, direct venography can then be performed to assure patency of this pathway to the right atrium. In our experience, access via direct or indirect puncture of the brachiocephalic vein provides one of the most durable catheter positions of all unconventional pathways, rivaling transjugular access for longevity and low complication rate. The procedure is completed as described for transjugular access, above. A tunneled catheter is preferred given that it is more stable, can remain in place for long periods, and is usually more comfortable since the catheter hub can be directed toward the child's shoulder or lateral chest. Promptly after the completion of the procedure a chest radiograph is obtained to check for the presence of a pneumothorax or hemothorax.

A catheter contrast study is performed to confirm catheter position and adequacy of flow for dialysis or infusion. The catheter is sutured in position and covered with a sterile transparent occlusive dressing and both lumens are heparinized. When the dialysis catheter or CVC is no longer required, the child is returned to the angiography suite and the catheter is removed under fluoroscopic guidance. The soft tissues surrounding the venous entry site are usually adequate to tamponade the venotomy wound, but placing the patient in an anti-Trendelenburg or seated position after removal will decrease risk of prolonged bleeding.

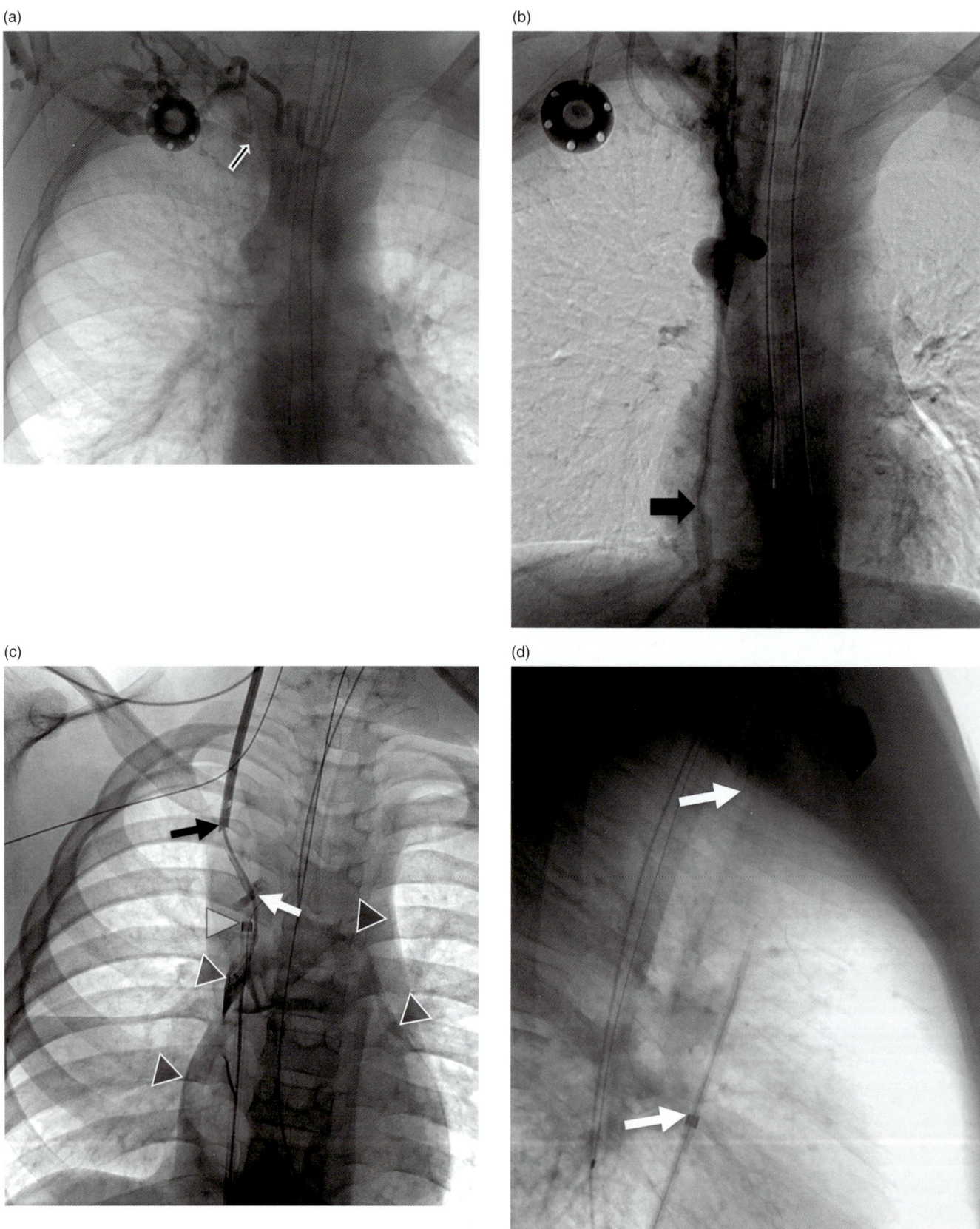

Figure 2.26 A 14-year-old boy was referred for severe facial swelling. (a) Right upper extremity venography shows complete occlusion of the proximal subclavian vein. The subclavian port catheter tip (*arrow*) had a 1 cm intravascular course. (b) Transjugular venography shows complete occlusion of the brachiocephalic vein and SVC with restricted retrograde drainage through azygos collaterals (*arrow*). (c) 10 French sheaths were placed from above (*black arrow*) in the right internal jugular vein and from below (*white arrow*) in the right common femoral vein. An attempt to pass bluntly from above resulted in dissection through the vein wall (*white arrowhead*) with self-limited extravasation into the pericardium (*black arrowheads*).

(e)
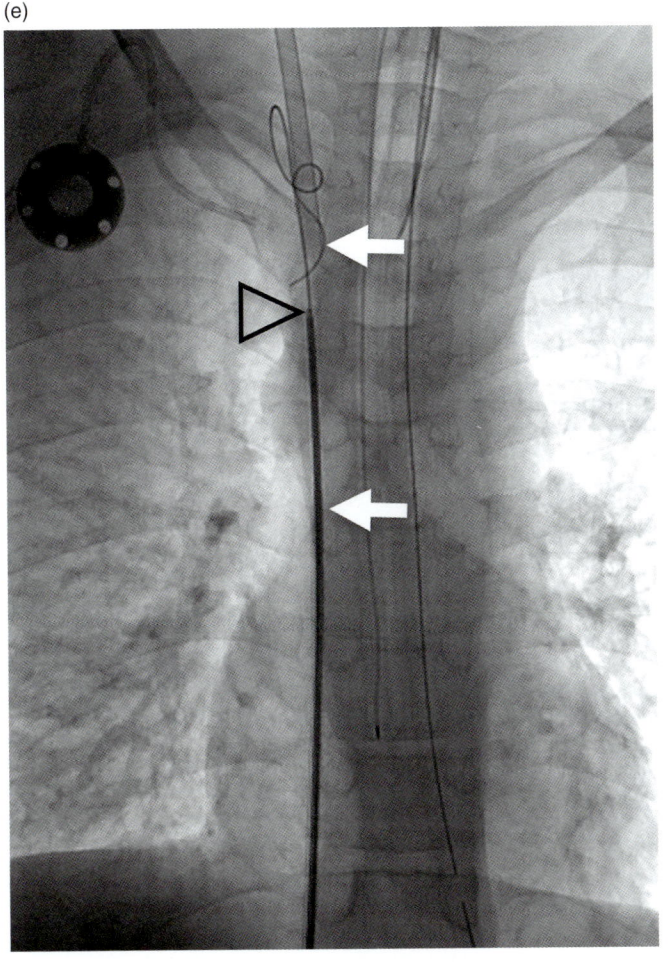

(f)
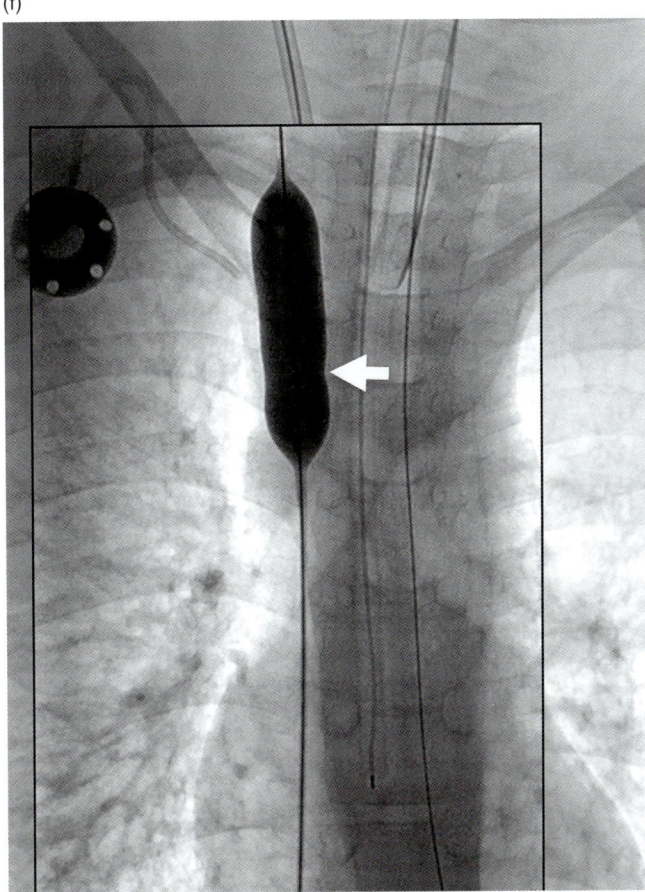

(g)
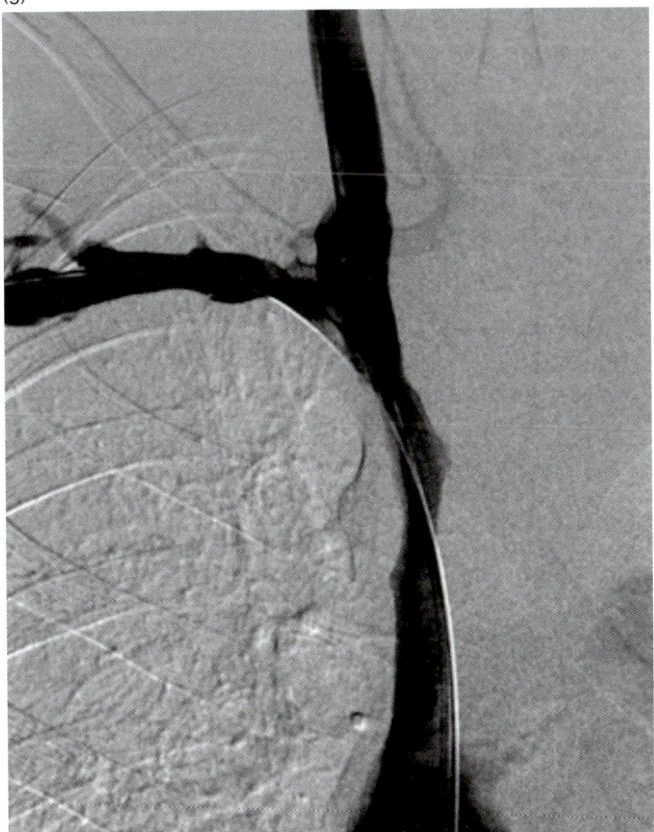

Figure 2.26 (*cont.*) (d–e) Simultaneous biplane fluoroscopy was used to guide a Colapinto needle (*arrowhead*; Cook, Bloomington, IN, USA) across the occluded region between the transfemoral and transjugular sheaths (*arrows*). (f) A super-stiff guide wire snared through the transjugular sheath provided a stable platform for venoplasty with serial non-compliant balloons up to 14 mm diameter (inset; *arrow*). (g) Two weeks later, a similar procedure was used to recanalize the right subclavian vein. Completion venography demonstrates patency of the treated vessels, which remained primarily patent at six-month follow-up.

Table 2.9 Procedure summary: transbrachiocephalic CVC insertion

- Obtain coagulation profile and other pertinent laboratory tests.
- Select entry site using US.
- Prepare and drape skin.
- Locally anesthetize skin at the entry site.
- Small skin incision.
- Insert sheathed or Chiba needle using real-time US guidance into the brachiocephalic vein or any large collateral vein near its connection to the brachiocephalic vein.
- Aspirate until free blood return. Confirm position with venography if necessary.
- Insert stiff guide wire and position tip in right atrium.
- Dilate tract as needed.
- Insert CVC or dialysis catheter.
- Create tunnel or subcutaneous pocket for a port.
- Inject catheter to confirm satisfactory position.
- Cover with occlusive dressing.
- Heparinize catheter.

Table 2.10 Procedure summary: translumbar/transhepatic CVC insertion

- Obtain coagulation profile and other pertinent laboratory tests.
- Select entry site using US.
- Prepare and drape skin.
- Locally anesthetize skin at the entry site.
- Small skin incision.
- Insert sheathed or Chiba needle using real-time US guidance into the IVC directly for translumbar access, or via the most vertical hepatic vein for transhepatic access.
- Aspirate until blood returns freely. Confirm position with venography if necessary.
- Insert stiff guide wire and position tip in distal IVC or right atrium.
- Dilate tract as needed.
- Insert CVC.
- Create tunnel or subcutaneous pocket for a port.
- Inject catheter to confirm satisfactory position.
- Cover with occlusive dressing.
- Heparinize catheter.

Standard technique: transhepatic access

In 1991, Kaufman et al. reported insertion of a central catheter via the transhepatic approach. We have adapted the technique described by Kaufman not only for insertion of CVCs but also for the placement of large-bore dialysis catheters and for transhepatic venography (see Chapter 5). Transhepatic placement of CVCs is indicated in patients who require acute or long-term central venous access but in whom all standard routes of venous access no longer remain. As with any transhepatic procedure, few absolute contraindications exist. A large vascular tumor or abscess within the liver parenchyma blocking access, uncorrectable coagulopathy, or clinical instability would probably preclude the procedure. However, with US a safe route can be sought and used if found. Relative contraindications are also the same as for any transhepatic procedure: coagulopathy, anemia, ascites, previous contrast reaction. In the case of massive ascites, we recommend placement of a peritoneal drainage catheter to drain as much fluid as possible prior to the procedure. Patients with known Budd–Chiari syndrome would, in most instances, not be candidates for this procedure.

Any cross-sectional imaging method may be used to survey the status of the hepatic venous system and IVC. However, in our setting contrast-enhanced CT or MR venography, augmented by US interrogation as indicated, is preferred. While any large vein that is in direct continuity with the vena cava or the IVC itself may be used, we prefer the hepatic veins (Table 2.10) over the IVC for short- or long-term venous access. A tunneled catheter is preferred given that it is more stable, can remain in place for long periods, and is usually more comfortable since the catheter hub can be directed toward the child's side.

The transhepatic approach for insertion of a CVC has been described by several authors. Insertion of a central line via the transhepatic route can be performed using local anesthesia and intravenous sedation, sedation, and paralysis in an intubated child, or general anesthesia. Children requiring a transhepatic central line or dialysis catheter tend to be more seriously ill. Thus these patients are more likely to require general anesthesia, or intubation and a combination of sedation and paralysis. The latter groups are usually in the intensive care unit and the procedure is performed in conjunction with an intensivist.

Preprocedural US is performed for route planning (Figure 2.4). The hepatic vein with the straightest course into the IVC (usually the middle hepatic vein) is selected if it is large enough to accept a 5 to 14.5 French catheter. Once the entry site is chosen the skin is marked. The entry site is usually intercostal. The right upper abdominal quadrant is sterilized, then covered with a large sterile drape. In the absence of general anesthesia the entry site is infiltrated with buffered lidocaine and a generous incision (8 to 10 mm) is made with a #11 scalpel blade.

Using real-time US guidance and a biopsy transducer, a 19-gauge translumbar aortography (TLA) needle, Yueh sheathed needle, or Chiba needle is inserted into the hepatic vein. Whenever possible a sheathed needle is used since it avoids the need for initial tract dilation and exchange of an 0.018-inch guide wire for an 0.035- or 0.038-inch guide wire that is often the most difficult step of the procedure. Once the needle is in place the metal stylet and stiffener are removed and a syringe and connecting tube are coupled to the sheath. When blood is freely aspirated a heavy-duty J wire, stiff Glidewire®, or Amplatz Super Stiff® guide wire is inserted via the sheath and maneuvered into the right atrium.

The next steps depend upon the type of catheter to be inserted. If a central line is needed, a 7 French double lumen catheter is usually selected. If a dialysis or apheresis catheter is planned, then a 7 French, 11.5 French, or 14.5 French catheter is used. For central line placement, the tract is dilated to 8 French so that a peel-away sheath can be positioned. In contrast, if a hemodialysis or plasmapheresis catheter is indicated, the tract is dilated only to the size of the dialysis catheter since it is nicely tapered and moves into position easily. In either case, catheter placement is monitored fluoroscopically in order to follow the course of the guide wire.

Alternatively, a Chiba needle can be substituted for a sheathed needle. Needle placement can be guided using real-time US using a freehand or guided approach. Since it is difficult to aspirate blood through a Chiba needle, dilute non-ionic contrast (~240 mg%) is injected as the needle is withdrawn. When the hepatic vein is entered contrast will flow toward the heart. A 0.018-inch guide wire is inserted and positioned in the right atrium.

A coaxial dilator is inserted and the 0.018-inch stiff guide wire is exchanged for a 0.035- or 0.038-inch guide wire. If the tract cannot be dilated over the 0.018-inch guide wire, alternative approaches may include exchange for a stiff 0.018-inch guide wire (Nitinol, stiff Glide wire, mandril), or use of the metallic stiffening cannula from a Towbin 5 French pigtail drain loaded into a 4 or 5 French 0.035- or 0.038-inch vascular dilator. This combination will create enough stiffness to facilitate entry into the hepatic vein. Once in position the cannula and 0.018-inch guide wire are removed and replaced with an 0.035- or 0.038-inch guide wire; or insert an 18-gauge needle over the guide wire into the hepatic vein. This will reduce the force necessary to pass through the tough connective tissue adjacent to the vein into the venous lumen.

Before inserting a CVC the length is tailored to the child's size. The preferred catheter position is from the junction of the IVC and upper right atrium. In addition, if the catheter is tunneled the length of the tunnel must be added. It is our policy to tunnel all transhepatic central lines since they are generally planned for long-term access and are better stabilized using this approach. Dialysis catheters are tunneled when needed. For children needing hemodialysis, a 7 French, 11.5 French, or 14.5 French double lumen catheter tip is positioned so the distal catheter tip and all of the side holes are within the right atrium. To accommodate the catheters and side hole the longest catheter tip is usually positioned in the upper third of the right atrium. Unfortunately, these catheters come in pre-determined lengths (e.g., Vas-Caths are available in 12.5 and 15 cm lengths) and cannot be tailored. Therefore the tunnel has to be planned carefully taking into consideration the cuff-to-tip length. We recommend that the operator add an addition 3 to 5 cm to the tract length to be sure that the cuff is well within the tunnel at the completion of the procedure. Soon after the completion of the procedure a chest radiograph is obtained to check for the presence of a pneumothorax or hemothorax.

A venogram is performed to confirm catheter position and adequacy of flow for dialysis or infusion. The catheter is sutured in position and covered with a sterile transparent occlusive dressing and both lumens are heparinized. When the dialysis catheter or CVC is no longer required, the child is returned to the angiography suite and the catheter is removed under fluoroscopic guidance. On removal, the catheter is exchanged over a wire for a sheath of appropriate size. The sheath is withdrawn until it is in the hepatic parenchyma. A directional catheter or vascular dilator is inserted for tract embolization. Extra-venous catheter position is confirmed by fluoroscopically monitored contrast injection.

Once the catheter is approximately 1 to 2 cm from the hepatic vein, Gelfoam® pledgets, Avitene® or Gianturco coils may be deposited in the tract as the catheter is withdrawn from the liver. When coils are chosen they should be larger than the diameter of the tract (e.g., when a 12.5 French catheter is used, at least 5 mm coils are deployed). Care is taken to avoid embolization of the hepatic vein branch. The last pledget or coil is deposited close to the liver capsule to protect against bleeding into the peritoneal cavity. To date, no child had suffered significant intraperitoneal hemorrhage in our experience.

Postprocedure and follow-up care

As is the case for other transhepatic procedures the main concern is postprocedural bleeding. In general the catheter will occlude the tract that the peel-away formed, but there can be some oozing around the catheter. The patient is closely observed for signs of blood loss and a CBC is drawn four to six hours after the line is placed. Otherwise no special precautions need be taken.

Standard technique: translumbar access

The technique for translumbar catheterization for central venous access (Table 2.10) was first reported by Kenney et al. in 1985. Subsequently, several reports have followed noting success using this technique in children of all ages and sizes. This approach, like the transhepatic route, is generally reserved for children with occluded subclavian, jugular, and femoral veins.

Like the transhepatic route, the translumbar approach is an excellent alternative to surgical cut-down (on saphenous or intercostal veins), thoracotomy with direct right atrial catheterization, catheterization of the azygos vein, or superior vena caval catheter placement. The potential risks of this technique include infection, pain, and inadvertent injury of a retroperitoneal or intra-abdominal organ, arterial or venous injury causing hemorrhage, and inferior vena caval thrombosis. To reduce the risk of injury, Denny and associates modified their technique by using a 21-gauge, rather than an 18-gauge needle for IVC puncture.

Preoperative evaluation of children for translumbar and transhepatic catheterization is usually identical. A PT, PTT, platelet count, and hematocrit are obtained. A bleeding time is ordered only in selected cases. An inferior vena cavogram or US is usually obtained to ensure IVC patency and evaluate its diameter. In our practice US is the preferred method for evaluation and guidance. Although the procedure can be accomplished under either local anesthesia with intravenous sedation or under general anesthesia, the latter is usually preferred in these children who are generally sicker and have more complex medical or surgical problems.

The technique used is similar to that described in the literature. A wide area extending from the lateral chest to the midline of the back is sterilely prepared and draped. The child is placed prone or with the right side slightly elevated. The entry site is selected at the level of the 3rd to 4th lumbar vertebra, lateral to the spinous process. In older children, an entry site 7 to 8 cm lateral to the spinous process may be acceptable as in adults; however, in younger children, the entry site is best selected in the region of the mid-scapular line. Volumetric assessment of the IVC, its patency, and its anatomic relationships can be accomplished with contrast-enhanced CT or rotational (cone-beam) CT. The latter modality can be used for semi-automated positioning of the angiographic C-arm for optimal fluoroscopic imaging during access.

Puncture of the IVC can be achieved without or with image guidance. The method most frequently described is to advance the needle at a 40- to 45-degree angle to the spine (in the axial plane) under fluoroscopic control until it is in contact with the third lumbar vertebral body. The needle is then withdrawn slightly and redirected anteriorly until blood return occurs. Some interventionalists inject contrast to confirm intraluminal position, others just insert a guide wire and if it moves freely in the expected anatomic path will proceed.

Our preference is to puncture the IVC using real-time US guidance (Figure 2.9). We believe that this approach is safest, fastest, and best reduces the risk of inadvertent puncture of adjacent structures (Figure 2.10). The guide wire selected is usually based on the operator's choice. Our preference is a stiff, non-kinking guide wire, i.e., a stiff Glidewire®, Nitinol®, or Amplatz Super Stiff® wire, which best accomplishes the task and minimizes technical problems. Once the guide wire is in a satisfactory position within the right atrium or distal IVC, the tract is progressively dilated and a peel-away sheath inserted. It is useful in such high-risk procedures to place a second "safety" guide wire outside the working sheath in case of inadvertent dislodgment of the working wire during the procedure (Figure 2.3e). The safety wire permits reacquisition of access with minimal risk and effort.

After the catheter length is measured, a single or double lumen tunneled catheter or port is inserted. The catheter tip is positioned above the cavoatrial junction in the inferior third of the atrium. After a tunnel or subcutaneous pocket is created, the peel-away is removed. The catheter is then sutured in place, and the site is covered with a dry, sterile, occlusive, transparent dressing. Before leaving the angiography suite, the catheter is injected confirming adequate position and all lumens are heparinized. A postprocedural chest radiograph is then obtained to exclude the presence of a complicating pneumothorax or hemothorax.

Technical variations

When the standard central and transhepatic and translumbar routes are not available esoteric sites must be considered. Collateral vessels may be identified by US or by injecting them with contrast. Using digital road mapping, directional catheters, and guide wires and, if needed, microcatheters, these indirect routes to the heart are in some instances navigable allowing placement of a CVC. If, however, placement of a CVC centrally is not possible, these catheters usually do not remain patent in the long term.

Another alternative may be found using cross-sectional imaging. Any suitable large vein (e.g., azygos, intercostal) may be punctured under real-time US guidance or with CT control. Depending on the size and location of the vessel and condition of the patient, a variable degree of increased risk may be anticipated. In these patients surgical intervention may be an appropriate option and transthoracic catheterization of the right atrium or other venous channel may be considered as a life-saving option. Direct transmediastinal catheterization of the distal SVC or right atrium may also be achieved under US guidance using the suprasternal notch as an imaging window.

Stabilizing the guide wire

Occasionally it is possible to pass a wire to or beyond the right atrium, but the catheter will not follow due to complex anatomy, compound angulation, or narrow regions in the venous pathway. Assuming the indication warrants and alternative pathways are not available, it may be necessary to improve the stability of the wire in order to complete the catheter insertion procedure. A variety of solutions to this problem can be formulated. A few representative approaches are outlined here under the more general rubric, "Stabilizing the guide wire." Such approaches are part of the core modular procedures that may be combined to solve both common and unusual challenges that present to the pediatric interventionalist (see "A modular approach to interventional radiology", in Chapter 1).

One tactic is to decrease resistance to passage of the catheter. Use of a hydrophilic guide wire (Glidewire®) is the simplest method. A smaller diameter catheter can be tried. A sterile lubricant (e.g., silicone spray or mineral oil) can be applied to the catheter surface and wire. Dynamic narrowing may respond to vasodilators. Static narrowing may respond to blunt dissection with a stiff dilator or to balloon angioplasty. Using a rotating hemostatic valve (Tuohy–Borst) attached to the catheter, forceful jets of saline may be used to lead the catheter tip forward.

Another approach involves stiffening the wire. If a stiff glide wire, a Nitinol®, mandril wire, or a stiff Amplatz® wire can be negotiated through the same pathway, it may hold its position with sufficient stability to pass the catheter over the same course. A stiffer catheter material (i.e., polyurethane rather than silicone) may aid catheter positioning.

Whenever possible the most effective way to stabilize a given wire is to hold it at both ends and provide tension. A gooseneck snare may be passed through an endovascular sheath from the opposite direction, e.g., if initial access is via the hepatic vein (HV) then the snare is inserted into the IJV. Using the snare to grasp the distal end of the exchange length wire, the guide wire is withdrawn through the sheath out to the skin surface. The CVC may now be advanced over the wire, pinning the wire at both ends and applying tension to maximize wire stability (and straighten the vascular pathway). When both ends of a wire are exteriorized (a technique affectionately known as "body flossing") a catheter may be pulled into position across a stenosis if desired. Care must be taken when employing this technique not to move the wire while it is stiffened, as it may slice through tissue.

Postprocedure and follow-up care

Except as noted, care of the patient receiving a CVC via alternate pathways is identical to that described above in "Technique: internal jugular CVC insertion." If the patient develops a significant drop in hemoglobin, evidence of hypovolemic shock, or chest, flank, back, groin, or abdominal pain (depending upon the pathway utilized), bleeding from the venous insertion site must be suspected and clinically investigated, including CT or US evaluation of the chest, peritoneum, or retroperitoneum as indicated.

Technique: venous recanalization

Children who have had multiple transvenous procedures are at risk for venous thrombosis, stenosis, fibrosis, and occlusion. Just one episode of intimal injury with a denuded epithelium can provoke platelet aggregation, thrombus formation, and fibrin deposition that may render the affected pathway. Recurrent or chronic injury results in wall thickening, calcification, perivenous inflammatory changes, venospasm, and scarring. Because the venous system is a highly redundant network of interconnected tributaries, with diffuse communications between deep and superficial veins and between systemic and somatic pathways, the venous system is incredibly adaptable to chronic and diffuse injury. The body has an amazing ability to recruit capsular, pericardial, portal, epidural, paravertebral and other somatic pathways to complete the venous circuit when the usual systemic pathways are impaired. However, when direct pathways from the periphery to the right atrium are compromised, it can be quite difficult to navigate the complex and tortuous residual pathways that serve to return blood to the heart for the purposes of central venous access.

In attempting to recanalize severely narrowed or closed venous pathways for central venous access, the first priority is to gain guide wire access across the affected segment. The associated challenge is to avoid dissecting the intima or perforating the vein wall proximal to the narrowed segment. There are two compatible objectives of recanalization: first, to permit placement of a venous catheter and, second, to establish long-term patency of the affected pathway. The former may be life saving and may allow life-preserving procedures such as hemodialysis and liver and small bowel transplantation. The latter is certainly desirable in the context of long-term preservation of venous capital but not necessary in every case. Perfect is the enemy of good.

Table 2.11 Equipment: venous recanalization

- Non-ionic contrast
- Connecting tubing
- Guide wires
  - 0.010- to 0.035-inch, angled, stiff, and superstiff
  - hydrophilic, nitinol, stainless steel
- 3 Fr–12 Fr vessel dilators
- 4 Fr–12 Fr endovascular sheaths, 5–50 cm, straight and angled
- 3 Fr–7 Fr directional catheters
- 2 mm–14 mm non-compliant angioplasty balloons, 12–30 ATM
- Trans-septal needle
- TIPS needle
- Stents, various

Equipment

The equipment (Table 2.11) necessary to redevelop a usable venous channel when a vein has become tightly stenosed or occluded will depend in part upon the cause of narrowing (e.g., thrombotic occlusion vs. chronic inflammation vs. external compression) and in part upon its duration (acute, subacute, or chronic). That is, the selection of equipment should be made in light of the intermediate objective (e.g., lysis of fresh clot, compared to microdissection of fibrotic thrombus or disruption of fibrotic perivenous inflammatory changes) and of the final objective (i.e., establishment of venous access vs. primary or secondary patency).

Patient preparation

There is no specific preparation necessary prior to a recanalization procedure. It is useful to correct a bleeding diathesis, and helpful not to perform the procedure in the face of an active systemic infection. Neither is an absolute contraindication. If balloon venoplasty or significant venous manipulation is anticipated, deep sedation or general anesthesia may be required, as stretching the vein wall can be painful and may provoke a vasovagal response.

Standard technique

Awareness of stenosis or occlusion often arises when during an attempted insertion of a central venous access device, the guide wire fails to advance centrally. Before attempting vigorous manipulation, it is appropriate to define the problem with venography. This may demonstrate occlusion with or without collateral pathways, or may show extravasation of contrast without clear definition of the intended path. The first principle of venous recanalization is to use the least invasive method necessary to gain purchase across the narrowed segment and to re-establish patency. If the stenosis or occlusion is peripheral and relatively distal, it may be best to attempt access either through an alternate vessel or more proximally in the same vessel. If the lesion is located more proximally or if the patient has a known history of occlusions and has a high likelihood of long-term need for venous access, then more assertive efforts may be in order.

One should begin to probe the pathway using blunt instruments, such as a reasonably compliant catheter/guide wire combination. Often, simply bringing the tip of a directional catheter near to the narrowed segment will provide sufficient support to allow advancement of the guide wire beyond the stenosis. If the stenosis is more resistant, it may be helpful to place a stiff angled catheter or an endovenous sheath with its dilator adjacent to the stenosis to support a stiffer angled guide wire. Alternating advancement of the catheter tip with the guide wire tip in small steps may produce a controlled microdissection through an occluded segment (Figure 2.27).

It is possible to use stiffer devices to cross recalcitrant occlusions, such as the back end of a guide wire or a sharp transvenous needle, such as a trans-septal needle or the puncture needle from a TIPS set. Such sharp recanalization procedures carry a significantly higher risk of inadvertent transgression of the vein wall and may lead to hemorrhage, pericardial tamponade, or hemothorax. This is especially so when blindly seeking for a patent lumen beyond the occlusion. If sharp recanalization is attempted, it is helpful to have a visible target toward which to direct the sharp device, and to visualize the needle path in two planes (Figure 2.26).

Once the guide wire has traversed the stenosis, a choice remains whether to attempt to restore long-term patency or to simply acquire central venous access. Recanalization using previously occluded venous pathways is one of the most durable approaches to preserving venous capital in these high-risk patients, and providing an effective route of access can often be life saving even in the absence of long-term venous patency (Figure 2.28). If guide wire access through a central venous pathway is achieved, but a CVC will not advance across the stenotic segment, the stenosis must be dilated. If a long fascial dilator with a tapered tip can reach the lesion, it may be possible to bluntly dissect across the stenosis. Alternatively, a non-compliant angioplasty balloon can be held with forward pressure and used to serially dissect across the stenosis (Figure 2.27) for the purpose of allowing passage of the CVC tip toward the right atrium.

If long-term venous patency is the objective of therapy, then larger balloons or balloons with higher nominal burst pressures may be necessary to disrupt the sometimes extensive inflammatory and fibrotic changes in and surrounding the affected vein wall, that may not be entirely apparent on venography. It is tempting to consider placing a bare metal stent or even a covered stent across the abnormal segment in the hope of extending the durability of venous patency. There is at this time no study that compares patency after recanalization with or without a stent in children, and likewise there is no study that defines a difference in either primary or secondary venous patency with a covered stent compared to an uncovered stent. Paclitaxel-coated stents have so recently been available in the USA that their potential application in the venous system is unknown. Our experience to date suggests that stenting in the venous system may be useful in limited applications, such as in conjunction with revascularization in May–Thurner syndrome, but generally does not prolong venous patency after recanalization and may often represent an impediment to future access.

Postprocedure and follow-up care

Patients should be observed closely for at least four to six hours after recanalization and venoplasty procedures for signs of hemorrhage, including early signs of hypovolemic shock. Although there are no well-constructed studies to rely upon, consideration may be given to a six-month course of anticoagulation or antiplatelet therapy following extensive recanalization and venoplasty procedures. If a CVL is placed after recanalization, it is prudent to perform venography both through the affected vein and through the catheter before removing the catheter for dysfunction or at the end of therapy, keeping a guide wire across the treated segment until its status is known. In this way, if there is residual stenosis the guide wire usually permits ready access for repeat venoplasty. Once the catheter is removed, if future access is required, repeat recanalization procedures may result in diminishing marginal success.

CVC removal

It bears repeating that central venous access devices are more easily removed than replaced. They can be left in place and heparin-locked with periodic flushes for days to weeks with small risk of complication (Appendix 2.D). Barring untoward events (e.g., catheter-related infection) it is helpful to be certain the endpoint of therapy has been reached prior to removal.

Uncuffed CVCs can simply be pulled out after removing any retention sutures, placing gentle compression at the venous entry point until hemostasis is achieved. A clean bandage is applied.

If extraction of the cuffed CVC is inhibited by fibrous ingrowth, it may be removed under sedation using a minor surgical procedure after the distal tract and exit site have been generously infiltrated with local anesthetic. The external component of the catheter and the area around the exit site are prepared and draped in sterile fashion. Using a small hemostat (mosquito), the exit site is dissected, opening the tract to the cuff, as previously described under "PICC removal," above. With gentle traction on the catheter, the cuff is brought into

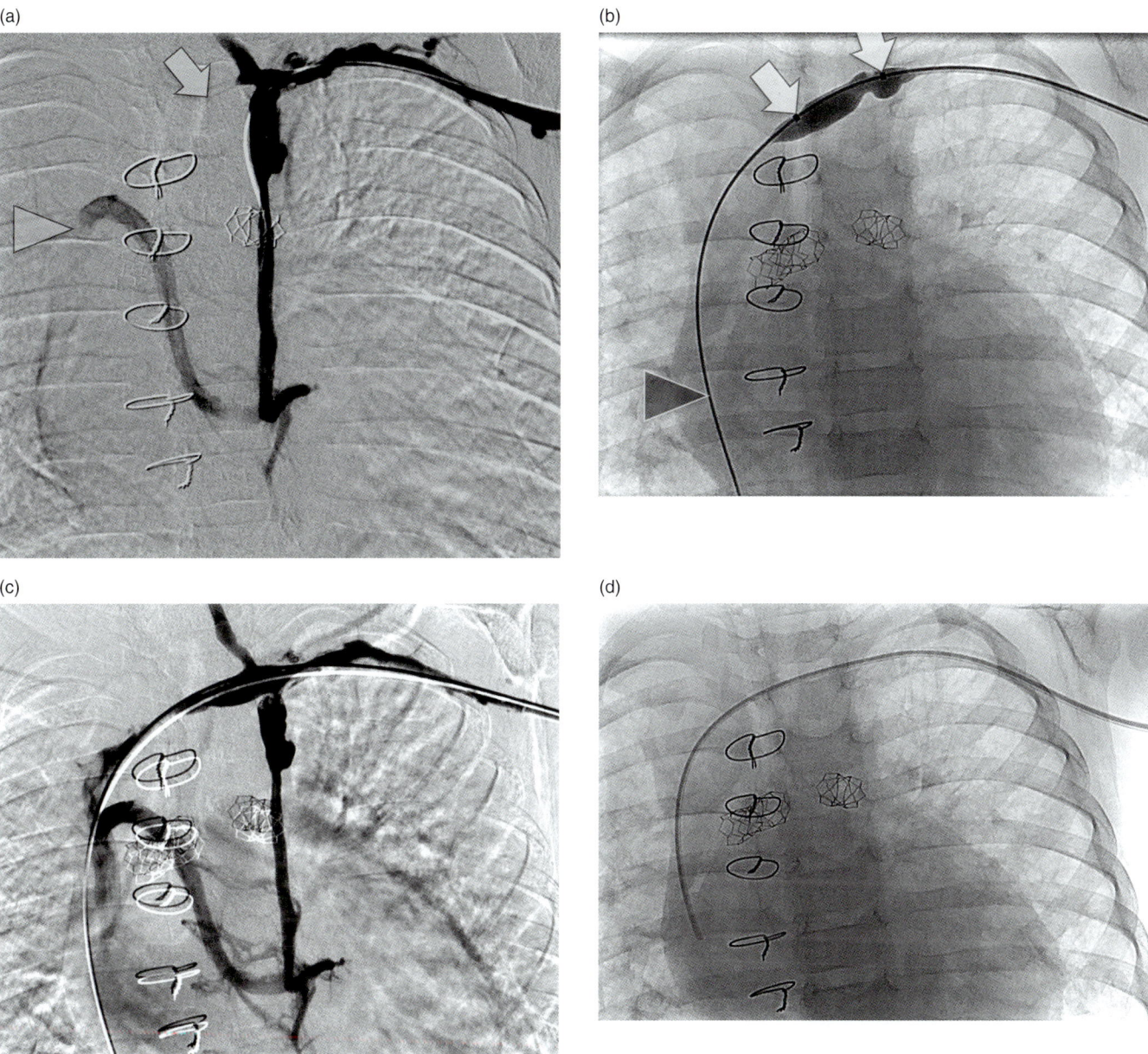

Figure 2.27 A three-month-old infant with congenital heart disease and proximal pulmonary artery stenosis has had multiple left subclavian venous catheters and now requires venous access. (a) A left brachial venogram shows left distal brachiocephalic occlusion (*arrow*) with drainage to the right atrium (*arrowhead*) via paravertebral and hemizygos collaterals to the azygos arch. (b) Initial microdissection was carried out by alternating advancement of a stiff 4 French directional catheter and a stiff hydrophilic guide wire (*arrowhead*), but the catheter could not be advanced beyond the proximal brachiocephalic vein. The catheter was replaced with a 4 mm × 2 cm 12 ATM balloon (*arrows*), and successive balloon dissections of the venous occlusion were performed. (c) Patency of the systemic pathway was restored. (d) A 4 Fr PICC was placed and functioned without complication to the end of therapy.

view. Using care not to tear the catheter, especially if the CVC is 5 French or smaller, the pseudo-capsule of connective tissue is dissected free from the catheter cuff with iris scissors or a scalpel. Remember, it may be important to obtain a sterile sample of the catheter tip for culture if infection is suspected. Once free, the catheter will pull out effortlessly. Gentle pressure at the venous entry site (not the skin exit site), combined with relative elevation of the site, will assist hemostasis. Once hemostasis is achieved, the exit wound is cleaned, bandaged, and left to heal by secondary intention. A suture is not placed, as the wound is considered "dirty."

Vigorous traction on the catheter should be avoided due to risk of catheter disruption and embolization. This is especially true for catheters in the smaller French sizes (5 French and smaller). If the cuff cannot be brought into view without undue traction or patient discomfort, or if the cuff is located too high in the tunnel to gain meaningful control, further attempts to free the cuff through the original tract may be abandoned in

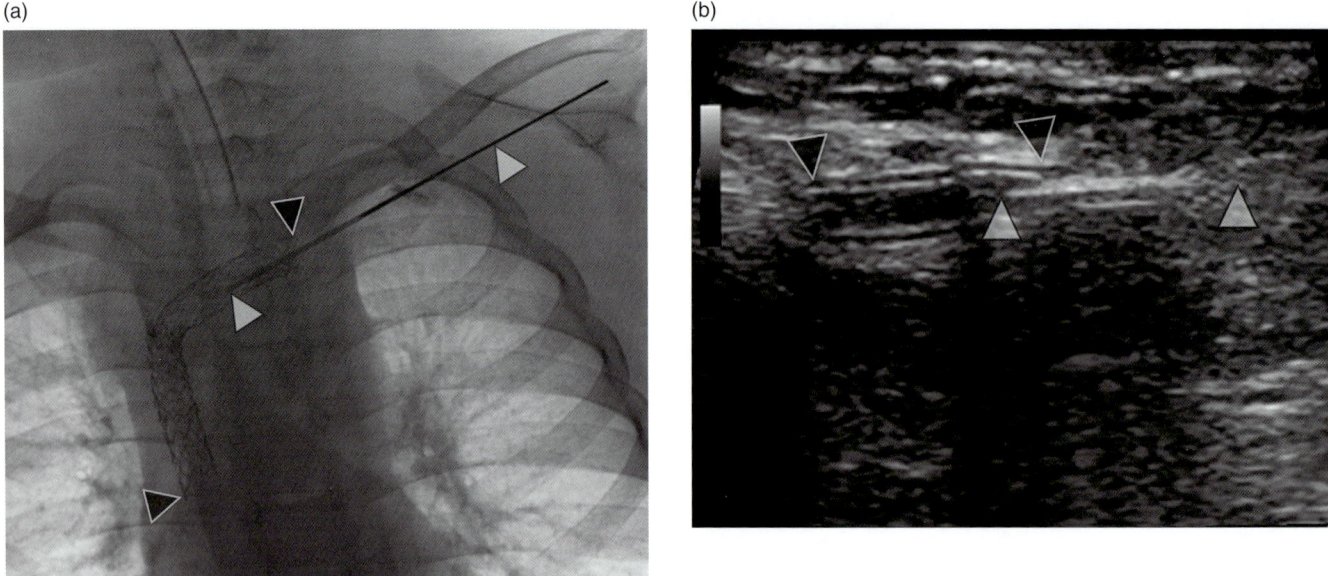

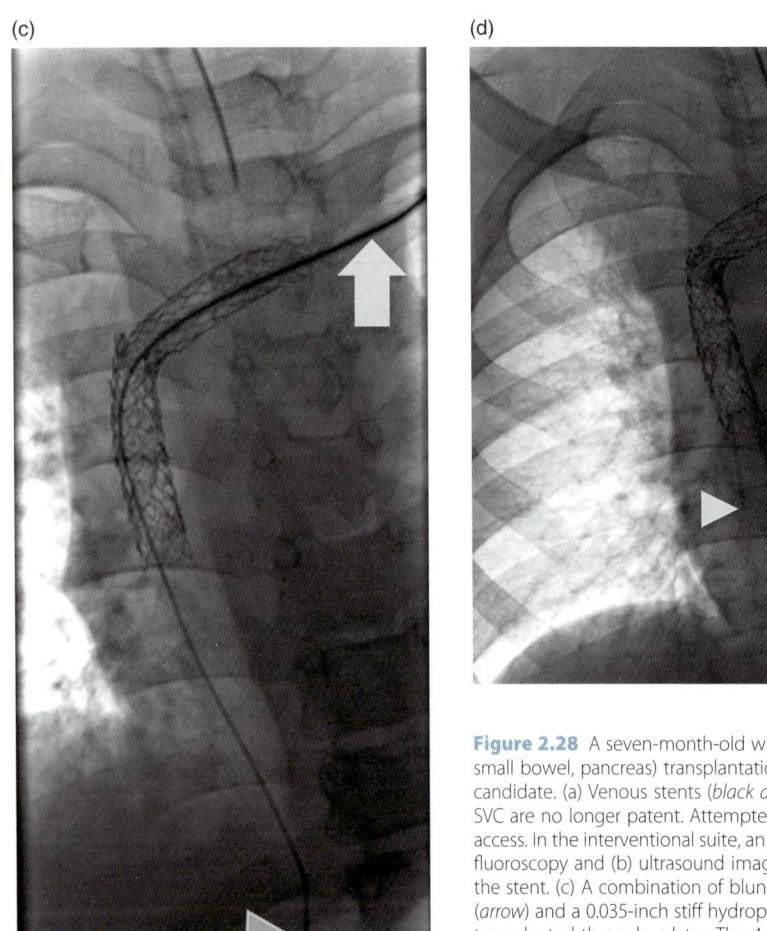

Figure 2.28 A seven-month-old with intestinal failure and cholestatic liver injury needs multivisceral (liver, small bowel, pancreas) transplantation, but with all named central venous pathways occluded, he is not a candidate. (a) Venous stents (*black arrowheads*) previously placed across the left brachiocephalic vein and SVC are no longer patent. Attempted replacement of a left subclavian CVC in the OR resulted in loss of access. In the interventional suite, an 18-gauge Chiba needle (*white arrowheads*) was guided with concurrent fluoroscopy and (b) ultrasound imaging across the thorax and mediastinum directly into the distal end of the stent. (c) A combination of blunt and sharp recanalization was used to advance a 5 Fr Kumpe catheter (*arrow*) and a 0.035-inch stiff hydrophilic guide wire (*arrowhead*) to the IVC. (d) The patient was successfully transplanted three days later. The 4 Fr single-lumen tunneled catheter projects with its tip (*arrowhead*) 2.5 vertebral bodies below the carina, beyond the end of the sheath. It remained in use without complication more than 21 months after insertion.

favor of a direct cut-down onto the cuff. The position of the cuff may be palpated through the skin, or verified by imaging.

Once the cuff is localized, the overlying skin is generously infiltrated with local anesthetic, and the area prepared and draped in sterile fashion, if not already included in the previous sterile field. A short (1–2 cm) incision is made through the skin transversely across the tract over the cuff, taking care not to cut the catheter. As described above, using a combination of blunt and sharp dissection, the pseudo-capsule of connective tissue is dissected from the circumference of the catheter both proximal and distal to the cuff. The catheter may now be easily removed through the original exit site. While the exit site is left to heal by secondary intention, the newly formed surgical wound is closed with a combination of deep interrupted and running subcuticular sutures and Steri-Strips®, and both wounds are bandaged. The CVC is inspected for defects, and the pertinent details of the procedure are recorded in the medical record.

Complications

It has been suggested that over 6 million CVCs are placed each year in the United States. Related complications have been conservatively estimated to occur in 10% of cases and include infection, occlusion, venous thrombosis, fragmentation, and migration. Most children have successful peripheral or central line insertion without any problem. However, both minor and major complications may occur in this group of patients. Since most minor complications require little or no therapy, they will not be discussed in detail. Minor problems identified include postprocedural pain and minor bleeding.

Major complications that have been observed can be classified into four groups: thrombotic, infectious, hemorrhagic, and mechanical. For radiologically placed tunneled central venous lines, a rate of immediate complications (including pneumothorax, air emboli, bleeding, and arterial puncture) of 3.8% was reported by Tseng and colleagues. The most commonly observed early complications are related to local trauma and include pneumothorax, hemothorax, subcutaneous emphysema, perivenous hematoma at the puncture site, arterial injury, and pseudoaneurysm formation (Figure 2.20), pleural effusion, brachial plexus injury, air embolism, and cardiac perforation (Figure 2.29).

Use of non-conventional pathways for access may entail additional risks. For example, like other transhepatic procedures the most likely complication of transhepatic access is bleeding, but surprisingly, we have rarely seen any cases of significant bleeding. Other possible complications include infection, bile leak, hepatic vein-to-hepatic artery fistula, and hemo- or pneumothorax. These complications are rare. Delayed complications include hepatic vein thrombosis, infection, and loss of the catheter secondary to the effects of respiratory and patient motion.

Late complications of central venous access procedures are most often related to infection, thrombotic and mechanical

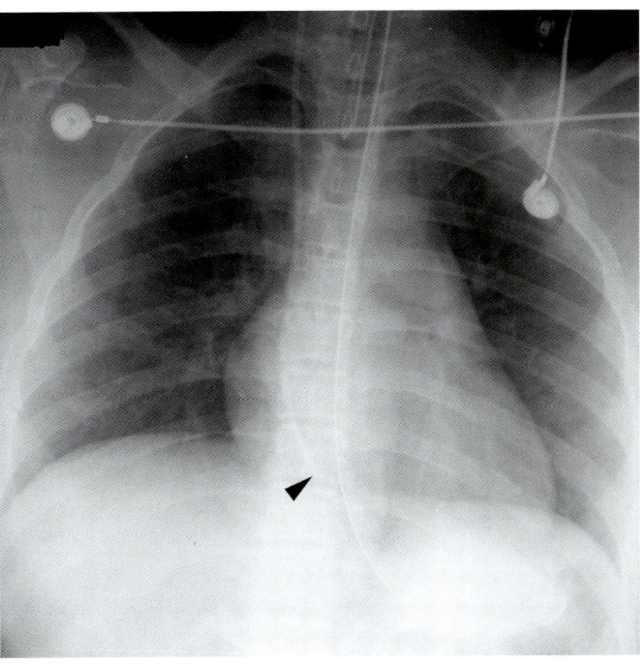

Figure 2.29 Eleven-year-old girl with bowel obstruction developed fatal cardiac tamponade following cardiac perforation related to malposition of the tip (*arrowhead*) of her temporary right internal jugular central venous catheter.

problems, although a variety of other significant but less common complications have been reported, including phrenic nerve palsy and hemidiaphragmatic paralysis, venobronchial and venocutaneous fistulae, syncope, and osteomyelitis. Certain patient groups are at significantly higher risk of CVC complications (e.g., ICU patients, renal failure, complex congenital heart disease, sickle cell disease, cancer, chronic pulmonary disease, transplant recipients, intestinal failure, neonates, burn victims) and deserve close monitoring and preventive care. With early recognition and appropriate intervention many CVC complications are preventable. The optimal treatment is prevention. Evidence-based guidelines are helpful when available, but are currently lacking for many situations relevant to central venous access in the pediatric population.

Infection

Infection, as a consequence of an indwelling CVC or PICC, has been reported in 7 to 16% of patients and up to 33% of those receiving hyperalimentation. Catheter-related bloodstream infection (CRBSI) is the second most common major catheter complication resulting from central lines, and involves a spectrum of disease including CRBL, exit site infection, tunnel infection, and septic thrombophlebitis. Infection may be a direct procedural complication (evidence of catheter-related infection within 48 hours of insertion) or occur later in the child's medical course. Identification of an infectious complication is extremely important and may be life saving. The first line of defense against early catheter

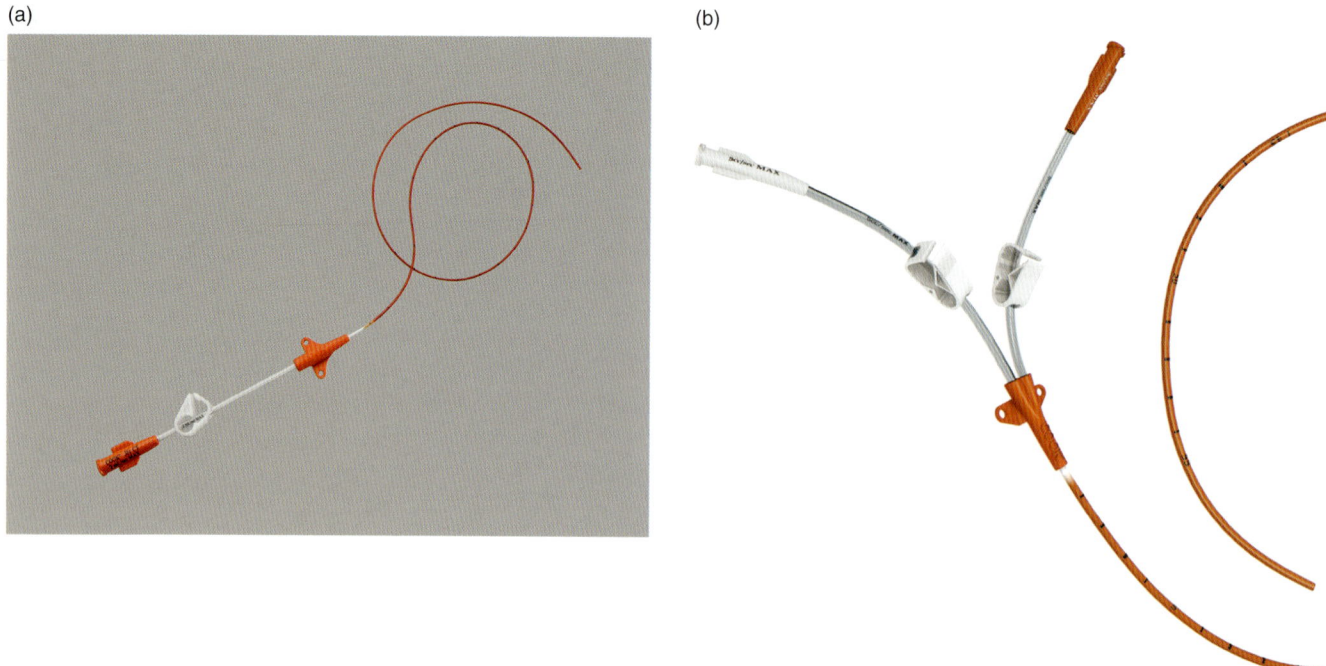

Figure 2.30 Spectrum minocycline-rifampin impregnated venous catheters (Cook Medical). (a) 3 French single lumen (b) 5 French double lumen.

infection or catheter-related sepsis is proper insertion technique carried out in a sterile environment. Some studies suggest that CVC implantation in a controlled theater (interventional suite or operating room) significantly reduces risk of infectious complications compared to insertion in the ICU, on the ward, or at the bedside.

Catheters are one of the most common causes of nosocomial infections and septicemia. Catheter-related infection is most often caused by coagulase positive and negative staphylococci, particularly slime-producing strains. It is these slime-producing organisms that often colonize catheters. The organisms embedded within and protected by this biofilm may become resistant to various agents and become a source of systemic infection. While it is possible to mechanically strip the colonized fibrin sheath from the catheter (see "Tip occlusion," below) or to disrupt the fibrin sheath with a balloon (Figure 2.3e), there is considerable current interest in bonding various agents to CVCs to help prevent such infectious or thrombotic complications. Pierce and colleagues have shown significant reduction in such complications with heparin-bonded CVCs. Others have recommended impregnating catheters with a variety of antiadhesive, antiseptic, and antimicrobial agents. Results to date are encouraging, demonstrating durability of antimicrobial activity and cost-effectiveness. Our experience suggests that antibiotic-impregnated central catheters (Figure 2.30), including both PICCs and tunneled central lines, yield as much as a 15-fold reduction in risk of infectious complications in high-risk children, although prospective evidence of similar effectiveness in the pediatric population is still needed.

Definitive diagnosis of catheter-related sepsis relies on positive quantitative cultures of the same microorganism from both the catheter and the bloodstream, or significantly higher colony counts from the catheter than from blood obtained from a peripheral vein. It is important to remember that a potential cause of false-positive cultures obtained through the catheter reflect colonization or contamination of the rubber-sealed cap at the catheter hub (the "clave"). The clave should therefore be changed before withdrawing a blood sample for catheter culture.

Methods for rapid diagnosis (less than 30 minutes) have been developed, and should be considered prior to catheter removal. Clinically apparent sepsis sometimes warrants removal of the CVC before these criteria are met, although documentation of a catheter-related infection remains epidemiologically critical and may be accomplished with a blood culture or culture of the removed catheter tip. Maki and associates consider a tip positive if it leads to greater than 15 colony-forming units. Cooper and Hopkins have described a technique for Gram stain of whole catheter segments (i.e., the catheter tip). It is important to remember that most suspected catheter infections are not proven, and most of those that are proven can be treated successfully without removal of the catheter. Erythema, swelling, pain, or discharge at or near the catheter entry site, the subcutaneous pocket, or tunnel tract should be considered presumptive evidence of infection. Since the central line is not always the source of bacteremia, a search for other sources of infection remains important.

It is essential to maintain sterile technique during the placement and care of the CVC in order to minimize catheter-related sepsis. Various investigators have reported the frequency of CRBSI to be between 10 and 30%, with a rate of 1.4 to 3.3 CRBSI per 1,000 catheter days. Implanted ports tend to have the lowest rate of CRBSI. Lorenz and colleagues reported a rate of 0.4 CRBSI per 1,000 catheter days in a series of chest ports placed in pediatric patients, which agrees with our experience in both chest and arm ports in children. PICCs may have a slightly higher rate of CRBSI, and higher still (up to 5 to 15 CRBSI per 1,000 catheter days) in patients at increased risk.

We have found the frequency of CRBSI to vary depending upon the medical characteristics of the population. For example, immune-suppressed children with organ transplants, children with immune suppression of depression, or underlying oncologic disease have a higher incidence of infection than do children with normal immune status. One study documented 7.4 catheter-related bloodstream infections per 1,000 catheter days in pediatric hematology–oncology patients, most of whom (75%) were severely neutropenic at the time they acquired their infection. In this group there was no significant difference between implanted infusion ports and tunneled catheters. We have found as many as 10 CRBSI per 1,000 catheter days in children with a history of intestinal failure and one or more occluded major central venous pathways. Low birthweight (14.5 CRBSI per 1,000 catheter days), duration of access, corticosteroid exposure, factor inhibition in children with congenital coagulation disorders (1.6 vs. 4.3 CRBSI per 1,000 catheter days) and other related events, including catheter thrombosis and multilumen lines, may also predispose patients to catheter-related infection. The rate of infection may be highest in burn patients, who may have as many as 30 CRBSI per 1,000 catheter days.

Infection in the immediate postoperative period is thought to be a procedural complication secondary to intraoperative contamination and the lack of a tunneled tract. To reduce this risk, some interventionalists cover the child with a broad-spectrum antibiotic for one or more doses after the catheter insertion. According to a study by Simon and colleagues in pediatric oncology patients, prophylactic antibiotics should neither be given during implantation nor during prolonged usage to prevent bacterial infection of a central venous access device, due to unproven efficacy and to the potential hazards of vancomycin-resistant gram-positive infections. In our practice, we do not routinely use prophylactic antibiotics at the time of a central catheter insertion procedure.

In most cases (50 to 70%), infection is caused by skin flora, which is thought to progressively extend from the skin to vein or from the catheter hub to venous lumen. Denny reports that the most common organisms identified are *Staphylococcus epidermidis* (25 to 50% of cases), *S. aureus* (25%), and *Candida* species (5 to 10%). For children with cancer, adding vancomycin to the flush solution (25 µg/ml in externalized catheters, 50 µg/ml in port catheters) may help protect against CVC-related *S. epidermidis* infections.

Most catheter-related infections can be successfully treated without catheter removal. Press and associates noted that only a small percentage of patients with exit-site skin infections required catheter removal while 70% of those with tunnel infections and all with septic thrombophlebitis or septicemia required removal of the line. Therefore it is imperative that the early signs of skin infection be actively looked for and, when found, treated aggressively. In many children, infection can be treated without removal of the line providing that the infection is not severe or life threatening, and if it can be cleared in 48 to 72 hours of intravenous antibiotic treatment, with eradication of the offending organism.

Historically, pseudomonas and fungal infections are hard to clear without removal of the catheter. According to Benjamin and colleagues, neonates with a positive culture for *S. aureus* or a gram-positive rod should have their CVC removed immediately. Patients should be treated with intravenous antibiotics for at least ten days to two weeks, or longer if fever and bacteremia persists for greater than 72 hours following removal (although this is itself evidence against a CRBSI, since signs and symptoms should resolve within 48 to 72 hours of catheter removal if the catheter was the primary source of infection). Similarly, catheter-related infections with *Candida* and *Bacillus* species in children are likely to require catheter removal. Medical management may be attempted for a culture positive for coagulase-negative staphylococcus, but if three serial cultures are positive, the line should be removed. Catheter-related infections associated with central venous thrombosis are especially refractory, and seldom resolve without catheter removal. Even a patient whose catheter-related coagulase-negative staphylococcal bacteremia is successfully treated without catheter removal may be up to three times more likely to experience recurrence than those whose catheters are removed.

Although the suggestion has been made that the use of a clear plastic occlusive dressing is associated with an increased rate of exit-site colonization and catheter-related infection, most interventionalists continue to use them (Appendix 2.E). In our experience we have not found occlusive dressings to increase the complication rate. In addition, the clear occlusive dressing serves as a barrier to the unwanted removal of the central line in the inquisitive or uncooperative child. It is, however, important to assure that the exit site is clean and dry before occlusive dressings are applied, and to change them if a significant amount of fluid or debris is found to accumulate under the dressing. In order to minimize the risk of site infection, we cover the exit site with a dry gauze dressing before covering it with the occlusive dressing. A chlorhexidine-impregnated dressing covered by a transparent polyurethane dressing, changed weekly, may also be used to protect the insertion site from infection, although local contact dermatitis may limit its application in some children.

In general, it is prudent to avoid implantation of a CVC during a period of symptomatic bacteremia or sepsis, since this may increase the risk of colonization of the newly placed CVC, or development of a catheter-related infection. It is our practice to delay placement of a new CVC until the infected patient has received 24 to 48 hours of antibiotic therapy. Intravenous therapy during this period may be provided through serial peripheral angiocatheters or, in certain cases, through a temporary CVC at a new site distant from the previously infected line. Use of an antibiotic-impregnated catheter may be a preferable alternative to this "catheter holiday" approach, as we have observed no measurable increase in the rate of CRBSI in patients who receive an antibiotic-impregnated catheter during a period of active infection compared to those who do not have an infection at the time of insertion. This strategy obviates insertion of an interim catheter, thus reducing the need for procedures and procedure-related sedation or anesthesia, as well as additional trauma to already overburdened venous systems. In fact, since we have observed a significant overall decrease in the rate of CRBSI in patients at higher risk of infection, including those with an active infection at the time of insertion, we would advocate for the use of these catheters for all central line insertions in high-risk children.

Malposition

Complications of CVC position fall into two classes: dislodgment and malposition. Accidental dislodgment may be partial or complete. Partial dislodgment is often difficult to recognize, especially if the bulk of the exterior portion of the catheter is hidden under dressings. Dislodgment is seldom threatening to the patient if it is recognized and corrected. Failure to recognize and correct this problem, however, can lead to thrombosis, fibrosis, and occlusion of major venous pathways. Patients and parents should be shown where in the neck or groin to apply pressure should a large-bore catheter be accidentally pulled out.

Unrecognized partial dislodgment increases the risk of central venous thrombosis, catheter occlusion, mechanical malfunction (tear, fracture, or separation), and extravasation. Changes in catheter position on serial radiographs are an important sign of impending or partial dislodgment, and should be brought to the attention of the primary care providers (and acted upon) promptly (Figure 2.31). Appearance of the catheter cuff at or outside the entry site of cuffed PICCs or CVCs ("traveling" cuff) should also be attended to immediately on recognition, before function is lost or impaired. Such partially dislodged but functioning catheters may be fixed in position for continued use if the tip is not malpositioned, or may be replaced.

Preventive care consists primarily in vigilant attention on the part of nurses, patients, and family members, who spend more time with the catheter than any other providers. The catheter should be dressed in a manner that protects it from being inadvertently snagged or pulled. Today, it is uncommon for us to suture a catheter in position since it increases the risk of infection. When possible the external portion of the catheter (especially PICC lines) may be doubled on itself under the dressing, so that accidental traction may be taken up by the loop so formed, rather than being transferred to the internal portion. We have found a Stat-lock® fixation device or

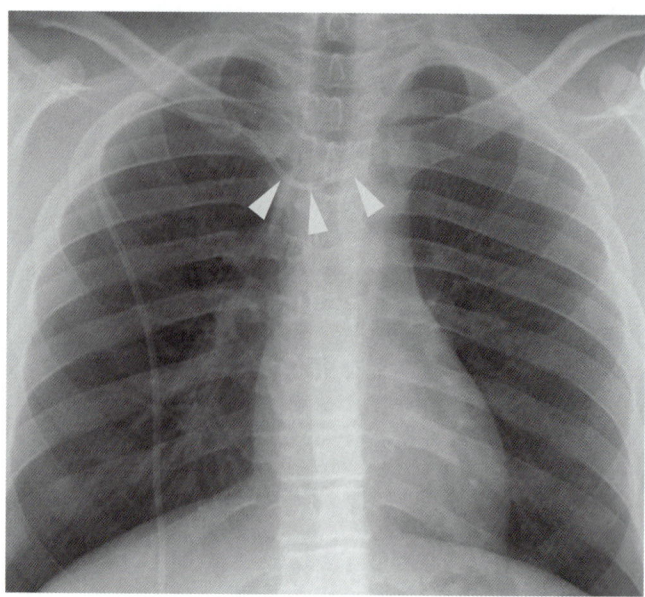

Figure 2.31 Seventeen-year-old boy with osteosarcoma had a right subclavian catheter inserted by the surgical service for chemotherapy. The original tip position was above the level of the carina. This chest radiograph obtained to investigate catheter dysfunction shows the tip (*arrowheads*) malpositioned in the contralateral brachiocephalic vein.

SorbaView® shield useful in preventing premature catheter removal. Particular caution should be employed during dressing changes, when the catheter is especially vulnerable to traction. Occasionally it is necessary to restrain mobility of the patient's arms to prevent accidental catheter dislodgment.

Catheter tip malposition, especially after surgical placement, occurs in up to 29% of CVC insertions and may go undetected for hours to weeks when postoperative radiographic confirmation of position is delayed or not performed, or when CVCs are placed by medical personnel not trained in radiologic interpretation (Figure 2.32). When CVCs are not placed under fluoroscopic guidance it is important to radiographically confirm tip position and complications within hours of the procedure. Malposition should be suspected whenever catheter dysfunction is noted. Common sites for the malpositioned tip include the contralateral brachiocephalic or subclavian vein (Figure 2.33), the jugular vein (Figure 2.34), or against the wall of the proximal SVC (Figure 2.35) for upper extremity and neck lines; and the iliac, paraspinal, or lower extremity veins, or hepatic vein for femoral or umbilical lines. However, there are a number of additional locations (e.g., azygos, vertebro-lumbar veins, brachiocephalic artery, persistent left SVC (Figure 2.13) or coronary sinus, even the subarachnoid space) for malpositioned tips that, while less common, may produce severe complications. A high index of suspicion must be maintained both during and following placement to detect and avoid or correct such complications.

Catheter malposition increases the risk of patient discomfort, catheter malfunction, vessel injury or perforation, venous thrombosis, or intraluminal fibrosis. In rare cases, more severe complications have been reported, including paraplegia,

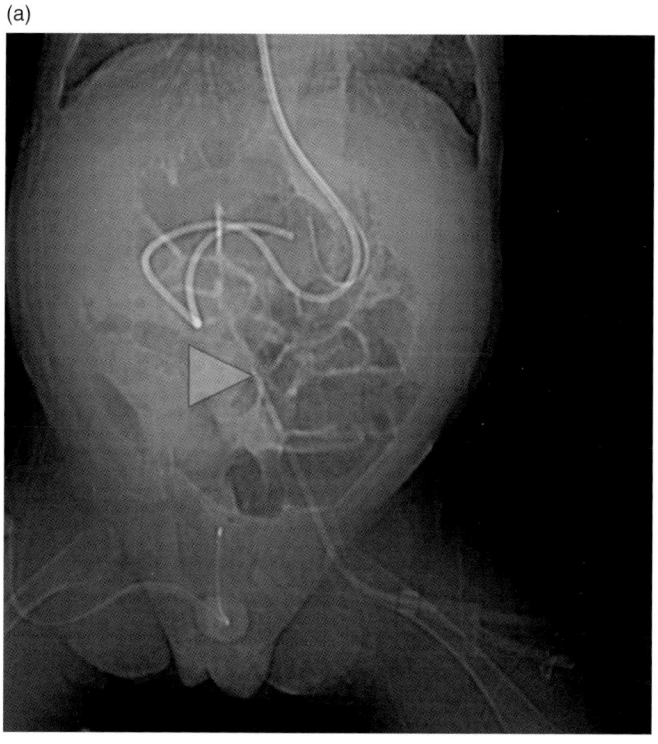 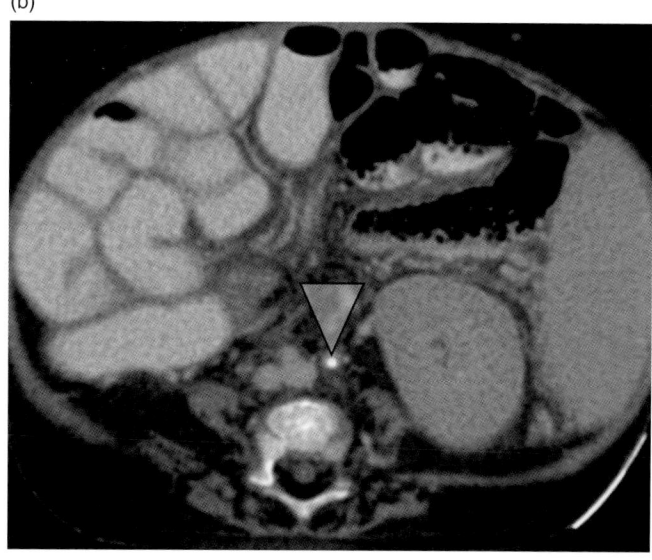

Figure 2.32 A left femoral double lumen catheter was placed urgently without image-guidance in the ICU in this three-week-old male infant. (a) On this postinsertion radiograph, the tip (*arrowhead*) projects over the midline at approximately the third lumbar vertebra. (b) On an axial CT image obtained five weeks later, the catheter tip (*arrowhead*) is malpositioned in the proximal left iliac artery.

cardiac tamponade, atrial thrombosis, mediastinal hemorrhage, and pulmonary infarction. Often, when the catheter tip has become malpositioned in an undesirable vessel (e.g., contralateral brachiocephalic or subclavian vein), it can be successfully repositioned by a rapid injection of saline through the catheter under fluoroscopic control (Figure 2.12). If this simple technique fails, the patient may be sedated and one of the techniques described below employed. Several such techniques have been developed to redirect catheters to a proper position in order to avoid premature catheter loss. It is important to remember that catheter position is a dynamic event. Documentation of appropriate position at insertion should not preclude continual reappraisal of position and function.

The venous entry site selected depends on the location of the malpositioned catheter. Since most malpositioned CVCs are in the upper chest veins, the femoral vein is used since it makes the repositioning technically easier. After the groin is prepared and draped in sterile fashion, local anesthesia is infiltrated into the skin over the femoral vein (usually right). A small skin incision is made and the vein is punctured using the Seldinger technique (Table 2.12). Successful venous access is confirmed when free-flowing blood is aspirated into the tubing attached to the syringe. A guide wire is inserted and a sheath with a hemostatic valve placed (Table 2.13). A directional catheter (JB-1) is inserted and positioned just above the malpositioned central line. A tip deflector wire is inserted through the 5 French catheter and the malpositioned catheter is hooked and pulled back into the desired position (Figure 2.33).

In the rare case when the deflector wire is not effective or when the malpositioned CVC is located in a position unsuitable for treatment using this technique, a loop snare can be substituted for the deflector wire (Figure 2.34). Variations of this technique have been described using other equipment such as a Simmons catheter, a "J" wire, and a Fogarty balloon catheter; however, these modifications have not been used in and are likely of no advantage in the pediatric population. Redirection of a malpositioned catheter may also be performed under US guidance.

Tip occlusion

The problem of a "fibrin sheath", tip thrombus, or intracatheter clot (histologically, a thrombus with or without a proteinaceous sheath) occluding the tip of a CVC (Figure 2.35) is considered when it becomes difficult to aspirate or infuse through the line. Prompt diagnosis and treatment is indicated to re-establish catheter function in order to minimize secondary infection, thromboembolism, or propagation of the clot resulting in a major venous thrombosis. Tip occlusion by fibrin sheath formation may also result in catheter rupture secondary to forceful injection with extravasation of caustic or chemotherapeutic agents or other material. Extravasation may lead to pain, tissue injury, hydro- or lipothorax, or lack of therapeutic effect.

Since most catheter occlusions are amenable to thrombolytic therapy, the diagnosis of tip occlusion may be suspected

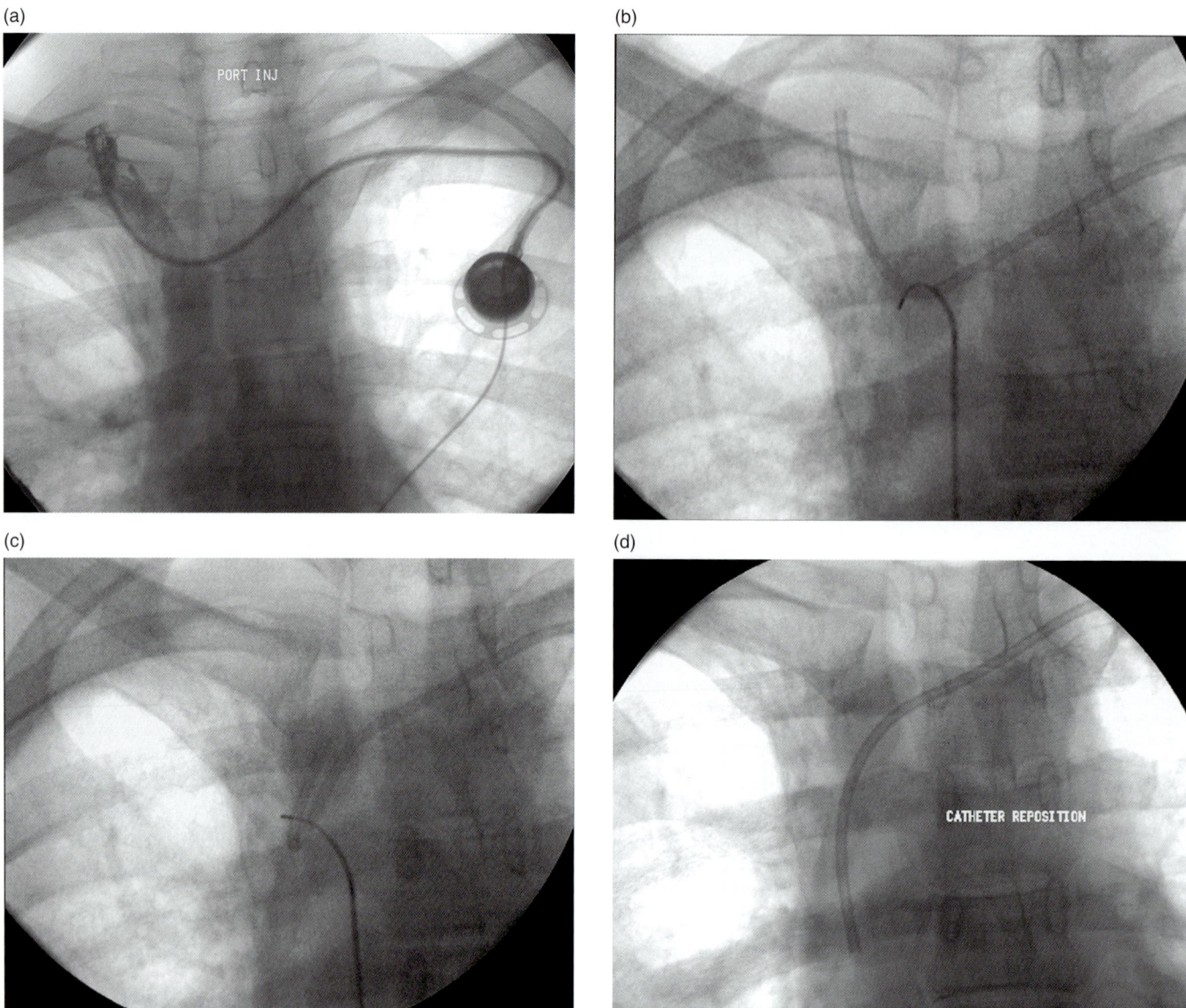

Figure 2.33 Twenty-one-year-old female with acute lymphoblastic leukemia with a subclavian port inserted for chemotherapy. (a) The initial image demonstrates the tip malpositioned in the contralateral jugular vein with related thrombosis. (b–d) The malpositioned port catheter is pulled back into the SVC with a tip deflector wire introduced through a transfemoral catheter.

clinically and treated with intracatheter tPA or confirmed by injection of contrast material. However, the next most common treatable cause of catheter occlusion is medication precipitation, which is not affected by thrombolytic therapy. Once the diagnosis of catheter dysfunction is suspected, a variety of approaches to treatment (Table 2.14) have been advocated.

For CVC declotting, several studies recommend tPA (e.g., alteplase). Davis and colleagues suggest an initial dose of 0.5 mg alteplase, escalating to 1 mg then 2 mg until the catheter is cleared. They found that 97% of catheter occlusions could be cleared with this protocol (Appendix 2.C). The tPA may be left in the catheter for 30 minutes up to four hours or more. The CVC is then aspirated. If blood flow is re-established, the line can be used or heparinized for later use. If flow is not re-established, a second dose of tPA per lumen is injected and left in the CVC for at least 30 minutes. If thrombolytic maneuvers fail, are contraindicated, too expensive, or not preferred, two alternatives are available: catheter removal or stripping of the clot with a loop snare.

Thrombolysis

When an indwelling venous or arterial catheter results in vessel thrombosis, several treatment options may be considered. In most cases, venous thrombosis is asymptomatic and goes unrecognized. If the asymptomatic child with a central venous occlusion is identified in the acute phase there is no literature experience to guide therapy. Therefore, we individualize each patient's care and try to make the best decision for the circumstances considering the risk–benefit relationship and cost factors. In cases where the patient is line dependent or symptomatic, more aggressive means may be warranted to re-establish and maintain vessel patency, including chemical or mechanical thrombolysis, sharp recanalization, and endovascular stenting. Thrombolytic therapy is the same approach used in veins as used for arterial thrombolysis.

Before catheter thrombolysis is initiated to treat vascular or graft occlusion, mechanical thrombolysis is utilized if possible. This can be accomplished with a variety of creatively designed tools (flow directed and mechanical). Mechanical thrombolytic devices that are effective in our experience include but are not limited to the Angiojet® Trellis device and Treratola® devices. Mechanical thrombolysis is performed through a vascular sheath with rotating hemostatic valve and can rapidly re-establish flow and remove a large clot burden. In addition, this

Table 2.12 Equipment: malposition

- Sheath with hemostasis valve.
- Directional catheter and guide wire.
- Deflector wire.
- Syringe and connecting tube.

Table 2.13 Procedure summary: malposition

- Prepare and drape the groin.
- Inject local anesthesia.
- Puncture vein.
- Insert sheath with hemostasis valve.
- Maneuver directional catheter into position adjacent to CVC.
- Remove guide wire and insert a deflector wire.
- Position deflector wire above malpositioned CVC, convert into J shape, and pull catheter into position.
- If deflector wire unsuccessful or not usable, use loop snare and pull CVC into position.

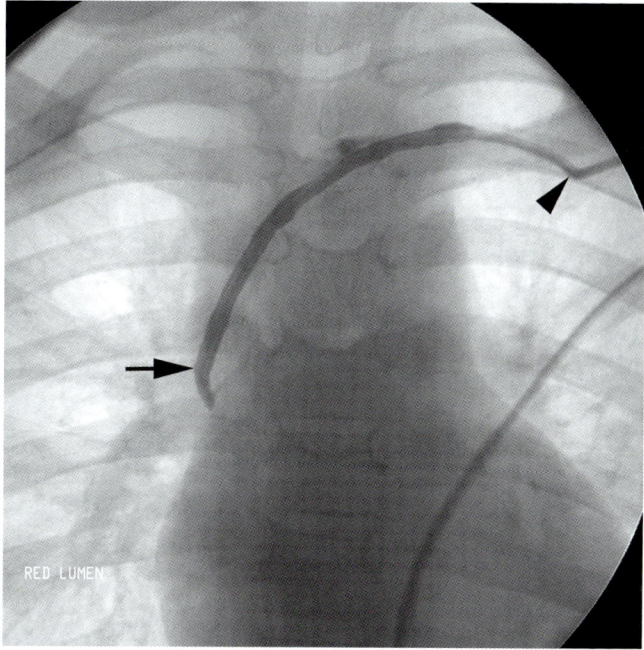

Figure 2.35 Eleven-year-old boy with acute lymphoblastic leukemia and central venous line dysfunction. The left subclavian catheter tip projects against the lateral wall of the SVC and has developed a long fibrin sheath from the tip (*arrow*) toward the venotomy site (*arrowhead*). The catheter was also infected with oxacillin-resistant *Staphylococcus epidermidis*, and was removed.

(a)

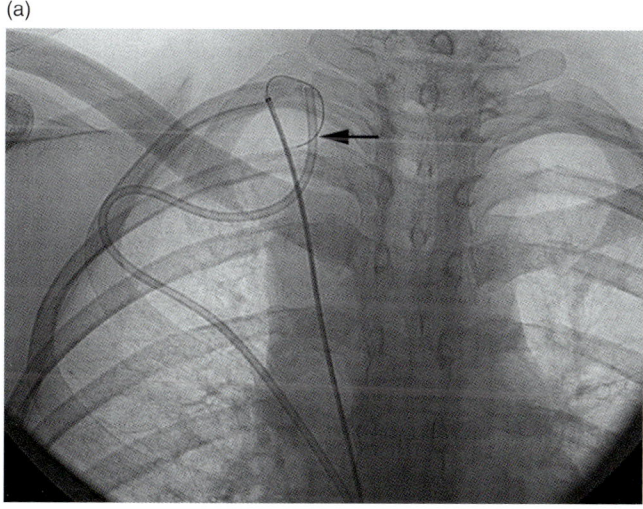

(b)

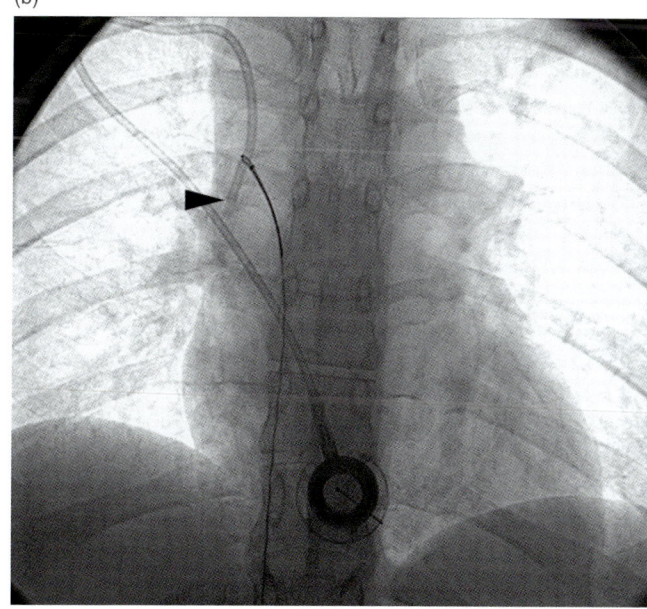

Figure 2.34 Nineteen-year-old female with Stage IIIb Hodgkin's lymphoma receiving chemotherapy, noted to have port dysfunction two months after insertion. (a) The malpositioned tip in the ipsilateral jugular vein is engaged by a nitinol loop snare (*arrow*) via a transfemoral catheter. (b) The catheter tip (*arrowhead*) has been repositioned, and remained functional until its removal at the end of therapy, ten months later.

Table 2.14 Procedural summary: fibrin sheath removal and catheter de-clotting

- Prepare and drape the groin in sterile fashion.
- Infiltrate local anesthesia at entry site.
- Puncture femoral vein or other entry vessel.
- Insert sheath with hemostatic valve.
- Position directional catheter and guide wire just above CVC.
- Exchange directional catheter for loop snare.
- Engage tip of CVC and tighten snare and strip off fibrin sheath.
- Remove intravascular equipment and compress vessel until hemostasis achieved.

approach will minimize or eliminate the time, need for hospitalization, systemic effects, risk, and expense of lytic drugs. With that said, it is not uncommon to also used lytic drugs, albeit for shorter periods of time, for "clean up" of residual mural thrombus. We have found the mechanical approach to be especially effective for treatment of hemodialysis graft de-clots and in most cases we do not use lytic drugs.

Whenever possible, a catheter designed for thrombolysis is chosen. In selected cases we have used a Katzen® wire, an end-hole catheter, or a straight catheter with end and side holes. However, the pulse spray catheter is currently used in most instances. These catheters may be used in children of all ages and sizes and are available in diameters as small as 3 French, with a wide variety of infusion lengths. In our practice we have been able to use this catheter for treatment of clots in the aorta, central veins, and vena cava, and intracranially in the sagittal sinus.

Urokinase (UK) was the drug of choice for intravenous or intra-arterial thrombolysis until it was removed from the market several years ago. It has returned for use in a recombinant form. Streptokinase is no longer used since it is less effective and has a higher incidence of complications. tPA has been used in children and it is an equally safe and effective drug. Hopefully, in the future there will be prospective studies to define the best strategies for treatment of catheter and vascular thromboses in children. When tPA is used for catheter clearance, a dose of 1 mg (1 mg/ml) is used, and may be repeated, although after two unsuccessful attempts, it is unlikely that additional attempts will be successful. This dose and volume may be proportionately reduced for catheters with a priming volume less than 1 ml.

There are no guidelines for thrombolytic infusion in children that have been scientifically validated, and given the infrequency of these procedures, there probably will not be in the foreseeable future. For tPA infusion in children, a starting dose of 0.1 to 0.5 mg/kg to an absolute maximum of 7 mg has been used as a bolus dose on the table for systemic loading or more often for pulse lysis of the thrombus, or during concurrent use of a mechanical thrombolytic device. Theoretically, larger bolus doses could be used without disrupting coagulation, if there is no continuous infusion planned following the acute procedure.

Following placement of an infusion catheter across the thrombus an hourly infusion of tPA can be given at a dose of 0.5 to 1 mg/kg/h for 24 h. If alterations in lab values are not prohibitive, and there is no evidence of frank bleeding, but adequate progress is not observed, the dose may be doubled up to 2 mg/kg/h. Interval follow-up every 12 to 24 hours using US, angiography, or venography is performed. Ultrasound is preferred for most situations where the lesion has been clearly and measurably observed by US at baseline.

The timing of the follow-up examination will depend on the location and extent of the thrombus as well as the response of the thrombus and child to the thrombolytic therapy. If significant bleeding or other complications occur, the infusion will be stopped. However, if there are no adverse signs or symptoms, then the infusion is continued and follow-up imaging is performed approximately every 12 to 24 hours. If clot lysis occurs, the infusion is continued until the clot has disappeared. Care is taken to maintain the catheter infusion zone within the body of the clot. If no significant progress is made with clot lysis, the infusion will be stopped after 48 hours or may rarely be extended as long as 72 hours. In cases where the thrombus is occluding critical organs e.g., bilateral renal arteries or other sites, one may increase the thrombolytic dose. We have arbitrarily used a maximum of 2 mg/kg/h of tPA. In most cases, thrombolytic infusion is combined with systemic heparinization; using a loading dose of 50 to 100 IU/kg followed by a heparin drip titrated to maintain the PTT 1.5 to 2 times normal. Labs should be checked at intervals of no more than four hours, with the first set drawn before the first administration of tPA. Standing orders should alert ICU staff to immediately notify the interventionalist *and* the intensivist of any abnormal values, bleeding, changes in neurologic status, or signs or symptoms of hypovolemic shock. Any of the clinical parameters should prompt immediate cessation of the infusion until the situation has been evaluated and a decision about further treatment has been made by the interventionalist. If hemoglobin drops by more than 10% or platelets fall below 100,000, consideration should be given to slowing or stopping the infusion. If fibrin split products (FSPs) drop below 300, the interventionalist and intensivist should be notified. If they drop below 200, the infusion should be slowed, and if below 100, the tPA infusion should be held. The values can be rechecked in four hours and a decision about whether to resume or increase therapy can then be made.

When a child arrives in the interventional suite, the catheter hub and entry site are sterilized and draped. If there is no flow, then recanalization may be attempted by pushing sterile saline through the catheter using a 1 ml or 3 ml syringe. If patency is not restored, a guide wire is inserted, if possible, and the occluding thrombus mechanically cleared. A hydrophilic wire works best in this setting. Ports cannot be manipulated with a guide wire. A tunneled line may be treatable depending on the tightness of the curve at the venous entry site. If any blood return is identified, the CVC is injected with contrast and images are obtained at a rate of one a second or one every other second. If blood cannot be aspirated or sterile saline injected, the line will need to be removed. In most instances, a fibrin sheath is demonstrated. When a fibrin sleeve is identified, it may be mechanically removed from the catheter. In most instances, clot removal is performed under local anesthesia and intravenous sedation via a transfemoral approach.

Mechanically stripping a fibrin sheath from a CVC begins with femoral vein puncture. After sterile preparation and draping, local anesthesia is injected and a small skin incision made. The femoral vein is punctured and a connecting tube is fitted onto the needle and suction is applied while withdrawing the needle. When blood is freely aspirated, a guide wire is inserted. If necessary, the tract is dilated to assist in placement of a sheath with a hemostasis valve. A directional catheter (usually a JB-1) and guide wire are used to position the catheter in the SVC just above the CVC. The catheter is then exchanged for a snare with a 5 to 10 mm loop. The snare is positioned around the CVC and the loop is closed loosely so that when it is pulled down, it will strip off the thrombus. In most cases, one or two passes are all that is necessary to re-establish flow in the CVC. Although it is possible, we know of no child who has become symptomatic secondary to a pulmonary embolus or other related complication from this maneuver.

Thrombosis

Moss and colleagues and Gray et al. reported the incidence of catheter-related thrombosis to range from 3.7 to 10% of patients. Massicote and colleagues found the incidence of catheter-related DVT to be 3.5 per 10,000 pediatric hospital admissions. In this study, 3.7% of children identified with CVC-related DVT died as a result of their thromboembolic disease. In most clinical settings, however, the exact incidence is unknown. Looked at another way, venous thromboembolic disease is most often diagnosed in hospitalized children, virtually always catheter-related in neonates, and catheter-related in about one-third of older children. Prospective studies of the efficacy and safety of prophylactic low-dose and low-molecular-weight heparin are currently underway.

It is likely that the actual incidence of catheter-related venous thrombosis is higher than generally appreciated and is dependent on multiple factors such as vessel diameter, flow velocity, venous position, the infusate, associated masses or conditions, and the methodology used to access the vessel. Clotting status (acquired hypercoagulability or congenital prothrombotic disorders) plays a less certain pathogenetic role. For example, percutaneous puncture is more likely to result in long-term venous patency than a cut-down. In order to maximize long-term venous patency it is important to pay careful attention to the early signs of developing thrombosis. The initial sign of trouble is often the inability to aspirate blood from the catheter. This may be the result of either a clot at the catheter tip or a fibrin sheath.

Venous thrombosis resulting from an indwelling venous catheter occurs frequently. Its clinical effect depends on the location and extent of the occlusion. In most instances of thrombosis of a peripheral vein, no significant problem results. Associated phlebitis (localized tenderness and redness) is often seen, but more serious events rarely occur. Central vein thrombosis is more serious and may result in clinical signs and symptoms and associated complications, including chest pain, recurrent DVT, postphlebitic syndrome (pain, swelling, discoloration, and ulceration), extensive collateralization of superficial veins, development of varicosities, SVC syndrome, IVC syndrome (lower extremity pain, swelling, back pain, weakness, and venous stasis ulceration), and pulmonary embolic disease. Central vein thrombosis is reported to occur in 4% to over 40% of patients. We suspect that this complication occurs more often than is reported since, in most instances, it is not associated with signs or symptoms. In addition, it is likely that the frequency of venous occlusion varies with the technique used for placement. For example, by definition there is a 100% rate of occlusion in patients undergoing a cut-down for catheter insertion. Although no long-term data is available, it is probable that percutaneously placed lines result in the highest long-term patency rates.

The rate of thrombosis increases with the duration of catheter stay within the vessel. Children with congenital coagulation disorders have some of the longest lived port catheters placed for intermittent factor and blood product replacement therapy, some bearing the same catheter for more than ten years. At least one study suggests that long-term thrombosis rates in this population are insignificant. However, our experience and that of other investigators suggests that nearly 50% of the subset of children with treated hemophilia develop extensive DVT over the lifetime of their catheters. This rate of occlusive complications is similar to the rate seen in patient populations with the "normalized" coagulation. A high rate of thrombotic complications has also been noted in other patient populations with long-term indwelling catheters and ports. It appears that venous thrombosis is a multifactorial problem that may be influenced by catheter material, the position of the line, venous endothelial damage during catheter insertion, and associated infection. It appears that polyurethane is the most thrombogenic while polyurethane coated with hydromer is the least thrombogenic. Silicone catheters are slightly less thrombogenic than polyurethane alone.

Hoshal and associates have described the sequence of clot formation on a CVC. Initially a fibrin sleeve forms on the catheter followed by clot build-up until it occludes the catheter and, in some cases, the vessel. Thrombus occurs most often in the brachiocephalic vein, SVC, and right atrium. Right atrial clots are more common in neonates receiving parenteral nutrition, pediatric patients receiving chemotherapy, and renal dialysis patients. Connors and colleagues noted that at autopsy, 60% of patients with indwelling CVCs had either microscopic emboli or emboli in a major pulmonary artery. Small mural thrombi usually adhere to the endothelium and so rarely cause distant emboli.

The position of a catheter may influence whether a thrombus will develop. Catheters positioned at the cavoatrial junction or in the distal SVC are purportedly the safest. However, in our experience, a CVC in the SVC, especially in the proximal two thirds, is not best from a functional point of view and is likely less safe than catheters positioned in the upper third of the right atrium as long as the catheter tip moves freely. In our experience, catheters positioned between the confluence of brachiocephalic veins and the cavoatrial junction are more prone to thrombosis. The catheters at greatest risk are those entering from the left internal jugular vein, left upper extremity, and to a lesser extent, left subclavian vein. As these left-sided catheters translate from a horizontal course (in the subclavian vein) to a vertical course in the SVC they will abut the lateral wall of the SVC. In a significant number of cases this leads to intermittent catheter malfunction and development of fibrin sleeves and intravenous clots. We believe that the contact with the lateral SVC wall is a factor in development of the thrombus especially if the catheter tip is pointing toward the wall. Therefore, it is our preference to place a CVC or PICC in the entrance (radiographically, the upper third) of the right atrium. As mentioned previously, the safest "landing zone" for a central catheter tip from above the diaphragm is between where the catheter crosses the inferior margin of the right mainstem bronchus and a point two vertebral bodies below the carina (Figure 2.1).

History of CVC insertion is the most prevalent predisposing factor related to development of DVT. If central catheter-related thrombosis is recognized the significant risk of related morbidity and mortality demands that definitive intervention is undertaken. Whereas in the past, this has meant early discontinuation of the catheter, today anticoagulation therapy without catheter removal may safely resolve the thrombosis in many cases. It is important to consider that catheter removal prior to definitive therapy may result in loss of that route for future catheter insertions. One alternative in cases that do not respond to anticoagulation is mechanical or chemical thrombolysis, with or without balloon venoplasty and stent placement, as described by several groups. Insertion of an IVC filter, preferably a retrievable venous filter, beyond the thrombus for the duration of thrombolytic therapy can be considered if pulmonary embolic events are of concern. Finally, in those cases where critical central thrombotic obstruction is otherwise impassable, various authors have described methods of sharp recanalization of central veins.

Mechanical malfunction

During the early days of percutaneous CVC placement, catheter fragmentation and intravascular migrations often occurred at the time of catheter insertion. Catheter fragmentation results from shearing of the distal component as the line was being positioned through a cutting needle, traction on the catheter hub, or fatigue of the catheter wall at stress points, as with repetitive bending at the elbow or wear between apposing bony structures. With the evolution of materials, techniques, and the use of image guidance, catheter insertion using either the percutaneous approach or a cut-down has made central line placement safer and easier. Today, catheter fragmentation and intravenous migration are seen infrequently. However, when it occurs, the most common etiologies are catheter "pinch off" and iatrogenic misadventure.

Catheter "pinch off" is a potentially dangerous problem and is reported to occur in 0.1 to 1.0% of cases, virtually always related to infraclavicular insertion of a subclavian catheter. Catheter fracture often results in distal migration and embolization to the right atrium or pulmonary artery, and may be associated with chest pain, palpations, or arrhythmias. The mechanism for the catheter damage has been shown to result from mechanical friction and material fatigue as the catheter passes between the first rib and clavicle (Figure 2.36). Numerous reports describe this problem, usually seen in patients having lines placed without image guidance using the standard infraclavicular approach whereby the entry site is medial to the mid-clavicular line. This complication may be avoided in most cases by locating the initial access more laterally, or selecting an alternative access pathway (e.g., internal jugular, femoral, or basilic veins).

The repetitive mechanical trauma to the CVC is related to the local anatomy of the costoclavicular space. This narrow space is bounded anteriorly by the clavicle and subclavius muscle and posteriorly by the first rib and anterior scalene muscle. The factor leading to catheter fragmentation is inadvertent passage of the CVC through the tough costoclavicular ligament, which spans the first rib and clavicle. Constant friction and motion eventually breaks the catheter. Entry in the lateral aspect of the mid-clavicular zone or preferably in the lateral third with image guidance will eliminate this problem by avoiding extravascular passage of the CVC through the costoclavicular space. Since the course of the subclavian vein is less predictable more proximally, imaging guidance using either contrast with fluoroscopic monitoring or real-time US is necessary. We have found US to be the best modality for localizing and guiding puncture of the subclavian vein. The use of image guidance also reduces the risk of needle puncture of the thorax with resulting pneumothorax or hemothorax. Lafreniere found that catheter fragmentation usually occurred at a mean of 6.5 months after catheter insertion. Clinically, one can suspect this problem when there is intermittent catheter malfunction in conjunction with evidence of catheter compression on a chest radiograph.

Hinke and colleagues have developed a scale for evaluating the severity of catheter compression and suggested recommendations for follow-up or removal of CVCs (Table 2.15). The authors suggest removal of CVCs with grade 2 or 3 distortion documented on a chest radiograph.

Table 2.15 Radiographic grading of catheter distortion

Grade	Catheter distortion	Significance	Recommendation
0	No distortion	None	Status quo
1	Mild without luminal narrowing	Uncertain	Close follow-up
2	Distortion with narrowing	Subsequent fracture likely	Remove catheter luminal
3	Fracture	Risk of migration	Remove promptly

Table 2.16 Procedural summary: foreign body retrieval

– Prepare and drape the groin in sterile fashion.
– Infiltrate local anesthesia at entry site.
– Puncture femoral vein or other entry vessel.
– Insert sheath with hemostatic valve.
– Position directional catheter and guide wire just above catheter fragment.
– Exchange directional catheter for loop snare.
– Single plane or biplane fluoroscopic guidance.
– Engage tip of catheter fragment, tighten snare, and remove.
– Remove intravascular equipment and compress vessel until hemostasis achieved.
– Discharge child from radiology department.

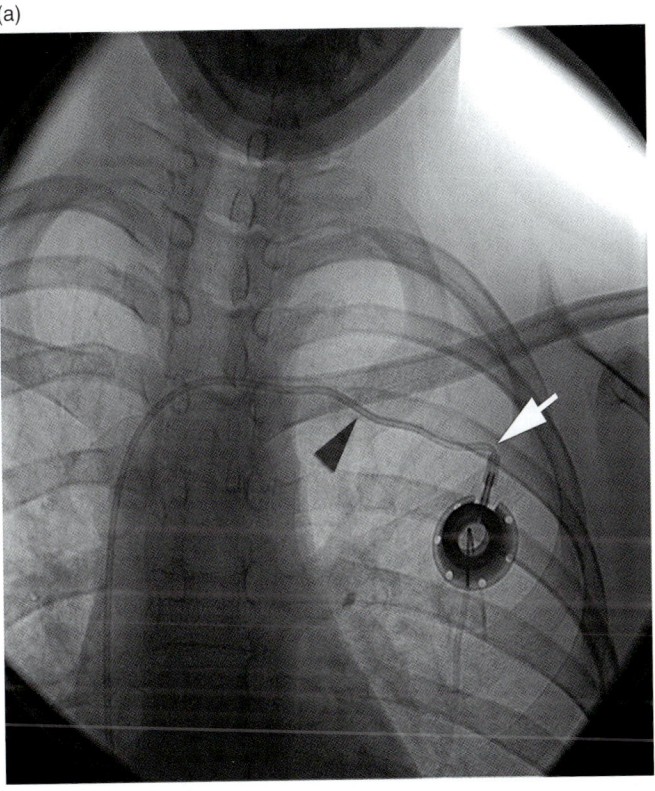
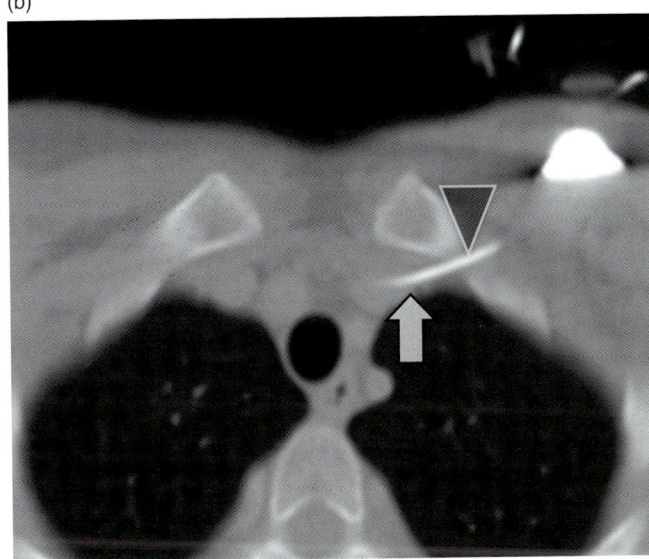

Figure 2.36 A 14-year-old girl with lymphoma and fungal pneumonia requires chemotherapy and other intravenous medications. (a) The left "subclavian" port placed in the operating room was functioning intermittently 22 days after insertion. There is a kink (*arrow*) at the catheter-hub interface due to poor positioning at insertion. The catheter has an irregular contour between the port and the venous insertion site (*arrowhead*), indicating fixation at two points. (b) The catheter passes between the clavicle and first rib, traversing the costoclavicular ligament (*arrowhead*), en route to the vein. This results in mechanical fatigue over time, leading to the catheter "pinch-off" sign. Of note, like many surgically placed "subclavian" lines, the catheter actually enters the brachiocephalic vein (*arrow*) medial to the subclavian vein. This port was explanted at 74 catheter days due to occlusion.

Intravascular foreign body

There are a variety of situations, which in recent years seem to be increasing in frequency, in which an object is lost with the vascular tree or non-vascular site. If this occurs all is not lost, and in most instances the object can be removed using image-guided interventional techniques (Table 2.16).

Before beginning the procedure, it is important to think through the options available and plan your approach.

Insertion of a sheath into the entry vessel is critical. A sheath with a hemostasis valve is inserted so that repeated access is possible. Also, the sheath protects the vein from trauma secondary to manipulation of the retrieval equipment and removal of the foreign body.

What size should the sheath be? In general, the smallest size that will accommodate the catheter is chosen. However, if the object cannot be grasped at its tip it will be necessary to fold it, thereby doubling its diameter, in order to remove it. If this

Table 2.17 Equipment: foreign body retrieval

- Endovascular sheath
- Guiding catheter

Snares
- nitinol snare, or
- tracter snare, or
- handmade snare using 0.018-inch guide wire

Baskets
- Dotter basket (reserved for the stomach or GI tract)
- Burhenne basket

outcome is likely, one must chose a sheath large enough to accommodate this larger size. In most cases, we have not been able to initially grasp the fragment at its end. When this occurs, we have learned to work the snare's loop to the proximal tip of the fragment by opening the loop just enough so that the guide catheter and loop can be withdrawn at tiny increments. When performing this maneuver, one should be aware of vascular pulsations so as to avoid disengaging the foreign body.

Localization of the catheter fragment is the initial step. Once identified, the best route to the foreign body is planned. For example, if the catheter were in the subclavian or pulmonary veins, a femoral vein approach would be best. A variety of different catheters and devices may be used for foreign body retrieval from the veins, arteries, or non-vascular lumens (Table 2.17). At this time we prefer gooseneck (e.g., Amplatz®) or trifoil (e.g., EnSnare®) endovascular snares as retrieval devices. The gooseneck snare design is particularly helpful since the soft, flexible loop projects at a right angle to the nitinol shaft, making grasping of the object easy in most instances. In addition, nitinol is a non-kinking material that is occasionally helpful especially in non-vascular applications. The trifoil design can simplify acquisition of the catheter tip especially when there is limited space to deploy and manipulate the snare loops.

We have found that initial catheterization of the vessel containing the catheter fragment is most easily accomplished using a directional catheter (e.g., JB-1) and guide wire (e.g., Glidewire®). The catheter tip is positioned distal to the object. For larger vessels (e.g., superior and inferior vena cava, internal jugular veins, and large arteries), a 5 or 10 mm snare works well. Regardless of the loop diameter the snare fits through a 5 or 6 French catheter with a 0.038-inch lumen. The snare is then pushed into the vessel lumen distal to the fragment and the directional catheter is then maneuvered so that the snare is positioned just at the tip of the fragment. The catheter is carefully pulled back in small increments as the snare sweeps the area (Figure 2.13). If necessary, in difficult cases, biplane fluoroscopy may be used to guide removal of the object. Although when needed biplane fluoroscopic guidance has been extremely helpful, it has not been necessary in most instances. Small catheter fragments that have embolized very distally in the pulmonary arterial tree may best be left alone, as the risks related to retrieval may outweigh the risk of leaving the fragment in place.

Indwelling infusaport (port) insertion

Introduction

For patients receiving long-term, intermittent intravenous therapy, such as intermittent chemotherapy or blood factor replacement, an indwelling venous access device (port) may be the preferred solution. The first such devices were intravenously located hydrocephalus shunts of the Ommaya type, described by Belin et al. in 1972 and Fortner and Pahnke in 1976. Since Niederhuber and colleagues described an implantable system specifically designed for intravenous therapy in 1982, numerous authors have described a variety of such devices, which share the same basic characteristics. Indwelling ports are implanted entirely beneath the skin, and are accessed as needed with a specially designed needle (Appendix 2.F). As with other central venous access devices, indwelling ports are as safely and quickly placed in the interventional suite as in the operating room, with lower cost and decreased complications, especially those related to access (including inadvertent arterial puncture and pneumothorax) and catheter position. Compared to tunneled central catheters and PICCs, ports carry a decreased risk of infection or dislodgment. With an improved cosmetic appearance and decreased restriction of activity, they also enjoy a high degree of acceptability to children and their parents.

Indications

The primary indication for implantation of a totally implantable port is the need for long-term, intermittent venous access (Table 2.2). Indwelling ports are predominantly used in children who require long-term (months to years) intermittent access, such as those on chemotherapy, children receiving frequent blood products such as hemophiliacs, children with chronic illnesses such as cystic fibrosis, and children with congenital abnormalities such as immune deficiencies requiring lifelong intravenous therapy. The disadvantages of using a port include its cost and the more extensive surgery necessary for placement and removal. Few absolute contraindications exist, and are similar to those for other venous access devices with two important exceptions. First, implantation of a metallic foreign body may be relatively contraindicated in patients, such as those receiving high-dose chemotherapy, who are expected to experience sustained and profound neutropenia or pancytopenia, both because of the risk of infection, and because of the risks associated with explantation of the device in this population should complications arise. Second, pain and anxiety related to recurrent access of the subcutaneous port may be a significant disadvantage. However, topical application of an anesthetic such as EMLA® cream at least one hour prior to needle puncture may ease this concern.

Technique

Equipment

Implantation of an indwelling port is a logical extension of the fundamental procedures, *initial vascular access*, and *tunneled catheter insertion*, when the anticipation of long-term intermittent therapy recommends internalization of the venous access port. Thus the equipment required for indwelling port insertion is, in the main, identical to the equipment necessary for other CVC insertions, with the addition of items specific to the creation of a subcutaneous pocket, and the port device itself (Figure 2.37). This equipment is outlined in Table 2.18.

Patient preparation

Except as noted, patient preparation required for indwelling central venous infusion port insertion is the same as for other CVCs, as described under "Technique: internal jugular CVC insertion," above. The right internal jugular vein is our strongly preferred access route, as it provides the most direct catheter course to the right atrium with the fewest mechanical and infectious complications in our experience. Alternative routes when the IJ is contraindicated include the basilic vein, femoral vein, and subclavian vein, in order of preference.

Creation of a subcutaneous pocket

Once the technique of central line insertion is mastered, then two additional options become available: creation of a subcutaneous tunnel, and creation of a subcutaneous pocket. The former was described in detail in the preceding section. In this section, the procedure for formation of a subcutaneous pocket and implantation of an indwelling port is explained (Table 2.19). A port is a tunneled central line that is completely skin covered. The port is accessed by inserting a needle through the skin into the metallic port usually through its diaphragm. Recently, a port without a diaphragm has been introduced, which can be accessed with standard sheathed needles used for IV access. The standard devices must be accessed with a special non-coring (Huber) needle. Peripherally accessed system (PAS) ports have been developed for placement in the upper arm or forearm. We have found these useful in older children, especially young women, who do not want a scar or bump in the chest region. Our experience has shown that the rate of complications for a peripheral port is the same as for a chest port. The only additional consideration is avoidance of the nerve and artery when using a transbrachial approach, as discussed with regard to PICC insertion, above.

Creation of a subcutaneous pocket is not too difficult but requires patience and comfort with surgical techniques. Although no specialized instruments are needed, it seems best to have a pack of surgical instruments available. We have found that a cut-down set has everything that is necessary. The instruments that are most helpful include a scalpel with #11 blade, pickups, hemostats, curved Kelley clamps, small retractors, a tunneling tool, a needle driver, and 3–0 and 4–0 self-resorbing sutures. Some operators find electrocautery useful for this procedure, if properly trained personnel are available to monitor the equipment. A disposable thermocautery device can also be used.

Development of the subcutaneous pocket begins with a choice of the skin site (Figure 2.38a). Again, it is important to use a site that is away from the nipple or breast bud. In most children either superomedial or superolateral to the breast is satisfactory. We prefer the superolateral position. In adolescent females with breast development the choice of site may be more difficult. In these young women an arm port or a port superolateral to the breast is preferred. If possible, avoid locations used for standard precordial lead sites, as well as usual locations used for sonographic windows (e.g., left fourth intercostal space). It helps to keep the tract short and the subcutaneous pocket as small as possible to limit movement of the port and subsequent withdrawal of the CVC as the patient becomes upright and active.

After a site for the subcutaneous pocket is selected, the area is generously anesthetized with buffered lidocaine or bupivacaine. In addition, the subcutaneous tissue through which the tunnel will run is also infiltrated using a Chiba needle. Some operators prefer to provide regional anesthesia as well, infiltrating the intercostal nerves at the level of the subcutaneous pocket, and one costal space above and below the pocket, a few centimeters lateral to the incision. For this purpose, bupivacaine is recommended, since the purpose is primarily to prevent postoperative discomfort.

The length of the incision depends on the diameter of the port but is generally 3 to 4 cm. The incision is carried down through the skin until subcutaneous fat is seen. Blunt dissection using a combination of hemostats, curved Kelley clamps, the back end of a pickup, and one's fingers, is performed until the pocket is enlarged just enough to accept the port comfortably allowing closure of the incision without tension on the suture line. Once the subcutaneous pocket is complete a tunnel is created and the port and CVC are pulled into position (Figure 2.38b). Although one can develop a subcutaneous pocket in any direction, it is our preference to keep the incision either at the most cranial or at the most caudal aspect of the pocket so that when it is closed, the needle can be inserted through intact skin corresponding to the center of the port. If the incision is made centrally, the port cannot be accessed until the incision heals and the suture line is more likely to fail. The port may be sutured to the chest wall at at least two points using 2–0 self-resorbing interrupted sutures (Figure 2.38c). The choice to suture the port in place is made if the device fits loosely within the subcutaneous pocket. Before closing the incision the catheter is trimmed to length using the bent guide wire technique as previously described, the catheter is inserted,

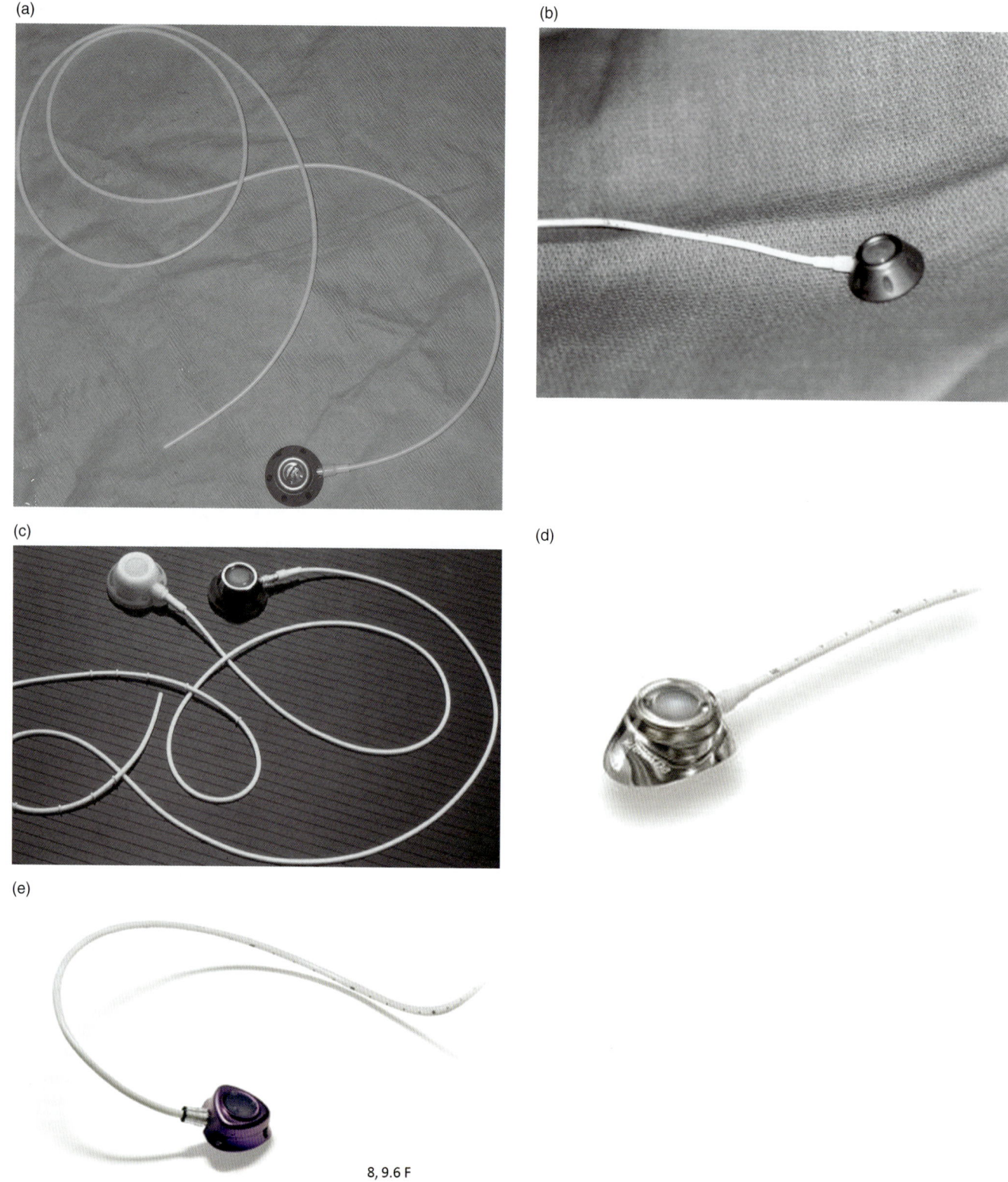

8, 9.6 F

Figure 2.37 (a–e) A low-profile port with a 5.2 French catheter.

Table 2.18 Equipment for indwelling port insertion

- Access needle
  - single wall needle
  - Potts–Cournand needle
  - Seldinger needle
  - micropuncture kit
- Tapered vascular dilators
- Peel-away sheath (3.5 to 17 French)
- Guide wire (Newton wire, "J" wire, Glidewire®, Amplatz Stiff® wire)
- Tunneling device
- Scalpel
- Cautery
- Port (petite, small, medium, large; single or double port)
- Huber needle (various lengths)
- Heparin (<10 kg = 1.5 ml 1:1,000, >10 kg = 3 ml 1:1,000)
- Suture (2-0, 3-0, 4-0 vicryl)
- Steri-Strips®
- Clear occlusive dressing

Table 2.19 Procedural summary: subcutaneous pocket

- Select site for port and tunnel placement.
- Prepare and drape site.
- Generously infiltrate skin with local anesthetic.
- 2 to 3 cm skin incision.
- Develop subcutaneous pocket.
- Create tunnel.
- Pull port and CVC into position.
- Insert CVC through peel-away sheath, remove sheath.
- Inject contrast to confirm satisfactory catheter position.
- Close pocket and CVC entry site.
- Cover with 4 × 4 gauze and occlusive dressing.
- Heparinize port and CVC.

and the position of the tip at the entrance to the right atrium is confirmed with fluoroscopy (Figure 2.38d).

The incision is closed using a two-layered approach. Initially, 3 to 5 deep interrupted absorbable sutures are placed perpendicular to the cavity to close the deep layer and to keep the port snugly in position. Then a subcuticular running suture is placed to approximate the skin margins (Figure 2.39). The skin about the incision is painted with liquid adhesive to make the skin sticky. The suture line is then reinforced with Dermabond® or Steri-Strips® to maintain good approximation of the skin margins. The Steri-Strips® are left on for seven to ten days or until they fall off. The site is covered with sterile 2 × 2 gauze and a clear occlusive dressing.

Technical variations

Arm port insertion

A low-profile arm port (Figure 2.40) has all the advantages of a central port without the risks of a central vein puncture. Several reports have demonstrated that bacteria that colonize the skin of the forearm are both less virulent and 100 to 1,000 times more prevalent than those of the skin of the chest in adults suggesting that one should expect a lower rate of CRBSI in peripheral ports compared to central ports. A similar study has not been reported in children. Our own experience suggests a similar rate of infections for the two routes of access, on the order of 0.3 to 0.4 CRBSI per 1,000 catheter days; a significantly lower rate than seen in other CVCs and PICCs, and favorably comparable to the rate of CRBSI from surgical chest port insertions. Peripheral ports essentially eliminate such risks as pneumothorax, hemothorax, or air embolism, especially important for patients with chronic severe pulmonary or cardiovascular disease in whom a pneumothorax or hemothorax could be life threatening. The risk of central venous stenosis is also substantially decreased, preserving the integrity of the central veins for future access needs. Like other central access insertions in the interventional radiology suite, same-day service, lower cost, ability to integrate access with other interventions in the same patient (biopsy, bone marrow aspirate, lumbar puncture, etc.) and the ability to perform the procedure with sedation in most cases makes this a resource-effective alternative to insertion in the operating room.

Patient preparation is identical to that for chest port insertion. Intravenous sedation is almost always satisfactory, with anesthesia reserved for those patients who failed sedation in the past, prefer anesthesia, or have a medical condition making anesthesia necessary. Whenever possible the non-dominant arm between the elbow and shoulder is selected for port insertion (Figure 2.41a). The arm is examined visually, with US and with venography, and the venous anatomy is defined from the entry point to the right atrium. The basilic vein is our entry route of choice. The cephalic vein is avoided if possible for the same reasons mentioned under "Peripherally inserted central venous catheter (PICC) insertion," above. The brachial vein may be used as an alternative, although there is a higher risk for paresthesia or pain due to nerve compression or injury at the venotomy site that usually requires port removal for resolution.

Ultrasound guidance is used exclusively in our current practice when the vein cannot be accessed by direct visualization and palpation. Access is obtained and secured with a guide wire just as previously described for other peripheral venous access procedures (Figure 2.41b). The entry site and area for the subcutaneous pocket is anesthetized using a 30-gauge, 1.5-inch needle to infiltrate the area generously with buffered lidocaine. The port is pressed firmly onto the skin to make an imprint in order to guide the initial incision for the subcutaneous pocket (Figure 2.41c). The incision, made with a #10 blade, should be about the same diameter as the port to insure that the pocket is tight. This obviates suturing the port into the pocket in most instances.

With the guide wire in stable position the access needle is removed and the tract dilated with a 6 to 7 French dilator. A similar sized peel-away sheath is then inserted over the guide

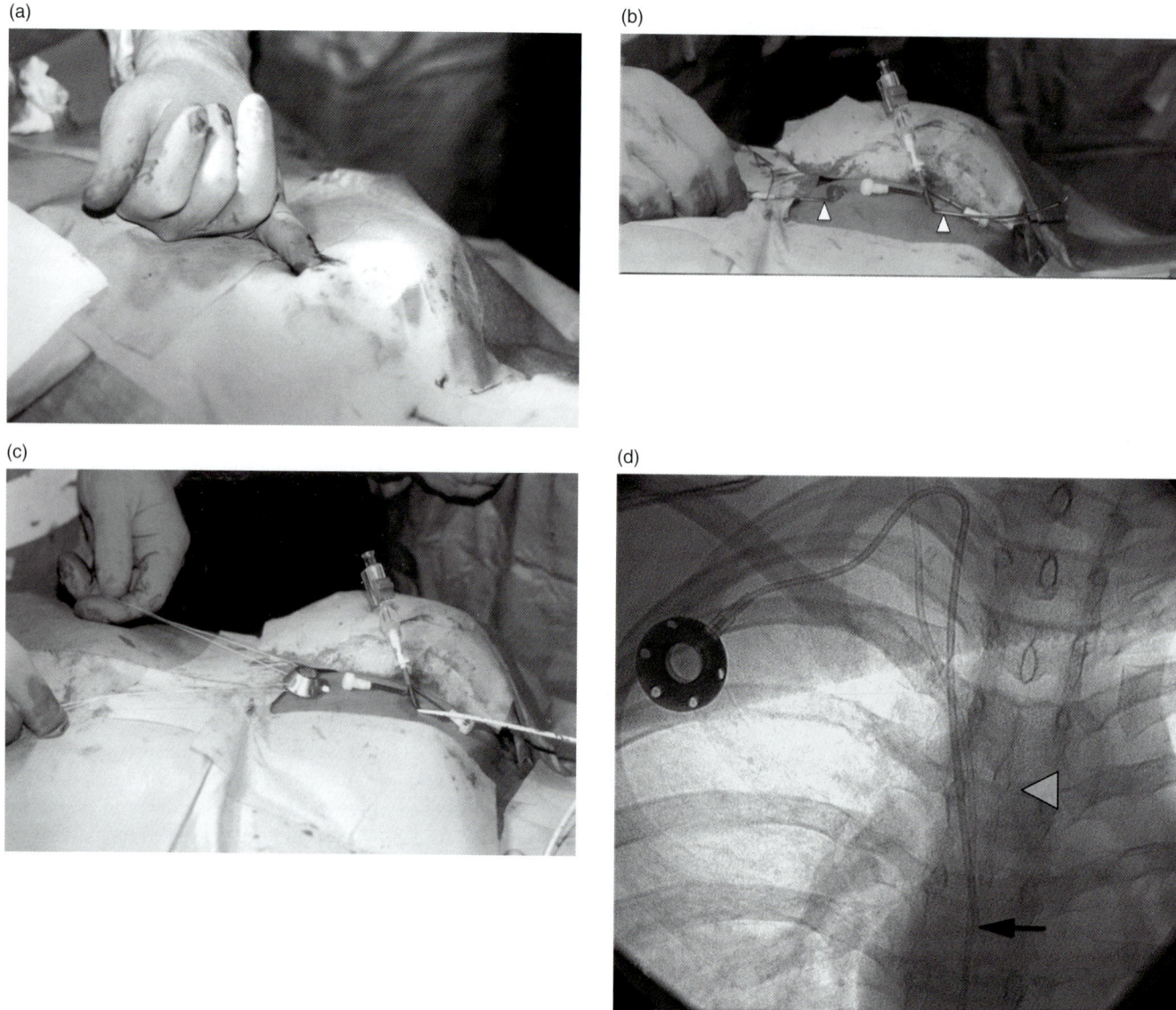

Figure 2.38 Sixteen-year-old with leukemia for indwelling chest port insertion. (a) The subcutaneous pocket is formed with a combination of blunt and sharp dissection. (b) The subcutaneous tunnel is created with a blunt dissector (*arrowheads*), such as a uterine sound. (c) If desired, the reservoir may be fixed to the muscle fascia with interrupted sutures. (d) After insertion via the right IJ, the catheter tip (*arrow*) is in satisfactory position, approximately 1.5 vertebral bodies below the carina (*arrowhead*).

wire into the entry vein (Figure 2.41d). The guide wire is advanced so that its tip is at the entrance to the right atrium as previously described. The bent guide wire technique is again used to determine the appropriate catheter length (Figure 2.41e–f). Since most peripheral ports are place in the non-dominant arm the usual adjustment should be made to assure that the final catheter length is not too short, so that the tip hangs freely at the entrance to the atrium, and does not abut or tent the wall of the vena cava.

Creation of a subcutaneous tunnel is elective. If preferred, it is formed 2 to 5 cm away from the venotomy site in the same manner as that described for central port insertion under tunneled catheter insertion, above. The port reservoir is placed in the pocket, and having been trimmed to length the catheter is advanced through the peel-away sheath (Figure 2.41g). After confirming that there is no kinking at the venotomy site, and that the tip is located in a satisfactory position, the peel-away sheath is removed and the pocket closed as described above (Figure 2.41h–i). The port is accessed with a Huber needle and heparinized with 1:1,000 IU heparin solution. The site is covered with a dry, sterile, occlusive dressing. The port may be used immediately. In addition to arm and chest ports, indwelling ports may be inserted through any access route used for any other central venous access, including the femoral or subclavian vein, or even such other routes as have been described in "Technique: difficult access," above. The port reservoir should be tunneled to a comfortable and accessible location.

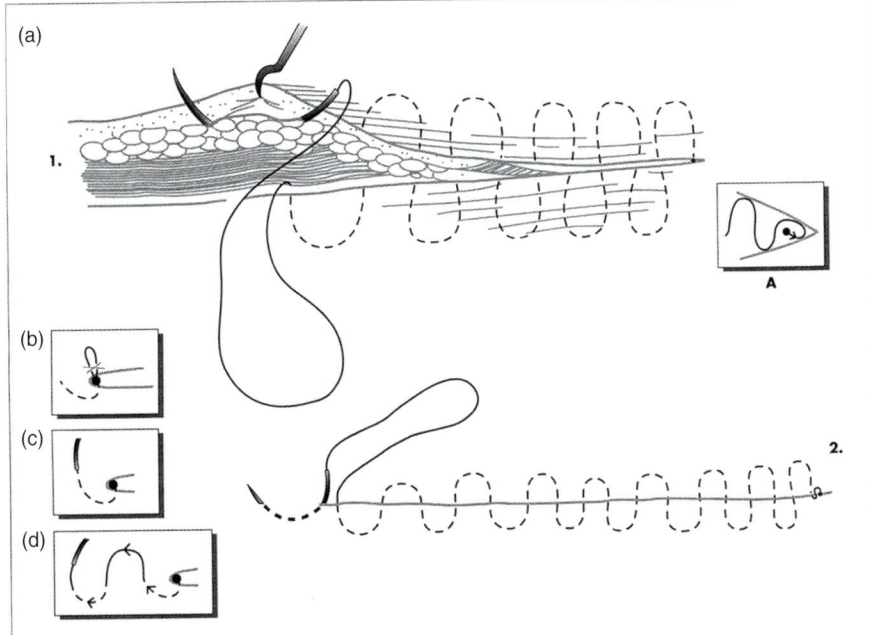

Figure 2.39 Subcuticular suture diagram. (a) An interior knot is placed at one end of the wound. In a running stitch, overlapping horizontal throws are taken on alternating sides of the wound, just at the superficial margin of the dermis, as shown in 1. The margins of the wound are gradually approximated, as shown in 2. (b) With tension on the suture a second interior knot is placed at the other extreme of the wound. (c) A length of suture may be "buried" beyond the wound margin once or (d) twice before cutting the absorbable suture. The wound may then be covered with Steri-Strips® or Dermabond®, and then a clean, dry dressing.

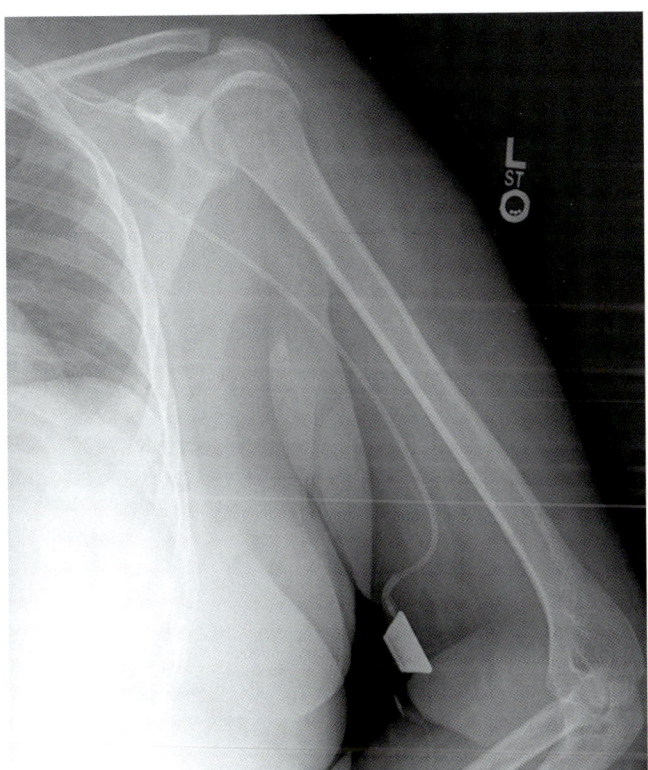

Figure 2.40 Thirteen-year-old girl with leukemia has an indwelling port placed via her left basilic vein with the reservoir located medially above the elbow.

Postprocedure and follow-up care

Care of the patient receiving an indwelling port is identical to that described above for "Technique: internal jugular CVC insertion." Port-specific issues are addressed in Appendix 2.G.

Technical problems and pitfalls

Although ports sutured to the chest wall are technically more difficult to remove, they are more stable within the subcutaneous pocket and resistant to inversion or migration of the port within the pseudo-capsule, which may occur with patient movement or secondary to repeated manipulation of the hub by the patient.

Port removal

When the endpoint of therapy has been achieved, or other conditions indicate, the port is removed using a procedure similar to the port insertion procedure described above. Explantation of the port can usually be accomplished with deep sedation or, in older children, generous infiltration of the soft tissues with a long-acting local anesthetic (such as 0.25% bupivacaine) allowing sufficient time for the anesthetic to take effect. The choice of incision site is solely dependent upon operator preference. We prefer to incise through the previous closure scar, although one may also avoid the previous incision, instead incising transversely across the center of the port or its caudal margin. The latter approach may protect against inadvertent transection of the port catheter, and allows rapid removal of the port once the pseudo-capsule has been opened. While reopening the original incision does require dissection through scar tissue and increased risk to the catheter, it may yield a better cosmetic result, especially in patients who receive several ports over their lifetime.

Regardless where the incision is made, the operator must accomplish three tasks. First, the port catheter is identified and controlled. Second, the port is freed from the tough, fibrous pseudo-capsule that characteristically surrounds it. Third, the port is freed from the chest wall. If sutures were placed

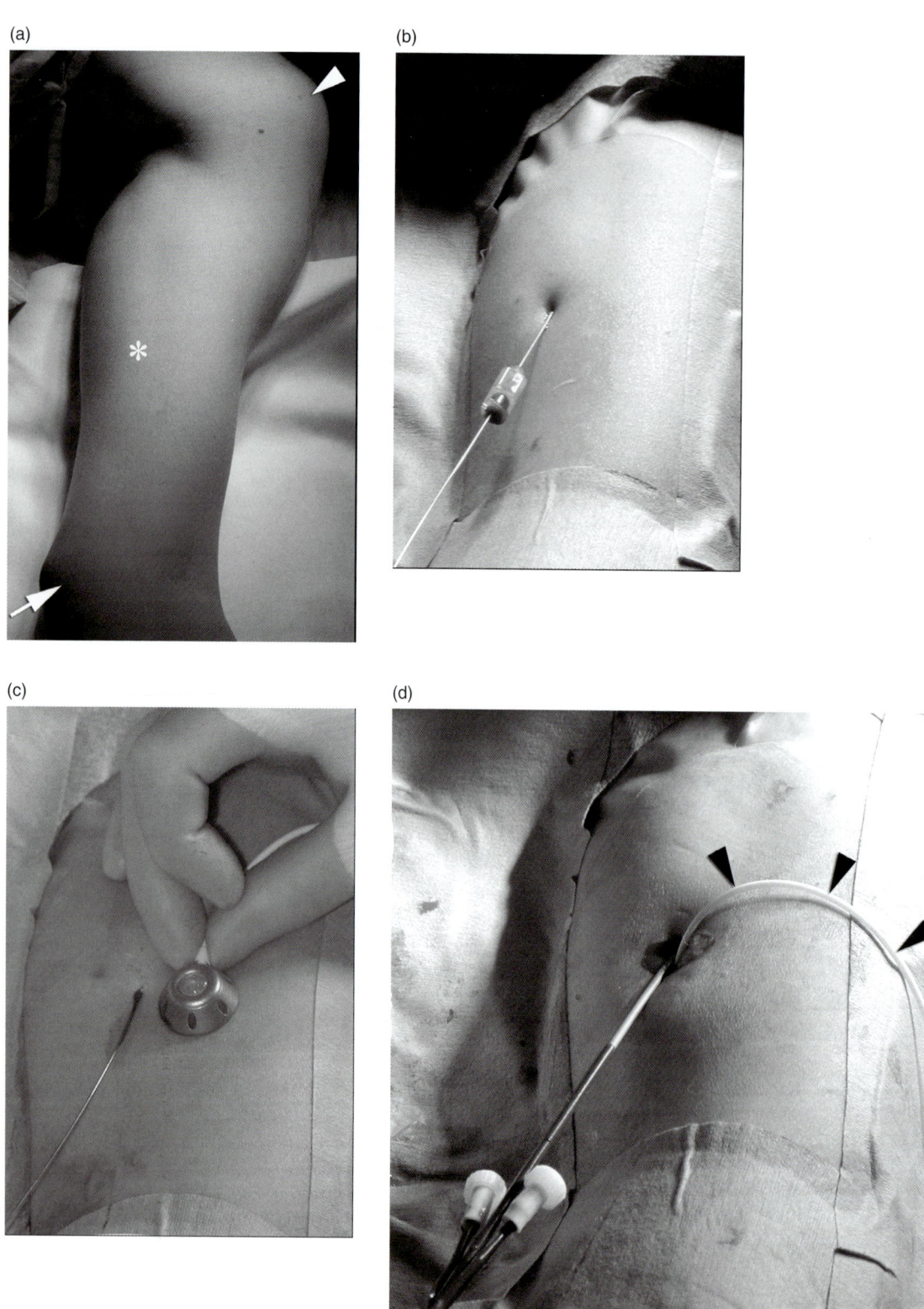

Figure 2.41 Peripheral (arm) indwelling port insertion. (a) With the patient supine and the elbow (*arrow*) flexed, the bicipital groove (*asterisk*) is accessible to the operator. A sterile field is prepared from the shoulder (*arrowhead*) to the elbow. (b) The basilic vein is the preferred access site. (c) The port reservoir will be centered over the wire, allowing sufficient space between the hub and the venotomy site to avoid kinking. (d) The reservoir may be positioned into the subcutaneous pocket either before (as in this case) or after dilation of the tract and insertion of the peel-away sheath over the wire. The port catheter (*arrowheads*) is seen here exiting the pocket. (e–f) The bent guide wire technique is used to measure the distance from the venotomy site to the entrance to the right atrium, under fluoroscopic control, and the catheter is trimmed to the appropriate length (*arrow*). (g–i) The trimmed catheter is advanced through the peel-away sheath and the sheath is removed. Once the final position of the catheter tip has been verified, the wound is closed in the manner described for chest port insertion.

(e)
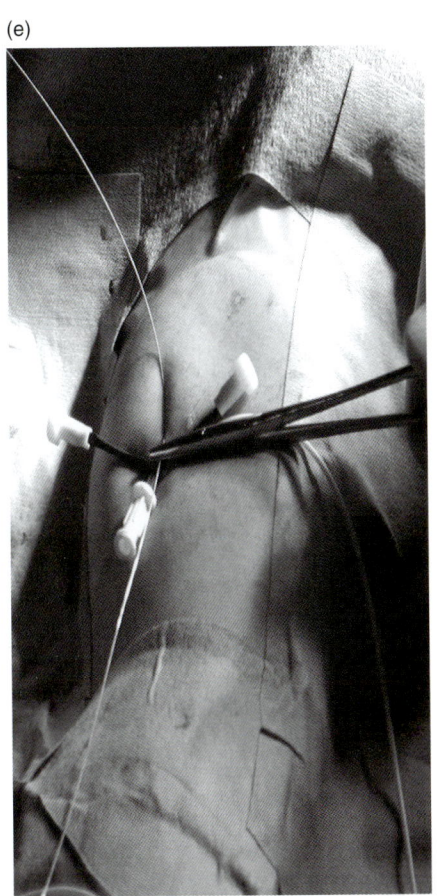

(f)
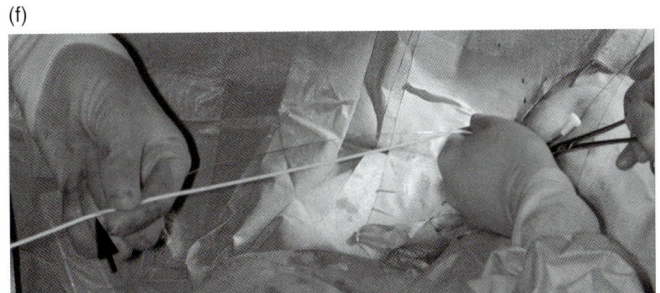

(g)
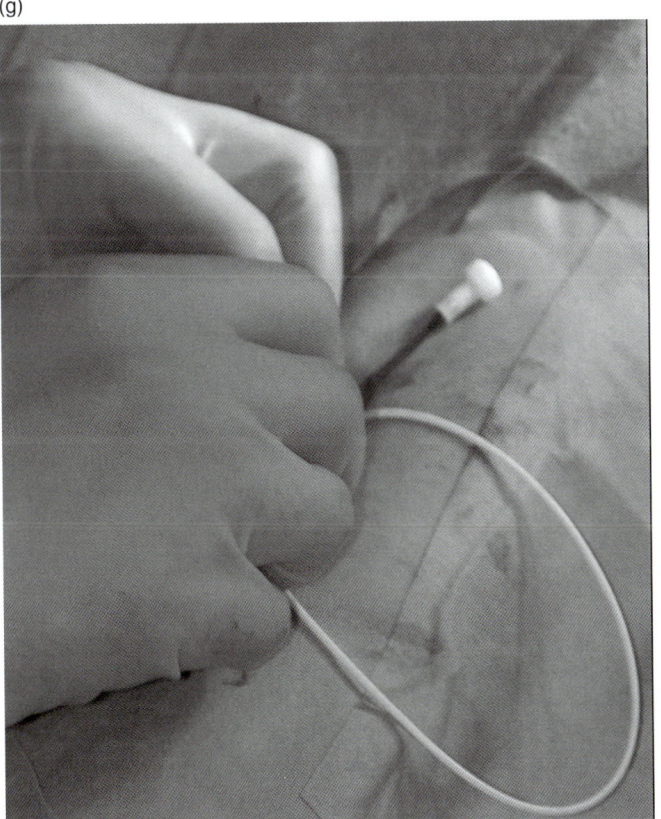

(h)
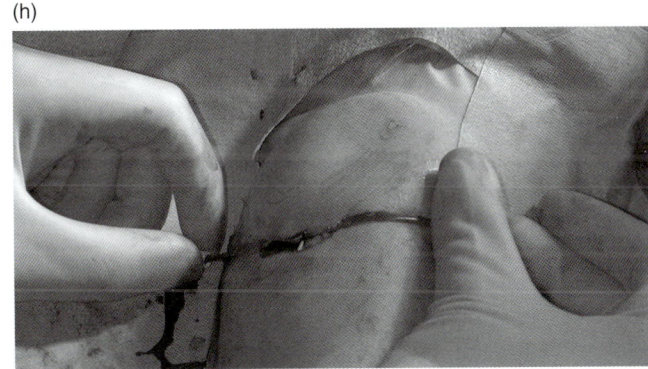

Figure 2.41 (cont.)

(i)

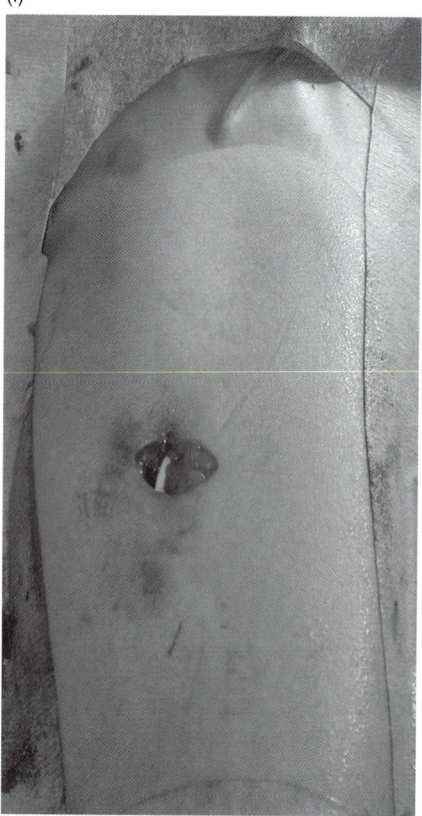

Figure 2.41 (cont.)

through the suture anchors embodied in the port, they are identified and removed. Placing the tines of a metal towel clamp through an unoccupied suture anchor in the port may simplify subsequent control and manipulation of the port. Once the port is free, with gentle compression on the venous entry point, the chamber and catheter are withdrawn. The subcutaneous pocket is closed with a combination of deep interrupted and subcuticular running sutures and Steri-Strips®, as previously described. As for any CVC removal, the catheter is inspected for defects, measured and compared with the length recorded at insertion, and the pertinent details of the procedure are documented in the medical record. If infection is suspected, the tip is sent for culture.

Conversion of port to CVC

Under certain circumstances (e.g., certain oncology and nephrology patients on transplant protocols) it may be helpful to convert an indwelling port to a CVC, or vice versa. Patient preparation and equipment required for the procedure are just as described in the sections on CVC insertion and port explantation, including the skin around both the venous insertion site and the prospective subcutaneous tract (if different from the port catheter tract) in the sterile field.

Once the port hub and distal catheter are under control, the operator must obtain access to the proximal arm of the catheter near the venous insertion site. Fluoroscopy is used to localize the skin entry site before a small (3–5 cm) incision is made. With a combination of blunt and sharp dissection the catheter is exposed. Two ligatures or hemostats are used to secure the catheter. The catheter is then cut close to the distal ligature.

A suitable wire is carefully advanced through the residual catheter into the right atrium or IVC, and the catheter fragment is removed over the wire and replaced with a peel-away sheath appropriate for insertion of the CVC selected. If the port is being exchanged for a large-bore catheter, tract dilation may be required prior to sheath insertion. Once venous access has been secured, a new tunnel is developed and the subcutaneous pocket is closed.

Complications

The most important complications related to indwelling ports are infection and thrombosis. In children with cancer, intensity of therapy (perhaps due to duration of neutropenia) and young age (less than four to seven years) increase the risk of port-related infection. Thrombosis is often associated with malposition, especially with failure to properly position the catheter tip at the entrance to the right atrium as previously described. These and other complications of CVCs have already been discussed in the relevant sections under both "Peripherally inserted central catheter (PICC) insertion" and "Central venous catheter (CVC) insertion," above. While the bulk of port-related complications are similar to those encountered in other central venous access devices, a few are particular to indwelling ports.

For example, several circumstances may lead to erosion of the port through the skin or wound dehiscence, including insufficient tissue superficial to the port at its insertion, vesicant drug extravasation (e.g., doxorubicin, mitomycin C, vinblastine), and pressure necrosis (e.g., from restrictive overlying clothing). Malposition or improper anchoring of the reservoir may lead to inversion of the reservoir or otherwise create a difficulty with periodic access. Reservoir dislodgment may also lead to kinking of the port catheter at the venous entry site (Figure 2.36) as well as malposition of the catheter tip (Figure 2.42). Malposition of the access needle is probably the single most common event leading to temporary port "dysfunction," but may also contribute to drug extravasation and skin breakdown. Poor or inattentive care of the access site, as well as hematogenous spread of remote infections, may lead to infection of the needle entry site or the subcutaneous pocket. Needle entry-site infections may be treated with removal of the access needle and a full course of intravenous antibiotics delivered through a site remote from the port. Infection of the subcutaneous pocket, defined as induration, erythema, and tenderness around the pocket with culture-positive material aspirated from the pocket, is most often due to Gram-positive organisms (usually *Staphylococcus aureus*) and usually necessitates port removal.

Chapter 2 Central venous access

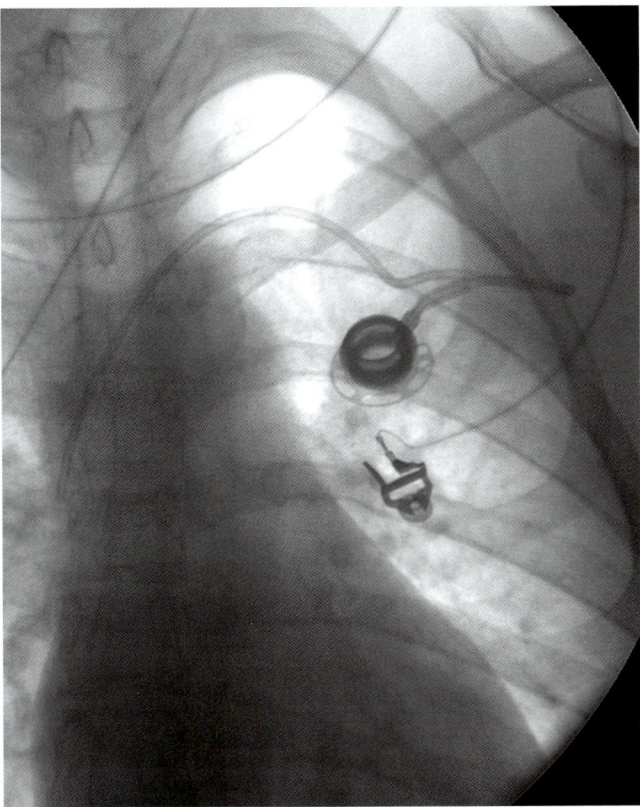

Figure 2.42 Chest port reservoir malposition with associated catheter malposition. With the proximal length of catheter dissecting into the axillary tissues, the catheter is intermittently kinking and the port is partially inverted.

diaphragm, and that the tip has been advanced to the bottom of the port chamber.

If the needle is properly situated, a contrast examination under fluoroscopy may be undertaken. The advancing contrast column is carefully observed in real time, because subtle evidence of extravasation may otherwise be missed. Filling of the port chamber is first documented, indicating the needle is properly positioned and patent, and that the chamber is not occluded with thrombus or precipitate. Next, extravasation in the region of the catheter attachment suggests either detachment or laceration of the catheter at the hub. Some ports are designed to have the catheter attached at the hub by the operator at the time of insertion (and are thus associated with a higher rate of catheter detachment). This design may allow revision of the attachment site without port replacement. In all other cases, the port is removed or replaced.

Future advances

New innovations in imaging equipment, access devices, and related instrumentation are ongoing. Recently, integrated image-guided interventional suites have been developed at several centers, combining fluoroscopy, US, and CT or MR in an OR quality room designed to be used on a multidisciplinary basis. Such developments encourage modality choices based on task performance rather than equipment availability or convenience.

Advances are progressing on other fronts as well. Investigators continue to develop and evaluate bonded catheters designed to help prevent catheter colonization and catheter-related thrombosis. Novel sites are being explored as alternatives in cases of difficult access or for specific therapeutic interventions, including portal veins, the spleen, and the medullary cavities of long bones.

With changes in the health care system, patients in tertiary care institutions are more acutely ill, and are admitted for an increasingly narrow portion of the acute phase of their illness. More care is pushed closer to home. The ability to safely and reliably deliver medications, fluids, electrolytes, nutrients, and blood products via central veins has played a pivotal role in this process. The complexity and acuity of the patient population so served extends well beyond the arbitrary boundaries of any one specialty. They demand organization and solutions that bridge conventional "islands of expertise" to take advantage of synergies in task-oriented management coordinating the many disciplines involved in CVC insertion and care. Such a coordinated cross-disciplinary strategy is severely challenged by fee-for-service reimbursement systems, although in the end it is most likely to stimulate a more appropriate and efficient allocation of resources that should benefit patients and caregivers alike. Institutional vascular access services serve as a nexus for communication, decision-making, scheduling, inventory control, management of complications, and information organization and dissemination that, in its optimal form, exemplifies true collegiality and patient-centered health care.

Because the port has no accessible external parts, evaluation of a dysfunctional port must rely primarily on imaging features. Evaluation of the dysfunctional port begins with visual inspection and, if necessary, sterile palpation of the access needle and needle entry site. Again, access needle malposition is the most common cause of port dysfunction. If the problem is not solved by repositioning or replacing the access needle, or other simple manipulations (such as unclamping the access catheter), the needle should be *left in position* and the patient sent to the interventional suite for further evaluation.

Fluoroscopic evaluation of a port should include the entire length of the catheter, using multiplanar imaging as required to fully evaluate both the reservoir and catheter course and position. Abnormalities of the catheter course and position are discussed in "Catheter dysfunction" under "Peripherally inserted central catheter(PICC) insertion," above. If the reservoir diaphragm is inaccessible, consider that the port may have flipped. If so, it must be repositioned or replaced. Even if it can be manipulated into a satisfactory position, there is a strong likelihood of repeated inversion. Fixation of the reservoir with stay sutures to the pectoral muscle fascia may avoid the need for port replacement. If the reservoir is in satisfactory position, the access needle should be evaluated in at least two imaging planes to assure that it is centrally located in the reservoir

Improvements in information management are coming somewhat more slowly than other technological innovations. After decades of database development centered around unique local solutions and sporadic application, information pertinent to vascular access procedures remains often distributed across each institution, isolated by ward, division, or department, sometimes in clinic files, sometimes in patient charts, occasionally in non-standardized electronic databases. A substantial proportion of important data is lost at the bedside, as it is simply not collected in any retrievable format. Truly prospective, randomized data, not filtered or biased by referral patterns or crippled by missing critical elements is essentially unavailable.

Such data, universalized across the institution and generalized across institutions is vital to the development of meaningful evidence-based strategies for improving access-related health care delivery. Choices regarding device type, access site, antibiotic and antithrombotic prophylaxis, dressing type and frequency of replacement, diagnosis and treatment of catheter-related infections, and strategies for thrombolytic and fibrinolytic therapy are just a few examples of the types of choices that would benefit from more reliable information.

We have presented an outline of data we believe useful to obtain on an institutional basis (Table 2.1), and anticipate that such data might be gathered on a much broader basis, perhaps through the development of a web-based national registry for pediatric vascular access. Considering the many lives and millions of dollars lost each year to access-related complications, even moderate reductions in complication rates and modest improvements in resource allocation would far more than offset the costs of such a system. Web-based resources could also be expanded to improve education and patient management (e.g., consent and assent, catheter care and troubleshooting, enabling care closer to home through set-top boxes for families and local providers) at the decision point of health care: the patient's bedside.

Controversies/issues

A number of controversial issues have currency in today's central venous access practice. The essential question of who should be responsible for primary insertion of CVCs, within what parameters, and in what location or locations, remains a politically and organizationally divisive concern dependent upon both economic and scientific influence. Objective cost/benefit analysis would help inform such questions, despite being difficult to obtain. Evidence suggests a significant shift of primary insertion referrals to the interventional suite when such services are available. At the same time, recruitment and training of non-physician providers (venous access nurses) as first-line responders to many vascular access problems may decrease cost and improve response time but also adds a layer of uncertainty and decentralization. This is not in itself undesirable, but further emphasizes the need for coordination and careful management of these services. An active institutional vascular access committee can provide this vital support, lead by an interventionalist well versed in delivery and care of venous access devices, broadly and collegially representative of the many services, specialties, disciplines, and providers who participate in the care of patients requiring central venous access.

Strategies for sedation, analgesia, and anesthesia can be particularly stressful for all involved. There are certainly times when access is required in a patient who is a poor candidate for anesthesia or deep sedation. Achieving access while providing the best comfort and safety possible for the child requires consideration and thorough understanding of the underlying issues by all participants. Frequent team-oriented planning and thoughtful discussion with patients and family assist this process. While use of general anesthesia is usually safe and effective, it is enormously costly and difficult to schedule, and should therefore be used with discretion. "Conscious sedation" is usually a misnomer in pediatric applications, and is seldom sufficient for painful procedures or those that require relative immobility. Deep sedation in children is often successful, but requires a highly trained and motivated staff to manage adequate sedation within safety margins given the narrow window of opportunity usually available for pediatric procedures. Newer solutions (e.g., use of propofol) and alternative therapeutic adjuncts (e.g., non-pharmacologic analgesia) are currently being explored, and may broaden the armamentarium of the interventional team in the future.

Despite substantial evidence of high complication rates, midline catheters continue to be used when obstacles arise making central location of a PICC difficult to achieve. This is especially true when insertions are attempted without image guidance, and when initial access is attempted via the cephalic vein. In fact, the frequency of thrombotic and other complications render midlines essentially equivalent to peripheral angiocatheters with one exception. Midlines located paracentrally (e.g., at the shoulder) may lead to DVT (for example, of the entire ipsilateral subclavian/brachiocephalic system), a complication very rarely seen with a peripheral angiocatheter. In addition to the untoward effects the occlusion of the subclavian or brachiocephalic vein is especially harmful to chronically ill patients because it simultaneously eliminates multiple potential sites of venous access. We have seen children who were candidates for an organ transplantation that could not be considered for this life-saving procedure because they no longer had patent central veins.

Uncuffed PICCs are quite susceptible to accidental dislodgment, either by the patient or, in a moment of inattention, by the health care professional, especially during dressing changes. Fixation of the catheter to the skin with stay sutures, while sometimes necessary, can be a source of substantial discomfort for the patient, especially for young children. A short, unprotected tract from the skin to the venous entry point may increase the likelihood of catheter-related infection. For catheters intended for less than two to three weeks of use, these are simply the realities of venous access. Unfortunately, no prospective randomized study of cuffed versus non-cuffed PICCs in a relevant pediatric population (e.g., patients receiving long-term total parenteral nutrition) has yet been performed.

Conclusions

The scope of indications for insertion of central venous access devices continues to expand in the pediatric population. Insertion of PICCs and CVCs in the interventional suite using percutaneous techniques is safe and effective. The success rates and complication rates are equal to or better than those seen with surgical insertion, with lower cost and more efficient resource utilization. It appears likely that the number of procedures will continue to increase and that a larger number of these patients will have their catheters inserted in the radiology department rather than the operating room. In most settings, placement of PICCs and CVCs outside of the operating room is cost effective since, in most cases, there is no need for general anesthesia, the recovery room, or expensive operating suites. We expect that in the future central access will become the most frequent procedure performed by pediatric interventionalists, and conversely that central access will almost exclusively be performed under the guidance of pediatric interventionalists where they are available.

Appendix 2.A: Blood drawing from a PICC or CVC

General guidelines

1. Discard blood standards:
   a. Under 10 kg: 1 ml
   b. Over 10 kg: 2 ml
   Discard blood not to be reinjected
2. Aseptic technique to be followed
3. Flush with sterile normal saline following blood removal:
   a. Under 10 kg: 0.5 to 1.0 ml/kg
   b. Over 10 kg: 20 ml

Note: modification of the amount of saline flush may be necessary in the fluid-restricted patient. In that case, the attending physician must specify the volume of flush. The amount must not be less than 0.5 ml/kg.

4. It is recommended that blood work be done only when the IV tubing is to be changed.
5. For children who have frequent blood draws, consult with the attending MD and lab for the volumes of blood required and the amount of flush and/or heparin to be administered.
6. If the PICC is not attached to an infusion, once blood is drawn, the line should be heparinized with the following amount:
   a. Less than 4 kg: 1.0 ml heparin (100 IU/ml)
   b. >4 kg to 10 kg: 1.5 ml heparin (100 IU/ml)
   c. Over 10 kg: 3.0 ml heparin (100 IU/ml)

Note: if blood draws are more frequent than twice per day, the line is capped and the heparin concentration should be 10 IU/ml.

Blood drawing from a PICC or CVC

Equipment:
1. Sterile gloves
2. Blood collection tubes
3. Syringes
4. Betadine preps
5. Alcohol preps
6. Saline (single dose without preservative)
7. Heparin (100 IU/ml)
8. Sterile needle (covered)
9. Cap (optional)
10. Clamp (optional)

Procedure:
1. Mask, wash hands and assemble equipment.
2. Prepare normal sterile saline.
3. Wash hands.
4. Put on sterile gloves.
5. Follow blood draw protocol for central lines.

Appendix 2.B Central venous catheter repair

General guidelines

1. Once a catheter leak is identified, the appropriate personnel or team, (i.e., the IV team or vascular access service), should be notified.
2. The interventionalist or surgeon responsible for device insertion should be notified.
3. Repair of the catheter must be performed as quickly as possible in order to prevent clotting or loss of the catheter, and to minimize the risk of infection.
4. Determine the size of the repair kit and order it from central sterile supply.
5. A minimum of two individuals will be necessary to perform the repair; one of whom has been trained in the procedure.
6. Once patency has been re-established the line may be used immediately after the repair.

Equipment

1. Single lumen and double lumen Broviac repair kit of appropriate size.
2. Sterile scissors (e.g., from suture removal kit).
3. Sterile gloves.
4. Alcohol preps.
5. Betadine preps.
6. Sterile 2 × 2 gauze.
7. Tongue blade.
8. Tape.
9. 3 ml syringes (× 4) with interlink caps.
10. Saline and heparin (100 U/ml) (volume appropriate for weight).
11. Sterile towels (× 2).
12. Broviac metal clamps.

Procedure

1. Gather supplies.
2. Wash hands.
3. Clamp the Broviac proximal to the fracture and as close as possible to the site of damage.
4. Open sterile gloves.
5. Prepare a sterile field by opening contents of the repair kit, suture removal kit, syringe needle, alcohol and Betadine wipes onto a sterile towel.
6. Put on sterile gloves.
7. Squirt adhesive into syringe barrel, then insert plunger and attach a blunt needle.
8. Prepare saline flush, having the second assistant hold the saline vial.
9. Flush the external replacement catheter with saline, leaving the syringe attached.
10. Using the Betadine preps, scrub the external segment of the catheter to be repaired. Finish scrub using two alcohol preps.
11. Using sterile scissors cut off the external portion of the damaged catheter using a straight, clean cut. Place a sterile towel under the catheter.
12. Insert splice segment of replacement catheter into white lumen of the catheter. Place a small amount of glue at area of the splice. Let this sit for 60 seconds.
13. Ease the sleeve completely over splice segment, inject adhesive under sleeve from both ends. Roll evenly between gloved fingers to properly disperse the glue. Wait 45 to 60 minutes for the glue to set.
14. Remove clamp and gently flush catheter with saline. If catheter successfully flushes then follow with heparin as per routine or restart infusion. Use catheter as stipulated in the general guidelines.
15. If the catheter does not flush and occlusion seems evident, secure order for urokinase or other thrombolytic and follow standard thrombolysis procedure.
16. Place catheter repair joint onto a tongue blade covered with gauze and tape to secure.

Documentation

1. Document in medical record the time fractured, time physician notified, time repair team notified, and the results of the repair.
2. Document time and name of physician notified that repair is completed and outcome of repair.

Appendix 2.C Procedure for CVC occlusion: complete or partial

If the line is newly occluded, a chest radiograph is recommended to verify line position prior to any procedural or pharmacologic intervention.

Mechanical occlusion

Assessment

1. External inspection of the catheter. Look for catheter kinking, suture occlusion, closed clamp, etc.
2. Consider contrast evaluation of the catheter under fluoroscopy. Follow contrast from the hub or Huber needle through each lumen to the tip. For indwelling ports, assure proper placement of the Huber needle in two planes.
3. If no mechanical cause is identified, proceed to "Medication precipitation," below.

Procedure

1. Relieve the source of occlusion if possible.
2. Otherwise, replace the catheter over a guide wire using sterile technique.
3. If a guide wire cannot be passed through the catheter from the hub, but the focal location of occlusion can be identified, it may be possible to pull the catheter back to this point, incise the catheter beyond the occlusion, and pass a guide wire through the remaining intravascular catheter to facilitate catheter exchange.

Medication precipitation

Assessment

1. The pharmacy and nursing histories should be evaluated for evidence of administration of medications known to precipitate, either alone or in combination with incompatible agents.
2. If a source for medication precipitation cannot be identified, proceed to "Clot lysis," below.

Procedure

1. Any agent used in an attempt to dissolve a precipitate or clot should be instilled in a volume ≤110% of the capacity of the venous catheter.
2. Lowering the pH toward the pK with 0.1 N HCl instilled into the catheter may dissolve precipitated calcium phosphate or acidic drugs (e.g., vancomycin).
3. For basic drugs known to precipitate (e.g., ticarcilllin, phenytoin), instillation of 0.1 N NaOH or $NaHCO_3$ may be effective. (These two interventions, HCl and $NaHCO_3$, should not be used one after the other, due to risk of thermal tissue injury.)
4. Lipid thrombi can be dissolved with either ethyl alcohol or 0.1 N NaOH.

Clot lysis

Assessment

1. Exclude mechanical causes of catheter dysfunction by careful inspection.
2. Exclude occlusion by precipitation of incompatible medications by review of pharmacy history.
3. Line is considered occluded if unable to aspirate blood and if unable to instill fluid into the line (use a 5 to 10 ml syringe). Attempts should be made changing positions and while the child is performing a Valsalva maneuver.

Equipment

1. 1 vial of alteplase (2 mg/2 ml)
2. 1 3 ml syringe
3. 1 5 ml syringe
4. 1 10 ml syringe
5. Normal saline (sterile)
6. Heparin 100 U/ml
7. Alcohol wipes

Note: dose of alteplase based on the size of the catheter, and calibrated to deliver 110% of the volume of the catheter up to a maximum of 2 mg. The following approximations may be helpful:
   3 to 4 French = 0.5 ml (0.5 mg)
   >4 French = 1–2 ml (1–2 mg)

Procedure

1. Use aseptic technique for accessing the central line, especially good hand washing. Obtain a vial of alteplase and dilute according to manufacturer's instructions. Be sure to use a preparation designated for treatment of venous catheter occlusion. Do not shake the solution – gently swirl.
2. Draw up 2.2 ml normal saline in a syringe and reconstitute alteplase in the single-use vial immediately before use.
3. Draw up the appropriate volume of reconstituted alteplase in a 10 ml syringe and instill into the occluded catheter.
4. Allow to dwell for at least 30 minutes, then attempt to aspirate.
5. If aspiration is successful, withdraw a small volume of blood to clear the catheter, then flush the catheter with normal saline.
6. Discard the unused portion of alteplase solution.
7. Repeat this procedure if the catheter remains occluded.

Appendix 2.D Heparin locking

General guidelines

1. Total heparin irrigation
   a. 1.0 ml for children less than 4 kg.
   b. 1.5 ml for children between 4 kg and 10 kg.
   c. 3.0 ml for children over 10 kg.
2. Concentration of heparin
   a. Heparin 100 U/ml if flushing Monday, Wednesday, Friday
   b. Heparin 100 U/ml if flushing daily; e.g., blood drawing
   c. Heparin 10 U/ml for more than two flushes per day
3. Children requiring continuous infusions or intermittent infusions
   a. Once medication is completed and the PICC or CVC is flushed with IV fluid, the catheter can be heparin locked. The line should be flushed with 1 to 3 ml of normal sterile saline for infants or 5 ml for older children.
   b. Heparin concentration is 10 U/ml.

Equipment

1. Syringe and proper-sized cannula
2. Alcohol wipe
3. New cap if changing
4. Heparin 100 U/ml, if irrigating per routine, 10 U/ml for multiple irrigations per day
5. Tape

Procedure for heparin locking

1. Wash hands.
2. Set up equipment. Draw up heparin dose.
3. Wash hands.
4. Clean cap vigorously with alcohol wipe and let dry.
5. Puncture cap with prepared heparin syringe and inject all but 0.5 ml of heparin. Continue to slowly inject the remaining 0.5 ml as the needle is pulled out of the cap.
6. Secure central line tubing to the child.

Procedure for cap change

1. Wash hands.
2. Prepare equipment. Draw up heparin dose and place the cap on the syringe.
   a. Open the sterile cap package
   b. Remove the cap in sterile fashion and do not touch cap top
   c. Puncture rubber stopper with syringe and needle
   d. Fill the sterile cap with about 0.2 ml of heparin.
   e. Place the syringe and cap back into sterile package.
3. Clamp tubing of the CVC or PICC.
4. Remove old cap.
5. Replace with new cap. Screw cap on tightly. Unclamp CVC or PICC.
6. Flush with remaining heparin dose, using the last 0.5 ml to inject cap as the syringe is pulled out.
7. Secure central line to the child.

Documentation

1. Document date and time cap changed.
2. Document the heparin dose given, date, and time.
3. Record patency of the catheter in the nursing record.

Appendix 2.E Dressing change

General guidelines
1. Dressing should be changed once per week. If it becomes wet, soiled, or loosened, dressing should be changed.
2. Small children will require two people to change a dressing. One person is to keep the child's hands and/or clothing from touching site and to help with distraction.
3. Older children may assist with part of the procedure but must wash hands and have adequate supervision.
4. Use a semi-permeable adhesive dressing with gauze 2 × 2 underneath is recommended. However, for some skin irritation problems, intermittent use of gauze covered by paper tape is acceptable.
5. Notify appropriate physician for redness, swelling, drainage, or pain at site.

Equipment
1. Central line dressing kit.
2. Transparent dressing.

Procedure
1. Ask visitors to leave the patient area.
2. Explain procedure to patient/caregiver.
3. Wash hands and take universal precautions.
4. Open dressing kit.
5. Remove old dressing
   a. Note condition of the site (sutures intact, line in place)
   b. Wash hands and put on gloves
6. Clean exit site of catheter with a hydrogen peroxide soaked swab starting at the catheter and moving in circular motion around catheter and out in spiral fashion for about 1 to 1.5 inches.
   Do not go back toward the catheter with the swab. Foaming may occur because of the action of the hydrogen peroxide on old skin and debris. This is normal.
   If foaming occurs or debris remains, the step can be repeated with a second, clean swab.
7. Use one dry swab to dry off the hydrogen peroxide and remaining foam/debris. Use the same circular, spiral motion.
8. Apply a Betadine® swab in the same motion as above. Allow skin to dry. Do not fan or blow dry.
9. Apply a dot of Betadine® ointment to the catheter exit site. Cover with 2 × 2 gauze (may fold in half to make a smaller dressing). Coil tubing if possible.
10. Remove gloves.
11. Cover gauze with adhesive dressing making sure of a good seal of at least 0.25 inches around the gauze.
12. Reinforce the edge of the dressing with paper tape where the catheter comes out of the adhesive dressing.
13. All tubing ends should be taped or secured to the child and not dangling so as to prevent pull on the tubing, accidental breakage, or contamination in underwear or diapers. If possible, tape the tubing ends upward.

Documentation
1. Date and initial the dressing.
2. Properly note in charts.

Appendix 2.F Accessing an implantable venous access device (IVAD port)

General guidelines

1. The interventionalist or surgeon must give approval before the *first* use of the device.
2. Aseptic technique must be followed.
3. Observe skin and tunnel tract before use to ascertain absence of edema, redness, or skin irritation. Notify MD of problems before accessing.
4. Non-coring Huber point needles are the *only* acceptable needles for use in such devices. They are available in several sizes: the 0.75-inch, 22-gauge, 90 degrees bent angle needle is preferred in most instances.

    Note: very thin or young children with pediatric-sized ports may need extra support padding as the 0.75-inch needle is the shortest available. Children with a thicker layer of tissue over the port may need a 1- to 1.5-inch needle.
5. Two people are usually required for accessing, particularly for young children.
6. The port septum has an expected half-life of 1,000 punctures.
7. The device may be used for the following reasons: chemotherapy, continuous IV infusion (TPN, intralipids), antibiotic therapy, blood drawing, and blood product transfusions.
8. When the port is not being used, it should be heparinized monthly using heparin 100 U/ml. Refer to chart for the proper amounts. Use the same volumes as for catheters with intermittent use.
9. The needle and dressing should be changed at least weekly when the port is used for continuous or intermittent heparin-lock purposes.
10. Checking for a blood return is indicated when
    a. unsure of needle position
    b. administering a tissue-damaging drug

    Note: blood return is not always present even if the system is patent.
11. Use a 3 ml or larger syringe. Do not use tuberculin syringe.
12. Only 10 ml syringes or larger should be used with mini ports.
    a. a 0.5-inch Huber needle is recommended
    b. blood products cannot be infused without a pump
    c. small volume medications should be diluted and put into a 10 ml syringe or infused via a port in a running IV.

Equipment

1. Standard port access kit.
2. Huber non-coring needle (0.75-inch 90 degree bend is usual).
3. Additional syringes as needed.
4. Sterile needles as needed.
5. Additional alcohol wipes for vials as needed.
6. Heparin 100 U/ml if not IV infusion.
7. Necessary IV tubing, pump, solution, medications.
8. Cap for tubing as needed.

Weight	Monthly	Daily	>Twice daily
4 kg	1.0 ml heparin	1.0 ml heparin	1.0 ml heparin
	100 U/ml	100 U/ml	10 U/ml
4 to 10 kg	1.5 ml heparin	1.5 ml heparin	1.5 ml heparin
	100 U/ml	100 U/ml	10 U/ml
>10 kg	3.0 ml heparin	3.0 ml heparin	3.0 ml heparin
	100 U/ml	100 U/ml	10 U/ml

Procedure: accessing the port

1. Gather equipment, assemble and prime IV bag and tubing.
2. Wash hands.
3. Open access kit; open and drop all ancillary equipment onto the sterile field using aseptic technique.
4. Glove.
5. Have helper prepare and hold heparin vial if needed.
6. Draw up appropriate amount of saline.
7. Prime needle with saline
   a. if using a double adapter, prime both tubes
   b. if drawing blood, prime all lumens
8. Leave syringe attached and clamp tubing(s). Use dry tubing if blood to be drawn.
9. Place child supine; must have a helper to hold unless the child is old enough to cooperate.
10. Cleanse skin with a suitable preparation, such as 2% chlorhexidine gluconate/70% isopropyl alcohol. Let dry.
11. Place a sterile towel on the skin below or around the port.
12. Locate the port diaphragm; position the port between two fingers and hold it firmly.
13. Hold the Huber needle at a right angle to the port and insert the needle through the skin, port diaphragm into the port. Press just until you feel the needle tip touch the back of the device.
14. Irrigate with normal sterile saline.
    a. under 10 kg: 1 ml/kg
    b. over 10 kg: 20 ml
15. For IV push medications:
    a. Slowly inject appropriate amount of normal sterile saline to assure that the needle is seated in the port.
    Note: if a sclerosant or caustic drug is to be administered, check for blood return prior to injection.
    b. Administer the medication using a 10 ml syringe if possible. Avoid using a tuberculin syringe (1 ml).
    c. Irrigate vigorously with normal sterile saline.
    d. Irrigate the port with appropriate amount and concentration of heparin (see chart) as the needle is withdrawn.
    e. Apply a small bandage.
16. Continuous infusion:
    a. Follow procedure for insertion of Huber needle as for IV push medication.
    b. Dress and support the angled Huber needle. Cover with a transparent dressing so that the site can be observed.
    c. Tape or pin tubing to prevent pull on the needle, allow slack in the tubing.
17. For intermittent infusion:
    a. Follow steps as per continuous infusion.
    b. Once Huber needle is inserted and the site dressed, the tubing is covered with a primed cap.
    c. Irrigate into the cap the appropriate amount and concentration of heparin using the standard technique.
    d. Follow the guidelines and the procedure for intermittent infusion via a central line using the appropriate amount of normal sterile saline before and after the medication.

Documentation

1. Record medications in appropriate section of the notes.
2. Record intactness of the needle, dressing applied, and blood work performed in the nurse's record.
3. Record the volume of irrigation in the I & O totals.

Procedure: de-accessing the port

General guidelines

1. Needles must be removed perpendicular to the port access site.
2. Two people are usually required.
3. If drawing blood prior to de-accessing, refer to blood drawing from a central line protocol.

Equipment

1. Alcohol.
2. Normal sterile saline syringe with cap.
3. Heparin.
4. Band-Aid.

Procedure

1. Gather equipment.
2. Wash hands.
3. Prepare syringes.
4. Loosen dressing.
5. Wash hands.
6. Clean tubing at the cap with alcohol.
7. Clamp tubing and remove.
8. Insert saline syringe into cap, unclamp, irrigate with appropriate volume of saline, clamp, and remove syringe.
9. Attach heparin syringe and unclamp.
10. Helper stabilizes port while second person irrigates with appropriate volume and concentration of heparin. When 0.5 ml remains, the needle is withdrawn from the port.
11. Inspect site for signs of skin breakdown or infection and apply a Band-Aid.
12. Documentation
    a. Record removal of needle and intactness of skin.
    b. Record irrigation volume in input and output record (I & O).

Appendix 2.G Critical management for implantable venous access devices (port)

Potential infection

1. Contamination of the line at or during the time of use is probably the most common cause of infection; therefore, strict attention to good hand washing and aseptic technique is absolutely necessary. It is of utmost importance that when the line is opened, the connection be cleansed prior to opening and the open end of the line held carefully so as not to be contaminated by non-sterile items. Change any portion of the line that becomes contaminated.
2. Signs and symptoms of infection. Physician must be notified.
   a. Fever with or without chills.
   b. Pain, erythema, edema or drainage at the site or tunnel.

Accessing

1. Occlusion should be dealt with immediately.
   a. First verify that the needle is in the port. If necessary, reaccess.
   b. If occlusion is suspected after reaccess, leave the needle in place and clamp the tube.
   c. Follow the procedure for CVC occlusion.
2. Swelling over or around the port during irrigation with saline.
   a. Stop infusion and check for blood return and needle placement (needle should not move around).
   b. If unsure, reaccess.
   c. If swelling continues, stop infusion of saline, leave needle in place, clamp, dress lightly, and call the interventionalist or surgeon.
3. Absence of blood return.
   a. Absence of a blood return does not necessarily indicate a non-functional or non-patent port. Do not reaccess before testing the function of the port.
4. During use (infusing blood or blood products).
   a. Packed red blood cells (PRBCs) should have a ratio of 1:4 normal sterile saline to PRBC (25 ml PRBC/100 ml normal saline solution (NSS)) piggybacked into the buretrol as a diluent.
   b. After the infusion, irrigate the line vigorously with the recommended amount of NSS and re-heparinize or reconnect to an infusion.
   c. For platelets, albumin, or fresh frozen plasma, no piggyback is necessary but the line must be irrigated vigorously with the recommended amount of NSS and either re-heparinized or reconnected to an infusion.
5. Occlusion alarm.
   a. Most often the cause of an occlusion alarm is that the needle has pulled slightly out and the tip is embedded in the port septum. Simply place one finger over the bent angle of the needle and press down firmly. If the needle continues to pull back, a new dressing may need to be applied to anchor it in place.
   b. If the needle tip seems to be in place and the occlusion alarm continues, reposition the child, raise his/her arms, turn the head, etc., and try to resume the infusion.
   c. Attempt to irrigate the port with a 3 ml or larger syringe of NSS. If resistance is met, again change patient position or have the child do a Valsalva maneuver as irrigation is attempted.
   d. Remove the needle from the port and reaccess the port.
   e. If occlusion is still evident, follow the procedure for CVC occlusion.
6. Infiltration, leak, needle completely out.
   a. The Huber needle can slip out of the port. It is important to check the dressing, area around the port, and the needle stability, and position frequently to verify correct placement.

Chapter 3

Thoracic interventions

Richard Towbin, Kevin M. Baskin, David Aria and Carrie Schaefer

History 98
Interventional radiology and thoracic interventions 98
Pleural fluid collections 98
Introduction 98
Pleural effusion 98
Empyema 99
Indications 100
Technique 100
Equipment 100
Patient preparation 101
Preprocedure imaging 101
Preprocedural lab studies 101
Standard technique 101
Management of parapneumonic effusion 101
Postprocedure and follow-up care 105
Catheter care 105
Postprocedural lab studies 107
Complications 107
Pneumothorax 108
Hemothorax 108
Chylothorax 108
Conclusions 108
Adjunctive transcatheter therapies in the thorax 108
Introduction 108
Indications 109
Technique 110
Equipment 110
Patient preparation 110
Standard technique 110
Intracavitary fibrinolysis 110
Chemical pleurodesis 111
Postprocedure and follow-up care 111
Complications 112

Conclusions 112
Intrathoracic abscesses 112
Introduction 112
Indications 112
Technique 115
Equipment 115
Patient preparation 115
Standard technique 115
Postprocedure and follow-up care 116
Complications 118
Conclusions 118
Mediastinal and pericardial fluid collections 118
Introduction 118
Indications 119
Technique 119
Equipment 119
Patient preparation 120
Preprocedural lab studies 120
Standard technique 120
Technical variations 121
Creating a mediastinal window 121
Percutaneous balloon pericardiotomy 121
Postprocedure and follow-up care 123
Complications 123
Conclusions 123
Biopsy of pulmonary and mediastinal lesions 123
Introduction 123
Indications 125
Technique 126
Equipment 126
Fine needle aspiration biopsy (FNAB) needles 126
Core biopsy needles 126

Pediatric Interventional Radiology, ed. Richard Towbin and Kevin M. Baskin. Published by Cambridge University Press. © Cambridge University Press 2015.

Patient preparation   128
Standard technique   130
Pulmonary nodules   130
Chronic lung disease   130
Imaging modalities   130
CT guidance   131
US guidance   133
Molecular imaging   133
MR guidance   133
Specimen handling   134
Technical variations   134
Coaxial and tandem needle techniques   134
Postprocedure and follow-up care   136
Complications   137
Pneumothorax   137
Conclusions   137
Marking lesions for resection   137
Introduction   137
Indications   138
Technique   138
Equipment   138

Patient preparation   138
Standard technique   138
Postprocedure and follow-up care   139
Technical variations   139
Complications   140
Conclusions   140
Tracheobronchial stent insertion   140
Introduction   140
Indications   141
Technique   144
Equipment   144
Patient preparation   146
Standard technique   146
Airway dilation   146
Tracheobronchial stenting   149
Postprocedure and follow-up care   149
Complications   149
Issues and controversies   150
Issues in using stents in the pediatric airway   150
Conclusions   150

History

In the past, relatively few thoracic interventional procedures were performed in the pediatric population. The majority of thoracic procedures have been performed by physicians and surgeons in their offices, on the wards, in emergency rooms, and in the clinics. This appears to be changing. Interventionalists, using image guidance, are now performing an increasing number of diagnostic and therapeutic procedures. Traditionally, most thoracic procedures involved diagnostic aspiration (thoracentesis), drainage of pleural fluid, or biopsy of pulmonary lesions. Recently, more complex interventions involving the tracheobronchial tree have become possible. The availability of high-quality ultrasound (US), computed tomography (CT), and to a lesser extent magnetic resonance imaging (MRI), has led to a wider range and larger number of procedures being performed each year.

Interventional radiology and thoracic interventions

To achieve maximal involvement, the interventionalist needs to play an active role in the patient care team. It is important to work closely with pediatricians, oncologists, cardiologists, pulmonologists, general and cardiovascular surgeons, and others, to clearly define the goals of each procedure and develop a treatment plan. As the treatment plan is tailored to each child's needs, attention to detail is critical for a successful outcome.

Three important features of the thoracic region bear directly on management decisions for image-guided therapy.

First, the bony thorax may limit the use of US. Therefore transducer selection is important. Whenever possible, use of a higher frequency transducer with a small footprint is recommended. Second, air-filled lung also limits sonographic visualization. Thus the risks associated with transgression of pleura and lung parenchyma may not be predicted with US guidance. However, there are situations where US can be useful, such as for visualization of pleural and subpleural lesions and mediastinal pathology, and for evaluation of pulmonary masses or other pathology when non-aerated lung is interposed between the target and the pleura. Regardless of the guidance approach, complications may ensue and potentially include pneumothorax, bleeding, dissemination of infection, and formation of bronchopleural or bronchocutaneous fistulae. To reduce these risks, an access route should transgress areas of pleurodesis or consolidated lung parenchyma whenever possible. To minimize the risks, careful route planning and a clear understanding of the procedural goals are important.

Pleural fluid collections

Introduction

Pleural effusion

Pleural effusions occur less commonly in children than in adults, with significant differences in cause, symptom presentation, character of the fluid, and techniques for diagnosis, treatment, management, and prognosis. Pleural effusions are most commonly a complication of bacterial pneumonia with the actual frequency and etiology varying widely. The most frequent bacterial organisms in otherwise healthy individuals are *Staphylococcus aureus*, *Streptococcus pneumoniae*, and *Streptococcus pyogenes*. In recent years the frequency of infection with methacillin-resisitant *Staphylococcus aureus* (MRSA) has increased. Disruptions in the normal equilibrium between filtration and absorption at the pleural surface may result from inflammation, direct damage to the pleural epithelium, increased vascular hydrostatic pressure, decreased plasma oncotic pressure, or interruptions in normal lymphatic drainage. Such disruptions may relate to a broad variety of underlying disorders, including infection, malignancy (e.g., leukemia), reactive (from thoracoabdominal infections), or parapneumonic inflammation, immune deficiency, prematurity, trauma, connective tissue disorders, and fistula formation (e.g., from pancreatitis).

As a result of the successful application of percutaneous drainage techniques and use of fibrinolytics, minimally invasive treatment of conditions involving the pleural space has gained in popularity. It is of interest that despite the availability of interventional techniques in many children's hospitals and the increased risk of hemothorax, perforation of intra-abdominal or intrathoracic organs, diaphragmatic laceration, empyema, pulmonary edema, and Horner's syndrome associated with surgical drainage, large-bore thoracostomy tubes placed by surgical services through a blindly created intercostal tunnel continues to be commonly used for removing air or fluid from the pleural space. Placement of smaller bore pigtail catheters using a percutaneous technique, without image guidance, has been advocated by some as an alternative to surgical placement of large-bore catheters. However, image-guided placement of pigtail catheters has been used effectively for thoracostomy and pleural drainage since its introduction in the 1980s, with limited complications. In fact, compared to conventional thoracostomy tube insertion, drainage via a pigtail catheter is associated with significantly improved results in children.

The optimal approach to the management of a pleural effusion depends on the type of fluid and the chronicity of the process. A percutaneously inserted drain can successfully treat most sterile, non-loculated pleural effusions in children. In most instances, an 8 to 10 French pigtail catheter is all that is necessary. On occasions when the effusion is fibrinous or bloody, a larger drain (12 to 16 French) is needed. Management of children with empyema is more controversial and a variety of approaches may be utilized. In the acute phase of empyema, percutaneous drainage and intravenous antibiotic therapy is the preferred initial therapy and is successful in most cases. As the fluid organizes and becomes fibrinous and loculated, percutaneous drainage alone is increasingly less likely to be successful. In addition, antibiotics are of questionable benefit. Traditionally, the favored approach to therapy has been open thoracostomy and more recently video-assisted thoracoscopic surgery (VATS) with debridement and irrigation of the pleural space to eliminate all fibrinous and infected material and to disrupt loculations and adhesions. Failure to successfully resolve the inflammatory process leads to further organization, which can only be treated by open, or more recently, thoracoscopic decortication. However, intrapleural fibrinolytics via an intrapleural pigtail catheter are also effective for treating loculated and complex pleural effusions.

Empyema

Since the 1990s, intracavitary therapies have been introduced, including the adjunctive use of urokinase (UK) or more recently tissue plasminogen activator (tPA) infusion through percutaneously placed drains, and the use of minimally invasive surgical techniques (e.g., VATS) for the management of empyema. Experience suggests that the combination of percutaneous catheter drainage and tPA infusion in the early fibrinopurulent phase is effective therapy (see "Adjunctive transcatheter therapies in the thorax," below). Alternatively, thoracoscopic debridement and irrigation can be used for treating these children in both the second and third stage of empyema. Open or VATS decortication is still accepted as the procedure of choice for late stage II and stage III disease. Staged protocols have been evaluated that progress from simple drainage to transcatheter fibrinolysis to early surgical drainage based on interval response with apparent success. Prospective studies are necessary to compare transcatheter and thoracoscopic approaches in children both medically and economically.

Infected pleural effusions may be treated empirically, with consideration for known bacterial pathogens in the community, and for the often polymicrobial progression of a maturing empyema. Culture and sensitivity tests may have a poor yield, especially if the child has been on antibiotics for more than 24 hours prior to sampling the pleural fluid. Immediate placement of a drainage catheter is recommended if the initial pleural fluid sample is frankly purulent, has a low pH (<7.2), is positive on Gram stain, or if the diagnosis is uncertain or there is a large effusion associated with sepsis.

Therapeutic options for treatment of a complex or loculated pleural fluid collection include thoracentesis, percutaneous pleural drainage tube placement without or with fibrinolysis, VATS and decortication, or thoracotomy and decortication. In the pediatric population, if minimally invasive measures fail or if the fluid collection begins to organize or is too viscid to drain, an open surgical decortication or VATS may be the best therapeutic approach. Recent reports in adults with empyema treated with 10 to 14 French percutaneously placed pleural drains have documented success rates ranging from 72 to 92%. In most instances, treatment failures have been the result of thick or viscid fluid that drains poorly, resulting in slow or incomplete resolution of the loculated collection.

Empyema in children occurs primarily in association with underlying pneumonia. Pleural fluid collections are classified as uncomplicated or complicated. Complicated fluid collections are defined as those that do not resolve without drainage, including large unilocular or multilocular parapneumonic effusions, empyemas, malignant effusions, and hemothoraces (sterile or infected). The temporal evolution of complicated exudative pleural effusions is classically divided into three stages. The first stage (Light's stage 1, exudative phase) is a thin, free-flowing exudate that is generally easily drainable with a catheter alone. The cellular and proteinaceous content of the fluid is minimal and the underlying lung and pleura remain pliable. The second stage (stage 2, fibropurulent phase) is characterized by fluid with increased cellularity and protein content. The protein in the fluid includes normal serum clotting factors that promote the formation of fibrin nets in the fluid, deposition of thin fibrin sheets on the pleural surfaces, and pleural loculations. These conditions lend themselves to catheter drainage with adjunctive fibrinolytic therapy. There is usually associated atelectasis of the underlying lung caused by both mass effect of the fluid and lung trapping by the relatively inelastic fibrin sheets. The third stage (stage 3, organizing phase) is characterized by ingrowth of capillaries and fibroblasts into the pleural membranes. This eventually leads to the formation of a mature inelastic fibrous pleural peel that is not amenable to fibrinolytic therapy. Progression from stage 1 to stage 2 can occur in as little as one day, whereas progression from stage 2 to stage 3 requires several weeks.

There is no appreciable difference in the history and physical findings of children with parapneumonic effusions compared to those with empyema. The lateral decubitus chest radiograph with the child lying on the affected side is the best view to determine the presence of an effusion and to obtain a rough estimate of its size. Computed tomography is useful for an overall assessment of complex pulmonary and pleural disease, including identification of primary loculations, associated masses or abnormalities, and pulmonary abscesses. Computed tomography does not reliably demonstrate secondary loculations, and will not always demonstrate a difference between pleural thickening and small pleural fluid collections. Sonographic evaluation will differentiate simple from complex fluid collections, with anechoic fluid or low level internal echoes visualized with simple pleural fluid collections, and complex fluid and mobile or fixed septations visualized with complex pleural fluid collections. Ultrasound may demonstrate an anechoic collection representing free fluid, with dynamic signs ("flapping" or "swirling") suggesting septations. Up to 40% of pleural fluid collections in adults will have an atypical appearance but, in most, dynamic signs will still help confirm pleural fluid. A small number of collections will produce diffuse internal echoes, have no dynamic signs, and will be indistinguishable from solid pleural lesions. It is expected that interval improvements in US technology and the higher proportion of parapneumonic effusions in children will lower this number. Ultrasound is the imaging modality of choice to guide therapeutic interventions for pleural fluid collections.

Indications

There are a variety of indications for percutaneous treatment of fluid collections involving the thorax (Table 3.1). There are almost no absolute contraindications to needle aspiration except possibly in children with an uncorrectable coagulopathy. Caution should be exercised when treating children with fungal infections of the lung and those with vasculitis because of their propensity for pulmonary hemorrhage.

Table 3.1 Indications for thoracic aspiration and drainage

Indications – aspiration
- Fluid for diagnostic evaluation
- Fluid for culture and sensitivity to guide antibiotic therapy
- Reduce size of fluid collection to diminish work of breathing, improve oxygenation, or improve blood return

Contraindications – aspiration
- Uncorrectable coagulopathy

Indications – drainage
- Infected fluid collection not responding to medical therapy
- Empyema (loculated and non-loculated)
- Lung abscess with associated pleurodesis
- Mediastinal abscess
- Preoperative

Contraindications – drainage
- Uncorrectable coagulopathy

Prerequisites for catheter drainage include: (1) a well-defined, unilocular collection with a cavity size of at least 3 cm; (2) a safe route for catheter placement; and (3) a normal coagulation profile or correctable coagulopathy. Children with thrombocytopenia or other bleeding diathesis are corrected prior to the procedure. Replacement therapy is often continued during and after the procedure in high-risk cases. Children with an uncorrectable coagulopathy may not be candidates for treatment if other therapeutic options are available.

Multiloculated collections may present difficulties for catheter drainage, as the inflammatory collection may not be completely treated with a single catheter. In these cases, manipulation of guide wires within the cavity to mechanically disrupt septations, multiple drainage catheters, or intracavitary (chemical) thrombolytics may be helpful. In the past, this type of collection was an indication for surgery. Currently, the decision to drain these collections percutaneously depends more on the number and location of loculations, wall thickness of the septations, and the clinical condition of the patient. In the case of multiple lung fluid collections or abscesses, collections that abut the visceral pleura (with pleurodesis present) or that are associated with pleural disease, are ideal for percutaneous treatment, even if multiple drains are needed. Pleurodesis markedly diminishes the risk of contaminating the adjacent, unaffected pleural space, preserving the potential for surgical cure if percutaneous drainage fails.

Technique

Equipment

No specialized equipment is needed for percutaneous drainage of thoracic fluid collections in children (Table 3.2). Percutaneous access is achieved with a thin needle or a sheathed needle (Figure 3.1) either for simple aspiration or for passage of a guide wire into the collection or both. The size of the drain

Table 3.2 Equipment for thoracic aspiration and drainage

- Sterile preparation and drape
- Sterile probe cover (if US guidance is used)
- Assorted syringes (1–60 ml)
- Coaxial end-hole introducer
- Access needle
  - 22- or 23-gauge Chiba needle, or
  - 16- to 19-gauge sheathed needle (Angiocath®, TLA), or
  - 4 to 5 French Yueh sheathed needle
- Guide wire, 0.035-inch to 0.038-inch (Glidewire® (standard and stiff), Newton®, Roadrunner®, Rosen®, Amplatz®, etc.)
- Luer Lock T-connector or other connecting tube
- Non-ionic contrast
- Fascial dilator sized to drainage catheter
- Drainage catheter
  - 8 French to 24 French locking pigtail catheter (APD, Dawson-Mueller), or
  - 18, 20, or 24 French Thal-Quick catheter
- Suture, 3–0 (or 2–0 non-absorbable suture for Thal-Quick catheter).
- Retention device (e.g., SorbaView® shield, StatLock®, Hollister® disc, tape bridge)
- Antibiotic ointment
- 4-inch × 4-inch gauze
- Mastisol® adhesive
- Tegaderm® or other transparent dressing
- Suction device (e.g., Pleur-evac®, Jackson Pratt®, or Hemovac®)
- Wall suction (–20 cm H_2O)

(Figure 3.2) selected depends on several factors including: (1) the viscosity of the fluid; (2) the size of the child; and (3) the proximity to organs or vessels. In general, we favor the smallest catheter diameter that successfully accomplishes the task and at the same time maximizes patient comfort. In most situations, this approach will be successful for treatment of pulmonary and mediastinal collections. However, pleural fluid in children with pneumonia is often thin in character but contains fibrin with a glue-like consistency. Patients with simple effusions can be successfully treated with an 8 or 10 French drain. A 6 French drainage catheter with a 1 cm pigtail loop may be adequate in small children (<10–20 kg). In children with viscid fluid, we prefer to use larger caliber catheters (range from 12–22 French) at the time of initial therapy. In order to maintain catheter patency and to provide optimal pleural drainage, the drain can be flushed three to four times per day with saline or tissue plasminogen activator (tPA).

Patient preparation
Preprocedure imaging
Suspected pleural fluid collections are often suggested on plain film, but a significantly increased yield of important information regarding etiology and complicating factors will be added by CT imaging. The volume and nature of the fluid collection (i.e., free, loculated, or multiseptate; thin or viscous) is often best evaluated using US. It is helpful to identify pleural fibrosis or infiltration to avoid futile attempts at drainage. Dynamic characteristics identified during US imaging can often help distinguish fluid collections from pleural thickening, including flow of particulate debris and flapping septations and atelectatic lung.

Simple transudates often resolve spontaneously and need only be evacuated if they become symptomatic through displacement of lung or mediastinum, or if drainage will prevent repeated thoracentesis. In our experience, stage 2 collections with a complex appearance by US have been easily drained. The re-intervention rate is significantly higher in children with parapneumonic effusions initially treated with aspiration alone when compared to those who receive primary drainage. Unless the collection is known to be a simple transudate, we prefer to place a thoracostomy drain at the initial procedure.

While frontal and lateral chest radiographs are usually the initial diagnostic images obtained and are satisfactory for a diagnosis of pleural and parenchymal abnormalities in most cases, plain film radiography is generally suboptimal for evaluation of mediastinal processes, route planning, and catheter placement. The availability of high-resolution CT and US has led to the widespread use of the percutaneous approach for the management of thoracic fluid collections in children. Computed tomography guidance is preferred for selecting the safest and most direct route and guidance for percutaneous drainage of parenchymal and mediastinal fluid collections. Real-time US guidance is preferred for drainage of pleural fluid collections.

No single imaging modality is used exclusively to guide percutaneous drainage. Whenever possible, real-time US guidance of needle insertion is utilized to gain entry into the fluid collection. Real-time US guidance is also helpful when performing a thoracentesis and for entry into parenchymal abnormalities with pleurodesis since no aerated lung is present to reflect the US beam. Although CT guidance alone is often utilized in the adult population to guide catheter insertion, we prefer to plan the procedure with CT but to guide needle insertion with US and monitor the placement of the guide wire and drains with fluoroscopy.

When CT is required to guide needle insertion, a guide wire is positioned within the abscess cavity and the catheter is inserted blindly over the guide wire (Figure 3.3). In rare instances, the child is transported to the interventional suite where the procedure is completed.

Preprocedural lab studies
Prior to any percutaneous procedure in the thorax, a coagulation profile (PT or INR, PTT, platelet count), and hemoglobin level are obtained. The child is kept NPO for at least four to six hours according to the anesthesia or sedation policy of the hospital. Antibiotics are given if the child is not already being treated.

Standard technique
Management of parapneumonic effusion
When aspiration without drainage of a pleural effusion or empyema is performed to obtain a diagnostic sample or as a

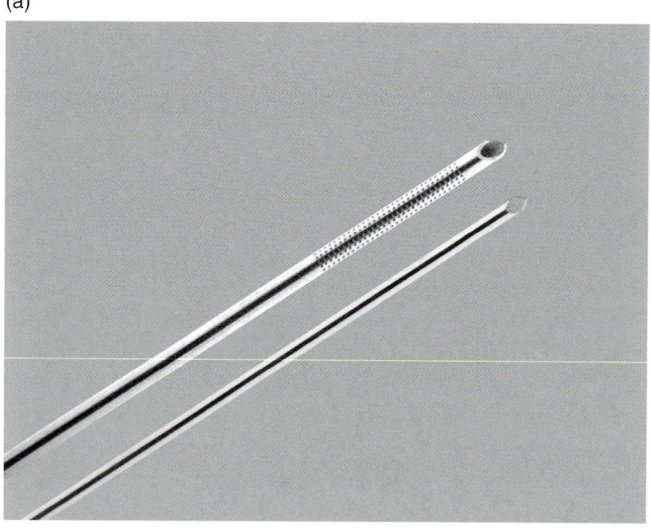
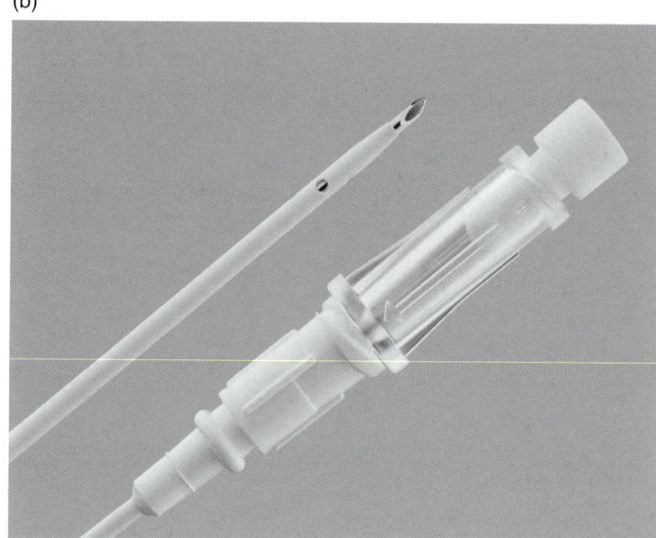
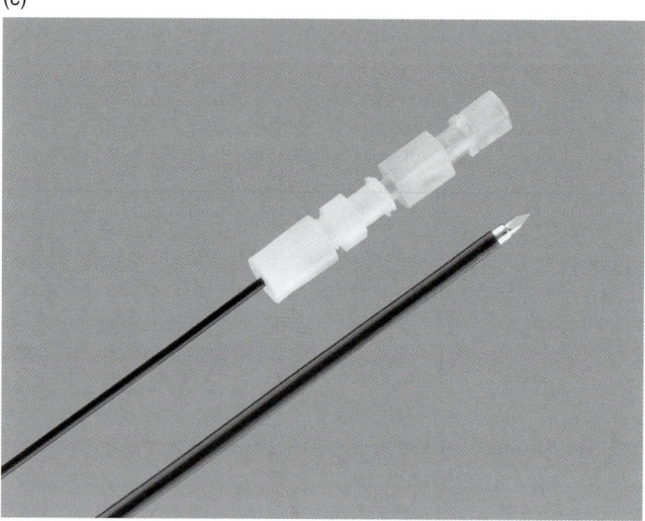

Figure 3.1 Access needles. (a) Chiba echo-tip needle (Cook Medical). (b) Yueh centesis sheathed needle (Cook Medical). (c) TFE sheathed needle with trocar stylet (Cook Medical).

means of therapy (usually for collections smaller than 3 cm), the modality selected for guidance depends on operator preference and ease of performance. In most situations a real-time US-guided approach is utilized. Fluoroscopic monitoring is not necessary in most cases, since guide wires and catheters are not being inserted.

If aspiration alone is indicated, for small fluid collections a 20 to 60 ml syringe is attached to the connecting tubing, and the fluid is removed manually. Larger (>500 ml) collections may be evacuated by attaching the connecting tubing via a Christmas tree adapter to either a wall or portable suction device. The suction device is usually set to −10 to −20 cm H_2O pressure.

When inserting a drain in a pleural fluid collection, a combination of US and fluoroscopic guidance is used in most instances. The child is usually positioned with the side to be drained elevated 30–45 degrees. Real-time US is used to guide needle access into the fluid collection. After preparing and draping the patient in sterile fashion, an entry site is chosen, usually from the third to tenth intercostal space in the posterior axillary line, with the patient in a supine position. A cooperative older child may be seated at the edge of the procedure table, leaning forward (over a pillow, for example), supported by a member of the interventional team. In this position, the pleural fluid tends to locate in the posterior costodiaphragmatic recess in the region of the eighth to the tenth intercostal space in the mid-scapular line.

The skin is anesthetized with buffered 1% lidocaine, keeping the thin (27- or 30-gauge) needle just superior to the rib to avoid the neurovascular bundle. The course of the access needle may then be observed under US to confirm a safe access route. A small skin incision is made and the subcutaneous tissue is bluntly dissected (Table 3.3). Depending on the size, depth, and location of the fluid collection, an 18- to 23-gauge Chiba needle (for central or deep collections) or a 19-gauge sheathed needle (for superficial or large collections) is inserted into the fluid collection.

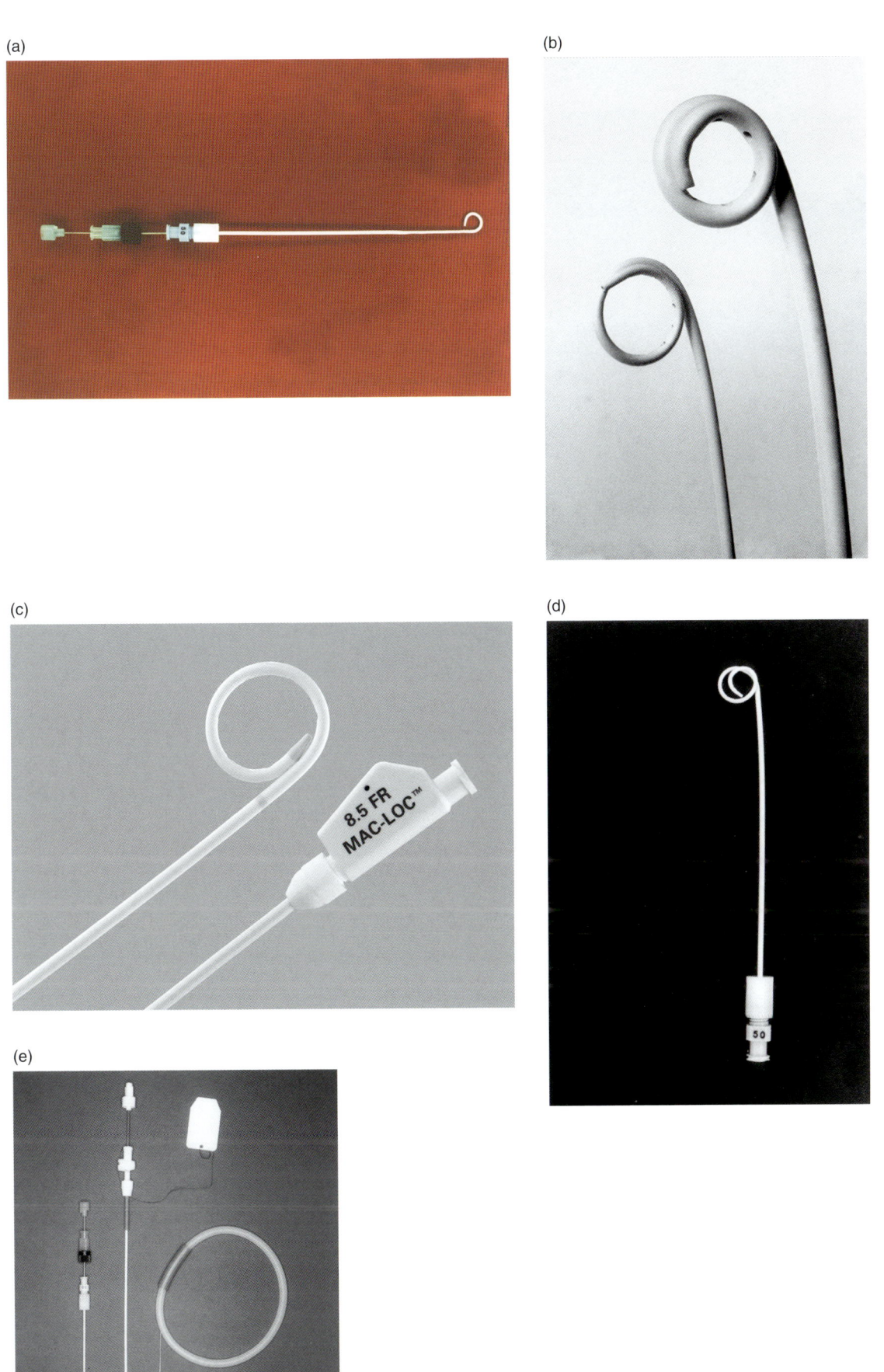

Figure 3.2 (a) 5 French drainage catheter. (b) "Pigtail" catheters. (c) Dawson–Mueller Mac-Loc™ 8.5 Fr multipurpose drainage catheter (Cook Medical). (d) 5 French pigtail. (e) 5 and 6 French drainage catheters (Cook Medical).

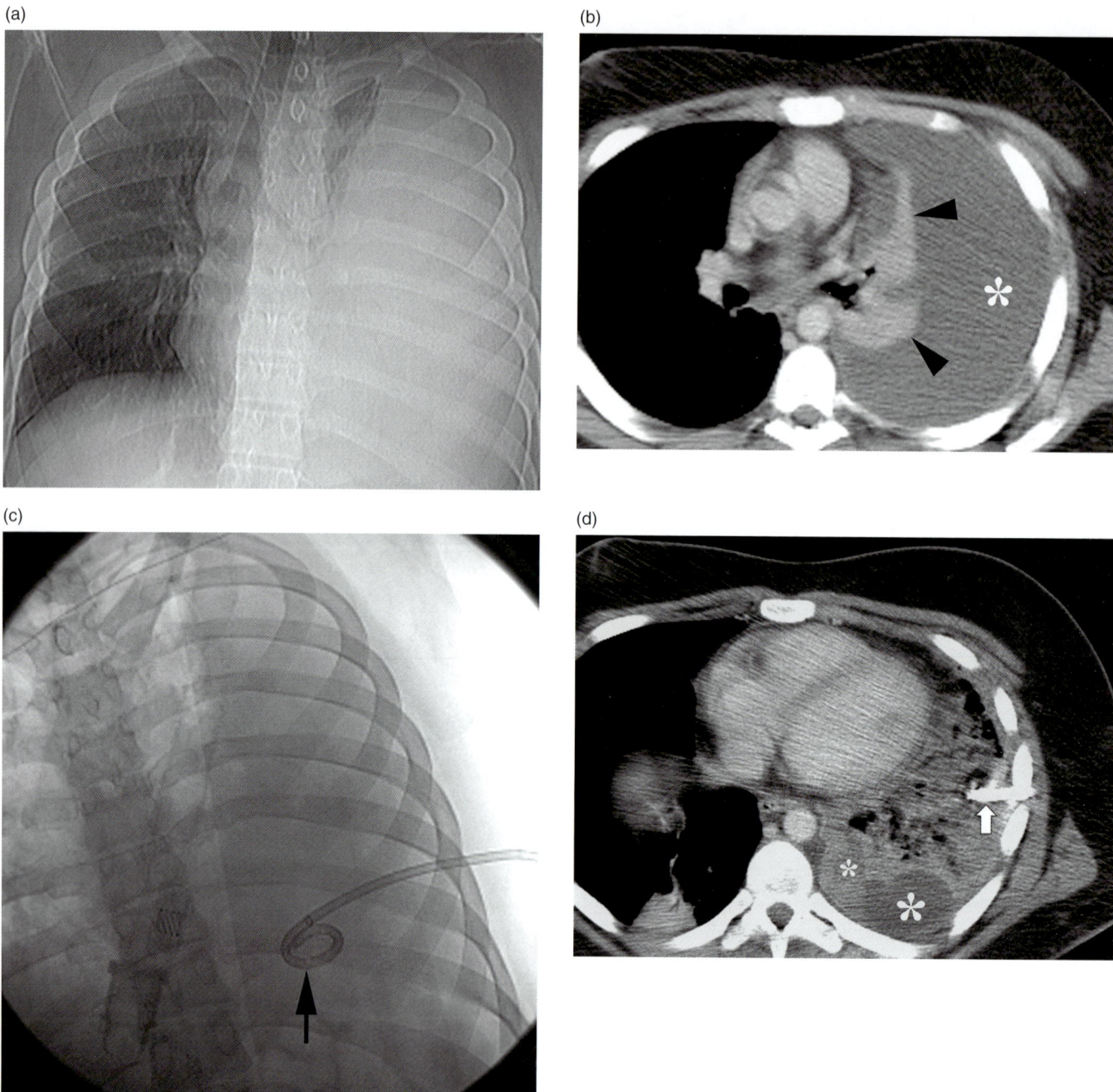

Figure 3.3 (a) Twenty-year-old male with synovial cell sarcoma has a large left pleural fluid collection seen here on a CT scout image. (b) The collapsed lingula and lower lobe (*arrowheads*) float freely in the large left pleural fluid collection (*asterisk*) demonstrated on a contrast-enhanced axial CT image through the mid-thorax. (c) A 14-French multipurpose drainage catheter has been inserted percutaneously into the collection under combined US and fluoroscopic guidance. At the time of insertion, the locked pigtail (*arrow*) is satisfactorily located in the mid-scapular line in a posterior position; that is, in the most dependent component of the free fluid collection. (d) A contrast-enhanced axial CT image shows that the catheter has been partially dislodged and the loop (*arrow*) is now neither in a gravity-dependent position nor is it within the remaining loculated collections (*asterisks*). Repositioning alone is unlikely to restore function.

The sheathed access needle is guided into the collection under real-time visualization and, once in the fluid collection, the sheath is advanced while pinning the stylet. Pleural tenting may give the false impression that the parietal pleura has been traversed. A short *thrust* with the needle will usually assure safe and successful passage. During expiration (or the inspiratory phase of positive pressure ventilation), the stylet is withdrawn and the sheath attached to the Luer lock T-connector. It is our practice to always attach connecting tubing, together with a flow switch (Meditech®), to the sheath or needle hub to avoid inadvertent dislodgment or retraction due to patient movement.

Table 3.3 Procedural summary: thoracic aspiration and drainage

1. Route planning.
2. Coagulation profile prn.
3. Sedation or anesthesia for procedure.
4. Prepare, drape, locally anesthetize.
5. Insert needle into abscess using image guidance.
6. Insert guide wire.
7. Dilate tract to size of the drainage catheter.
8. Insert drain.
9. Secure drain with suture and retention device.
10. Suction collection device prn.
11. Postprocedure chest radiograph.
12. Follow-up contrast injection of cavity prn.

At this point, samples of the pleural fluid are obtained to avoid accidental contamination or forgetting to submit a specimen. As small a sample as necessary for planned laboratory analysis should be obtained so that enough fluid is left to form the loop of a locking drainage catheter. If the aspirate appears non-purulent, the fluid is sent for an immediate Gram stain. If results are significantly delayed, or there is a question concerning the nature of the fluid, or the collection is large, a drainage catheter is left in place until the results of the culture are known or the child is asymptomatic.

If the material obtained is purulent, malodorous, or cloudy, a drain is placed. Intrapleural location of the sheathed needle is confirmed by aspiration of fluid or injection of a small amount of contrast. The distribution of contrast should be evaluated if a loculated or septated collection is suspected. Next, a guide wire is advanced until a substantial amount of the stiff portion of the wire is in the pleural space. If a sheathed needle (e.g., Yueh) is selected for initial puncture of the collection, a 0.035-inch or 0.038-inch guide wire can be placed into the collection directly after removal of the stylet. This approach is taken whenever possible, since it reduces the complexity of the procedure and the time required for completion. The wire may be swept through the collection for mechanical dehiscence of septations to encourage more complete drainage. The sheath may then be exchanged over the wire first for the appropriately sized fascial dilator, then for the drainage catheter. Overdilatation of the tract, useful during drain insertion into abdominal fluid collections, is not recommended for pleural drainage because of the increased risk of pneumothorax, leakage of fluid, and contamination of the pleural space.

The diameter of the internal locking pigtail drainage catheter should be selected based upon the viscosity, or fibrous nature, of the fluid obtained. We have found that it is generally best to use larger drains for treatment of pleural effusions than would be used for drainage of abdominal fluid collections. Simple transudates and uncomplicated exudates are drained through a 10 or 14 French catheter, while very thick collections may most effectively be drained through a large bore catheter such as the Thal-Quick. When intracavitary fibrinolysis is employed, the viscosity of the fluid can be expected to decrease substantially in most cases. Once in place, the catheter should be advanced and then fed off the stiffener until the last sidehole is within the pleural space. After the stiffener and guide wire have been removed a small amount of contrast may be injected to confirm intrapleural placement. Proper location in two imaging planes should be confirmed if fluid is not freely obtained or a complication is suspected. Careful attention should be directed to the possible demonstration of a sinogram during contrast instillation, indicating a bronchopleural fistula. The catheter can be secured using a variety of methods. Currently, we use a SorbaView® dressing and may also suture the drain in place. Alternatively, we have found the StatLock® covered with an occlusive dressing (such as Tegaderm® or Opsite®) is also satisfactory. In small infants, we may use a tape bridge (Figure 3.4) covered with a transparent dressing to secure a catheter since it can be easily tailored to size and is more comfortable for the patient. The Thal-Quick catheter may be secured with a subcutaneous purse-string suture, wrapping the free ends of the suture around the catheter at the skin exit site before tying. This suture may be used to close the exit wound when the catheter is removed.

After securing the drainage catheter, it should be immediately connected to an underwater sealed vacuum drainage system, such as the Pleur-evac®, at -20 cm H_2O pressure. In the absence of respiratory distress or concern for electrolyte or fluid shifts, large collections should be slowly drained (in aliquots not exceeding 60 ml/kg) to avoid electrolyte imbalances or re-expansion pulmonary edema. If re-expansion pulmonary edema occurs, it should be treated with supplemental oxygen and diuretics.

Postprocedure and follow-up care
Catheter care

When the pleural space is drained, the catheter is attached to a closed drainage system and placed to continuous suction or gravity drainage, depending upon the type of fluid encountered. When the fluid is thick or viscous, the Pleur-evac® is set at approximately -20 cm H_2O, and continuous suction is applied. Pertinent details of the procedure are recorded in the patient's chart, and orders entered (e.g., regarding management of the catheter and any suction devices). It may be helpful to both patient care and ongoing quality assurance to maintain pertinent demographic and procedure-related data in an electronic database. Suggested items for data management are included in Table 3.4. It is our practice to observe a child for at least two hours after a chest procedure on an outpatient basis to make sure that no complication has occurred. In addition, anteroposterior and lateral chest radiographs are obtained to confirm the absence of complications before discharge. The same routine is performed for asymptomatic inpatients.

If an associated bronchopleural fistula or pneumothorax is present, a Pleur-evac® is used with suction set to -20 to -30 cm

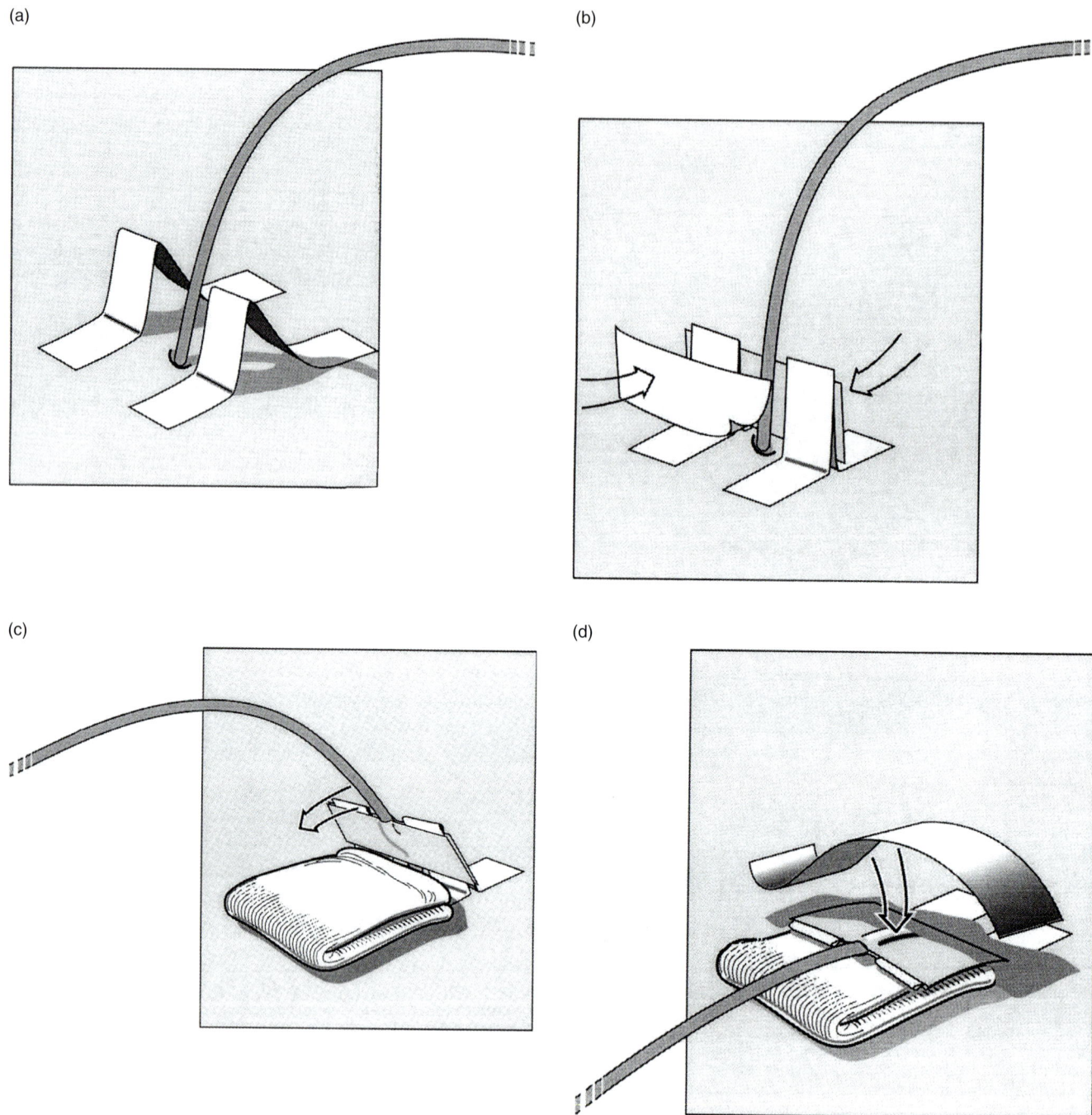

Figure 3.4 Tape bridge illustration. (a) The skin is prepared with mastisol to enhance tape adhesion. Then two pieces of tape of the same length are folded at the halfway point. The tape is stuck together for half of its length. The legs are created by folding the final quarter in opposite directions. The legs are then adhered to the skin so the pieces form "goal posts" on either side of the catheter exit site. (b) The uprights and drainage catheter are then joined by a bridging piece of tape on both sides (*arrows*). Any tug on the catheter is now transferred through the tape bridge to the skin, helping to prevent accidental dislodgment. (c) The adjacent skin is padded with gauze and the tape bridge is folded down (*arrow*). The direction must be consistent with the original angle of entry of the access needle, or the catheter will tend to kink. (d) The tape bridge is secured to the skin with adhesive tape (*arrow*).

H_2O to aid tract closure. Larger air leaks may require a larger chest tube (such as an 18 to 22 French Thal-Quick) or multiple tubes to successfully evacuate the air leak. If closure cannot be achieved after several weeks of drainage, the surgical service is consulted. Irrigation of the catheter is performed at least twice per day when thick or viscous fluid is noted but not routinely for thin fluid. In addition, intracavitary thrombolytic agents are considered as an adjunctive therapy when drainage is

Table 3.4 Outcome measures for thoracic procedures

To improve outcome and quality assurance analysis, it may be helpful to record the following information for each thoracic interventional procedure performed:

- Demographic information (patient name, unique identification number, date and time of procedure, age, sex, weight, date of birth, etc.)
- Primary diagnosis
- Reason for procedure; referring service and provider
- Anticipated endpoint
- Primary provider responsible for procedure (interventionalist, pulmonologist, surgeon, etc.)
- Collaborating provider(s)
- Procedure location (interventional suite, operating room, ICU, bedside, etc.)
- Provider(s) responsible for anesthesia/sedation (interventionalist, anesthesiologist, nurse, etc.)
- Preprocedural evaluation (e.g., coagulation profile, pulmonary function studies)
- Preprocedural interventions (e.g., antibiotics, blood products, imaging)
- Initial access
  - access needle
  - guidance (anatomic landmarks, US, fluoroscopy, CT, MRI, etc.)
  - operative site
  - device (e.g., APD, Dawson-Mueller, Thal-Quick, Palmaz® stent, etc.)
  - number of attempts
  - reason for deferral, discontinuation or failure, if procedure not completed
- Access drainage device and position
  - manufacturer, type, diameter, length
  - tip position
- Equipment and supplies used
- Procedure time
- Type and adequacy of anesthesia/sedation/analgesia
- Procedural complications (e.g., pneumothorax, bleeding) and management
- Adjunctive procedures (e.g., intracavitary tPA, dose, dwell time)
- Complications (major or minor), including
  1. Procedure-related discomfort (include dates)
     a. type
     b. management (e.g., NSAIDs, narcotics)
     c. outcome
  2. Pulmonary complications (include dates)
     a. type (e.g., air leak, fistula, dissemination of pathology)
     b. method of diagnosis
     c. management (e.g., observation, intervention, surgery)
     d. outcome
  3. Bleeding and vascular injury (include dates)
     a. type (e.g., hemorrhage, hemothorax, arteriovenous (AV) fistula, or pseudoaneurysm)
     b. method of diagnosis (e.g., hemoglobin, CT scan, arteriogram)
     c. management (e.g., observation, transfusion, embolization)
     d. outcome
  4. Dislodgment or malposition (include dates)
     a. method of diagnosis or documentation
     b. management
     c. outcome
- Other procedure-related complications or interventions
- Outcome at follow-up (method and date; endpoint achieved?)
  - postprocedural lab studies (e.g., fluid pH, culture, or biopsy findings)
  - response (e.g., reduction in fever, dyspnea, debilitation, discomfort)
  - results (e.g., daily volume of fluid drained, radiographic evidence of resolution, hospital days)
  - treatment failure (e.g., residual pleural "peel", recurrent pneumothorax)
  - change in pulmonary function

incomplete, or the fluid is thick, viscid, loculated, or fibrinous (see "Adjunctive transcatheter therapies in the thorax," below). The catheter is left in place until all significant drainage has stopped (less than 10 ml/day), and resolution or significant improvement of signs and symptoms has been achieved.

An important and desirable endpoint of therapy is re-expansion of the associated lung and re-establishment of normal pulmonary function. Failure to observe the lung re-expand may indicate restriction by an organized pleural peel, intrinsic lung disease, presence of an endobronchial lesion, ineffective drainage (Figure 3.3d), or airway compression by an extrinsic lesion.

Postprocedural lab studies

Because the fluid obtained at thoracentesis or thoracostomy tube placement is sampled from an otherwise normally sterile space, examination of the fluid may provide information necessary to make a diagnosis of the underlying abnormality. This sample should be handled with care, without inadvertent contamination or introduction of bacteriostatic agents (i.e., through mixture with bacteriostatic saline or contrast). A Gram stain of the sample should be performed and aliquots distributed to the microbiology laboratory for culture (e.g., aerobic and anaerobic bacterial, tuberculosis and fungal cultures), cell count, and differential analysis. Biochemical analysis should include pH, glucose, lactic dehydrogenase (LDH), protein, and amylase. Simultaneous serum pH, glucose, LDH, and protein should be determined. In the proper clinical setting, rheumatoid factor and antinuclear antibody titers may be helpful. Additional special lab studies may be indicated in specific clinical situations (e.g., adenosine deaminase and gamma-interferon in suspected TB; pleural fluid cytology in suspected pleural malignancy).

Complications

As with any drainage procedure, mechanical dysfunction is not uncommon, including catheter kinking, accidental dislodgment (Figure 3.3), iatrogenic suture ligation of the catheter, and inadvertent closure of valves or stopcocks. In our experience, serious complications occur in less than 2% of cases. The main risks of aspiration and drainage of the thorax include symptomatic pneumothorax, hemothorax, pyothorax, pyopneumothorax, pulmonary hemorrhage, injury to intercostal and other vessels, and contamination of the pleural space. Pleural contamination may occur when draining a lung or mediastinal abscess in the absence of pleurodesis. In spite of these risks, serious untoward effects infrequently occur.

Pneumothorax

Free communication between the pleural space or pulmonary perivascular space and the atmosphere, either from alveolar or chest wall trauma, allows for the development of air collections in the pulmonary interstitium (pulmonary interstitial emphysema), the hilum and mediastinal space (pneumomediastinum), or the intrapleural space (pneumothorax). From these spaces, air may dissect into the peritoneal cavity (pneumoperitoneum), the soft tissues (subcutaneous emphysema), or the pericardium (pneumopericardium). Massive continued air leak may lead to elevation of the pressure (tension) in the air-containing space. This may produce compression of vital structures, including the lungs, heart (tamponade), and major vessels, with concomitant cardiorespiratory compromise. Measures taken to improve ventilation in these patients often exacerbate the tension. Children with a small or asymptomatic air collection may be treated with 100% O_2 ("nitrogen washout"). This will produce a differential partial pressure in the air-containing space that should hasten its reabsorption, in the absence of continuing air leak.

In the face of a clinical situation consistent with tension pneumothorax with cardiorespiratory compromise, immediate decompression is essential. This is most easily accomplished empirically with a 16- to 20-gauge angiocatheter or needle advanced perpendicularly through the skin just superior to the second rib in the midclavicular line, without prior imaging or image guidance. Prompt radiographic confirmation should be sought after this procedure. If the patient is stable enough for preprocedure imaging, or if emergent needle aspiration is positive for air or fluid, a chest tube should be placed in the interventional suite under fluoroscopic guidance, using the same technique outlined above for drainage of pleural fluid. Percutaneous catheter placement enables safe and effective drainage of pneumothoraces with rapid restoration of vital capacity, oxygenation, and lung re-expansion. The catheter should be connected to an underwater seal and suction applied at –5 to –15 cm H_2O. Where loculated or multiloculated pneumothoraces or pneumatoceles are unstable or cause cardiopulmonary compromise, especially those located in regions technically difficult to reach by conventional approaches, CT guidance may offer a safe and accurate alternative for percutaneous placement of small-bore thoracostomy catheters.

Hemothorax

In the face of frank bleeding at the time of thoracostomy tube placement, transcatheter embolization or direct surgical repair of bleeding vessels should follow immediate vascular volume expansion. Most often, children developing a hemothorax require chest tube drainage to decompress the pressure effects and reduce the chance of future obliteration of the pleural space.

Chylothorax

Accumulation of chyle in the pleural space may cause life-threatening cardiopulmonary complications. This should be treated with immediate thoracentesis, repeated as necessary. Often, chylothorax will respond to a single thoracentesis with complete evacuation, followed by medical management directed at reducing chyle production and supporting nutritional losses. Direct surgical intervention may be avoided by embolization of the thoracic duct and any major collaterals guided by fluoroscopic pedal, or direct nodal, lymphangiography and cannulation of the cisterna chyli. Alternative methods of draining the thoracic duct to a neck port or to the esophagus are being explored in animal models. Surgical therapy may also be considered.

Conclusions

Image-guided aspiration and drainage is the treatment of choice for most abnormal fluid collections involving the pediatric thorax, eliminating or markedly reducing the need for open surgical or thoracoscopic intervention. With the use of image guidance, needles and catheters can be accurately and safely inserted into fluid collections in all compartments of the thorax. Adjunctive therapies, such as intracavitary fibrinolysis or pleurodesis (see below), further expand the scope of problems amenable to image-guided therapies. As is the case for other anatomic sites, percutaneous drainage may be used in lieu of or as an adjunct to surgical drainage. The use of these interventional techniques will likely reduce postprocedural morbidity, shorten hospital stays, and decrease costs in the pediatric population.

Adjunctive transcatheter therapies in the thorax

Introduction

The insertion of a drainage catheter in the pleural space or within a pathologic intrathoracic cavity (e.g., pulmonary abscess or necrotic tumor) provides the means for introduction of various adjunctive therapies. While simple pleural effusions can easily be treated with catheter drainage, complex pleural collections may require more intensive therapy, including instillation of fibrinolytic agents, in order to break up fibrinopurulent barriers and to decrease the viscosity of the fluid component. Similarly, a simple pneumothorax may be satisfactorily treated by suction applied through a catheter. However, patients with recurrent pneumothoraces may require more definitive therapy, such as chemical pleurodesis. Intracavitary chemotherapeutic treatments, such as delivery of antifungal and antineoplastic agents, are also possible using a preexisting catheter. In each case, successful adjunctive transcatheter therapies may avoid more invasive and costly alternatives. Intracavitary fibrinolysis serves as a prototypical transcatheter therapy and will be discussed in detail. Other transcatheter therapies will be briefly introduced.

Image-guided therapy, using US, fluoroscopy, or CT, alone or in combination, permits definition of, access to, and drainage of free or loculated empyemas with a high rate of success and substantially reduced risk. Preprocedure imaging, whether plain radiograph, CT, or US is poorly predictive of the likelihood of success of catheter drainage alone, although US provides the most accurate evaluation of the nature of the parapneumonic collection (anechoic, complex non-septated, or complex septated). Selecting the best therapeutic strategy for children with empyemas is a controversial decision and is often dependent on individual experience and preference. Although antibiotic therapy has significantly reduced the incidence of empyema associated with pneumonia, 50% of all empyemas are still a complication of bacterial pneumonia.

Adjunctive therapy with fibrinolytic enzymes may be used to decrease the viscosity of almost any type of proteinaceous collection and to improve drainage of loculated collections, thick pus, or blood. In 1949, Tillet and Sherry used streptokinase to treat fibrinous pleurisy, bacterial empyema, and hemothorax. One year later, Sherry and associates described the use of streptokinase and streptodornase for treatment of loculated hemothorax and empyema. Since then, many others have reported the use of streptokinase for the treatment of empyema, thereby avoiding a thoracotomy. However, the use of intracavitary thrombolytic agents did not gain favor until Vogelzang and colleagues reported the first use of urokinase (UK) for the treatment of infected extravascular hematomas. Hemorrhagic complications with intracavitary fibrinolysis have been reported, but are rare. In 1989, Moulton and associates reported their experience with intracavitary UK for the treatment of loculated pleural collections. This report and others have led to the use of adjunctive fibrinolysis in the pediatric population. When UK was temporarily removed from the market, other thrombolytic agents, especially tPA, gained widespread use for intracavitary thrombolysis. Our experience and that of others with the intrapleural instillation of fibrinolytic agents has shown that it is a good alternative to surgery during the acute phase, prior to organization of the pleural fluid collection.

Multiloculated fibrinopurulent empyemas and fibrinous effusions are difficult to treat because of the difficulty lysing the internal fibrin septations. In the past, this limited the efficacy of tube drainage, often necessitating operative intervention or the insertion of large-bore chest tubes. When percutaneous drainage with smaller tubes (≤ 8 French) was performed and septations were identified, the interventionalist would try to mechanically lyse the septations by maneuvering a guide wire within the pleural space, flushing with saline to unplug the catheter, or inserting multiple drains into the major loculations. In spite of these approaches, complete and prompt drainage of complex collections was often not accomplished, leading to prolonged hospitalization with or without surgery for decortication. Currently, tPA is the lytic agent of choice and is well tested with good results in children.

Indications

In the pediatric population, the indications and contraindications for the use of intracavitary thrombolytic agents are somewhat arbitrary since limited prospective studies have been performed. In our opinion, the use of fibrinolytic therapy (Figure 3.5) is indicated during stage 1 of a pleural effusion, especially if there is fibrinous pleural fluid, hemothorax, collections draining more slowly than anticipated, thick or viscid fluid collections, or children in whom imaging suggests thin septations within the pleural space (Light stage 2) (Table 3.5). Patients known to have a thickened visceral pleural peel, pleural fluid pH <7.2, LDH >1,000, or glucose <40 mg/dl may be considered for early referral for surgical management although some pediatric interventionalists recommend that all children, regardless of the stage, be treated with percutaneous drainage and those with stage 2 or 3 effusions also receive a trial of intracavitary fibrinolysis. Then, only those children who fail therapy should be referred for VATS. At this time, there are no prospective studies to turn to for guidance.

Intracavitary thrombolytic therapy may be contraindicated in children with a known sensitivity to the fibrinolytic agent, recent intrapleural or intracavitary bleeding, children who have had major thoracic or abdominal surgery within ten days, a history of hemorrhagic stroke, intracranial neoplasm, cranial surgery or head trauma within 14 days, and in the presence of a bronchopleural fistula, to avoid recurrent hemorrhage or reopening of the fistulous connection. Moulton and colleagues recommend at least a three-day wait before intracavitary instillation of thrombolytic agents after an intrapleural bleed. Although we have worried about the potential of systemic effects, several studies have suggested that intracavitary instillation of fibrinolytic agents does not result in a systemic fibrinolytic effect. To date, we have not identified adverse effects resulting from intracavitary fibrinolysis of complicated pleural effusions in children. Also, there has been no prospective study to investigate the incidence of uncovering a bronchopleural fistulae with fibrinolytic agents, although we have seen instances of this complication.

Chemical pleurodesis is indicated to treat chronic or recurrent air leaks, such as occur in patients with recurrent spontaneous pneumothorax, cavitary pneumonias, or chronic

Table 3.5 Indications for adjunctive transcatheter therapies in the thorax

Indication:
1. For drainage of a pleural (parapneumonic) fluid collection, if:
   a. acute collection (Light stage 1), or
   b. fibrinopurulent collection (Light stage 2)
   c. trial of therapy for organized collection (Light stage 3)
2. To decrease viscosity of thick pus or blood, including infected hematoma
3. To assist drainage of complex, loculated, or septated collections
4. Treatment of infectious or neoplastic disease, e.g.:
   a. bacterial or fungal infection – antibiotic or antifungal
   b. malignant effusion – antineoplastic
   c. echinococcal cyst – antiparasitic and sclerosant
   d. thoracic lymphocele – sclerosant

Contraindications:
1. Uncorrected coagulopathy or known bleeding diathesis
2. Frank blood return from chest tube, or recent intrapleural or intracavitary hemorrhage
3. Major thoracic or abdominal surgery within ten days
4. Hemorrhagic stroke, intracranial neoplasm, cranial surgery or head trauma within 14 days
5. Active or recent bronchopleural fistula
6. Thickened visceral pleural peel (Light stage 3)

obstructive pulmonary disease. It may also be useful in patients with symptomatic malignant pleural effusions that have previously responded to thoracentesis. A similar approach has been described for ethanol sclerosis of pericardial cysts. Directly instilling antifungal agents into the pleural space or cavity may be considered when fungal pneumonias are associated with evidence of chest wall, cavitary pulmonary disease, or pleural involvement. For example, amphotericin B has been instilled in the pleural space for treatment of aspergillus and pulmonary mucormycosis, with variable results.

Technique
Equipment
With a preexisting intrapleural catheter in place, no special equipment is required for adjuvant therapies.

Patient preparation
If the use of inflammatory agents is contemplated during intracavitary therapy, pain management specialists may be of assistance during and following the procedure in order to avoid unduly severe or prolonged patient discomfort.

Standard technique
Intracavitary fibrinolysis
Our current approach to intracavitary fibrinolysis in children follows the approach described in the adult literature, as

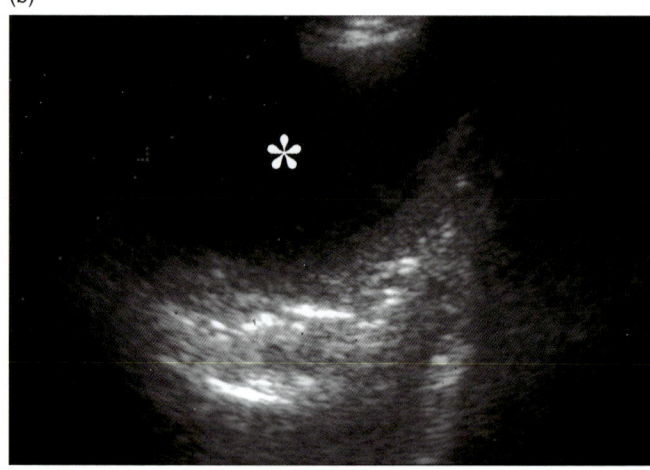

Figure 3.5 (a) A PA chest radiograph of a 4.5-year-old boy with pneumonia shows a right pleural fluid collection. (b) Ultrasound examination prior to thoracostomy tube drainage assisted by fibrinolysis reveals a 10.9 cm loculated fluid collection (*asterisk*) that is anechoic except for subtle internal septations.

Table 3.6 Procedural summary: intracavitary fibrinolysis

1. Chest radiograph or chest CT for diagnosis and planning
2. Sedate or anesthetize child
3. Chest drain insertion
4. Inject tPA 2 to 5 mg in 50 to 150 ml of normal saline depending on patient size
5. Clamp drain for one to three hours
6. Gravity drainage, suction device, or wall suction at −20 cm H_2O
7. Follow-up chest radiograph or chest CT
8. Repeat treatment as needed or use twice-daily approach

modified for children (Table 3.6). Given the intermittent availability of UK, we now use tPA, 5 mg dissolved in 25 to 150 ml sterile saline, as appropriate to the volume of the pleural space. If UK is used, up to 250,000 U may be dissolved in 250 ml sterile normal saline. The optimal volume of fluid injected appears to relate to distribution of the agent in the pleural space. Therefore the unit dose of fibrinolytic should be delivered in a volume sufficient to achieve adequate distribution without compromising cardiopulmonary function.

After instillation of a volume appropriate to the size of the patient, divided among the drainage tubes if multiple loculations are being treated simultaneously, the chest tube is clamped for a minimum of one hour during which time the patient is asked to change position frequently in order to bathe the entire pleural surface in the solution. Fluid is then aspirated, the net output recorded, and the catheter reopened to suction drainage. After one hour of drainage (−20 cm H_2O) the process may be repeated two to four times daily. Although some grossly bloody output may be observed without clinical significance, active bleeding into the pleural space is considered an absolute contraindication to intracavitary fibrinolysis.

Chemical pleurodesis

Chemical pleurodesis provides a means to treat recurrent pneumothoraces or persistent air leak when conventional therapy has failed. This often includes children with spontaneous pneumothorax as well as pneumothoraces secondary to a variety of conditions such as congenital cystic lung disease, barotrauma, diffuse lung disease, connective tissue disease, and some metastatic neoplasms. Spontaneous pneumothorax has a high rate of recurrence in patients over nine years of age. Because children under nine years of age have a lower rate of recurrence, they may be safely managed conservatively. Tube thoracostomy offers a minimally invasive therapy for simple pneumothorax but is less often effective in preventing recurrence of spontaneous pneumothorax and its related complications (e.g., air leak, contralateral spontaneous pneumothorax, and tension pneumothorax). Definitive therapy involves obliteration of the potential space by obtaining permanent apposition of the two pleural layers (i.e., pleurodesis). The same approach can be applied to recurrent pleural effusions refractory to other forms of treatment. This may be achieved by a variety of methods including open thoracostomy with apical pleurectomy, mechanical pleurodesis (gauze or brush abrasion), pleural irritation with laser or cautery, or chemical pleurodesis via instillation of an inflammatory agent into the pleural space.

Open surgical pleurodesis is associated with significant morbidity, including prolonged hospital stay, bleeding, and chronic postoperative pain. In the past decade, VATS has become an alternative to open thoracotomy for the performance of mechanical pleurodesis. Closed tube drainage with transcatheter instillation of chemical sclerosants offers a minimally invasive alternative for the prevention of recurrent pneumothorax or effusion and has been performed using a variety of inflammatory agents, including talc, doxycycline, bleomycin, acromycin, tetracycline, OK-432, autologous blood patch, silver nitrate, olive oil, fibrin glue, and other agents. Of these, talc has been the most effective agent in our experience. Approximately 2 to 4 g of sterile talc may be suspended in 100 ml normal saline and injected into the pleural space. Alternatively, 500 mg doxycycline may be mixed in 100 ml normal saline, or 60 IU bleomycin may be mixed in 100 ml of 5% dextrose in water (D_5W) and the solution instilled into the pleural space. The pleurodesis agent is allowed to remain in the pleural space for one hour, after which the catheter is returned to water suction for at least 24 hours.

Re-administration on the second and third treatment days is frequently required. The pleural space should be prepared by pre-administration of 20 ml of 0.25% bupivacaine into the pleural space, 20 to 30 minutes prior to instillation of the pleurodesis agent. Deep sedation or general anesthesia is required during the period so that the pleurodesis agent remains in the pleural space, as the resulting inflammation can be acute and painful. Once the agent is evacuated, the painful stimulus usually recedes quickly. No single method or agent is perfectly reliable, but the recurrence rate following pleurodesis by whatever method is significantly lower than thoracostomy without pleurodesis. Transcatheter chemical pleurodesis can be as effective, safe, and rapid as surgical alternatives, especially in patients with bullae <2 cm in diameter. Long-term sequelae may include recurrence, pain, pleural thickening, and fibrothorax.

Postprocedure and follow-up care

It may be helpful to both patient care and ongoing quality assurance to maintain pertinent demographic and procedure-related data in an electronic database. Suggested items for data management are included in Table 3.4. The result of treatment is monitored by chest radiographs and intermittent chest CT. A chest CT is useful in gauging the effects of therapy. If loculated fluid remains, the procedure may be repeated, additional drains inserted, or the patient may be referred for surgical debridement. No studies are yet available that outline the optimal approach to therapy. If no significant residual remains, the patient would be maintained on suction until they were asymptomatic with less than 10 ml of drainage over a 24-hour period. At this point the chest tube(s) are removed.

Complications

Potential complications associated with adjunctive therapy usually relate to the primary procedure (i.e., catheter insertion). Bleeding complications are rare, but fibrinolytics should be held in the face of frank bleeding or recent surgery. Occasionally, intracavitary fibrinolysis may uncover a previously occult bronchopleural fistula. Treatment failure may be seen in late stage 2 and stage 3 disease, including the inability to evacuate viscid material and intractable pleural thickening. These children may best be treated by early referral for surgical intervention.

Conclusions

Clearly, a delay in the definitive therapy of childhood empyema carries a significant risk for an unfavorable outcome, including recurrent empyema with lung abscess, scoliosis, restrictive lung disease, bronchopleural fistula, sympathetic pericardial effusion, and septicemia. However, it remains unclear which definitive therapeutic intervention, catheter drainage with early intracavitary fibrinolysis, VATS, or thoracotomy and decortication of both the parietal and visceral pleural peel, will prove to optimize outcome, cost, and resource allocation. In our opinion, aggressive closed chest interventions with early adjunctive intracavitary fibrinolysis should be attempted in parapneumonic effusions up to four to six weeks old. Later than this, it is likely that chronic inflammation and mature fibrous thickening (stage 3) will require VATS or other surgical approaches.

The dosage of fibrinolytic drug is arbitrary, and few prospective trials have been performed in either adults or children. Therefore the adult dose is usually used and either the volume of fluid infused is reduced proportional to patient size, thereby reducing the total drug dose, or the total drug dose is given in a smaller fluid volume. The latter approach is more frequently used in organizing effusions or those resistant to treatment. Catheter drainage with intracavitary fibrinolysis may obviate need for thoracoscopic or surgical pleural drainage techniques.

Intrathoracic abscesses

Introduction

Before the advent of antibiotic therapy, a lung abscess was a common outcome of pneumonia in children. Prior to the availability of percutaneous management, pulmonary abscess in children with pneumonia or other preexisting conditions caused greater than 90% mortality. With advances in antibiotic therapy, it has become a rare complication, most commonly related to *Staphylococcus* or *Haemophilus influenzae*. In an otherwise healthy child, pulmonary abscess is usually a solitary lesion, tending to occur early in the course of disease while the patient is clinically ill. Multiple scattered abscesses are usually due to septic emboli from bacterial endocarditis. The high prevalence of immunologic impairment in children presenting with a pulmonary abscess increases the risk of a poor outcome and the urgency for prompt intervention.

Complications of an untreated lung abscess may include compression of vital structures, cardiorespiratory compromise, spontaneous rupture with spread of infection to other parts of the lung, disseminated sepsis, and death. Chest CT is usually helpful in the identification of multiple abscesses, in the distinction of lung abscess from emphysema, in the characterization of the intrinsic nature of the abscess and its proximity to the pleura, and in the evaluation of a safe access window for percutaneous drainage. Good results have also been achieved in the percutaneous treatment of mediastinal, chest wall, and intraparenchymal abscesses. Most loculated abscesses (Figure 3.6), regardless of their location, require some form of drainage. In older children, lung abscesses often respond to chest physiotherapy or to transbronchial aspiration. However, children less than seven years of age are unlikely to drain spontaneously and require more aggressive therapy.

Successful percutaneous diagnosis and treatment of intrapulmonary abscesses can be achieved in children. Lacey and Koslosky have described the use of a local pneumonostomy (mini-thoracostomy) to drain peripheral lung abscesses in children who have failed to respond to medical management. Their success was aided by the presence of pleurodesis (fusion of the visceral and parietal pleural layers) adjacent to the abscess. Since approximately 90% of lesions abut a pleural surface, pleurodesis often facilitates percutaneous drainage of lung abscesses. Creation of the catheter tract through a region of pleurodesis prevents inadvertent contamination of the pleural space and progression to empyema and minimizes the risk of a pneumothorax. Centrally located intraparenchymal abscesses still represent a management problem and may require a thoracotomy and wedge resection for treatment. With the precise anatomic localization available with CT, these collections can now be considered for percutaneous therapy in most instances. Each case should be considered individually and the treatment tailored to each situation.

Indications

As in adults, abscess formation in children most commonly results from aspiration of mouth flora. However, lung abscesses in younger children are less likely to drain spontaneously or to respond to antibiotics. The presence of congenital or acquired immune disorders, impairment of normal protective mechanisms, prematurity, endocarditis, cerebral palsy, poor oral hygiene, or congenital pulmonary abnormalities such as sequestration may result in a predisposition to chronic or recurrent aspiration, or to an extensive or severe bronchopneumonia due to staphylococcal or Gram-negative organisms. Arising from ineffective clearance of infective

Chapter 3 Thoracic interventions

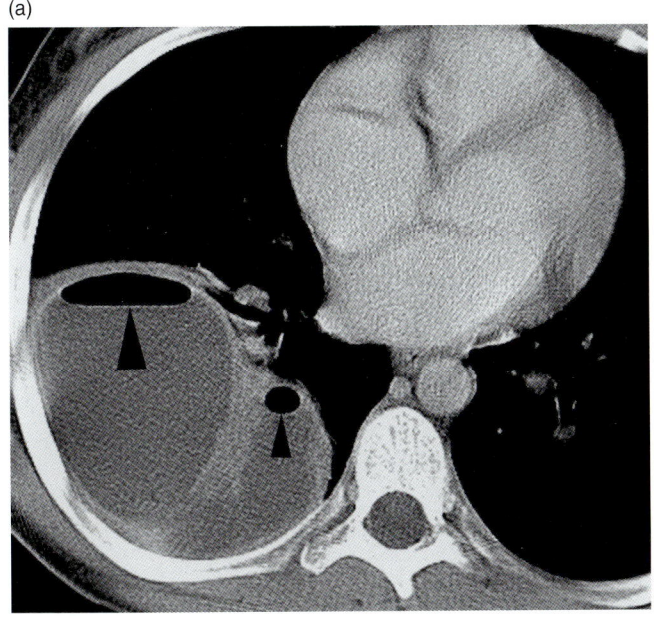

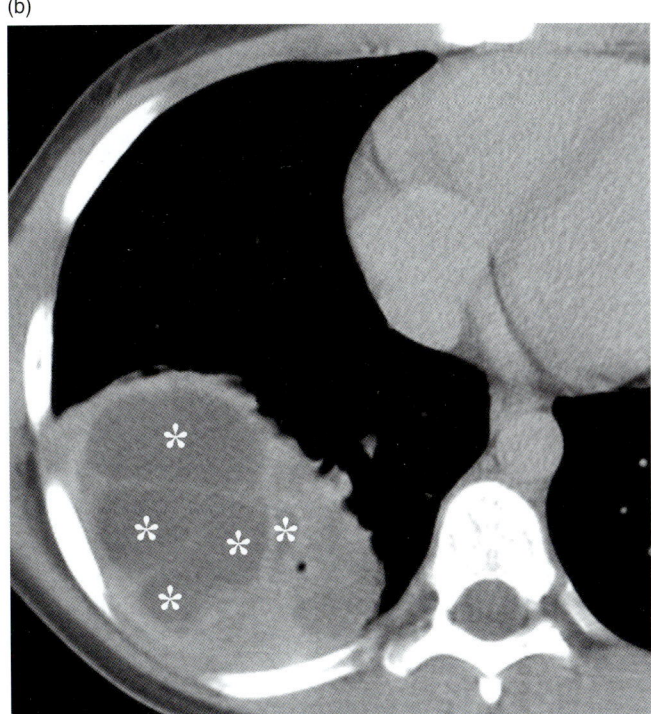

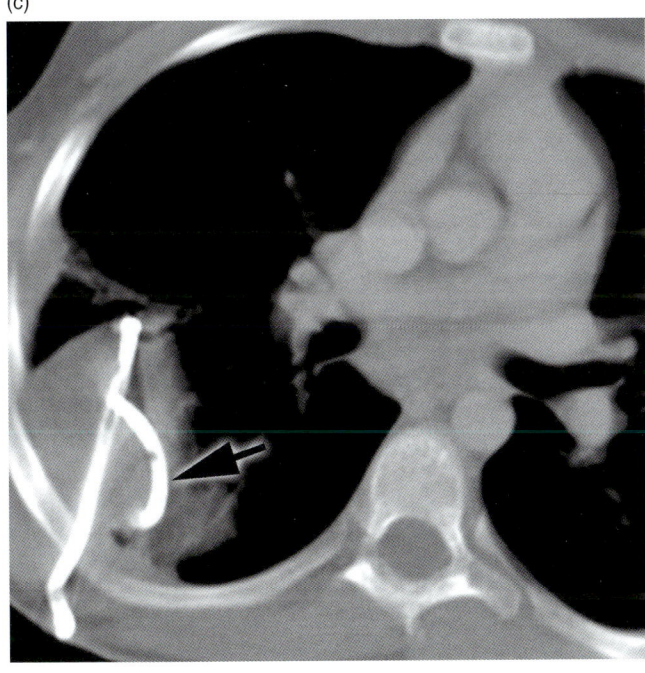

Figure 3.6 (a) This 12-year-old girl presented with a five-day history of fever and cough. A contrast-enhanced axial CT image of the thorax demonstrates a multiloculated right middle lobe abscess containing non-dependent gas collections (*arrowheads*). (b) A second axial CT image through the same collection suggests that multiple internal septations divide this collection into several loculated compartments (*asterisks*). (c) A postprocedure supine axial CT image demonstrates partial evacuation and collapse of the cavity. Despite its loculated appearance, mechanical disruption of the internal septations allowed the entire collection to be successfully drained through a single locking pigtail catheter (*arrow*). Samples obtained at the time of insertion grew non-typable *Haemophilus influenzae*. The 10 French drainage catheter was removed on the fifth postprocedure day.

organisms or incomplete treatment of pneumonia, a phlegmonous consolidation of infected lung parenchyma may progress to necrosis and formation of a circumscribed cavity containing necrotic parenchyma and purulent fluid.

Once it drains through a bronchial communication, a mature lung abscess may have the classic imaging appearance of an enhancing (or echogenic) thick-walled (5–15 mm), irregular cavity (2–20 cm in diameter), filled with variable amounts of fluid and air, forming an acute angle with the pleura (Figure 3.7). This appearance is not specific. The differential diagnosis of pulmonary cavities in children includes pulmonary abscess, loculated empyema, traumatic pseudocyst, pneumatocele, echinococcal cyst, solitary (congenital) cyst, adenomatoid malformation, cavitary tuberculosis, cavitating pneumonia (cavitary necrosis), cavitating hematoma, cavitating infarct, foregut cysts, cystadenomatous malformation and sequestration, and lymphangioma of the lung. Under certain circumstances (such as an inability to mount a normal

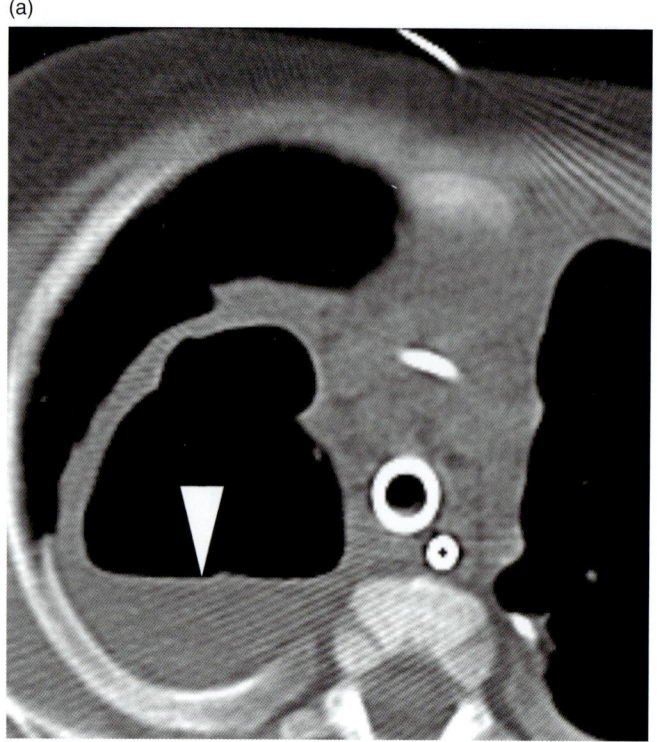
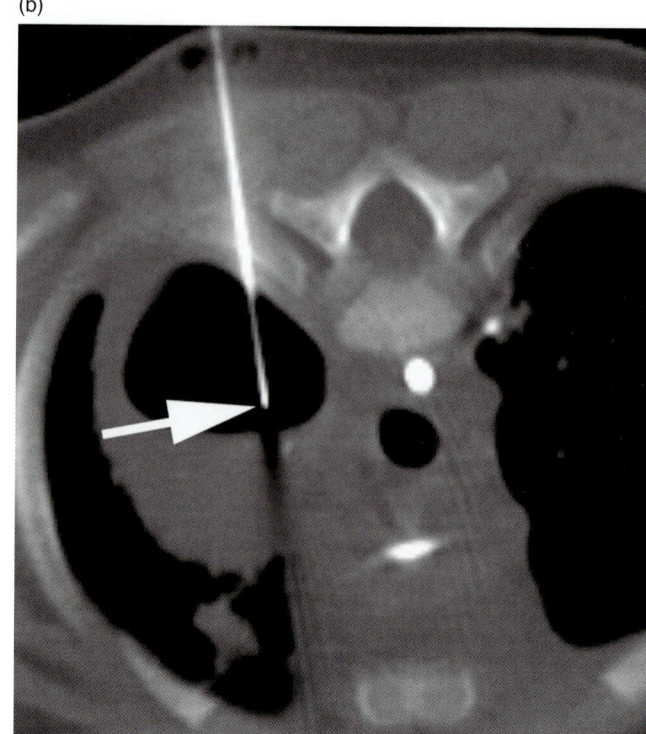
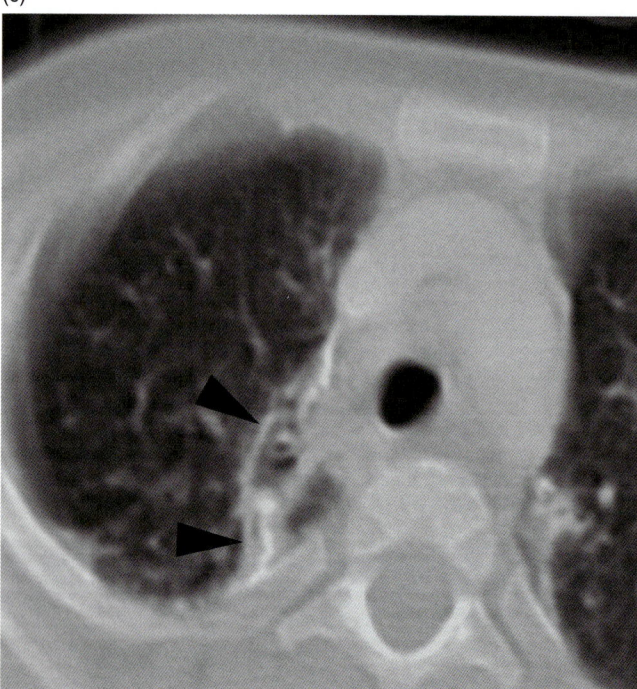

Figure 3.7 (a) Four-year-old girl with a surfactant deficiency who has had a lung transplant now demonstrates a right upper lobe pneumatocele on this unenhanced axial CT image through the thorax. The pneumatocele developed a bronchopleural fistula with a gas–fluid level (*arrowhead*). (b) Under CT guidance in a prone position, access to the collection is achieved with a 19-gauge needle (*arrow*). 2 ml of fluid was aspirated. Microbiologic examination demonstrated *Pseudomonas aeruginosa*. (c) After drainage through an 8.5-French Dawson–Mueller drainage catheter and appropriate antibiotics, a follow-up CT image nine months later shows interval resolution of the bronchopleural fistula and the fluid collection, with residual pleural scarring and calcification (*arrowheads*).

inflammatory response in the immunocompromised patient), a pulmonary abscess may not be surrounded by a thick wall, may not cavitate, or may become grossly distended with air.

A parapneumonic pulmonary collection of known bacterial origin and imaging features characteristic of an abscess, as well as a cavity larger than 3 cm in diameter and a location abutting a region of pleurodesis without overlying aerated lung, is an ideal candidate for percutaneous drainage (Table 3.7). Abscesses that are centrally located, multiple, fungal, progress despite catheter drainage, or develop persistent bronchopleural fistula are particularly challenging and may be candidates for a combined interventional and surgical approach, including thoracostomy and surgical resection. Aspiration through a thin (e.g., 18- to

Table 3.7 Indications for percutaneous treatment of intrathoracic abscess

Indications
- Pulmonary abscess (abscesses >3 cm, especially those abutting the pleura or subjacent to pulmonary consolidation)
- Chest wall and mediastinal abscesses
- Thoracic pancreatic pseudocyst

Contraindications
- Uncorrectable coagulopathy
- Platelet count <50,000 (unable to correct)
- Unsafe access route
- Fungal disease (controversial)

Table 3.8 Procedure summary: intrathoracic and mediastinal abscess drainage

1. Preprocedural work-up (include CT with contrast)
2. Route planning. Mark entry site on the skin surface
3. Sterile preparation and draping
4. Locally anesthetize entry site
5. Small skin incision
6. Image-guided (CT or US) puncture
7. Move to fluoroscopy suite if necessary to monitor remainder of procedure
8. Insert guide wire and coil within cavity
9. Dilate tract
10. Insert locking pigtail catheter
11. Secure catheter to patient
12. Apply a dry, sterile dressing
13. Consider Pleur-evac® set to –20 cm H_2O

22-gauge Chiba or sheathed) needle (Figure 3.7b) is sometimes considered for diagnosis of a presumed fluid collection of uncertain etiology or for evacuation of a collection too small (i.e., less than 3 cm) to hold a drainage catheter, too deeply located, or with too much overlying aerated lung to be safely drained.

As Lee and colleagues demonstrated in a neonatal series, aspiration alone can be curative with minimal risk. However, aspiration alone is substantially less likely to be curative in infected collections large enough to accept the pigtail of a drainage catheter. Unless they can be shown to interconnect, multiple abscesses or multilocular collections may require a separate drain for each locule. All collections should be either drained or aspirated and separate samples sent from each for microbiologic analysis to help select the most appropriate antibiotic coverage. If any discrete collections cannot be safely accessed, surgical incision and drainage may be indicated.

Absolute contraindications to abscess drainage include an uncorrectable bleeding diathesis or unsafe route for drainage. In select cases, fluid collections in these patients may be safely aspirated. A suspected fungal abscess, which can be quite invasive, may be considered a relative contraindication to percutaneous drainage, although some advocate for percutaneous evacuation of intrapulmonary mycetomas. Usually, surgically treated fungal abscesses are preferentially resected rather than drained. Local adjuvant therapy with intracavitary instillation of antifungal agents may provide a viable therapeutic alternative in select cases.

Technique

Equipment

The size, nature, and location of the collection must be identified as well as the safety of the access route guide catheter. Equipment for aspiration and drainage of intrathoracic abscesses is the same as that used in other thoracic collections, as presented in Table 3.2. A Seldinger technique is virtually always preferred over the trochar method.

Patient preparation

All patients have a contrast-enhanced CT scan prior to being referred for the procedure. Coagulation profiles and platelet counts are routinely performed in all patients. A platelet count of at least 50,000 is preferred for the procedure. Any coagulation abnormality is corrected if possible. Admission is planned for those patients with a history or laboratory values suggesting abnormal coagulation or with an ASA classification greater than 2. Procedures are performed under deep sedation with local anesthesia or under general anesthesia. General anesthesia is planned when medically indicated or for patients in whom respiratory control is needed for lesion stability. All patients are kept NPO according to relevant hospital sedation and anesthesia policy prior to the procedure.

Standard technique

A contrast-enhanced CT scan of the chest is most likely to demonstrate the number and character of pulmonary fluid collections, their relationship to vessels and other vital structures, and potential access routes (Table 3.8). If a lesion is in the lung periphery US guidance may be considered. Even if US guidance is contemplated, CT localization can define an optimal approach and suggest a likely sonographic window, and then can be used to confirm satisfactory placement at the end of the procedure. It can therefore be useful to have access to US in the CT suite.

If an adequate and sufficiently current preprocedure CT is available to characterize the collection and suggest an appropriate window, focused diagnostic US examination to confirm the presence of an appropriate sonographic route of access can be performed (Figure 3.8). In fact, for many pleural-based collections the entire procedure can be performed using US guidance, with final confirmation of tube position and function using fluoroscopy (Figure 3.9).

Otherwise, CT guidance must be employed. When CT is utilized, either the entire procedure is completed in the CT suite or, if necessary, the guide wire is coiled within the cavity

Chapter 3 Thoracic interventions

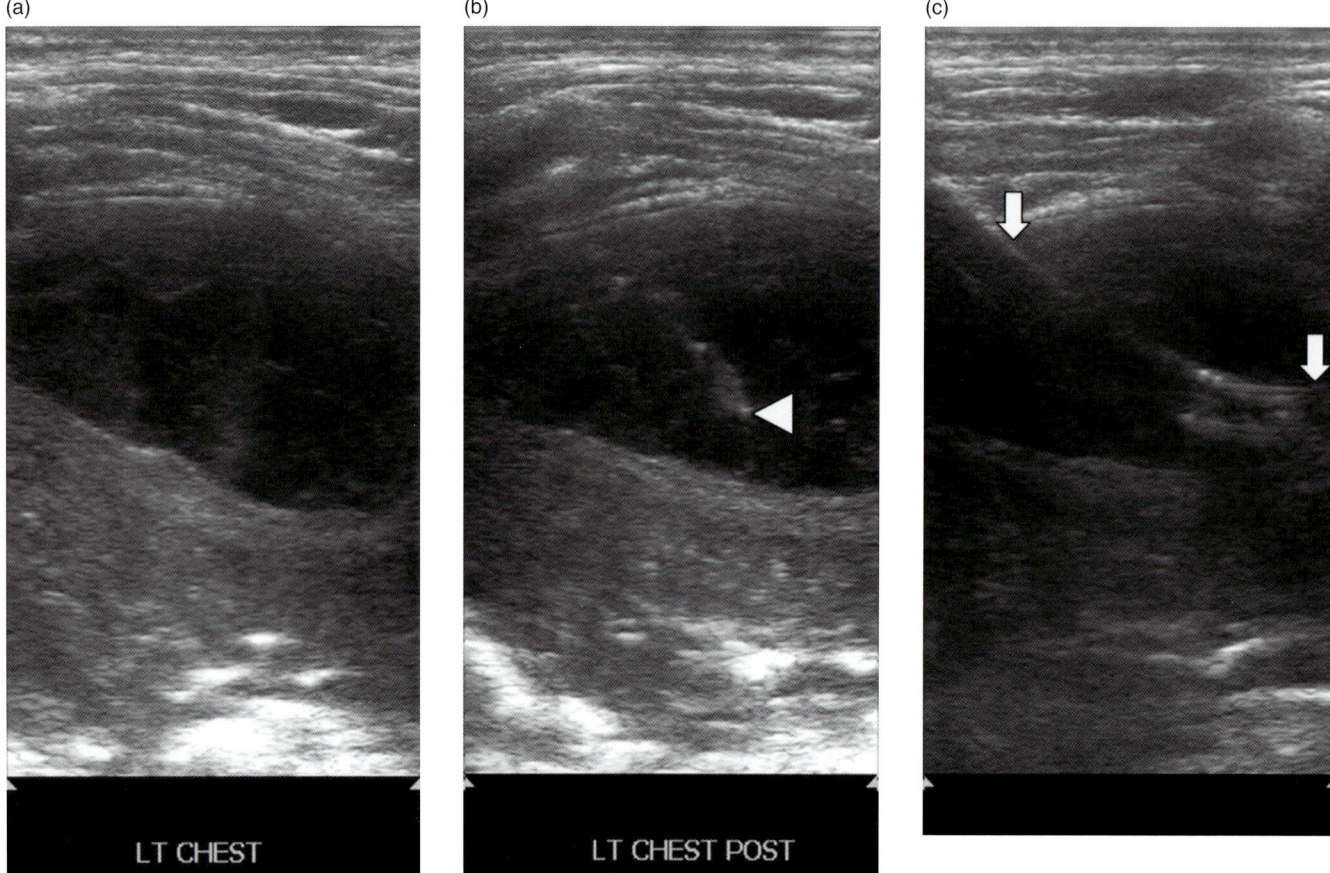

Figure 3.8 (a) Seven-year-old female with respiratory compromise and pain was found to have a left chest pleural-based elliptical fluid collection as demonstrated on this gray-scale US image using a high-frequency linear transducer. (b) Ultrasound-guided needle access was performed using a 5 French sheathed needle (*arrowhead*). (c) After tract dilation, an 8.5 French pigtail drainage catheter was advanced into the collection with postprocedure US showing catheter position (*arrows*).

and the patient is transported (while still sedated or anesthetized) to the interventional suite for completion of the procedure using fluoroscopic guidance. In practice, the latter is rarely necessary. Drainage of the abscess can be accomplished using either a Seldinger or trochar technique. Direct puncture with a trochar catheter is seldom used in our practice because there is little room for error in small infants and children, and a misdirected pass may result in injury to adjacent structures. However, this technique may be considered for children with superficial or large collections.

If a Chiba needle is selected for puncture of the abscess cavity (Table 3.9), a 0.018-inch guide wire (e.g., Glidewire®, Newton, Mandril) is inserted and coiled within the cavity. To exchange for a 0.035-inch or 0.038-inch guide wire, a coaxial introducer or micropuncture set can be used. The inner cannula and 0.018-inch guide wire are removed and exchanged for a stiff, non-kinkable 0.035-inch or 0.038-inch (e.g., Glidewire®, Amplatz®, Roadrunner®) guide wire.

There are now a variety of guide wires that are helpful. Amplatz Stiff® and Superstiff®, Roadrunner®, Rosen and nitinol guide wires are available in sizes ranging from 0.018-inch to 0.038-inch and lengths from 60 cm and longer. These stiff, kink-resistant guide wires are important in cases in which a 0.018-inch guide wire is used because of the inability to deform the guide wire. When a guide wire kink occurs, positioning of a catheter is considerably more difficult and time consuming and may lead to loss of target access. In older and obese children, these guide wires are also helpful because of their kink resistance and the support they provide, enabling easier and faster tract dilation and catheter insertion. One caveat, however; it may be difficult to coil a stiff guide wire within an abscess cavity, especially one of small diameter. In addition, there is a greater tendency for the guide wire to spring out of the cavity if it is not held in position at skin level. To reduce the opportunity for wire loss, we often will secure the wire at skin level with a hemostat when making exchanges. Thus, in these situations, it may be best to compromise and use a less stiff guide wire to avoid rupture of the cavity or loss of guide wire position.

Postprocedure and follow-up care

Pertinent details of the procedure are recorded in the patient's chart and orders entered (e.g., regarding management of the

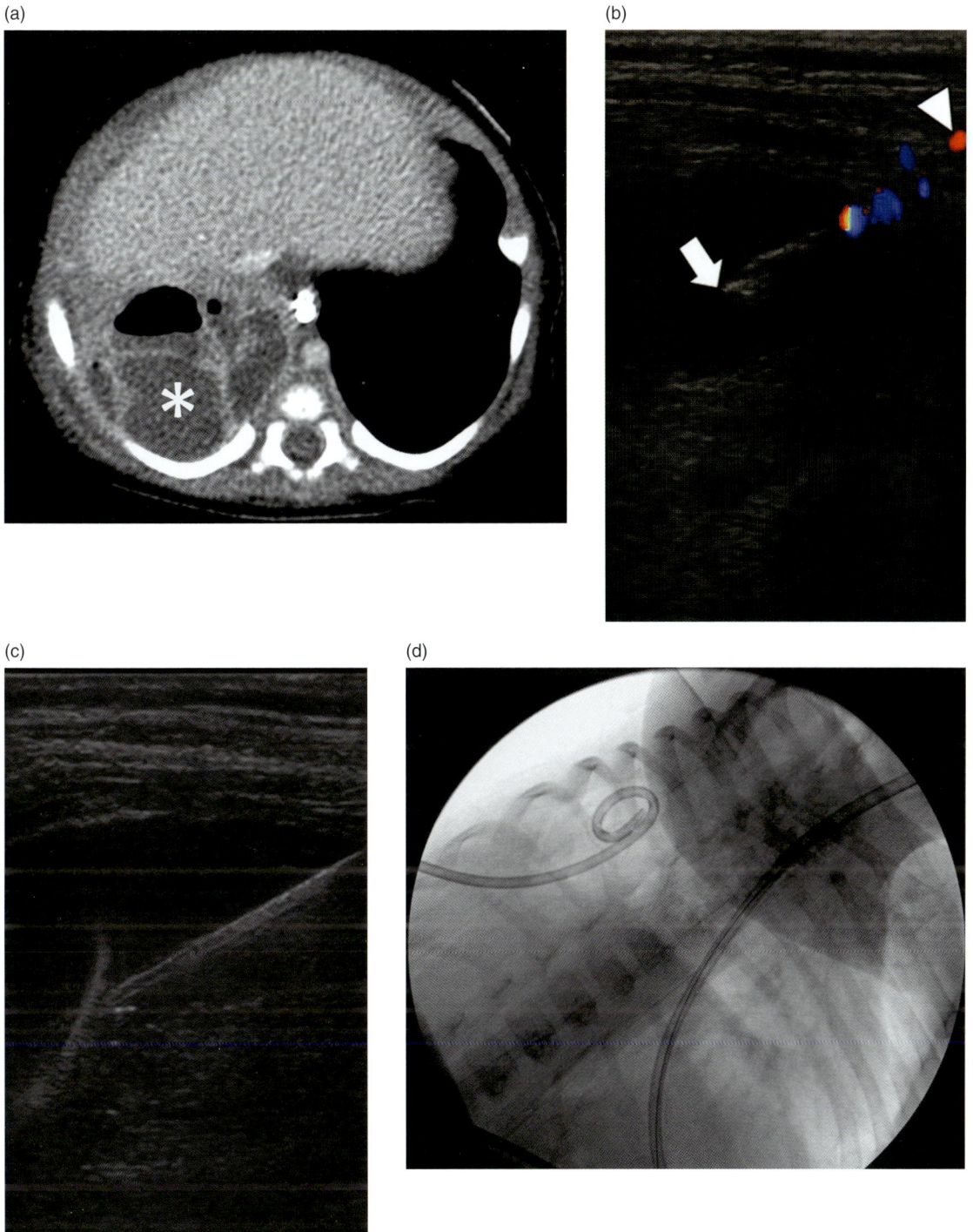

Figure 3.9 (a) Preprocedure chest CT with vascular contrast in this three-month-old female shows a right-sided light stage 2 parapneumonic effusion with an associated multiloculated abscess (*asterisk*). Air in the collection suggests the possibility of a spontaneous bronchopleural fistula. (b) With the patient in a left-side-down decubitus position, a 7 cm 5 French Yueh centesis needle (*arrow*) was used to access the abscess collection. Color Doppler imaging was used to assist avoidance of the subcostal artery (*arrowhead*) in the narrow infantile intercostal space. (c) Under continuous US guidance, the stylet was exchanged for a 0.035-inch stiff Amplatz® wire (*shown*), over which a 7 French Dawson–Mueller pigtail catheter was advanced with its stiffener. (d) The stiffener and guide wire were removed, and the drainage catheter formed and locked. 50 ml of thick, purulent, blood-tinged fluid was aspirated. Aspiration of air confirmed the bronchopleural fistula. The abscess and effusion resolved without sequelae with tube thoracostomy drainage alone.

catheter and any suction devices). It may be helpful to both patient care and ongoing quality assurance to maintain pertinent demographic and procedure-related data in an electronic database. Suggested items for data management are included in Table 3.4. When there is no communication with the tracheobronchial tree, drainage of large mediastinal or pulmonary abscesses may be assisted (Figure 3.10) with a Hemovac®, while a bulb suction device (e.g., Jackson Pratt) is used for

Table 3.9 Equipment for percutaneous treatment of intrathoracic and mediastinal abscess

- Chlorhexidine gluconate (0.5%) with 70% isopropyl alcohol solution skin prep
- Sterile US cover
- Angiocatheter, 16- to 22-gauge or Yueh disposable catheter needle (4 and 5 French, with side holes) or Chiba highliter needle, 22-gauge (5, 10 or 15-cm)
- Neff introducer system
- Coaxial end hole introducer system
- All purpose drains, 6 to 14 French or Thalquick drainage catheter, 12 to 24 French or Duan drainage catheter with 1 cm loop for neonates/small infants, 5 French
- Dilators, 5 French to 22 French (Coons, standard vascular)
- Abscess drainage bag, Pleur-evac®, Hemovac®
- Adhesive bandage
- Catheter retention device: SorbaView®, StatLock®, Hollister®, tape bridge

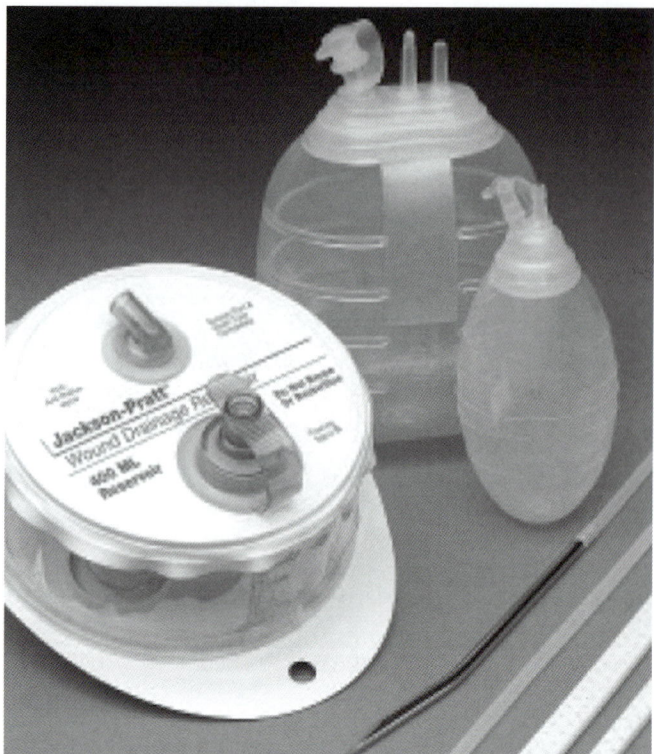

Figure 3.10 Suction devices. A Hemovac® suction drain (*lower left*) is used to assist drainage of larger collections, while Jackson–Pratt bulb suction devices (*upper right*, (both from Medline Industries, Mudelein, IL)) are used for smaller collections.

smaller collections. If an associated bronchopleural fistula or pneumothorax is present, a Pleur-evac® is used with –20 to –30 cm H_2O suction pressure to aid fistula closure. If closure cannot be achieved after several weeks of drainage, a surgical consultation is obtained. Outpatients are routinely admitted if significant or symptomatic postprocedural complications (i.e., large or tension pneumothorax or substantial bleeding) are identified.

Irrigation of the catheter is performed at least twice per day when thick or viscous fluid is noted but not routinely for thin fluid. In addition, intracavitary thrombolytic agents are considered as an adjunctive therapy when there is poor drainage or the fluid is thick, viscid, loculated, or fibrinous. The catheter is left in place until all significant drainage has stopped (less than 10 ml/day) and resolution or significant improvement of signs and symptoms has been achieved. For children with pulmonary or mediastinal abscesses, a contrast injection is performed before catheter removal or when the postdrainage course is atypical to document cavity size, catheter position, and to look for possible fistulous communications or undrained collections. Chest CT may be performed to document interval change or resolution of the abscess.

Contrast material is injected slowly until the cavity is filled and contrast begins to reflux along the catheter tract indicating that the cavity is completely filled. Fluoroscopic spot images are then taken in one or more projections. If drainage persists for more than two to three days, the volume of drainage remains high, or symptoms persist, repeat chest CT is performed. The catheter is left in place until all significant drainage has stopped (less than 10 ml/day) and resolution or significant improvement of signs and symptoms has been achieved.

Complications

Complications associated with the percutaneous management of pulmonary abscesses in children include catheter dislodgment, chest pain, hemorrhage or hemothorax, infection of other compartments (e.g., aspiration pneumonia, empyema), bronchopleural fistula, pneumothorax, abscess recurrence, and ongoing or overwhelming sepsis. Serious complications related to catheter drainage of pulmonary abscesses are infrequent in the pediatric population.

Conclusions

Percutaneous management of pulmonary abscesses refractory to conservative therapy has been shown to be safe, simple, and efficacious in most circumstances. The goals of therapy include resolution of the infection (cure), stabilization of the patient (palliation), or facilitation of a definitive procedure (temporization). Failure to achieve these goals is usually avoidable. The first element of success is appropriate patient selection. Patients with an infected hematoma, infected necrotic tumor, phlegmon or necrotizing pneumonia are less likely to respond to catheter drainage alone. In these patients, adjunctive therapies or surgical debridement may be necessary to achieve complete resolution.

Mediastinal and pericardial fluid collections

Introduction

In the past, mediastinal and pericardial fluid collections were primarily treated surgically. Depending on the location of the collection a thoracotomy, median sternotomy, suprasternal mediastinoscopy, or subxiphoid approach was often required for treatment. The principles used successfully for the percutaneous treatment of fluid collections elsewhere in the thorax have also been effectively applied for these collections.

Indications

Potential causes of mediastinal and pericardial fluid and gas collections are numerous and may represent any of a broad spectrum of traumatic, postsurgical, infectious, inflammatory, or congenital etiologies (Table 3.10). While the frequency of any single entity in pediatric practice is low, causes may include chest wall injury, infection, inflammation, neoplastic disease, pulmonary disease (e.g., pneumonia, asthma), uremia, descending necrotizing mediastinitis (a potentially life-threatening complication of an oropharyngeal infection), stab wound, iatrogenic esophageal perforation or Boerhaave syndrome, PTFE graft leak, mediastinitis, *Mycobacterium tuberculosis* (TB) infection, metabolic disease, lymphatic leak (e.g., idiopathic chylopericardium), mediastinal surgery (postpericardiotomy syndrome), or as a complication of central venous catheterization, congenital mediastinal cyst, or even thoracic pancreatic pseudocyst. Morbidity and mortality are high if treatment is not rapid and effective.

Widening of the mediastinum in the face of a retropharyngeal abscess or suitable surgical, infectious, or traumatic history should be considered as strong evidence of a mediastinal abscess for which the best therapeutic option is aggressive cervico-mediastinal and transthoracic drainage combined with broad-spectrum antimicrobial therapy. This may require a subxiphoid incision, debridement via a parasternal approach with resection of cervical fistula or a right thoracotomy, or perhaps VATS. Where marked improvement is achieved after retropharyngeal drainage, a minimally invasive, image-guided approach to the mediastinal abscess may be advised.

In the postoperative patient, fever, sternal tenderness, erythema, purulent drainage, and bone destruction may signal mediastinitis due to *Staphylococcus aureus*, coagulase-negative staphylococci, or gram-negative bacilli. Again, immediate and suitable drainage, debridement, and postoperative irrigation via a surgical incision should accompany appropriate antibiotic therapy.

The chronic accumulation of pericardial fluid may be reasonably well tolerated, while in the acute setting, even relatively small volumes of pericardial effusion may lead to rapid hemodynamic compromise and death. Patients with thoracic malignancy, postpericardiotomy syndrome, or other conditions with postoperative fluid accumulation or pericarditis may present with clinical deterioration or hemodynamic compromise secondary to tamponade, or may develop a large asymptomatic pericardial effusion. Pericardial fluid collections in children may be safely treated by aspiration alone or by pigtail catheter drainage under image guidance from either an intercostal or subxiphoid approach.

Certain patients will present with collections for percutaneous drainage that are not optimal for surgical management, with mediastinal abscesses (especially those that descend below the fourth thoracic vertebral level), as well as infected tumors and non-infected mediastinal or pericardial collections (Figure 3.11). Tailored use of techniques similar to those described elsewhere for drainage of abdominopelvic (see Chapter 4) and pulmonary (see above) collections should permit evacuation of most of these collections.

Technique

Equipment

Percutaneous treatment of mediastinal and pericardial fluid collections makes use of similar equipment and methods to those used for pleural collections (Table 3.9). In some cases

Table 3.10 Indications for mediastinal and pericardial drainage

Indications
- Abnormal fluid or gas collection due to congenital cystic lung disease
  - Congenital adenomatoid malformation
  - Bronchogenic cyst
  - Intrathoracic pancreatic pseudocyst
- Pneumomediastinum due to increased intrathoracic pressure
  - Asthma
  - Cystic fibrosis
  - Foreign body with air trapping
  - Bronchiolitis
- Abnormal fluid collection due to infection or postsurgical change
  - Mediastinal abscess
  - Broncho-mediastinal fistula
  - Peri-graft (e.g., Blalock–Taussig shunt) leakage
  - Intrathoracic lymphocele, hematoma, seroma
  - Reactive pericardial effusion
  - Pericardial tamponade
- Pneumomediastinum due to congenital diffuse pulmonary disease
  - Langerhans cell histiocytosis
  - Tuberous sclerosis
  - Marfan's disease
  - Ehlers–Danlos disease
  - Alpha-1-anti-trypsin disease
- Metastasis (e.g., osteogenic sarcoma)
- Trauma
  - Iatrogenic
  - Blunt

Contraindications
- Uncorrectable coagulopathy
- Platelet count <50,000 (unable to correct)
- Unsafe access route
- Fungal disease (controversial)

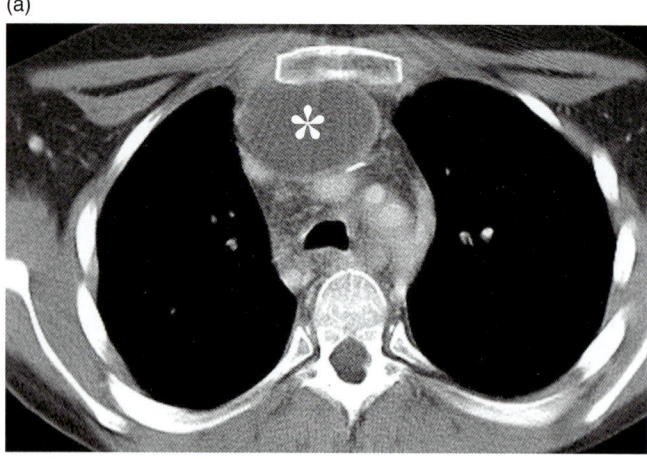 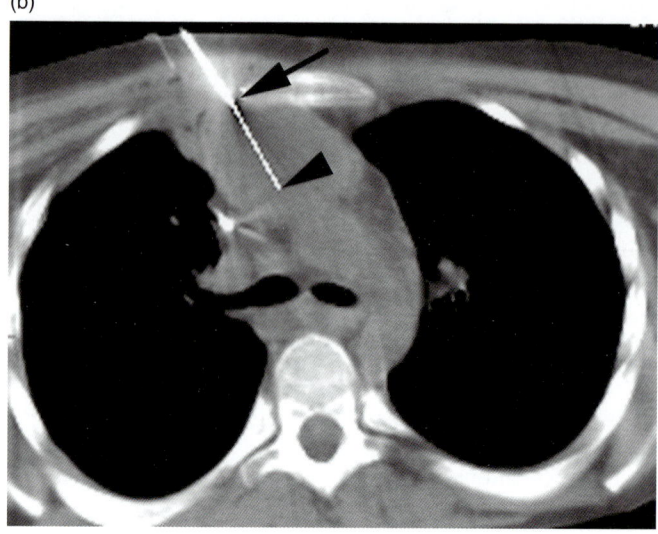

Figure 3.11 (a) Fourteen-year-old boy, six months after initial diagnosis and treatment of mediastinal lymphoma. Contrast-enhanced axial CT imaging through the thorax shows a rim-enhancing soft tissue lesion (*asterisk*) in the anterior mediastinum. (b) An axial CT image at the same level shows a coaxial guiding needle tip (*arrow*) at the anterior margin of the target lesion. A dotted line (*arrowhead*) shows the anticipated course of the sampling needle. An attempt at CT-guided aspiration produced no drainable fluid. Core biopsy of the lesion margin showed necrosis. Microbiological analysis showed no organisms. The region resolved without further specific treatment.

(e.g., mediastinal collections in neonates), smaller catheters (5–6 French with 1 cm loops) may be necessary, although the risk of catheter occlusion may increase. In general, we favor the smallest catheter diameter that successfully accomplishes the task and, at the same time, maximizes patient comfort. Drainage catheters are available in a wide range of sizes and shapes. Locking pigtail catheters are the drains of choice in most instances and are used to treat pleural fluid collections and, more rarely, pulmonary and mediastinal abscesses.

Patient preparation

Suspected mediastinal collections are usually first evaluated by CT. If there is any evidence of current or potential airway compromise related to the mediastinal or pericardial process under consideration for intervention, consultation with the anesthesiology service should be obtained and appropriate precautions taken, including endotracheal intubation.

No single imaging modality is used exclusively to guide percutaneous drainage. In our practice, CT has been preferred preprocedurally for selecting the safest and most direct route, and US or CT used to guide percutaneous drainage of mediastinal fluid collections. Ultrasound with an echocardiographic imaging package and a packed array transducer (4–7 MHz) from a subxiphoid or parasternal intercostal approach has often been used to access pericardial collections. In a given situation, the imaging guidance selected is based upon which modality provides the interventionalist the best view of the needle, the target, and any intervening or surrounding structures at risk.

Preprocedural lab studies

Prior to any percutaneous procedure in the thorax, a coagulopathy profile (PT or INR, PTT, platelet count, and bleeding time if necessary) and hemoglobin level are obtained. The child is kept NPO for four to six hours. Preprocedural antibiotics are given if the child is not already being treated.

Standard technique

Preprocedure CT imaging of the mediastinum, with vascular contrast if possible, is usually essential to adequately define cardiac, pleural, pericardial, and mediastinal structures and plan a safe interventional approach. However, real-time control during needle guidance into the mediastinum, via US (or CT fluoroscopy, if available), may increase safety and accuracy in select cases. In this respect, use of a high-quality US machine with a full array of transducers assists imaging performance. For pericardial drainage, an US machine with a cardiac package and a suitable small packed-array transducer (4–7 MHz) may be helpful in obtaining an adequate intercostal imaging window. Real-time imaging and color Doppler enhancement of vascular structures may assist the interventionalist in avoiding complications when working near the beating heart and great vessels. When the fluid collection is related to an esophageal leak, fluoroscopic guidance with esophagography, supplemented by catheter-directed injection of contrast at the level of the esophageal tear, may assist localization.

Once access to the collection is achieved, usually with a micropuncture set, the initial 0.018-inch wire may be exchanged for a 0.035-inch or 0.038-inch standard or stiff wire (Amplatz®, Rosen, Glide®) via an introducer set prior to

Table 3.11 Procedure summary: mediastinal and pericardial drainage

a. Preprocedural work-up (include US).
b. Route planning. Mark entry site on the skin surface.
c. Sterile preparation and draping.
d. Locally anesthetize entry site.
e. Small skin incision.
f. Consider creation of a fluid window if vital structures are interposed between skin and the target lesion.
g. Ultrasound-guided puncture.
h. Aspirate fluid. Insert drain if purulent fluid removed.
i. For drain placement, insert guide wire and coil within cavity.
j. Dilate tract.
k. Insert locking pigtail catheter.
l. Secure catheter to patient.
m. Apply a dry, sterile dressing.
n. Gravity drainage or suction. Consider Jackson–Pratt.

dilation of the tract and placement of a suitable pigtail catheter. Formation of a paraspinal or paramediastinal extrapleural window (see "Creating a mediastinal window," below) with a saline–lidocaine mixture may improve extrapleural access to mediastinal collections (Table 3.11).

Cardiac tamponade may be treated emergently via blind subxiphoid needle pericardiocentesis, but this carries a risk of ventricular puncture, coronary artery laceration, cardiac arrhythmia, and pneumothorax. Open surgical alternatives include emergent left thoracotomy or median sternotomy accompanied by pericardiostomy or pericardiectomy. Video-assisted pericardioscopy has been suggested as a less invasive alternative, but this procedure requires general anesthesia and deflation of one lung, which may be poorly tolerated in a hemodynamically unstable patient. Percutaneous catheter drainage of the pericardium (Figure 3.12) offers an effective alternative to blind or open surgical approaches for life-threatening cardiac tamponade if an interventionalist skilled in US-guided access is immediately available.

Under appropriate circumstances, especially in the hemodynamically stable patient, percutaneous pericardiocentesis and catheter drainage may be performed under fluoroscopic or CT control, although it is our preference to use US if an adequate imaging window is available due to its ability to demonstrate cardiac anatomy during needle advancement. The pericardium may be imaged transthoracically via a parasternal intercostal window, or from a subcostal window, while a 16- to 18-gauge angiocatheter or 4 to 5 French sheathed (Yueh) needle is advanced at an angle of 20 to 30 degrees from the abdomen from a subxiphoid or apical approach under real-time imaging control. A 22-gauge Chiba needle and 0.018-inch Cope mandril wire may be useful for initial access in neonates and infants, exchanging for a larger wire prior to catheter placement using one of the introducer sets in Table 3.2.

Once fluid is returned, the needle is withdrawn from the sheath, and an adequate volume of fluid aspirated from the pericardium to restore hemodynamic stability. A sample is submitted for culture and cytologic analysis, Gram stain, and other assays as required, as for other thoracic fluid collections. If fluoroscopy is available, intrapericardial position of the sheath may be confirmed by instillation of a small volume of iodinated contrast, and the procedure may be completed under fluoroscopic control. Otherwise, sonographic contrast (e.g., agitated saline or microbubble solution) may be instilled under US control.

In children as in adults, recurrence rates are dramatically lower if four to five days of catheter drainage are employed rather than pericardiocentesis alone. Therefore a guide wire is then advanced through the sheath into the pericardium, followed by a dilator, and then a 5 to 8 French pigtail catheter. Pericardial fluid may then be fully drained. Treatment of patients with malignant pericardial effusions or purulent pericarditis that require intrapericardial administration of sclerosants, antimicrobial agents, or fibrinolytics is facilitated by the percutaneous catheter as well. In general, these patients will be managed in collaboration with the cardiologist.

Technical variations
Creating a mediastinal window

Obtaining access to the mediastinum or medial aspect of the lung may be challenging due to the proximity of vital vascular structures and intervening lung. To minimize the possibility of complications and maximize the safe space available to approach and drain fluid collections or to perform a biopsy, development of a "mediastinal window" can be helpful. Widening may already be present in the form of a pleural effusion or pneumothorax. If not, a larger access route may be formed using US or CT guidance.

A mediastinal window is created by injection of sterile saline mixed with local anesthetic (9:1 concentration) into the extrapleural space adjacent to the mediastinum in the area through which the needle will course (Figures 3.13, 3.14). This fluid creates a mass effect and will tend to displace adjacent structures laterally allowing for safer and easier access to the target lesion. In most instances, approximately 25 to 75 ml of fluid are required. Although the absolute volume is not important, the interventionalist should carefully observe the child's vital signs during the injection. If significant changes are noted, the injection should be discontinued. In our experience, this technique works best for access to the anterior and middle mediastinum. Posterior mediastinal fluid injections seem to diffuse and do not widen the mediastinum as readily. Therefore larger injected volumes may be required to create a useful window.

Percutaneous balloon pericardiotomy

For patients with recurrent effusions, long-term catheter drainage may increase the risk of infection. In these patients, percutaneous balloon pericardiotomy may offer a suitable therapeutic alternative. In this procedure, a non-compliant monofoil balloon catheter (e.g., 20 to 30 mm diameter, 3 cm long; Mansfield Scientific, Mansfield, MA) is advanced over a

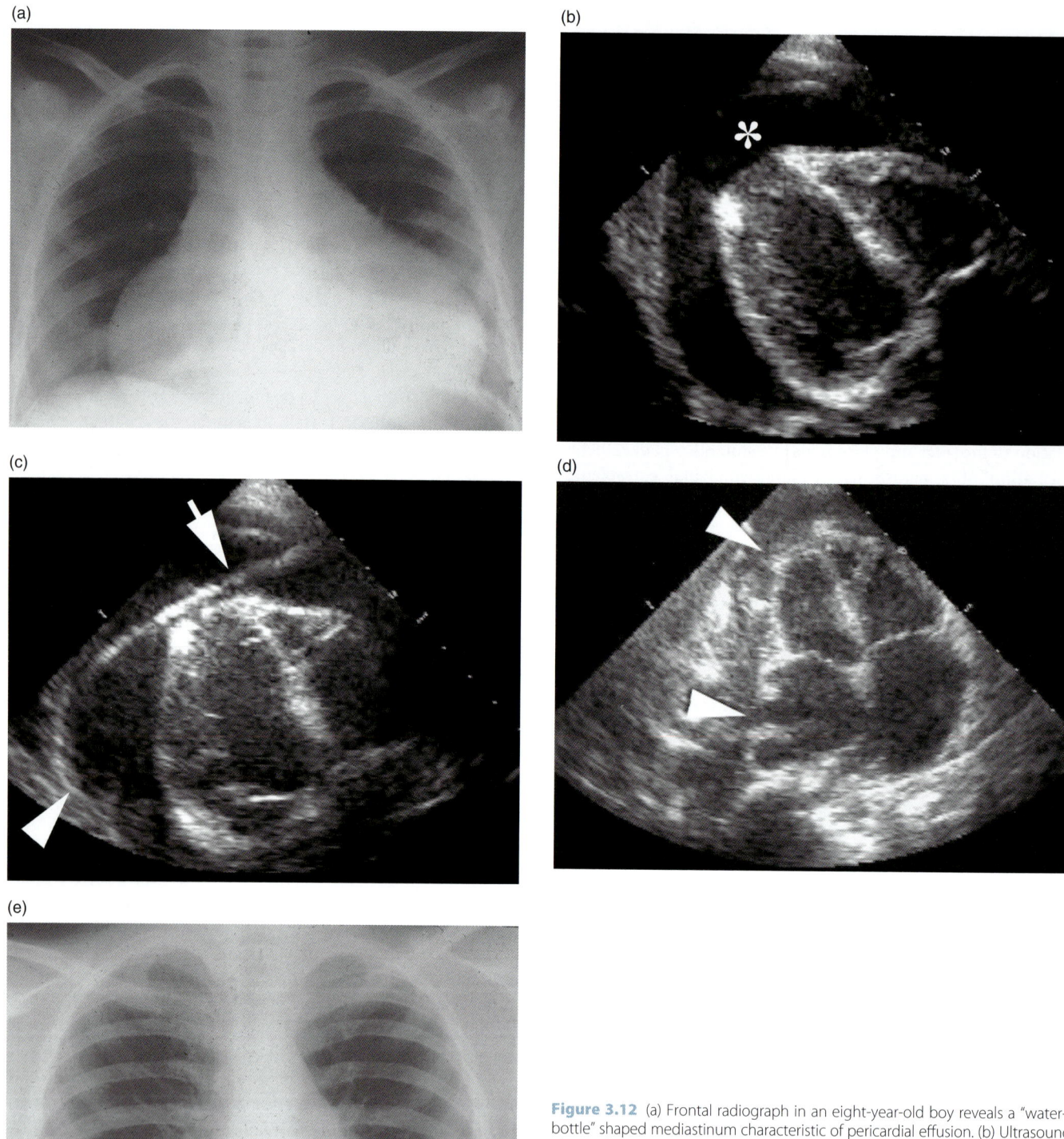

Figure 3.12 (a) Frontal radiograph in an eight-year-old boy reveals a "water-bottle" shaped mediastinum characteristic of pericardial effusion. (b) Ultrasound obtained using a 3.5 MHz vector transducer with echocardiographic software, from a subxiphoid window, demonstrates the heart in a four-chamber (long-axis) view surrounded by fluid in the pericardial space (*asterisk*). (Image courtesy of Jack Rychik, MD.) (c) After achieving access with a 22-gauge Chiba needle, a 0.018-inch mandril guide wire (*arrowhead*) was used to advance a 6 French drainage catheter (*arrow*) into the pericardial effusion. (Image courtesy of Jack Rychik, MD.) (d) The catheter was removed after aspiration of approximately 150 ml of clear fluid. A postprocedure US demonstrates complete evacuation of the pericardial space (*arrowheads*). (Image courtesy of Jack Rychik, MD.) (e) A frontal chest radiograph obtained after pericardial drainage shows normalization of the mediastinal contour.

Chapter 3 Thoracic interventions

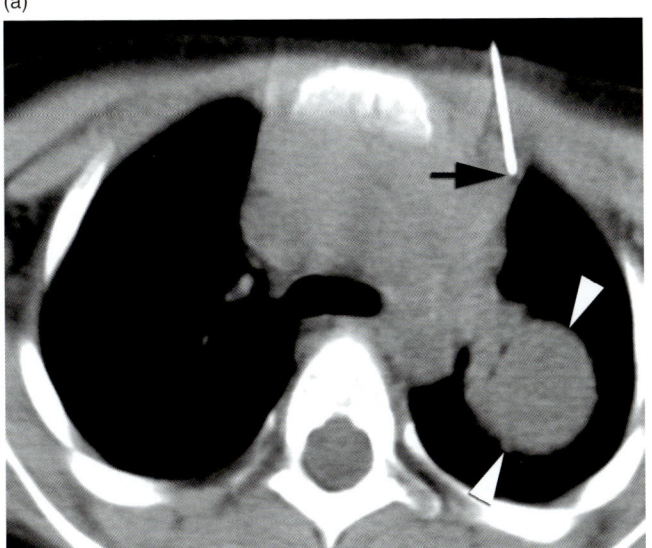 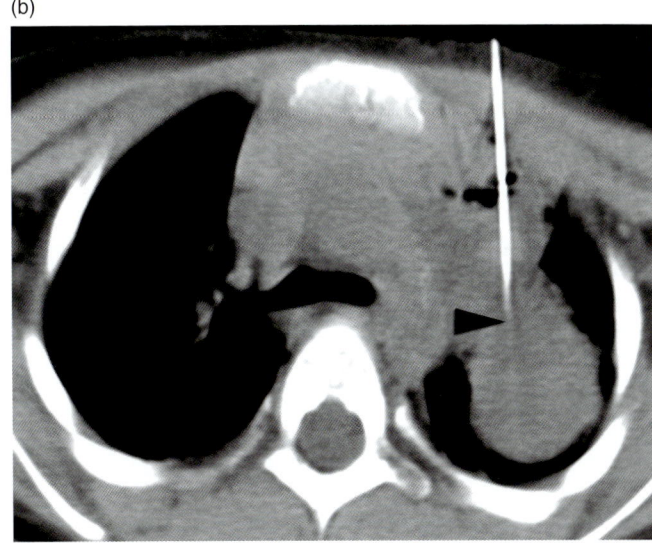

Figure 3.13 (a) A non-enhanced axial chest CT demonstrates percutaneous insertion of a fine needle (*arrow*) in the left mediastinum of this five-year-old girl with a left upper lobe mass. The mass (*arrowheads*) is surrounded by aerated lung. (b) After injection of approximately 25 ml of sterile saline, a window has been created allowing percutaneous access to the lesion (*arrowhead*) without traversing aerated lung. An 18-gauge core biopsy was obtained from the lesion, which demonstrated bronchiolitis obliterans with organizing pneumonia. There was no evidence of pneumothorax or other complication on postprocedure imaging.

wire until it straddles the parietal pericardium. Inflation of the balloon creates an opening from the pericardium into the pleural space, thus greatly increasing the surface area available for reabsorption of the effusion.

Postprocedure and follow-up care

It may be helpful to both patient care and ongoing quality assurance to maintain pertinent demographic and procedure-related data in an electronic database. Suggested items for data management are included in Table 3.4. Catheter management follows the same principles previously enumerated (see "Catheter care," above). Postprocedure care centers around monitoring vital signs, especially to detect evidence of cardiopulmonary compromise by compression of vital structures, or hemorrhage through vascular laceration or erosion. In children with mediastinal and pericardial pathology, imaging follow-up with chest radiographs and intermittent CT or US is recommended.

Complications

Retrospective outcome analyses of percutaneous image-guided pericardial drainage compared to subxiphoid pericardiostomy in adults have been equivocal, although studies agree that it is the preferred method for patients with hemodynamic instability. In children, this procedure has been demonstrated, over the past two decades, to be safe and effective by many centers, even in the face of hemodynamic compromise or underlying neoplastic disease. In a more stable patient (i.e., with chronic pericardial effusion), preprocedure CT may improve resolution of cardiac, pleural, pericardial, and mediastinal structures compared to US, although hemopericardium may appear isoattenuating with blood and myocardium. In theory, there is the potential for injury to the cardiovascular structures and tracheobronchial tree when a mediastinal collection is drained. In addition, it is possible for a catheter to erode into adjacent structures resulting in exsanguinating hemorrhage. Although possible, these complications have rarely been identified in pediatric practice.

Conclusions

The ability to safely and accurately deliver adequate drainage of mediastinal collections using percutaneous, image-guided techniques may obviate the need for thoracotomy and more invasive surgical management in select cases. Adjunctive intracavitary therapy may be considered in those who do not respond to medical management.

Biopsy of pulmonary and mediastinal lesions

Introduction

The diagnosis and management of an intrathoracic mass is tailored to the individual child's presentation. When a chest wall or intrathoracic lesion is identified, percutaneous core biopsy is often the initial invasive procedure considered. Image-guided biopsy offers a safe, cost-effective alternative to surgical biopsy and is the method of choice in most cases. Since the initial report of CT-guided biopsy in 1976 by Haaga and Alfidi, technical improvements have continued to expand the scope of lesions that may be approached. The same is true

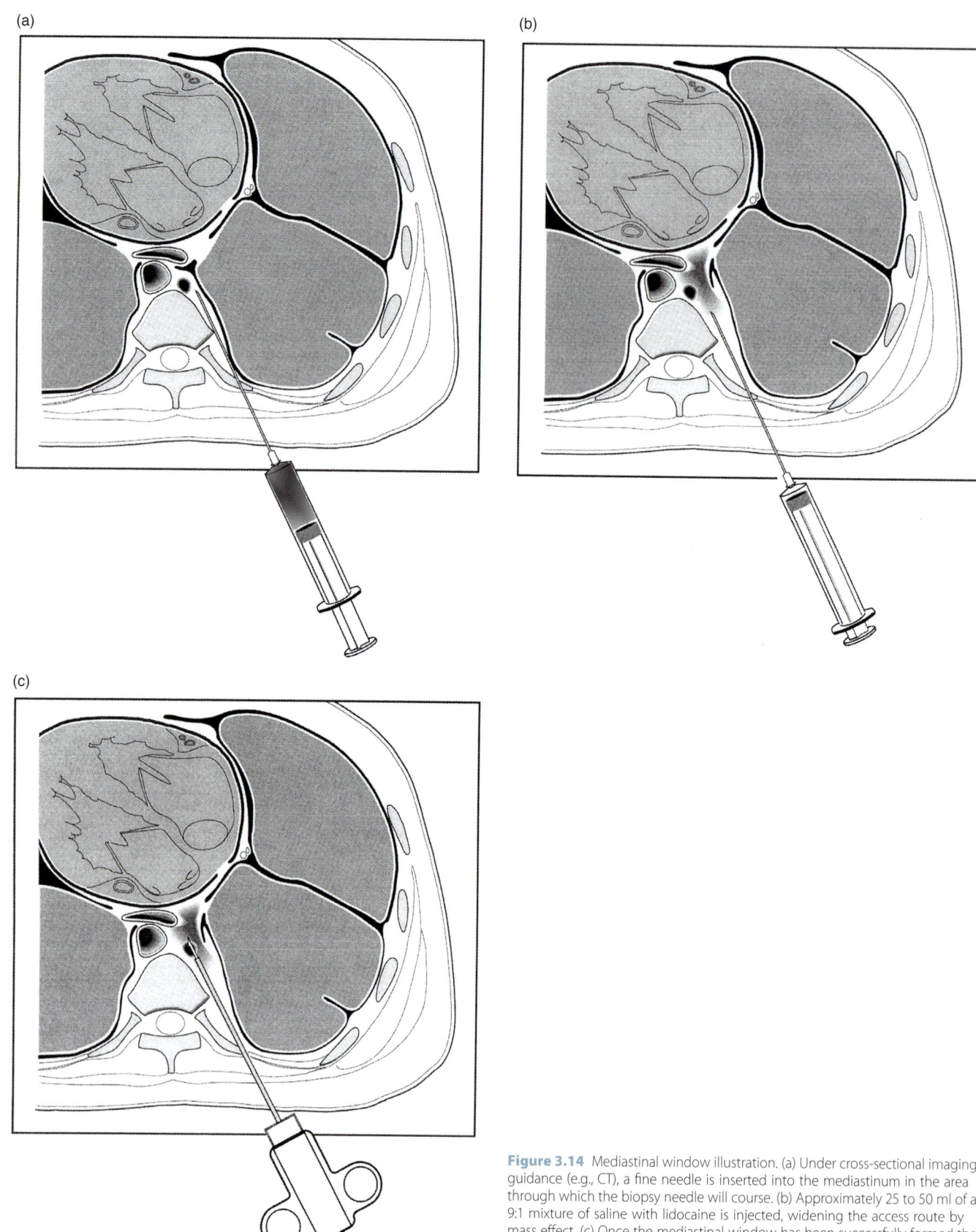

Figure 3.14 Mediastinal window illustration. (a) Under cross-sectional imaging guidance (e.g., CT), a fine needle is inserted into the mediastinum in the area through which the biopsy needle will course. (b) Approximately 25 to 50 ml of a 9:1 mixture of saline with lidocaine is injected, widening the access route by mass effect. (c) Once the mediastinal window has been successfully formed the lesion may be sampled using core biopsy or aspiration techniques without transgressing the pleura.

for US-guided biopsy in the thorax, described in 1976 by Chandrasekhar and colleagues. Both US equipment and biopsy instruments have improved dramatically over the intervening years, and today, even small (3 mm) peripheral pulmonary nodules can be biopsied percutaneously under image guidance with acceptable diagnostic reliability.

Over the years, fine needle aspiration techniques have been infrequently used in children because of the lower rate of primary or metastatic neoplasm involving the lungs; relative inexperience making a pathologic diagnosis using cytopathologic techniques in children's hospitals; and because children are often affected by less differentiated neoplasms that are more difficult to characterize with cytopathologic techniques. This results in the general preference of pediatric pathologists for core biopsy specimens. In recent years, experience with cytopathologic diagnosis and improved safety of core biopsy techniques have substantially increased the use of percutaneous biopsy techniques and confirmed their value.

If only cellular information is needed (especially for evaluation of recurrence or metastasis), fine needle aspiration biopsy (FNAB) can provide a rapid diagnosis, has a low rate of complication, and is cost-effective. In most instances, FNAB can be performed in an outpatient setting under local anesthesia and intravenous sedation.

A core biopsy is preferred in most pediatric situations, although the diagnostic yield can sometimes be increased by obtaining both core and FNAB samples. In most cases, a core biopsy can be obtained for lesions involving the chest wall and mediastinum. Pulmonary lesions have been treated more conservatively. Because even a small amount of hemorrhage around the intraparenchymal biopsy tract may obscure small lesions, it is best to plan as if the first pass may be the only pass achievable. For children with lesions up to 1 cm in diameter, an FNAB is sometimes preferred; lesions between 1 and 2 cm may undergo core biopsy using a biopsy gun with a 1 cm throw if the needle can be safely positioned within the mass (e.g., using a BioPince® automated end-cutting needle or a Temno® semiautomated sidecutting needle). For lesions greater than 2 cm in diameter, a core biopsy is performed whenever possible.

It has been shown that percutaneous biopsy techniques are safe and effective in the pediatric population, yielding an answer to the clinical question in over 90% of cases. These techniques should be used in lieu of open biopsy as long as a safe access route is available and the operator is familiar with pediatric indications and contraindications. The percutaneous approach has advantages over open biopsy including the ability to perform the procedure under local anesthesia and intravenous sedation or general anesthesia, with lower morbidity, fewer complications, and lower cost. Biopsy is not a therapeutic procedure, and the outcome depends on the ability of the sample obtained to answer the specific clinical question posed. It is therefore important to clearly define the clinical question in consultation with the referring service, and to assure the sample is optimized with regard to quantity, character, and handling, through consultation with the pathologist who will interpret the results, prior to obtaining the sample. If the opportunity is available, it is often helpful to have the pathologist in attendance or readily available to receive and process the sample and to assure its adequacy for diagnosis, and even to review touch-prep or frozen section samples with the pathologist before concluding the procedure.

Indications

In children, the indications for percutaneous biopsy of the chest wall, lung, or mediastinum are fewer in number than in adults (Table 3.12). In general, percutaneous biopsy should be considered when: (1) a tissue or bacteriologic diagnosis may modify therapy; (2) diagnosis is needed to direct therapy in high-risk patients unable to undergo a surgical procedure; and (3) analysis of recurrent or metastatic tumor is required. In selected cases, architectural information may not be required to refine the diagnostic quality of the sample. In such cases, fine needle aspiration may be sufficient (Table 3.13).

Table 3.12 Indications for percutaneous biopsy in the thorax

Indications
- Pulmonary lesions (lesions >3 mm, abutting the pleura or just subpleural)
- Chest wall and mediastinal lesions
- Skeletal lesions
- Coalescent pulmonary lymphoproliferative disease

Contraindications
- Uncorrectable coagulopathy
- Platelet count <50,000 (unable to correct)
- Unsafe access route
- Inadequate visualization of the lesion
- Severely compromised pulmonary function
- Pulmonary hypertension
- Vasculitis
- Fungal disease (controversial)

Table 3.13 Indications for intrathoracic fine needle aspiration biopsy

Indications
- Pulmonary nodules
- When a tissue or bacteriologic diagnosis could modify therapy
- Possible metastatic disease
- Diagnosis needed to modify therapy in a high-risk patient

Contraindications
- Uncorrectable coagulopathy
- Platelet count <50,000 (unable to correct)
- Lack of a safe access route
- Inability to visualize the lesion during the needle insertion
- Pulmonary hypertension
- Severely compromised pulmonary function
- Vasculitis and fungal disease

Table 3.14 Equipment: intrathoracic biopsy

Fine needle aspiration biopsy
– Chiba needle (22- or 23-gauge)
– Coaxial lung biopsy set
– Spinal needle

Core needle
– Automated (1 or 2 cm throw); side or end cut
– Semi-automated or manual biopsy needles

Biopsy guide for US transducer (optional)
1% lidocaine buffered with sodium bicarbonate (8:2 mixture)
Formalin or sterile test tubes or containers for specimens

Contraindications are uncommon but include rare situations where there is no safe access route, inadequate visualization of the lesion, or an uncorrectable coagulopathy. Rarely, the presence of severely compromised pulmonary function and pulmonary hypertension (e.g., when biopsy of a hilar mass is contemplated) may make a pulmonary biopsy unwise. When an intrathoracic mass compresses or threatens to compress the airways or vital vascular structures, a pediatric anesthesiologist should be consulted prior to the procedure to assure protection of cardiopulmonary function. Fungal disease or vasculitis may be a relative contraindication because of the greater likelihood of pulmonary hemorrhage in these individuals.

Technique

Equipment

A variety of needles are available for aspiration (cytologic) and core (histologic) biopsy. The needles can be grouped by the type of biopsy being performed (Table 3.14). Chiba (thin) needles, cutting needles, and automated systems (biopsy guns) are available in a spectrum of diameters, lengths, levels of automation, and lengths of the biopsy channel (throw). In addition, either aspiration or core techniques can be performed directly or coaxially through a guide needle (see "Technical variations," below). The latter approach is especially useful for intrapulmonary lesions and has the advantage of facilitating repeated access without multiple individual punctures of the pleura, lung, or mediastinum. This leads to a shorter procedure time, fewer CT images for localization and monitoring of the biopsy passes, a lower complication rate, and a higher percentage of quality specimens. In addition, the biopsy tract is protected from deposition of malignant cells or exposure to infection.

Fine needle aspiration biopsy (FNAB) needles

Aspiration needles are used to obtain samples for cytopathologic analysis (Figure 3.15). Aspiration needles are characteristically thin, ranging from approximately 18- to 24-gauge. Examples of aspiration needles include spinal and Chiba types. Both have central stylets with beveled tip angles of 24 and 30 degrees respectively. The 24-degree bevel angle has been found to be optimal for cytologic sample collection in the laboratory. Spinal needles have smaller central bores with thicker walls when compared to the Chiba (Figure 3.15d (inset)), making it easier to control during placement. The smaller bore does not significantly decrease sample volume. Aspiration needles demonstrate increased yield with increasing gauge and decreasing bevel angle.

In adults, FNAB is common as samples are primarily used for cytologic analysis. In the pediatric population, indications for this technique are more limited and ultimately rely on the availability of a pediatric pathologist experienced in the interpretation of cytologic specimens. When FNAB is to be performed, our needle of choice is a 22- or 23-gauge Chiba needle (Figure 3.1a). The thin-walled construction makes the Chiba needle safe for use in virtually any location in the lung. A Chiba needle is malleable and frequently does not track in a straight line even when an US biopsy guide is used. This may be especially problematic when the distance to the target is long (≥ 5 cm), when the tissue is firm, or when the consistency of the tissue varies along the course of the needle. Little can be done to overcome this problem, except to make several passes and try to correct the tracking error. Other needles, such as a spinal needle, can be substituted; however, these stiffer needles with cutting tips are more dangerous and should be used with caution.

Core biopsy needles

Cutting needles (Figure 3.16) tend to be larger in size (14- to 19-gauge) and are divided into end- (e.g., Biopince®) or side-cutting types (e.g., Temno®, Quick-Core®, Max-Core®). End-cutting needles are like aspiration needles with the tip design modified to increase yield. Manual needles (e.g., Turner and Franseen) obtain samples by rotating the tip while advancing the needle after removing the stylet. Suction, as from a syringe, may assist the operator in obtaining a suitable sample. The Turner needle is thin-walled with a 45-degree tip that is circumferentially sharpened and with a secondary bevel. The Franseen needle has a trephine (serrated) end to aid in obtaining histologic material in firm lesions while reducing crush artifact. Side-cutting needles operate by shearing the tissue sample. The Temno®-type needle is a semi-automated side-cutting needle. The central portion containing a 0.7 to 2.0 cm recessed channel is introduced into the lesion. A cutting outer cannula is subsequently introduced trapping the sample in the notch. The sharp tip of semi-automated devices does not move forward during activation, increasing safety when vital structures are in the "line of fire." The Westcott needle has a cutting notch in the outer cannula. The choice of needle depends on the lesion, location, and personal preference. In our experience, side-cutting needles are more effective with soft, gelatinous masses. End-cutting needles tend to give better samples with firm lesions. The defining advantage of all core biopsy needles is that they provide both architectural and cytologic information, an especially important consideration for accurate diagnosis of the common pediatric sarcomatous tumors.

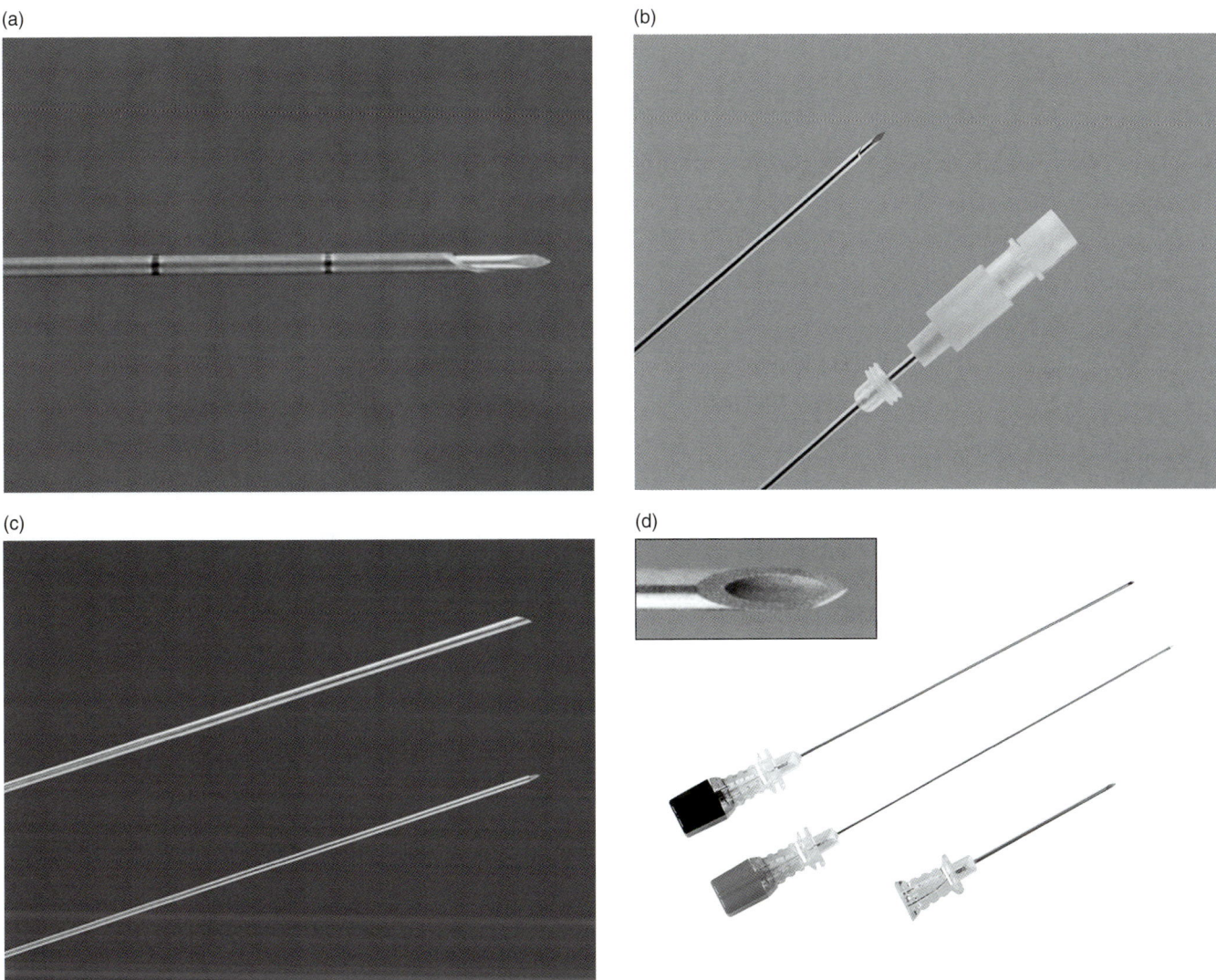

Figure 3.15 Fine needle aspiration biopsy needles. (a) Menghini (Invivocorp, Gainsville, FL). (b) Turner (Cook Medical). (c) Greene lung aspiration needle (Cook Medical). (d) Quinke spinal needles (Becton Dickenson Medical, Franklin Lakes, NJ). (Inset) The wall of the spinal needle is thicker than most other needles used for access or aspiration.

Larger sizes (smaller gauges) give greater stiffness, control, and increased yield at the risk of increased bleeding complications. Increased bleeding may be expected when biopsies are performed with smaller gauge (larger diameter) needles. Multiple needle passes increase risk of complication but also increase yield. Coaxial systems protect the tract from seeding and aid in decreasing injury related to multiple passes but limit the sampling volume from a given position. Simply changing the angulation of the guiding needle without otherwise repositioning allows greater sample variation without a substantial increase in risk.

Since the introduction of automated biopsy devices in the early 1980s, numerous variations have become commercially available. Once the device has been cocked, on activation they thrust the biopsy channel or chamber forward a predetermined distance, quickly followed by a shearing outer cannula (or, in the case of the end-cutting BioPince®, a shearing device at the rear of the sample chamber). The purpose of these devices is to increase ease and reliability of core biopsies, resulting in higher yields and shorter procedures, while providing high-quality specimens. Most of these devices allow the operator to select the "throw" length. Some are single-use devices, while others combine a reusable handle with disposable needles of varying diameter and length.

Since the introduction of the automated biopsy gun, core biopsies have become much easier to perform. However, ease of firing does not make a gun safe. Critical determinants of success, such as where to aim, when and how often to fire, how best to avoid injury to adjacent structures, and prompt recognition and treatment of complications, still require the skill of an experienced interventionalist. Core needles used in our practice range in size from 22-gauge to 14-gauge with the 15- and 18-gauge needles most often selected. In general, the 15-gauge needle is chosen when the lesion is large (usually >5 cm) and easily accessible, and no unusual risk factors are present. Risk

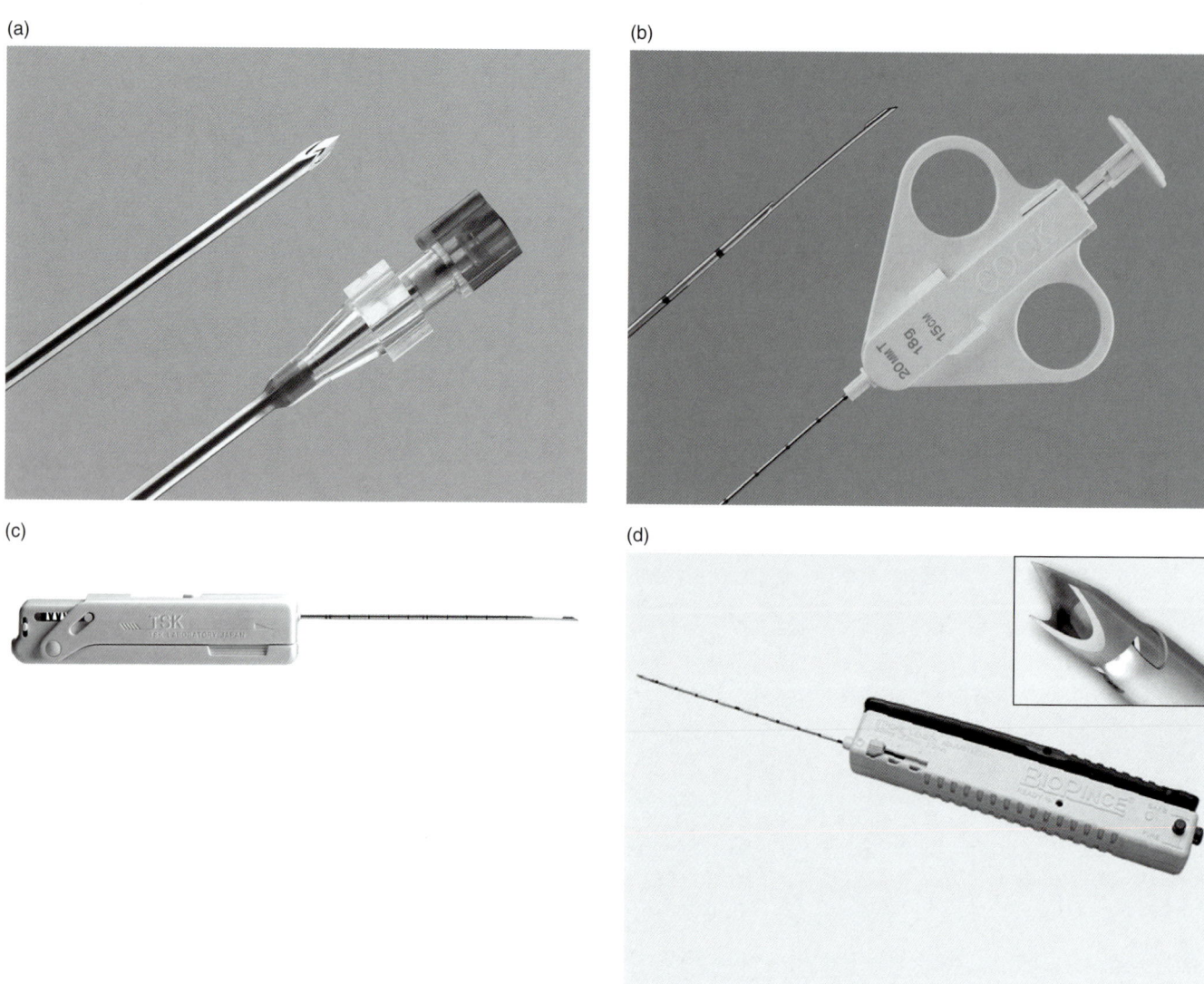

Figure 3.16 Core biopsy needles. (a) The Franseen needle (Cook Medical) has a serrated or "crown" tip designed to manually cut a core in lung parenchyma or pulmonary lesions. (b) The Quick-Core® needle (Cook Medical) is a semi-automated Temno-type side-cutting needle with an etched tip to facilitate visualization with ultrasound. (c) The ACECUT® (TSK Laboratories, Vancouver, BC, Canada) is an automated side-cutting needle. (d) The BioPince® needle (Argon Medical Devices, Plano, TX) is an automated end-cutting device. The tip (inset) is designed to shear the full-core specimen off its pedicle.

factors include a low platelet count <50,000, an elevated PT, PTT, or prolonged bleeding time (e.g., children on Depakane® or Depakote®), and history of a treated coagulopathy or unfavorable anatomy (e.g., adjacent vessels or vascular organs). When such risk factors are present, an 18-gauge needle is preferred. Twenty-one gauge needles are available but provide limited tissue samples or require multiple passes and are rarely used. In cases where there is a high risk of postprocedural bleeding, either because of the type of lesion being biopsied or abnormal coagulation studies, a coaxial technique may be used. In these cases, the biopsy is performed and the cutting needle containing the biopsy specimen is removed, leaving the outer cannula in place. If bleeding is observed or if there is significant concern of bleeding, tract embolization can be performed by inserting Gelfoam® pledgets or slurry, Avitene®, or embolization coils through the guide (outer) needle cannula.

When an US biopsy guide is used, an additional 5 cm of needle length is needed. The length of the biopsy channel (throw) is an important consideration. Whenever possible, a needle with a longer throw (e.g., 2–3 cm) is chosen to improve yield. However, a shorter (e.g., 1 cm) throw needle is used for lesions less than 2 cm in diameter or close to critical structures. Coaxial needles are generally 18- to 19-gauge and are safe for children of all ages and sizes.

Patient preparation

Optimally, a member of the interventional team should assess patients before scheduling the procedure to determine if sedation or general anesthesia (GA) will be required. This decision is based on multiple criteria including patient age, compliance, cooperation, lesion location, and size. A procedure in a young,

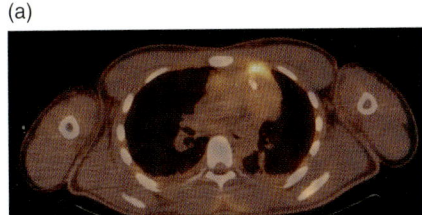
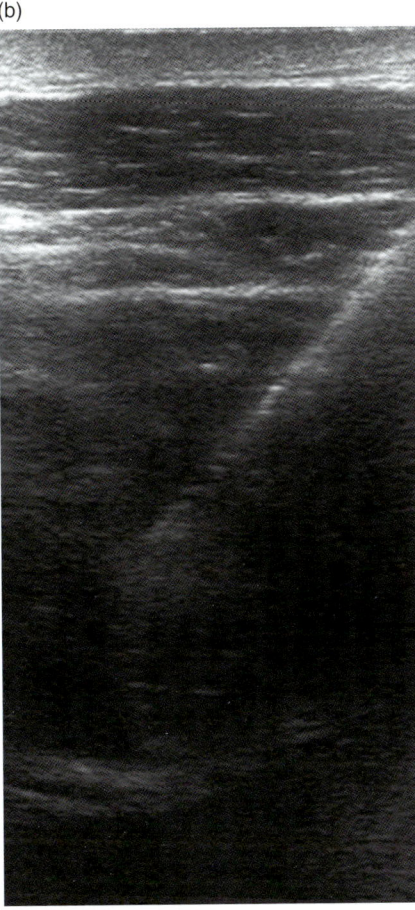

Figure 3.17 (a) Sixteen-year-old male who presented with chest pain was found to have an abnormal chest radiograph, which led to further cross-sectional imaging. This PET/CT fusion image demonstrates an FDG-avid anterior mediastinal mass. Note coarse calcifications. (b) Ultrasound was used to direct a 16-gauge core biopsy needle into the mediastinal mass. Core specimens revealed a diagnosis of malignant teratoma with yolk sac tumor.

potentially uncooperative patient may need to be performed under GA, whereas the same procedure in an older patient may be performed with only local anesthetic and intravenous sedation. Biopsy of a subset of small lesions may require respiratory control to manage position of the lung and pleura and thereby position of the lesion *vis a vis* intervening structures such as ribs and sternum that may otherwise obscure access. If respiratory control is required the procedure must be performed under GA with pharmacologic paralysis of the patient. It is helpful to plan this with the anesthesiologist in advance.

Children initially evaluated by frontal and lateral chest radiographs are usually referred for chest CT if interventional therapy is considered. Computed tomography enables accurate route planning, identifies potential problems, and determines optimal patient positioning for the procedure. If it is known in advance that a biopsy is to be performed immediately following the diagnostic CT, the anticipated entry site is marked so the biopsy may be performed at the same sitting. If the target nodule is adjacent to the pleura, or in the chest wall or mediastinum, US may also be helpful for route planning or procedural guidance (Figure 3.17).

Routine laboratory testing is not performed. However, a coagulation profile, including a PT, PTT, INR, CBC, and platelet count, is usually obtained. If the patient is known or suspected to have a bleeding diathesis, a bleeding time may be performed, although this is not recommended as a routine part of preprocedural screening. Medications known to interfere with coagulation should be withheld according to the schedule recommended in Chapter 1: "Preprocedure medications." If possible, coagulopathies should be corrected prior to or during the procedure. If this is not possible, the indications for the procedure and potential benefit of a tissue diagnosis must be weighed against the risk of hemorrhage. While the preprocedure work-up may include determination of clotting factors and correction of any coagulopathy, abnormal clotting factors are not a good predictor of hemorrhage.

If there is any evidence of current or potential airway compromise related to the mass under consideration for intervention, consultation with the anesthesiology service should be obtained and appropriate precautions taken, including endotracheal intubation if indicated. No other special preparation is required. As usual, the child should have nothing by mouth prior to the procedure (according to relevant hospital sedation and anesthesia policy). Antibiotics are not routinely given. The pathology service should be notified prior to commencement of the procedure so that the pathologist can assist in preliminary evaluation, special handling, or sample preservation.

Standard technique

The patient is placed in the appropriate position, and the biopsy area is cleansed and draped in sterile fashion. If the procedure is performed under sedation, the skin and tract are infiltrated with a local anesthetic such as 1% buffered lidocaine. Even when the patient is under GA, a long-acting local anesthetic such as bupivacaine can be administered when necessary to decrease discomfort after the procedure. Local anesthetic with epinephrine can be used to prolong the anesthetic effect and decrease bleeding. This approach is to be avoided in areas with end-organ blood supply (e.g., the digits and nose). Pain associated with administration of local anesthetic can be decreased by using a thin gauge needle (e.g., 30-gauge) and buffering the solution with sodium bicarbonate or preparing the area with a topical agent such as ELA-Max®, EMLA® or 1% buffered lidocaine via a J-Tip® for rapid skin anesthesia. A small skin incision is made, and the needle or biopsy device is introduced.

The needle is advanced under image guidance and, when in proper position, the sample is obtained (Figure 3.18). If both aspiration and core biopsy samples are obtained, aspiration is performed first. As mentioned previously, multiple samples increase yield. Multiple passes into the same lesion can be performed in a variety of ways. Each pass can be performed separately or the initial needle can be used as a guide by placing a second needle in tandem along the tract (see "Technical variations," below). Coaxial systems allow a larger outer guiding needle to be placed near the lesion with multiple samples obtained through a smaller central needle (see "Technical variations," below). Multiple biopsies can then be performed without having to localize the lesion again, decreasing trauma and the chance of seeding from multiple passes. As in other systems, we generally limit ourselves to three passes at any one location to minimize the risk of bleeding. After obtaining adequate tissue, the samples are sent to pathology. It is also important to document that the biopsy specimen was obtained from the target lesion and to incorporate data relevant to the procedure into the medical record and the interventional database (Table 3.4).

For FNAB, aspiration and non-aspiration methods of sampling have been described. The aspiration method involves the use of suction obtained by attaching a 10 to 20 ml syringe to the needle. Suction is applied when the needle is in the lesion and is either maintained during removal or is discontinued if blood appears in the needle hub. Blood in a sample limits sensitivity. When the needle is within the lesion some authors advocate gently moving the needle in and out and rotating it to increase yield. The non-aspiration method involves placing the needle into the lesion and allowing capillary action to draw cells into the needle. Utility of each method varies with the organ and tumor being sampled.

Pulmonary nodules

There are many causes of lung nodules including infection, neoplasm, post-transplant lymphoproliferative disorder (PTLD), arteriovenous malformation, and autoimmune disorders. Confirmation of metastatic disease in a patient with a newly diagnosed or known tumor substantially changes treatment and prognosis. The utility of biopsy of multiple lung lesions in adults with a known primary neoplasm has been questioned. While FNAB is standard in adults, the higher prevalence of sarcomatous neoplasms in children necessitates attempts at obtaining additional material by way of cutting-needle biopsy. Percutaneous biopsy can also be helpful in obtaining a diagnosis in infectious diseases and PTLD.

At our institution, central parenchymal nodules greater than 3 mm are biopsied with CT guidance, usually using a coaxial system. This has been demonstrated to be safe and the resulting sample is adequate for definitive identification in almost all patients. Hilar disease may be amenable to CT-guided biopsy if a safe route can be defined (Figure 3.19). Peripheral nodules that abut the pleural surface (Figure 3.20) are sampled using US guidance when possible. Nodules that are too small for percutaneous biopsy may be amenable to thoracoscopic or open resection after localization with CT-guided placement of a hook wire (see "Marking lesions for resection," below).

Chronic lung disease

Percutaneous biopsy has been used as an alternative to open lung biopsy in the diagnosis of chronic lung disease. High resolution CT is used to confirm interstitial lung disease and optimize the biopsy site. CT-guided biopsy with a 14-gauge cutting needle biopsy device has been shown to be safe and accurate.

Imaging modalities

There are a variety of successful approaches to percutaneous biopsy of the lungs, mediastinum, and chest wall. The imaging modality chosen for guidance depends upon the size and

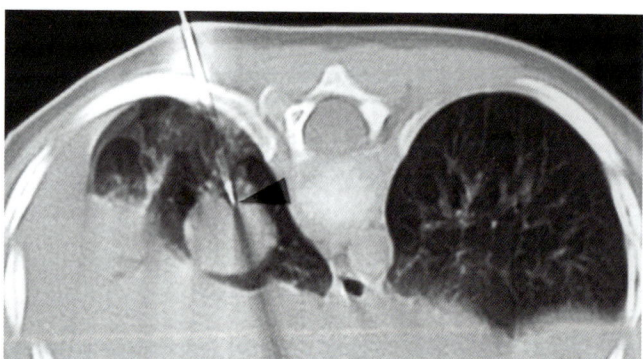

Figure 3.18 A two-year-old boy with a pulmonary nodule surrounded by aerated lung was referred for percutaneous biopsy. An unenhanced CT image through the chest with the patient in a prone position shows the entire length of the guiding coaxial needle in the imaging plane, with the tip at the margin of the target lesion (*arrowhead*). The 18-gauge core biopsy resulted in a diagnosis of metastatic mesoblastic nephroma. There was no evidence of complication following the procedure.

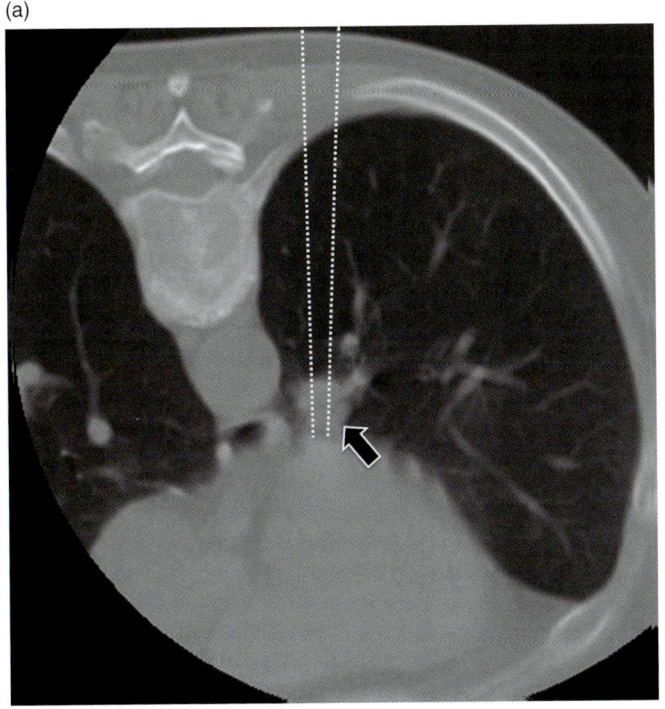 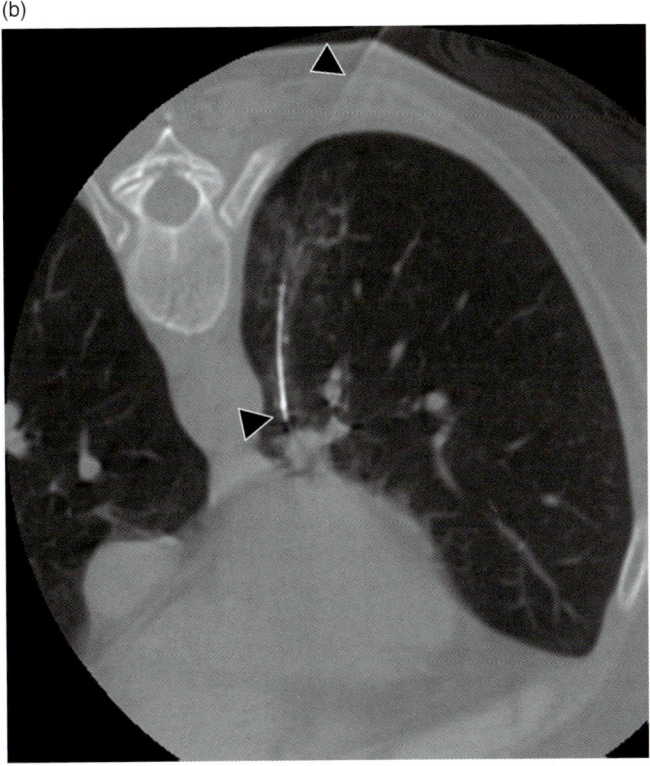

Figure 3.19 (a) Prone chest CT without contrast in an older patient shows a single pulmonary nodule in the hilum (*arrow*). Vascular and bony structures limit the available percutaneous biopsy pathways to a narrow region (between the *dashed lines*). (b) In order to more easily avoid surrounding vascular structures, a semi-automated side-cutting needle (*arrowheads*) was curved by hand, then iteratively advanced until the sample channel was across the lesion. The device was then activated, and an adequate sample for diagnosis was obtained without complication.

location of the lesion and the imaging device that best demonstrates the target lesion and its relationship to surrounding structures. Today, fluoroscopy is infrequently used for guidance. Computed tomography with or without injection of intravenous contrast is in many ways ideally suited to thoracic interventions, as it offers excellent two-dimensional visualization with high resolution that is not limited by the presence of air or bone (Figure 3.21). Computed tomography is excellent for route planning and guidance of needle placement. Although CT is the preferred modality for guidance, difficulties do exist. Computed tomography is not a real-time technique. Needle movement is unobserved, requiring additional time for repeated CT imaging to evaluate iterative changes in the needle position.

CT guidance

The child is positioned, as determined by prior imaging, so that the most direct approach to the lesion can be taken (Table 3.15). A limited scan is performed through the region of interest to locate the lesion. If sedation is used, we have found it to be best to sedate the patient at this time so that the depth and rate of breathing will be the same as during the biopsy. Radio-opaque markers are placed on the skin and several contiguous axial images are obtained, centered on the lesion (Figure 3.22). A safe pathway from the skin to the lesion is determined using the markers as a reference point or grid.

As is true elsewhere, a route should be planned so as to avoid transgressing (and potentially contaminating or seeding) more than one compartment whenever possible. An optimal path would lie in an axial plane.

The distance from the skin to both the superficial and deep aspects of the lesion is measured to determine how deeply the biopsy needle should be passed to obtain the desired sample. Image postprocessing software may also allow calculation of the angle, from perpendicular, that the needle should be directed from the skin entry site to the lesion. The chest wall is prepared and draped in sterile fashion and 1% buffered lidocaine slowly injected into the skin with a thin gauge (30-gauge) needle. The needle is then advanced toward the lesion, taking care not to enter the lung or pleural space, or to draw near vital structures, before verifying the needle trajectory. At least three contiguous axial images are obtained, centered on the lesion. Ideally, a single slice should contain the entire needle, including tip (streak) artifact and the bulk of the lesion in line with each other, without intervening vital structures. The effects of partial volume artifact and potential respiratory motion must especially be considered during this phase of the procedure.

Small corrections to the needle trajectory may be made during advancement. However, if substantial corrections are needed, the needle should be withdrawn to the tip and corrections made before re-entering the tissues. If the needle alignment and anticipated pathway are appropriate, the needle may

Chapter 3 Thoracic interventions

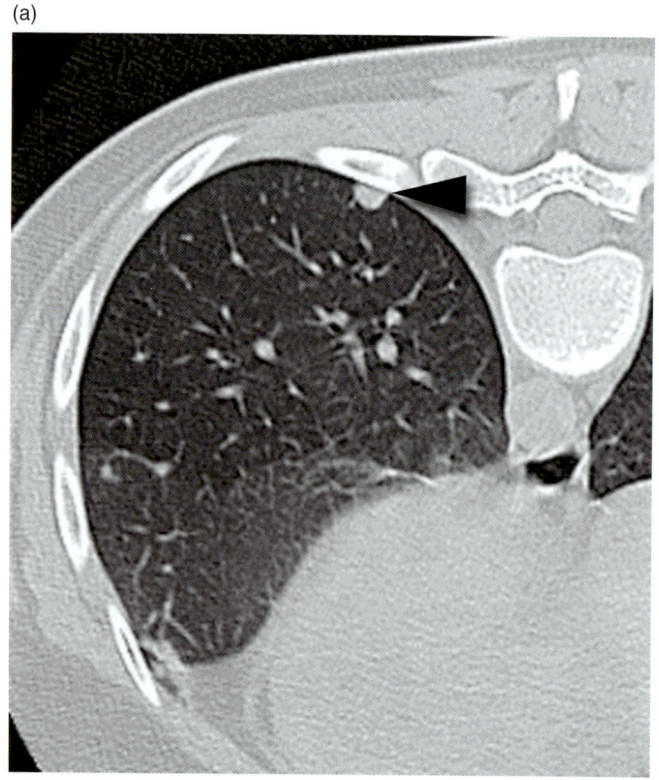

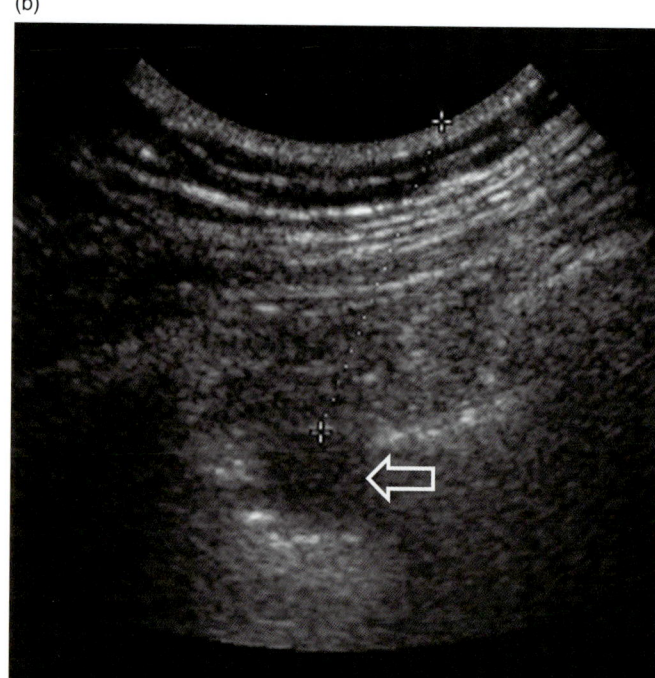

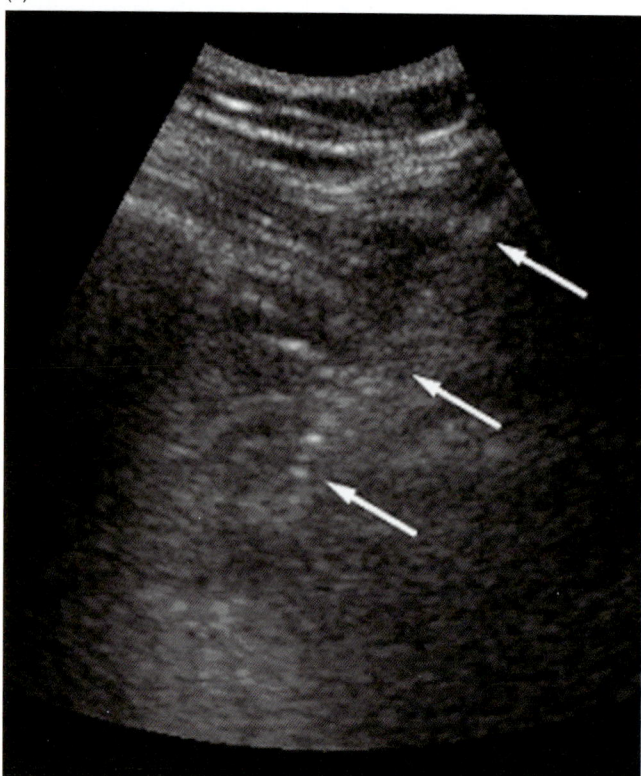

Figure 3.20 (a) An axial CT section through the chest of a 14-year-old boy with a presacral primitive neurectodermal tumor demonstrates a 4 mm × 7 mm pleural-based nodule (*arrowhead*). Biopsy was requested for staging. (b) Under real-time ultrasound, respiratory control is used to move and maintain the lesion (*arrow*) into an accessible position with respect to potentially obscuring bony structures. The depth from skin surface to lesion is calculated using the measurement tool on the ultrasound machine following the anticipated biopsy route (*dashed line*). This aids the operator in determining the appropriate needle length. In a similar fashion, a measurement of the lesion will aid in determining the amount of throw if an automated biopsy device is being used. (c) Ultrasound imaging allows visualization of the needle (*white arrows*) in real time as it enters the target lesion, assuring that the sample has been obtained from the desired location.

be further advanced toward the lesion, and position again verified. When the needle tip is adjacent to the lesion, such that the throw of the needle will extend into or through the lesion without endangering vital structures beyond the lesion, a sample or samples should be obtained. Routinely, we obtain two to three samples per lesion. At the completion of the procedure a portable chest radiograph is obtained to identify any complication.

US guidance

The principal goals of imaging during biopsy are to identify the target lesion, to avoid intervening vital structures, to visualize the biopsy needle in plane with the lesion during advancement, to confirm passage of the sample chamber through the lesion, and to evaluate for potential complications following biopsy. In many situations, US fulfills these goals exceptionally well. The general principles of US guidance for interventional procedures are presented in Chapter 1 (Figure 1.1).

Ultrasound has had a limited role in the guidance of lung or mediastinal biopsies since optimal visualization of the lesion is often limited by intervening aerated lung or bone. However, US has been successfully incorporated into a multimodality approach to interventions in the thorax that can often overcome these potential limitations. For example, CT can help localize a lesion, can suggest likely US imaging windows, and can assist the operator to correctly identify the lesion, improving accuracy and saving considerable time compared to searching for the lesion with US alone. With improved US equipment, including development of high-quality linear transducers with a small footprint, and with intraprocedural respiratory control, core biopsy or FNAB of peripheral or pleural-based pulmonary lesions and even deep mediastinal lesions can be safely performed with a high diagnostic yield (Figures 3.20, 3.23).

Table 3.15 Procedure summary: intrathoracic biopsy

- Diagnostic and planning CT.
- Select entry site.
- Prepare entry site for biopsy.
- Image-guided biopsy.
- Obtain at least two to three specimens per lesion.
- Work with pathologist to properly handle the specimens.
- Follow-up chest radiograph.

Molecular imaging

For biopsy to be useful, a sample of tissue must be selected, obtained, processed, and evaluated that is most representative of the underlying disease process, that will yield the most accurate prognosis, or that will most reliably guide a plan of management to optimize outcomes. This depends upon correctly identifying and accurately sampling the suspicious tissue based upon imaging characteristics and, at open biopsy, upon visual and palpable tissue characteristics. It remains difficult under any conditions to differentiate vital tumor from necrosis, fibrosis, and hemorrhage, and to avoid biopsy of equivocal tissue. Using standard CT or US cross-sectional imaging it is often not possible to selectively target the most physiologically active tissue, or to know that samples obtained accurately represent an underlying neoplastic process. Physiologic imaging (e.g., PET, SPECT) offers insight into the biologic nature of the target lesion that is not available from anatomic imaging alone. However, it does not allow adequate target resolution or visualization of surrounding structures necessary for the safe performance of percutaneous biopsy techniques. Combined anatomic–physiologic imaging gives both targeting biologic data and guiding anatomic localization. Although there is limited experience to date, we have found that the use of image fusion such as PET-CT imaging for procedure planning and, where appropriate, for percutaneous biopsy guidance, can improve patient outcomes compared to conventional techniques in select cases (Figures 3.17, 3.23).

MR guidance

At present, interventional MRI is in its infancy and is not yet being used on a widespread basis. Specially designed, open MR units and non-ferromagnetic equipment are required.

(a)
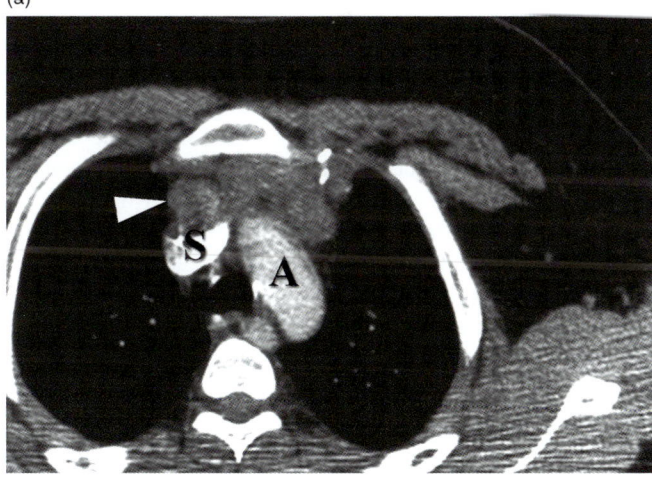

(b)
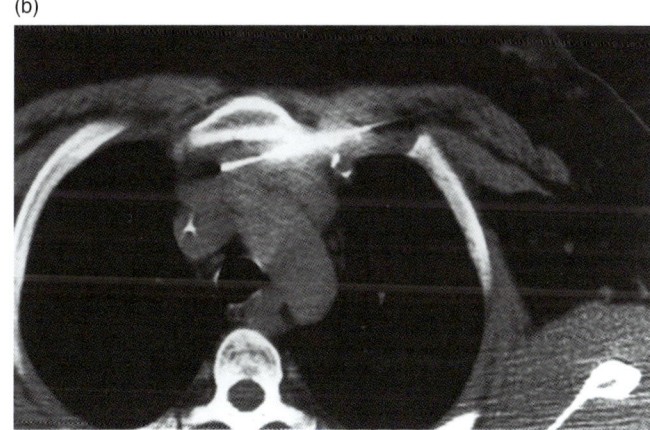

Figure 3.21 (a) Contrast-enhanced axial CT through the chest of a 16-year-old male with a history of heart transplant shows anterior mediastinal adenopathy. The nodules (*arrowhead*) were just anterior to the superior vena cava (*S*) and aorta (*A*), and overlying sternum impaired US visualization. (b) Computed tomography-guided biopsy using a retrosternal approach with an 18-gauge automated core biopsy needle was diagnosed as an inflammatory nodule.

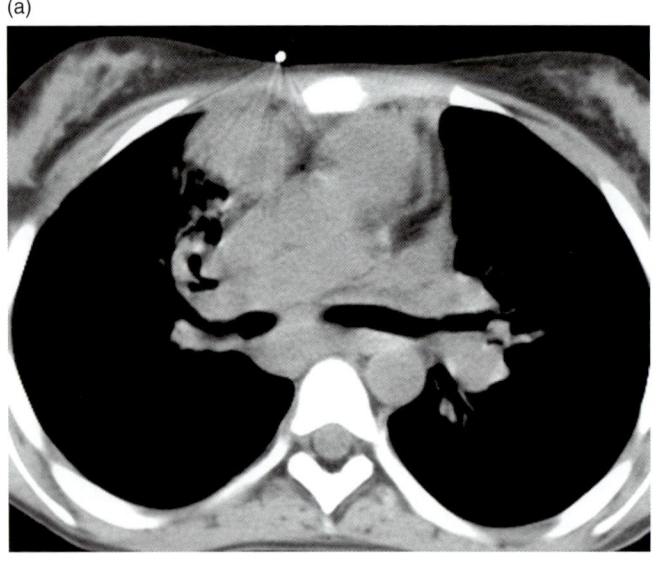 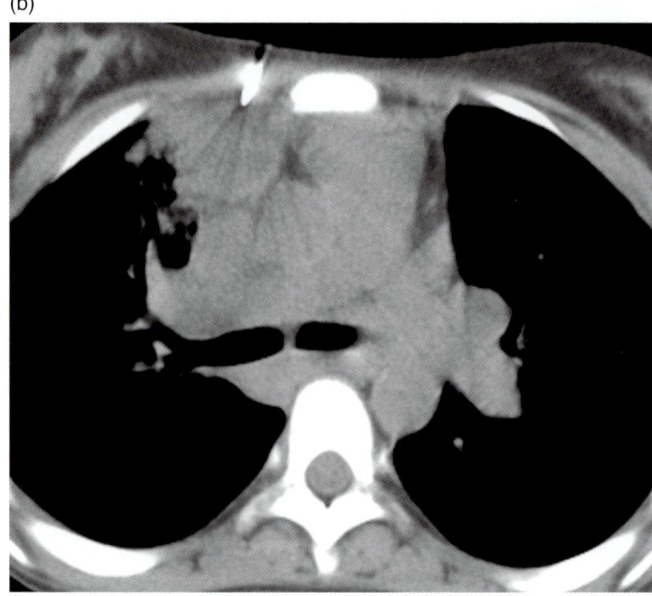

Figure 3.22 (a) This 15-year-old girl presented with a history of congenital autoimmune disease, now end-stage, complicated by multiple opportunistic infections, including *Pneumocystis carinii*, *Herpes zoster*, and disseminated *Mycoplasma avium intracellulare*. Computed tomography obtained as part of a work-up for acute weight loss demonstrated anterior mediastinal adenopathy. In this image obtained in a supine position a Beekley® spot identifies the planned entry site for percutaneous biopsy. (b) Four passes were made with an 18-gauge Tru-Cut® core biopsy needle through the 16-gauge coaxial system shown here. The samples were negative for neoplastic disease, bacteria, fungus, or acid-fast bacilli, and showed only non-specific inflammatory changes. The lesion resolved without further specific therapy.

Specimen handling

Once the specimen is obtained it must be appropriately prepared for transit and subsequent analysis. For cytological preparations, the cells are spread onto a slide and evaluated by the pathologist to determine if an adequate sample has been obtained. Histologic samples are placed onto a Telfa® pad or suspended in normal saline or formalin depending on the specific pathologic question and the laboratory analysis that is anticipated. It is helpful to discuss the biopsy with the pathology service beforehand to determine which suspension is preferred. An adequate volume of saline should be used to avoid evaporation in transit, which may cause unintended alteration of the sample.

For the best results, there should be close cooperation between the interventionalist and pathologist. It is often preferable that the pathologist be present or easily accessible to receive and process the specimen. In select cases a wet reading is helpful to confirm the adequacy of the material while the patient is still under sedation or anesthesia. If needed, additional specimens can be obtained during the same session. This approach is helpful for the patient and family since it minimizes apprehension, increases efficiency, and contributes to a timely diagnosis. In select cases, a biopsy procedure may be performed on an outpatient basis.

Technical variations

Coaxial and tandem needle techniques

In certain cases, it is helpful to either improve control or limit the number of needle passes through part or all of the prospective access pathway. For example, multiple passes through the pleura may increase the risk of symptomatic pneumothorax or bronchopleural fistula. The target lesion may be in close proximity to vital structures. Initial approaches to a small lesion with a large needle may provoke enough hemorrhage to obscure the target. Seeding of the biopsy tract from fragmentation or translation of pathologic (e.g., malignant or infectious) material may complicate an otherwise successful procedure. In order to increase the opportunity for a meaningful sample and to decrease the risk of complication, coaxial or tandem needle techniques may be used alone or in combination.

For *coaxial* guidance, a larger caliber guiding needle with a diamond stylet is advanced to one of two positions. For sampling a pulmonary nodule or mass, where multiple passes through the pleura are undesirable, a guiding needle may be advanced from the subcutaneous tissues through the pleura deeply enough that respiratory motion will not dislodge the needle into the pleural space but not beyond the superficial limit of the lesion. For sampling a lesion adjacent to or partially obscured by a vital structure, the guiding needle may be positioned in gradual steps to a position that, when the stylet is removed, provides safe and unobscured access to the lesion. In either case, once having cleared the obstacle, the guiding needle may be left in this position or advanced to the perimeter of the target lesion as circumstances dictate. In general, we prefer to position the guiding cannula just within the lesion margin. The caliber of the guiding needle must be sufficient to allow passage of the biopsy needle when the stylet is removed. Additionally, the exact distance the biopsy needle can extend

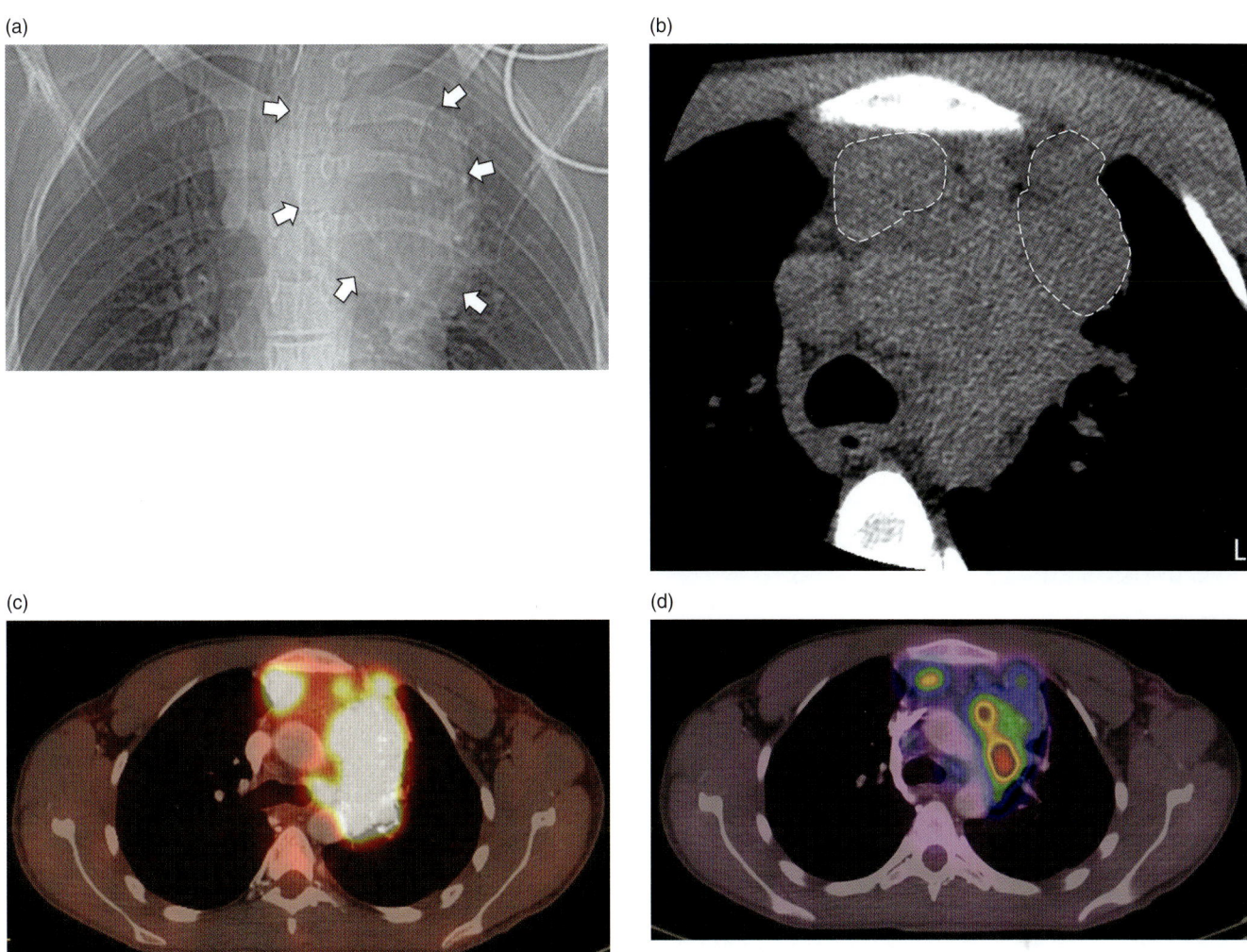

Figure 3.23 (a) A CT-topogram of the chest in a 16-year-old male with a history of Hodgkins lymphoma treated with chemotherapy now with recurrent symptoms and an enlarging mediastinal mass (*arrows*). (b) Computed tomography without contrast through the mediastinum shows undifferentiated bulky adenopathy. Under CT guidance, ten passes were made through the two outlined regions (*dashed lines*). The samples yielded only small pieces of friable tissue that were necrotic on pathologic examination. (c) 18-F FDG-PET/CT fusion with a conventional continuous SUV distribution shows supra-physiologic uptake in the regions of interest but does not suggest a more specific target for biopsy. (d) Reformatting of the PET-CT fusion image with a stepwise algorithm shows the highest uptake in two foci adjacent to the aortic arch, deep in the mediastinum. (e) The reformatted molecular imaging was used to plan the route shown by the *dashed line* on the CT section shown in (b). (f) Two 18-gauge Temno® core (*arrows*) specimens were obtained under US guidance using a 5–3 MHz curvilinear transducer. The color Doppler sampling region was kept as small as possible to improve the image refresh rate, allowing selection of a needle path in real time that avoided vascular structures. (g) This composite image, overlaying the PET-CT fusion image with intraprocedural US shows the 20 mm specimen channel across the target tissue. Touch-prep of the small tissue fragments obtained confirmed Reed–Sternberg cells diagnostic of Hodgkins recurrence.

from the guiding needle when fully engaged must be known in order to calculate how far the biopsy needle should be advanced prior to sampling.

Once the guiding needle is in position, it must be fixed in place in alignment with the lesion and maintained at a constant depth while the stylet is exchanged for the biopsy needle, and the sample is obtained. If multiple samples are required and the lesion is sufficiently large, the angle of the guiding needle may be varied between passes in order to sample different portions of the lesion. To minimize complications, the stylet is usually returned to the guiding needle between passes. When an adequate sample has been obtained, the biopsy needle and guiding cannula may be removed as a unit. The same guiding cannula may of course be used to obtain FNAB and core samples from the same lesion. If brisk hemorrhage is noted or bronchopleural fistula formation is suspected during the biopsy procedure, the tract may be embolized through the guiding cannula after removal of the biopsy needle.

There are two basic principles of tandem needle guidance. First, it is safer and easier to manipulate a thin needle rather than one of larger caliber. When the angle from the skin to the target lesion is difficult to gauge or risky, passing a thin needle and confirming appropriate alignment with imaging provides a visual "pointer" to the lesion. The biopsy needle, or guiding needle if using a coaxial approach, can then be advanced in a parallel orientation alongside the thin needle. If local anesthetic is to be infiltrated along the prospective tract, the thin needle used for this purpose may easily be detached from the

Chapter 3 Thoracic interventions

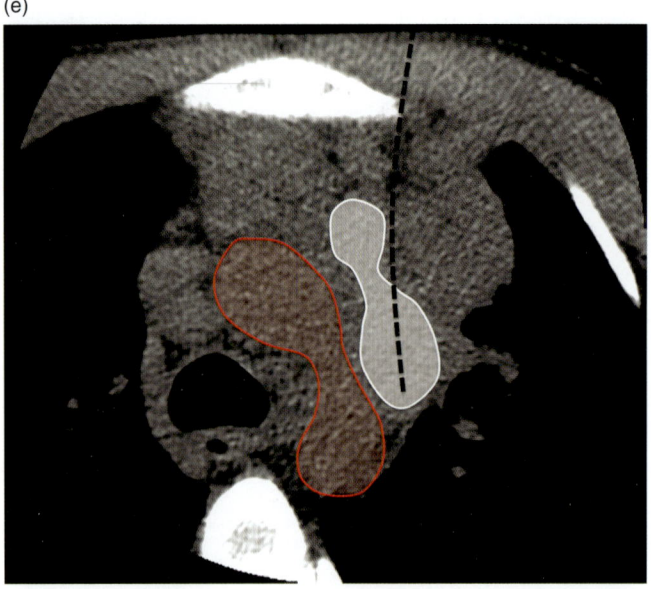

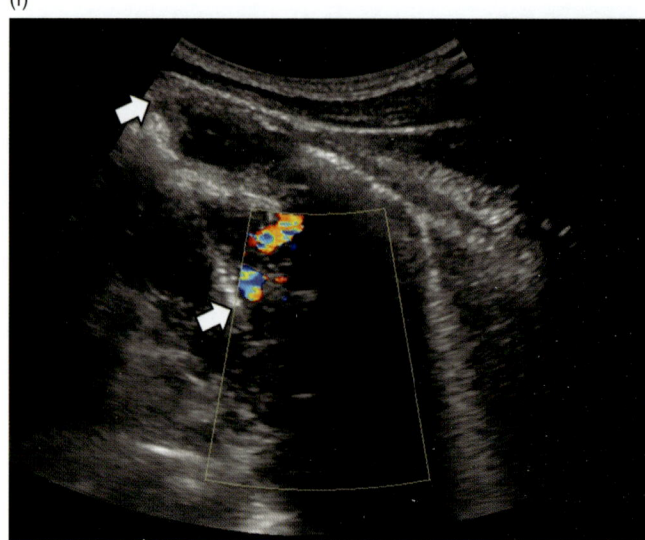

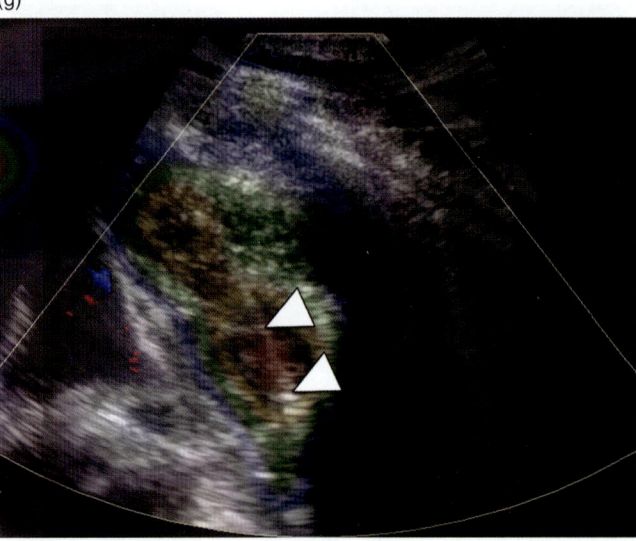

Figure 3.23 (cont.)

hub of the anesthetic syringe and left in place during final lesion localization to provide "first pass" tandem needle guidance.

Second, it is better to pass close to (or even through!) a vital structure with a very thin needle than with one of larger caliber. A thin needle can be used as a "guard rail" to avoid straying from the intended pathway. By keeping to the "safe" side of the thin needle, the biopsy or coaxial needle can then be passed with less risk of complication. If there are multiple vital structures at risk, additional thin needles may be placed to "guard" them.

Postprocedure and follow-up care

Children who undergo a percutaneous biopsy do not tend to present any special management problems in the postbiopsy period. Postprocedural care centers around recovery from sedation or anesthesia, pain management, and, rarely, treatment of complications. For recovery when sedation and local anesthetic were used, oxygen is administered by mask, nasal cannula, or blowby, for oxygen saturations <95%. Outpatients who have their biopsies performed under sedation generally recover in the radiology department. Inpatients usually return to their wards for monitoring. Regardless of the location, our protocol includes vital signs every 15 minutes × 2, every 30 minutes × 2, and then every hour until the child is alert and able to tolerate oral fluids. In addition, all sedated children will have their oxygen saturation continuously monitored until they are awake or easy to arouse. Outpatients are discharged to home when they are alert and can drink. Children who have had general anesthesia are monitored in the recovery room and are cared for by the anesthesiologist. Prior to discharge, a chest X-ray is obtained.

Postprocedural pain is uncommon and, when it occurs, is usually minor and controlled with oral acetaminophen or ibuprofen. Occasionally, more potent pain relievers are required. We prefer intravenous ketorolac tromethamine (Toradol®). If necessary, narcotics including fentanyl citrate or meperidine hydrochloride may be used. Upon discharge, a prescription for oral acetaminophen with codeine may be given.

Complications

The two potential complications of most immediate concern following a percutaneous biopsy procedure in the thorax are pneumothorax (discussed below) and shock (discussed in Chapter 1). Other complications may include pain, hemo- or pneumomediastinum, hemothorax or hemopneumothorax, intrapulmonary hemorrhage (especially in children with a vasculitis or fungal infection), hemoptysis, air embolism, and neoplastic seeding of the biopsy tract.

Pneumothorax

Pneumothorax occurs most commonly following transthoracic lung biopsy (Figure 3.24) but can also occur following biopsy of liver, spleen, adrenal gland, or mediastinum.

Small lesion size, deep location, and preexisting parenchymal disease or emphysematous changes are indicators of increased risk. Maneuvers to decrease the likelihood of pneumothorax include decreasing the number of needle passes, limited transgression of the pleural surfaces, avoiding transgression of aerated lung, oxygen administration, and possibly placing the patient biopsy site down.

Small pneumothoraces in asymptomatic patients with normal respiratory reserve can be treated expectantly. Nitrogen washout with 100% oxygen is effective when used. Treatment of symptomatic patients usually includes hospital admission and placement of a chest tube. Treatment alternatives include use of a Heimlich valve and simple aspiration. Such methods can decrease hospital stay or allow outpatient treatment decreasing overall costs.

A pneumothorax is the most commonly identified complication of transthoracic biopsy, reported in 8 to 61% of cases. Some authors suggest that the increasing depth of a lung lesion increases the risk of pneumothorax. Cox found the risk of pneumothorax was 15% for pleural-based lesions and 50% for parenchymal lesions, independent of depth.

In our experience, the rate of symptomatic pneumothorax in children is considerably less (<5%) than that reported in the adult literature. This lower rate of pneumothorax may be due to healthier lung tissue, or the size and location of abnormalities sampled. However, the actual frequency depends on a variety of factors including the size and location of the lesion being sampled, needle diameter, the number of passes, and the technique employed. Fortunately, when present, most pneumothoraces are small in size and asymptomatic. Postbiopsy pneumothorax may often be successfully treated with simple aspiration, nitrogen washout, or expectant observation. Less than 5% of children require insertion of a chest tube. Permutt and associates emphasize that most significant pneumothoraces necessitating treatment present within the first hour after biopsy and that pneumothoraces are rarely identified more than four hours after completion of the biopsy. Therefore we get a chest radiograph a minimum of one hour postprocedure before deciding to discharge an outpatient.

Conclusions

Percutaneous image-guided biopsy of the thorax can be safely performed in children of all ages and sizes. Standard needles and techniques can be used, although in some instances shorter needles are easier to maintain in position. Core biopsy specimens are preferred whenever possible. The most important components of successful percutaneous biopsy include refining the clinical question to be answered and close consultation between the interventionalist and both the pathologist and referring clinician. Careful route planning (including appropriate selection of imaging modality) before the procedure and expectant observation, with close monitoring of vital signs for the first several hours after the procedure, should promptly identify complications and potential problems. Use of percutaneous techniques can often provide a satisfactory answer to the clinical question with minimal discomfort and morbidity, decreased cost, and improved resource allocation compared to surgical alternatives.

Marking lesions for resection

Introduction

Over the last several years, there has been an increase in the number of requests to identify small pulmonary lesions (e.g.,

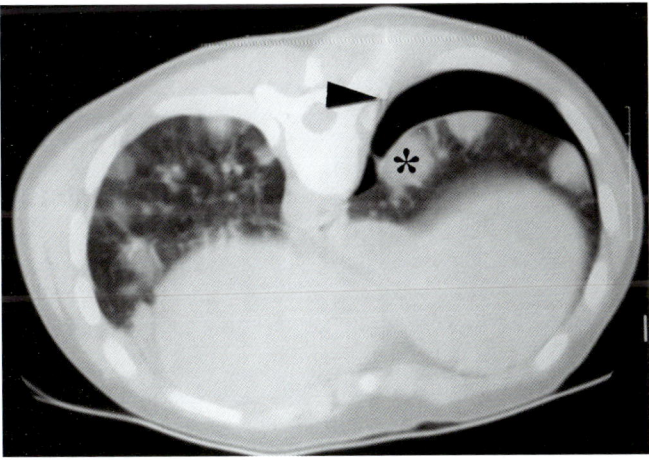

Figure 3.24 After coaxial core biopsy of a pleural-based pulmonary nodule (*asterisk*) in this 17-year-old male with known osteosarcoma, an axial CT image through the chest with the patient in a prone position demonstrates a significant pneumothorax. The coaxial guiding needle (*arrowhead*) remains in the paraspinal soft tissues.

Table 3.16 Indications: preoperative marking

Indications
- Possible pulmonary metastases.
- Lesion requiring surgery but not anticipated to be visible or palpable at the time of surgery.
- Surgeon's preference.

Contraindications
- Uncorrectable coagulopathy.
- Obliterated pleural space.

Relative contraindications
- Vasculitis.
- Pneumothorax.
- Inaccessible anatomy.

Table 3.17 Equipment: preoperative marking

- Beekley® skin marker or other marking method.
- 1% lidocaine buffered with sodium bicarbonate (8:2).
- Breast localization needle (Kopans).
- Sterile methylene blue.

Table 3.18 Procedural summary: preoperative lesion marking

1. Localize lesion.
2. Position child on the CT table.
3. Mark entry site on the skin (Beekley® skin marker or other device).
4. Prepare and drape skin.
5. Locally anesthetize with 1% buffered lidocaine.
6. Insert breast biopsy needle adjacent to the lesion.
7. Confirm needle position with CT.
8. Inject methylene blue into Kopans needle then blow out gently with air, then insert breast biopsy localizing hook needle into needle.
9. Confirm hook needle position.
10. Transport to operating room.

suspected metastases, fungal infiltrates, or PTLD) for thoracoscopic removal. Lesions larger than 1 cm and those abutting or near the pleural surface are amenable to transthoracic image-guided biopsy, as described above. Smaller and more deeply located nodules have in the past required open thoracotomy and lobectomy for successful resection and diagnosis. In most instances, the surgeon is unable to determine the location of these small lesions by inspection or palpation since they generally do not distort the lung or pleural surface. Likewise, the most common reason necessitating conversion from thoracoscopy to thoracotomy is failure to localize the lesion. In order to assist the surgeon, we have modified the technique used for CT-guided lung biopsy. By marking lesions with a localization wire, they can be subsequently excised under VATS. In addition, this strategy allows for a minimally invasive approach and a limited resection of pulmonary tissue.

Indications

Small pulmonary nodules (<10 mm), particularly those distant from the pleural surface (>5 mm), are most likely to be undetected at surgery without preoperative localization. Marking lesions is especially beneficial when it permits a less invasive intervention to be performed in patients whose illness or underlying condition places them at higher risk for open surgical procedures. As is true for other intrathoracic procedures, every effort should be made to correct a bleeding diathesis prior to the planned intervention (Table 3.16).

Technique

Equipment

The equipment required for marking pulmonary lesions prior to surgical resection is fairly simple (Table 3.17), including a localization needle (e.g., Kopans breast biopsy needle, Cook®) and sterile methylene blue dye.

Patient preparation

The work-up for marking of a pulmonary lesion is similar to that discussed for lung biopsy. However, frontal and lateral chest radiographs are usually not helpful in most cases. High-resolution CT is the diagnostic method of choice. In addition, CT is necessary for selecting the safest and most direct route, and for guidance of needle placement.

As is the case for image-guided biopsy of the thorax, no special preparation is required. As usual, the child should have nothing by mouth according to the relevant hospital anesthesia and sedation policy. Antibiotics are not routinely given. Needle localization of pulmonary lesions requires planning and coordination with the surgical service and OR. The procedure is performed under general anesthesia (GA) and the child then needs to be transported to the OR immediately after needle placement for thoracoscopic removal of the lesion(s). Rapid transport to the operating room decreases the likelihood of a growing pneumothorax, migration of the localization needle, and diffusion of the methylene blue.

Standard technique

The technique used for marking a pulmonary lesion for surgical removal is similar to that used for biopsy (Table 3.18). Computed tomography, usually without injection of intravenous contrast, is the modality of choice for guidance. Selected images through the lesion are obtained and the section best demonstrating the lesion is chosen. Using the laser light, the level is traced on the skin with a marking pen. The entry site is determined and a line perpendicular to the axial line is made. A skin marker (Beekley® spot; Beekley®, Bristol, CT) is positioned over the crosshatch and three contiguous images are obtained to confirm a satisfactory skin entry site.

The chest wall is prepared and draped in sterile fashion and 1% buffered lidocaine is slowly injected into the skin with a 30-gauge needle. The biopsy needle is filled with methylene blue

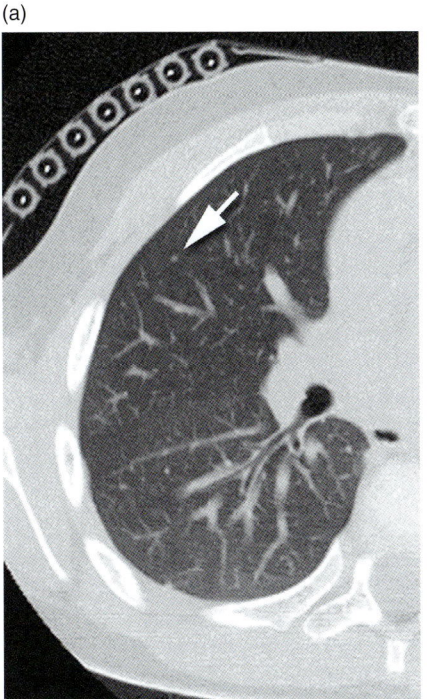 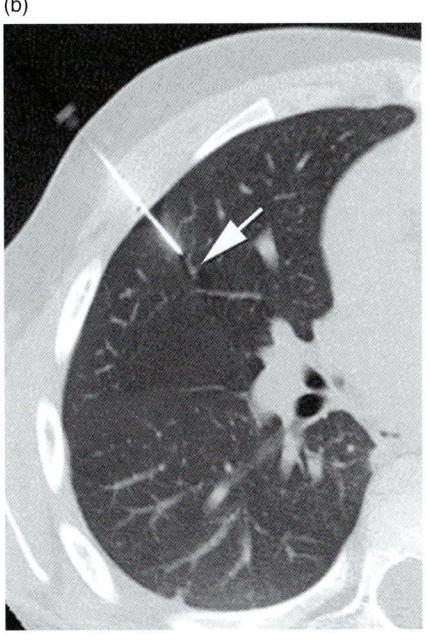 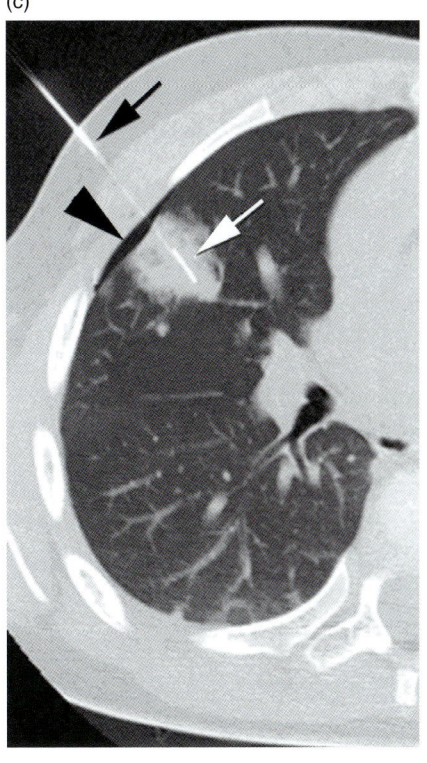

Figure 3.25 (a) Computed tomography-guided biopsy in an immunocompromised patient. Radio-opaque markers are used to identify the entry site. In this case, the pulmonary nodule (*arrow*) was considered too small for biopsy so placement of a Kopans hookwire prior to surgical resection was requested. The entry site was marked between the second and third lateral markers (needle hubs) at this axial level. (b) The needle is introduced. Images may be obtained during placement to assure the needle is taking the correct path to the lesion. If a coaxial biopsy were being performed, the guiding needle could be advanced to the margin of the target lesion (*arrow*) and a sample obtained. (c) This is a composite image of two sequential axial sections demonstrating the hookwire in place (*white arrow*) after the guiding needle (*black arrow*) has been partially withdrawn. The opacity surrounding the hookwire is hemorrhage. Once hemorrhage occurs, visualization of the lesion is lost. A small pneumothorax (*arrowhead*) is also present. Surgical resection of the lesion resulted in diagnosis of *Candida albicans*.

then flushed with air to minimize the volume remaining in the needle. Deposition of methylene blue at the needle tip location identifies the area to be resected if the hooked needle migrates or becomes dislodged, which sometimes occurs. Then, using the previously determined depth and angle, the breast biopsy needle (e.g., Kopans) is inserted so that the tip is adjacent to and 1 to 5 mm deep to the lesion (Figure 3.25). The guide needle is removed as if doing a catheter exchange. The external component of the hook needle is then taped to the skin and covered with gauze and a transparent dressing. More than one lesion may be marked during the same session by this method. A series of three images is obtained to confirm needle tip position. It is valuable to position the needle in the desired location on the first pass. Pneumothorax or pulmonary hemorrhage may move or obscure the lesion if this is not achieved. The child is then moved to the stretcher and immediately transported to the OR for thoracoscopic removal of the lesion (and hook).

It is important to realize that only a *tiny* volume of methylene blue is needed. If too much is injected, a large volume of lung parenchyma turns blue, and its value for localizing the lesion is lost. In addition, the interventionalist should understand that methylene blue stains skin and clothing and will **not** wash off.

Postprocedure and follow-up care

Postprocedural care is provided by the anesthesia and surgical services since the child is immediately transported to the OR for thoracoscopic resection of the lesion(s) and guide needle. It is important to communicate the position of the needle to the anesthesiologist, and to advise the anesthesiologist of the potential for pneumothorax following the localization procedure.

Technical variations

A number of creative strategies have been reported for the preoperative localization of small pulmonary nodules. To avoid accidental migration or dislodgment of the localization wire, alternative devices have been explored, including embolization microcoils attached to a trailing suture. Nomori and colleagues report marking lesions with lipiodol, while marking the nearby pleural surface with collagen colored with methylene blue. The radio-opaque marking allows the lesion to be reacquired up to days later under fluoroscopy for subsequent removal under VATS. Boni *et al.* describe a similar approach using ^{99m}Tc-labeled human serum albumin microspheres to mark the nodule hours before surgery, for later intraoperative identification with a gamma-probe through the VATS trocar.

There is not enough experience with these diverse and innovative approaches in children to comment upon them specifically. However, it is important to remember that the objective is to mark the lesion as safely, expeditiously, and economically as possible. Elegance and sophistication are optional.

Complications

In our experience, there has been a small to moderate pneumothorax in almost all cases. In most children the pneumothorax is not under tension and does not cause difficulty in either oxygenating or ventilating the child. A large pneumothorax may dislodge the needle and make replacement impossible. Although possible, neither pulmonary infection nor empyema has occurred in our patients. Other untoward effects that might be identified include pneumomediastinum, hemothorax, and bronchopleural fistula. Self-limited pulmonary hemorrhage usually occurs along the wire tract, as it does along the biopsy needle tract after lung biopsy, but this is considered an expected outcome of the procedure that is simply more conspicuous due to the air/fluid interface.

Conclusions

Computed tomography-guided lesion localization and marking is a safe technique in children, with a high diagnostic yield following thoracoscopic resection, and a low complication rate. Such a minimally invasive alternative to open thoracotomy is emblematic of the successful collaboration possible between surgical and interventional services. Multidisciplinary procedures completed without moving the patient (i.e., performing the interventional and surgical procedures in an interventional suite outfitted for CT guidance and thoracoscopy) may maximize the yield from this procedure while minimizing complications.

Tracheobronchial stent insertion

Introduction

Stenting of the tracheobronchial tree is now feasible for the treatment of strictures involving the adult and pediatric airway. In 1965, Montgomery reported the use of silicone stents. Since that time, several types of silicone stents have been used for the treatment of tracheobronchial stenoses.

Metallic stents were initially designed for intravascular use and have since been used in the biliary tree, esophagus, urinary tract, and, most recently, in the tracheobronchial tree. In 1986, Wallace and colleagues reported the usefulness of expandable metal stents for treatment of stenoses following tracheobronchial reconstruction. Since then, several groups have described the successful placement of metallic stents for treatment of a variety of conditions affecting the airway. When an airway stenosis is identified, there are a variety of therapeutic options available. Bronchoscopy with dilation, laser therapy, endobronchial resection, fluoroscopically guided balloon dilation, and stenting all may be helpful depending upon the clinical setting. The relative indications for each therapeutic approach have changed with technical advances.

Currently, surgical resection of an airway stricture is recommended whenever possible. However, surgery is not always feasible. The risks and technical limitations of surgical resection and tracheobronchial reconstruction make the use of stents and other techniques appealing for management of these difficult patients. The location of the stenosis, postoperative recurrence(s), uncorrectable coagulopathy, or poor surgical candidacy due to the severity of underlying disease may all mitigate for a minimally invasive alternative. The use of stents represents an advancement in the management of otherwise inoperable patients and, in these settings, may be a life-saving procedure. In the absence of an active inflammatory process, placement of a metallic stent may be the best option.

When active inflammation is present, a combination of medical therapy (e.g., inhalation and intravenous or oral steroids), balloon dilation (as a primary treatment or temporizing measure), or placement of a silicone stent may be selected. When the inflammation subsides, a metal stent can be deployed if necessary. In the past, the most frequent type of stent utilized was made of silicone rubber. However, expandable metallic stents have become more widely used and seem to be the approach of choice in many instances.

Silicone stents were initially designed for use as T-tubes and were modified for use in other areas. Today, the Dumon stent is the most widely used silicone endoprosthesis, similar to the Westaby and Cooper–Hood prostheses. Silicone stents were the first to be used in the airway and offer several advantages. They are easily inserted, can be modified into a variety of shapes and lengths and are generally well tolerated. They are efficacious for treatment of inflammatory and malignant strictures. The plastic prevents in-growth of granulation tissue and tumor into the tracheal or bronchial lumen although there is tissue growth between the stent and airway wall. Perhaps the biggest advantage of this material is its ease of removal.

Unfortunately, disadvantages also exist and tend to outweigh the advantages. Silicone stents are a non-tapered, high-friction material. Their construction makes it difficult to position them in individuals with tight strictures. These stents are prone to displacement (approximately 10%) and expulsion from the airway; they have relatively thick walls and narrow lumens that are apt to obstruct (approximately 4%) with mucus and other secretions; and are subject to complication by granuloma formation (approximately 8%). These complications can be especially problematic in children with smaller airways. Being solid, these stents interfere with normal mucociliary action and clearance of secretions. Patients with a silicone stent deployed require constant pulmonary toilet. Use of a silicone stent is contraindicated if the lesion crosses a bronchial orifice since it would result in obstruction of a lung segment. Thus, when used in children, silicone stents tend to be only a short-term solution.

Metallic stents have several advantages over silicone stents, especially their low profile, expandability, flexibility, and the ability to become epithelialized. Regardless of type, metal stents have thinner walls with significantly larger lumens than equivalent-sized silicone stents. With their low profile, metallic stents are easily positioned across a stricture without significant trauma. Because of their open mesh design, they can be placed across a bronchial origin without obstructing it. Finally, metallic stents are more stable and are less likely to become dislodged. These physical characteristics reduce the amount of specialized care required after stent placement.

In spite of the positive features of metal stents, problems do exist. In general, metal stents can be deployed accurately. However, on occasion, they may be inadvertently malpositioned. If this occurs, repositioning may be difficult or impossible. Also, the open mesh design does not protect against tissue in-growth into the lumen with secondary stent compression. Perhaps covered stents will help in some situations; however, no experience is yet available to answer this question. In the long term, if the stent is no longer needed or is causing problems, it may be difficult or impossible to remove.

Although stent removal is not generally recommended, Filler and colleagues have removed 11 of 30 stents in a pediatric population. They state that using a twisting motion, stent removal and withdrawal can be accomplished in less than 30 seconds so that significant airway obstruction does not occur. A small amount of mucosal bleeding was noted in all cases, which stopped spontaneously in a few minutes. These authors did note, however, that one child died during an attempted stent removal because it was welded into the tracheal wall by fibrous reaction. Nashef and colleagues and others have also removed stents without sequelae. Nashef and associates describe removal of Gianturco stents as a process similar to rolling spaghetti on a fork, but much more difficult and time consuming. Others have removed Palmaz® and wall stents by cutting them with lasers to affect removal. Stents have been intentionally temporarily deployed in several patients with chemo- or radiosensitive malignancies with success. Thus, although some stents have been removed, it is clear that the current generation of stents is intended for permanent deployment. Therefore it may be the best strategy to consider tracheal stents as permanent at this time.

Indications

Airway obstruction unresponsive to medical or surgical therapy is the primary indication for stent placement in childhood (Table 3.19). The most common conditions requiring stent insertion are malacia, stricture, and airway compression (e.g., from infection, thoracic or mediastinal masses, vascular abnormalities, etc.). A number of conditions may lead to narrowing or obstruction of the pediatric airway (Table 3.20). However, severe tracheomalacia or bronchomalacia, unresponsive to standard therapy, and postoperative strictures, have been the most common indications to date. Tracheobronchomalacia,

Table 3.19 Indications for tracheobronchial stent insertion

Congenital abnormalities
- Tracheomalacia or bronchomalacia unresponsive to conventional therapy.
- Vascular compression with or without secondary tracheobronchomalacia unresponsive to operative repair or medical management especially if ventilator dependent.
- Vascular compression secondary to normal anatomic variations or congenital heart disease e.g., pulmonary artery sling with associated airway anomalies, transposition of the great vessels, unresponsive to surgical (pexy procedure or correction) and/or medical management.
- Severe tracheomalacia resulting from esophageal atresia and tracheoesophageal fistula.

Acquired conditions
- Stricture after single or double lung transplantation.
- Following tracheal surgery or bronchoplasty.
- Chronic inflammatory strictures.
- Chondritis.
- Extraluminal masses for palliation or cure.
- Post-tracheostomy strictures.
- Tracheobronchial stricture in a patient in poor medical condition and not a surgical candidate.
- Unresectable lesion.

Table 3.20 Causes of pediatric airway narrowing

- Extrinsic
  - Pulmonary masses
  - Mediastinal masses
  - Mediastinal or hilar lymphadenopathy
  - Congenital vascular rings and slings
- Intrinsic
  - Iatrogenic (multiple intubations)
  - Traumatic
  - Infectious
  - Congenital (tracheal stenosis, tracheomalacia)

whether primary or secondary, is often seen in young children. The condition may be outgrown, managed by supportive medical therapy, or less commonly managed surgically. Children with severe malacia requiring ventilation and those who are debilitated may be considered for stent placement. This is an ideal group of patients for this therapy since the underlying pathophysiology is excessive collapsibility of an airway segment without underlying inflammation. To date, these children have responded well to stent insertion and their respiratory distress is promptly and often dramatically improved (Figure 3.26). The long-term effect of a stent on tracheal growth, development, and wall integrity remains unknown.

Strictures involving the airway are the second most common indication for stenting. In younger children, postoperative strictures secondary to tracheoplasty or other surgical procedures are most common. In older children, strictures resulting from lung transplantation increase in prevalence

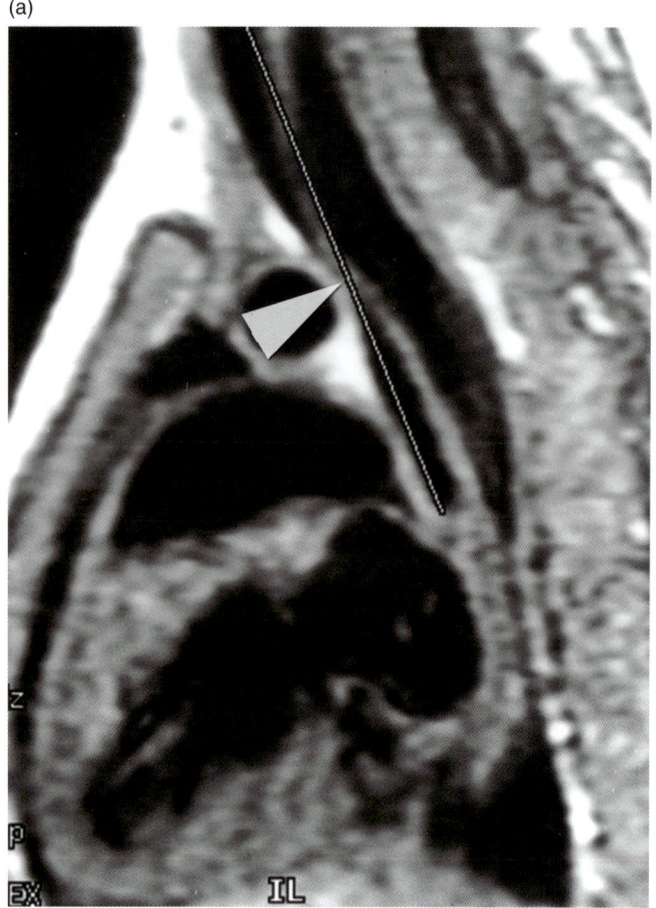 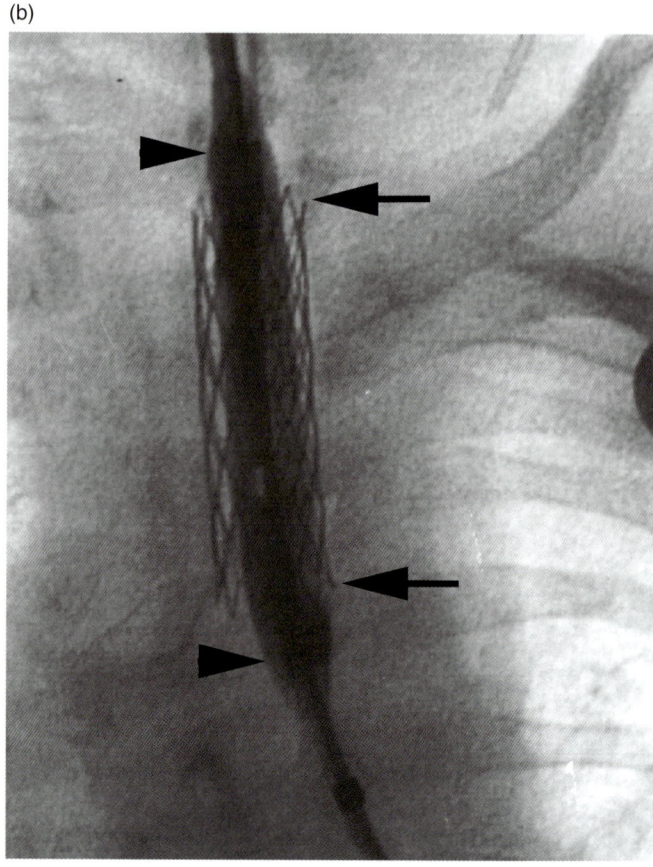

Figure 3.26 (a) A midsagittal non-enhanced T1-weighted MR image through the chest in a six-month-old boy with prematurity and VACTERL syndrome. The patient was ventilator dependent in the intensive care unit. The tracheal narrowing (*arrowhead*) at the level of the aortic arch is consistent with the history of severe tracheomalacia. The line along the long axis of the trachea was used to estimate the distance to the carina. (b) In this PA fluoroscopic image, a Palmaz® stent (*arrows*) is positioned across the region of tracheal stenosis and dilated over a non-compliant angioplasty balloon (*arrowheads*). The infant demonstrated dramatic and immediate resolution of his airway obstruction. He was discharged to home from the intensive care unit two days after this procedure. Lateral (c) and PA (d) chest radiographs obtained the day of the procedure show the stent in satisfactory position. (e) PA chest radiograph almost ten years after the stenting procedure demonstrates the stent in good position with a well-maintained airway.

(Figure 3.27). Airway management following lung transplantation is a complex issue. Successful lung transplantation has been hindered by a relatively high incidence of airway complications. Postoperatively, the bronchial anastomosis is dependent on the pulmonary circulation for healing. Collaterals from the bronchial circulation usually develop over several weeks. In spite of improvements in operative techniques, peri-anastomotic airway problems still account for 12 to 40% of all postoperative complications. Unlike the bronchial anastomosis, the tracheal anastomosis is much less prone to stricture because of its built-in collaterals from the coronary arteries. Anastomotic complications range from mild to severe and include anything from mucosal webs to frank necrosis with associated obstruction or dehiscence. The management of these ischemic complications may be challenging and include airway debridement via an endoscope, balloon dilation, and silicone or metal stent placement (Figure 3.28).

Currently, the treatment of choice for tracheobronchial strictures is surgical resection with an end-to-end anastomosis. However, this approach may not be feasible because of the location of the stricture and extent of the narrowing, the underlying etiology, and the general health of the individual. Non-operative, palliative techniques are well suited for children with severe tracheomalacia, unresectable disease, or prior extensive tracheal or bronchial resection.

The list of indications for which placement of a stent may be efficacious in the pediatric population seems to be slowly growing. In general, in spite of the allure of this therapeutic option, the long-term effect of stenting an airway in a growing child is still unknown. Thus, at this time, it is our feeling that stent placement should be reserved for treatment of conditions that are not responding to conventional forms of management. Although in time it may be shown that stenting of a child's airway is safe, effective, and the approach of choice, it is probably wise to take a conservative view until more data

Chapter 3 Thoracic interventions

(c)
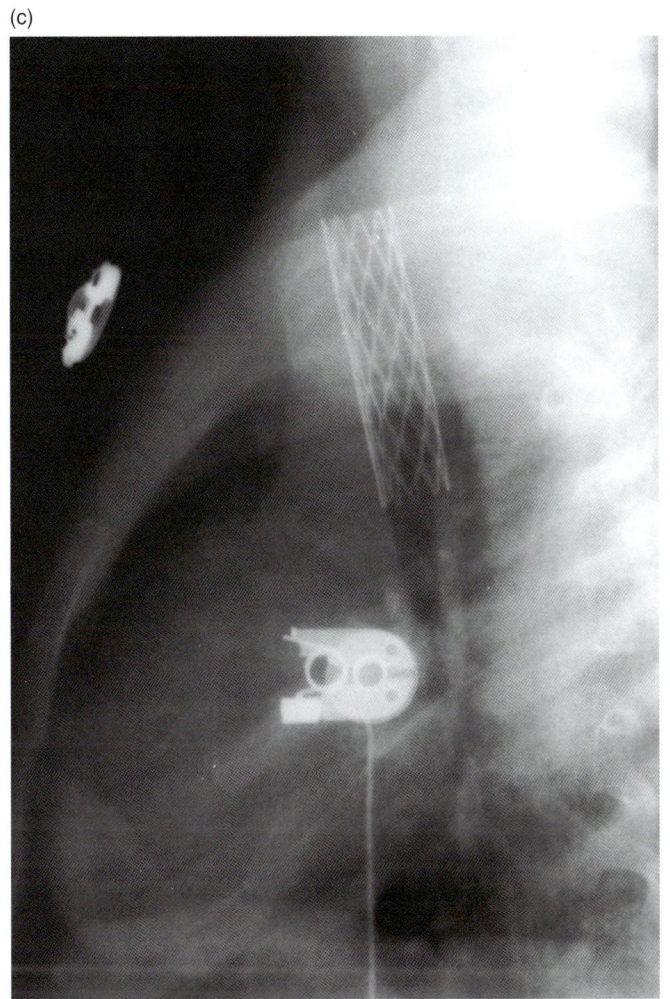

(d)
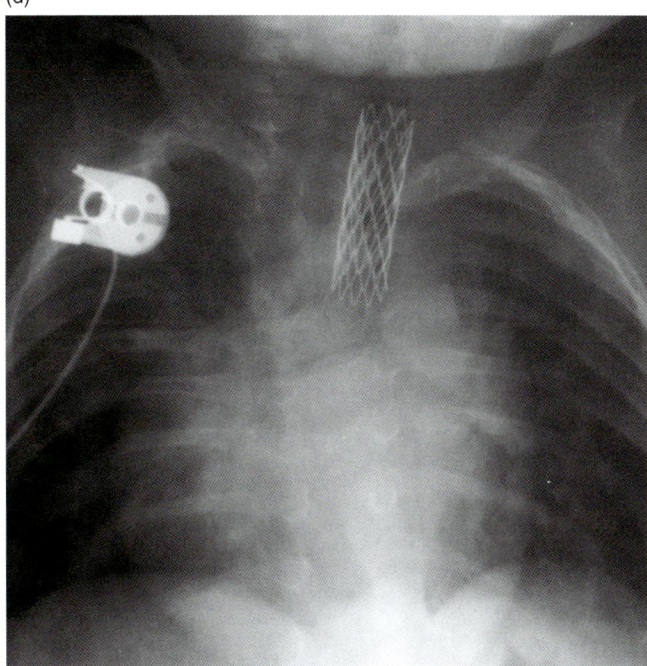

(e)
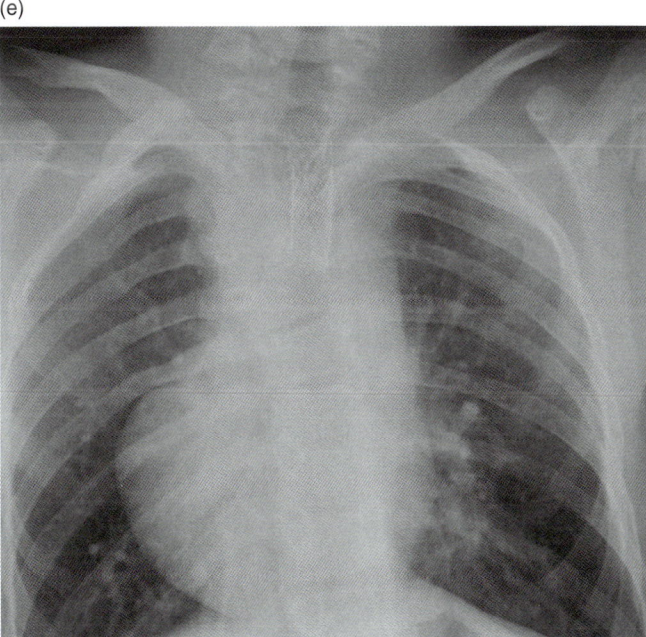

Figure 3.26 (cont.)

143

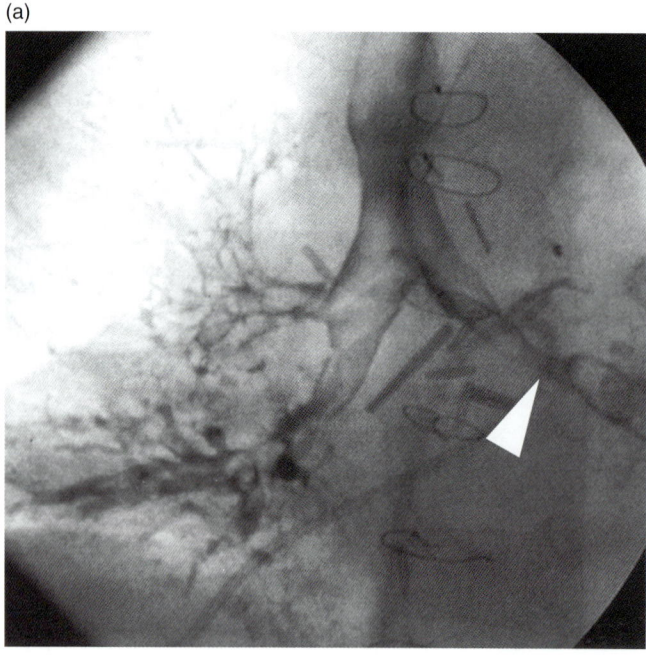
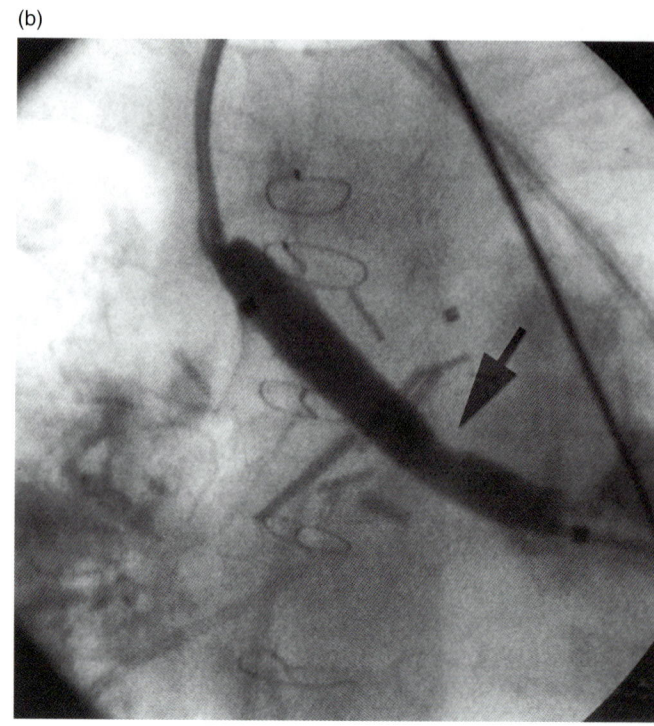

Figure 3.27 (a) A bronchogram performed with non-ionic contrast in a three-year-old boy with a lung transplant shows a focal stenosis (*arrowhead*) of the left mainstem bronchus. (b) Contrast in the non-compliant angioplasty balloon on this frontal fluoroscopic image obtained during bronchial dilation demonstrates a partial "waist" at the stenosis (*arrow*). This was ablated with further dilation, and the patient demonstrated complete resolution of his symptoms.

becomes available. Having said this, it has already become obvious that tracheobronchial stenting may be life saving and should be offered to patients whose conditions are not amenable to surgery.

The preliminary results of tracheobronchial stenting suggest the long-term results of airway stenting depend upon the underlying etiology of the stricture. In patients with narrowing secondary to fibrosis, those with tracheobronchomalacia or extrinsic compression, stenting is an excellent therapeutic option. However, children with fibroinflammatory disease with active inflammation and proliferation of granulation tissue usually have more difficulties. These patients have a high incidence of restenosis that may necessitate stent removal. In these individuals, it may be best to delay insertion of a metallic stent until the inflammation subsides, if possible. If stenting is necessary during this acute phase, a silicone stent may initially be placed until the inflammation subsides since this type of stent does not allow in-growth of granulation tissue. Later, a metallic stent can be inserted, if needed. Alternatively, insertion of a metallic stent in combination with aggressive medical therapy aimed at treating the airway inflammation may be effective.

It appears that placement of a metal stent for treatment of an airway stricture can be accomplished safely and effectively in the majority of cases. Certainly, successful stent deployment can be facilitated by either bronchoscopy or fluoroscopy and a catheter-based stent system. Fluoroscopic guidance appears to have advantages over bronchoscopic guidance including: (1) the ability to simultaneously visualize the stricture and the stent in order to facilitate accurate deployment of the stent and avoid inadvertent crossing of a bronchial orifice; (2) a lower profile system enabling treatment of patients with tighter strictures; (3) the ease of treating bronchial lesions since the stent can track around steep angles; and (4) the smaller size of the catheter – ideal for the pediatric population and technically easier and less traumatic.

Contraindications to the placement of a stent in the airway of a child are difficult to elucidate at this time due to the lack of experience with this technique. However, patients with a breach in the integrity of an airway wall or with abnormal airway anatomy may be more prone to stent erosion and secondary complications. Nashef *et al.* reported a case of massive fatal hemoptysis resulting from penetration of a Gianturco Z-stent into a pulmonary artery. Children with the combination of a mucosal proliferative process and a tracheobronchial stricture have a high risk of recurrent strictures. Thus, in these children, placement of a metallic stent may be a relative contraindication. In this subgroup, medical therapy, a silicone stent or a covered metal stent may be preferable.

Technique

Equipment

Currently, there are several types of stents available, which are potentially useful for treating children with narrowed airways, including the Palmaz® stent, the Wallstent®, the Gianturco

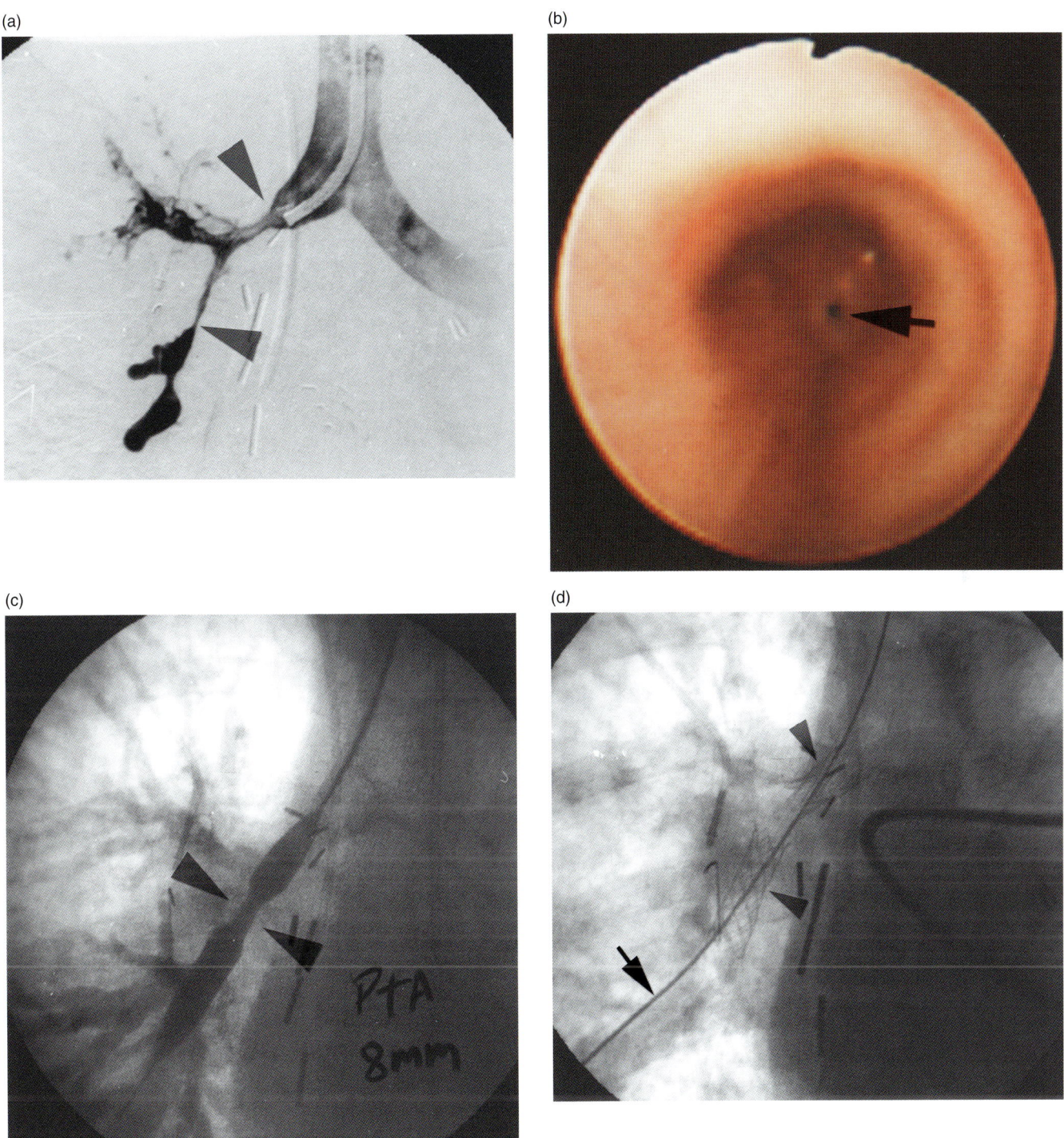

Figure 3.28 (a) A 17-year-old woman with cystic fibrosis presented with recurrent pneumonias after lung transplantation. Bronchography with non-ionic contrast shows stenoses (*arrowheads*) of the right mainstem and lower lobe bronchi. (b) Preprocedure bronchoscopy demonstrates the tight stenosis (*arrow*) in the right lower lobe bronchus. (c) Contrast in the 8-mm non-compliant angioplasty balloon demonstrates a "waist" at the location of the right lower lobe bronchial stenosis (*arrowheads*). With further dilation this was effaced. (d) With the safety guide wire (*arrow*) still in place, this postprocedure frontal chest radiograph shows the Palmaz® stents (*arrowheads*) in satisfactory position. (e) Follow-up bronchoscopy shows the stent in position with a patent airway.

Z-stent, and the nitinol stent (Table 3.21). Each stent has a different design with differing physical characteristics and perhaps different indications. The interventionalist should review the various stents that are available and choose the one that best fits the clinical indication. Currently, we prefer Palmaz® stents and wall stents. In general, we select Palmaz® stents for use in the trachea, mainstem bronchi, and often the bronchus intermedius. Wall stents are used in smaller airways, tortuous

(e)

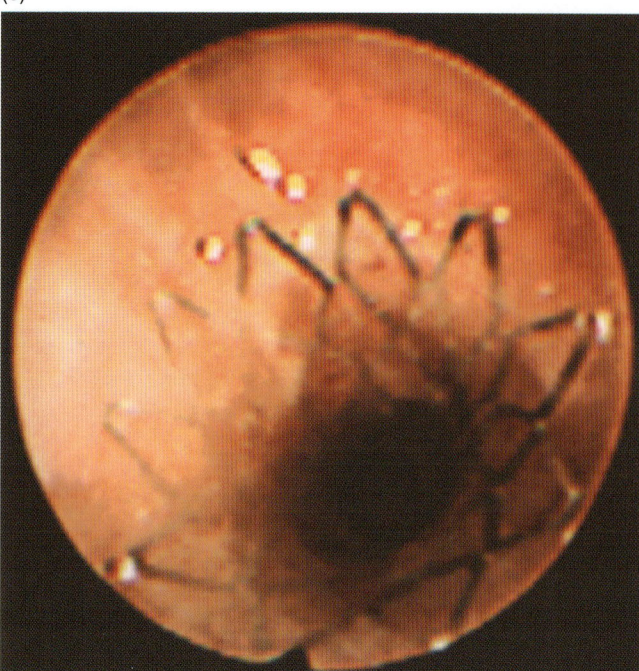

Figure 3.28 (cont.)

Table 3.21 Equipment: tracheobronchial stenting

- Ventilator with associated equipment in the care of anesthesiology or critical care
- Slit-valve to be inserted in the ventilator circuit for entry of catheters, wires, stents, etc.
- JB-1 or other directional catheter
- Directional non-hydrophilic guide wire
- Non-ionic contrast
- PTA catheter of appropriate diameter
- Stent

Table 3.22 Procedural summary: tracheobronchial stenting

- Position directional catheter proximal to the stricture.
- Perform a bronchogram with non-ionic contrast.
- Measure diameter of the normal airway and stricture.
- Maneuver JB-1 catheter distal to the stricture.
- Exchange guide wire for a stiff guide wire.
- Dilate or stent stricture site. A conservative approach to stenting is suggested.
- Postprocedural bronchogram or bronchoscopy.
- Chest radiograph and possibly CT.

airways, airways that have a significant caliber change, and when a bronchial orifice is crossed because of its more open design.

Patient preparation

In general, before a child is considered for treatment of tracheobronchial pathology using a stent, they should be thoroughly evaluated by the appropriate medical and surgical services. Conventional therapies should be considered or attempted prior to consideration of stent placement. However, when the patient becomes a candidate for stent placement, preoperative evaluation will usually include one or more of the following procedures: frontal and lateral chest radiographs, bronchoscopy, chest CT, chest MRI, and, in children with tracheomalacia, fluoroscopy or dynamic CT to evaluate the dynamic nature of the tracheal collapse.

Before stent insertion, a detailed evaluation of the type, location, and extent of the airway pathology is essential. Measurements of the airway diameter are also made at the level of the stenosis, of the stricture length, and of the diameter of the airway proximal and distal to the stricture. In some instances, three-dimensional reconstructions are useful. This preoperative imaging aids in the selection of the type, of the ideal diameter, and length of the endoprosthesis. Insertion of a tracheal or bronchial endoprosthesis is a relatively simple and atraumatic procedure. However, in most instances, these children are ill and require greater levels of intraprocedural support. Therefore the endoprosthesis is usually inserted under general anesthesia or in an intubated child using a combination of sedation and paralysis. All children who have tracheostomies or who are intubated are mechanically ventilated. We have found that inclusion of a side arm adapter with slit valve at the level of the ventilator connection facilities entry into the tracheobronchial tree making the procedure technically easier.

Standard technique
Airway dilation

Initially, a directional catheter (JB-1) and guide wire (Bentson, Newton) system is positioned in the airway proximal to the stricture. A bronchogram is performed (Table 3.22) via a catheter using non-ionic contrast (>240 mg %). The midpoint of the airway narrowing (Figure 3.29a) is marked on the skin surface with a radio-opaque marker (e.g., Beekley® spot) or a hemostat fastened to the drapes. If a tight stricture is present, a directional catheter/guide wire system is maneuvered past the stricture (Figure 3.29b). The directional guide wire is then exchanged for a stiff guide wire (e.g., Amplatz Super Stiff®, Roadrunner®, or Rosen guide wire), to facilitate positioning of the angioplasty balloon (Figure 3.29c). Due to rapid drying with airflow, a hydrophilic guide wire is not useful in this setting. The diameter of the normal trachea or bronchus above and below the stricture, the length of the lesion, and the diameter of the stricture, are measured. In general, the percutaneous transluminal angioplasty (PTA) balloon selected is usually 2 mm larger than the normal luminal diameter. When tight strictures are present, the initial balloon diameter selected is usually not less than one half the final diameter. We have had the best results using high atmosphere (>17 ATM) PTA balloons whenever possible and noted postoperative strictures

Chapter 3 Thoracic interventions

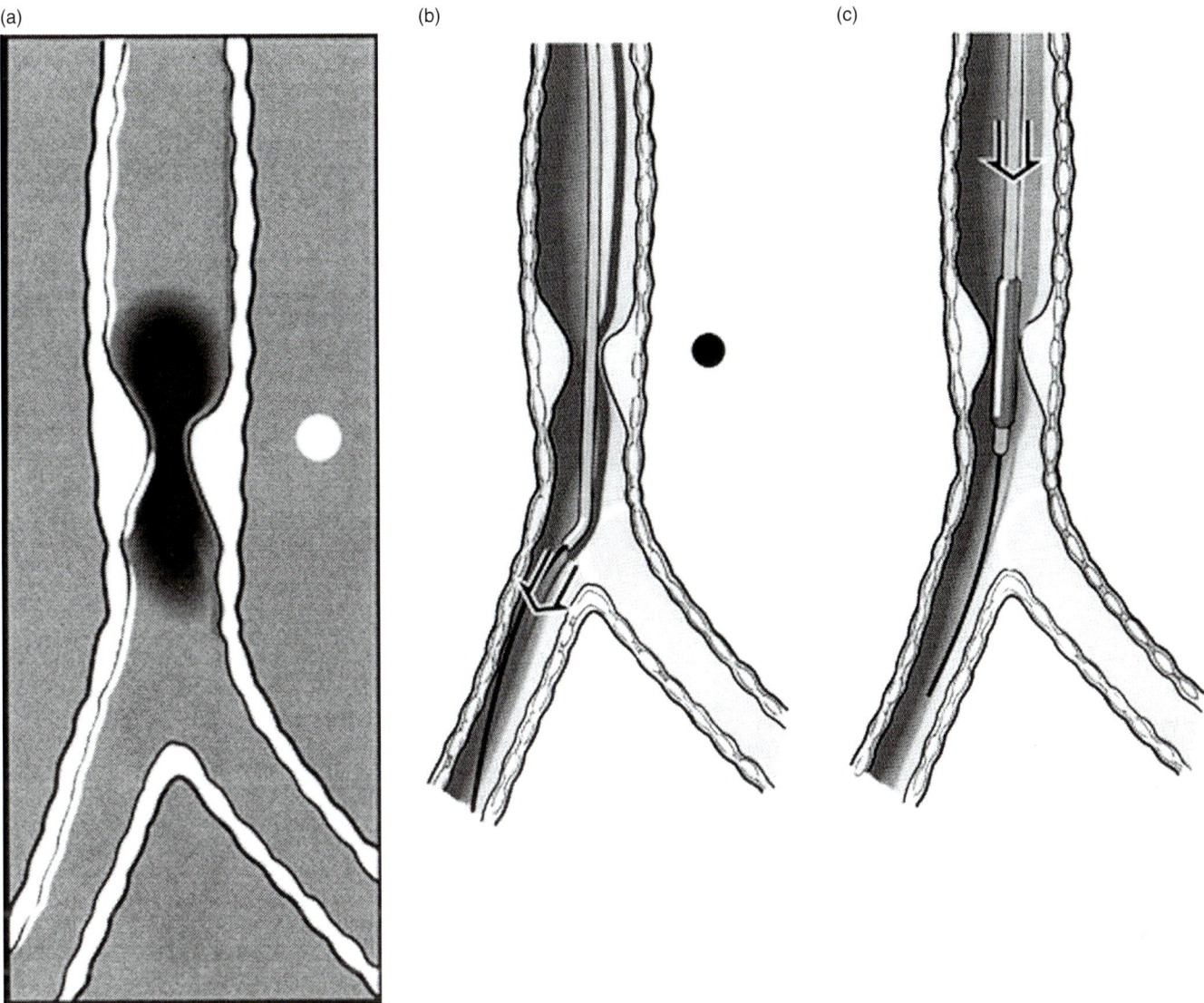

Figure 3.29 Tracheal stent illustration. (a) The midpoint of the tracheal narrowing is marked on the skin surface with a radio-opaque marker or a hemostat. (b) A directional catheter/guide wire system is maneuvered past the stricture. (c) A non-compliant angioplasty balloon is positioned over a stiff guide wire. (d) Once in position, the balloon is inflated for three to five minutes as long as the oxygen saturation and vital signs are satisfactory. If a waist remains, the balloon will be reinflated an additional one or two times. (e) The stent is centered over the stricture under fluoroscopic guidance. (f) Once in position the stent is enlarged by inflating the balloon. (g) Once the stent is in place, a postprocedural bronchogram is performed to assess the results. If needed, additional dilation with larger balloons can be performed to enlarge the stent.

to be resistant to dilation below 10 to 12 ATM in many instances.

Once in position, the balloon is inflated with dilute water-soluble contrast using a pressure gauge to monitor balloon pressure. We prefer to maintain inflation for three to five minutes as long as the oxygen saturation and vital signs remain at the preinflation baseline. If a waist remains, the balloon will be reinflated an additional one or two times until the waist decreases or disappears (Figure 3.29d). If, after a second inflation, the waist is still present, a larger balloon or one with higher inflation pressure is considered. If the waist disappears, no further dilation is performed. If an exchange is made for a larger balloon, the catheter is examined. If there is gross blood on the balloon no further dilations are performed that day. At the completion of the procedure, a follow-up bronchogram is performed to document the results.

The radiographic result may look suboptimal immediately post-PTA; however, further improvement may occur as the edema and submucosal hemorrhage resolves. Therefore it is imperative to follow these children clinically, by bronchoscopy, and with imaging to assess their outcome as needed. In the early stages of treatment, repeat balloon dilations are usually necessary every two to four weeks to maintain the desired airway diameter. Later, as the larger luminal diameter

Chapter 3 Thoracic interventions

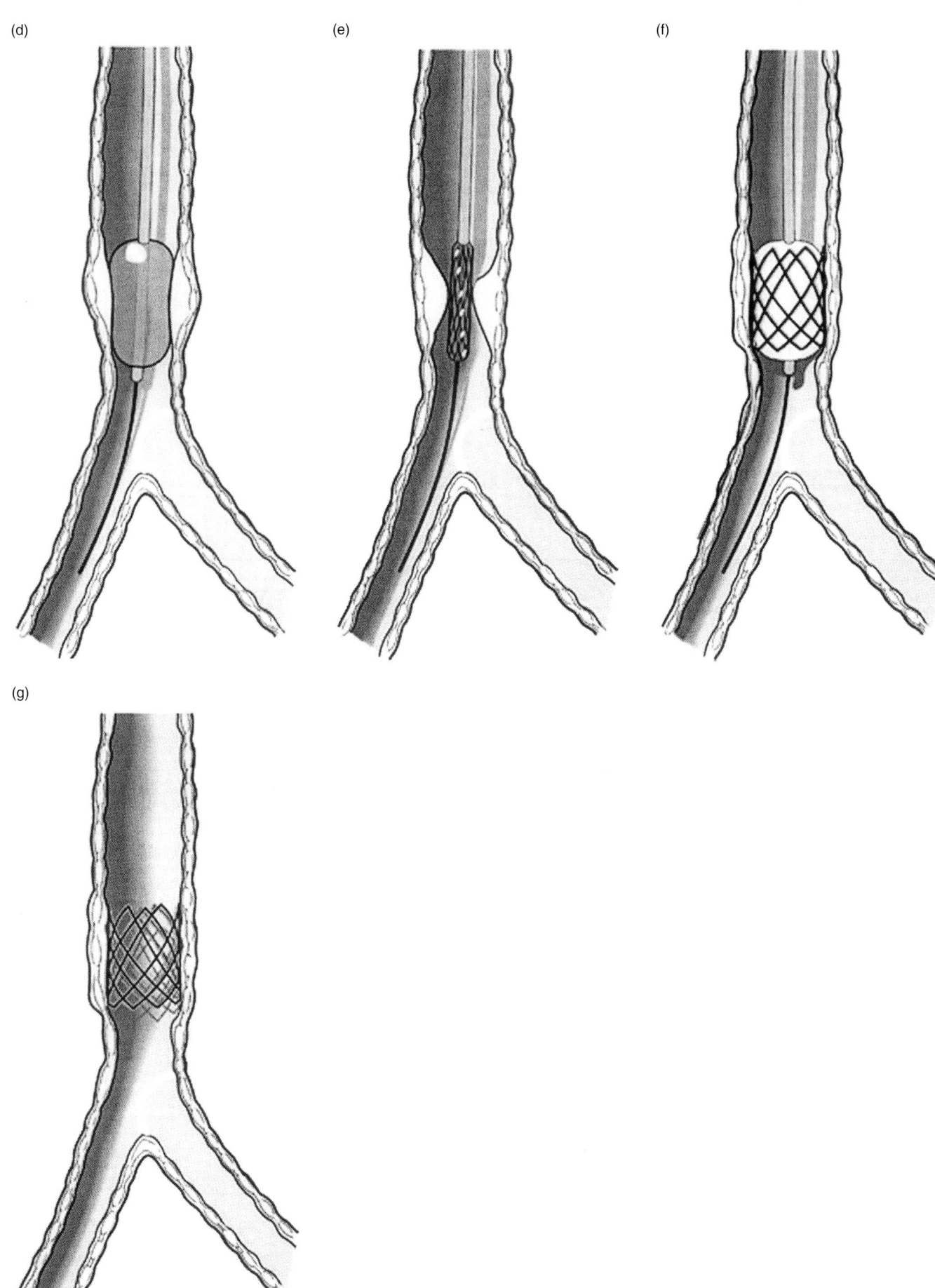

Figure 3.29 (cont.)

stabilizes, the interval between dilations increases significantly, often to a one- to three-month interval. Whenever possible, the stricture is dilated to its maximal size with the first inflation to minimize cost and keep procedure time as short as possible. It is our habit to clean and save all functional equipment (balloons, catheters, wires, etc.) for future use in the same patient.

Tracheobronchial stenting

Once the decision to stent the trachea or bronchus is made, bronchography is performed, usually following bronchoscopy, with the level of intended stent placement marked and tracheobronchial measurements made. The length and diameter of the stent is tailored to the individual situation; however, in young children, we generally prefer a stent at least 2 mm larger than the normal airway proximal to the narrowing to allow for future airway growth.

With the catheter proximal to the airway pathology, nonionic contrast (240 to 320 mg%) is injected and the airway anatomy delineated. The midpoint of the stricture is identified and marked on the skin surface using a Beekley® spot or with a hemostat on the gown. Many factors influence the type of stent selected for insertion. Unfortunately, there are currently no scientifically determined guidelines that aid in the selection of the endoprosthesis. Currently, we feel factors to consider are the underlying cause of the stricture, the location of the stricture, and, perhaps most importantly, the child's age.

To date, a Palmaz® stent or wall stent has been most often used. We are uncomfortable using the Gianturco Z-stent because of the higher reported incidence of complications. The Palmaz® stents and wall stents are interchangeable in most instances. Since the wall stent is more flexible and has thinner monofilament wires making up its walls, it probably has a lower likelihood of obstructing secondary to airway secretions. Thus the wall stent is preferred when a lesion crosses a bronchial origin or in those patients who have tortuous or angulated airways. In contrast, the Palmaz® stent is used when greater radial strength is needed, such as in patients with post-transplant strictures when precise deployment is necessary and when significant patient growth is anticipated. Using successively larger angioplasty balloons, the stent diameter can be progressively enlarged. Currently, it appears to be the preferred stent for treating tracheal lesions, while the wall stent is more frequently used for bronchial pathology. For children with tracheomalacia, either stent will likely be successful. Preliminary experience with nitinol stents is encouraging, in that it may offer a reasonable compromise between mechanical reliability and ease of removal in life-threatening or inoperable stenosis or compression of the trachea and main stem bronchi in children.

Once the directional catheter is positioned distal to the stricture, a stiff guide wire is inserted and the directional catheter exchanged for the catheter/stent device. The stent is then deployed. A Palmaz® stent, with the greatest range of diameters, is selected so that it can be enlarged as the airway grows. This stent is easy to insert (Figure 3.29e–g). It is merely centered over the stricture and enlarged by inflating the balloon. If a wall stent is deployed, the stent is initially positioned with about 70% of the stent length distal to the stricture. The stent is released approximately halfway to allow for shortening as the stent exits its protective canister. The inner catheter is then retracted until it is again in contact with the stent so that it can be pulled proximally and centered. The rolling membrane is then retracted until about 75% is exposed. At this time, the last positional adjustments are made and the endoprosthesis is centered across the stricture. Once the stent is in place, a postprocedural bronchogram is performed to assess the results. If needed, additional dilation with larger balloons can be performed to enlarge the stent. Follow-up chest radiographs and bronchoscopy are performed if the child's symptoms persist or recur.

Postprocedure and follow-up care

A chest radiograph is obtained following the procedure to confirm and document stent position and to evaluate for complications (see below). The child is otherwise treated expectantly, monitoring vital signs closely until the patient returns to baseline, at which time the child can be discharged or returned to the ward as appropriate.

Complications

At this time, it seems that almost all metallic stents can be accurately and atraumatically deployed. In the reported cases, there is nearly a 100% success rate. Acutely, minor complications occur in less than 20% of cases, with an irritating cough; mild, self-limiting hemoptysis; dysphagia; mucosal edema; restenosis; and infections being most commonly reported. Major complications are unusual and rarely occur at the time of stent placement. The most common stent-related complication that causes moderate to severe symptoms is ingrowth of granulation tissue, especially in patients with fibroinflammatory strictures. These patients may become severely dyspneic and require endobronchial ablation of the granulation tissue by laser therapy, cryotherapy, or some other form of treatment. However, we feel that whenever possible, angioplasty should be the initial treatment. This approach is less traumatic and tends to limit the postprocedural recurrence of granulation tissue. Steroids may also be of use to reduce granulation tissue recurrence. Operative ablation using lasers is reserved for children who remain symptomatic.

In patients with fibroinflammatory strictures, stent removal is sometimes required. Other major complications which have been reported include massive fatal hemoptysis secondary to stent erosion into a pulmonary artery in a patient with necrosis of an airway wall, a tracheo-innominate artery fistula, erosion into a brachiocephalic artery with massive bleeding resulting in death, and fatal respiratory distress. These latter severe complications have all occurred with the Gianturco Z-stent and have been due to perforation by the stabilizing hooks. In addition, Rousseau and colleagues have reported a 31% (6/19) incidence of stent migration or breakage. Therefore, it appears that the Gianturco stent, although suitable for maintaining luminal patency, presents a higher risk for major complications primarily by perforation of the tracheobronchial tree by its hooks. This is problematic in any age group; however, in children with thinner tracheobronchial walls, it seems advisable to avoid using this device in the airway until its safety is proven. Similarly, a combination stent (steel spring coated with silicone rubber) has also been reported but has demonstrated a tendency for dislodgment and tissue reactivity, and is not recommended for use at this time.

Issues and controversies

Issues in using stents in the pediatric airway

There are no long-term studies available in children that assess the effect of a stent on the circumferential and longitudinal growth of an airway. Thus it seems prudent to avoid stent insertion, especially those devices that might be more likely to tether or injure a growing tracheobronchial tree. It is currently our practice to select only those children who have severe symptoms and who have failed conventional therapy before considering insertion of a metallic stent. In these severely affected children with tracheobronchial strictures, balloon dilation is the initial therapy of choice. Balloon dilation will be repeated if restenosis occurs as long as PTA relieves the child's symptoms. Stenting is utilized if PTA is unsuccessful in alleviating symptoms or symptomatic restenosis occurs rapidly. In the rare child with tracheomalacia who is ventilator dependent, primary stenting is the procedure of choice.

Conclusions

Management of tracheal or tracheobronchial compromise benefits from a strongly collaborative multidisciplinary approach, making use of the complementary strengths available in the skill sets of interventionalists, pulmonologists, otolaryngologists, intensivists, cardiothoracic surgeons, and others involved in airway management. The development of the metal stent has been a major advancement in the treatment of strictures and malacia of the airway, accounting for a significant improvement in forced expiratory volume at one second (FEV1). Although there is still relatively small experience in the pediatric population, it seems clear that metallic stents can be used safely and successfully. Children with postoperative anastomotic strictures, children with anastomotic or non-anastomotic strictures who have undergone lung transplantation, children with primary or secondary tracheomalacia, and children with extrinsic airway compression secondary to vascular compression appear to be the best candidates. At this time, the most difficult questions to answer are how to best select children for stent placement and what will be the long-term effect of metallic stents on the growing airway.

Chapter 4

Abdominopelvic interventions

Kevin M. Baskin and Richard Towbin

Introduction 153
Gastrostomy and related procedures 153
Introduction 153
Enterostomy care 154
Indications 154
Technique 157
Equipment 157
Patient preparation 157
Standard technique 159
Nasojejunal tube insertion 159
Antegrade gastrostomy 160
Retrograde gastrostomy 165
Percutaneous gastrojejunostomy 167
Technical variations 168
The "push–pull" gastrostomy for infants 168
Percutaneous jejunostomy 168
Bowel decompression 168
Postprocedure and follow-up care 168
Postoperative orders and initial tube care 168
Catheter exchange and reinsertion 170
Gastrostomy button or button jejunostomy 172
Technical problems and pitfalls 174
Avoiding transcolonic puncture 174
Inability to access the gastric lumen 174
Deep structures at risk 174
Difficult delivery of the retention device or J tube 175
Treating inadvertent dislodgment 175
Complications 175
General considerations 175
Tract and skin surface complications 178
Peritonitis, tube dislodgment, and bowel perforation 181
Occlusion and leakage 181
Intussusception 182
Controversies/issues 183
Conclusions 183
Percutaneous cecostomy 183
Introduction 183

Indications 184
Technique 184
Equipment 184
Patient preparation 184
Latex sensitivity 185
Preprocedure imaging 185
Standard technique 185
Technical variations 186
Postprocedure and follow-up care 187
Catheter fixation 187
Catheter exchange and reinsertion 187
Technical problems and pitfalls 187
Primary placement of the trapdoor catheter 187
Patient support 187
Complications 187
Primary tube malposition 188
Peritonitis, skin infection, and abscess formation 189
Granulation tissue 190
Occlusion and leakage 190
Dislodgment 190
Controversies/issues 190
Future advances 190
Conclusions 191
Percutaneous aspiration and drainage of fluid collections 191
Introduction 191
Indications 191
Technique 193
Equipment 193
Image guidance 194
Ultrasound 195
Fluoroscopic imaging 195
Computed tomography 196
Other modalities 198
Patient preparation 198

Pediatric Interventional Radiology, ed. Richard Towbin and Kevin M. Baskin. Published by Cambridge University Press. © Cambridge University Press 2015.

Chapter 4 Abdominopelvic interventions

Standard technique 198
Regional considerations 199
  Paracentesis 199
  Access to deep pelvic collections 199
  Peri-appendiceal abscesses 201
  Subphrenic and lesser sac collections 203
  Solid organ abscesses 203
  Pancreatic pseudocyst drainage 205
  Renal cysts 205
  Cholecystic and pericholecystic collections 209
Technical variations 210
  Sclerotherapy and lymphocele drainage 210
  Abscess drainage in high-risk populations 210
  Non-linear and curvilinear pathways 210
Postprocedure and follow-up care 210
  Specimen handling 212
  Catheter fixation and drainage 212
  Catheter removal 212
Technical problems and pitfalls 213
Complications 214
Conclusions 214

Percutaneous biopsy 215
Introduction 215
Indications 215
Technique 215
Equipment 215
  Biopsy needles 216
Image guidance 216
  Ultrasound guidance 216
  CT guidance 217
  Molecular imaging 217
  MR guidance 217
Patient preparation 217
  Preprocedure care 218
  Pathologic considerations 218
Standard technique 220
  Percutaneous liver biopsy 220
  Right lobe biopsy 221
  Left lobe biopsy 222
  Tract embolization 222
  Transvenous biopsy: transjugular approach 223
  Renal biopsy 223
  Splenic biopsy 223
  Pancreatic biopsy 224
  Biopsy of nodules and masses 224
  Neuroblastoma 224
Technical variations 226
  Coaxial and tandem needle techniques 226

Molecular imaging guidance 227
Postprocedure and follow-up care 227
  Specimen handling 227
Complications 228
  Hemorrhage 228
  Tract seeding 228
  Bile leakage and bile peritonitis 228
Controversies/issues 228
  Outpatient liver biopsy in children 228
Conclusions 229

Dilation of hollow viscera 229
Introduction 229
Indications 231
  Congenital esophageal stenosis 231
  Acquired esophageal strictures 232
  Other gastrointestinal strictures 235
Technique 235
Equipment 235
Patient preparation 235
Standard technique (esophageal dilation) 236
Technical variations 237
  Management of eccentric stricture and pseudodiverticulum 237
  Colonic dilation 237
Postprocedure and follow-up care 237
Technical problems and pitfalls 238
  Balloon rupture 238
  Stiffening the balloon delivery platform 239
  Positioning for colonic dilation 239
  "Kissing" balloons 239
Complications 239
Conclusions 239

Foreign body retrieval 239
Introduction 239
Indications 240
Technique 242
Equipment 242
Patient preparation 243
Standard technique 243
Technical variations 245
  Variable balloon inflation 245
  Magnetic foreign body removal 245
Postprocedure and follow-up care 247
Complications 247
Conclusions 247

Introduction

Patient problems in the abdomen and pelvis demand the fullest expression of clinical interventional radiology. From acute trauma to chronic renal failure, from solid organ biopsy to dilation of hollow viscera, from gastrojejunostomy tube exchange to transgastric drainage of a pancreatic pseudocyst, abdominopelvic interventional procedures can challenge practitioners on every level: intellectually, technically, emotionally, and ethically.

Virtually any problem in this region can be solved by distinctly different methods and with use of a variety of imaging approaches. For example, a pelvic fluid collection may be accessible from transrectal, transgluteal, or percutaneous access, using ultrasound, CT, or fluoroscopy, or a combination of multiple modalities. One may use a straight needle, a curved needle, or no needle at all (in the case of trocar access). These and many other choices are available to the interventionalist, and solutions must be individualized to each patient presentation.

Perhaps one of the most essential questions the interventional radiologist must answer is to what degree he or she will become integrated into the patient's total care. One can limit a practice to the provision of technical expertise in the performance of procedures on demand. It is our belief, professed throughout this text, that our involvement in patient care should ideally begin with consultation for assessment and planning at the time of initial presentation, and should end when the problem for which we have been consulted has been resolved, for problems that fall within our scope of practice, in a manner and by a process that is indistinguishable from any other procedure-based practitioner. It is to this end that this chapter is directed.

Gastrostomy and related procedures

Introduction

Adequate nutrition is essential for normal growth and development. In order for children with chronic illnesses or those who are unwilling or unable to take in adequate calories or essential nutrients to thrive, nutritional supplementation is necessary. In children with normal digestive function it is preferable to utilize the gastrointestinal (GI) tract for feeding to avoid hyperalimentation and its complications. To maintain normal nutritional status in the face of short-term or long-term nutritional deficiency, several strategies may be enlisted and tailored to the individual patient's need.

In our practice children who are expected to require short-term nutritional support (for approximately six weeks or less) are advised to get their nutrition by intravenous hyperalimentation, nasogastric (NG) or nasojejunal (NJ) tube feeding, or a combination of these techniques. However, when longer periods of nutritional support are anticipated, or for children with significant failure to thrive, a more permanent means of nutritional support is preferred. Children in this large group are candidates for a percutaneous gastrostomy (PG) or percutaneous gastrojejunostomy (PGJ).

Although Egeberg first proposed the operative gastrostomy in 1837, it was not until 1876 that Verneuil performed the first successful surgical gastrostomy (SG) in a human. In 1897, Stamm modified the prevailing surgical technique. This modified technique has become today's operative standard. By the 1950s, the procedural modifications and the coincident improvements in anesthetic techniques significantly reduced the associated procedural morbidity and mortality of surgical gastrostomy insertion. This has resulted in a progressive broadening of the indications for insertion of a gastrostomy and increased its safety and efficacy. As a result, the SG became one of the most commonly performed operations in the pediatric population and central to the care of critically ill and nutritionally deficient children of all ages.

An alternative to SG did not appear until 1979, over 100 years after the initial operation performed by Verneuil. In 1979, Sacks and Glotzer introduced the concept of PG insertion using fluoroscopically guided placement of a gastric feeding tube through a healed Stamm gastrostomy site. Shortly thereafter, Gauderer, Ponsky, and Izant described and popularized the percutaneous endoscopic gastrostomy (PEG) that fundamentally changed pediatric medical and surgical practice.

In the short time since the introduction of the PEG, it has essentially replaced the SG in most situations. In the early 1980s, the PEG technique was modified so that a PG could be inserted under fluoroscopic guidance (FPG).

Over the next few years, fluoroscopically guided placement of gastrostomy tubes became well established in adult patients. However, little was known about the safety and efficacy of the percutaneous technique in children. In the late 1980s, Keller, Towbin, and others described the antegrade approach for PG and PGJ insertion and the first large series of children receiving these devices was reported. Since that time, the safety and utility of the PG and PGJ in children has been clearly demonstrated, and many technical modifications have been devised.

Currently, there are two different methods for placement of a fluoroscopically guided PG: the retrograde (push) and antegrade (pull) approaches. In addition, we have developed the push–pull technique, a hybrid approach for insertion of feeding tubes in small infants. Regardless of the approach selected, PG appears to be highly successful and well suited to large segments of the pediatric population. In the time since its introduction, the percutaneous approach has become recognized as a safe and cost-effective alternative to the SG and PEG.

The SG is one of the oldest abdominal operations in continuous use. Gastrostomy feeding has gained in popularity over the years because of the advantages of enteric alimentation over parenteral nutrition and the introduction of percutaneous techniques for tube placement. Since 1980, with the introduction of the PEG and subsequently the FPG, the percutaneous techniques have demonstrated numerous advantages over the open operative approach. A percutaneous gastrostomy can be inserted under local anesthesia and intravenous sedation avoiding general anesthesia. The percutaneous approach thus decreases overall procedure time, requires a shorter hospital stay, allows for easier conversion to a gastrojejunostomy, has a lower rate of complications, and is less expensive.

Importantly, the FPG is generally better positioned in the stomach. In most SGs and PEGs, the tube is in the middle third of the stomach and directed toward the esophagus and to the left of the lesser curvature (Figure 4.1). In this position the lesser curvature is interposed between the gastrostomy stoma and the pylorus. This makes jejunostomy tube insertion time consuming, more technically difficult, and associated with a higher incidence of gastroesophageal reflux (GER). The SG also has a greater incidence of skin problems secondary to leakage of gastric contents, and a higher rate of jejunostomy tube loss. As a result of these numerous advantages, the percutaneous approach, especially PGJ, has become the preferred method for tube placement in many situations. Whether the retrograde or antegrade route is chosen, the high likelihood of success (84 to 100%) and low rate of major (2 to 5%) and minor (12 to 16%) complications compare favorably with the operative approach. In 1995, the first reports of laparoscopic gastrostomy were presented. This approach has gained popularity over the ensuing years and has the advantage of the ability to insert a G-tube or G-button under direct visualization. Like the open surgical approach potential disadvantages include increased cost, increased incidence of GER (e.g., from iatrogenic organoaxial rotation of the stomach), and positioning the feeding device in the mid to distal stomach making insertion of a gastrojejunostomy more difficult.

The gastrostomy button (GB), a simple, skin-level, nonrefluxing gastrostomy device, was also introduced in the early 1980s as a substitute for conventional gastrostomy tubes. The intended use was for replacement of gastrostomy tubes in patients with established tracts that had been inserted surgically or endoscopically. Shortly after its introduction, other reports appeared supporting the use of the GB and stressing the positive features of the device and the high level of patient satisfaction. Since that time, the use of GBs for long-term nutritional support has grown tremendously and the GB is now the most commonly used feeding device for individuals who require prolonged assisted feeding.

As a result of the widespread acceptance of the GB, there has been increasing interest in using it as a primary device, thereby avoiding the initial step of gastrostomy tube insertion. The one-step insertion has been advocated as an efficient approach to feeding and avoiding the need for a second procedure and its attendant risks and costs. Several series have been presented demonstrating the safety and effectiveness of this method. Today, placement of a primary GB is most often performed using the laparoscopic approach.

When a primary gastrostomy or gastrojejunostomy has been performed, exchange for a low-profile device can be performed as a second procedure at a later date (usually six to twelve weeks later). In 1994, Towbin developed a button jejunostomy. Subsequently, a button gastrojejunostomy became available. Both devices are useful in patients with GER. It is likely that the area of percutaneous feeding will continue to evolve with minimally invasive techniques replacing open surgery whenever possible.

Enterostomy care

In some settings, such as home care and chronic care facilities, ostomy care may be episodic, with complications or tube dysfunction requiring trips to emergency departments or tertiary facilities with varying experience in the management of ostomy catheters and stomas. In some hospitals, ostomy care may be provided by an advanced practice nurse or ostomy nurse, while in others a pediatrician surgeon, gastroenterologist, or interventional radiologist may direct care of these patients. In facilities where primary insertion of gastrostomy catheters is performed, this care tends to be distributed under the auspices of multiple services, medical, surgical, and interventional, with varying degrees of coordination between services. For example, primary insertion may be performed by gastroenterologists or surgeons, but diagnosis and management of catheter-related complications falls to the radiologist, ostomy and skin care or ostomy nurses, and nutritional management to dieticians, with limited communication between providers.

Where experienced pediatric interventionalists are available, over time there is a tendency for ostomy care to centralize under the supervision of the interventional service, from primary insertion to continuing care. This may even take the form of a multidisciplinary enterostomy team, with highly coordinated care provided by those services already mentioned as well as admission and discharge planners, occupational therapists, educational nurses, and other providers. Such a team can offer a single point of contact for patient and parent education, referral, assessment, and prioritization of enterostomy patients, as well as for information management, quality assurance, and outcome analysis related to these patients. An organized approach to management of this large patient group remains an opportunity to improve patient care and decrease costs (Table 4.1).

Indications

Since the introduction of the percutaneous approach to placement of feeding tubes, there has been a steady increase in the number of indications in the pediatric population (Table 4.2). At this time, it can be said that any child with a need for medium- to long-term nutritional support who has a functioning GI tract is a candidate for PG. It can be broadly stated that the indications are failure to thrive, inability to take adequate calories and essential nutrients by mouth, need for chronic

Chapter 4 Abdominopelvic interventions

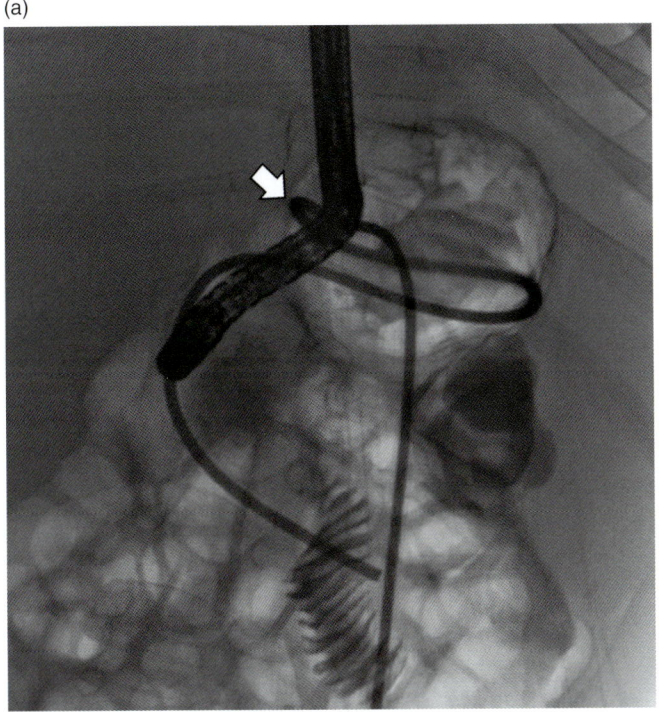

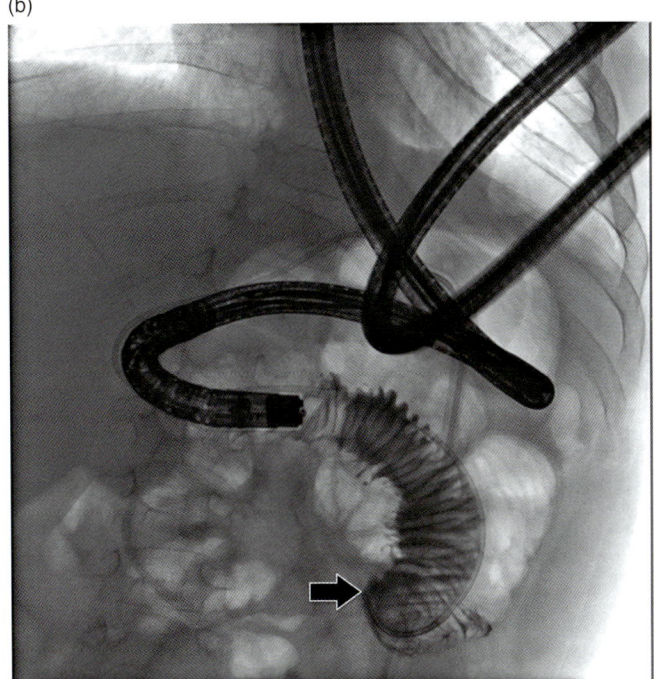

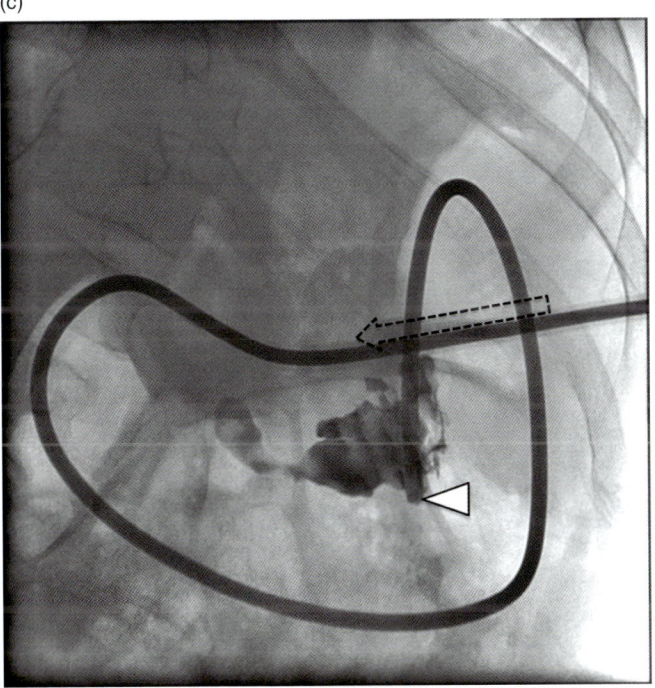

Figure 4.1 (a) Due to the location of this surgically created gastrostomy in the proximal fundus, the transgastric jejunostomy tube became coiled in the gastric lumen. Because the stoma is directed toward the left side of the lesser curvature (*arrow*), it was not possible to advance the catheter through the pylorus without protracted effort and undue exposure to ionizing radiation. An endoscope was used to redirect the jejunostomy catheter into the duodenum but could not uncoil the Waltman's loop in the stomach. (b) The jejunostomy catheter was removed, and a 5 French angled catheter was directed by a combination of endoscopic and fluoroscopic guidance. The endoscope traverses the esophagus, stomach and pylorus, with the tip in the third part of the duodenum. The catheter tip (*arrow*) was advanced to the proximal jejunum, and a small amount of contrast instilled through it to confirm position. (c) A stiff guide wire was advanced through the directional catheter, and the catheter was exchanged for a new transgastric gastrojejunostomy catheter, taking care to keep the catheter directed (*arrow*) toward the pylorus. The tip (*arrowhead*) was located in the proximal jejunum.

gastric decompression or drainage, and rarely for associated procedures such as esophageal dilation. Common underlying conditions in candidates for percutaneous feeding include neurologic disorders (e.g., cerebral palsy), cystic fibrosis, and underlying malignancies. With increasing complexity and acuity of patients, and improved survival of patients with severe metabolic, congenital cardiac, and other diseases as well as solid organ and bone marrow transplantation, there is a continually growing population of candidates for placement of either a PG or PGJ.

Few contraindications to PG exist; however, an uncorrectable coagulopathy, instability of vital signs, and inaccessible anatomy may make placement of a PG unwise. Addressable coagulopathies and bleeding abnormalities should be corrected prior to gastrostomy insertion (see Chapter 1). Cardiorespiratory abnormalities that limit deep sedation or general

Table 4.1 Outcome measures

To improve outcome and quality assurance analysis, it may be helpful to record the following information for each abdominopelvic procedure:

- Demographic information (patient name, unique identification number, date and time of procedure, age, sex, weight, date of birth, etc.)
- Primary diagnosis (underlying disease), patient acuity, comorbid illness, ASA class, competence of patient or primary caregiver
- Any contraindicating or complicating factors
  - Coagulopathy
  - Infection, immunodeficiency, nutritional status, cardiorespiratory compromise
  - Skin or mucosal abnormality (e.g., cellulitis, epidermolysis bullosa)
  - Limitation to access (e.g., micrognathia, microgastria, intervening vital structure or mass)
- Reason (indication) for procedure; referring service and provider; inpatient or outpatient status
- Anticipated endpoint
- Primary provider responsible for procedure (interventionalist, gastroenterologist, surgeon, etc.)
- Collaborating provider(s)
- Procedure location (interventional suite, operating room, ICU, bedside, etc.)
- Provider(s) responsible for anesthesia/sedation (interventionalist, intensivist, anesthesiologist, nurse, etc.)
- Preprocedural evaluation (e.g., coagulation profile, creatinine, amylase, etc.)
- Preprocedural interventions (e.g., antibiotics, blood products, imaging, endoscopy)
- Initial access
  - Guidance (anatomic landmarks, US, fluoroscopy, CT, MRI, PET fusion, endoscopy, etc.)
  - Operative site or pathway (e.g., percutaneous (location), transoral, transrectal)
  - Number of attempts/passes
  - Reason for deferral, discontinuation or failure, if procedure not completed
- Access device and position
  - Manufacturer, type, diameter, length, other pertinent characteristics
  - Tip or target position
- Equipment and supplies used
- Procedure time, fluoroscopy time, or estimated radiation dose
- Type and adequacy of anesthesia/sedation/analgesia
- Procedural complications (e.g., pneumothorax, unintended gastrointestinal perforation or rupture, bleeding) and management
- Adjunctive procedures (e.g., bowel decompression, intracavitary sclerotherapy, tract embolization)
- Complications (major or minor), including
  - Procedure-related discomfort (include dates)
    - Type
    - Management (e.g., NSAIDs, narcotics)
    - Outcome
  - Gastrointestinal catheter complications (include dates)
    - Type (e.g., transcolonic puncture, lumen perforation or rupture, peritonitis, granulation tissue, intussusception)
    - Method of diagnosis
    - Management (e.g., observation, intervention, surgery)
    - Outcome
  - Bleeding or vascular injury (include dates)
    - Type (e.g., hemorrhage, AV fistula or pseudoaneurysm, thrombosis)
    - Method of diagnosis (e.g., hemoglobin, US, CT scan, arteriogram)
    - Management (e.g., observation, transfusion, embolization, thrombolysis)
    - Outcome
  - Dislodgment or malposition (include dates)
    - Method of diagnosis or documentation
    - Management
    - Outcome
- Other procedure-related complications or interventions
- Complications, additional details
  - Major
    - Admission to hospital for therapy
    - Unplanned increase in level of care
    - Prolonged hospitalization
    - Permanent adverse sequelae
    - Death
  - Minor
    - No sequelae
    - Nominal therapy
    - Short hospital stay (for observation)
  - Procedurally related (within 24 hours)
  - Early (within 30 days)
  - Late
- Removal or replacement (reason and date; endpoint achieved?)
- Outcome at follow-up (method and date; endpoint achieved?)
  - Postprocedural lab studies (e.g., fluid pH, culture or biopsy findings)
  - Response (e.g., reduction in fever, dyspnea, debilitation, discomfort)
  - Results (e.g., daily volume of fluid drained, radiographic evidence of resolution, hospital days)
  - Treatment failure (e.g., recurrent abscess, gastroesophageal reflux, dysphagia)

anesthesia may require local anesthesia augmented by careful use of intravenous or inhalational sedation, usually with the assistance of cardiac anesthesiologists.

Specific maneuvers (described under "Technical variations," below) or time may adequately resolve anatomic barriers to safe access such as dilated loops of bowel. In a small number of children, abnormalities such as severe scoliosis, high horizontal orientation of the stomach, an incompetent pylorus (preventing adequate gastric insufflation), abdominal masses or organomegaly may represent fixed obstacles to

Table 4.2 Indications: enterostomy insertion

Percutaneous gastrostomy
Neurologic disorders
    Static encephalopathy
    Progressive encephalopathy
    Brain tumors
    Coma
Pulmonary disease
    Cystic fibrosis
    Recurrent aspiration
Bronchopulmonary dysplasia (severe)
    Chronic pulmonary disease (severe)
    Respiratory failure
Head and neck
    Swallowing and chewing disorders
    Malignancy
    Macroglossia secondary to amyloid or other condition
    Syndromes
Gastrointestinal
    Short gut syndrome
    Esophageal dysfunction
    Inflammatory bowel disease
    Motility disorder
    Epidermolysis bullosa
Miscellaneous
    Failure to thrive
    Prematurity
    Pre or post liver transplantation
    Anorexia and cachexia (e.g., cystic fibrosis)
    Severe congenital heart disease
    Metabolic stress (e.g., trauma, burns)
    Inflammatory myopathy
    Connective tissue diseases
    Storage diseases

Percutaneous gastrojejunostomy
– Children at risk for aspiration
– Children with proven GER
– Poor gastric emptying
– Superior mesenteric artery syndrome
– Small intestinal motility disorder
– Partial obstruction of the stomach or duodenum
– Pancreatitis
– Static or progressive encephalopathy
– Need to simultaneously vent the stomach and feed
– Abnormal gastric function

successful percutaneous access and mitigate for surgical or endoscopic alternatives. While coexistence of a ventriculoperitoneal (VP) shunt is not in itself a contraindication to gastrostomy insertion, an access site should be chosen well away from the shunt to minimize the chance for shunt infection. In addition, elective percutaneous transgastric procedures should not be performed within 30 days of VP shunt placement or revision, as this is the most vulnerable period for development of a VP shunt infection. In our experience, children with VP shunts, peritoneal dialysis, or Crohn's disease may otherwise safely receive a PG. To encourage effective maturation of the tract, dialysate or ascitic fluid should be drained prior to the procedure.

The antegrade (pull) gastrostomy cannot be safely performed if the esophagus is too small in diameter to permit atraumatic passage of the device, or if there is an esophageal obstruction or a pathologic process such as epidermolysis bullosa that makes passage of a tube through the esophagus dangerous or unwise. Of course, with the exception of a small esophageal diameter in infants <5 to 7 kg, these problems rarely occur in children and in many cases can be circumvented by using the retrograde, push–pull, or the antegrade approach using a retention device with a smaller diameter.

Surgical anti-reflux procedures have failure and complication rates in the range of 8 to 12% and approaching 20%, respectively. These problems are especially prominent in children with neurologic problems and those with repaired esophageal atresia with or without tracheoesophageal fistula. There have been discussions and disagreements over the issue of whether GER contraindicates placement of a PG in favor of an SG. In children with severe encephalopathy and GER, or those with the propensity to develop GER, it is better to insert a PGJ than to perform an SG and fundoplication in most instances. Percutaneous gastrojejunostomy has the advantages of a lower major complication rate, shorter hospitalization, and a less costly procedure. The cost differential is about 5:1, with the SG and fundoplication averaging about US$25,000 per patient and the PGJ about US$5,000, at the time of writing. An initial PGJ appears to be a good strategy since most children tolerate feedings and gain weight. In our experience, only a small percentage of children (<8%) have problems that require subsequent fundoplication.

Technique

Equipment

The equipment selected depends on the operator's approach to tube insertion: antegrade versus retrograde versus push–pull technique. However, in general, the procedure is relatively simple to perform and the majority of the equipment used is similar regardless of approach save for the PG type selected (Table 4.3).

Patient preparation

Clinical and radiological evaluation of children prior to the PG insertion is important in order to identify those individuals who will benefit from this approach to feeding. The evaluation should focus on identifying children requiring at least six weeks of total or near-total nutritional support, for whom long-term nutritional support may offer substantive benefit. Patients should be excluded who have anatomic or functional abnormalities likely to preclude safe and successful PG

Table 4.3 Equipment: enterostomy insertion

Antegrade gastrostomy
- Monitoring equipment (pulse oximeter, blood pressure monitor, and other monitors prn).
- Oral barium meal four to six hours prior to PG insertion *or* barium enema at the time of the PG.
- 8 to 10 French feeding tube for NG placement.
- Topical anesthetic (e.g., EMLA®, ELA-Max®)
- Bite block or side mouth gag to keep mouth open in uncooperative children who might bite *or* those who will not voluntarily open their mouths.
- 8 to 10 French feeding tube with end cut off to create an end-hole catheter *or* a 5 French JB-1 catheter.
- 0.035- or 0.038-inch Bentson guide wire.
- 34 mm nitinol snare (Microvena, White Bear Lake, MN)
- Betadine or other skin prep.
- 1% lidocaine or other local anesthetic.
- Ross-Flexiflo® peg kit (Ross Products Division, Abbott Laboratories, Columbus, OH)
  . 18-gauge needle
  . Scalpel with #10 or #11 blade
  . 0.038-inch, 260 cm guide wire
  . 14 to 16 French Corpak Antegrade gastrostomy tube (Corpak Med Systems, Buffalo Grove, IL) with:
    – Outer friction lock disk to stabilize PG at the skin surface.
    – Yellow adapter to connect to the feeding pump or syringe.
- Water-soluble contrast.

Retrograde gastrostomy
- Monitoring equipment (oximeter, blood pressure, electrocardiogram, other monitors prn).
- 8 to 10 French feeding tube *or* 5 French JB-1 catheter.
- Betadine or other skin prep.
- 1% lidocaine or other local anesthetic.
- Pediatric gastrointestinal suture anchor set.
- Syringes and needles, including a 27-gauge, 1.5 inch needle for administration of local anesthetic.
- 18-gauge single wall puncture needle.
- Slip-ring extension set.
- Low-osmolar contrast (e.g., iohexol 300 mg I per ml).
- 70 cm non-Teflon coated 0.035-inch guide wire
- Dilators appropriate for the size of the gastrostomy tube selected.
- Peel-away sheath appropriate for the catheter/tube selected.
- Gastrostomy tube (e.g., Dawson–Mueller Mac-Loc™ ultrathane catheter, 15 cm, 8.5 to 12 French, Cook, Inc.).

Percutaneous gastrojejunostomy
- Obtain percutaneous gastric access as described under **Antegrade gastrostomy** or **Retrograde gastrostomy**.
- Jejunostomy tube (e.g., 8 French Frederick–Miller (FM) tube modified by cutting off its weighted tip creating an end hole catheter, a 6 French Corpak® or a 9 French FlexiFlo® tube), *or*
- Unibody transgastric gastrojejunostomy tube (16–18 French)
- Directional catheter (e.g., 5 French JB-1, Kumpe or Berenstein catheter)
- Bentson 0.035- or 0.038-inch guide wire
- Silicone spray (Rusch Silkospray, Willy Rusch AG, Rommelshausen, Germany), mineral oil, Pam vegetable spray, or K-Y Jelly (Roxane Laboratories, Inc., Columbus, OH).

insertion or function, including those with abnormal gastric emptying. Those children with GER, poor gastric emptying, or risk of aspiration of gastric contents, should be considered for a PGJ (Table 4.2). A PG is preferred whenever possible since it is easier to care for, is less apt to clog or be prematurely dislodged, and allows for eventual bolus feeding. Both PGs and PGJs can be converted to a low profile device at a later date.

Currently, only the rare child with complicated GER is primarily referred for an SG and anti-reflux surgical procedure. The vast majority of children are considered for PG or PGJ insertion. Thus the question of the optimal and most cost-effective work-up to help decide the appropriate feeding procedure(s) becomes important. While there is no prospective study to suggest the best approach to preoperative evaluation, a variety of diagnostic tests are available. Children who are candidates for a PG or PGJ may be examined with an esophagram and upper gastrointestinal series (UGI series), nuclear gastric scintigraphy, pH probe to identify and grade GER, and endoscopy.

We have found the esophagram and UGI series to be adequate for preoperative decision-making prior to PG or PGJ insertion. The esophagram and UGI series is performed using barium, and images of the esophagus are obtained in frontal and lateral projections. An image is obtained with a scoliosis ruler in the field so that the esophageal diameter can be measured. Measurement can also be made electronically if digital fluoroscopy is available. The remainder of the UGI series focuses on the size and position of the stomach, gastric emptying, and the presence of GER. The position of the duodenojejunal junction is noted to exclude a malrotation, and the proximal small intestines are visualized to rule out the possibility of a malabsorption syndrome and motility disorder.

If necessary, gastric scintigraphy, using sulfur colloid in milk, can be performed. This examination can more accurately assess and quantitate gastric emptying and GER, but does not permit measurement of the esophageal diameter and evaluation of the anatomy. Therefore fluoroscopic examination is preferred, especially in young children in whom esophageal size is important for procedural planning. Diagnostic evaluation using a pH probe and endoscopy are utilized in selected cases.

In our experience, antibiotics do not need to be routinely given unless the child: (1) is immune depressed or immune deficient; (2) has a history of postoperative infections; or (3) has a procedural complication or visualization of free intraperitoneal air on postprocedural abdominal radiographs. This approach, however, is not universally accepted and some groups prefer to give prophylactic antibiotics to all patients, or to additional specific subgroups such as patients with ventriculoperitoneal shunts. A similar approach is taken toward the use of routine preoperative laboratory testing. It is our preference *not* to obtain a routine CBC and coagulation profile or other blood tests unless there is a specific history or risk of bleeding abnormality (see Chapter 1). Those laboratory tests obtained are tailored to the child's specific clinical problems.

In most cases, preparation for insertion of a PG or PGJ is relatively straightforward. The child is kept NPO according to hospital policy for sedation and anesthesia. Whenever possible, a barium meal is given prior to gastrostomy insertion so that the transverse colon is opacified at the time of the procedure. If an esophagram and UGI series is not needed and a barium meal cannot be given, then a thin barium contrast enema is carried out at the time of the PG. When an UGI series is necessary, we find that it is most efficient to complete the contrast study the morning of the procedure so that contrast will be in the transverse colon in the afternoon at the time of the PG insertion. When the child arrives in the department, the details of the procedure are reviewed with the patient, parents, or guardian and last minute questions are answered.

Standard technique
Nasojejunal tube insertion

Although a large number of children need nutritional support, not all require a PG or PGJ. In the short term, in a child with a functional GI tract, temporizing with a nasogastric (NG) or nasojejunostomy (NJ) tube may be sufficient. There are no definitive guidelines to suggest the optimal time period for these measures and each patient should be considered individually. It is our policy to consider children for a PG or PGJ if it is expected that they will require nutritional support for about six weeks or longer. If the expected need is less than six weeks, an NJ tube is recommended.

Nasogastric tubes are usually inserted at the bedside by the clinicians caring for the child unless a problem or anatomic variation makes fluoroscopic guidance preferable. Nasojejunostomy tubes may also be inserted without guidance by using a weighted tube and keeping the child in the right lateral decubitus position to encourage passage through the pylorus into the small intestine. Unfortunately, it may take days for the tube to get into the duodenum. In our experience, these tubes usually do not get distal to the second portion of the duodenum. We do not recommend the bedside approach since it is both costly and usually delays the onset of nutritional support. The high cost of bedside placement is due to the need for multiple chest radiographs and longer hospitalization resulting from delayed feeding. Therefore if rapid deployment of an NJ tube is desired, it is done in the IR suite with fluoroscopic guidance.

Although a relatively mundane procedure, it is one that is commonly requested in the pediatric population and serves as practice for other catheter-guide wire manipulations, e.g., vascular interventions. There are a variety of catheter-guide wire combinations that can be used successfully; however, we prefer the combination of a 4 or 5 French directional catheter and a 0.035-inch guide wire (e.g., Bentson guide wire) for all gastrointestinal procedures and at this time rarely use anything else (Table 4.4). If a patient comes to the radiology department

Table 4.4 Equipment: nasojejunal tube insertion

- Directional catheter (JB-1, Berenstein).
- Floppy tipped guide wire (Bentson, J wires).
- 8 or 9 French jejunostomy tube (8 French Frederick–Miller, 9 French Flexiflow).
- Silicone spray (Rusch Silkospray, Willy Rusch AG, Rommelshausen, Germany), mineral oil, Pam vegetable spray, or K-Y Jelly (Roxane Laboratories, Inc., Columbus, OH).
- Tegaderm®, Opsite®, micropore tape to secure NJ to upper lip or gastric tube (GT).
- Restraints: sock mittens, no-no's.

with an NG tube, it will usually need to be removed since it has only side holes. Attempts to advance a feeding tube are usually unsuccessful and may entail considerable radiation exposure, so beginning with a directional system is advisable.

Using a directional system, a >99% success rate and virtually no complications can be expected. Once the catheter is in the distal stomach, the tip is directed first superiorly and then inferiorly while the Bentson guide wire is used as a probe (Table 4.5). It is important to extend the guide wire out of the catheter until it becomes J shaped and slightly coiled. This allows the guide wire to search for the pylorus and duodenum. In some instances, the guide wire coils in the duodenal bulb. If this occurs, it is best to advance the catheter to that point and then retract the guide wire back into the catheter.

The catheter should then be pointed inferiorly and the Bentson pushed out into the duodenum. If this maneuver is repeated a few times without success, it is best to inject contrast and distend the lumen. In addition, the C-arm can be rotated into the right anterior oblique (RAO) position to profile contrast in the pyloroduodenal junction. Likewise, the patient may be rotated into the RAO position to encourage contrast to fill the bulb. These maneuvers usually aid rapid positioning of the guide wire distally. These steps are repeated until the guide wire is maneuvered into the proximal jejunum. At this point the JB-1 is exchanged for a modified 8 French Frederick–Miller tube cut to length for the patient. The same approach is utilized for insertion of a GJ tube since the same anatomic problems are encountered.

The NJ tube is secured to the skin by making a tape moustache. Before the tube is fixed in place the skin is treated with a skin adhesive such as benzoin or Mastisol® then covered with tape, Tegaderm® or Opsite®, cut to the proper size and shape. The tube is brought across the cheek and put behind the child's ear to minimize the chance for accidental dislodgment. The entire length of NJ tube on the face is secured by covering it with tape or occlusive dressing strips. In children who are prone to pull tubes out, additional protective measures can be used to keep the tube in place. Arm and hand movement can be restricted with sock mittens, 'no-no's' or other devices can be positioned over the elbows to dissuade the child from pulling out the tube.

Chapter 4 Abdominopelvic interventions

Table 4.5 Procedure summary: nasojejunal tube insertion

- Advance a 5 to 8 French directional catheter over a 0.035- to 0.038-inch guide wire via the naris to the stomach.
- Monitor initial insertion through the nasopharynx and hypopharynx to proximal esophagus with intermittent fluoroscopy.
- Monitoring during passage through the esophagus is not necessary.
- In the event of coughing or decreased oxygenation on oximetry, confirm non-tracheal position of the catheter tip.
- Once in the stomach, turn catheter tip toward the right upper quadrant and advance toward the pylorus.
- If the catheter tip does not easily engage the pylorus, a small amount of dilute contrast may be used to define the antral and pyloric anatomy.
- Rotating the catheter tip and translating it forward and back will usually enable engagement of the pylorus.
- Angling the tube may assist visualization of relationships in the gastric outlet, but will not change those relationships.
- Rotating the patient *will* change relationships, and may permit alignment of the catheter tip with the pylorus in difficult cases.
- Probing the pylorus with small, gentle movements of the wire and catheter tip is preferred.
- Pylorospasm, sometimes caused by repeated or ungentle instrumentation of the pylorus, may significantly degrade success.
- Once the catheter tip has passed the pylorus, the catheter and guide wire are iteratively advanced until they are beyond the ligament of Treitz.
- The internal catheter length is measured by marking the catheter where it exits the naris, and the catheter is then exchanged over the wire for an 8 French Frederick–Miller tube trimmed to appropriate length.
- Confirm appropriate position with a small amount of contrast.
- The NJ tube is fixed to the skin of the face from the naris to the ear with micropore tape on the skin and over the tube, then the tube is positioned out of reach of the child. Precautions may be necessary (including no-no's if indicated) to prevent the child from accidentally dislodging the tube.

Antegrade gastrostomy

The antegrade placement of a gastrostomy tube begins with a limited abdominal ultrasound (Figure 4.2). The left lobe of the liver is identified and its position is outlined on the anterior wall with an ink marker. A line is also drawn one to two fingerbreadths below the left inferior costal margin. The transverse colon is opacified by a prior barium meal or retrograde enema, so that it may be avoided (Figure 4.3). A nasogastric (NG) and an orogastric (OG) tube are inserted. We find that in most instances it is fastest and easiest to use a 5 French JB-1 catheter and 0.035- or 0.038-inch Bentson guide wire to ease passage of both tubes through the oropharynx into the stomach (Table 4.6).

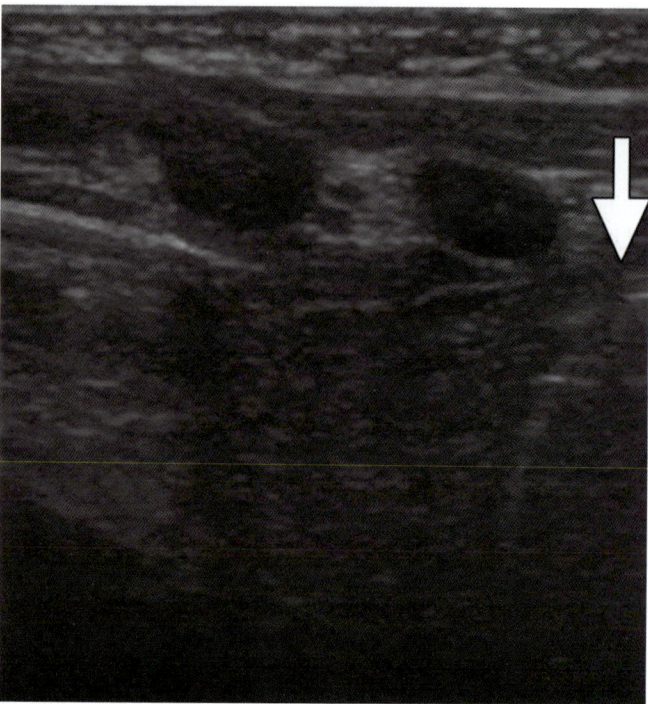

Figure 4.2 Linear ultrasound is used to determine the inferior margin of the liver (*arrow*), which is marked on the skin surface.

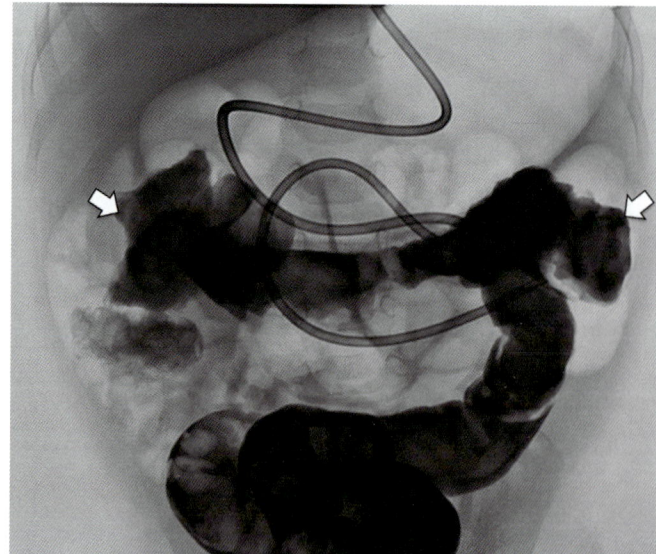

Figure 4.3 Thin barium or water-soluble contrast solution is administered by way of a transrectal enema. Once contrast reaches the transverse colon (between *arrows*), the flow is reversed and as much contrast as possible drained to avoid obscuring structures. A nasojejunal tube will be pulled back until the tip is in the stomach and used to insufflate the stomach with air after administration of glucagon and prior to percutaneous puncture.

Once the wire is coiled in the stomach, the OG tube is exchanged for a 5 French Teflon® sheath to guide the nitinol snare (Figure 4.4). The guide wire is removed and replaced with a large (25 to 34 mm) nitinol gooseneck snare. Once the

Chapter 4 Abdominopelvic interventions

Table 4.6 Procedure summary: enterostomy insertion

Antegrade gastrostomy
- Ultrasound abdomen and identify the left lobe of liver. Mark liver and costal margins on skin surface.
- Barium meal (four to six hours prior to procedure) or enema to identify transverse colon.
- Insert NG and OG tubes.
- Exchange OG tube for 34 mm nitinol snare.
- Inflate stomach via NG tube.
- Puncture stomach under fluoroscopic guidance after transverse colon is cleared.
- Insert, grasp, and retrieve guide wire via the mouth.

For "push–pull" method, continue at * below
- Position antegrade PGT over guide wire and pull through anterior abdominal wall.
- Insert outer retention disc over GT and hub fitting onto GT.
- Coaxially insert JT if needed.
- Secure JT to GT with Tegaderm® or other device/method.

"Push–pull" method (* continues from above)
- Position antegrade PGT over guide wire and pull through anterior abdominal wall until 14 French portion of dilator is visible.
- Position 14 French balloon-tipped GT retrograde over guide wire and tightly couple to dilating tip of antegrade PG.
- Simultaneously *pull* back PGT at the mouth while *pushing* the balloon-tipped PGT at the skin surface until the balloon-tipped tube is in the esophagus.
- Visualize the balloon-tipped PGT in the mouth and uncouple the tubes.
- Partially inflate the balloon with dilute contrast and using fluoroscopic guidance, pull the balloon into the stomach and fully inflate it with water (3 to 7 ml).
- Leave guide wire in position and inject contrast to confirm intragastric PG position.
- Coaxially insert JT, if needed.
- Secure JT to GT with Tegaderm®.

Retrograde gastrostomy
- Antibiotics, if preferred.
- Identify left lobe of liver and transverse colon.
- Insert NG tube.
- Inflate stomach.
- Insert T-fasteners.
- Inflate and puncture stomach.
- Maneuver guide wire into stomach or small intestines.
- Insert peel-away sheath, if desired.
- Dilate tract.
- Insert pigtail, unibody GJT, or other catheter type as preferred.
- Place catheter to suction for 24 hours.
- Cut retention sutures in one week.
- Later, sequentially dilate tract as needed.

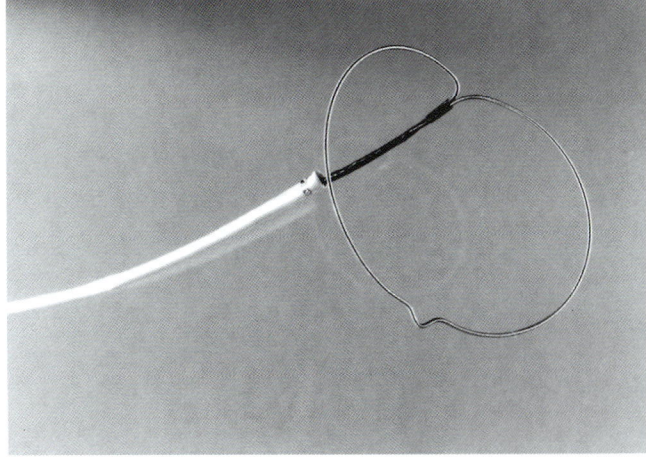

Figure 4.4 The nitinol snare loop opens when advanced beyond the snare catheter.

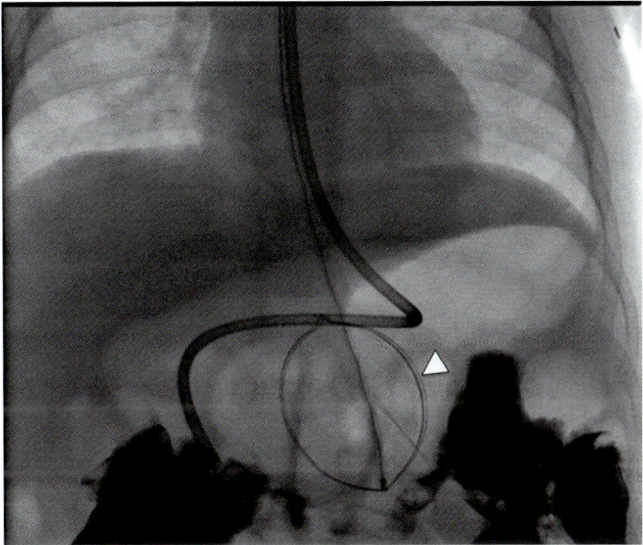

Figure 4.5 A large (34 mm) gooseneck snare (*arrowhead*) is delivered transorally to the gastric body just proximal to the antrum, where it is opened and directed to serve as a target for percutaneous transgastric puncture.

snare is in the gastric lumen, it is kept in the open position adjacent to the greater curvature (Figure 4.5). Occasionally, depending on gastric shape, a more posterior location of the snare is preferable. To accomplish this, the snare may be positioned closer to the esophagogastric junction. The best position depends on the needle position and angle, and on the gastric anatomy.

In most patients, the PG puncture site is selected just lateral to the margin of the rectus abdominus muscle, inferior to the left lobe of the liver (if it is in the area), and one to two fingerbreadths below the costal margin (Figure 4.6). The potential entry site is confirmed by placing a hemostat on the skin surface and observing its relationship to the transverse colon, the liver, and the snare. In children with a transverse, midline, or high stomach, a sub-xyphoid entry site may be necessary. Puncture through the rectus abdominus muscle is not preferred since it may cause cramping discomfort and may place the inferior epigastric artery at risk of injury. However, when necessary, a transmuscular approach may be used.

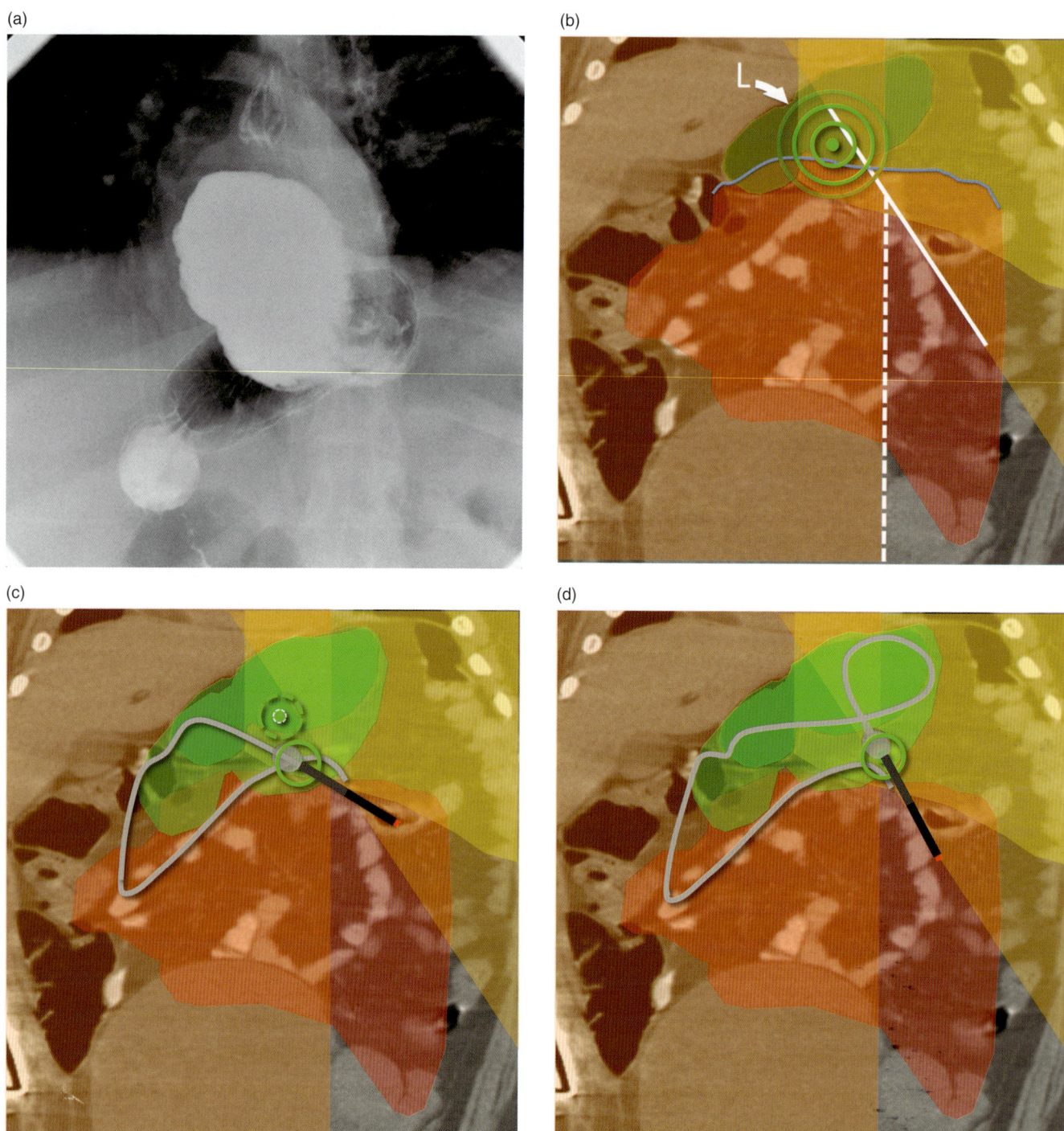

Figure 4.6 (a) An anteroposterior image shows a large hiatal hernia and organoaxial rotation of the stomach, which is partially filled with contrast. As a result, the inferior margin of the stomach is at the level of the inferior costal margin, making percutaneous access difficult. (b) Coronal CT from the same patient shows the inferior borders of the liver (*L*) and spleen (not shown), the costal margin (*solid line*), the lateral margin of the rectus abdominus muscle (*dashed line*), and, when it lies anterior to the stomach (*green-shaded region*), the superior margin of the transverse colon (*blue line*). These borders together define the safest region (target) for percutaneous puncture of the gastric wall. (c) When the stomach is distended with air (*light-green shaded region*) through a nasogastric tube prior to puncture, the altered anatomic relationships frequently provide a more optimal safe zone (solid target). This allows a stoma site and angle that directs the gastrostomy tube (*black line*) and jejunostomy tube (*gray line*) toward the gastric outlet. (d) A choice of site and angle, common to surgical and endoscopic placement, that directs the gastrojejunostomy tube (*gray line*) to the left of the lesser curvature and toward the gastric inlet, often leads to formation of a Waltman loop and to inexorable and frequent dislodgment. (e) During surgical gastrostomy in this patient, the stomach was pulled inferiorly to reach the gastrostomy site, distorting the already abnormal gastric anatomy. (f) Anteroposterior and (g) lateral contrast studies of the newly placed gastrostomy obtained due to irregular vital signs demonstrated extragastric position of the gastrostomy retention balloon (*arrow*).

(e)
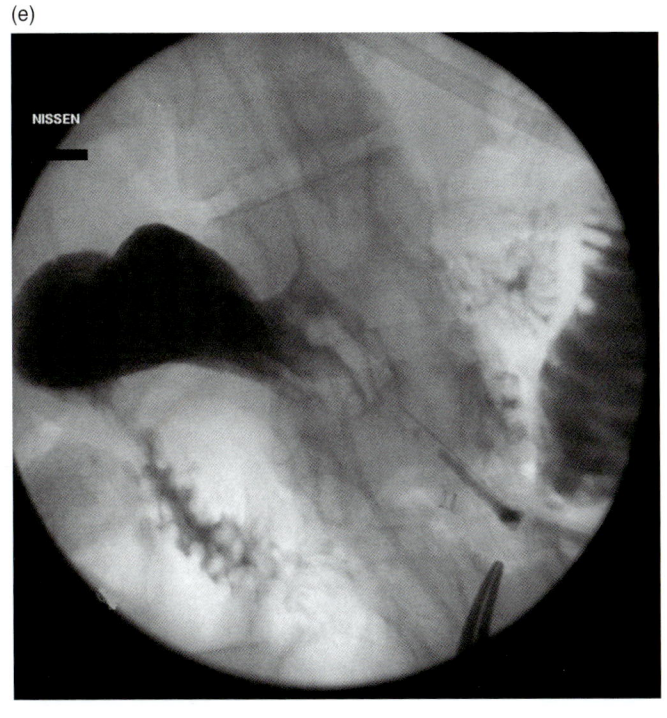

(f)
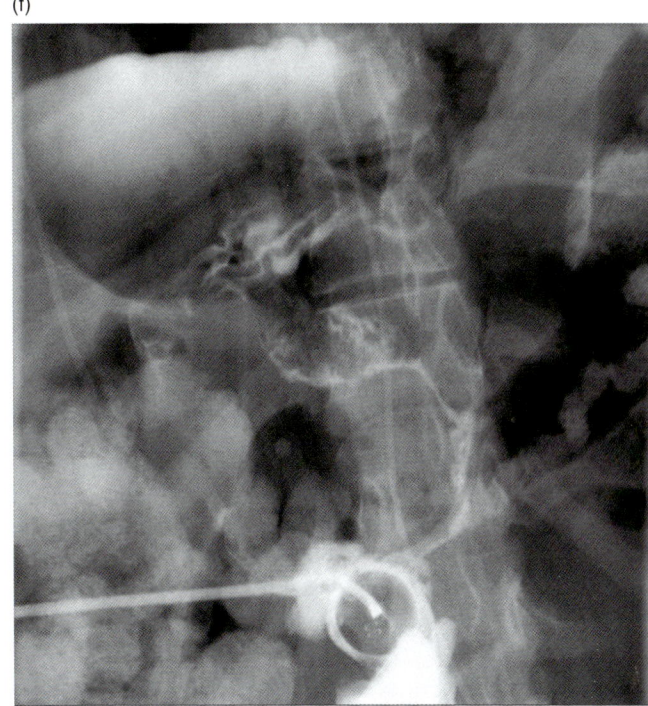

(g)
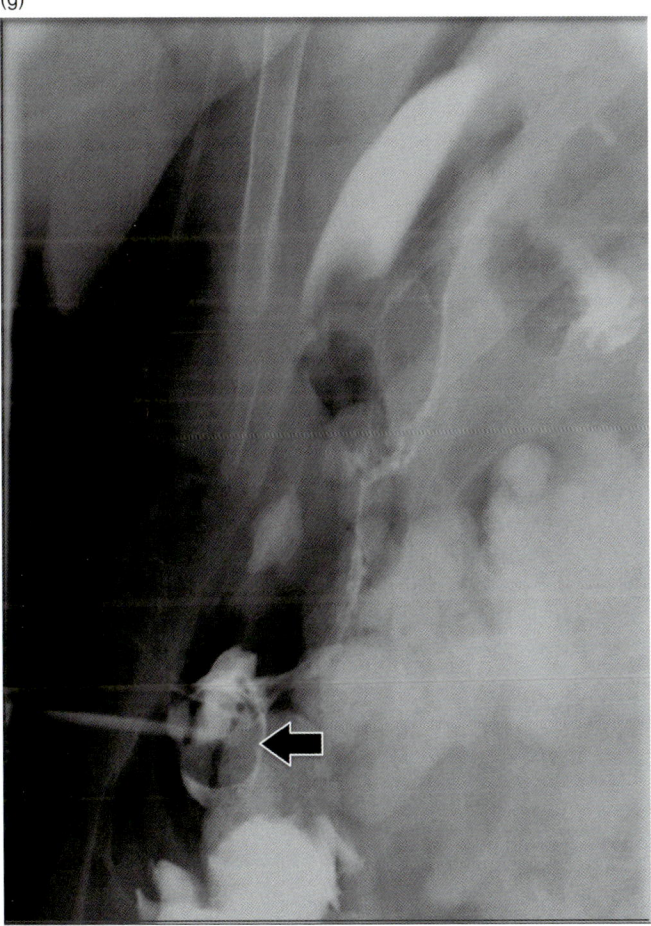

Figure 4.6 (cont.)

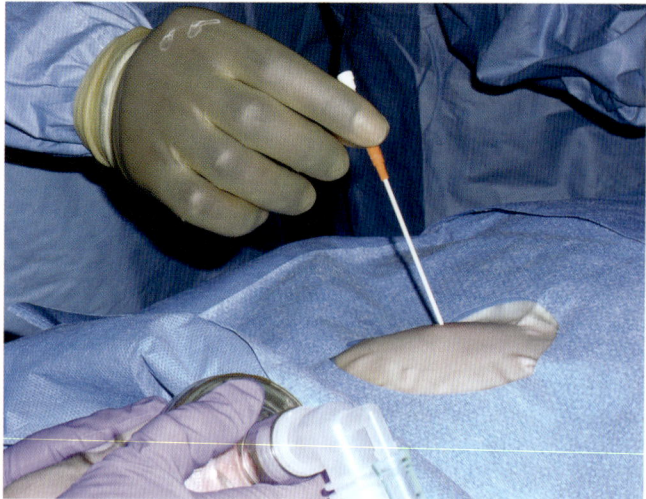

Figure 4.7 After the gastric lumen has been distended with air, the access needle is directed toward the gastric outlet and advanced with a sharp jab. Angulation of the C-arm may be necessary to confirm an entry point within the scope of the snare loop.

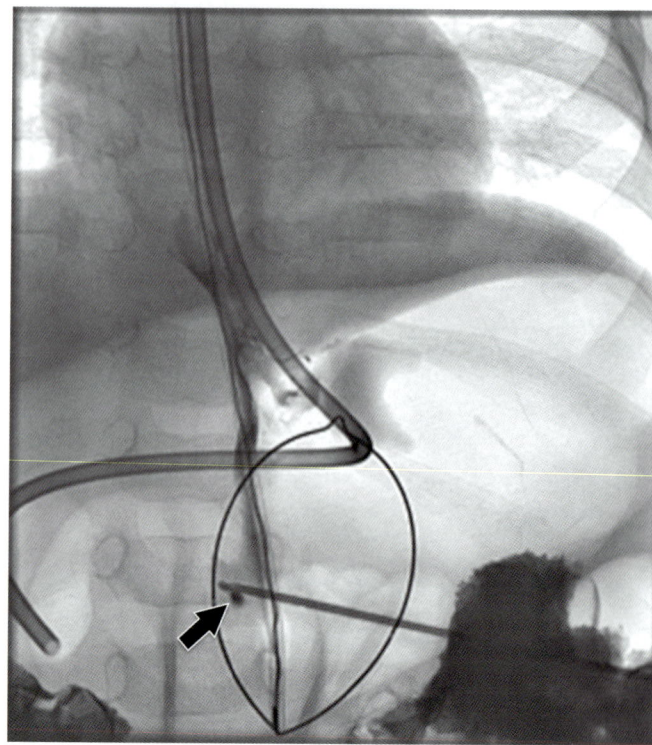

Figure 4.8 A "hanging drop" (*arrow*) of non-ionic iodinated contrast falling through the lumen confirms intraluminal position of the access needle prior to deployment of the retention suture and guide wire.

The entry site is prepared in sterile fashion and then draped. The skin at the entry site is anesthetized with a *slow* injection of 1% lidocaine buffered with sodium bicarbonate (8 ml/2 ml mixture) using a 27- to 30-gauge, 1.5 inch needle to minimize discomfort.

Once the child is sedated or anesthetized and the skin adequately anesthetized, a 1.0 to 1.5 cm skin incision is made at the previously selected entry site with a scalpel blade. The incision is purposely made larger than the diameter of the PG tube so that the possibility of ischemia leading to fasciitis is reduced in the rare case of postoperative infection of the abdominal wall. The subcutaneous tissue is then bluntly dissected to make passage of the GT easier. Some interventionalists prefer to administer glucagon at this point in an IV dose of 0.1 to 0.5 mg, in order to increase the tone of the pylorus and decrease the risk of air escaping into the small bowel during percutaneous access.

Under fluoroscopic guidance, the stomach is inflated with air via the NG tube. The 18-gauge needle is inserted into the incision in an almost vertical orientation with the tip pointed toward the pylorus (Figure 4.7). When the needle tip is observed to clear the transverse colon it is *thrust* into the gastric lumen as if throwing a dart (rapid needle acceleration). In cases where there is uncertainty that the needle will clear the transverse colon, it is helpful to angle the C-arm in a caudocranial direction to confirm a satisfactory route. Once the anterior gastric wall has been punctured, intragastric position of the tip may be confirmed with a small amount of contrast. This is most easily achieved if a syringe of contrast is attached to the access needle with a T-connector prior to puncture. Observation of a drop of contrast freely falling through the gastric lumen provides positive confirmation of successful puncture (Figure 4.8). At this point, the tip of the needle is redirected toward the center of the open snare.

The puncture of the stomach and capture of the guide wire is easily accomplished in most instances using single-plane fluoroscopic guidance alone. However, for problem cases, biplane fluoroscopy is helpful since it enables more precise needle positioning, makes puncture of the stomach easier, especially for patients with a high or horizontally oriented stomach, and assists grasping the guide wire if the process is not progressing quickly or smoothly. When using biplane guidance, the trick is to be sure that the needle is directed toward the center of the snare in *both* planes. Once the needle is in the stomach, a 260 cm guide wire is advanced through the snare until it deflects off of the posterior gastric wall. This also positively confirms intragastric position of the needle.

Once the snare is closed around the guide wire (Figure 4.9), it is pulled up through the esophagus and out of the mouth. Nearly the entire length of wire is fed through the needle so that there is enough length for the PG tube. A 16 French (a larger tube is rarely necessary) over the wire or pull type gastrostomy tube is fitted onto the wire, liberally lubricated, and advanced until the needle is pushed out of the puncture site indicating that the dilating tip of the GT (Figure 4.10) exits the puncture site and is visible. The dilating tip is grasped with one hand while the other hand is placed on the skin surface to apply counter-traction (Figure 4.11). Counter-traction is applied to the skin surface and the GT is then quickly pulled out through the anterior abdominal wall until there is resistance to further forward movement. This indicates that the retention disc is up against the anterior gastric wall.

Chapter 4 Abdominopelvic interventions

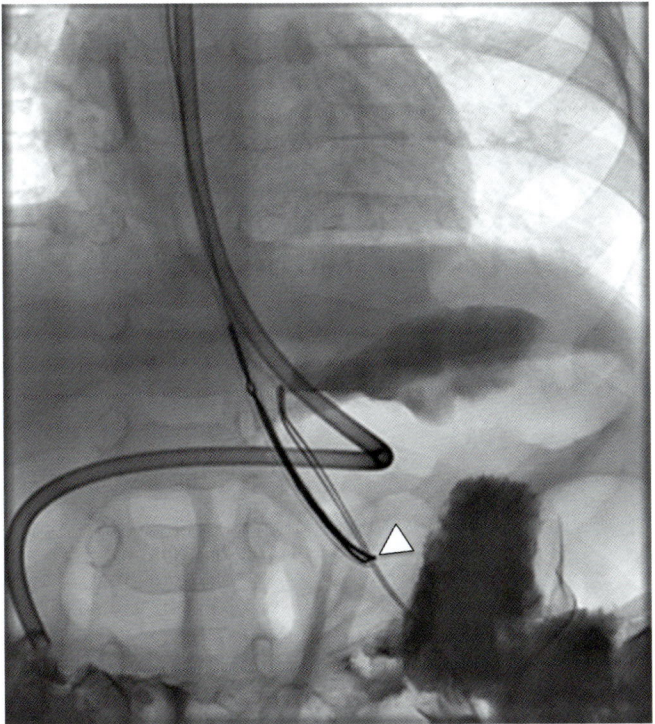

Figure 4.9 The guide wire is advanced through the access needle and through the snare loop. It is then snared (*arrowhead*) and exteriorized in retrograde fashion through the mouth.

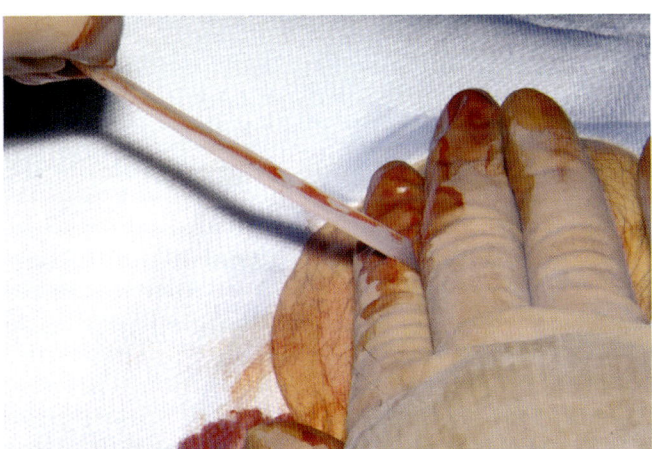

Figure 4.11 The tapered tip of the gastrostomy tube is grasped with one hand while the other hand is placed on the skin surface to apply countertraction as the tube is pulled externally.

When the GT is in place, before the dilating segment is cut off, a friction lock is slid over the GT until it rests loosely (2 to 3 mm from the skin surface) against the anterior abdominal wall (Figure 4.12). It is important not to pull the PG tube too tightly against the skin. When this occurs, there is a greater chance over time for the disc to ulcerate the gastric mucosa and become embedded within the gastric wall by granulation tissue. No sutures are necessary to stabilize the GT. Contrast is injected via the PG to confirm intragastric position and

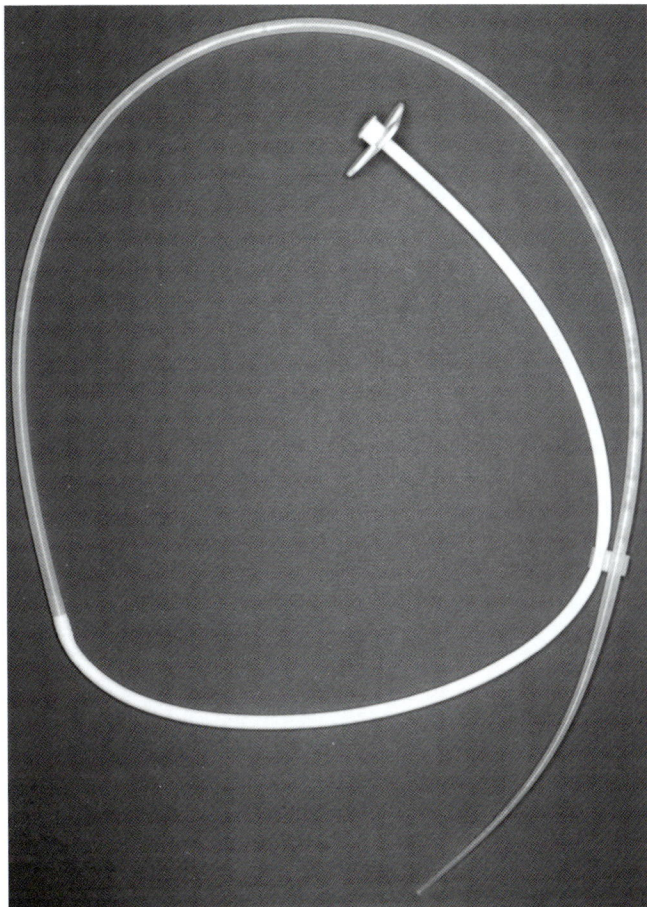

Figure 4.10 The primary gastrostomy tube has a tapered tip that dilates the newly created stoma as it is gently pulled forward until the internal bumper brings the anterior gastric wall in apposition to the anterior abdominal wall.

exclude a gastric leak. Postoperatively frontal and, if necessary, cross-table lateral radiographs are taken to evaluate the abdomen and exclude free intraperitoneal gas or gastric leakage (Figure 4.13). With antegrade placement there is less than a 1% chance for this to occur. Even if free air is identified it is not indicative of imminent peritonitis or other complications. In spite of this, when free intraperitoneal air is observed, these children are usually given 24 to 72 hours of a broad-spectrum antibiotic.

Retrograde gastrostomy

The retrograde or push technique was introduced by Gauderer and colleagues in 1980 and is used in children and adults. The push technique was popularized by Russell in 1984 and subsequently used for both endoscopic and fluoroscopic gastrostomies. Over the years, interventionalists have selected this approach most often for placement of a PG. However, relatively few reports of the retrograde technique have been published in the pediatric population.

In general, the procedure is similar to that outlined for antegrade gastrostomy insertion. The primary difference is the use of anchor sutures. In addition, the initial tube inserted is

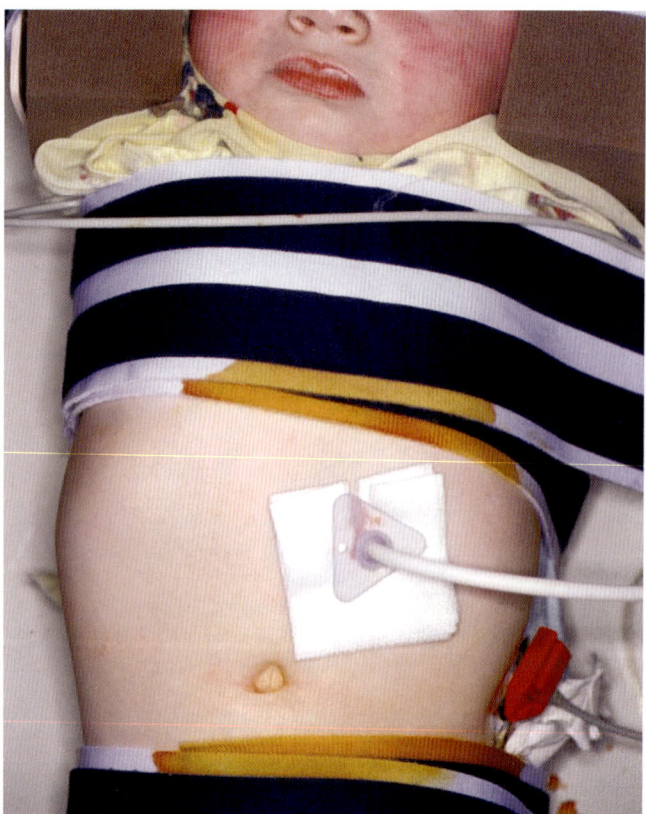

Figure 4.12 The primary gastrostomy tube is dressed with a slotted gauze between the skin and the external bumper. The tube is left open to atmosphere or to low wall suction until bowel sounds return.

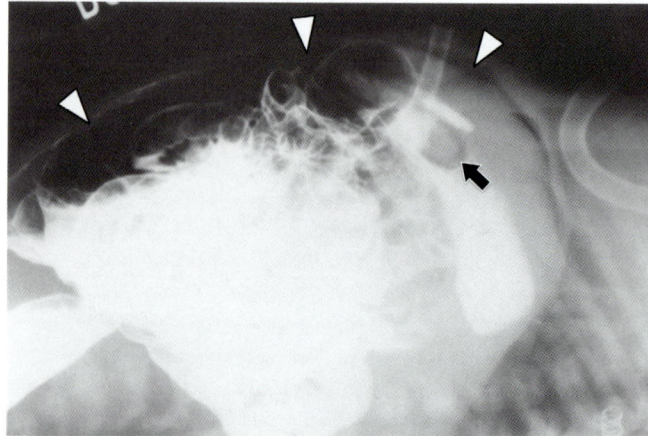

Figure 4.13 The balloon internal retention bumper (*arrow*) of a freshly placed percutaneous antegrade gastrostomy is seen in satisfactory position in this 27-day-old male with adrenal leukodystrophy. Placement is complicated by extensive free intraperitoneal air (*arrowheads*). The patient was kept NPO and placed on a course of triple antibiotics. Feeding was resumed uneventfully after three days.

often smaller. Otherwise, the approach to monitoring and localization of the left lobe of liver and transverse colon is the same.

Primary retrograde gastrostomy insertion in children may be performed using intravenous sedation and local anesthesia or under GA. In most series, a single dose of antibiotics (e.g., cefazolin 40 mg/kg) is given intravenously. Intravenous glucagon may be given (0.1 to 0.3 mg) to relax (close) the pylorus and deter loss of insufflated air into the duodenum. The position of the left lobe of the liver is identified using US and marked on the skin surface. The transverse colon is opacified and an NG tube is inserted. The stomach is insufflated with air to bring it into firm contact with the anterior abdominal wall.

At this point, access is obtained with an 18-gauge single wall needle in the same manner described for antegrade insertion, above. The needle can be preloaded with an anchor suture near the tip, and connected through a T-connector to a syringe containing half-strength contrast. When the needle has been "darted" through the abdomen and anterior wall of the stomach, intraluminal position is verified with a small amount of contrast, and the guide wire deployed. As the guide wire is advanced it pushes the preloaded anchor suture ahead. When the needle is removed, the external strands of the anchor suture are grasped with a hemostat and gentle traction maintains apposition of the stomach and abdominal wall

throughout the remainder of the procedure. Some practitioners prefer to insert one to three anchor sutures first to fix the stomach in position against the anterior abdominal wall. Under fluoroscopic guidance, the stomach can then be punctured between the retention sutures and the guide wire coiled within the stomach or proximal small intestine.

In either case, the tract is then dilated to the size of the intended catheter and an 8 to 12 French locking pigtail catheter is inserted. It is important during both tract dilation and catheter insertion to *push* with the dilator or catheter rather than *pull* the anchor sutures. Exerting substantial traction on the anchor sutures may cause them to pull through the stomach wall, with potential loss of the newly formed tract. Intragastric position of the catheter is confirmed with injection of contrast material. If needed, a peel-away sheath may be inserted to aid in catheter placement or to protect the fresh tract while other manipulations, i.e. JT insertion, are performed. The GT is placed to drainage for 24 hours.

Initial follow-up is at one week to cut the retention suture(s) and check the ostomy site. If a button is planned, the locking pigtail drain is exchanged for a 12 French balloon catheter at six weeks. Thereafter, serial catheter changes to 14 to 18 French are performed over the next six weeks. At three months the child is brought back and a button inserted. Alternatively, the child can be scheduled three months post-gastrostomy insertion for tract dilation using either progressive dilators (our preference) or a 5 to 7 mm angioplasty balloon, depending on the size of the button selected. Button insertion is generally performed on an outpatient basis. If tract dilation is needed, it is usually performed using local anesthesia and intravenous sedation. The patient is kept NPO for a minimum of six hours and a button inserted. The latter approach is our preference since it is less costly and requires

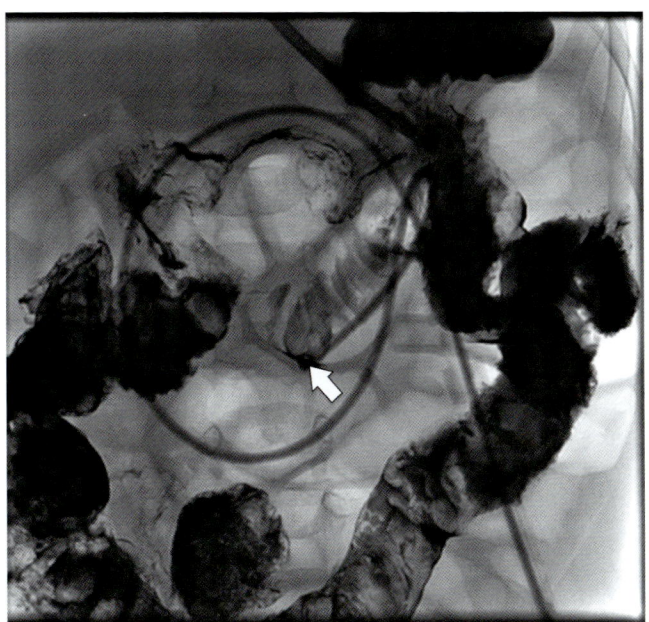

Figure 4.14 In select patients, a jejunostomy tube can be placed at the time of primary transgastric access, through the newly placed percutaneous gastrostomy tube. The tip (arrow) location in the proximal jejunum is confirmed with a small amount of contrast.

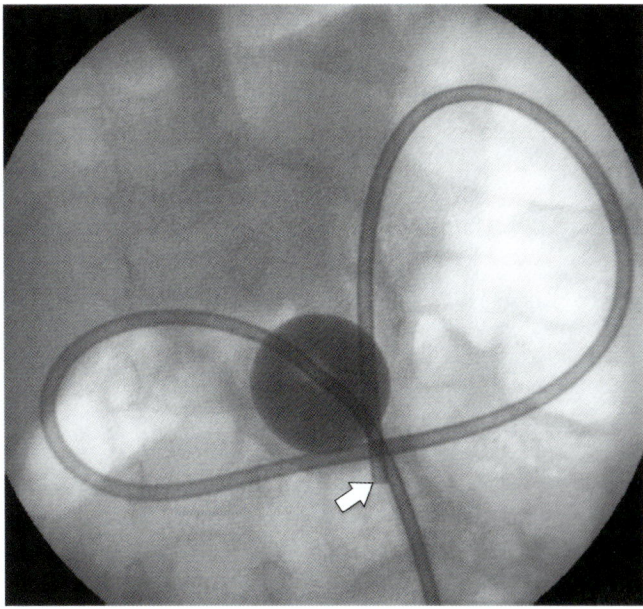

Figure 4.15 Four-month-old male with a replacement transgastric gastrojejunostomy system comprised of a 14 French balloon-tipped end-hole gastrostomy (Ross FlexiFlo®) and an 8 Fr shortened Frederick–Miller jejunostomy tube (Cook Medical) coaxially inserted with the tip in the proximal jejunum (arrow).

fewer steps. Subsequent care is on an as-needed basis for treatment of skin problems or replacement of jejunostomy tubes.

The retrograde gastrostomy inserted without the use of retention sutures has the disadvantage of not pulling the stomach into close contact with the anterior abdominal wall. If this occurs, the fibrous tract that develops may be long. This can predispose to tract perforation and communication with the peritoneal space during button insertion.

Percutaneous gastrojejunostomy

When indicated, a gastrojejunostomy may be inserted following dilation of the gastrostomy tract. If needed, a jejunostomy tube (JT) may be inserted coaxially through the GT either at the time of *antegrade* GT placement (Figure 4.14), or at a later date (Figure 4.15). Currently, we are using three tubes for jejunostomies: an 8 French Frederick–Miller (FM) tube modified by cutting off its weighted tip creating an end-hole catheter, a 6 French Corpak® or a 9 French Flexiflow tube. In most situations, the FM tube is preferred because of its combination of stiffness, easy pushability, its tendency to harden without straightening out, and its durability. The 6 French Corpak® is used for children less than 10 kg with smaller lumen GTs and the 9 French Flexiflow JT is softer and has a greater tendency to kink.

To expedite JT placement, a 5 French JB-1 catheter and Bentson guide wire are used to maneuver through the pylorus into the proximal jejunum just distal to the ligament of Treitz. After JT position is confirmed by contrast injection, the tubes are secured to one another. Initially, the tubes are coated with benzoin or Mastisol® to enhance their adhesiveness. Then the GT and JT are bound together by wrapping them with Tegaderm® or Opsite®.

A PGJ may also be placed directly through the PG tract, again either at the time of *retrograde* access or at a later date (perhaps following an unsuccessful trial of GT feeding). In this case, the GJ tube of choice is usually an 8.5 or 10.2 French unibody gastrojejunostomy catheter with a proximal fixation loop, balloon or malecot retention device in the stomach, and a straight or non-locking pigtail silicone catheter positioned within the small bowel.

If primary PGJ is planned, a glide wire of suitable length is used rather than the 70 cm non-Teflon® wire. This wire is guided through the duodenum to the proximal jejunum using a directional catheter. The guiding catheter is exchanged for the PGJ catheter. Once the catheter tip reaches the proximal duodenum it may be carefully advanced off the stiffener until the tip is securely in place past the ligament of Treitz. The intragastric retention device is secured and a small amount of contrast injected to demonstrate that the tip is in good position and that there is no intragastric leak of contrast. (Since most patients referred for PGJ are at risk for reflux and aspiration, intragastric leak defeats the purpose.) A high level of caution must be exercised throughout to assure that control of the newly formed tract is not inadvertently lost during manipulation of the wire and catheters. Regardless of the type of tube inserted, an NG tube is often left in place for 24 hours to drain the stomach and to reduce the risk of leakage. The postoperative orders are the same as those described for gastrostomy.

Technical variations
The "push–pull" gastrostomy for infants
The push–pull method of percutaneous gastrostomy insertion is considered for most infants less than 7 kg or those with an esophageal diameter less than approximately 1.2 cm. Although an antegrade gastrostomy tube has been successfully inserted in children weighing as little as 2.3 kg, we have found that in this subgroup of children there is a chance that the retention device at the end of a gastrostomy tube may traumatize the esophagus during passage into the stomach. In these children, the problem is usually the diameter of the normal anatomic narrowing at the level of the cricopharyngeus muscle or thoracic inlet. To solve this problem, we have developed an alternative: the push–pull method. The push–pull approach is usually employed either electively in small infants or, if excessive tension is appreciated, while attempting an antegrade gastrostomy. Alternatively, an antegrade PGT with a smaller disc can be used.

When utilizing the push–pull method, the initial steps of the procedure are the same as for the antegrade technique. The colon is opacified and the left lobe of the liver is identified with US and marked on the skin surface. An NG tube is placed into the stomach. An OG tube is then inserted and the guide wire exchanged for a 34 mm nitinol snare. While observing with the fluoroscope, the stomach is inflated with air and punctured as soon as the transverse colon is moved away. The percutaneous guide wire is snared and exteriorized at the mouth.

The tube is pulled through the anterior abdominal wall until its dilating segment has enlarged the skin tract to 14 French. Then, a 14 to 16 French balloon-tipped Flexiflo GT is back-loaded over the guide wire onto the dilating segment of the antegrade gastrostomy tube until it is firmly engaged. The tubes are simultaneously maneuvered. The antegrade gastrostomy tube is *pulled* back at the mouth while the Flexiflow GT is *pushed* at the skin surface of the abdominal wall until the GT passes into the stomach coming to rest in the esophagus. The Flexiflow catheter is pushed back until it is out of the mouth, facilitating separation from the antegrade gastrostomy tube.

The balloon catheter is pulled into the upper esophagus and the balloon is inflated with 1 to 2 ml of contrast to confirm its position. With the balloon partially inflated, the GT is pulled back into the stomach where the balloon is inflated with 5 to 10 ml of water. A Christmas tree adapter is connected to the GT while the wire is maintained in position and contrast is injected to confirm that the balloon is in the gastric lumen. Once proper position is confirmed, the guide wire is removed. It is essential *not* to remove the guide wire until satisfactory tube position is confirmed.

In most instances, the procedure is easily accomplished. However, if the GT cannot be pushed into the stomach, several maneuvers can be used to safely get the GT into place: (1) the tract can be dilated in retrograde fashion to 16 to 20 French with progressive dilators or a PTA balloon and the push–pull technique repeated; (2) a tapered pigtail (8 to 10 French) or other catheter can be inserted without further dilation; (3) retention sutures can be placed followed by either choice (1) or (2); or (4) the skin incision can be enlarged by sharp dissection down to the fascia. In most cases, option (4) is the best solution.

Percutaneous jejunostomy
Occasionally, transgastric access to the small bowel for long-term feeding may be impeded by a proximal stricture or obstruction of the duodenum or other contraindications. In such a situation, direct percutaneous access to the jejunum may be obtained by a technique similar to that described for retrograde gastrostomy, above. Several authors have described direct jejunostomy, either as a primary procedure or as an alternative to gastrojejunostomy. This procedure is facilitated by the presence of a dilated segment of proximal jejunum. In the absence of this fortuitous finding, identification of a proximal loop of jejunum can itself be problematic. Even once identified, selective dilation of such a loop is inhibited by the absence of any functional sphincter.

Bowel decompression
Interposition of transverse colon or a dilated loop of bowel between the abdominal wall and the anticipated entry point into the gastric wall (or other planned access) can result in cancellation or delay in the planned procedure (Figures 4.16 and 4.17). If angulation of the fluoroscope or alteration in the patient's body position is unsuccessful in moving the bowel away from the tract, then deflation of the interposed bowel loop may permit continuation of the procedure. This is accomplished by percutaneous puncture with a thin (27-gauge) needle, and subsequent aspiration of the gas from the bowel lumen. A small amount of contrast can be used to confirm deflation of the bowel loop. This maneuver can provide a safe route of access to the stomach, jejunum, cecum, or other targets of percutaneous access obstructed by an overlying loop of distended bowel.

Postprocedure and follow-up care
Postoperative orders and initial tube care
Postoperative orders are generally minimal regardless of the tube inserted. Vital signs are initially obtained every 15 minutes for the first half hour, every 30 minutes for one hour, then every one hour for a minimum of two hours or until the child has returned to baseline. Depending on the hour of the day the procedure is completed, the child is usually kept NPO and given nothing by GT for a minimum of six hours. Children with PGJs are kept NPO for at least two hours. Fluids and medications are given intravenously. In general, full PG or PGJ feeding is initiated at 08:00 the morning after tube insertion provided bowel sounds are normal.

Prior to initiating feeding, dietary and home care consultations are obtained. Initially, a consultation from the dietary service is obtained so that the child's ideal caloric requirements

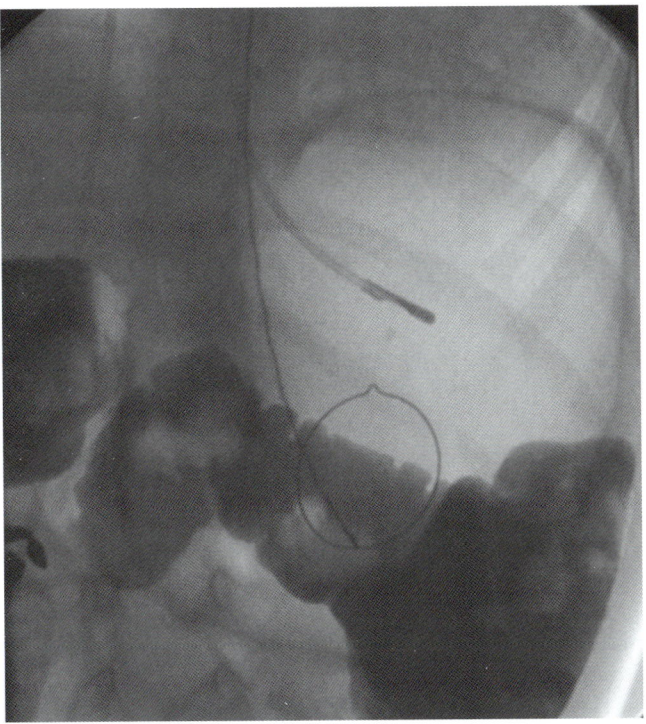

Figure 4.16 In this 12-year-old male, fluoroscopy shows a nasogastric tube tip and orogastric snare placed in preparation for percutaneous gastrostomy. Thin barium contrast in the transverse colon projects over the open gooseneck snare. An orthotopic view is required to determine whether the colon is posterior to the gastric lumen, permitting the procedure, or interposed between the anterior abdominal wall and the targeted portion of the anterior gastric wall, as was found in this case.

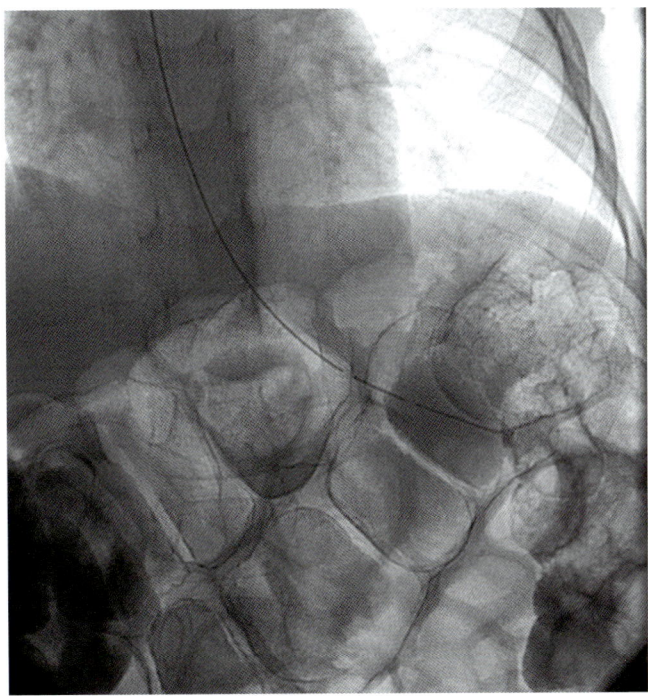

Figure 4.17 Multiple loops of air-filled bowel are interposed between the abdominal wall and the stomach in this anteroposterior radiograph of the upper abdomen in a 14-year-old candidate for percutaneous gastrojejunostomy. The procedure was delayed until a subsequent radiograph demonstrated a safe access path.

and preferred formula can be determined. Whenever possible, the dietary service is notified prior to the insertion of the PG or PGJ so that the feeding recommendations can be prepared and in place on the first day after gastrostomy insertion. The home care service is consulted in order to facilitate a timely hospital discharge. An infusion pump, a supply of formula, the assorted tubes and syringes, and the home services are all arranged so that a smooth transition from hospital to home can be made. The home care provider is expected to educate the caretakers on the proper use of the equipment. The radiology nurse or others familiar with proper PGJ feedings and care will teach the family about the care of the tubes, give discharge instructions, and provide written instructions, including telephone numbers to call for future appointments and emergency services. Currently, in uncomplicated cases, children are discharged to home approximately 36 hours after PG or PGJ insertion.

All patients are initially fed by continuous pump infusion. Feeding is started with a clear electrolyte solution (e.g., Pedialyte®) to test the system. The volume of infusate is calculated at 1/24th the total daily caloric requirement. For example, if the child is to receive 1,200 ml of formula per day, then Pedialyte® would be started at a rate of 50 ml/h. If this initial feeding with Pedialyte® is tolerated for one to two hours without difficulty, the recommended daily volume of full strength formula is given by continuous feeding over 24 hours. Reduced hourly rates or use of dilute formula (e.g., ½ strength concentration) is rarely necessary and is reserved for those children who have feeding problems that make them unable to tolerate full strength formula.

We have found that nearly all children who have previously tolerated feeding, albeit at reduced volumes, do well with this regimen. This approach obviates a gradual build-up of calories or volume that may prolong hospitalization, makes care more complex and tedious, and takes longer for the child to get into positive nitrogen and calorie balance.

If postoperative day one feeding is tolerated, on day two the rate is increased. The calculated daily volume is now infused over an 18-hour period, e.g., again using the example 1,200 calories per day, if a volume of 1,200 ml of a 1 Calorie/ml formula is selected, the rate will be increased to 67 ml/h for 18 hours. This adjustment can be made incrementally or as a one-time change. Thus there will be a six-hour period each day during which the child can be off the feeding pump. Currently, most children are discharged in the afternoon of the second postoperative day if they have tolerated the 18-hour rate without problems. The remainder of the volume progression is carried out from home following the prescribed feeding regimen.

The 18-hour rate is maintained for the remainder of the first week. At the end of this time the infusion is increased to a rate that delivers the recommended daily volume in 15 hours, with 9 hours off the pump each day. This rate is maintained for one to two weeks. Again, if tolerated, the rate is advanced to allow 12 hours on and 12 hours off the pump each day. Children fed through a PG (but not those fed through a PGJ) are candidates for bolus feeds. Patients with PGJs are kept on pump feedings and not advanced past 12-hour rates since they would be at increased risk for developing a dumping syndrome secondary to osmotic diuresis.

When bolus feeds are instituted, the total volume of daily formula is divided into multiple portions and generally given to the child at the family's meal times, snacks, and before bed. In children who are able to tolerate oral feeding, solid food can be started to partially replace tube feeding. As the child becomes able to take a significant amount of calories by mouth, the pump feedings are reduced proportionally and used only as a supplement. In most cases, a significant volume of formula is given while the child is asleep. We have found that it is best to first establish successful feeding by pump before adding a significant amount of calories by mouth. Therefore it is important to closely monitor the child's weight gain and growth during these first few months of gastrostomy feeding. The child's primary care physician usually provides this follow-up.

The interventionalist often manages the child's care while an inpatient. However, upon discharge, the interventionalist remains involved in the technical management of the tubes, skin care, and performing normal and emergency tube maintenance. In addition, depending upon the preference and expertise of the primary care physician, the interventionalist may play an active role in the management of the child's feeding regimen.

In the early stages of our experience it is our preference to electively replace transgastric JTs every three months to avoid the risks of tube hardening and potential bowel injury. However, we have not seen any children who have sustained bowel injuries so we now replace the JTs on an as-needed basis. The GTs are only changed if necessary, and usually last at least 9 to 12 months. All parents are instructed to clean their child's skin with ½ strength hydrogen peroxide or mild soap at least once per day and carefully dry it in order to keep the skin from becoming inflamed or infected.

Catheter exchange and reinsertion

With the large number of children with gastrostomies, it has become increasingly common for patients to require gastrostomy tube replacement or conversion to a gastrojejunostomy because of GER, equipment failure, or inadvertent removal. In addition, children with gastrojejunostomies (GJ) may require gastric venting. There are now a variety of tubes, in a range of sizes that are available to the interventionalist for these purposes (Figure 4.18). In addition to gastrostomy tubes through which a jejunostomy can be coaxially inserted, there are unibody gastrojejunostomy tubes. Both tube types have their pros and cons and the ultimate choice should be tailored to the needs of the child tempered by the experience and preference of the interventionalist. The coaxial replacement GTs are technically easy to insert and the same approach is used as described for NJ or GJ insertion. In general, we prefer the coaxial system since it is more flexible and less costly. However, these GJs do *not* vent well when a 14 to 16 French GT and 8 French JT are used. When venting is a priority, it is usually best to substitute a gastrostomy >18 French for the 14 French GT or use a different stoma for the PG or PGJ tube. The length of the JT is customized so that its tip is positioned at, or distal to, the ligament of Treitz. This position is favored since it minimizes reflux of feedings into the duodenum and stomach, reduces the likelihood of vomiting and aspiration pneumonia after feeding, and best stabilizes the JT minimizing the frequency of JT malposition and dysfunction.

Today, the button GJ tubes (Figure 4.19) have become the tube of choice for long-term GJ feeding. They are low-profile devices that parents prefer and have the advantage of being easily vented and inserted in a single step. However, they may be problematic in small children and toddlers because the gastric component is too long and stiff and often projects into and deforms the distal stomach or duodenal bulb. This results in discomfort and may predispose the child, especially infants, to ulceration or perforation of the stomach or duodenum. In addition, the jejunostomy component is generally longer and of a larger French size than needed and therefore requires shortening. In some children, especially infants less than 10 kg, the jejunostomy produces gastrointestinal discomfort and, on occasion, obstruction of the gastric outflow tract. It is possible that symptoms are due to tube-related small bowel irritability or intermittent small bowel intussusceptions. Also, GJ button tubes may not move easily over a guide wire. In these situations, a hydrophilic guide wire, silicone spray, or other lubricant (e.g., sterile mineral oil), may be needed.

When replacing a GT or converting it to a GJ, it is most convenient and the least invasive, to use the same tube size as the primary GT. However, if the GT is less than 16 French, we have found it best to enlarge the tract to at least this size to minimize the chance of clogging. A GT larger than 16 French is rarely used if feeding is the only goal. When necessary, however, GTs of 18 French to 24 French are utilized. Other indications for >14 French GT include replacement of a large tube already in place, as is often the case when replacing surgical gastrostomies, or when the ostomy site is leaking and the skin is inflamed.

An unexpected source of referrals for GT or GJ replacement is to care for children with skin breakdown secondary to gastrostomy leakage. This problem has most often resulted from gastrostomies that have developed an asymmetric hole (usually an SG), gastrostomies too small for the hole that has been created, and from ostomies that have rapidly enlarged due to inflamed skin. When this occurs and gastric contents begin to leak, it is imperative to treat this promptly to resolve skin inflammation and allow the hole to reduce in size. With successful treatment, the problems of secondary infection, discomfort, and further ostomy enlargement with the potential

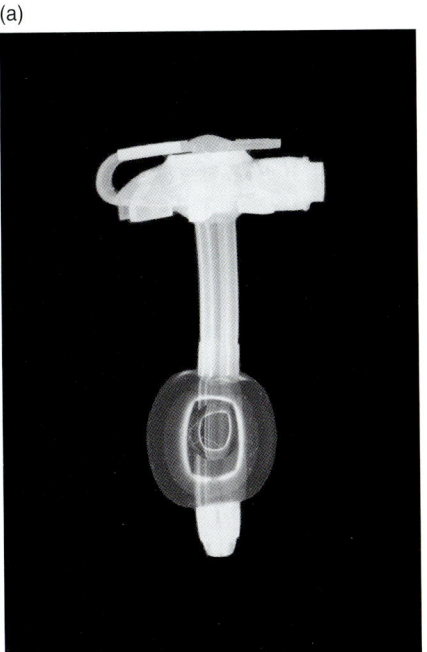
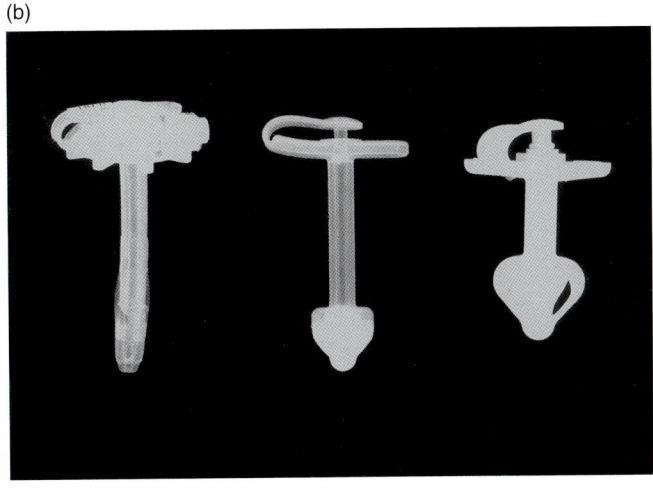

Figure 4.18 (a) This low-profile gastrostomy device has an inflated balloon internal retention bumper. These devices come in a variety of shaft diameters and lengths. (b) Deflated balloon (left), mushroom (middle), and Malecot (right) internal retention bumpers are shown. There are numerous variations commercially available.

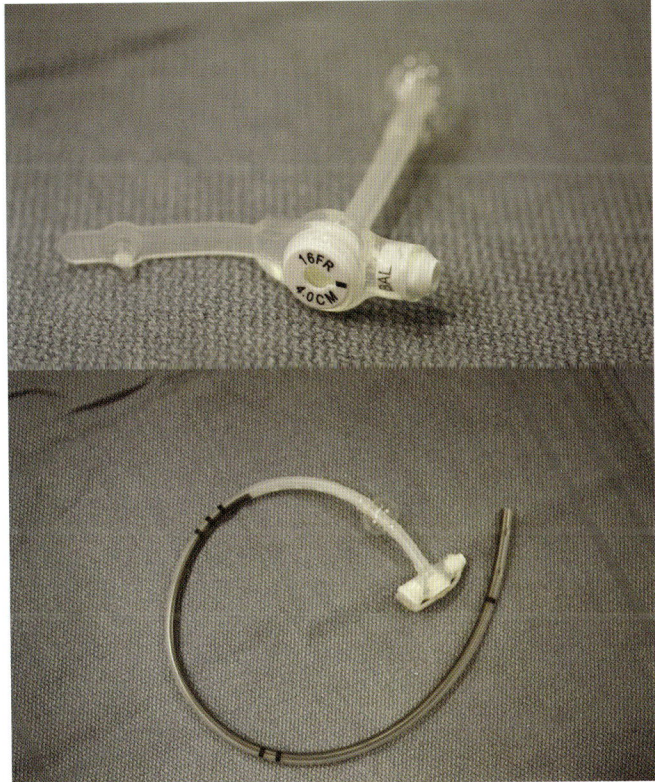

Figure 4.19 Low-profile button gastrostomy tube (top) and button gastrojejunostomy (bottom). Examples of connection tubing for low-profile gastrostomy tubes. Straight connectors have a larger volume and therefore better flow rate, but tend to kink. The angled tube has a narrower caliber but resists kinking.

of gastric mucosal herniation requiring surgical repair, can be avoided.

Replacement gastrostomy tubes and primary gastrostomies inserted using the retrograde technique may be secured by a balloon-tipped catheter, which has a high resistance to accidental dislodgment when the balloon is inflated, and essentially no resistance to dislodgment when the balloon is deflated or ruptures. They are less commonly retained by a mushroom-tipped catheter, for which resistance to accidental dislodgment is less but constant (cannot be deflated) and requires a device to stretch the mushroom in order to deliver or retrieve the device (Figure 4.20). Both types are prone to premature loss, so it is important to educate the caregiver how to safely reinsert the tube. To safeguard against the inability to replace a lost GT, outpatients are given a Foley catheter 2 French smaller than the gastrostomy. This enables the caregiver to place the temporary tube at home to help avoid the risk of ostomy closure before the GT can be replaced. The caretaker is instructed to initially attempt reinserting the tube that has come out before inserting a smaller tube. It must be stressed that the ostomy will shrink in size rapidly, thus replacement at home is strongly preferred. If the retention balloon has ruptured and a smaller tube is not available, the 14 to 16 French system should be reinserted and secured to the skin with tape.

If the GT is not replaced or if a smaller tube is utilized, the tract probably will have to be enlarged at the time of reinsertion. This can be accomplished using a PTA balloon or progressive dilators. We prefer the latter approach since it is less expensive. We have found that it is usually necessary to dilate

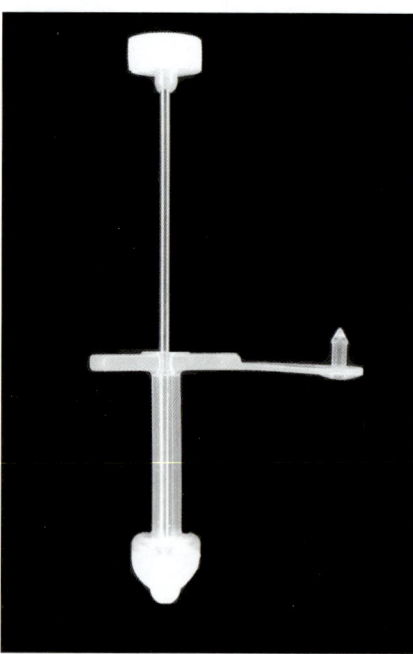

Figure 4.20 An obturator is passed through the gastrostomy lumen, stretching the button body and narrowing the internal mushroom-type retention device to allow the device to be passed through the gastrostomy stoma during insertion and removal.

replacement there is no associated discomfort, and sedation or local anesthesia is usually not required. Therefore there is no need for an intravenous line nor is the child changed into a gown. The shirt is pulled up to expose the gastrostomy or gastrojejunostomy site and the clothing is covered with a chuck to keep them dry and clean. No special equipment is needed in most cases. If the tract has reduced in size, it will require dilation with progressive dilators or a PTA balloon.

If there is a mature tract, the GT or GJ may be removed without any special precautions. If the tube has been in place for less than two weeks, there is a known problem with wound healing, malnutrition, or there is a question concerning the integrity of the gastrostomy tract, it is safest to remove the preexisting catheter over a guide wire. Removal of a primary tube may be as easy as deflating the balloon tip or may require an over the guide wire technique as described above in the section for removal of a gastrostomy retention disc. If a mature tract is present, the GT can be removed without guide wire insertion and a new GT with an end hole reinserted. If a JT is required, a directional catheter and Bentson guide wire is used to catheterize the proximal jejunum or fourth portion of the duodenum. The catheter is marked at the level of the hub of the GT to record the tube length and is then removed. The JT is measured from the mark on the catheter and is cut to the desired length. The JT is lubricated with mineral oil, silicone spray, or K-Y jelly and inserted through the GT. The JT is then secured to the GT using a cable tie and covered with tape to prevent skin abrasions.

Gastrostomy button or button jejunostomy

Regardless of the method of insertion, all patients with gastrostomies without gastrojejunostomies are candidates for replacement with a gastrostomy button. In the past, children requiring GJ were ineligible for buttons since there was no good method for securing a low-profile JT and preventing significant leakage of gastric contents. Today, there are several types of low-profile devices (Figures 4.18 and 4.21). The button type selected is dictated by the needs of the child. In general, the button has become the tube of choice for all long-term feeding.

The gastrostomy button is a soft, 14 to 24 French, low-profile tube with a one-way valve. This device has several advantages over other types of gastrostomies. First and foremost the button is low profile, which is much preferred by patients since it is less noticeable, does not move around as much with activity causing less irritation and reactive granulation tissue, and is easy to use. The one-way valve effectively prevents leakage of gastric contents. The button jejunostomy and gastrojejunostomy tubes are also low-profile devices. The button jejunostomy has a single jejunostomy lumen that may be tailored to length. The device is accessed in the same way as a gastrostomy button. However, there is no available lumen into the stomach. The button gastrojejunostomy has two lumens. Today, the button GJ is most commonly utilized.

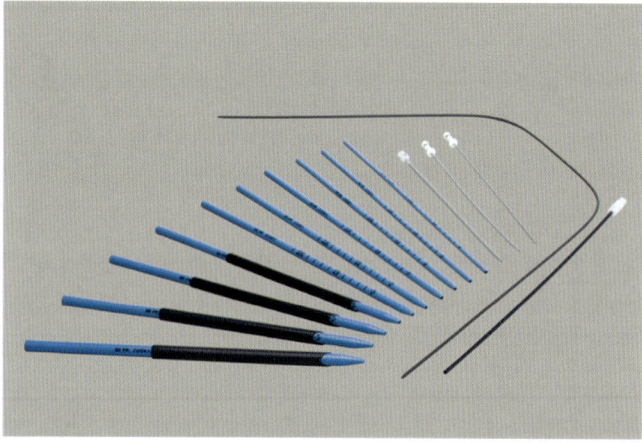

Figure 4.21 Amplatz® progressive dilators and sheaths (Cook Medical) provide a 6 to 30 French working channel from the skin to the renal collecting system through which endoscopes, balloon catheters, and other equipment can be passed. They can also be used to serially dilate a percutaneous tract, such as a gastrostomy or cecostomy stoma.

the ostomy to about 2 to 4 French larger than the replacement GT. In order to ease the GT reinsertion, the balloon-tipped GT is lubricated with sterile mineral oil, silicone spray, or K-Y jelly. If a "knitting needle" type 10 French guide catheter is used with Amplatz® dilators (Figure 4.21), one may insert the replacement gastrostomy catheter (or button) over it making tube reinsertion easier.

No special preparation is necessary. Since the technique of tube insertion is relatively easy, the procedure can be completed in less than 15 minutes in most instances. With

It is important to understand that a replacement button should not be electively inserted until the GT tract is mature. Although this may be in as little as two weeks, we prefer to wait six to twelve weeks before electively inserting a button. Insertion of a balloon-tipped button is an easy task and relatively atraumatic to the child (Table 4.7). After removal of a primary gastrostomy or if a child has gained weight, a calibrated balloon-tipped measuring device (Figure 4.22) is inserted into the stomach to determine the length of the tract (Table 4.8). The balloon is inflated with water and gentle traction is applied. The distance from the skin surface to the anterior gastric wall is determined by the markings on the measuring device. The button selected is generally the same French size as the GT removed. If the gastrostomy tract is less than 14 French or a diameter that is non-standard, either the tract must be dilated or in the case of tracts greater than 14 French, a smaller button can be inserted. If the option of a smaller shaft diameter is chosen, one must be careful that there is no leakage of gastric contents onto the abdominal wall. If this occurs, the ostomy will not reduce in size, and progressive skin injury and tract enlargement may result. This problem is easily prevented by using the next larger button shaft diameter.

Regardless of the button size, to insert it, the tip is lubricated and with gentle forward pressure, is pushed into the stomach until it is flush with the skin. The balloon is inflated with water, usually to a total of 5 ml, depending on patient size. The balloon should never be inflated with air since it is

Table 4.8 Equipment: enterostomy exchange or replacement

Replacement gastrostomy tube
– Replacement gastrostomy (e.g., Flexiflow 14 French, 16 French, 18 French, 20 French, 24 French), *or*
– Unibody tube
– Progressive dilators or PTA balloon

Conversion to a percutaneous gastrojejunostomy
– 5 French JB-1 catheter
– 0.035- or 0.038-inch Bentson guide wire
– Benzoin
– Tegaderm® or Opsite®
– 8 French Frederick–Miller tube (Cook, Inc., Bloomington, IN)
– Plastic hemostat

Gastrostomy button or button jejunostomy
– Sound (depth gauge)
– Gastrostomy button (balloon-tipped or mushroom type) or GJ button
– Dilators (if mushroom type used)

Table 4.7 Procedure summary: gastrostomy tube exchange or replacement

– Remove preexisting PG or PGJ over a guide wire if the tract is not mature.
– Insert replacement GT into gastric lumen.
– Dilate tract if necessary.
– Using directional catheter and Bentson guide wire maneuver system into distal duodenum or proximal jejunum.
– Exchange catheter for modified 8 French Fredrick–Miller JT.
– Secure JT to GT.
– Inject contrast via JT to confirm satisfactory tube position.

(a)

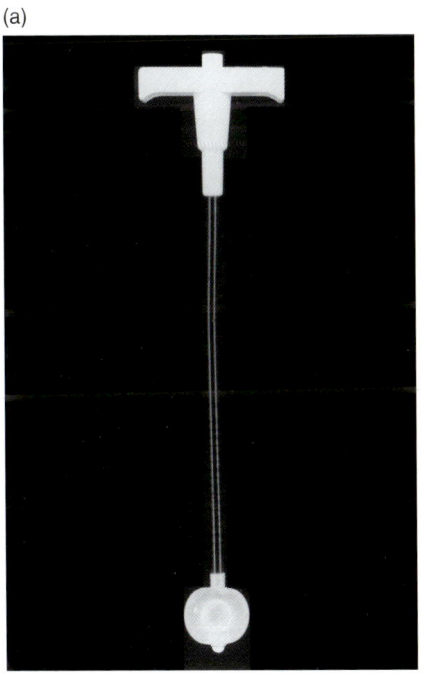

(b)

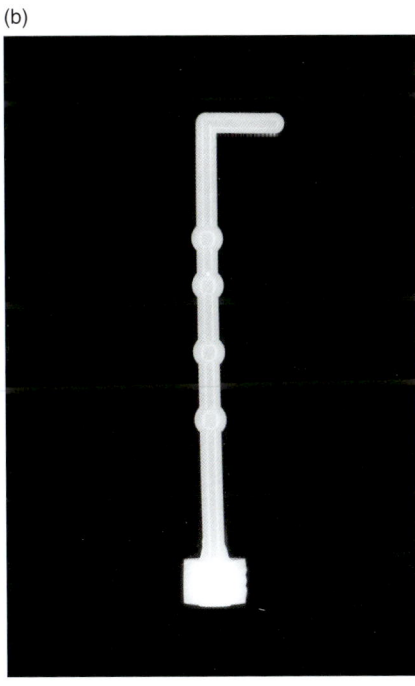

Figure 4.22 Various devices are available to measure the stoma length to select an appropriate shaft length for gastrostomy buttons, e.g., (a) balloon type and (b) sound type.

semi-permeable and will deflate over the next several hours. Intragastric position of the gastrostomy button is confirmed with contrast injection.

In contrast, the placement of a mushroom-tipped button requires tract dilation in most cases. If the tract is larger than 18 French (e.g., a surgical gastrostomy), insertion of a 14 French button may be attempted without predilation. If the attempted insertion does not go smoothly, the attempt is abandoned and further enlargement of the tract is performed. For replacement of a 14 French gastrostomy tract, dilation is generally needed. To accomplish this, a guide wire is introduced into the stomach directly through the ostomy or via a vascular dilator. Progressive dilators or a PTA balloon (usually not used because of the cost) may be used to enlarge the tract to 18 or 20 French. An L-shaped measuring device (Figure 4.22b) is inserted into the gastric lumen and the tract length is determined. In order to insert a mushroom-tipped button, an obturator is introduced into the button lumen so that the shaft is elongated and deformed (Figure 4.19), making the tip smaller in diameter. The stretched button is then placed into the dilated tract, and using moderate downward force, pushed into the gastric lumen. When the button is seated the operator will notice a substantial decrease in resistance. The obturator is removed and the intragastric position confirmed by contrast injection. Because of the considerable force required, there is a higher incidence of separation of the stomach from the anterior abdominal wall. Because of the related discomfort sedation or general anesthesia may be needed.

Regardless of the type of button utilized, feeding is initiated in the same manner. A specially designed connecting tube is fitted into the button. The selection of pump infusion or bolus infusion is of no importance from the technical standpoint and is the choice of the team managing the child's nutrition.

Technical problems and pitfalls

Avoiding transcolonic puncture

We have found asymptomatic transcolonic gastrostomy tube location over a year after insertion during routine tube exchanges. Accidental transgression of the colon during primary insertion can also occur and leads to peritonitis or to bowel obstruction. Brief fluoroscopic observation of mucosal movement and the relationship to surrounding structures during anesthetic injection and again during percutaneous transgastric puncture can verify the safety of the proposed tract. If movement of contrast in the transverse colon is seen during manipulation of the anesthetic needle or the transgastric access needle, it is possible the needle is transgressing the transverse colon and a different angle of approach should be used (Figure 4.23).

Inability to access the gastric lumen

Occasionally, the stomach is difficult to puncture and, as a result, the guide wire is extragastric in location. Incomplete

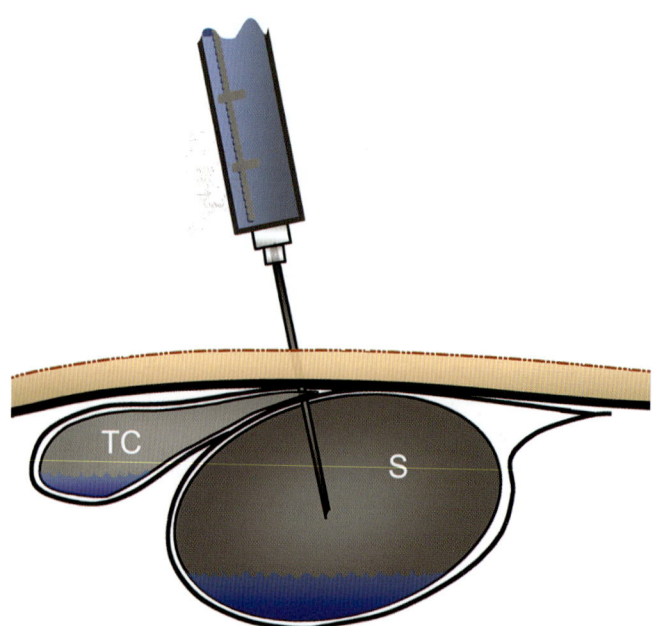

Figure 4.23 Contrast in the transverse colon (*TC*) and in the gastric lumen (*S*) may appear to be separate in an anterior projection, yet the access needle may transfix the decompressed portion of the transverse colon where it depends from the gastrocolic ligament and drapes across the greater curvature, before it enters the stomach, as illustrated.

penetration of the gastric wall can be anticipated if one sees a subtle, grayish, curvilinear interface at the needle tip, which likely represents the gastric mucosa being displaced by the needle embedded within the serosa, or if the needle and guide wire are lined up in both frontal and lateral planes but the wire cannot be grasped. Lateral fluoroscopy will quickly confirm this impression. Anatomic issues such as malrotation, microgastria, an enlarged or midline liver, spleen, or colon, gastric position above the inferior costal margin, or incompetent pylorus allowing air to escape into the small bowel can all lead to inability to access the stomach. If such issues cannot be corrected the procedure will need to be abandoned in lieu of an open or laparoscopic gastrostomy, although the risk of malposition still exists despite a surgical approach if the stomach must be mobilized over a distance to reach the anterior abdominal wall (Figure 4.6e–g). We have, on occasion, used a catheter with a large toy balloon attached to inflate the stomach. The balloon is popped when the needle enters the stomach.

Deep structures at risk

Be mindful that the pancreas and its vessels, the IVC and the aorta, and the kidney may lie deep to the needle pathway during gastric access procedures and may be placed at risk from overly aggressive puncture attempts. Conversely, slow and ineffectual acceleration of the needle tends to compress the anterior gastric wall against the posterior wall, making it difficult to achieve gastric puncture without advancing to whatever structure lies deeply at that point. Adequate inflation of the gastric lumen, a satisfactory skin incision, and a short sharp thrust of the needle through the anterior gastric wall will significantly reduce risk.

Difficult delivery of the retention device or J tube

On the occasions when the fascia is tough or the GT tip is difficult to deliver through the puncture site, it is helpful to dilate the skin tract with a 6 or 7 French vascular dilator in retrograde fashion. The GT will then advance easily. When advancing the GT, there are usually two areas of increased resistance encountered: first at the junction of the stiff dilating section and softer feeding component of the GT, and second as the retention disc passes the region of the cricopharyngeus muscle and thoracic inlet.

In small children (<7 kg) with esophageal diameters less than about 1.2 cm, the collapsed retention disc of the PGT may not pass through the esophagus. If significant resistance occurs, it is best to abandon the antegrade approach and use a device with a smaller retention disc, e.g., Corpak PGT, or the modified (push–pull) or retrograde techniques for gastrostomy placement.

A problem that is commonly encountered, especially in children with an SG inserted in the mid or distal third of the stomach, those with a horizontally oriented stomach, those in whom the GT is directed toward the fundus, or patients with gastric distention, is the tendency for the JT to buckle and loop as it exits from the GT into the stomach. When this occurs, it may become a frustrating and time-consuming problem. The best solution is early identification of the potential for this occurrence and its prevention by carefully pulling back and rotating the catheter in the appropriate direction (usually counter-clockwise) to uncoil the JB-1 catheter and recreate the preferred arc-like configuration of the catheter–guide wire system. It is important to firmly pin the guide wire to eliminate all slack while advancing the catheter. Laxity of the catheter or guide wire is the most common source of difficulty in creating a gastric loop with secondary problems positioning the JT in the proximal jejunum. If there is still difficulty moving the JT into position, here are a few tricks that may help. First, you can use short piston-like movements to assist a tube moving around a bend and if this is not successful exchange for a Roadrunner® or other stiff guide wire. If a stiff guide wire is used, one must be careful to avoid injury to the bowel wall.

Treating inadvertent dislodgment

If access is inadvertently lost at the time of primary insertion or before the tract has matured, it is safe to repeat the procedure and make a second puncture and tract as long as no variance from the child's baseline vital signs is noted. If a second tract is made, we recommend: (1) keeping the child NPO for at least 24 hours; (2) keep an NG tube in the stomach. Attach the NG to suction in order to keep the stomach empty and to minimize the chance of leakage; and (3) insert a GJ or NJ to bypass the stomach so that the unused insertion tract has a chance to heal. Arbitrarily, we maintain GJ feeding for at least three days in the absence of peritoneal signs, and begin the child on antibiotics to minimize the chance of peritonitis.

If access is lost after tract maturation, it is often possible to regain access, although the window of opportunity is time limited and of uncertain duration. Patients and families should be prospectively advised to keep a small-caliber blunt tube, such as Foley or red rubber tube, in case the percutaneous transgastric device is dislodged and cannot be *easily* replaced. The caretaker should be counseled against persistent or vigorous attempts to replace the tube, either by family or by medical staff without real-time image guidance and adequate experience. This event should be considered an urgent indication for intervention. Our technique for re-establishing a closed or probe patent track is the same for any ostomy or fistula. In the case of a closing gastrostomy or cecostomy track, a 3 French dilator and 0.018-inch glide wire is used to *gently* probe (Figure 4.24). It is essential to avoid creating a false lumen. If this occurs, successfully re-establishing the gastostomy or cecostomy is unlikely. If there is any resistance or buckling of the guide wire, injection of small amounts of contrast under fluoroscopy is recommended to create a road map. Once access to the gastric lumen is positively confirmed, the wire can be upsized and a stiffer wire used if needed to suit the device. We have found it convenient to use a coaxial dilator e.g., a 3 to 4 French dilator in the micropuncture set or a directional catheter to complete the wire exchange. If access cannot be regained, then the guidelines above for formation of a second tract may be followed on an elective basis.

Complications

General considerations

Percutaneous gastrostomy is a safe and effective technique in the pediatric population as documented by numerous reports. Successful percutaneous insertion of a PG or PGJ occurs in over 98% of cases, and has been performed in patients of all ages, ranging from 800 g to >80 kg. Postprocedural complications occurring within the first 30 days have been reported in 3 to 12% of patients. In our experience, major complications have been identified in approximately 3% while minor complications have occurred in about 8%.

The major complications that have been described include erosion with catheter migration, acquired gastrocolic fistula (Figure 4.25), occult transfixation of small bowel or colon (Figure 4.23), gastric or small bowel perforation or intraperitoneal leakage, peritonitis, anterior abdominal wall abscess, infectious or non-infectious stoma ulceration, esophageal laceration, gastric herniation through an enlarged ostomy, and exacerbation of respiratory distress and congestive heart failure in children predisposed to these problems. At least one death has been reported following duodenal perforation (Figure 4.26). Minor problems have included tract granulation (Figure 4.27), localized cellulitis, pneumoperitoneum, premature tube loss, intermittent intussusception (Figure 4.28),

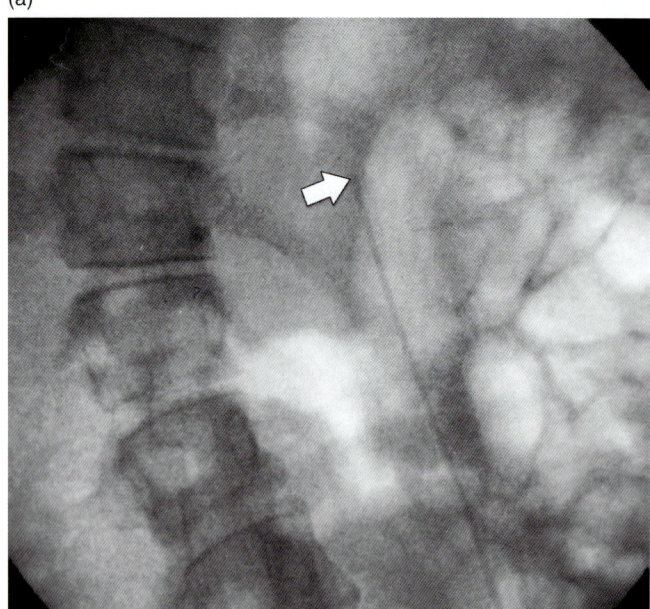 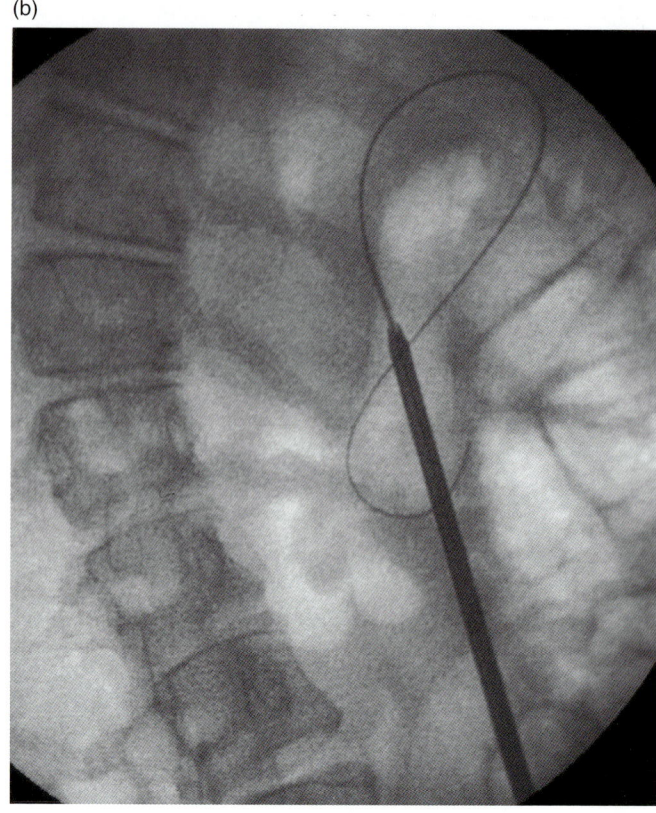

Figure 4.24 (a) A probe-patent tract may be gently tested with a narrow-caliber (e.g., 22-gauge or 3 to 4 French) cannula (*arrow*) in an attempt to regain the gastric lumen. An angled hydrophilic wire and a small amount of contrast may also be useful to define and regain the abandoned tract after accidental dislodgment of a gastrostomy tube. (b) Once the cannula is within the lumen, a guide wire is coiled within, then the cannula exchanged for dilators of serially increasing diameter (see Figure 4.20) until the tract is large enough to admit a new gastrostomy tube.

malposition of the tube (Figure 4.29) or the retention device (Figure 4.30) and localized pain.

The results of the percutaneous technique compare favorably with the operative and endoscopic approaches. Like with the PEG, the morbidity and mortality of the PG is lower than with surgical gastrostomies. Comparison of the PEG and PG is more difficult. However, comparison of large series suggests that major complications were as much as two times more common with the endoscopic approach, and minor morbidity as high as three times more frequent. Although there are many similarities between the endoscopic and fluoroscopic techniques, fluoroscopic guidance offers many advantages. First, fluoroscopic guidance does not require the presence of an endoscopist and surgeon skilled in PEG and an anesthesiologist. Therefore, the fluoroscopically guided procedure is easier to perform and less costly. In addition, the identification of adjacent organs, such as the left lobe of liver with US and colon with contrast, is accurately made and minimizes the risk of adjacent organ injury. Also, the fluoroscopic approach enables placement of a PGJ at the time of initial feeding-tube insertion. Lastly, but perhaps most significantly, the fluoroscopically guided GT is usually positioned in the lateral third of the gastric body while PEG, laproscopic, and surgical gastrostomies are usually located in the antrum making conversion to GJ technically difficult and mechanically unstable (Figure 4.6). These patients often have a higher incidence of JT loss due to recoil of the tube into the stomach. Although extreme measures may be used to replace these tubes into the small bowel (Figure 4.1), the need for increased frequency of hospital visits, increased exposure to radiation, and cost mitigate for abandoning the initial site and creation of a new stoma more suitably located and directed for the purpose of gastrojejunostomy.

The SG has the additional disadvantages of a greater frequency of skin problems secondary to leakage through irregularly shaped or ovoid ostomies. The PEG, laproscopic, and open surgical methods may have a higher incidence of GER. A prospective study is needed to answer this question. We speculate that when the child is anesthetized and the stomach becomes flaccid the stomach falls into the abdominal cavity making it difficult to determine the *in situ* gastric position. Without gastric distention, when the stomach is approximated to the anterior abdominal wall, it does not always lie in anatomic position. This results in an alteration of the relationship of the esophagogastric junction leading to GER.

Since G and GJ buttons are usually inserted into mature tracts to replace indwelling tubes, complications are less frequent. Interestingly, there appears to be a relationship between

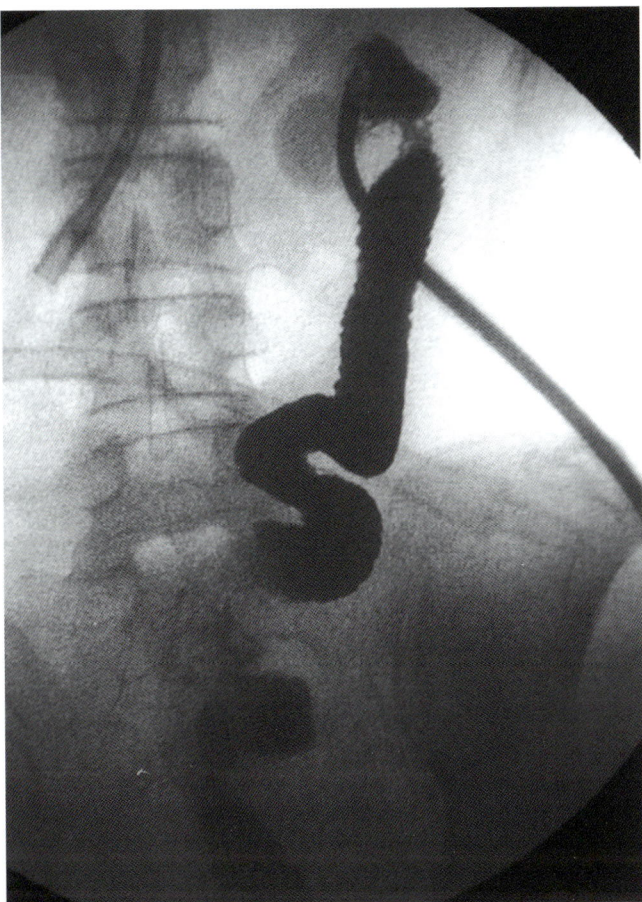

Figure 4.25 A contrast fluoroscopic study is performed in a 14-year-old boy with severe neurologic sequelae of anoxic brain injury who has been expressing feces through a long-term percutaneous transgastric gastrojejunostomy tube. Injected contrast through the gastric port is immediately apparent in the descending colon, indicating a gastrocolic fistula.

initiation of feeding. If feeding occurs into the abdominal cavity, serious morbidity or mortality can occur.

In addition to tract perforation and potential leakage, other complications have been reported. Approximately 25% of patients complain of mild abdominal discomfort that usually resolves within a week after gastrostomy placement. Treatment with analgesics is rarely necessary. Skin irritation beneath the wings of the device may occur, especially in a child who sweats a lot or whose skin remains damp after bathing. This is easily averted by keeping the skin dry and, when necessary, placing a slotted gauze between the button and skin. Also, the button can be rotated 45 degrees daily so that it does not chronically create the same footprint. Leakage around the tube causing skin irritation may occur. Again, treating this problem in a timely manner to prevent further skin injury with subsequent tract enlargement is important.

Accidental dislodgment of the button occurs. This is more common with balloon-tipped buttons than with mushroom-tipped buttons. If the button is replaced quickly there is usually no problem. However, if there is a delay in reinserting a catheter, the tract will rapidly begin to close. We have seen children with tracts that have become pinhole in size in less than eight hours after tube loss. Therefore it is now our practice to give the caretaker a Foley catheter 2 to 4 French smaller in size to insert if an unexpected dislodgment occurs. It is for this reason that we prefer the balloon-tipped buttons.

There are several strategies that may be used if a button or gastrostomy is unexpectedly lost. First, if the child has a button, a prescription for a second button can be given to the caretaker at the time of discharge. We ask that a second button (balloon tipped) is kept in the house or care facility. When the indwelling button fails, the new one can be easily reinserted by lubricating the tip and with mild to moderate forward pressure, pushing it back into the gastric lumen. If this cannot be accomplished, the interventionalist on call is contacted and the button is replaced in the interventional suite. In children, even those whose tracts are small and difficult to visualize, the ostomy can be re-established with a 3 French dilator (Figure 4.24). The dilator is used to probe the center of the old ostomy. In most instances, a tiny opening will be identified into which the dilator can be advanced. Then, a 0.018-inch glide wire is advanced into the stomach. In most cases, the tract can then be easily enlarged using progressively larger vascular dilators until the desired tract diameter is attained. Another button is then inserted. Before discharge, contrast is injected to confirm satisfactory placement.

Failure of the anti-reflux valve remains a problem and may occur in 10% or more cases. This problem is usually identified after six months of use although we have seen buttons last for considerably more than 12 months. If it occurs in the first weeks after insertion, a defective product should be considered. When valve failure occurs, button replacement is required.

the length of the tract and the potential risk of button insertion. The longer the tract length, the greater the risk. Tracts longer than approximately 4.5 cm have a high failure rate. The button, especially mushroom tipped, can be misdirected and perforate the tract leading to failure to successfully insert the button into the stomach. This failure of placement elevates the risk of peritonitis and may result in the need to redo the gastrostomy. However, loss of gastrostomy access can be prevented if this problem is anticipated. In patients with long tracts, suggested by unexpectedly long tube shaft lengths, the feeding tube can be exchanged over a guide wire. The 10 French dilator from the Amplatz® progressive dilator set or an 8 French or 10 French catheter with its hub cut off, is positioned over the guide wire and coiled in the stomach. A 14 French balloon-tipped button can be fitted over the catheter and guide wire and guided into the stomach. If the button cannot be easily inserted the tract should be dilated 2 French to 4 French larger than the button shaft diameter selected. Once the button is assumed to be in position it should be injected with contrast to confirm intragastric positioning prior to

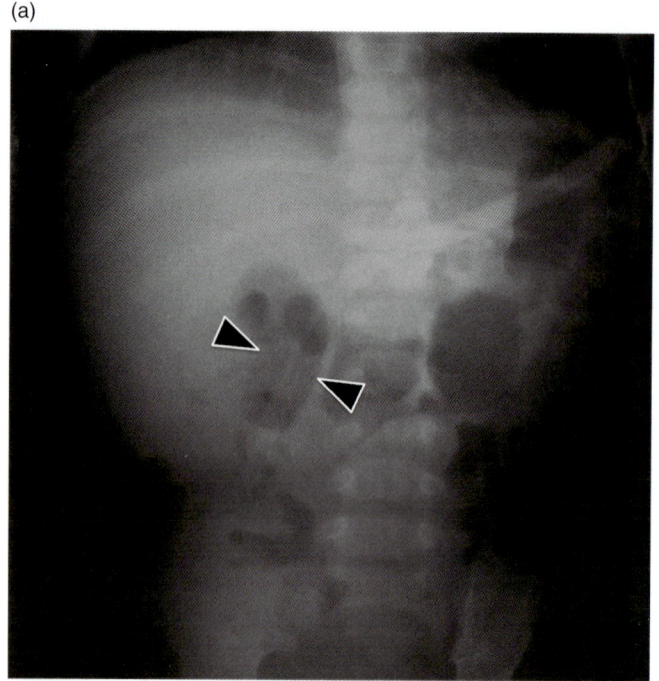
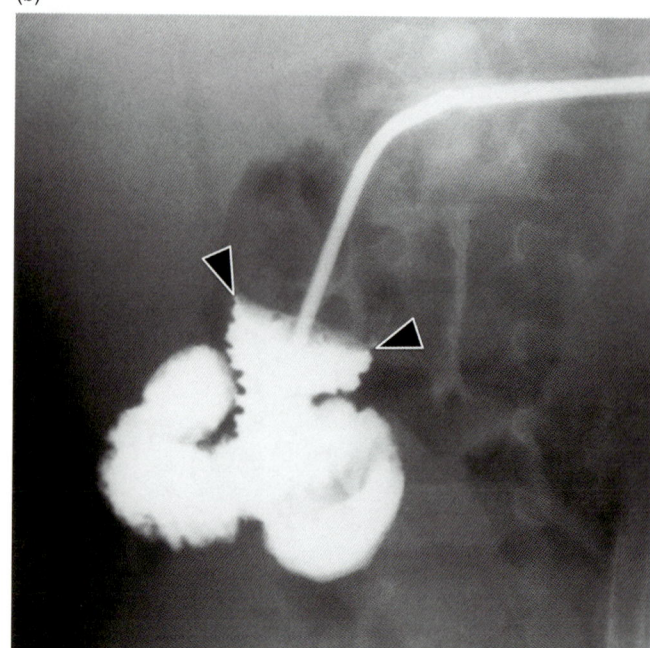
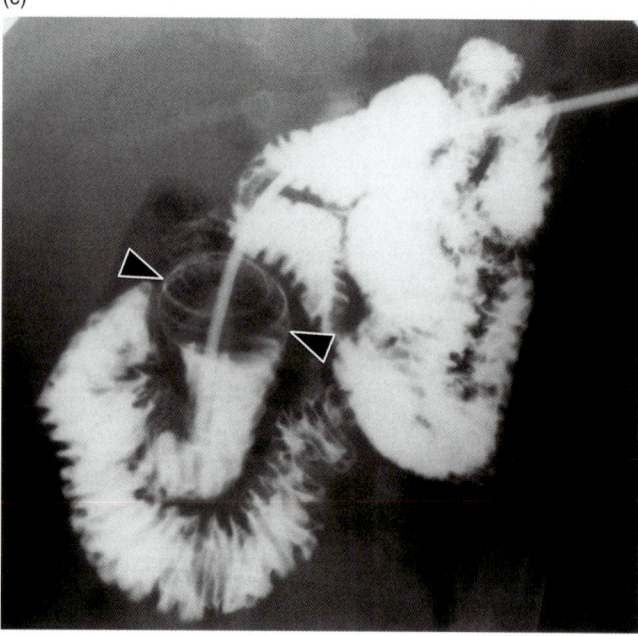

Figure 4.26 (a) An 18-month-old female with cerebral palsy has a surgical gastrostomy tube for enteral nutrition. The internal retention balloon (*arrowheads*) is evident on this plain radiograph of the abdomen. She presented with symptoms of small bowel obstruction. (b,c) Contrast injected into the small bowel through the gastrostomy tube outlines the retention balloon (*arrowheads*), which has migrated into the first part of the duodenum.

Tract and skin surface complications

There are a few minor but nagging problems that are seen in children with long-standing GTs that require brief discussion. In the rare instances when an infection does occur, normal skin organisms are the most common agents. However, fungal infection should also be considered if the skin appears dry and scaly or if routine antibiotic therapy is unsuccessful. When a bacterial infection is present, there may be associated erythema, mild induration, and occasionally expressible pus. If an abscess is present, with or without systemic signs and symptoms, the abscess is incised and debrided and oral antibiotics are begun along with standard skin care. In rare instances, the child is admitted to the hospital for intravenous antibiotics. If a minor infection is suspected, treatment with hydrogen peroxide and an antibiotic ointment, such as mupirocin, is initiated three to four times per day. If this is ineffective, the site is cultured and an oral broad-spectrum antibiotic is given.

In our experience, secondary skin infection with a yeast is occasionally identified. Clinically, these children have erythematous, dry, flaky skin without an associated purulent

Chapter 4 Abdominopelvic interventions

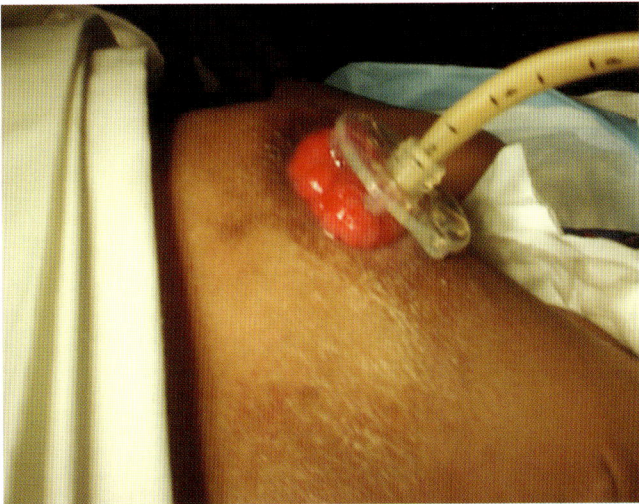

Figure 4.27 Granulation tissue at the stoma margin. This was treated successfully with topical application of silver nitrate.

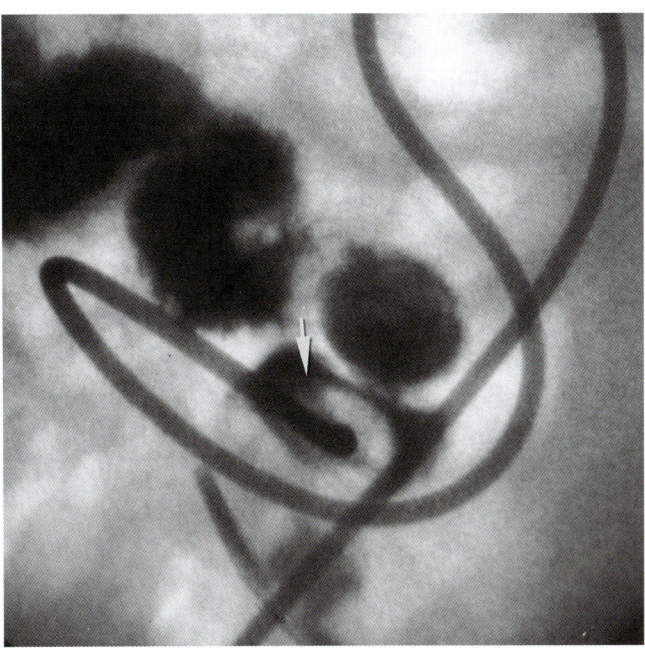

Figure 4.28 In a 30-month-old female with cerebral palsy and a transgastric gastrojejunostomy tube, a contrast fluoroscopic study was obtained to investigate the cause of fussiness. Intermittent small bowel intussusception is seen as effacement of the contrast by the intussusceptum (*arrow*).

discharge. In these instances, treatment with a topical antifungal cream is usually successful.

In general, it is important to keep the skin around the ostomy dry and clean. Once the skin becomes reddened, inflamed, and gastric contents begin to leak, there is a rapid skin breakdown and discomfort. The result will be enlargement, sometimes quite rapidly, of the gastrostomy tract and more serious leakage of gastric contents. To prevent this cycle, it is important to identify and treat this complication as early as possible. Children who perspire a lot, those with granulation tissue with associated serous secretions, or whose skin is not carefully dried after cleaning, are also prone to develop irritation and skin breakdown. To prevent these problems, the skin must be kept dry and granulation tissue treated. To accomplish this, attention to detail is important with frequent observation of the skin and, if needed, a slotted 2 × 2 cm gauze or DuoDERM® is positioned between the disc and skin surface.

Erosion and ulceration of the stoma may occur with or without fungal infection. Especially where the gastrostomy tip is proximal to a functional gastric outlet obstruction, increased intragastric pressure or loosening of the stoma relative to the tube may lead to chronic exposure of the peristomal skin to gastric secretions, leading to irritation or ulceration. This may become superinfected, often with fungus, and may lead to profound excavation of the stoma (Figure 4.31). Restoration of skin integrity and of a useful stoma can be accomplished, but requires skilled wound care and may take weeks to months of inpatient care to heal. During this time it is helpful to replace the usual tube with a narrow-caliber transgastric jejunostomy tube to maintain access.

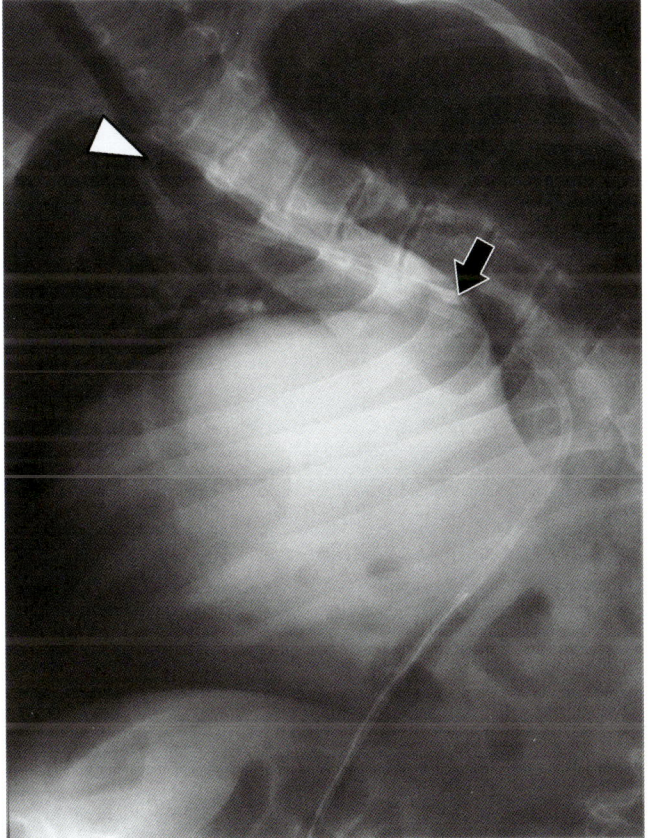

Figure 4.29 In this 14-year-old male with severe kyphoscoliosis, the surgical gastrojejunostomy tube enters the antrum, directed toward the gastric inlet. The body (*arrow*) and tip (*arrowhead*) are malpositioned in the esophagus. Poor choices in position and orientation may lead to organoaxial rotation of the stomach with increased reflux, as well as creating a significantly more difficult angle for conversion to a gastrojejunostomy, with increased frequency of tube loss, dysfunction or, as in this case, malposition.

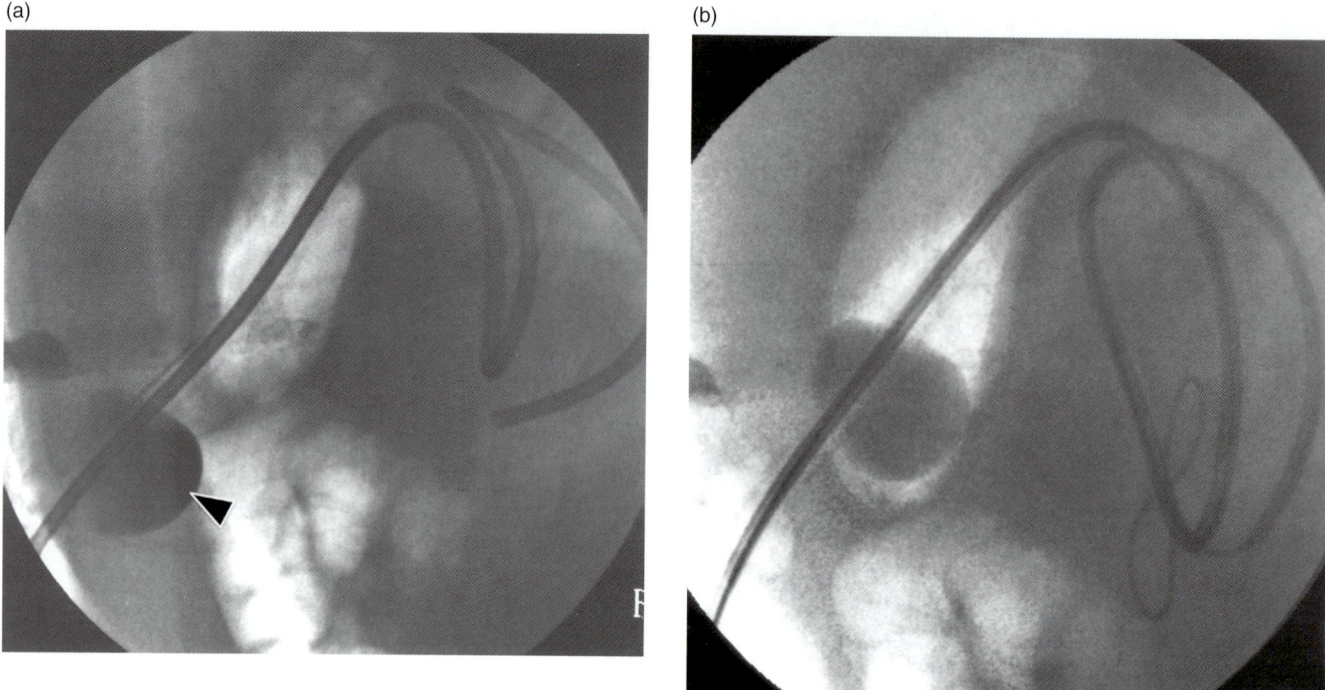

Figure 4.30 A 32-month-old neurologically devastated infant presented with grimacing and fussiness. (a) A cross-table lateral view demonstrated the contrast-filled retention balloon (*arrowhead*) malpositioned in the gastrostomy tract. (b) The tube was easily repositioned.

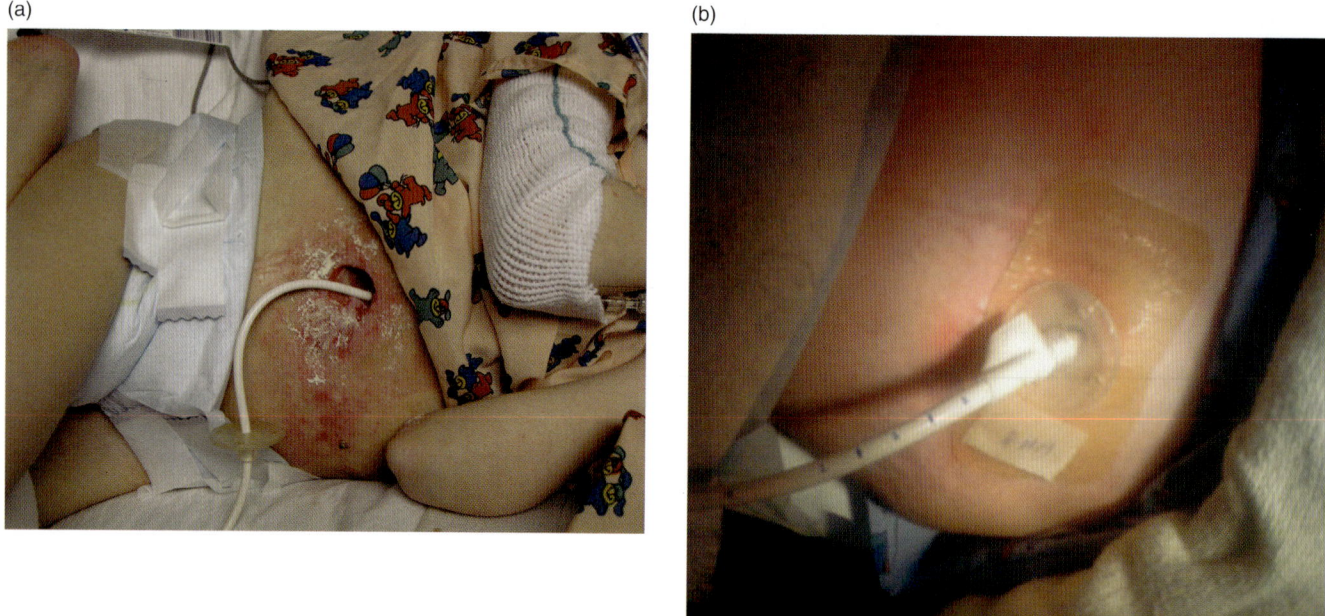

Figure 4.31 (a) Iatrogenic gastric plication caused by the surgically placed gastrostomy in this 14-year-old boy with cerebral palsy resulted in poor gastric emptying and chronic leakage of gastric contents from the stoma. He developed ulceration and erosion of the stoma margin and fungal superinfection. The original gastrostomy and transgastric jejunostomy tubes have been exchanged for an 8 French jejunostomy tube shown here, to allow the stoma to heal to a small diameter. (b) Three months of intensive inpatient wound management by the interventional nurse practitioner and the stoma nurse were required to heal the stoma and surrounding skin. This allowed restoration of the original feeding tube, although re-siting the stoma will ultimately be necessary to avoid the effect of the iatrogenic deformity.

When the skin is injured or other skin problems have developed, the skin may be protected by covering the affected area with REPLICARE® or DuoDERM®. These products are non-allergenic, colloidal suspensions that create a barrier to further injury while allowing the damaged skin to heal. As a secondary benefit this also will help secure the GT so that it will be positioned perpendicularly to the skin surface and will not freely move and further enlarge the ostomy site. The

REPLICARE® or DuoDERM® is cut to size so that all of the abnormal skin is covered. In addition, a second piece may be placed over the GT skin disc to stabilize it. If further tube stabilization is needed, a Hollister® disc is utilized. The REPLICARE® or DuoDERM® is left on for several days until it becomes wet or falls off. In most cases, this will help the skin irritation to resolve and, more importantly, allow the enlarged GT tract to heal and again become water-tight. Control of leakage of gastric contents is critical for skin healing. If the above does not work then the gastrostomy tube should be removed and exchanged for a tube large enough to fill the ostomy and stop the leakage. In the rare instance when this approach does not work, several options remain. The GT may be removed and the site covered with an occlusive dressing allowing the ostomy site to shrink. The site should be examined every 12 to 24 hours to make sure that it does not close completely. In addition, an NG tube can be inserted and placed to suction, and drugs to reduce gastric secretion may be given. As a last resort, the site may be surgically closed and a new GT inserted.

In summary, the key to treatment is to stop the leak of gastric acid and protect the skin to avoid secondary problems. An approach that we have found to be effective is to make the ostomy round by putting in a button or replacement gastrostomy tube that is large enough to completely fill the hole. Once the skin inflammation subsides the ostomy size is reduced with successively smaller tubes (2 to 4 French each one to two weeks), then the skin should be treated. If the skin is not infected the entire area of abnormal skin is covered with DuoDERM®. If infection is suspected it may be cultured then treated with oral antibiotics and covered with DuoDERM®.

A question that is often asked by parents or caretakers is, can the child have a bath or go swimming? We recommend that they do not take a bath or swim for a minimum of six weeks so that the tract can completely heal and seal itself. In children in whom wound healing is suspect (such as the severely neutropenic and those on chronic systemic steroids), a minimum of 12 weeks is suggested. After this time we ask the parent to first place the child in bath water and watch for bubbles. If none are identified then we assume that the GT site is water-tight and bathing or limited swimming is allowed. An additional precaution that can be taken is to cover the ostomy site with a clear, waterproof, occlusive dressing (e.g., Tegaderm® or Opsite®) to further minimize any potential problems. For older children taking a shower is usually no problem.

A significant percentage of children develop a granulation tissue collar around the GT ostomy site. This tissue is highly vascular, may grow to a size of 1 to 2 cm or more, and secretes a yellow or yellow-green fluid that may be mistaken for purulence. In the vast majority of instances, no infection is present and cauterization is all that is needed. In most situations, the granulation tissue is treated with silver nitrate sticks until the tissue appears gray-black. It is important to avoid cauterizing normal skin or into the tract so as not to cause skin injury or tract enlargement. This procedure is repeated as needed.

Peritonitis, tube dislodgment, and bowel perforation

Peritonitis following primary gastrostomy is rare, albeit under-reported. Causes include inadvertent colonic puncture, leakage of gastric contents during access maneuvers, and leakage of feedings into the peritoneal cavity due to tube malposition, tract elongation, or elevated intragastric pressure. Symptoms may include prolonged or severe pain after the gastrostomy procedure, pain during feeding, or external leakage of gastric contents. Unexplained changes in vital signs following the procedure should raise suspicion of peritonitis. Retching during the early postprocedure period may also cause leakage of gastric contents into the peritoneal cavity. If peritonitis is suspected, feedings should be held immediately. A contrast study under fluoroscopy or CT may help confirm the diagnosis.

Intraperitoneal leakage of gastric contents usually causes a chemical peritonitis, but a course of broad-spectrum antibiotics with coverage for common gastrointestinal pathogens is prudent. If free intraperitoneal fluid is observed, a sample may be obtained for culture and sensitivity to help guide appropriate coverage. Presuming the reason for leakage has been corrected and the gastrostomy tube is properly positioned, feeding can usually be safely resumed on the third day of antibiotics.

Intraperitoneal tube malposition or disruption of the gastrostomy tract may be suspected if after exchanging the tube through a mature tract there is difficulty or pain while injecting water through the new tube. Similarly, if the existing tube was accidentally dislodged, a low threshold for suspecting complication should be maintained. In such cases a contrast study under fluoroscopy should be performed to positively confirm appropriate position and function of the new tube. If peritoneal contamination is suspected, feeding should be stopped and the patient treated with broad-spectrum antibiotics as described above. If access to the gastric lumen cannot be safely regained through the old tract, the gastrostomy may have to be re-sited.

If bowel transgression is suspected, after the tract has matured the tube can be removed over a guide wire and a catheter with a caliber large enough for injection of contrast around the wire can be introduced into the gastric lumen. Contrast may be injected under fluoroscopy during withdrawal of the catheter (leaving the safety wire coiled in the stomach), looking for contrast escaping into the colon or peritoneal cavity to confirm the diagnosis (Figure 4.25). If bowel transgression is proven, the gastrostomy should be re-sited.

Occlusion and leakage

Although virtually no technical expertise is required to unclog a blocked feeding tube, the interventionalist is frequently called upon by their patients to either replace or re-establish flow in feeding tubes of all sizes. A variety of materials cause tube

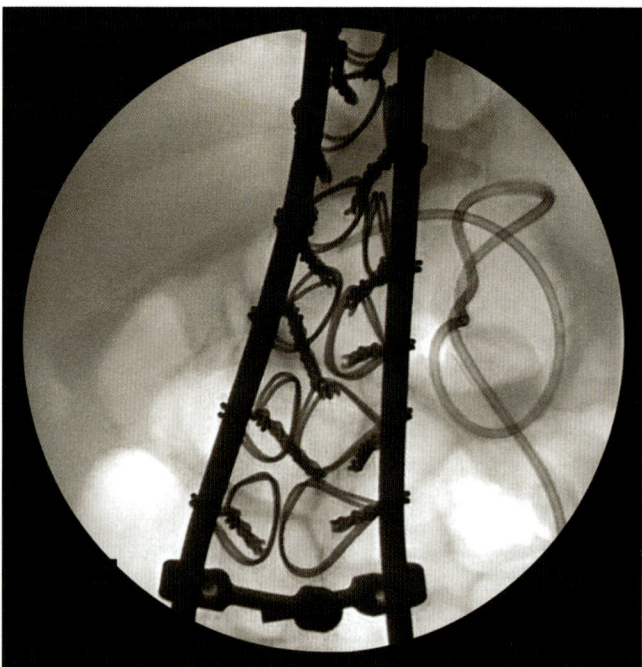

Figure 4.32 Turning the hub while attaching flush syringes can cause the catheter to "corkscrew," as shown here, resulting in accidental dislodgment of the tip from the small bowel into the stomach.

obstruction. In our experience, the most common causes are formula or other foods and medications such as crushed lansoprazole (Prevacid®) tabs. The tubes that are most prone to clogging are jejunostomy catheters since they are usually 8 to 9 French in diameter. Larger tubes, such as gastrostomies and buttons, can become blocked but much less frequently. Regardless of the type of tube, the approach to re-establish luminal patency is the same. Since there is a large number of children who are dependent on feeding tubes for their nutrition, dealing with obstructed tubes is a common problem and often comes to attention in the evening hours. Over the years, we have developed an approach that is successful in the vast majority of cases.

The best treatment for a clogged feeding tube is prevention. Parents and caretakers are instructed to flush the tube after each use with a clear carbonated diet soda, warm tap water, or other liquid that does not contain sugar. For children on continuous 24-hour feeding, we recommend flushing the tube two to four times per day. Caregivers are also advised to avoid rotating the tube while attaching and removing syringes used for flushing, as rotation over time will cause the tube to twist and will eventually dislodge the jejunostomy component from the small bowel (Figure 4.32).

In addition to the above, it is suggested that all medication be ground into fine particles or diluted into 5 to 15 ml of liquid if possible. This approach will maximize tube life. In spite of even the most meticulous care, a tube clog may occur. If this happens, the tube is flushed with a 1, 3 or 5 ml syringe with one of the recommended liquids until the tube function returns to normal. If tube patency is not rapidly returned to normal, a regimen of flushing with syringes of decreasing size is begun. Initially a 5 ml syringe is filled with a carbonated or other liquid and forcefully injected. If the obstruction is not cleared, then the procedure is repeated with the 3 ml and 1 ml syringes. In our experience, the 3 ml syringe is the one that most effectively clears the catheter.

If this maneuver fails, then a flowswitch is connected and a forceful injection is repeated with the 3 ml syringe. When peak pressure on the syringe plunger is achieved, the flowswitch is closed creating pressure within the tube. The flowswitch is left closed for 30 to 60 minutes. At the end of this time the flowswitch is opened and alternating suction and injection is applied using 60 ml and 3 ml syringes respectively. This procedure may be repeated several times. If the tube remains obstructed, Zap-it, an enzymatic cleaner, may be injected into the tube to digest the food or other material obstructing the tube. This material appears to work for a variety of material especially food. Zap-it is not used earlier since it costs >US$20 per unit. If these measures fail, the tube will need to be replaced.

The timing of tube replacement may become a significant issue with the parent or caregiver. Our approach is to consider tube replacement elective in most instances. Therefore, it is usually replaced the next working day. To help this policy work effectively, it is important to explain this in detail after the initial tube insertion, provide the caregivers with written instructions, and repeat the discussion at each tube change. Indications for non-elective tube replacement are children less than 10 kg who can become dehydrated, those with metabolic problems requiring continuous calories or glucose, and children with severe gastroesophageal reflux (GER) unable to tolerate any fluid in the stomach. Feeding children with less severe GER is approached by reducing the volume of formula or other fluids to half their usually hourly volume or, at minimum, providing the equivalent of insensible fluid loss. In addition to reducing the hourly rate of infusion, the child is fed in a sitting or upright position or prone oblique position to avoid aspiration if vomiting or GER occurs.

Whenever a gastrostomy tube (alone or with a jejunostomy) inadvertently comes out, it must be replaced as soon as possible to avoid closure or marked reduction in the ostomy. Gastrostomy sites may reduce in size or close rapidly. Reductions in ostomy size preventing reinsertion of the GT may occur in as little as one hour. Whenever possible, instructions are given by telephone to aid the parent or nurse in replacing the tube. If the parent is unable to or refuses to replace it, the child is brought to the interventional suite and the tube(s) replaced. Alternatively, the patient may be treated in the emergency room although they will not be able to insert a jejunostomy, thus requiring another hospital visit.

Intussusception

It is possible for the jejunostomy tube to act as the lead point in development of small bowel intussusception (Figure 4.28). This condition is usually transient, and may cause intermittent sharp cramping discomfort for the child. The most common situation in which this occurs is when the jejunostomy tube terminates in a modified tip, such as a Cope loop or pigtail. The prevalence of intermittent small bowel intussusception in children with such devices may approach 30%. The diagnosis can be made with transabdominal ultrasound, although the search is most likely to be successful when the patient is acutely symptomatic. Potential solutions include trimming the tip of the tube or using a different device.

Controversies/issues

Since its introduction, there has been rapid and widespread acceptance of the gastrostomy button for use in both children and adults requiring long-term nutritional support. Several authors have explored the potential for insertion of a gastrostomy button as a single-step procedure. These authors suggest that the single-step insertion technique has the advantages of avoiding a second procedure and any associated risk and cost. A number of studies have shown that this procedure can be performed safely.

The technique initially described employed endoscopy for button insertion with sedation and local anesthesia. In an alternative approach to single-step button placement the gastrostomy button is delivered transorally, coaxially fitted to a tapered silastic tube. More recently, retrograde single-step insertion has been performed radiographically by advancing the button and measured tube through a telescoping sheath that is removed once the gastrostomy has been delivered. Other technical modifications for one-step button insertion have also been described.

In all cases, accurate measurement of the prospective tract is an essential component of the insertion procedure. There are tract-measuring devices, or a balloon catheter can be advanced coaxially over a guide wire through the fresh tract, and the balloon inflated within the gastric lumen. The balloon is pulled back until it is in contact with the anterior gastric wall and the balloon catheter is marked at the skin exit. The balloon is deflated and removed, then reinflated. The distance from the proximal end of the balloon to the mark is the tract length. In most cases the button selected has a catheter length 0.5 cm longer than the measured tract length.

The one-step approach, while a potentially attractive alternative, suffers from several potential problems. The complication rate is higher than percutaneous endoscopic or fluoroscopic gastrostomy techniques. The complication rate ranges from 3 to 30% for PEGs and 5 to 15% for fluoroscopically inserted tubes. The complication rate with the one-step button may be as high as 17 to 29%. The most common complication is peristomal wound infection, occurring in 5 to 30% of PEG insertions and less than 5% using the fluoroscopic method. The advantages of a low-profile device and significantly decreased risk of accidental dislodgment or tube clogging can be obtained through conversion from a tube gastrostomy to a button placement after the tract has matured,

with negligible delay. Nevertheless, primary insertion of the low-profile device remains attractive to many referring providers and caregivers.

Conclusions

Percutaneous feeding techniques have rapidly become established as safe and effective methods. In a relatively short period of time they have become the procedure of choice for placement of feeding tubes in most situations. Today the interventionalist is routinely consulted for placement of PGT, PGJT, gastrostomy buttons, and NJT. These assisted feeding techniques have now become one of the most often performed procedural groups in the pediatric population. It is likely that their frequency will continue to grow in the near future.

Percutaneous cecostomy

Introduction

The number of people, young and old, with loss of bowel control or fecal soiling is quite large. Spina bifida, the most common underlying disorder in children with fecal incontinence, occurs in about 1/1,000 births. Patients with other underlying diagnoses, such as imperforate anus, cloacal abnormalities, sacral agenesis, paraplegia, and cerebral palsy may also be at risk for fecal soiling. There may be as many as 3 million people with fecal incontinence in North America.

Bowel control depends on a normal internal sphincter, normal external sphincter, sensation, peristalsis, a normal ano-rectal angle, psychosocial factors, and the absence of scarring. Normally, stool enters the rectum and results in relaxation of the internal anal sphincter. This is independent of the central nervous system. Voluntary contraction of the external sphincter is needed to contain flatus or feces. When any component of this system fails, or is not normally developed, this may result in "fecal incontinence," or the inability to control bowel function. Treatment of fecal incontinence may include spontaneous defecation, dietary modification, laxatives, manual expression, disimpaction, bowel training, biofeedback, suppositories, electrostimulation, and large volume enemas delivered via a special rectal balloon catheter.

Antegrade colonic enemas have been described as a surgical procedure where the appendix is used to form a cutaneous cecostomy for fluid irrigation (Malone Antegrade Colonic Enema – MACE). Transcolonoscopic extraperitoneal cecostomies have also been described. A percutaneous approach to the placement of a cecostomy catheter was described for colonic decompression in adults, and was adapted for the introduction of antegrade enemas in pediatric fecal incontinence by Chait and Shandling.

Placement of the cecostomy tube involves two different procedures that take place about six weeks apart. In the first, a temporary cecostomy catheter (C-tube) is inserted into the patient's colon through the skin usually in the lower right part

Table 4.9 Indications: percutaneous cecostomy

Indications
- Fecal incontinence (especially secondary to spina bifida)
- Refractory colonic pseudo-obstruction (Ogilvie's syndrome)
- Cecal volvulus
- Cecal dilation (greater than 10 cm)
- Distal colonic obstruction

Contraindications
- Bowel ischemia
- Cecal perforation

Table 4.10 Equipment: cecostomy insertion

- Non-latex gloves and supplies
- Topical anesthetic (e.g., ELA-Max®, EMLA® (AstraZeneca))
- Chlorhexidine gluconate 0.5% solution with 70% isopropyl alcohol
- #11 scalpel blade (Becton-Dickenson)
- Local anesthetic (1% lidocaine, AstraZeneca,)
- Syringes
- 18-gauge, 1.5-inch needle to draw local anesthetic
- 27-gauge, 1¼-inch needle for local anesthetic infiltration
- Glucagon (Lily)
- Low-osmolar contrast (Omnipaque (Iohexol) 300 mg I/ml, Nycomed)
- 22-French silicone (non-latex) Foley catheter (Rush, Canada)
- 60-ml Luer lock syringe for inflation of the Foley catheter
- Insufflation bulb (EZEM Whispering, NY)
- 18-gauge single wall puncture needle (BSDN, Cook Medical)
- Pediatric GI suture anchor set (Cook Inc.)
- Slip ring extension set (Benlan), attached to a syringe filled with contrast.
- 125-cm Teflon®-coated 0.035-inch Amplatz® guide wire
- Small mosquito clamp
- Lubricating jelly (bacteriostatic Muko®, Ingram and Bell)
- 8-French Coons dilator (Cook Medical)
- 15 cm, 8.5 Fr Dawson–Mueller Mac-Loc™ (non-latex) catheter
- Antibiotic ointment (Polyderm (bacitracin zinc + polymyxin B sulfate) Taro)
- Gauze bandage (2 × 2)
- Mefix adhesive bandage (Hypafix Dressing Retention Sheet, Smith and Nephew)
- Drainage bag (Holister U bag)
- Methylmethacrylate glue (non-sterile)
- K-lock adhesive catheter retention device (Zefon Medical Products)

of the abdomen, to encourage maturation of a short, straight tract. Approximately six weeks later, a more permanent tube is exchanged over the wire in a brief outpatient procedure. The C-tube insertion procedure is designed to provide a comfortable, convenient way to deliver a small-volume enema to periodically cleanse the colon. By emptying the colon in this regular, predictable way potentially embarrassing accidents are avoided and the patient often gains freedom to pursue activities previously prevented by fear of incontinent episodes. After their C-tube insertion, some patients are able to give their own enemas and thus manage a significant component of self-care for the first time. All of our patients have described almost complete resolution of their fecal incontinence with few unexpected accidents.

Indications

A potential candidate for C-tube insertion may experience fecal incontinence with troublesome soiling, or not respond well to rectal enemas, or wear diapers (Table 4.9). Patients may not be candidates for C-tube insertion if they have had previous surgical procedures, coagulopathies, or known medical problems that unduly increase risk during the procedure or sedation. Although many of our patients are older, feedback from patients and parents indicates that the optimal time for primary cecostomy placement is before they first attend school (age four to six years).

Technique

Equipment

We normally place a 15-cm, 8.5-French locking pigtail catheter for primary C-tube insertion. Use of latex-free equipment is recommended for patients predisposed to latex allergy (e.g., spina bifida), as well as for those with known latex sensitivity. In our practice we use latex-free equipment routinely. A detailed list of additional equipment necessary for primary percutaneous cecostomy insertion is provided in Table 4.10.

Patient preparation

Most patients who have a C-tube placed are in otherwise good health, except for their fecal incontinence. For this reason, we do not routinely order preoperative laboratory studies on this patient population. In select cases, where the medical history is unknown or raises a suspicion of a bleeding diathesis, a coagulation profile, platelet count, and hemoglobin level are obtained. Because C-tube insertion is an elective procedure, an uncorrectable coagulopathy is an absolute contraindication.

Candidates for C-tube placement are maintained on a strict clear fluid diet for two days prior to the procedure to help assure a clean bowel preparation. Up to 45 ml sodium phosphate oral solution (four- to six-year-olds: 10 ml; seven- to nine-year-olds: 20 ml; ten years and older: 45 ml) is administered the night before the procedure (or per NG tube for patients that can't tolerate oral administration). The patient is admitted to the hospital on the morning of the procedure with a repeat dose of sodium phosphate as needed according to the results of the preprocedure abdominal radiograph. Patients fasting for a procedure should not become dehydrated, and orders for maintenance intravenous fluids should be part of the preprocedure order regimen.

A topical anesthetic preparation such as ELA-Max® or EMLA® is applied topically to the prospective tube insertion site two hours prior to the procedure. A rectal dose of acetaminophen (15 mg/kg) is given one hour prior to the procedure. Patients are given a combination of gentamicin (2.5 mg/kg), ampicillin (50 mg/kg), and metronidazole (10 mg/kg) as a single preprocedure dose, and continue the same dosage three times per day for several days following the procedure.

Latex sensitivity

Because children with symptomatic spina bifida have many spinal, genitourinary, and gastrointestinal procedures performed during infancy and childhood, they have traditionally been exposed to and develop hypersensitivity to latex medical products including gloves, tubes, etc. Patients, family members, and medical staff exposed to latex may develop life-threatening airway complications or inflammation that threatens other tissues. Since there are now satisfactory alternatives to virtually all latex medical devices, equipment, and supplies, it is sensible to consider making all interventional suites and clinics "latex-free" zones.

Preprocedure imaging

The cecostomy tube insertion procedure is performed on a C-arm fluoroscopic interventional table. After US is performed to identify the liver, gallbladder, and urinary bladder margins, a 22-French silicone catheter or appropriately sized enema tip is introduced into the rectum and the retention balloon filled with air from a 50 ml Luer lock syringe. In patients with a ventriculoperitoneal shunt, special care is taken to look with US for and to avoid any intraperitoneal fluid collection that might be associated with shunt drainage. The abdomen is prepared and draped in sterile fashion using a chlorhexidine solution. The sterile equipment and local anesthetic is prepared and readily available prior to administration of glucagon. Up to 1 mg glucagon is given intravenously and the colon inflated with air via the rectal catheter. It is important to intermittently monitor the progress of insufflation from the rectum to the cecum, as occasionally redundant segments of colon at the flexures or even in the sigmoid region may mimic the appearance of the cecum and may otherwise be unwittingly punctured accidentally. The position of the cecum is assessed and the prospective tract site is determined (Figure 4.33a).

Lidocaine 1 to 2% (to a maximum of 0.25 ml/kg) can be infiltrated under fluoroscopic control into the skin and soft tissues down to the cecal wall, using a transperitoneal approach. One should see evidence of tenting of the cecal mucosa by the needle tip, and often a small bulge can be seen from deposition of anesthetic into the wall itself.

Standard technique

The cecal access procedure (Table 4.11) is similar to the percutaneous gastric access procedure previously described. After sufficient local anesthetic has been given a small skin incision is made with a #11 scalpel blade. An 18-gauge single wall

Table 4.11 Procedure summary: cecostomy insertion

- Obtain CBC with differential, electrolytes, and coagulation profile
- Clear fluids only on the day prior to procedure
- NPO after midnight prior to procedure
- Picosulfate sodium-magnesium oxide citric acid (PICO-SALAX®) at 09:00 and 15:00 on day prior to procedure
- Cefoxitin IV 30 minutes prior to procedure (alternatively, gentamicin and metronidazole)
- KUB (kidney, ureter, and bladder X-ray) prior to procedure
- General anesthesia or moderate to deep sedation as appropriate
- Insert 22 French Foley catheter in rectum, inflate 30 ml balloon, obtain seal
- Consider glucagon, 0.5 to 1.0 mg IV five to ten minutes prior to rectal insufflation
- Insufflate air, observe intermittently under fluoroscopy until air reaches cecum
- Inject local anesthetic from skin to cecal wall along prospective percutaneous access route
- Prepare an 18-gauge single wall needle preloaded with two gastropexy retention sutures and attached to a 10 ml syringe of non-ionic contrast via a slip-tip extension tubing
- Advance the access needle, preferably by a retroperitoneal route from the flank, into the cecum
- Try to locate the skin entry point at a position that will be comfortable for and accessible to the patient, but covered by normal clothing
- After thrusting the needle tip into the cecum with a short sharp jabbing motion, confirm intraluminal position with a small amount of contrast
- Advance a 0.035- to 0.038-inch Bentson guide wire into the cecum, deploying the retention sutures
- With gentle traction on the retention sutures, dilate the tract with 8 to 14 French fascial dilators
- Advance a 12 French Dawson–Mueller pigtail catheter with its stiffener over the wire until the tip of the catheter is well within the cecal lumen
- Advance the catheter off the stiffener, remove the stiffener and wire, lock pigtail
- Confirm position with a small amount of contrast, pull pigtail up to wall gently
- Dress retention sutures and external catheter securely
- Leave catheter open to atmosphere until bowel sounds return

puncture needle, preloaded with two pediatric retention sutures is connected to a T-connector and a syringe filled with sterile water-soluble contrast. The needle is advanced through the skin and soft tissues until tenting of the cecal wall is again observed. Air should be insufflated as needed to maintain distension of the cecum. Under fluoroscopic guidance, the needle is rapidly advanced into the cecum with a single thrust (Figure 4.33b). Contrast is then injected to confirm the position of the needle within the colon.

Under fluoroscopic control, a stiff 0.035-inch guide wire is advanced through the needle to deploy the retention sutures

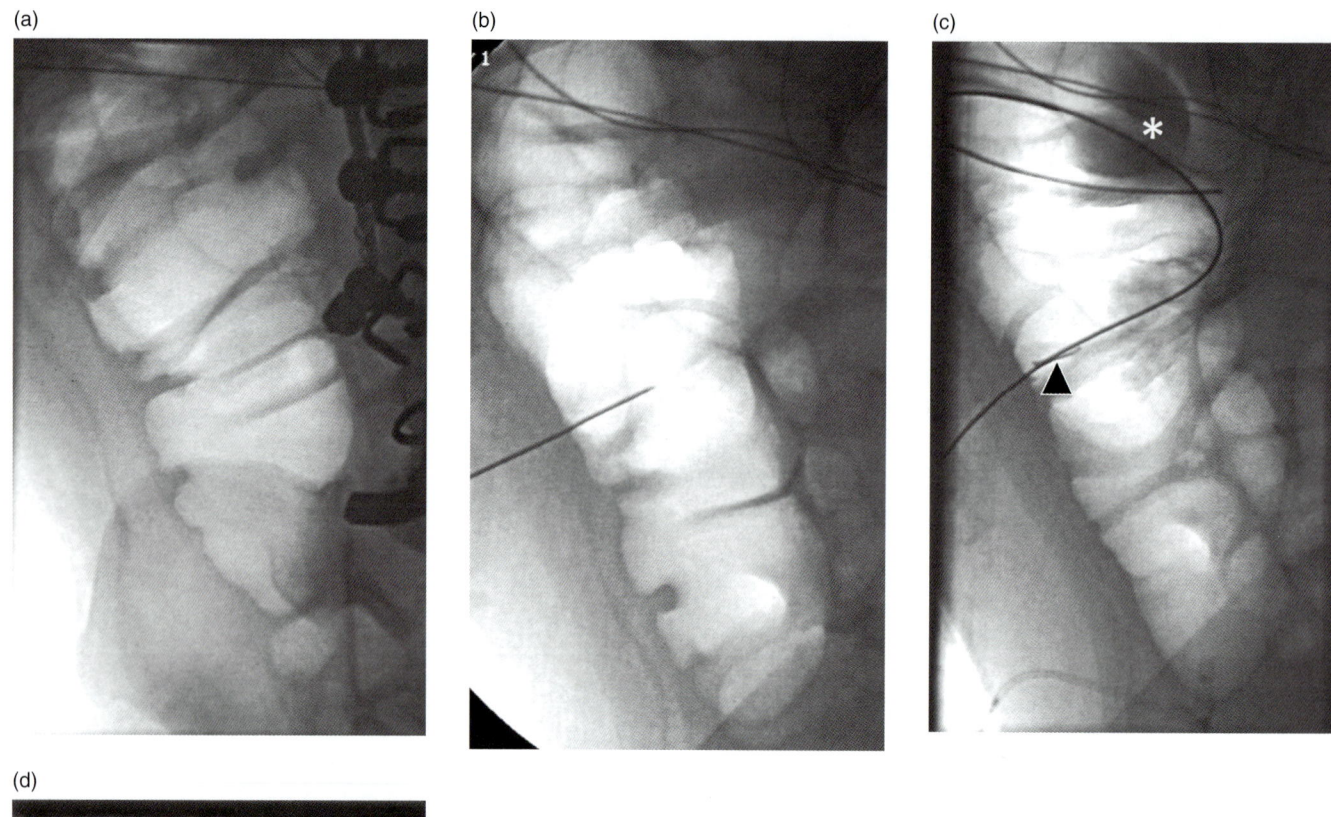

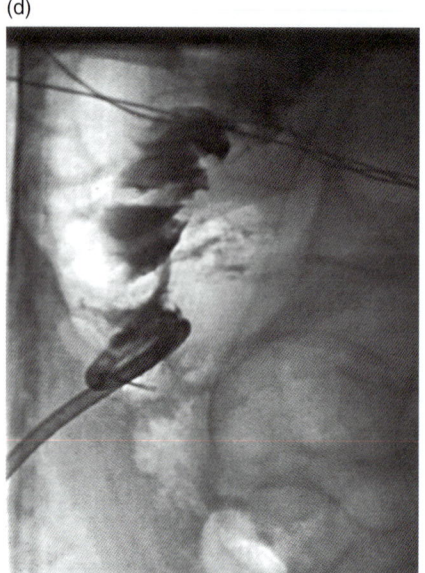

Figure 4.33 (a) In this plain radiograph of the right lower quadrant in a young teenager with spina bifida and fecal incontinence, air instilled via a rectal tube insufflated the cecum. Intravenous glucagon helped prevent passage of air into the ileum, which might otherwise obscure the access pathway. (b) After anesthetizing from the skin surface to the anterolateral cecal wall, the access needle was advanced from the right flank under fluoroscopic control until "tenting" of the cecal mucosa was evident. At that point, the needle was darted forward with a short, quick jab to puncture the wall of the cecum. (c) A small amount of contrast injected through the access needle is seen pooling in the cecum (*asterisk*), confirming intraluminal position. The guide wire was advanced through the needle, which had been preloaded with gastropexy sutures (*arrowhead*). (d) While holding gentle counter-traction on the retention sutures, the tract was first dilated with appropriate fascial dilators passed over the guide wire. Then a Cope loop catheter with its stiffening cannula was passed over the wire until the tip was well within the lumen, then the catheter was advanced off the stiffener and the Cope loop was formed and locked. Additional contrast was instilled to confirm position, then the Cope loop was pulled back gently to bring the cecal wall in apposition to the flank wall.

(Figure 4.33c). The wire should be advanced until the stiff portion is well within the lumen. The needle is then removed leaving the wire in place and the two sutures are clamped with a mosquito forceps. Gentle tension on the sutures will appose the cecum against the anterolateral abdominal wall. An 8-French fascial dilator is introduced over the wire, maintaining gentle tension on the retention sutures. This is followed by introduction of an 8.5-French Dawson–Mueller Mac-Loc™ 15-cm catheter or other locking pigtail catheter. The catheter is locked and its position within the cecum is confirmed in two planes with a small amount of contrast (Figure 4.33d).

The locked "pigtail" of the catheter is pulled up against the anterior wall of the cecum, and the retention sutures are anchored to a small roll of gauze and fixed to the skin with adhesive tape. The skin at the tube exit site is dressed with a 2 × 2 gauze dressing and antibiotic ointment and covered with a non-occlusive dressing. The catheter is then left to drain to a drainage bag.

Technical variations

Occasionally air introduced into the rectum does not fill the cecum. Placing the patient in the left side down or lateral decubitus position usually allows good filling of the cecum. Rotation of the C-arm may be necessary to separate loops of bowel that overlie the cecum. We have had one patient whose procedure was delayed because of very distended sigmoid overlying the cecum. The procedure was repeated and the cecum was clearly separated from the sigmoid and a successful procedure performed. Ventriculoperitoneal (VP) shunts are avoided if possible, although evidence indicates that the procedure is safe even in this patient group. As discussed with regard to gastrostomy, it is sensible to avoid primary insertion within 30 days of VP shunt insertion or revision. Occasionally the cecum is high and just below the ribs and a more lateral and superior approach is used. It is important to examine the borders of the liver, spleen, and gallbladder with US in case this situation is present. If the retention sutures break during the procedure, we replace the suture prior to further dilatation. Safe access obstructed by dilated loops of bowel may be improved by percutaneous needle decompression.

Postprocedure and follow-up care

Analgesia is provided in the form of intravenous morphine sulfate (0.05 mg/kg each four hours for 24 hours), followed by oral acetaminophen (15 mg/kg every three to four hours as needed). The patient is allowed to ambulate as tolerated. Clear fluids are initially given until the patient has normal bowel movements and bowel sounds. The gentamicin, ampicillin, and metronidazole are continued with the same dosages three times a day for 48 hours and then the metronidazole is changed to an oral dose and given for a further five days.

The patient is usually discharged at two days post procedure with orders to flush through the catheter twice daily with 10 ml of saline. The preprocedural rectal enema regimen is continued for nine days after the procedure at which time the antegrade enemas are begun. The retention sutures are cut at the skin by the parents two weeks following the procedure. The patients are provided with a contact list of physicians and nursing staff who deal with any troubleshooting.

Catheter fixation

It is not necessary to fix the catheter externally to the skin. The external component of the initial Cope loop catheter can be taped to the skin for convenience if desired. The trapdoor catheter, once placed, also does not require external fixation. If desired, a small dressing may be placed over the trapdoor catheter to keep it from catching on clothing or furniture.

Catheter exchange and reinsertion

Approximately six weeks after primary tube insertion, the tract has matured and the catheter is changed for a Chait Trapdoor™ catheter (Figure 4.34). This is performed as an outpatient procedure and seldom requires sedation. No antibiotic coverage is given for this exchange. The position of the existing tube is checked and once the new tube has been placed over a wire, position of the internal coil is confirmed with contrast (Figure 4.35). The trapdoor device provides a low-profile catheter that is easily hidden under clothing or a small dressing, allowing the patient to lead a normal life. These catheters have been left in place up to three years between changes, but may become concreted and more difficult to remove over time.

We currently recommend replacing the catheter at least yearly. Our current technique for exchanging the trapdoor device is to introduce a stiff wire with a floppy tip into the colon, and exchange the old catheter for a new one. Alternatively, the old trapdoor may be clamped, the head of the catheter cut off, and a wire inserted. Then the new catheter can be inserted pushing the old catheter into the colon where it will pass in the feces. We prefer the former approach.

Technical problems and pitfalls

Primary placement of the trapdoor catheter

There has been a tendency for non-radiologist operators to place the trapdoor catheter as a primary device, bypassing placement of an initial Cope loop drainage catheter. While this does save a step, the pigtail portion of the trapdoor catheter often causes the maturing tract to become elongated and tortuous (spiraled). If the tract matures in this fashion, it makes every subsequent catheter exchange significantly more difficult. We therefore recommend against this practice.

Patient support

In our experience, the most frequent cause of catheter failure has been difficulty obtaining access to knowledgeable personnel at the time a problem is perceived. The population at risk for this procedure have often experienced protracted frustration searching for a successful approach to managing fecal incontinence prior to referral for the cecostomy procedure. While some patients and their families have no difficulty in transition to antegrade enemas through the cecostomy, many patients experience at least one obstacle during transition that impedes success. Virtually always, this difficulty can be easily managed with encouragement and additional education from the interventional staff. However, if the problem arises during off hours and knowledgeable personnel cannot be reached, the resulting frustration and anxiety can be enough to cause patients to abandon the catheter. Having a strong support infrastructure in place is the single best way to minimize complications and improve satisfaction of patients, families, and referring providers.

Complications

We have successfully placed hundreds of cecostomy tubes since 1994. We have found that in the initial period, learning to use the tube effectively can be quite stressful for the patient and family. A few patients have had their catheters removed due to emotional complications. Early complications include some pain at the insertion site, which is successfully treated with oral analgesics. Several patients have developed local

Chapter 4 Abdominopelvic interventions

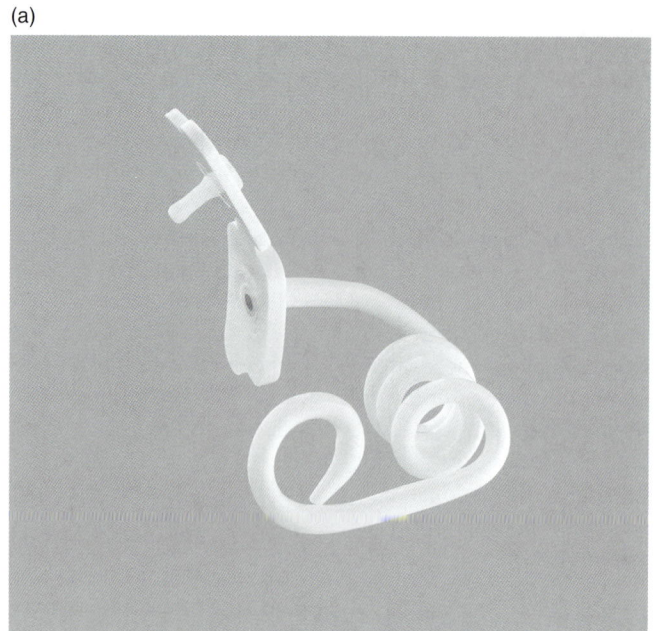

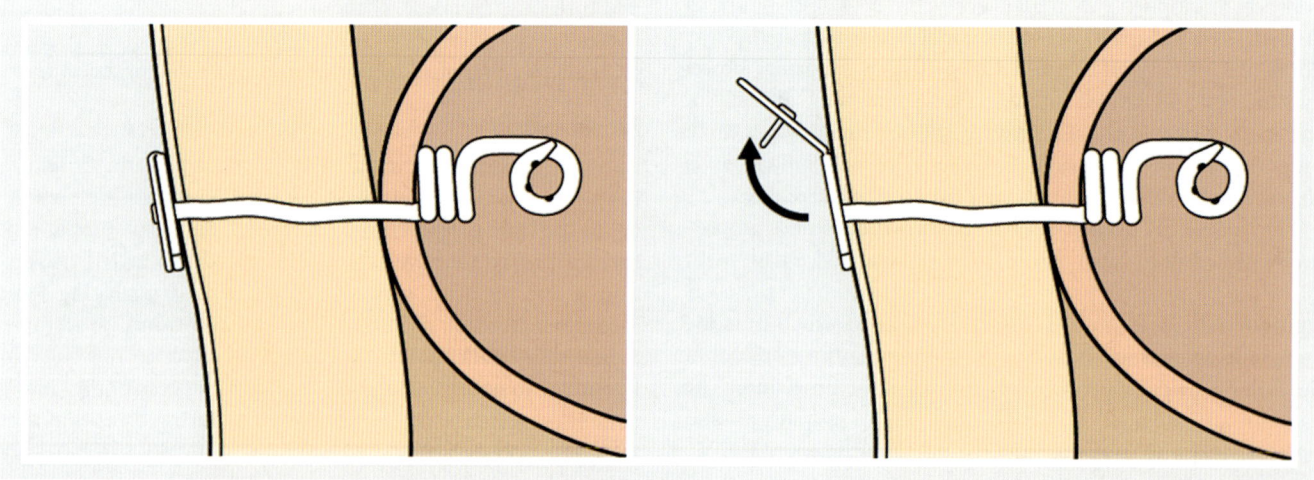

Figure 4.34 (a) The Trapdoor catheter (Cook Medical) is placed after the primary tract has matured. It has a low-profile hub with a locking cap. The body has a shaft available in several lengths, selected according to the tract length. The internal portion of the body is formed in a soft corkscrewing pigtail to retain the catheter atraumatically within the cecal lumen. (b) Cecostomy illustration. The Trapdoor is a low-profile device. The closed device (left) sits flush with the skin surface, while the pigtail is retained in the cecal lumen. The device is opened (right) for use.

tenderness and required IV antibiotics for a total of five days. We have seen no incidence of cellulitis, but have treated one patient for deep soft tissue abscess by percutaneous drainage. Late complications may occasionally be directly related to the volume of the phosphate enema. Therefore we recommend the smallest volumes that are appropriate for patient size. If problems occur, further reduction of enema volume usually alleviates symptoms such as vomiting. Several patients have pulled the catheters out inadvertently. Temporary Foley catheters were placed by the parents at home. Later, the catheters were electively replaced with permanent catheters in the interventional suite. If patients develop constipation, a high fiber diet and stool softeners will often solve this problem.

Primary tube malposition

Occasionally, a redundant loop of bowel may be mistakenly accessed during the primary insertion procedure. This risk is elevated when the cecum is retroflexed or positioned elsewhere than the right lower quadrant, reinforcing the importance of careful observation of cecal position during air insufflation. If this error is noted at the time of initial access, the needle can,

Chapter 4 Abdominopelvic interventions

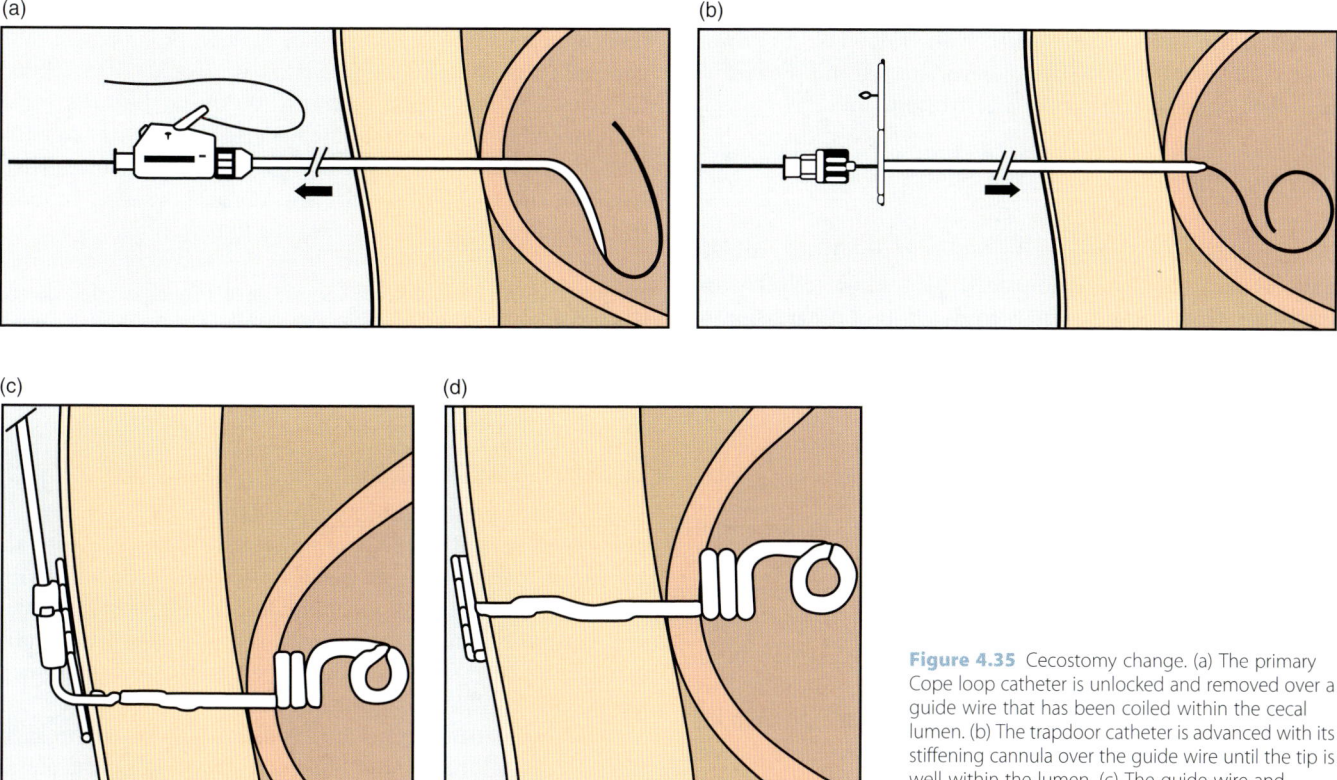

Figure 4.35 Cecostomy change. (a) The primary Cope loop catheter is unlocked and removed over a guide wire that has been coiled within the cecal lumen. (b) The trapdoor catheter is advanced with its stiffening cannula over the guide wire until the tip is well within the lumen. (c) The guide wire and stiffener are withdrawn, allowing the pigtail to form within the lumen. A small amount of contrast is instilled to confirm intraluminal position. (d) The "trapdoor" is closed between uses. Usually, no other external fixation is required.

in most cases, be withdrawn and appropriate access obtained, although there should be heightened surveillance for evidence of chemical peritonitis (see below). If the error is noted after tract dilation, the tract should *not* be peremptorily abandoned. Rather, the primary drainage tube should be placed in the accessed loop and left in place for a sufficient time to allow the tract to mature (usually, three to six weeks). The cecum should then be positively identified and may be accessed without delay according to the procedure described above. The only exception is that the new access should be placed at least 2 cm from the erroneous access. Once the erroneous access tract has matured, the tube can be removed, and the iatrogenic enterocutaneous fistula will normally close without further complication. If there is concern about bowel obstruction from the malpositioned tube, an extremely uncommon event, the tube can be removed surgically with concurrent repair of the enterostomy.

Peritonitis, skin infection, and abscess formation

Peritonitis or local skin infection following primary cecostomy is rare. Causes include leakage of cecal contents during access maneuvers, and contamination due to tube malposition, tract elongation, or elevated intra-abdominal pressure. Symptoms may include prolonged or severe pain after the cecostomy procedure, pain during enemas, or external leakage of cecal contents. Unexplained changes in vital signs following the procedure should raise suspicion of peritonitis. If peritonitis is suspected, enemas should be discontinued and a contrast study under fluoroscopy or CT may help confirm the diagnosis. A course of broad-spectrum antibiotics with coverage for common gastrointestinal pathogens is prudent. If free intraperitoneal fluid is observed, a sample may be obtained for culture and sensitivity to help guide appropriate coverage. Once the reason for leakage has been corrected and the cecostomy tube is properly positioned, enemas can usually be safely resumed on the third day of antibiotics.

Intraperitoneal tube malposition or disruption of the cecostomy tract may be suspected if after exchanging the tube through a mature tract there is difficulty or pain while injecting contrast or water through the new tube. Similarly, if the existing tube was accidentally dislodged, a low threshold for suspecting complication should be maintained. In such cases a contrast study under fluoroscopy should be performed to positively confirm appropriate position and function of the new tube. If peritoneal contamination is suspected, enemas should be stopped and the patient treated with broad-spectrum antibiotics as described above. If access to the cecal lumen cannot be safely regained through the old tract, the cecostomy may have to be re-sited.

If an abscess associated with the cecostomy tract is suspected, it can easily be confirmed with US or CT. If such an abscess is identified, it should be evaluated and treated as described above for abscess of a gastrostomy tract.

Granulation tissue

Approximately 60% of percutaneous cecostomy recipients develop granulation tissue at the insertion site. This is usually painless and may be accompanied by a clear to yellowish discharge. Granulation tissue is treated with a progression of saline soaks, hydrogen peroxide soaks, topical calcium carbonate, and silver nitrate cauterization as indicated. Surgical excision is very rarely required.

Occlusion and leakage

Cecostomy tubes may occasionally become narrowed or occluded with inspissated fecal material or calcified concretion. Although tube occlusion is seldom seen if tubes are exchanged yearly, the longer they are left without exchange, the greater this risk becomes. If tube blockage prevents admission of an exchange guide wire, and the tract is mature, the tube may simply be removed, a guide wire carefully directed through the tract with a dilator, and a new tube placed after confirmation that the guide wire is clearly within the cecal lumen. Removal of a concreted tube may require firm traction. Consideration should be given to injection of local anesthesia along the tract for patients who have sensation in this region. Some bleeding may be expected, but is usually brief and self-limited. If the tract is not mature and tube blockage cannot otherwise be remedied, an exchange dilator and 0.018-inch hydrophilic wire may be carefully advanced alongside the tube under fluoroscopic guidance until the cecal lumen is reached. Injection of contrast through the dilator can confirm appropriate placement. The occluded tube can then be removed, the guide wire exchanged for a 0.035-inch stiff guide wire, and a new tube placed.

Dislodgment

If the cecostomy tube is partially dislodged at home, the tube may be taped in place by the patient or caregiver. If the tube is completely dislodged from a mature tract, the patient or caregiver should place a Foley catheter through the tract and tape it securely in place. In either case, the patient should have a new tube placed in the interventional suite. If the tube is dislodged from an immature tract, vigorous attempts to regain access by caregivers or medical personnel unfamiliar with this device should be discouraged. The patient should be expeditiously transported to the interventional suite, where an attempt to regain access can be made in a manner similar to that described above for gastrostomy tube dislodgment. If such attempts are not clearly successful, the tube may have to be re-sited. Antibiotics are usually not required for dislodgment from a mature tract, but should be considered if access is lost from an immature tract and cannot be regained. Lastly, if the tract appears to be closed it may still be probe-patent. We approach this in the same way that we would for a "closed GT tract" or any closed osteomy. We begin by inserting a 3 French dilator and a 0.018-inch angled glide wire and gently push the catheter as far as it will go without resistance. Then we insert the angled glide wire and advance the wire. In most instances the guide wire will find the lumen. If that is not the case, a sinogram is performed. If the guide wire cannot simply be directed intraluminally a short 3 or 4 French angled directional catheter is substituted for the dilator. If these maneuvers are unsuccessful the procedure is abandoned and a new tube insertion is scheduled.

Controversies/issues

The percutaneous cecostomy procedure is an alternative to other non-surgical methods of bowel maintenance in patients with fecal incontinence. It is most effective for patients with normal bowel tone but an inability to detect feces in the rectal vault and to evacuate voluntarily. It is probably not an appropriate alternative for those with hyperactive bowel tone, such as patients with Hirschsprung's disease.

The percutaneous procedure is also an alternative to such surgical procedures as the antegrade cecostomy that either surgically or laparoscopically creates a mucocutaneous fistula from the skin through the appendix for antegrade enemas. The percutaneous procedure has the advantage of shorter postprocedure hospitalization, shorter time to tract maturity, and preservation of the vermiform appendix for other reconstructive procedures, such as appendicovesicostomy, that may be useful in the same patient population.

Future advances

As is also the case for transgastric gastrojejunostomy, the need for separate procedures and devices for primary tract formation and placement of a long-term, low-profile device is not ideal. Some of the newer gastrostomy devices that might be repurposed for primary percutaneous cecostomy insertion require primary development of a tract 24 French or more in diameter. Development of a successful low-profile device that can be safely and simply inserted in a primary procedure without an excessively large tract would be welcomed by patients, families, caregivers, and providers.

Although an increasing number of centers offer this procedure, the majority of patients with fecal incontinence must travel long distances not only for primary insertion and tube exchanges but also for assessment of relatively routine potential complications and issues. This is but one of many examples where telehealth solutions that allow distance surveillance, education, and consultation by expert centers would facilitate better and more cost-effective care closer to home with fewer disruptions of family, work, and school.

Conclusions

Fecal incontinence is a difficult problem to treat. Most forms of treatment have been unsatisfactory, unsuccessful, esthetically unappealing, or difficult for the child to administer without assistance. Administration of small-volume antegrade enemas via a percutaneously placed cecostomy is a safe and effective alternative for the treatment of fecal incontinence with excellent patient response and acceptance and minimal complication, resulting in increased independence and mobility. In addition to the social benefits of alleviating incontinence, patients have reported decreased constipation, improved urinary bladder capacitance (with decompression of the colon and rectum), and decreased halitosis following insertion of their cecostomy tube.

Percutaneous aspiration and drainage of fluid collections

Introduction

Abscess drainage using percutaneous techniques has been performed for more than eighty years. More recently, percutaneous aspiration and drainage has become the first-line therapy for evaluation or evacuation of most sterile and infected fluid collections in the abdomen, pelvis, chest, musculoskeletal system, and soft tissues. In many institutions the percutaneous approach has replaced surgical incision and drainage.

When percutaneous techniques first became available image-guided abscess drainage was confined to well-circumscribed, solitary collections that were easily accessible without traversing uninvolved organs or compartments. Over the past 20 years, enabled by substantial improvements in cross-sectional imaging modalities (especially US and CT), safety and accuracy of needle and catheter placement have been proven. In comparison with surgical management, interventional procedures generally have lower morbidity and mortality, require shorter hospital stays, and are less expensive. As a result of these innovations and experiences aspiration and drainage using percutaneous techniques has gained widespread acceptance within the surgical and medical communities. Preprocedural imaging and planning, adequate monitoring and sedation during the procedure, and selection of equipment appropriate for a child maximizes the chance for a successful outcome.

Indications

There are numerous indications for aspiration or drainage of fluid collections in the pediatric population (Table 4.12). In most instances aspiration is considered for diagnostic sampling of a fluid collection of uncertain etiology to guide medical or surgical therapy (Figure 4.36). If a drain cannot be safely placed, aspiration may be helpful to reduce the volume of small (<2 to 3 cm) or poorly accessible fluid collections.

Table 4.12 Indications: percutaneous aspiration and drainage

Indications
- Discriminate between fluid and solid tissue or phlegmon
- Diagnostic sampling of abnormal fluid, including:
  - bacterial
  - fungal
  - atypical organisms
  - parasitic
  - viral
  - malignant
  - biliary
  - CSF
  - lymphatic
  - hematoma or seroma
  - urinary
  - gastrointestinal (e.g., salivary, duplication cyst)
  - reactive/inflammatory
- Decompression or evacuation of a fluid collection
- Decompression or evacuation of a viscus organ obstruction or pseudo-obstruction
- Provide continuous drainage of infected collections (abscesses)
- Provide drainage of chronic sterile collections, including:
  - lymphatic malformation/lymphocele
  - ranula
  - other cervico-facial cysts
  - pseudocyst (e.g., pancreatic, CSF)
  - biloma
  - urinoma
  - effusion
- Provide a pathway for intracavitary delivery of medication:
  - fibrinolysis (tPA)
  - chemotherapy agents
  - antibacterials
  - antifungals
  - sclerosants

Contraindications
- Uncorrectable coagulopathy
- No fluid or liquefiable component
- No safe pathway for percutaneous or transmucosal access
- Inadequate volume for formation of a pigtail drain (for drainage procedures)

However, aspiration alone is substantially less likely to be curative in infected collections large enough to accept the pigtail of a drainage catheter.

Percutaneous drainage of fluid collections is usually preferred for treatment of larger fluid collections (>2 to 3 cm), loculated collections, and abscesses or infected fluid collections. Fluid collections may be drained through a single catheter if unilocular or interconnected. In our experience, one drainage catheter is all that is needed in most children. Injection of radiographic contrast or dynamic sonographic evaluation of fluid flow patterns can often demonstrate whether complex collections are isolated or communicating. If the septations can be disrupted with a guide wire or

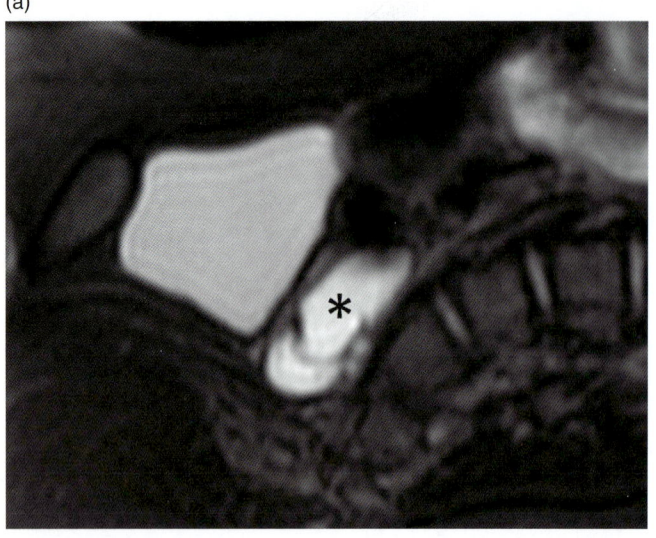
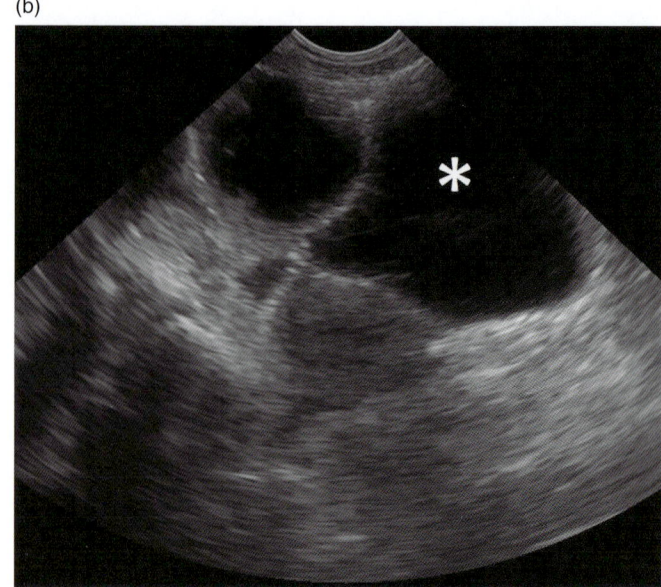
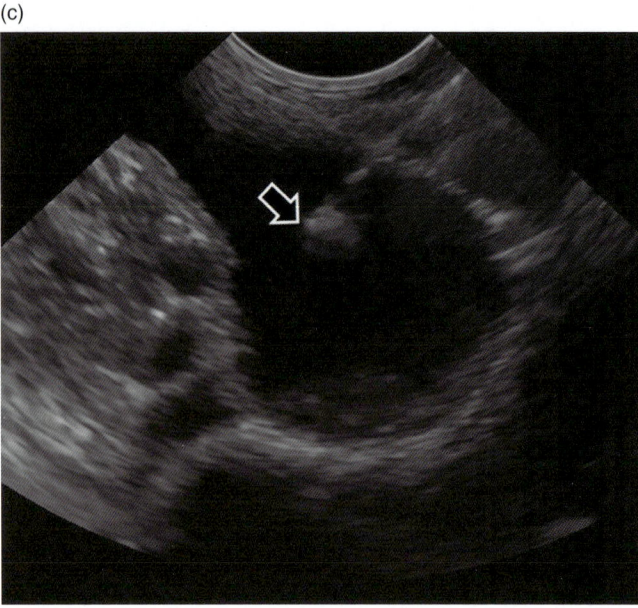

Figure 4.36 A five-year-old with abdominal discomfort. (a) Sagittal T2 MRI through the pelvis shows a septated fluid collection (*asterisk*) adjacent to the left ovary. (b) Transabdominal US shows a similar view of the ovarian cyst (*asterisk*). (c) A 5 French Yueh sheathed needle (*arrow*) is used to aspirate the cyst under US control.

catheter, multiseptate collections may also be drained through a single catheter. Multiple isolated collections and multiloculated cavities may require insertion of a separate drain into each significant sized locule (Figure 4.37). Alternatively, if an access tract can be planned so as to serially span multiple locules, side holes can be cut along the shaft of the drainage tube to allow simultaneous drainage of multiple collections through a single tube. If this is done, care should be taken to make the side holes no larger than those in the pigtail, and to space them spirally around the tube rather than linearly along the shaft, so that the structural integrity of the tube is not unduly impaired.

All non-communicating collections should be either drained or aspirated, and separate samples sent from each for microbiologic analysis to help select the most appropriate antibiotic coverage. If any discrete collections cannot be safely accessed surgical incision and drainage may be indicated.

Absolute contraindications to abscess drainage include an uncorrectable bleeding diathesis or an unsafe route for drainage. In our experience the latter has become a rare occurrence in recent years. In select cases, fluid collections in these patients may be safely aspirated through a thin needle (e.g., Chiba, see Figure 3.1). Suspected fungal abscess, which can be quite invasive, may be considered a relative contraindication to percutaneous drainage, unless local adjuvant therapy with direct injection of antifungal agents is anticipated. Interloop abscesses are also difficult to treat percutaneously and

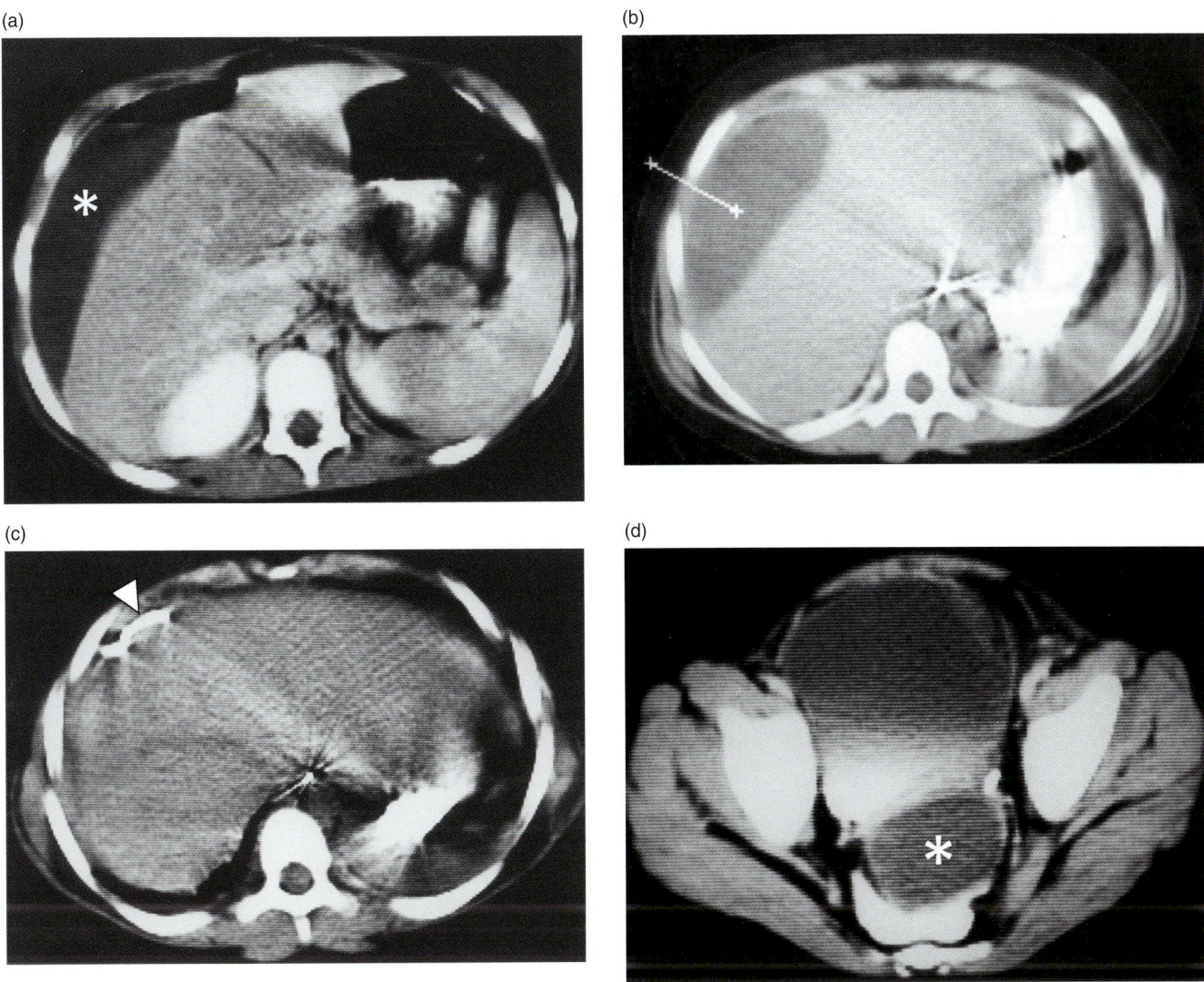

Figure 4.37 (a) A nine-year-old girl developed a right paracolic gutter abscess extending to the extrahepatic space (*asterisk*), seen on this contrast-enhanced CT, after appendiceal rupture and subsequent appendectomy. (b) Computed tomography is useful for identifying a safe route of access and measuring the distance to related vital structures. (c) Following placement of an 8 French drainage catheter (*arrowhead*), the collection is completely evacuated. (d) A second collection (*asterisk*) is seen in the pouch of Douglas, from which the same organism was cultured. This collection is amenable to either transrectal or transgluteal drainage.

aspiration with a thin needle may be all that is possible. The maximum number of drains that can be safely inserted into a child has not been established (Figure 4.38). In practice it is the condition of the patient, the ability of the patient to undergo a surgical procedure, and the experience of the interventionalist that usually determines the approach to therapy.

Technique

The approach to percutaneous abscess drainage in children differs from that in adults, mainly with respect to equipment and sedation. Although CT is often used for preoperative evaluation in children with suspected abscess collections, it is seldom used for guidance during the procedure. Instead, US is usually used for abscess localization and access, while fluoroscopy is used for final placement of the drainage catheter. Also, a trocar technique for direct insertion of a drainage catheter is generally not preferred.

Equipment

Although the approach to drainage is somewhat standardized the equipment selected varies considerably and depends on the preference of the interventionalist, the clinical problem to be solved, and the size of the patient. Access is usually accomplished with a Chiba needle over a stylet or a sheathed needle over a trocar (see Figure 3.1). Currently there are many companies producing a wide variety of devices that are suited for drainage of fluid collections (see Figure 3.2). Our preferences are listed in Table 4.13.

Chapter 4 Abdominopelvic interventions

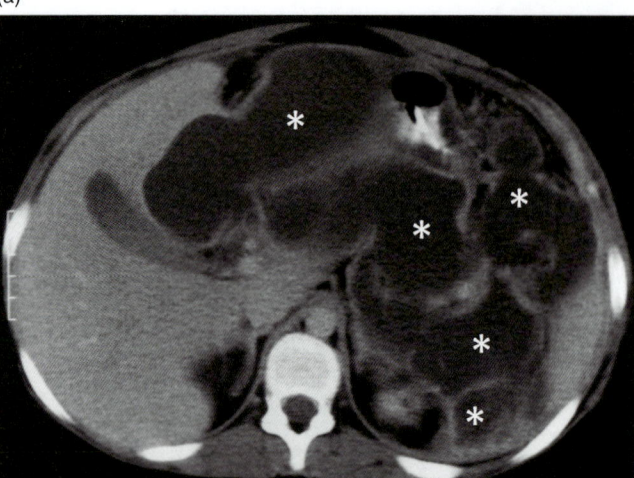
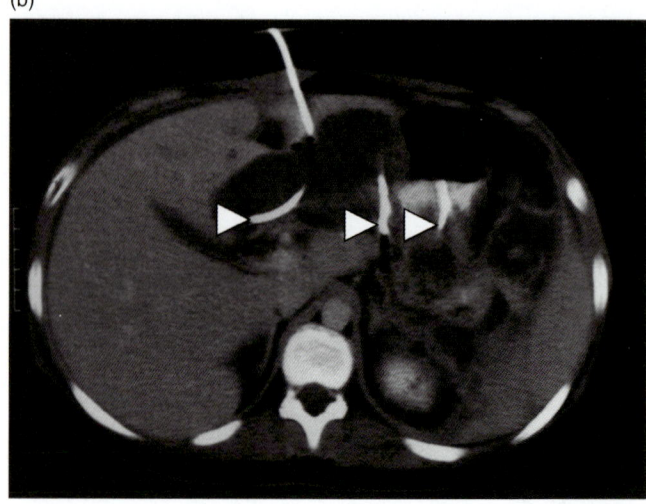

Figure 4.38 (a) A CT section with vascular and enteric contrast enhancement shows multiple abnormal fluid collections (*asterisks*) in this 14-year-old female with a family history of hyperparathyroidism and a history of congenital renal cystic disease and recent ingestion of a large volume of alcoholic beverages. (b) With placement of three percutaneous drains (*arrowheads*), the infected pancreatic pseudocysts resolved, as did the related pancreatic duct fistula.

Table 4.13 Equipment: percutaneous aspiration and drainage

Preparation and draping
- Chlorhexidine gluconate (0.5%) with 70% isopropyl alcohol solution (SoluPrep™ (tinted), Solumed Inc., Laval, Quebec)
- Betadine solution
- Isopropyl alcohol
- Sterile US cover (Civco Medical Instruments, Kalona, IA)
- Drapes (aperture drapes are preferred)

Puncture needles
- Angiocatheter, 16–24 gauge (Becton Dickenson, Sandy, UT)
- Yueh centesis disposable catheter needle, 4 and 5 French, with side holes (Cook Inc.)
- Chiba needle, 22 gauge (5, 10 and 15 cm, Highliter, Inrad, Michigan)
- Seldinger needle, 19 gauge (Cook Inc.)
- Single wall puncture needle, 18 and 19 gauge (2.5, 4, 7 cm) (BSDN, Cook Inc.)
- Trochar needle, 18 gauge (11 and 20 cm) (Cook, Inc.)

Introducer systems
- Neff introducer system (Cook Inc.)
- AccuStick™ introducer system (Boston Scientific, Meditech, Boston, MA)
- Cope introducer (Cook, Inc.)

Dilators
- Coons dilator, 5 French to 22 French (Cook Inc.)
- Vascular dilators (0.018–0.038 inches, 3 French–18 French)
- Angioplasty balloons of appropriate diameter

Drainage catheters
- All purpose drains, 6 to 14 French (Meditech)
- Pigtail drainage catheter, 8 to 24 French (Cook Inc.)
- Duan (Towbin) drainage catheter, 5 French (Cook Inc.)

Miscellaneous supplies
- Abscess drainage bag (Medics Inc. Hilliard, OH)
- Mefix™ adhesive bandage (Hypafix™ dressing retention sheet, Smith and Nephew, Lachine, Quebec)
- K-Lock adhesive catheter retention device (Zefon Medical Products)
- Jackson–Pratt suction
- Hemovac® suction
- Stat-Lock®

Image guidance

Cross-sectional imaging is usually requested early in the evaluation of patients presenting with clinical signs and symptoms of an abscess or fluid collection. Clinical history and prior imaging are reviewed in close consultation with referring physicians to determine the likely source and nature of abnormal collections, and additional preprocedure studies are obtained as required. Etiologic considerations for suspected fluid collections should include abscess, sterile fluid collection (hematoma, seroma, biloma, urinoma), congenital cyst or malformation, lymphocele, malignant fluid collection, pancreatic pseudocyst, aneurysm or pseudoaneurysm, and fluid-filled loops of bowel. Typically, contrast-enhanced CT is performed to identify the extent of the problem, to establish a diagnosis when possible, and to exclude a vascular mass or malformation.

It is important to confirm the presence and number of fluid collections, to distinguish a mature abscess (which is drainable) from a phlegmon (which is not), to assess for the presence of an associated tumor, and to determine the availability of a safe access route. It is important to distinguish inflammatory tissue or cellulitis from a mature abscess, as drainage of inflammatory tissue without fluid is not possible. A combination of contrast-enhanced CT and US may be

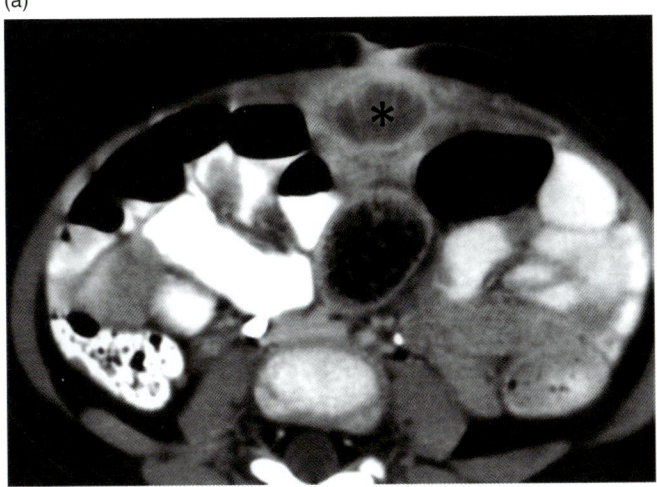
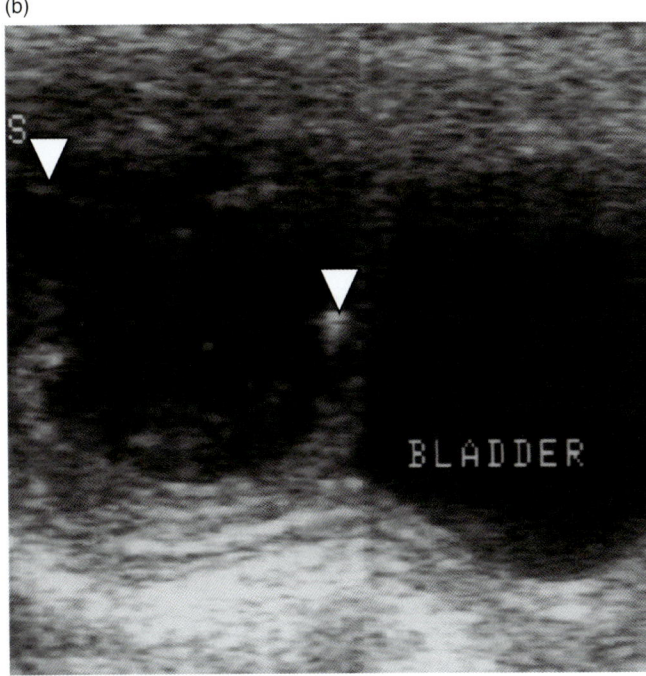

Figure 4.39 (a) A three-year-old boy presented with abdominal pain and fever. A CT scan shows a cystic structure (*asterisk*) in the extraperitoneal soft tissues between the umbilicus and the bladder. (b) Sagittal ultrasound confirmed an urachal cyst, and guided percutaneous access with a 22-gauge Chiba needle (*arrowheads*). The needle tip shows a classic "comet tail" artifact.

needed at times to differentiate these conditions. For example, color flow by Doppler imaging or contrast enhancement by CT in the center of a mass suggests a phlegmon rather than a fluid collection.

Ultrasound

Treatment of a fluid collection may be regarded as a two-stage procedure. The first stage, *confirming the diagnosis*, requires analysis of a fluid sample obtained from the abnormal area identified on preprocedure imaging. In the case of small or poorly accessible collections, this may be accomplished with a Chiba needle under US guidance. Larger sterile collections (except lymphoceles and pancreatic pseudocysts) may be evacuated through a 16-gauge angiocather or a sheathed needle with side holes such as a Yueh centesis catheter needle or an 18-gauge single wall puncture needle under US guidance. A one-step needle aspiration and saline lavage technique has been described using an 18-gauge needle under US or CT guidance to successfully treat both simple and multiloculated abdominal and pelvic abscesses, using either percutaneous or transrectal access. However, redirection of the same needle into multiple collections does risk cross-contamination. Ultrasound can also be used to differentiate abnormal collections from normal structures (Figure 4.39). If drainage is anticipated, interval US and fluoroscopy is usually performed directly on the C-arm fluoroscopic table (Figure 4.40). As soon as a safe route of access is determined, the site is identified and marked, and the child is prepared and draped in sterile fashion.

A sterile cover is placed over the US probe for intraprocedural guidance. Most experienced interventionalists prefer a "freehand" technique, especially where fluid collections are small or deeply situated, where the needle and US probe are distant from each other or where the ultrasonographic window is very small. In this way the movement of the needle is observed throughout its course. This is best accomplished if the fluid collection is eccentrically located within the scanning field, so that most of the field of view is available for observing the motion of the needle (see Figure 1.1). Finally, it is a helpful rule of thumb to never move the needle and the transducer at the same time. The most common US transducers useful for image guidance are 8, 7, or 5 MHz vector or small hockey stick probes. There is no substitute for a high-quality US machine in image-guided applications. Hand-held US machines are often inadequate for guidance.

Larger, symptomatic or infected collections will usually require progression to the second stage, catheter drainage. While the second stage is usually completed under fluoroscopic control or, less often, under CT control, continued access to US can assist disruption of septa within complex collections, confirm optimum positioning of the guide wire and catheter, and document evacuation of the collection at the conclusion of the procedure.

Fluoroscopic imaging

Having secured needle access to the fluid collection under US guidance, a guide wire is passed into the collection and the tract dilation and catheter insertion is completed under

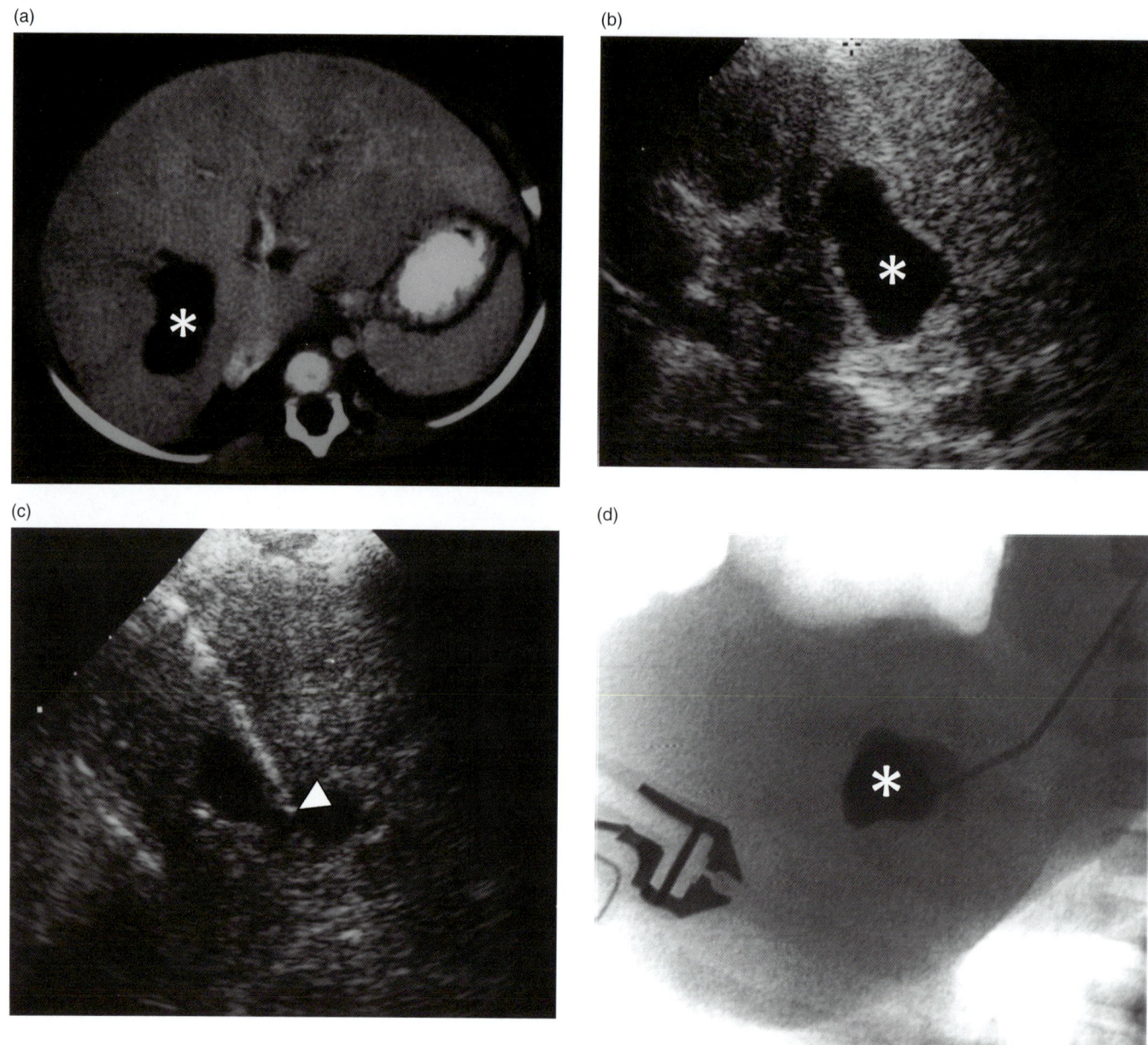

Figure 4.40 (a) In a six-month-old after a Kasai procedure for biliary atresia, CT with vascular and enteric contrast shows an intrahepatic biloma (*asterisk*). (b) Right upper quadrant ultrasound confirms the intrahepatic collection (*asterisk*). (c) A 21-gauge Chiba needle has been advanced percutaneously toward the biloma, and the tip (*arrowhead*) is seen to tent the anterior margin of the collection in this image. (d) Once access was achieved under US guidance, the remainder of the drainage procedure was completed under fluoroscopic control. In this image a small amount of contrast (*asterisk*) injected through the drainage catheter shows the limits of the biloma.

fluoroscopic control. Initial access under fluoroscopic guidance is possible in gas-containing collections, but is rarely the procedure of choice with abdominal collections.

Computed tomography

Computed tomography guidance is indicated to access fluid collections for which no adequate sonographic window can be identified. In children this is more often related to collections obscured by overlying gas or bone or for transgluteal drainage of pelvic abscess drainage. Computed tomography guidance may be especially advantageous in small, deeply situated lesions in larger patients, where the target is adjacent to vital structures, or where the lesion is obscured by overlying echogenic structures (e.g., lung, bowel gas, bone). During CT-guided approaches for biopsy, it is helpful to orient the needle perpendicular to the skin within the imaging plane, as compound angulation is difficult to perform. Angulation of the gantry is occasionally useful for lesions that are otherwise difficult to reach (Figure 4.41). Multiple imaging modalities are being integrated with imaging archives, other data sources,

Chapter 4 Abdominopelvic interventions

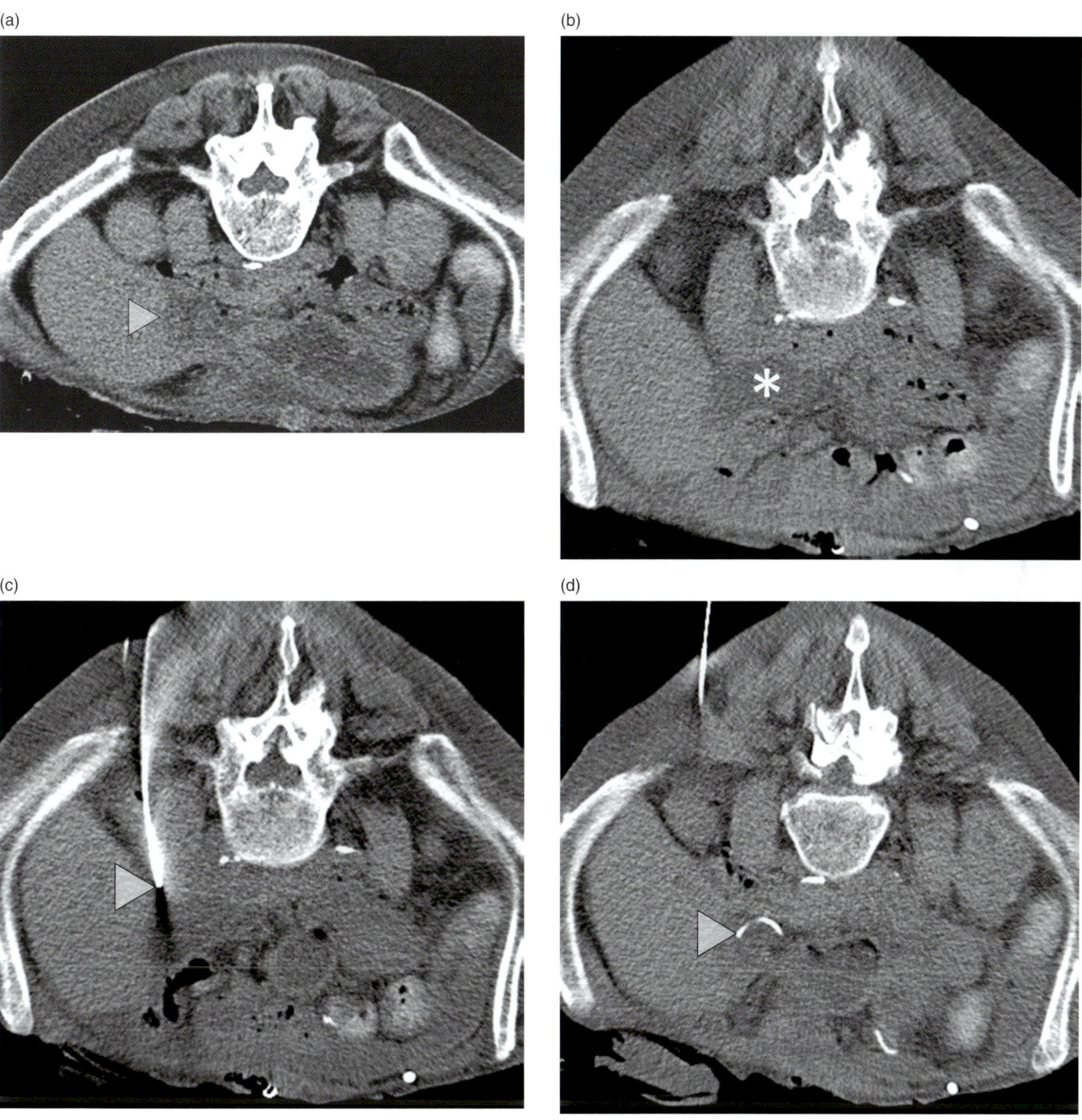

Figure 4.41 (a) In an older female patient, a postoperative pelvic fluid collection (*arrowhead*) visualized on prone CT is completely surrounded by bony pelvis and spine, loops of bowel, inferior pole of the right kidney, and pelvic vessels. (b) Placing the patient over a bolster and 23 degrees caudal angulation of the CT gantry opens a pathway through the lumbosacral space to the collection (*asterisk*). (c) Curving the 18-gauge Chiba access needle (*arrowhead*), avoids transgressing the psoas muscle and associated structures while advancing to the collection. (d) The floppy tip of the super stiff guide wire (*arrowhead*) is coiled within the collection. (e) A 12 French Mac-Loc™ drainage catheter (Cook Medical) has its Cope loop (*arrowhead*) coiled within the pelvic collection on this CT topogram. (f) The postoperative abscess (*arrowhead*) was completely evacuated and after five days the drain was removed.

and image processing and analysis software, into interventional suites (most notably at present in neuroimaging and intervention). As this field matures, practitioners will be more likely to select image guidance by task, based on safety and efficacy rather than convenience and availability. For example, diagnosis, procedure planning, and initial access for select collections may be performed under CT or cone-beam CT guidance, the catheter placed under fluoroscopic guidance, and evacuation of the cavity confirmed with US as a continuous procedure without moving the patient.

(e) (f)

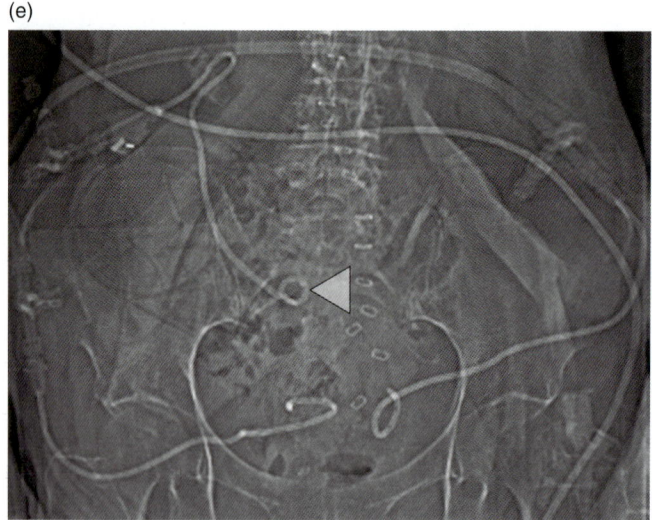
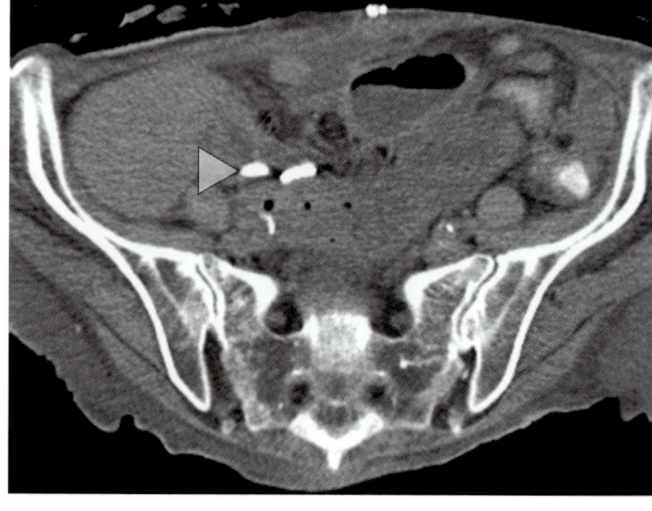

Figure 4.41 (cont.)

Other modalities

A variety of features including fine anatomic and physiologic detail, cross-sectional, multiplanar and volumetric image rendering, and near real-time capability would make interventional MRI a desirable modality for image-guided procedures. However, there is not yet any proven advantage of MR over other modalities, and issues of cost and availability still limit its applicability in practical terms. Similarly, nuclear scanning using gallium or white-blood cell labeled agents offers high sensitivity for the detection of infectious and inflammatory processes, but very limited anatomic detail. In the future devices such as PET-CT may change our approach to the diagnosis and treatment of these patients. As economic concerns are addressed, and when this technology can be integrated into an interventional suite, one would anticipate that some of the more difficult procedures would be shifted to this environment.

Patient preparation

The interventional radiology team monitors the patient closely during the procedure with pulse oximetry, intermittent blood pressure monitoring, and continuous electrocardiography. Usually, pediatric patients are sedated or anesthetized for drainage procedures, although in cooperative teens this may not be necessary depending upon the depth of the collection, the proximity of vital structures, the intricacy of the planned procedure, and the clinical status of the patient. Combined with local anesthetic this approach allows for successful completion in most cases. Administration of general anesthesia by a pediatric anesthetist may be preferred by the interventionalist, and paralysis may be desirable especially if the need for respiratory control is anticipated. In select cases, local anesthesia alone will suffice.

The procedure is performed using sterile technique, unless the operative field is obviously contaminated, as in a transrectal procedure. Most procedures are performed in an interventional suite equipped with modern C-arm fluoroscopy and high-quality US. The skin entry site is marked with washable ink. When planning percutaneous drainage of an upper abdominal collection, care should be taken to avoid the pleural space. Accordingly, the access site should be below the eighth rib anteriorly and the twelfth rib posteriorly. A posterior approach often requires cranial angulation of the access needle. In these situations, transabdominal US may allow visualization of the access needle entering posteriorly with the patient in the decubitus position. Then the skin is prepared with a suitable agent and sterile drapes are placed. Buffered 1% lidocaine solution (9 ml:1 ml lidocaine and bicarbonate) up to 0.5 ml/kg is infiltrated into the subcutaneous tissues and along the prospective tract with a 27- or 30-gauge needle.

Standard technique

The size and type of needle used for initial access depends upon the size, location, and the expected viscosity of the collection. In large collections that are easily accessible a 16-gauge angiocatheter, a 5-French Yueh sheathed needle, or a 19-gauge single wall needle is used under US guidance. After sampling the contents of the collection, a 0.035-inch wire can be passed coaxially. For deeper or riskier collections, a 22-gauge Chiba needle is advanced using US guidance to avoid loops of bowel or vital structures and safely enter the collection. Aspiration of the fluid confirms its character, and guides subsequent management decisions. If drainage is required, a 0.018-inch glide wire is placed through the Chiba needle and is then exchanged for a coaxial introducer system (Table 4.14).

Table 4.14 Procedure summary: percutaneous aspiration and drainage

- Preprocedural work-up (include CT with contrast)
- Route planning
- Sterile preparation and draping
- Locally anesthetize entry site
- Small skin incision
- Image-guided puncture
- Insert guide wire and coil within cavity
- Dilate tract
- Insert locking drainage catheter
- Secure catheter to patient
- Dry sterile dressing

The inner dilator and guide wire can then be replaced with a larger and stiffer (e.g., Amplatz®, Rosen, Glide®) guide wire, over which a suitable drainage catheter may be inserted. Direct access with a trochar catheter system is less precise and seldom used in the drainage of intra-abdominal abscesses unless they are very large and superficial. After obtaining samples for microbiologic or pathologic analysis, contrast is introduced through the needle or the sheath to outline the walls of the collection. This allows the introduction of a 0.035-inch guide wire into the fluid cavity without perforating the cavity walls.

Regional considerations

Paracentesis

Children requiring diagnostic or therapeutic drainage of peritoneal fluid often present with abdominal distension and elevation of the diaphragm, which in rare instances can become a relative contraindication to general anesthesia or deep sedation due to potential respiratory compromise. Application of a topical anesthetic such as ELA-Max® or EMLA® prior to the planned procedure, and light sedation and analgesia are usually sufficient to alleviate discomfort for this procedure. It can be helpful to place the patient in 15- to 20-degrees anti-Trendelenburg position to allow freely flowing ascites to reach a gravity-dependent position within the abdomen. Careful pre-procedure US scanning is essential, as suspected ascites is not always present by the time the procedure is requested, and because fluid collections may occasionally be loculated and more difficult to access.

After infiltration of local anesthetic along the prospective tract, initial access is most easily achieved with a 16- to 18-gauge angiocatheter or 5-French sheathed (e.g., Yueh) needle under US control. One must look for and be careful to avoid transgressing the epigastric artery within the rectus abdominus muscle at the junction of the mid and lateral thirds. The parietal peritoneum has a tendency to "tent" or drape over the tip of the needle. A short sharp jabbing motion with the needle is usually sufficient to pass into the peritoneal cavity, but failure to aspirate fluid after apparent passage of the needle should call this factor to mind. As direct a line as possible should be maintained during needle entry, without sharp changes in direction, else the catheter is likely to kink in the irregular tract upon withdrawal of the stylet.

Once fluid is returned, the stylet is removed, and the catheter attached via a three-way stopcock to an extension tube. Be aware that removing large volumes of fluid at once may result in the development of unintended electrolyte imbalance. Therefore it is important to carefully monitor vital signs and provide intravenous replacement fluid and electrolytes when necessary. However, based on patient symptoms, malignant or recurrent ascites may be drained serially as above or with a cuffed, tunneled indwelling catheter e.g., 15.5-French PleurX® catheter, designed for long-term use.

Access to deep pelvic collections

Pelvic abscesses are usually deep and may be obscured by overlying bowel, vessels, urinary bladder, and bony pelvis. If they are superficial and easily visualized with US or CT, they are easy to drain using the transabdominal approach described above. Children with pelvic abscess (most often the result of complicated appendicitis) may be treated with either a transgluteal or transrectal approach (Figure 4.42). The transgluteal approach is accomplished using CT guidance for route planning. The entry site is usually selected 1 to 4 cm lateral to the lumbar spine. The shortest route to the fluid collection that does not transgress vital structures is selected (Figure 4.43). Once the entry site is chosen and marked the puncture may be completed and the catheter inserted in standard fashion on the CT table. Although never proven in a pediatric series there has been a suggestion that there is a higher incidence of pain, bleeding, nerve damage, and other complications related to the transgluteal route. However, transgluteal pelvic drainage in children through the greater sciatic notch is generally well tolerated. Our experience supports the use of either the transrectal or the transgluteal route based on the individual characteristics of the target collection. Similar techniques may be used for transvaginal or transperineal access to pelvic fluid collections, but these are seldom employed in the pediatric population.

If the transrectal approach is used (Figure 4.44) the patient is positioned in the left side down decubitus position. A transvaginal or transrectal probe fitted with a needle guide may be used for transrectal imaging during needle insertion. Alternatively, a digital rectal examination is performed while scanning through the anterior abdominal wall with US, usually with a curvilinear transducer using ob/gyn settings with the full bladder as a sonographic window (when imaging through the full bladder through-transmission may result in overwhelming echogenicity using routine abdominal settings). The examining digit is visualized within the rectum, and the relationship between the rectal wall and the fluid collection is defined. For lesions higher up in the pelvis, an enema catheter

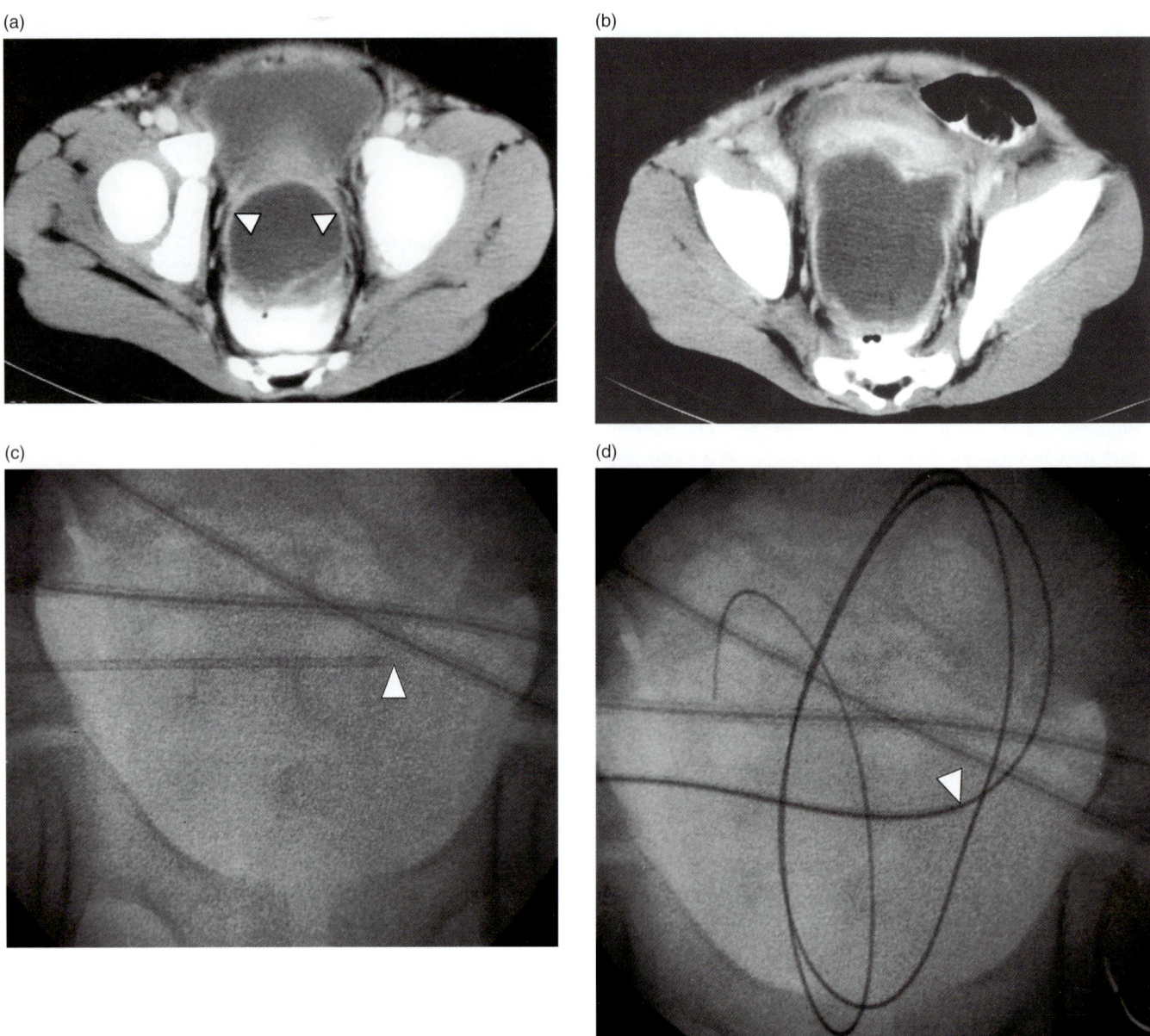

Figure 4.42 (a) A CT section through the pelvis with vascular and enteric contrast enhancement shows a rim-enhancing fluid collection (*arrowheads*) in this 12-year-old female after appendectomy for ruptured appendix. (b) The large collection is easily accessible to either a transrectal or transgluteal approach. (c) After gaining access under CT guidance, the patient was transferred to the angiography suite for completion of the procedure. In this posteroanterior view of the pelvis, the needle (*arrowhead*) is visualized projecting over the pelvis. (d) A superstiff guide wire was passed through the needle and coiled within the collection, and the needle was exchanged for a fascial dilator (*arrowhead*). (e) A Cope loop internally locking 12 French drainage catheter was placed within the collection, and the abscess was evacuated. (f) Contrast injected through the catheter outlines the limits of the abscess.

is used to protect the mucosa from the sharp needle tip during introduction of the needle.

Under US control, a long 18-gauge trochar needle is advanced either along the gloved index finger or protected within the enema tip. In either case, the needle tip is advanced into the abscess collection under real-time US imaging. The collection is aspirated and fluid sent for laboratory assessment. Pus from a ruptured appendiceal abscess, a common indication for transrectal drainage, has a characteristically foul odor.

Under fluoroscopic control a small amount of contrast is instilled to define the limits of the abscess cavity, and a 0.035-inch Amplatz® guide wire is advanced through the needle into the collection. The tract is dilated and an appropriately sized drain inserted over the guide wire.

Percutaneous and transrectal management of pelvic fluid collections may be performed safely in children with inflammatory bowel disease (IBD). Such treatment may alleviate the need for open surgery during the active phase of disease

Chapter 4 Abdominopelvic interventions

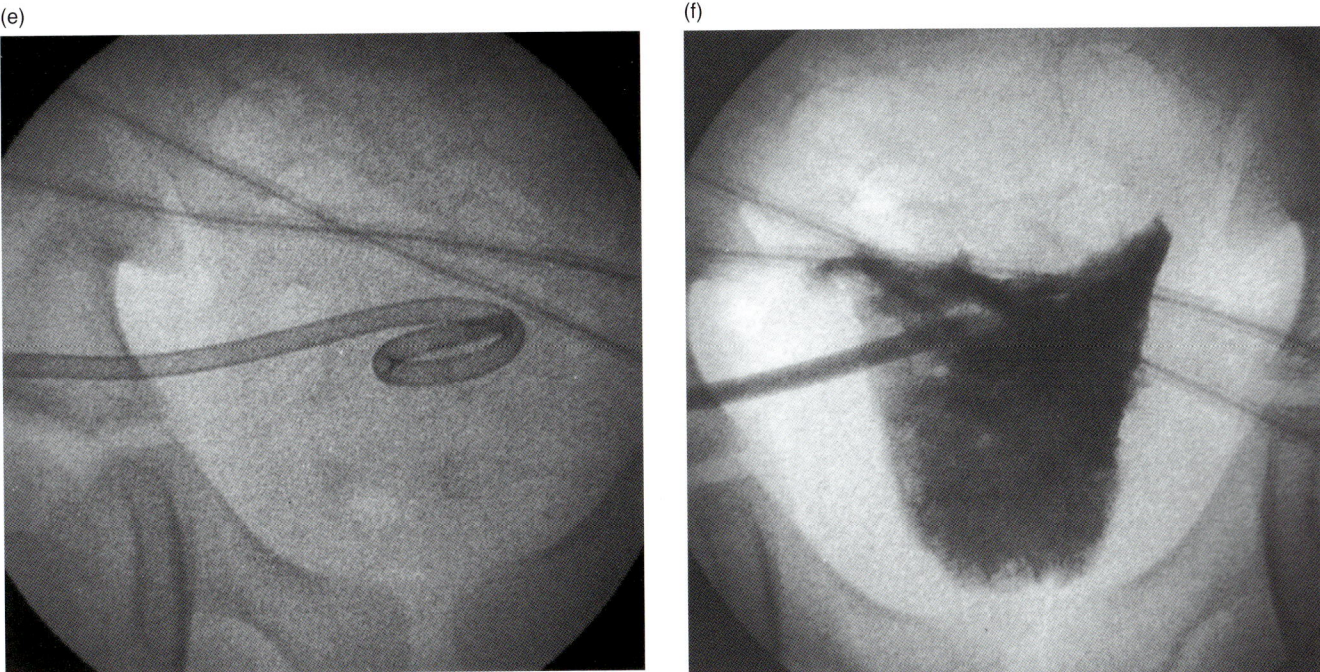

Figure 4.42 (cont.)

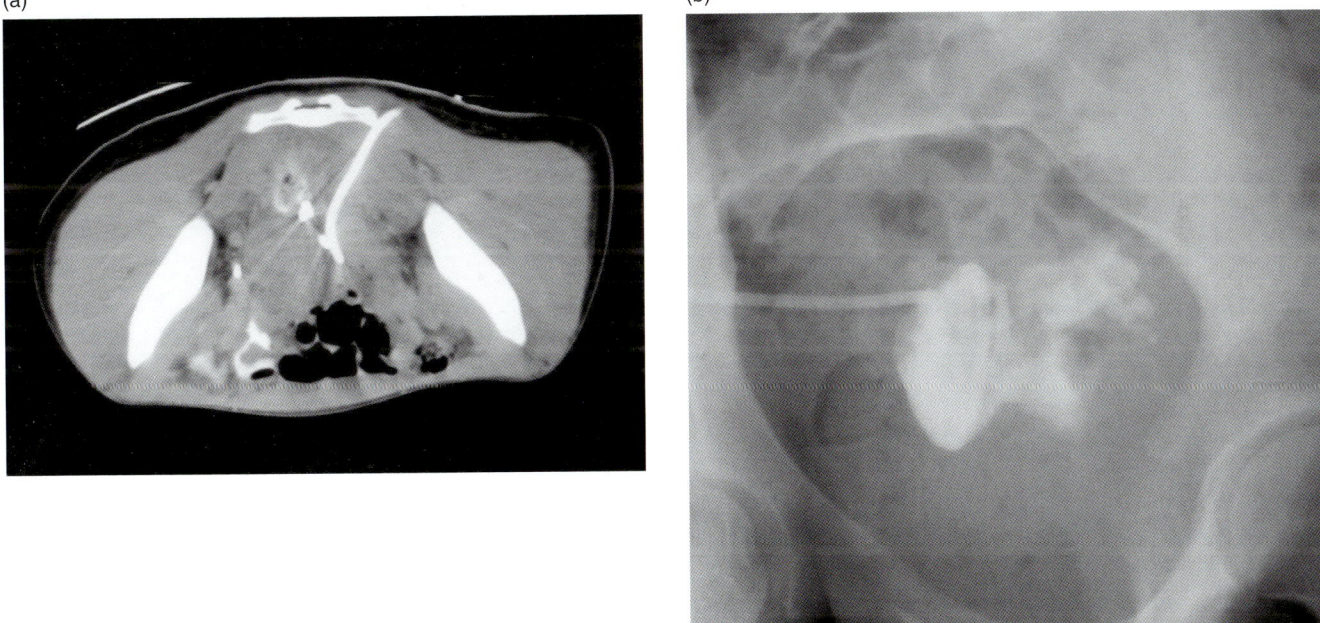

Figure 4.43 (a) Prone CT shows drainage of a pelvic abscess secondary to ruptured appendix in a 13-year-old girl. (b) A contrast fluoroscopic sinogram through the drainage catheter obtained several days later shows that the abscess is incompletely resolved.

and may reduce the morbidity of subsequent surgical intervention. In our experience enterocutaneous fistulae are extremely unlikely following percutaneous or transrectal drainage in children with IBD. One preexisting fistula did not resolve with percutaneous intervention alone.

Peri-appendiceal abscesses

Following acute appendicitis or ruptured appendiceal abscess, the high risk of recurrent abscesses and postoperative adhesions is a relative contraindication to immediate appendicectomy. As a result initial treatment with percutaneous drainage

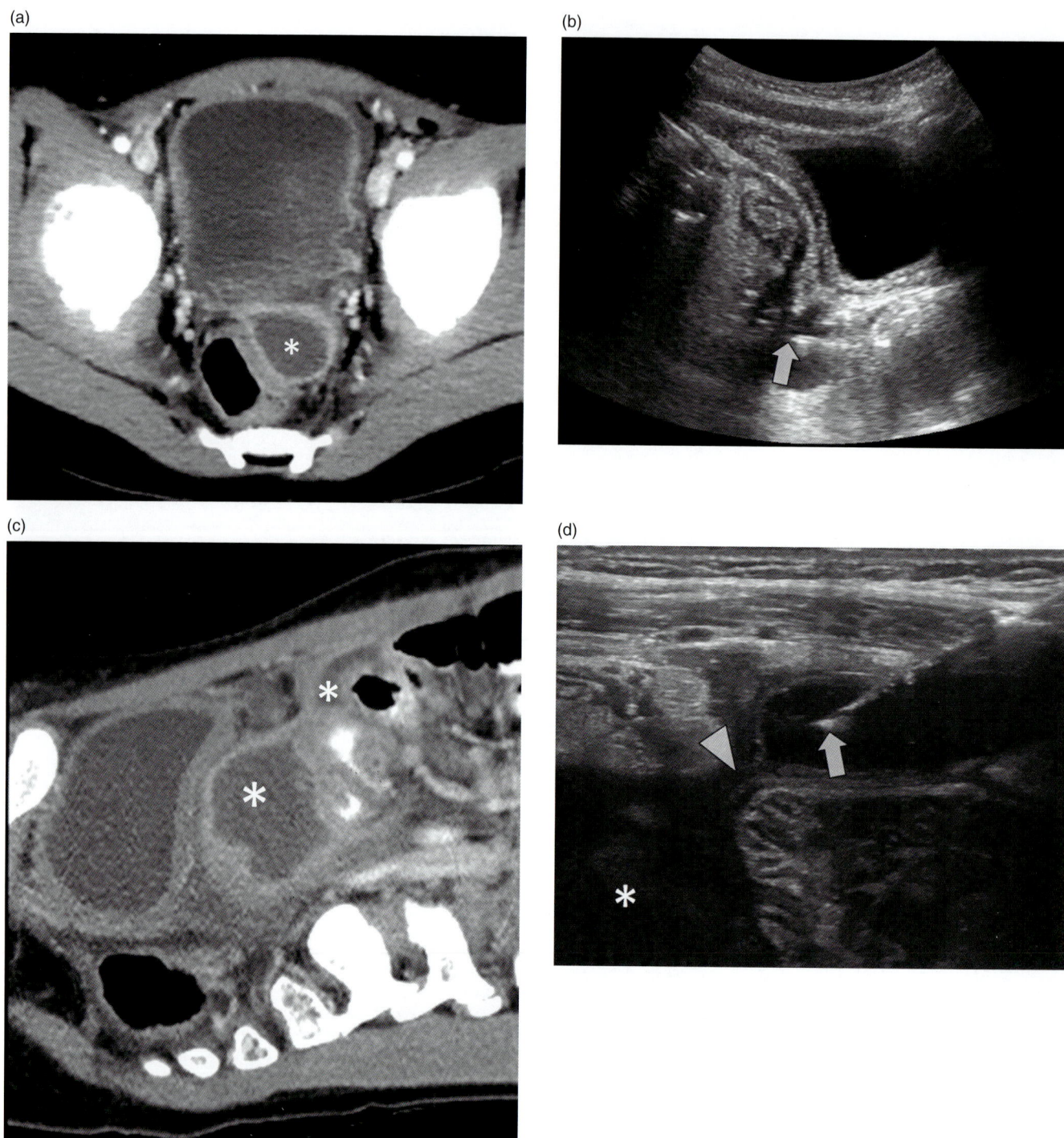

Figure 4.44 (a) Computed tomography with vascular contrast enhancement in a six-year-old male after appendectomy shows a 2.4 cm fluid collection (*asterisk*) with an enhancing wall between the rectum and the bladder. (b) With the patient in a left side down decubitus position, a 20 cm 22-gauge Chiba needle (*arrow*) was advanced through an enema tip used to protect the mucosa into the fluid collection under transabdominal US guidance. (c) A sagittal reconstruction of the CT shown in (a) demonstrates an abdominal fluid collection (*asterisks*) that extends from the anterior peritoneum between loops of bowel to the posterior pelvic wall. (d) After marking the inferior epigastric artery, a 5-French Yueh needle (*arrow*) was advanced percutaneously into the more superficial component of the abscess. A 0.035-inch stiff guide wire was advanced through the sheath and manipulated bluntly through the narrow channel (*arrowhead*) into the most gravity-dependent portion of the abscess (*asterisk*). (e) 8.5-French pigtail drains were placed, respectively, in the pelvic collection (*arrowhead*) and in the abdominal collection (*arrow*) as shown in this fluoroscopic image.

(e)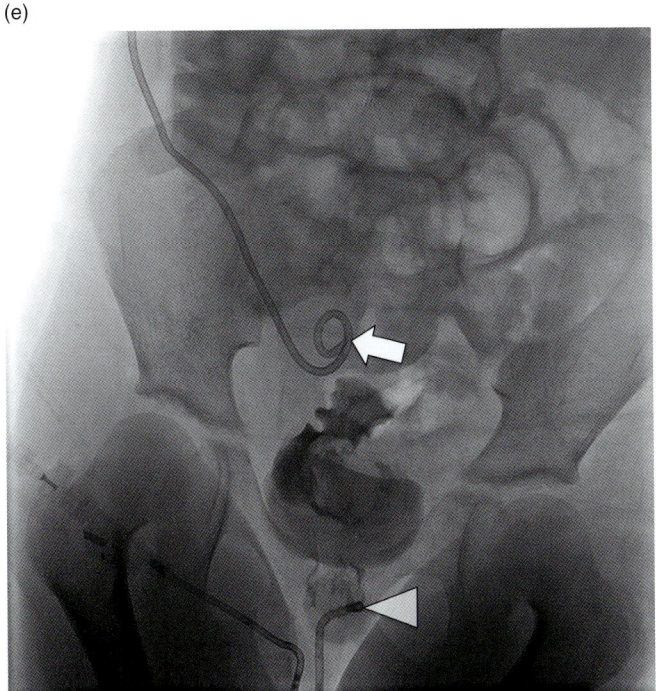

Figure 4.44 (cont.)

is the preferred treatment of localized collections presumed to be due to a ruptured appendix. It is helpful to prepare patients and families for the likelihood that additional abscesses may become apparent after antibiotics are discontinued despite appropriate treatment of all visualized abscesses after appendiceal rupture.

By their nature, interloop abscesses are surrounded by bowel and are often difficult to access or to drain completely. These children may require image-guided aspiration, several drains, repeated procedures and a good deal of patience to achieve success (Figure 4.45). In some instances surgical drainage is the preferred approach. Aspiration with a 20- or 22-gauge Chiba needle is an accepted treatment for collections that cannot be safely drained. If the location of a large interloop abscess is known from CT, this information can be used to guide percutaneous access under US control between loops of bowel using non-linear techniques. Similarly, collections that are not amenable to direct percutaneous access due to interposed vital structures may still be accessible under either US or CT using a curvilinear approach (see "Non-linear and curvilinear pathways," below).

Subphrenic and lesser sac collections

Subphrenic abscesses are usually seen as a postoperative complication or in children with a ruptured appendix. Because of lower cost and morbidity, a percutaneous rather than a surgical approach is preferred for drainage of these abscesses. They are often difficult to access and may require a transhepatic subcostal approach or an intercostal approach. In these cases the use of both US and CT guidance may be necessary to access these collections. Fluoroscopy may be needed for final tube placement. Seeding of the transhepatic tract and subsequent hepatic abscess formation is one of the possible complications of this procedure.

Fluid in the lesser sac is often associated with pancreatitis and is typically drained transgastrically (Figure 4.46), in a manner similar to pancreatic pseudocysts, as described below. If there is a clear window to the fluid collection under US, direct drainage or aspiration may be performed and is the preferred route. In some cases where access has been limited by surrounding structures transintestinal and transsplenic routes have been utilized. However, when possible these more complicated and risky approaches should be avoided.

Solid organ abscesses

Primary hepatic abscesses are uncommon in the pediatric population. However, pyogenic abscesses are most commonly seen in the immunocompromised patient, patients with chronic granulomatous disease, and following abdominal trauma. Occasionally, they complicate appendicitis (septic emboli), portal vein thrombosis, umbilical catheters in neonates, or liver infarction (as in sickle cell disease or tumor necrosis). Depending upon their size, pyogenic abscesses are aspirated or drained. Small lesions can be aspirated with a 22-gauge Chiba needle or small sheathed needle with US guidance. For larger collections, standard drainage technique is used with access under US guidance followed by contrast, guide wire placement, tract dilation, and drainage catheter insertion under fluoroscopy. Alternatively, a collection can be localized with CT, accessed and drained under US, then drainage can be confirmed with CT (Figure 4.47). Just as for liver biopsy, a choice of access route that interposes normal liver tissue between the liver capsule and the collection will help prevent hemorrhage and, in this case, intraperitoneal contamination.

Percutaneous drainage plays an important role in the management of children with infected collections occurring after liver transplantation. Retransplantation has been avoided in some children after successful drainage of infected bilomas secondary to hepatic arterial thrombosis. In the immunecompromised patient, focal microabscesses are often seen as a consequence of fungal infection. These are usually too small to allow for drainage but may be aspirated (or biopsied) for diagnostic purposes.

The multiloculated cysts with satellite cysts characteristically seen on CT (or by 3D-sonography) with *Echinococcus granulosa* infection are preferentially treated with antibiotics (albendazole) alone. The persistence of symptoms for greater than two weeks while on appropriate medical therapy is an indication for percutaneous management. Standard access technique is used to catheterize the cysts, and portions of the cyst fluid are exchanged with equal volumes of hypertonic saline until the entire cyst volume has been replaced. This replacement technique avoids intraperitoneal spillage of

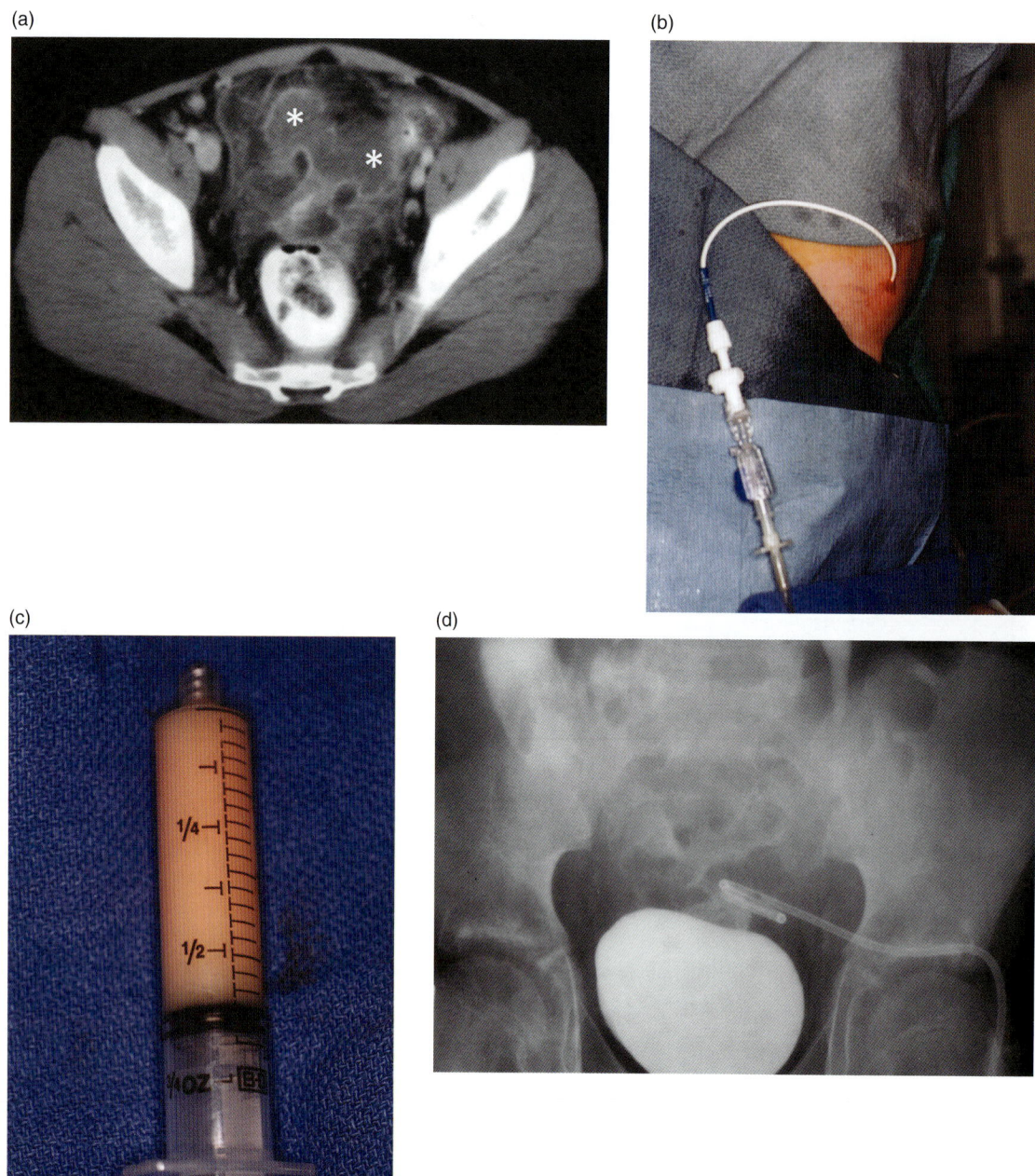

Figure 4.45 (a) Percutaneous CT through the pelvis obtained with vascular and enteric contrast shows multiple interloop abscesses (*asterisks*) as well as omental and bowel wall inflammatory changes in this nine-year-old boy after appendiceal rupture. (b) The external portions of the 7-French drain are seen projecting from the patient's flank. (c) Frank pus was aspirated from the abscesses with a creamy white to pale green color and foul odor characteristic of peri-appendiceal abscess. (d) These interloop abscesses were successfully resolved with a single percutaneous drain shown on this fluoroscopic image of the pelvis.

infected fluid during the procedure. At this point, the cyst is completely evacuated and left to gravity drainage. If the cyst is intact (without connection to the biliary tree) and greater than 5 cm in diameter, it may be helpful to sclerose the cyst lining with absolute alcohol or silver nitrate solution. Antibiotic therapy is continued for eight weeks or until the catheter is removed.

Patients who have immigrated from or traveled in underdeveloped areas, particularly in Africa, South America, and Asia are at increased risk for amebic liver abscesses. They present as single or lobulated masses, usually in the right lobe and are most often treated conservatively. Percutaneous drainage is indicated for failed antibiotic therapy or imminent rupture.

The optimum approach to splenic abscesses is controversial. There are concerns about the safety of trans-splenic percutaneous interventions. However, experience in both adult and pediatric patients suggests that percutaneous drainage of

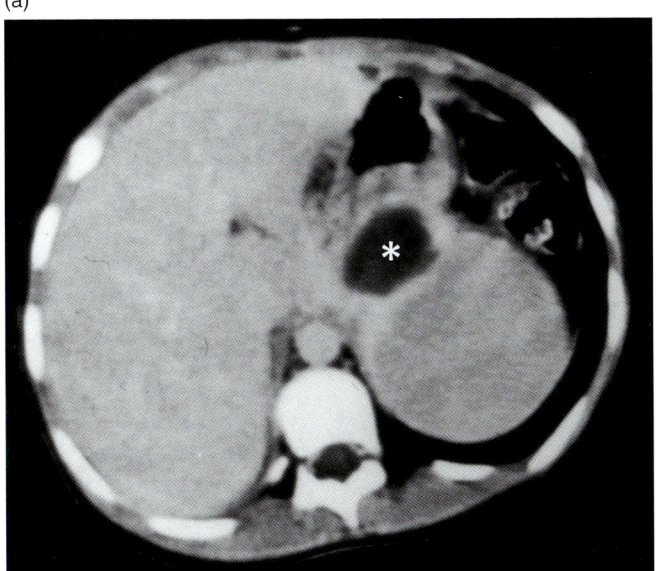 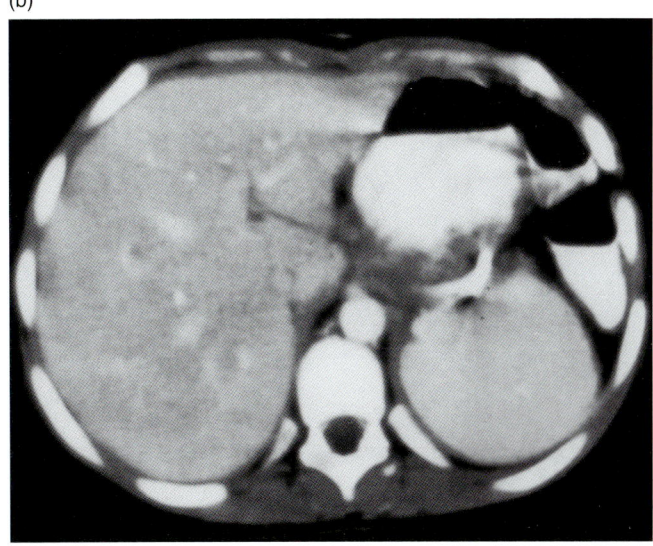

Figure 4.46 (a) Computed tomography with vascular and enteric contrast enhancement in a four-year-old after appendectomy shows a rim-enhancing fluid collection (*asterisk*) in the lesser sac. Compare this with the lack of contrast in Figures 4.49 and 4.50 that differentiates most pancreatic pseudocysts from abscess. (b) A postprocedure CT shows complete evacuation of the abscess through a percutaneous transgastric drain.

splenic abscesses can be performed safely and effectively. Percutaneous drainage offers the advantage of preserving splenic function, important for host immune response. Percutaneous aspiration may be indicated in any size collection in the spleen. Drainage with a catheter should be considered in a significantly sized lesion that is not complex and is not close to any large vascular structures (Figure 4.48).

Pancreatic pseudocyst drainage

Percutaneous drainage of pancreatic fluid collections is indicated in the case of infected, symptomatic, or persistent pseudocysts. Pancreatic phlegmon, peripancreatic necrosis, or the presence of pseudoaneurysms or varices are relative contraindications to percutaneous management.

Pancreatic abscesses are rare but may be seen, particularly in immune-compromised children. Depending on their size, position, and accessibility, they may be aspirated with a Chiba needle or drained. If small or difficult to access because of the deep position of the pancreas, aspiration is usually performed as the initial procedure. For larger pseudocysts drainage is preferred if an access route is available.

Pseudocysts usually develop as a result of acute pancreatitis from whatever cause. They may present as an upper abdominal mass, which appears hypoechoic on US, with or without debris. Computed tomography confirms the appearance of a low-density collection, which usually arises close to the pancreas in the region of the lesser sac (Figure 4.49). Clinically, most pseudocysts will resolve with bowel rest and parenteral nutrition. However, persistent symptomatic collections require treatment, preferably by transgastric or direct drainage. After defining the extent of the cyst on preprocedure CT, drainage is usually performed under combined US and fluoroscopic control. In some instances more than one catheter is needed for resolution of multiple, unconnected collections.

Pancreatic pseudocysts may be drained by a transgastric route (Figure 4.50). With the stomach deflated, the margins of the cyst are identified with US and marked on the skin. Next, the stomach is inflated and accessed (as for a percutaneous gastrostomy), and a retention suture and safety wire placed in the stomach. The stomach is now deflated and a second needle advanced through both walls of the stomach and into the pseudocyst itself. A sample of fluid is aspirated and some contrast is introduced to outline the extent of the cavity. After dilation of the tract a drainage catheter is inserted and left to gravity drainage. Contrast is injected once drainage ceases or symptoms resolve to redefine the extent of the pseudocyst(s) and to search for the presence of a fistula to the pancreatic duct. Normally, the catheter is left in position for at least six weeks to allow the tract between the stomach and the cyst to mature. This decreases the risk of enterocutaneous fistula formation by allowing the cyst to continue draining into the stomach until it resolves. If longer term drainage is required, a short "double-J" stent may be placed between the pseudocyst and the stomach to provide completely internalized drainage. When the pseudocyst has resolved, the stent can be snared and recovered transorally. Alternatively, a combined percutaneous–endoscopic approach may also be used for placement of an internal stent between the pseudocyst and the duodenum.

Renal cysts

Renal cysts are common in adults but rare in children. The incidence and size of simple renal cysts will increase as age advances, with approximately 5% by the fourth decade and

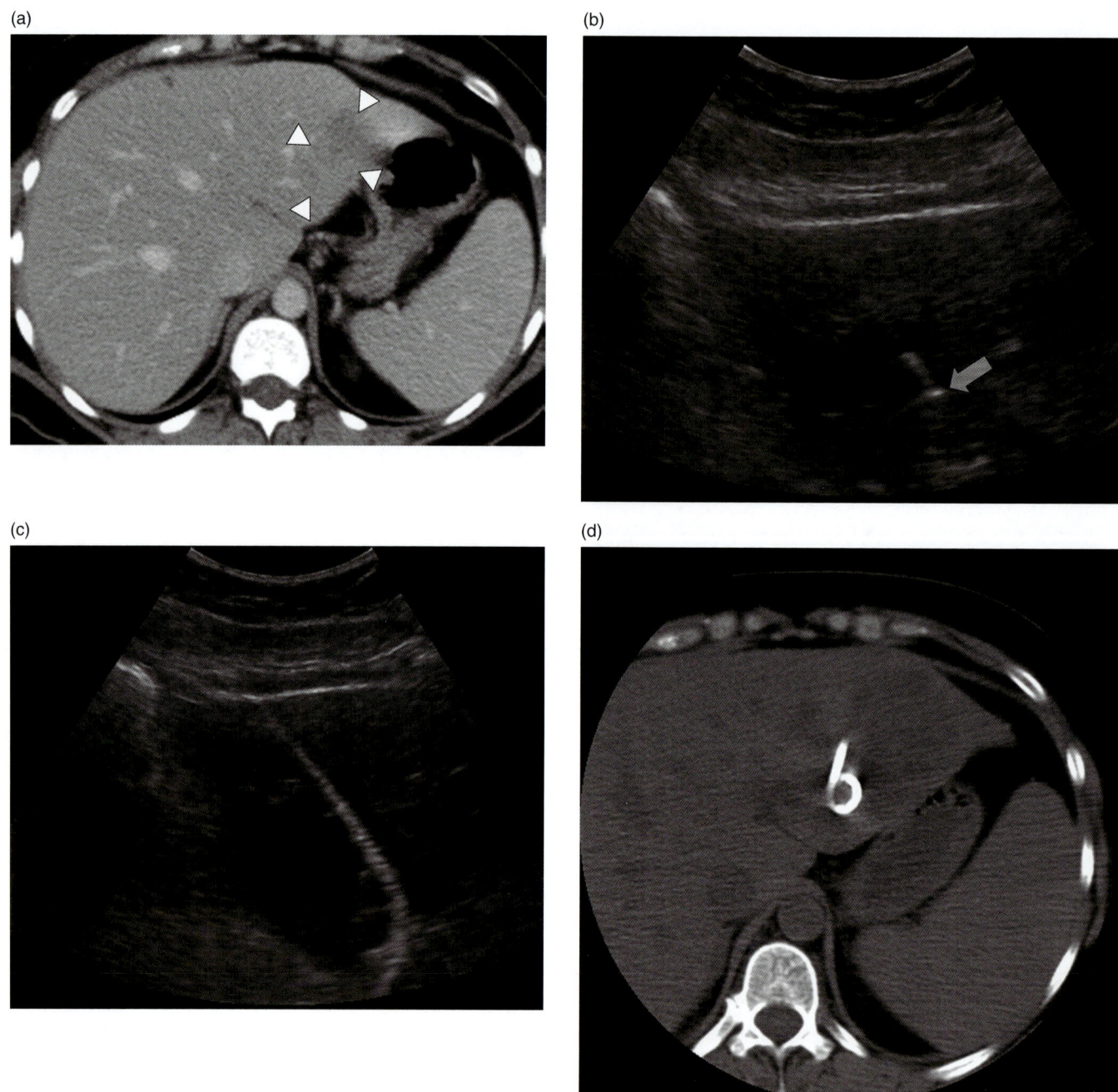

Figure 4.47 (a) A CT scan with vascular contrast enhancement shows a poorly defined avascular mass in segment three of the left lobe in this previously well 15-year-old female with abdominal pain and fever (*arrowheads*). (b) After localization with CT, US was used to define an abnormal fluid collection, and then to access the collection percutaneously with an 18-gauge Chiba Echotip® needle. Note the comet-tail artifact at the needle tip (*arrow*). (c) The insertion of a drainage catheter over a stiff guide wire was completed under US guidance in the CT suite. (d) Limited CT sections through the target region at the conclusion of the procedure and aspiration of frank pus confirmed appropriate location of the 8.5-French drainage catheter, limiting radiation dose.

over 35% by the eighth decade of life. In addition, cysts increase in both size and number, although the growth rate declines with time. The prevalence of simple cysts in children on routine screening US is significantly lower (much less than 0.5%), and may range in diameter from 3 mm to 7.0 cm. Most cysts are located in the right upper pole. In children, symptomatic cysts are rare. There are no data indicating how many incidentally discovered cysts will become symptomatic.

Associated symptoms that have been reported include pain, hematuria, ischemia, recurrent infection, obstructive uropathy, and hypertension.

The diagnosis of a benign renal cyst is usually made on the basis of the typical radiologic findings plus normal surrounding parenchyma, normal renal function, and absence of associated systemic illness or disease. In making the diagnosis of a simple renal cyst it is important to rule out a malignant or

Chapter 4 Abdominopelvic interventions

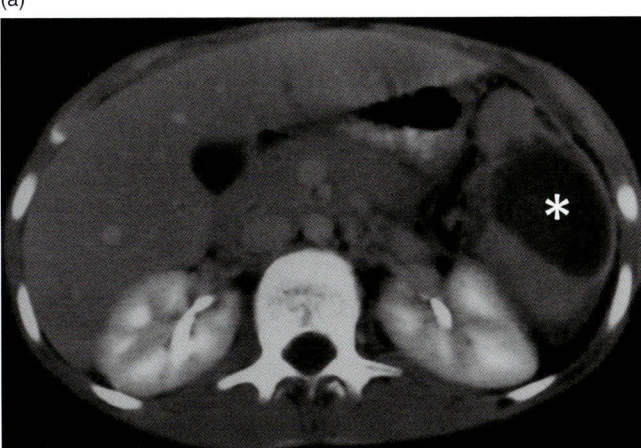

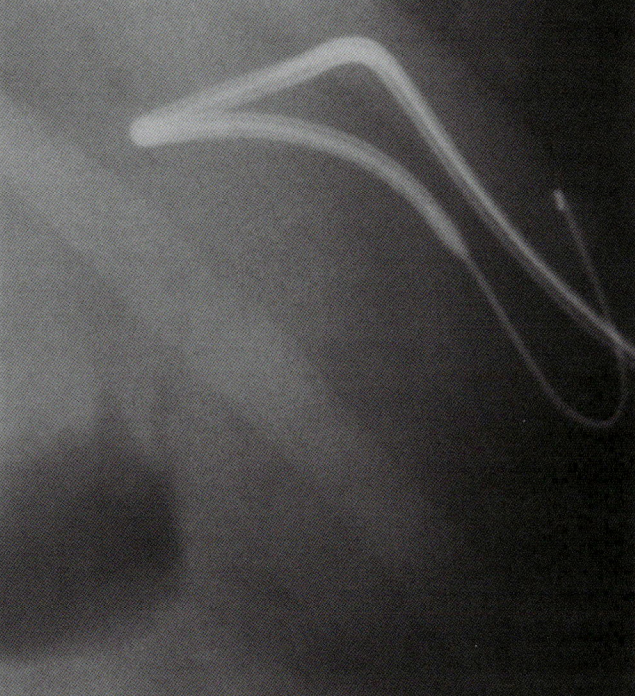

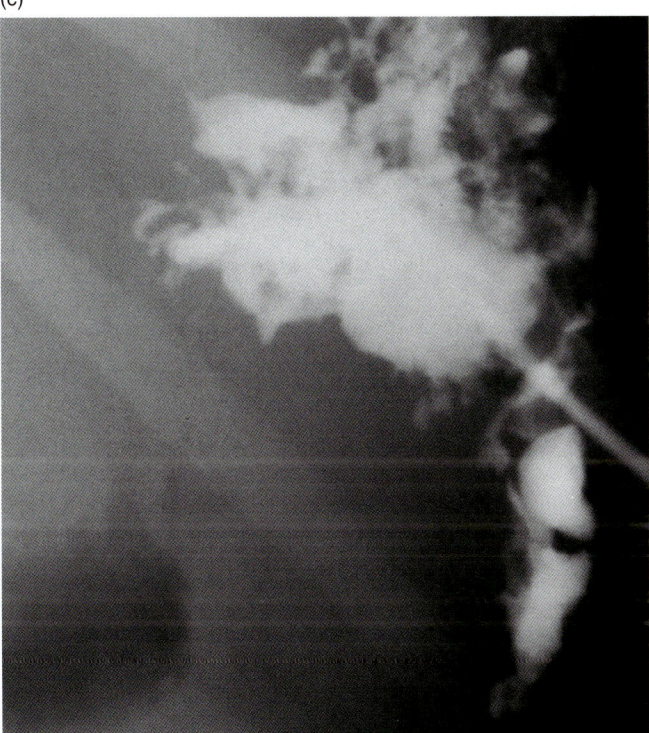

Figure 4.48 (a) A nine-year-old male presented with fever and left shoulder pain. A chest radiograph showed a sympathetic pleural effusion. Computed tomography with vascular and enteric contrast enhancement shows a low-attenuation splenic fluid collection (*asterisk*). (b) After US-guided percutaneous access, an 8-French drainage catheter is advanced over a stiffener and guide wire into the collection using fluoroscopic control. (c) Injection of contrast through the drain outlines the splenic abscess and fills the proximal descending colon via an enteric fistula. Both the abscess and the fistula resolved with this single drain.

aggressive process. Although this is of concern in adults because of the risk of cystic malignancy, the risk of a misdiagnosed malignancy in childhood is small. However, to minimize the risk of a misdiagnosis the interventionalist should keep in mind the imaging features of a benign renal cyst. The differential diagnosis of a cystic renal mass in a child consists of polycystic disease, tuberous sclerosis, cystic duplication, cystic Wilms tumor, and previously treated malignancy.

Treatment is usually reserved for children with symptoms thought to be the result of the renal cyst. The treatment options that are currently available are open surgical ablation, laparoscopic cyst ablation, retrograde marsupialization, flexible ureteroscopy and nephroscopy, and percutaneous aspiration with or without sclerotherapy.

Surgical treatment of a simple cyst may include decortication, marsupialization of the cyst, hemi-nephrectomy or a complete nephrectomy. The advantage of the surgical approach is that it allows direct visualization of the pathology. Thus if there is any doubt of the correct diagnosis a biopsy can be obtained and the proper procedure performed based on the pathologic diagnosis. In addition, other pathology or problems can be taken care of during the same operative procedure. Unfortunately, the perioperative complication rate is approximately 33% making effective alternatives desirable. The

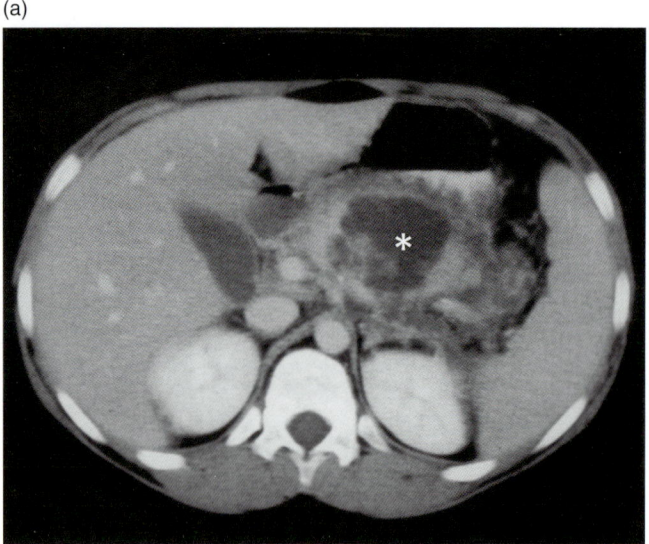 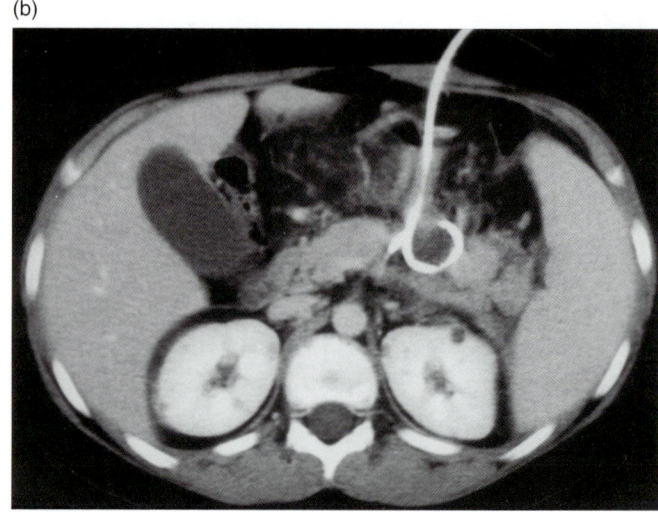

Figure 4.49 (a) Computed tomography with vascular and enteric contrast enhancement shows a non-enhancing lesser sac complex pseudocyst (*asterisk*) in a 12-year-old boy with hyperparathyroidism. (b) The pancreatic pseudocyst resolved after prolonged transgastric drainage, but an associated pancreatic duct fistula required surgical repair.

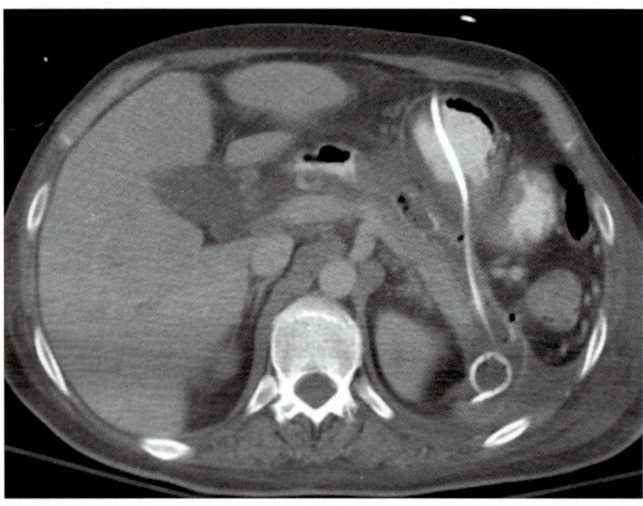

Figure 4.50 This CT section with enteric contrast enhancement was obtained at the conclusion of percutaneous transgastric drainage catheter insertion. The Cope loop is positioned in the most gravity-dependent component of the pancreatic tail pseudocyst. If, as is often the case, prolonged drainage is required, the catheter can be exchanged for a double-J catheter for direct enteric drainage of the pseudocyst.

perioperative complications include wound infection, problems associated with immobilization, urinary retention, atelectasis, pneumonia, and venous thrombosis. In addition, the procedure has significant postoperative pain and a relatively long convalescence.

Retrograde marsupialization and flexible ureteroscopy and nephroscopy is a less invasive alternative than open surgery. As a result the postoperative morbidity is minimized. However, there are several disadvantages to this approach including a moderate to high degree of technical difficulty, an ability to treat only peri-pelvic cysts and not exophytic cysts, a limited endoscopic view of the internal cyst wall, creation of a large nephrostomy tract and the need for a stent postoperatively, associated pain and discomfort, a potential for electrolyte disturbance secondary to the large volume of infusate used during the procedure, and the need for a second procedure to remove the ureteral stent.

Laparoscopic cyst ablation has the advantage of minimal postprocedural pain, no significant scarring, minimal blood loss, and a short hospital stay. This approach allows treatment of multiple renal cysts at the same operation including peripelvic and exophytic cysts, without the need for stents and drains at the completion of the procedure. Disadvantages of this approach include longer procedure times, need for expensive equipment and significant technical expertise, risk of injury to bowel and other organs, limited long-term results, and misdiagnosis of a benign cyst as a malignancy. A prospective comparison of laparoscopic surgery and percutaneous therapy (see below) has not yet been performed, but would be helpful in more clearly defining the role of these minimally invasive approaches.

Image-guided percutaneous aspiration with or without injection of a sclerosant has an extremely high technical success rate and may be the least invasive alternative. With US or CT guidance, one or more cysts can be selected and accurately entered with a needle or small catheter. Once within the cyst cavity a sterile sample of the fluid can be obtained for laboratory and microbiology analysis. If desired, contrast material can be exchanged for cyst fluid and the internal anatomy of the cyst examined.

At the same procedure the cyst can be treated by either complete aspiration or sclerotherapy. At this time there are several sclerosing agents that can be used including absolute alcohol, hypertonic saline, minocycline, tetracycline, sodium tetradecyl sulfate, sodium morhullate, Betadine®, acetic acid, talc, glue, and Ethibloc®. Unfortunately, there are no prospective studies available to guide us as to what is the best agent. At this time our preference is dehydrated alcohol. In general the results are somewhat disappointing with complete cyst ablation in approximately 10% of cases and reduction in size in another 30 to 40%. If the cyst is still present but the patient is asymptomatic the therapy is considered a success and the patient is observed and followed. If the cyst remains symptomatic, sclerotherapy sessions may be repeated for two consecutive days, followed by a period of two to three weeks' observation to evaluate effect.

The main disadvantage of percutaneous therapy is the relatively high recurrence rate of over 50%. In addition, recurrent pain in the early phase of recovery occurs in approximately 15% of patients, with an 8% rate of other complications including cyst hemorrhage.

The equipment needed to perform a cyst aspiration and sclerotherapy is minimal and depends upon the interventionalist's preference, and, if sclerotherapy is to be performed, the agent to be infused. In most cases the cyst is punctured using US guidance and on occasion CT guidance. The needles utilized are most often a 22- or 23-gauge Chiba needle or a sheathed (e.g., Yueh) needle.

Depending on the approach selected the interventionalist may choose to drain the cyst before sclerosant is injected and later drain out the material. In these cases either the sheath can be left in position or the needle exchanged for a guide wire, the tract dilated, and a drainage catheter (locking pigtail) is inserted. In these cases the guide wire selection is most important.

If a floppy-tipped guide wire is selected one must be careful to ensure that the entire floppy segment can coil inside the cyst cavity so that the stiff portion of the guide wire is used to enlarge the tract. If the floppy segment is left crossing the cyst wall it may be difficult or impossible to gain catheter access to the cyst. If the child is large or obese it is helpful to use a stiffer guide wire. Thus several guide wire types should be available. The tract is dilated with standard dilators to the size of the catheter.

Finally, the catheter chosen is usually a standard pigtail ranging in size from 5 to 8.5 French. It is important to keep in mind that the larger the drainage catheter the larger the hole in the cyst wall will be when the catheter is removed. This may be a source of hemorrhage into the abdominal or retroperitoneal spaces, or of leakage and potential injury to the tissues adjacent to the hole.

There is more than one approach that may be safely and successfully utilized. When the goal is simply aspiration of the cyst contents to acquire fluid for laboratory analysis a 22- or 23-gauge Chiba needle or sheathed needle can be utilized. An entry site is selected on the skin surface after US examination. The most direct route to the cyst is selected whenever possible. The skin is marked and the site is prepared and draped in sterile fashion. The entry site is locally anesthetized with a 30-gauge, 1.5-inch needle using 1% buffered lidocaine and a small incision is made with a #10 scalpel blade. Using freehand technique the needle is advanced into the cyst. The stylet is removed and the needle is connected to connecting tubing and a fluid sample obtained using sterile technique. The cyst is emptied until drainage stops and the needle is removed.

If the goal of the procedure is sclerosis of the cyst a sheathed needle is used. Once the cyst has been entered, only the minimum necessary amount of fluid is removed for culture and laboratory analysis so that the cyst does not collapse. In the usual case a glide wire is inserted and coiled within the cyst while monitoring with fluoroscopy. The needle is then exchanged for a vascular dilator and the tract enlarged and a small drainage catheter is inserted. In children who weigh less than 10 kg a 5- to 6-French drain is used while in those more than 10 kg a 6- to 8.5-French drain might be used.

When the catheter is secured the cyst fluid is drained completely before the sclerosant is injected. Initial volume of alcohol should be at least half the volume of the cyst, to a maximum of 1 ml/kg or less than 50 ml total. Regardless of the agent selected the child is positioned so that the entire cyst wall is exposed to the sclerosant with the hope of destroying the cyst wall and preventing continued secretion of fluid. In theory, the longer the contact between the cyst wall and the alcohol the lower the likelihood of recurrence, so the sclerosant is kept in the cyst for about one to four hours before being allowed to drain. A second injection may be given within a 48-hour period to reduce the possibility of recurrence and is similar to our recommendations for treatment of perinephric lymphoceles (see below). This approach can be used to treat other forms of renal cystic disease such as adult polycystic kidney disease or cysts of other solid organs such as the spleen.

At the completion of the treatment the drain is removed and a dry sterile dressing placed. If no problems or complications have occurred the child is discharged home after an additional 30 to 60 minutes of observation. If a second procedure is desired the patient is either admitted or scheduled to return the next day. In these individuals the drain is left in place and covered to maintain sterility and reduce the chance of inadvertent removal.

Pain in the early phase of recovery occurs in approximately 15% of patients. Acquired stricture of the uretero-pelvic junction (UPJ) secondary to injury by the sclerosant has been reported in as many as 2% of cases and the overall rate of major and minor complications is reported to be 1.4% and 10%, respectively. Other risks include renal or peri-renal hemorrhage, extravasation of urine or sclerosant, injury of adjacent structures, and technical misadventures. While not a complication, some patients note slight inebriation when treated with alcohol as a sclerosant.

Cholecystic and pericholecystic collections

See Chapter 5.

Technical variations

Sclerotherapy and lymphocele drainage

Lymphoceles are most commonly seen in renal transplant patients, and may result in impaired graft function or infection. Many asymptomatic lymphoceles resolve without intervention. Of the lymphoceles we have treated since 1991, approximately half required percutaneous aspiration or drainage, and a quarter were treated with transcatheter sclerosis with tetracycline, ethanol, povidone-iodine, or a combination. Although these patients often require treatment over a period of months to years, they are usually able to avoid surgery. Frequent (two to three times per week) instillation of sclerosants may help obliterate the cavity more quickly. No complications, other than pain, were associated with percutaneous treatment in our experience.

Abscess drainage in high-risk populations

Hepatic abscess is a known but rarely reported complication associated with umbilical venous catheter (UVC) placement and from hematogenous spread. Umbilical venous catheters are used almost routinely in very low birthweight (<1,000 g) infants. Regardless of etiology, percutaneous treatment of hepatic abscesses, even in very low birthweight infants, can be performed safely, with gentle technique and small (5- or 6- to 8.3-French) catheters, and may represent a desirable alternative to conservative treatment.

Successful percutaneous management of fluid associated with a hematoma or necrotic tumor, especially if infected, is usually not achievable. Instillation of a thrombolytic agent (such as tissue plasminogen activator) as adjuvant therapy in the management of an uninfected hematoma may increase the likelihood of success.

The presence of a foreign body within a collection may result in recurrent abscess formation. Nevertheless, percutaneous drainage should be regarded as first-line therapy, in close consultation with the referring clinician. Infected collections associated with VP shunts may be aspirated percutaneously or drained surgically. The VP shunt is then surgically re-sited.

Non-linear and curvilinear pathways

When a collection is visualized with cross-sectional imaging but intervening structures such as the bony pelvis, bowel loops, vessels, or other vital structures do not allow a direct percutaneous pathway to be defined, a non-linear or curvilinear approach may be successful. In the non-linear method, the access needle is advanced under real-time guidance beyond the intervening structure at risk. At this point, the needle may be redirected toward the target, levering the intervening structure out of the way with the needle shaft. The pathway should be planned so that there is less than 30 degrees between the initial path and the final path to avoid bending the needle or kinking the drainage catheter. If needed, needles with exchangeable blunt stylets are available. Once the target collection is entered, the needle is exchanged for a stiff guide wire, and the procedure is completed according to the usual method. If a catheter will be left *in situ* at the conclusion of the procedure, care should be taken to assure that the vital structure is not injured or incapacitated due to compression by the catheter shaft, although there is usually enough flexibility in the drainage catheter that this is unlikely to be a problem.

The curvilinear method involves curving the access needle to match a path that preprocedure cross-sectional imaging indicates will allow the needle to be advanced from the skin to the target structure without transgressing important intervening structures (Figure 4.51). It is important to note that manufacturers in general do not recommend post-market curving of needles, and that such use may fall outside approved use of the device. The needle should be curved into a smooth and continuous arc, with the bevel facing away from the center of the arc. If the bevel faces any other direction it will tend to drive the needle out of the access plane, or to progressively flatten the arc that the needle follows. Compound curves are generally not useful. Once the needle curve has been formed, the operator should assure that the stylet moves easily (or that the needle fires properly, if a semi-automated biopsy needle is curved). The curved needle should be held in plane with the tip perpendicular to the skin entry point, and advanced in-plane, taking care to allow the needle to follow its own curve. Advancement of the needle should be monitored with frequent cross-sectional images as intervening structures are approached and passed, until the needle enters the target. Very little adjustment of the needle's trajectory will be possible during advancement. If the needle veers more than a little off course, it is usually best to withdraw the needle almost completely, redirect the needle, then re-advance. This method has been used to safely, accurately, and successfully access targets deep in the pelvis and anterior to the spine in locations usually inaccessible to percutaneous techniques. If this method is used to access a target that can be visualized with fluoroscopy, simultaneous biplane imaging can also facilitate success (e.g., Figures 2.28d–e).

Postprocedure and follow-up care

Analgesia is provided in the form of intravenous ketorolac (0.5 mg/kg IV followed by a bolus of 1 mg/kg each six hours or continuous infusion of 0.17 mg/kg/h, to a maximum of 90 mg per day, for no more than two days) or morphine sulfate (0.05 mg/kg every four hours for 24 hours), followed by oral acetaminophen (15 mg/kg every three to four hours as needed). The patient is allowed to ambulate as tolerated. Clear fluids are initially given until the patient has normal bowel movements and bowel sounds. The drainage catheter is left to gravity drainage or to a Jackson–Pratt type suction device (see Figure 3.9). A three-way valve is usually placed on the catheter system. Depending on the type of drainage, saline lavage of the cavity (5 to 10 ml, three to four times per day) followed by gentle irrigation (5 ml of normal saline flushed through the tube after aspiration of the lavaged fluid, two to three times a

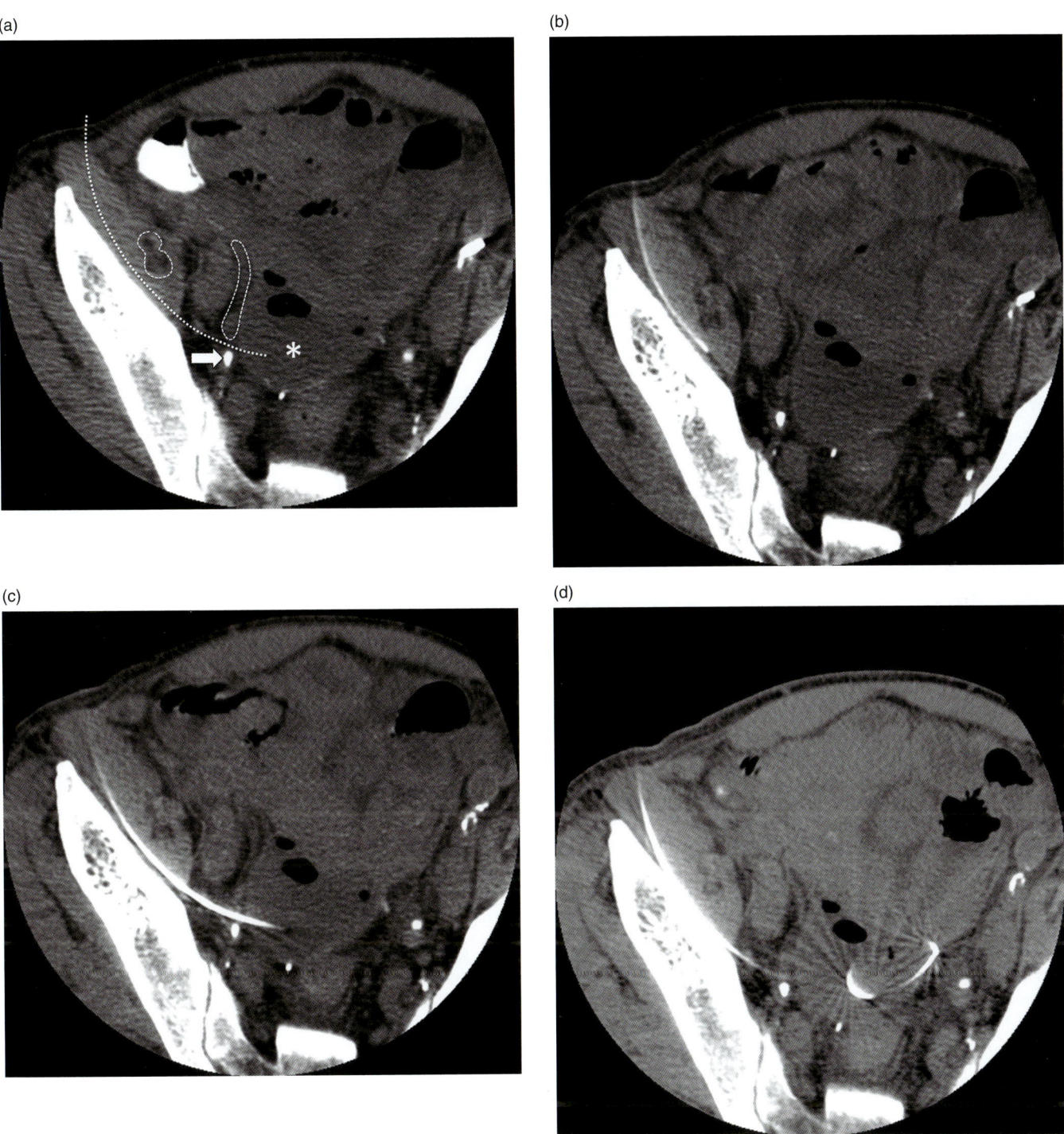

Figure 4.51 (a) A CT section in a 17-year-old male shows a postoperative fluid collection (*asterisk*) surrounded by bony pelvis and fluid-filled loops of bowel. The ureter (*arrow*) and neurovascular structures (*dashed regions*) are along a direct route between skin and the collection. The target lesion is too high in the pelvis for a transrectal or transgluteal approach. A safe curved pathway was calculated from the skin through the iliacus muscle to the collection. (b,c) The calculated pathway was used to prepare a curved 18-gauge needle, which was advanced in a stepwise fashion, maintaining the needle within the imaging plane, until the needle entered the collection and a small amount of pus was aspirated. (d) Once the needle tip was within the collection, the floppy tip of a super stiff guide wire was coiled within it. (e) This CT topogram shows the 8-French drainage catheter *in situ* in the right pelvis. (f) Injection of contrast through the drainage catheter shows complete evacuation of the abscess, but also shows an enteric fistula to adjacent bowel. The abscess and fistula resolved uneventfully, and the catheter was removed a week later without recurrence.

(e) 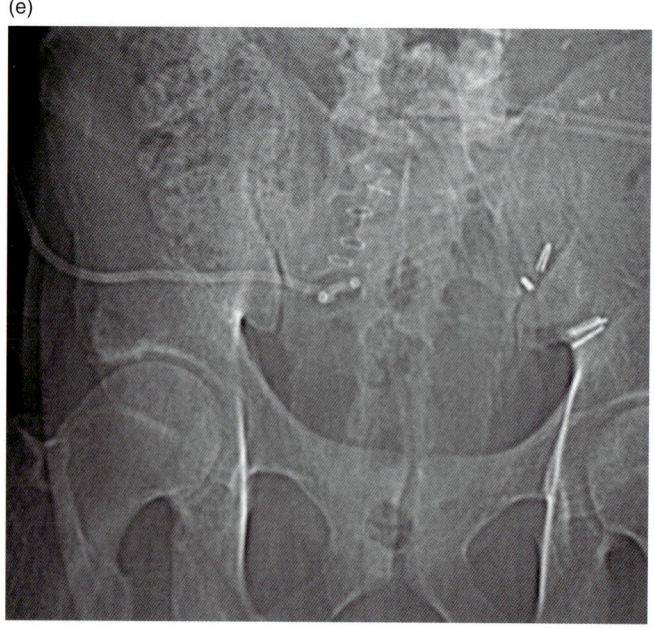 (f)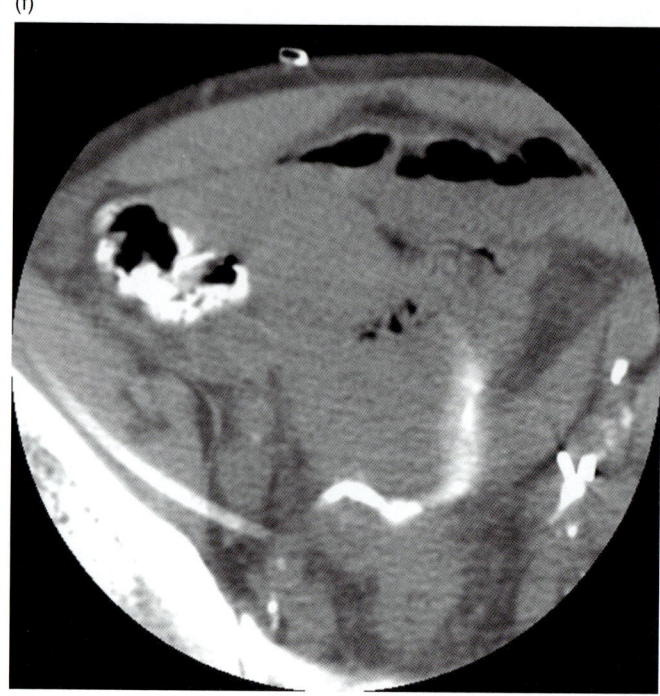

Figure 4.51 (cont.)

day) may be performed. The volume of output from the tube, less irrigant, is recorded each shift.

Specimen handling

Fluid samples obtained at initial access should be placed in a sterile container and transferred immediately to the microbiology laboratory for distribution, special stains, and preparation for culture. In most cases, the decision to drain a collection is made on the basis of size, location, and visual appearance of the fluid. For this reason, an immediate Gram stain may be reserved for particularly difficult or hazardous cases, where the diagnosis remains in doubt after initial aspiration. If no fluid is obtained a small amount of non-bacteriostatic saline may be infiltrated through the needle to lavage the suspected site of infection. Any fluid then aspirated should be sent to the laboratory in the syringe in a sealed sterile container. Additionally, biopsy specimens from the region of the "dry" tap may be obtained for pathologic analysis. Not all dry taps are undrainable, and a large-bore catheter combined with a lytic adjuvant (such as tissue plasminogen activator) may assist drainage of symptomatic viscous fluid collections including thick pus and maturing hematoma.

Catheter fixation and drainage

Once having secured access to the collection with a guide wire, the tract is enlarged with an appropriate series of fascial dilators. Lubricant (sterile mineral oil, silicone oil, or Surgilube®) may be used to assist passage of the dilator. After successful dilatation, a drainage catheter appropriate to the size, viscosity, and location of the collection is inserted under fluoroscopic guidance with a stiffener. Catheters range in size from as small as 5-French up to 22-French. For simple non-viscous fluid drainage an 8-, 10-, or 12-French locking pigtail catheter with side holes is usually used. For a larger or more viscous collection, a sump or Thal-Quick drain can be used. The stiffener is released from the catheter as it enters the collection and the catheter is advanced so all side holes lie within the collection.

Most catheters used for this purpose have an internal locking mechanism that is secured, and the catheter is connected to an abscess drainage system. The catheter is fixed in position by a Stat-Lock® or SorbaView® shield and not sutured to the skin. In our experience sutures are not long lasting and predispose to skin infection.

Catheter removal

In children without an impairment of healing, symptoms should resolve substantially within three to five days following catheter placement. If symptoms persist or worsen, the collection continues to drain or a contrast study reveals a fistula, further investigation is needed (Figure 4.52). Specifically, a search should be conducted for evidence of undiagnosed or undrained collections, an associated fistula to bowel or other hollow viscus organs (Figure 4.53), foreign bodies, distal obstruction, or undiagnosed tumor that could account for continued symptoms or drainage. If imaging studies cannot document clear resolution, the catheter may be clamped for

Chapter 4 Abdominopelvic interventions

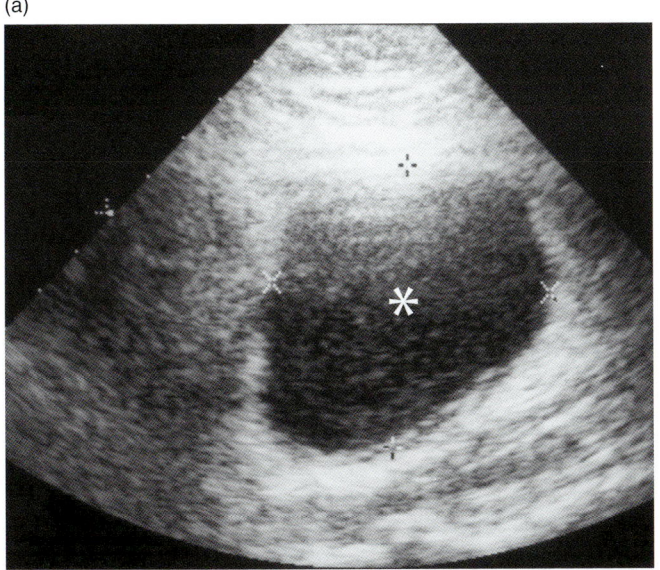
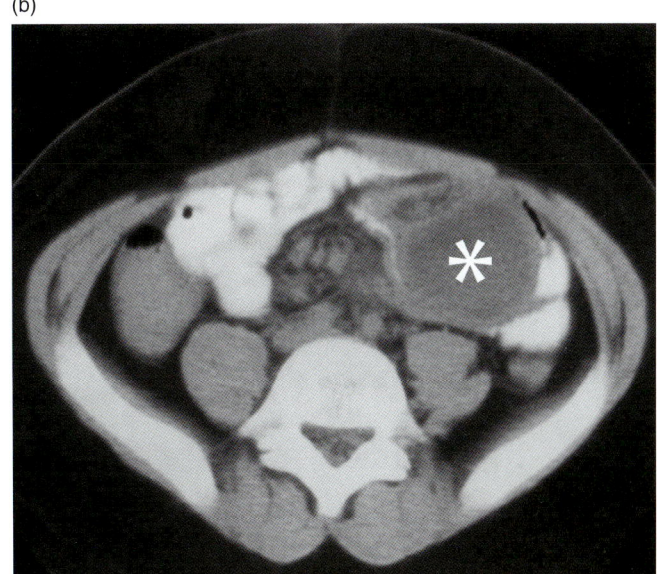
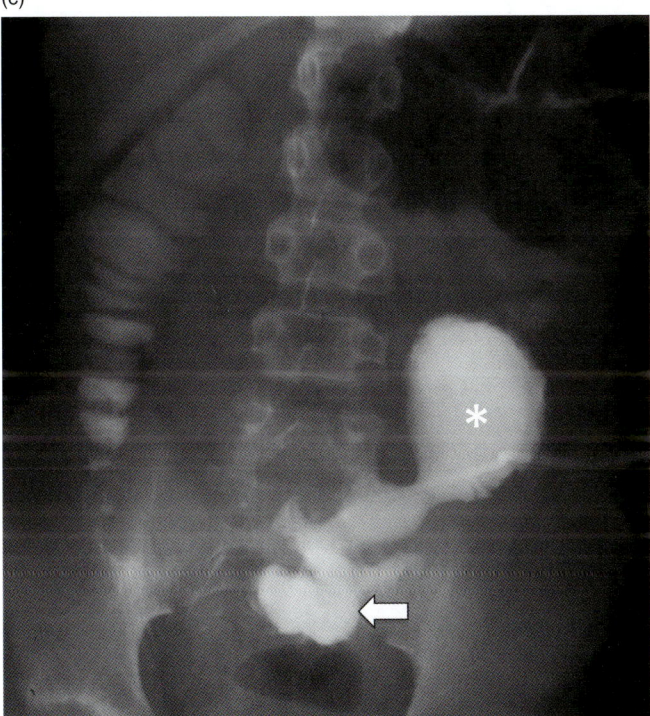

Figure 4.52 (a) After appendectomy, an eight-year-old boy developed recurrent fever and diffuse abdominal pain. Computed tomography with enteric contrast enhancement shows a right paracolic gutter low attenuation mass (*asterisk*). (b) Ultrasound confirmed the diagnosis of abscess (*asterisk*), and was used to guide percutaneous access. (c) Fluoroscopy was used to guide completion of drainage catheter insertion. Injection of contrast shows that the Cope loop (*arrow*) of the drainage catheter has migrated through an enteric fistula from the abscess (*asterisk*) into a loop of bowel. The catheter was pulled back into the abscess cavity, and both the abscess and the fistula resolved without further event.

one to several days to evaluate for reaccumulation prior to removal.

Progress may be assessed at 48 to 72 hours with US. If the patient is asymptomatic, laboratory parameters (e.g., white cell counts) are returning to normal, negligible outputs are recorded from the catheter and imaging (usually US) shows resolution of the collection, no further examinations are required and the catheter can be removed. Most drainage failures are mechanical, attributed to undrained collections, catheter blockage or kinking, poor catheter position, or early removal of the catheter. Specific orders should be left not to remove the catheter without consulting the interventional service.

Technical problems and pitfalls

Perhaps the most serious complications that occur during or following drainage procedures result from inadvertent transgression of non-target structures, such as vessels or bowel. Unless a collection is superficial and not in proximity to known vessels, it is reasonable to review the region if a recent contrast study is available, or to evaluate the prospective tract

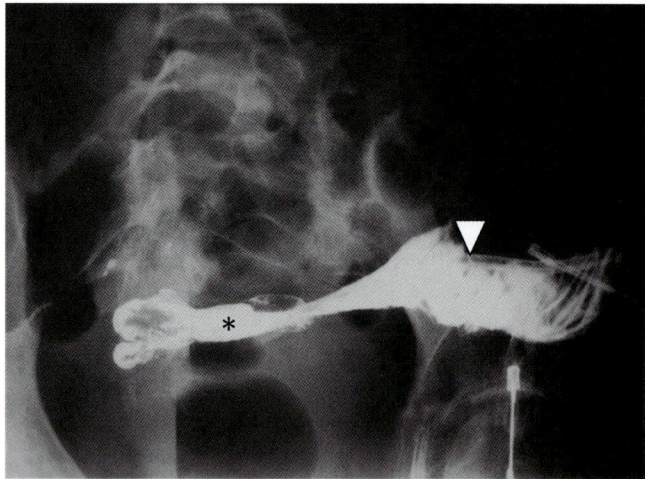

Figure 4.53 Injection of contrast through a drainage catheter placed in a left lower quadrant abscess (*arrowhead*) in a six-year-old female demonstrates a fistula to left Fallopian tube with contrast filling the immature uterus (*asterisk*).

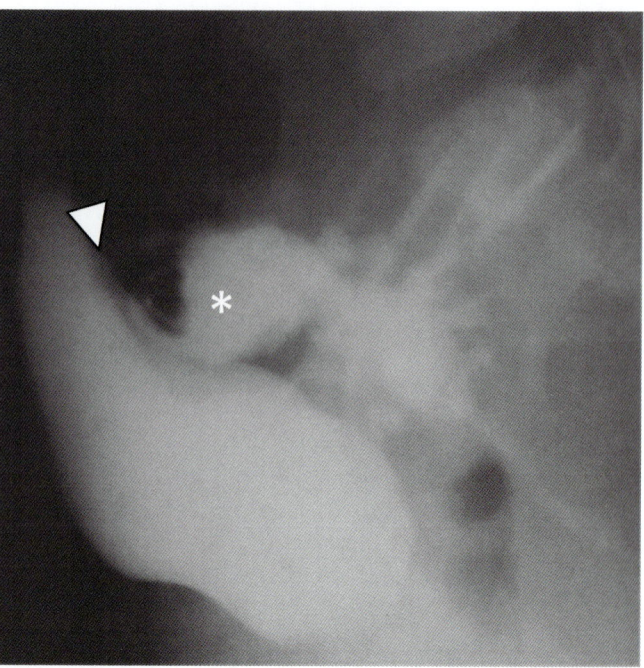

Figure 4.54 On a lateral radiograph of the pelvis, a percutaneous drainage catheter projects with its Cope loop (*asterisk*) formed in an upper pelvic abscess. The catheter shaft (*arrowhead*) transgresses the superior aspect of the urinary bladder. The drainage catheter was left *in situ* for three weeks, until the abscess had resolved and the transcystic tract had matured. The catheter was first withdrawn into the bladder lumen, then a few days later was withdrawn completely without sequelae.

with color Doppler US. Vessels known to pose risk, such as the epigastric artery, can be marked or monitored in real-time at the time of initial access.

Bowel loops can pose a more difficult problem. They shift with changes in patient position and move with peristalsis, so their position on preoperative imaging cannot be relied upon. Additionally, when decompressed and hypoactive they can be very difficult to identify despite concerted effort. The risk of bowel perforation or transgression should be prospectively discussed as part of the consent process for almost any abdominopelvic procedure. In the event that inadvertent bowel transgression is discovered after the tract is dilated or the drainage catheter is placed, access should not be removed precipitously. The drainage catheter should be left in place until the enterocutaneous tract has matured, at which time it can usually be removed without ill effect. Such catheters rarely pose risk of bowel obstruction. However, if this or other concerns warrant, the tube may be surgically removed with concurrent repair of the iatrogenic enterostomy.

Complications

Complications of percutaneous drainage are infrequent and usually minor. Fever shortly after initial drainage may represent bacteremia as a result of manipulation or lavage, especially of an immature abscess cavity. Severe hemorrhage occurs infrequently and is either related to unsuspected coagulopathy, laceration of a vessel or pseudoaneurysm related to pancreatic inflammation. Transgression of the pleural space during percutaneous drainage of subphrenic, hepatic, or splenic collections may result in pneumothorax, hemothorax, pyothorax, or empyema. It is possible to contaminate other spaces, by traversing them during drainage, such as the subphrenic and subhepatic spaces during drainage of a hepatic abscess.

Similarly, generalized peritonitis may develop due to perforation of an abscess cavity. Rarely, bowel perforation or transgression of other non-target structures (Figure 4.54) may occur at the time of initial puncture (see "Technical problems and pitfalls," above) or due to catheter erosion. Overall, morbidity associated with image-guided percutaneous drainage is significantly lower than with operative drainages, predominately related to the advantages of real-time US control. Mortality is extremely rare in children treated by percutaneous aspiration or drainage, and is more often related to underlying pathology and the clinical status of the patient than to the drainage procedure itself.

Conclusions

This multidisciplinary, multimodality approach has made percutaneous abscess drainage a safe and effective procedure in the pediatric population. Advances in imaging technologies (e.g., CT fluoroscopy, interventional MRI, laparoscopic US) and novel approaches (including combined laparoscopic, endoscopic, surgical, and interventional techniques) in a multipurpose image-guided therapy suite outfitted for both open and percutaneous procedures will likely increase the range and effectiveness of minimally invasive procedures in the future.

Percutaneous biopsy

Introduction

Biopsy is one of the most commonly performed procedures in pediatric interventional radiology practices. Since the initial reports of CT-guided biopsy in the mid-1970s improvements in equipment and technique have continued to expand the scope of lesions that may be sampled by a percutaneous approach. Image-guided biopsy offers a safe, cost-effective alternative to both surgical and endoscopic biopsy and is the method of choice in most situations. This section details the progression of a biopsy from preprocedure work-up to postprocedure care and covers selection of imaging modality, biopsy devices, technical variations, and specimen handling. A description of biopsy procedures in specific locations follows.

Indications

The primary indication for percutaneous image-guided biopsy is the diagnosis of malignancy (either primary or metastatic) or the characterization of diffuse parenchymal disease (Table 4.15). Additional indications include confirmation of a benign diagnosis, investigation of non-malignant pathology (e.g., transplant organ rejection, graft-versus-host disease, biliary atresia, neonatal hepatitis, sclerosing cholangitis), and acquisition of fluid or tissue for culture or other laboratory studies. The relative frequency of each indication may vary substantially based on the population served in a given institution. In general, percutaneous image-guided biopsy should be considered whenever a tissue diagnosis might confirm the diagnosis and modify therapy.

There are no absolute contraindications to percutaneous biopsy except an uncorrectable coagulopathy. The decision to obtain a biopsy should be made with consideration for the relative risks and benefits of the procedure and any alternatives in each patient. However, percutaneous biopsy should not be employed when the result will not influence management or when surgical intervention is planned regardless of the percutaneous result. Relative contraindications include coagulation abnormalities that might increase the risk of postprocedure bleeding, and absence of a safe pathway from the skin to the target site. A transvenous approach for core biopsy or fine needle aspirate (FNA) biopsy, or percutaneous biopsy with tract embolization may be useful alternatives in patients with an uncorrectable bleeding diathesis. Transgression of a hollow viscus or other non-target solid organs is generally avoided if alternative pathways are available.

Although FNA is considered relatively safe under almost any condition, its use is currently limited by the scarcity of pediatric pathologists experienced in interpretation of the resulting cytopathologic specimens. For this reason, and the complex nature of neoplasms in childhood, core samples that include both cellular and architectural information are preferred in most institutions.

Technique

Equipment

A variety of needles are available for aspiration (cytologic) and core (histologic) biopsy (see also "Biopsy of pulmonary and mediastinal lesions" in Chapter 3). Biopsy needles (see Figures 3.14 and 3.15) can be grouped by diameter, length and length of throw, by the type of biopsy being performed (Table 4.16), by the mechanism of activation, by the nature

Table 4.15 Indications: abdominopelvic biopsy

Indications
- Diagnosis of malignancy
  - primary
  - metastatic
  - recurrent
  - secondary
- Characterization of diffuse parenchymal disease
- Confirmation of a benign diagnosis
- Investigation of non-malignant pathology
  - transplant organ rejection
  - graft-versus-host disease
  - biliary atresia
  - neonatal hepatitis
  - sclerosing cholangitis
- Acquisition of tissue or fluid for culture or other laboratory studies

Contraindications
- Uncorrectable bleeding diathesis
- Results will not alter management or outcome (relative)

Table 4.16 Equipment: abdominopelvic biopsy

Preparation and draping
- Chlorhexidine gluconate (0.5%) with 70% isopropyl alcohol solution (SoluPrep™ (tinted), Solumed Inc., Laval, Quebec)
- Betadine® solution
- Isopropyl alcohol
- Sterile US cover (Civco Medical Instruments, Kalona, IA)
- Drapes (aperture drapes are preferred)

Fine needle aspiration biopsy needles
- Angiocatheter, 16 to 24 gauge (Becton Dickenson, Sandy, UT)
- Yueh centesis disposable catheter needle, 4 and 5 French, with side holes (Cook Inc.)
- Chiba needle, 22 gauge (5, 10 and 15 cm, Highliter, Inrad, Michigan)
- Seldinger needle, 19 gauge (Cook Inc.)
- Single wall puncture needle, 18 and 19 gauge (2.5, 4, 7 cm) (BSDN, Cook Inc.)
- Trochar needle, 18 gauge (11 and 20 cm) (Cook, Inc.)

Core biopsy needles
- Angiocatheter, 16 to 24 gauge (Becton Dickenson, Sandy, UT)

Miscellaneous supplies
- Abscess drainage bag (Medics Inc. Hilliard, OH)

of the sample chamber, and by special modifications for particular tissue types and circumstances.

Biopsy needles

Safe acquisition of sufficient tissue for a specific diagnosis without undue artifact or sampling error remains the central objective of all biopsy techniques. Fine needle aspiration biopsy (FNAB) may maximize safety. If a pathologist skilled in cytopathology is available for preliminary diagnosis in the procedure room, sufficient yields for specific diagnoses may rival alternative techniques, especially for documentation of metastases or tumor recurrence in patients with known primary malignancies. Sampling error and a low negative predictive value (given a high false-negative rate and the high prevalence of malignancy in tertiary centers) continue to be limiting features of the FNA technique.

Thin-walled, small-gauge (22- to 14-gauge) core biopsy needles with a variety of tip configurations facilitate the collection of larger tissue specimens necessary for histologic and immunohistochemical analysis for specific diagnosis of certain tumors such as sarcomas or the small round blue cell tumors that are more prevalent in the pediatric population. A coaxial system (using a larger needle to control the target lesion and through which a thinner needle is passed for sampling) may improve both safety and yield in select cases.

A variety of needles may be used for tissue acquisition. In general, they may be divided between non-cutting and cutting needles. Cutting needles may be further subdivided into manual, semi-automated, and automated devices. Non-cutting (aspiration) needles (Chiba and spinal needles with bevels of 25 degrees and 45 degrees, respectively, see Figure 3.1) allow for sampling of cells and fluids for cytopathologic and microbiologic analysis. Manual cutting needles include end-cutting (e.g., Menghini, Turner, Jamshidi®, Surecut®, Madayag, Greene, Franseen) and side-cutting needles (e.g., Travenol Tru-Cut®, Manan™ Pro-Cut™, Westcott, Stylet-Gap). These have various tip configurations, from smoothly beveled to serrated, each of which offers a particular advantage in specific situations. For example, a needle with a serrated tip (such as the Franseen) may assist tissue acquisition in a firm, resilient lesion while minimizing crush artifact. Semi-automated needles, such as the Quick-Core®, allow manual advancement of the stylet with its sampling channel across the target tissue, then spring-loaded firing of the cannula to shear the specimen. When fired, the sharp needle tip does not move, so this device is often useful when sampling adjacent to a vital structure.

Automated systems include end-cutting (BioPince® and Angiomed Autovac™, both single use) and side-cutting devices (Bard Biopty® and Manan™ Pro-Mag™, both reusable devices with disposable needles; and Monopty®, spring-loaded biopsy, and ASAP, all single-use devices). They allow a variable distance between the "cocked" and "fired" positions so that the "throw" (and therefore the length of the specimen) can be adapted to the specific patient problem. In our practice we try to match the length of the throw to the diameter of the lesion so that the sample obtained is limited to the lesion itself. Unless aspiration cytology is needed, automated end-cutting needles are currently our needles of choice for firm lesions and parenchymal samples, while semi-automated side-cutting needles are usually preferable for more friable or less well-organized tissue. Currently available end-cutting needles have a variable throw and can obtain 1.3, 2.3, or 3.3 cm cores. A 3.3 cm, 18-gauge core specimen may provide sufficient tissue for parenchymal analysis with a single pass. More material may be required for solid lesions, especially where cell biomarker and immunofluorescence studies are planned. The amount of material required should be discussed with the referring clinician and the pathologist prior to the procedure in such cases.

Needles also vary by gauge. Thin needles (20 to 25 gauge) are more often used for obtaining aspiration cytology and microbiology specimens or for core specimens in locations where there is a risk of entering vital structures, bowel loops, or blood vessels. Middle-gauge needles (18 to 20 gauge) are used to obtain core (histologic) material and thicker fluid or phlegmon samples for microbiology. Larger needles (less than 18 gauge) are used in the pediatric population for biopsy of larger and less vascular lesions (especially when a childhood sarcoma or lymphoma is suspected) and for bone biopsy procedures.

Ultimately, the experience and preference of the operator and the nature of the target lesion determine needle selection. Special needles are manufactured for specific applications, including needles designed for easy visualization within the US beam (see Figure 3.1), needles designed for sampling in the bony skeleton, non-ferrous needles for MR-guided procedures, kits for the performance of transvenous biopsies, and needles designed for vacuum-assisted acquisition. Although expensive, these needles are quite helpful for their dedicated purposes.

Image guidance

There are a variety of successful approaches to percutaneous biopsy. The imaging modality chosen for guidance depends upon the size and location of the lesion and the imaging device that best demonstrates the target lesion and its relationship to surrounding structures. Today, fluoroscopy is almost never used for imaging guidance. Computed tomography is most frequently used for image-guided biopsies in the thorax; however, US offers an ideal modality for most image-guided procedures in the pediatric abdomen, retroperitoneum, and pelvis. Ultrasound has the advantages of a real-time, cross-sectional technique limited only by the presence of air (such as in gas-filled loops of bowel) and bone (such as in the transgluteal approach to pelvic masses). Occasionally, a lesion may be too deep for adequate tissue resolution using US, in which case CT may prove a valuable alternative.

Ultrasound guidance

The principal goals of US imaging during biopsy are presented in Chapter 1. In summary, they are to identify the target lesion, to avoid intervening vital structures, to visualize the biopsy needle in plane with the lesion during advancement, to confirm passage of the sample chamber through the lesion, and to evaluate for potential complications following biopsy. Linear, curvilinear, or sector transducers are most useful for US-guided biopsy. Transducer frequencies ranging from 18 to 2.5 MHz can be used depending on the situation.

In our hands, sonographically guided biopsy is performed using a freehand method (see Figure 1.1). The target lesion should be unequivocally identified and the anticipated pathway interrogated for intervening vital structures. Use of color Doppler imaging allows vascular structures to be avoided during needle insertion. The needle is introduced and constantly monitored during advancement toward the lesion. The entire needle (including the characteristic "comet tail" tip artifact, see Figure 4.39) must be contained in the imaging plane to assure control of the tip position.

CT guidance

The child is positioned, as determined by prior imaging, so that the most direct approach to the lesion can be taken. For CT-guided biopsy a scan is performed through the region of interest to locate the lesion. If sedation is used, we have found it best to sedate or anesthetize the patient at this time so that the depth and rate of breathing will be the same as during the biopsy. There are two main approaches to marking the entry site of the needle. Radio-opaque markers may be placed on the skin and several contiguous axial images are obtained, centered on the lesion. A safe pathway from the skin to the lesion is determined using the markers as a reference point or grid. Alternatively, once the target is identified the ideal slice location for skin entry is selected. Then using the positioning laser this level is traced on the skin and a Beekley® spot is used to mark the entry spot. We prefer the latter approach. As is true elsewhere, a route should be planned so as to avoid transgressing (and potentially contaminating or seeding) more than one anatomic compartment whenever possible. An optimal path would lie in a line normal to the skin in both an axial and parasagittal plane. Angulation of the gantry may be useful when the safest apparent path to the lesion does not lie in an axial plane. As a general rule, compound angulation of the biopsy needle (in other words, along a path that crosses the imaging plane rather than lying within it) should be avoided.

The distance from the skin to both the superficial and deep aspects of the lesion is measured to determine how deeply the biopsy needle should be passed to obtain the desired sample. Image postprocessing software may also allow calculation of the angle from perpendicular that the needle should be directed from the skin entry site to the lesion. The skin is prepared and draped in sterile fashion and 1% buffered lidocaine is slowly injected with a thin (e.g., 30-gauge) needle. With the coordinates in mind, the guide needle (coaxial technique is used if more than one specimen is desired) is then advanced into the lesion. The needle position is confirmed with three contiguous axial images. Ideally, a single slice should contain the entire needle, including tip (streak) within the lesion (Figure 4.55). The effects of partial volume and motion artifact must especially be considered during this phase of the procedure.

Small corrections to the needle trajectory may be made during advancement. However, if substantial corrections are needed, the needle should be withdrawn to the tip and corrections made before re-entering the tissues. To decrease radiation dose and procedure time, CT may be used intermittently to monitor the needle tip position when it is passing vital structures. If the needle alignment and anticipated pathway are appropriate, the needle may be further advanced toward the lesion, and position again verified. The amount that the needle can safely be advanced at each iteration is dependent on the experience of the interventionalist and the nature of the intended pathway. When the needle tip is in proper position such that the throw of the needle will extend into or through the lesion without endangering vital structures beyond the lesion, a sample or samples should be obtained. Routinely, we obtain two to three samples per lesion.

Molecular imaging

Physiologic imaging offers insight beyond anatomy into the biologic nature of tissue. PET and SPECT imaging, for example, can demonstrate tissue with abnormally high metabolic activity characteristic of malignant and, to a lesser extent, inflammatory processes. This may allow more accurate sampling of suspicious tissue based upon imaging characteristics and to differentiate vital tumor from necrosis, fibrosis, and hemorrhage, as well as helping to avoid biopsy of equivocal tissue. However, achieving adequate target resolution and visualization of surrounding structures necessary for the safe performance of percutaneous biopsy techniques requires fusion with a modality that can represent anatomic relationships with adequate spatial resolution to guide a safe approach to tissue acquisition. We have found that the use of image fusion such as PET-CT imaging for procedure planning and, where appropriate, for percutaneous biopsy guidance, can improve patient outcomes compared to conventional techniques in select cases (Figure 4.56).

MR guidance

At present, interventional MRI is in its infancy and is not yet being used on a widespread basis.

Patient preparation

Prior to the procedure, the patient's imaging studies and medical history should be reviewed with the referring physicians and surgeons to determine a likely clinicoradiologic diagnosis and to discuss the potential risks and benefits of the image-guided approach. Close consultation with the pathologist is important to determine the need for histologic specimens, the amount of tissue required for specific diagnosis, and the desired transport medium and handling procedures for the

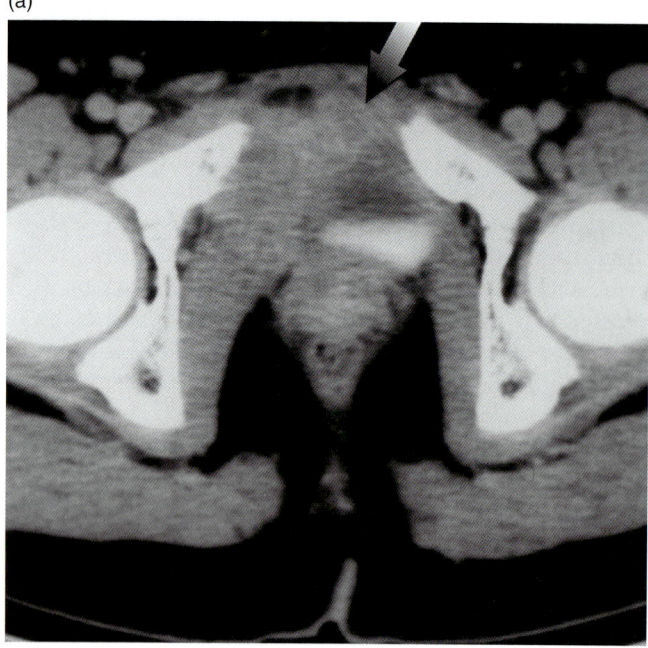 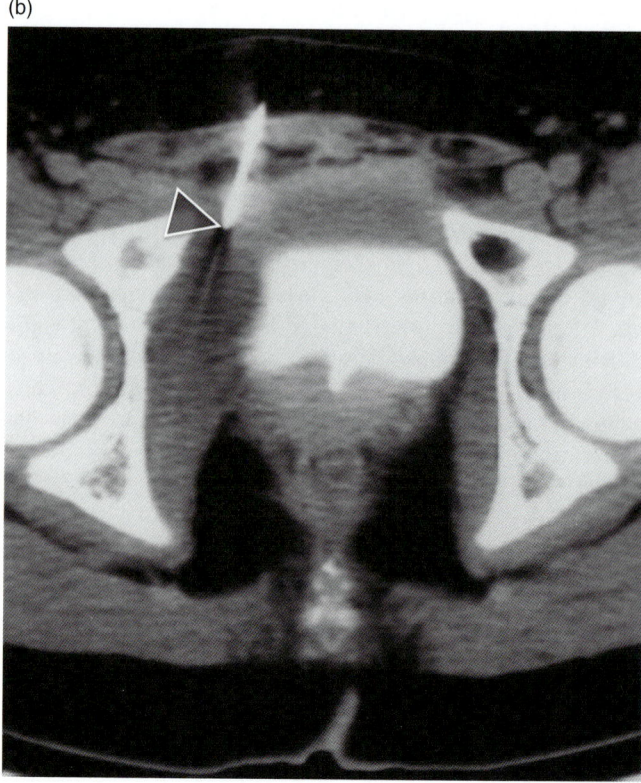

Figure 4.55 (a) Pelvic CT without contrast in a 15-year-old male who presented with difficulty urinating shows abnormal soft tissue in the region of the prostate extending to the right pelvic wall and involving the pubic ramus. (b) A 16-gauge coaxial guiding needle is seen in the imaging plane with tip artifact extending beyond the needle tip (*arrowhead*). Several 18-gauge core biopsy specimens were obtained through the coaxial needle, and led to diagnosis of recurrent prostatic rhabdomyosarcoma.

biopsy material. Patient preparation is otherwise similar to that of other interventional procedures in children. When sampling small lesions or lesions adjacent to vital structures in the epigastrium, general anesthesia with control of respiration at a fixed point in the cycle (e.g., mid- or end-expiration) can be of considerable benefit in minimizing motion artifact and respiratory misregistration.

Preprocedure care

Patients fasting for a procedure should not become dehydrated, and orders for maintenance intravenous fluids should be considered for patients fasting overnight. For outpatient procedures under sedation in otherwise healthy children this may not be required. Secure intravenous access should be maintained throughout the procedure and postprocedure period of close medical observation. Patients should be evaluated for bleeding risk and appropriate corrective actions should be taken when needed, as described in the guidelines in Chapter 1.

When either sedation or general anesthesia is planned, patients' intake must be restricted from solids based on hospital policy. All patients who require sedation or anesthesia must have adequate intravenous access. Emergency cases may require deviations from these guidelines and must be considered on a case-by-case basis.

Pathologic considerations

There are strengths and weaknesses to both cytological and histological examinations, depending upon the pathologist's experience as well as on the suitability of samples as representative of the target lesion or tissue. For the interpretation of cellular changes in the cytoplasm, nuclei, nucleoli, and chromatin, FNA biopsy may suffice; but FNA requires specific expertise in cytopathology on the part of the pathologist, and it benefits from the presence of the pathologist in the procedure room. Expertise in classic histologic interpretation is more readily available but depends upon preservation of both cellular morphology and architectural organization (including the intercellular matrix and supporting stroma) in the sample for proper diagnosis. Sampling the desired lesion has become more reliable as imaging modalities, especially US, have improved. However, non-representative sampling from the target tissue may occur due to the presence of central necrosis, intense inflammatory reaction, or hemorrhage. Stains that characterize subcellular architecture and cellular biochemical products, immunocytochemical subclassification of mesenchymal malignancies (such as lymphomas), and ultrastructural analysis by electron microscopy all improve the diagnostic accuracy of core biopsies but may require a greater mass of sampled tissue and will certainly add to the overall cost of the procedure. However, with core biopsy techniques, the

Chapter 4 Abdominopelvic interventions

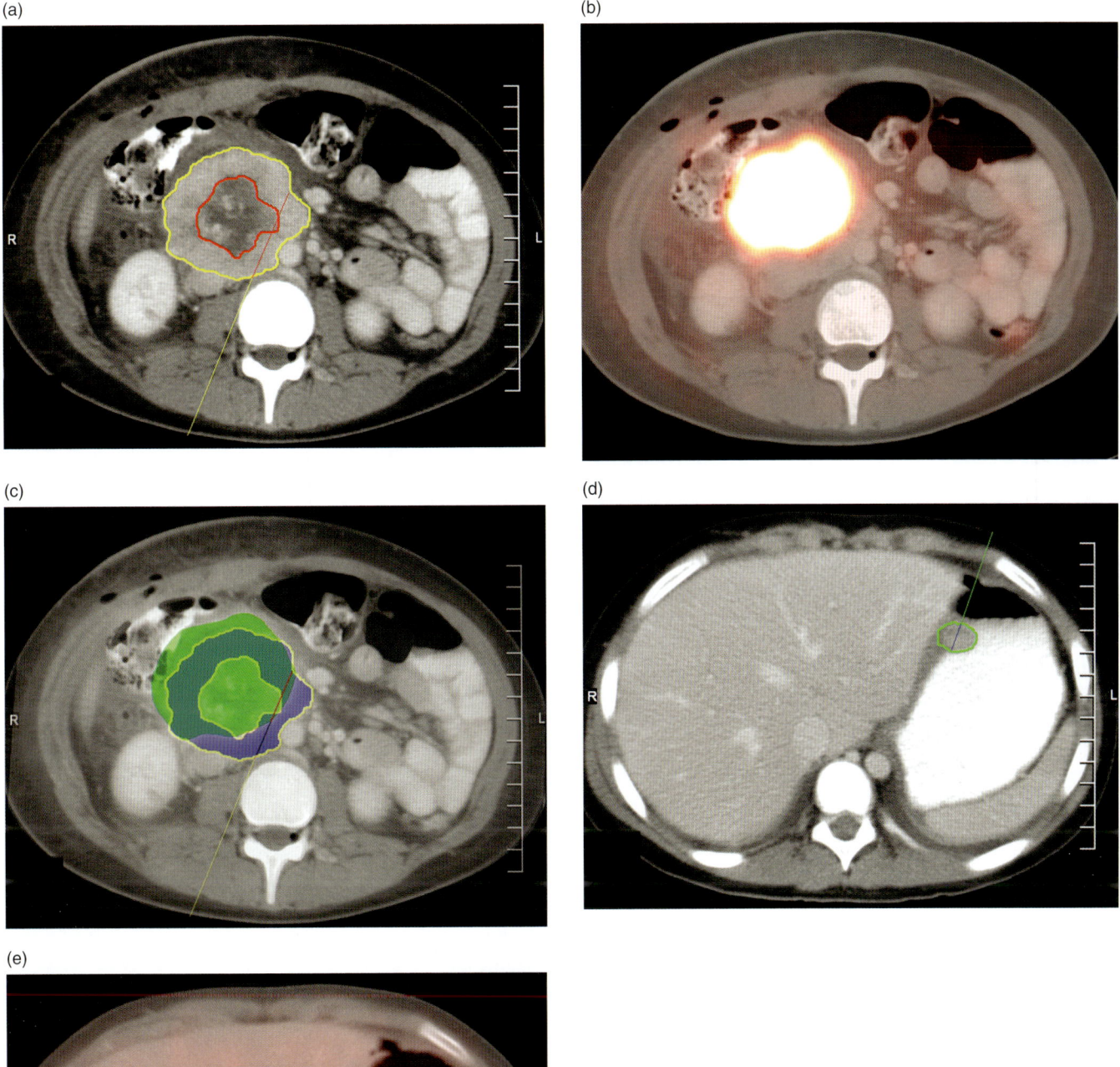

Figure 4.56 (a) Abdominal CT with vascular and enteric contrast enhancement in an 11-year-old female with vague abdominal discomfort and a palpable mass shows a moderately enhancing 6 cm mass with tumor vasculature in the low-attenuation (necrotic) central region. Surgical changes are noted. (b) 18-F FDG PET-CT fusion reconstructed with a continuous ("hot metal") algorithm shows intense uptake throughout the mass, suggesting that biopsy anywhere within the lesion would be equally representative of the tumor's biologic activity. (c) When the same study is reconstructed with a stepwise algorithm, the highest uptake is clearly confined to the region of CT enhancement. If percutaneous samples were obtained, they should target this region. Surgical biopsy showed malignant gastrointestinal stromal-cell tumor (GIST). (d) A CT section more superiorly located than (a) shows a soft tissue nodule (*outlined in green*) at the lesser curvature that was not noted in the original interpretation. (e) This nodule showed intense uptake on PET-CT fusion imaging, and was later diagnosed as a non-functioning paraganglioma, part of an incomplete Carney triad (no pulmonary chondroma was detected), a specific type of multiple endocrine neoplasia.

improved accuracy in analysis of mesenchymal malignancies and the improved ability to make a specific benign diagnosis increase the negative predictive value to nearly 100%. Since this may eliminate the need for repeat biopsies or open surgery in follow-up of negative results in these patients, the relative value of histologic material from core biopsy specimens in the pediatric population should not be underestimated.

Intraoperative evaluation of either fresh specimens or frozen sections with nucleic acids and proteins stained according to usual protocols (e.g., with hematoxylin-eosin or similar stains) with the pathologist is an often overlooked alternative in interventional suites, although this is common practice in most surgical departments. The potential benefits are multifold: such analysis virtually assures that useful tissue is obtained before the conclusion of the encounter, improves communication between the referring clinician, the interventionalist, and the interpreting pathologist, reduces the frequency of false-negative and inadequate biopsies, reduces the need for repeat biopsies by other methods (such as open surgical or laparoscopic), permits performance of related procedures under the same anesthesia or sedation when evidence of pathology is conclusive (such as central venous catheter insertion), and improves the credibility of the interventionalist within the clinical community. Perhaps most importantly, it connects the interventionalist to the outcome of biopsy procedures, providing for ongoing education and continuous quality improvement. Evaluation of frozen sections especially may require carrying the specimen to the pathology lab and a longer procedure time but, especially in cases where the target is small or difficult to reach, the delay is worth the advantages obtained.

Standard technique

Although the general elements of percutaneous biopsy are modular in nature and apply across virtually all applications within the abdomen and pelvis (Table 4.17), considerations in each organ and space encourage focus on the specific conditions that pertain to each situation.

Percutaneous liver biopsy

Historically, liver biopsy has been performed as an inpatient procedure either surgically (open wedge biopsy, or laparoscopic wedge, or core biopsy), medically (core biopsy as a non-guided procedure, with or without prior imaging of the prospective percutaneous site), or interventionally (core or FNA biopsy under real-time US guidance or CT). Percutaneous biopsy has been performed in children since the 1940s. The introduction of the "one-second" technique by Menghini improved the accessibility of this procedure and significantly lowered associated morbidity and mortality. However, the unguided technique of percutaneous biopsy is known to elevate risk of pleural puncture, gallbladder or bowel transgression, perforation of a large central vessel, unintended biopsy of kidney or pancreas, or perforation of the liver capsule in the

Table 4.17 Procedural summary: abdominopelvic biopsy

1. Obtain preprocedural laboratory studies: CBC plus platelets, coagulation profile.
2. Preprocedural cross-sectional imaging: evaluate anatomy, identify ascites if present.
3. Child is immobilized and sedated *or* under general anesthesia.
4. Sterile preparation and draping.
5. Imaging guidance to assist needle placement. Ultrasound is preferred whenever possible.
6. Use of single needle or coaxial needle approach. Coaxial approach favored for children who have ascites, are at high risk for bleeding, or who have large masses that benefit from multiple specimens and reduce risk for tumor seeding.
7. Track embolization requires coaxial approach.
8. Postprocedural US.

presence of unsuspected free ascites. Unguided biopsies also have a higher rate of hospitalization for pain, hypotension, or bleeding, and require more passes to obtain adequate tissue, compared to those performed under US guidance.

Image guidance, especially real-time US guidance, has significantly increased the diagnostic yield, safety, and comfort of this procedure. Careful preprocedure screening, targeted preprocedure preparation, and provision of specialized and experienced postprocedural care with a low and clearly defined threshold for admission have allowed percutaneous US-guided liver biopsies to be safely performed as an outpatient procedure in select cases. Development of tract-embolization and transvenous techniques for patients at higher risk for hemorrhagic complications has further reduced the risk of severe complications from this procedure. In the end, care should be individualized to the specific patient.

Liver biopsy is performed to diagnose suspected malignancy, to characterize diffuse hepatocellular disease (e.g. fibrosis, cirrhosis), to manage patients after liver transplant, or to monitor iron content in patients requiring regular blood transfusions. Blind (non-image-guided) liver biopsies are still performed regularly despite the fact that image guidance is cost effective while significantly reducing complications. Complications include bleeding or other vascular trauma (pseudoaneurysm, arteriovenous or arteriobiliary fistula), bowel perforation, pneumothorax, and hemothorax. It is difficult to justify non-guided liver biopsy in a time when interventional radiologists trained to provide this technique safely and comfortably are ubiquitously available.

Conventionally, one of two approaches is used to gain access to the hepatic parenchyma for sampling: a right interior subcostal approach, or a subxiphoid approach to the left lobe. Focal lesions often require more elaborate route planning to maximize the opportunity for a successful sample while limiting risk of hemorrhage, injury to non-parenchymal structures, and contamination of additional compartments. Focal liver lesions as small as 3 to 4 mm can be reliably sampled (Figures 4.57 and 4.58). It is helpful to choose an approach that interposes a rim of normal tissue between the liver capsule and

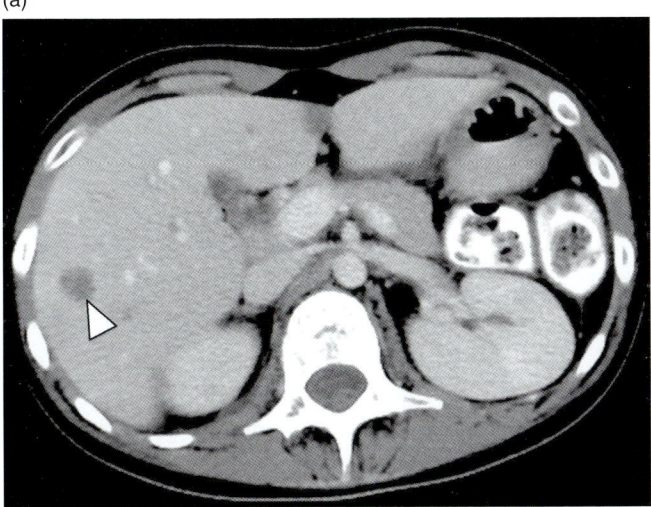
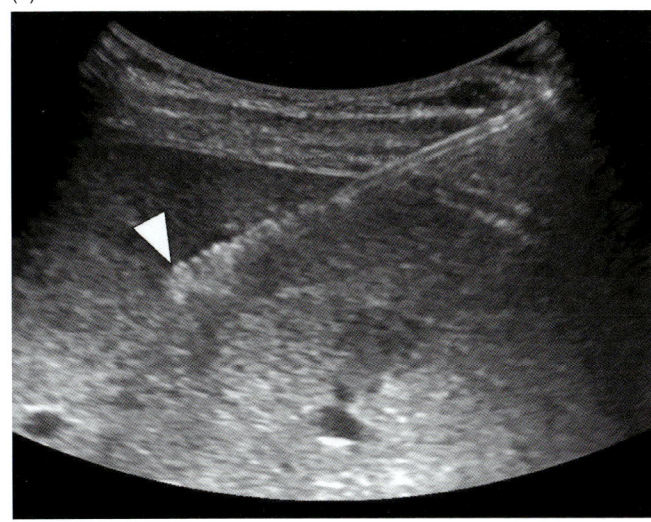
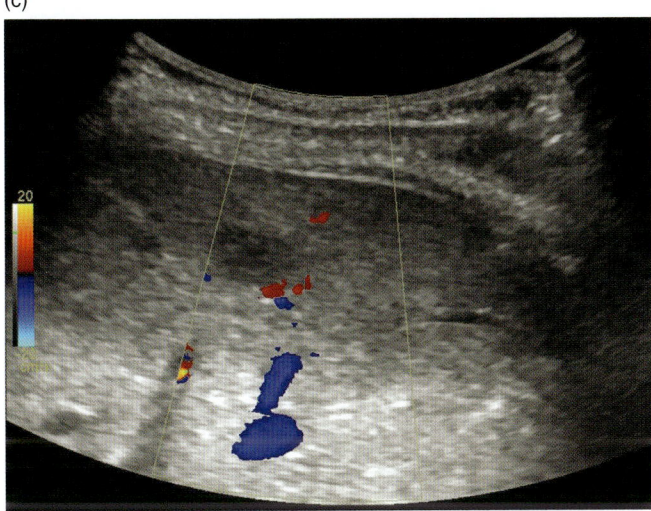

Figure 4.57 (a) Multiple low-attenuation lesions with rim enhancement are seen in this abdominal CT with vascular and enteric contrast in a 16-year-old female with abdominal pain while receiving chemotherapy for acute lymphocytic leukemia. The Couinaud segment 6 lesion (indicated by the *arrowhead*) was selected for its size, accessibility, and presence of hepatic parenchyma between the lesion and the liver capsule. (b) Two core biopsy specimens were obtained under US guidance with an 18-gauge automated needle (*arrowhead*). (c) Postbiopsy color Doppler US image through the biopsy site shows no evidence of complication.

a lesion in order to minimize bleeding. Occasionally, CT guidance is required for lesions that are not well visualized with US. Ascitic fluid present at the time of planned biopsy may increase the risk of hemorrhagic complications by preventing the normal tamponade offered by tissues compressed against the transcapsular entry site. It is both advisable and a simple matter to aspirate or drain the ascites prior to biopsy (Figure 4.59).

Right lobe biopsy

The patient is placed in a partial left decubitus position (right side elevated approximately 30 degrees from the table-top using high-density foam wedges). With the patient adequately sedated or anesthetized, screening US is performed. A suitable entry site is selected and marked on the skin. If possible, the site will be located in the mid-right lobe in a relatively hypovascular area, with a generous amount of parenchyma between the site and both the porta hepatis and the free edge of the liver. The entry site will usually be intercostal, and is optimally between the anterior and midaxillary line to minimize the risk of pleural transgression. From this approach, puncture anterior to the anterior axillary line significantly increases risk of hemorrhage from injury to vessels in the porta hepatis.

After sterile preparation and draping of the skin around the entry site, buffered local anesthetic is injected slowly but generously with a thin gauge (i.e., 27- or 30-gauge) needle. A small skin incision is made with a scalpel blade. Depending on the anticipated risk of the procedure a coaxial technique may be selected as this approach has several advantages including: one hole in the liver capsule, limits most biopsies to one needle pass, facilitates obtaining two to three specimens in short order, and allows for tract embolization whenever desired. As described above, US guidance is used and the biopsy needle is visualized through the entire course through the liver parenchyma to the desired location (Figure 4.60). After obtaining adequate specimens, the site is once again evaluated with US to look for evidence of postprocedure hemorrhage.

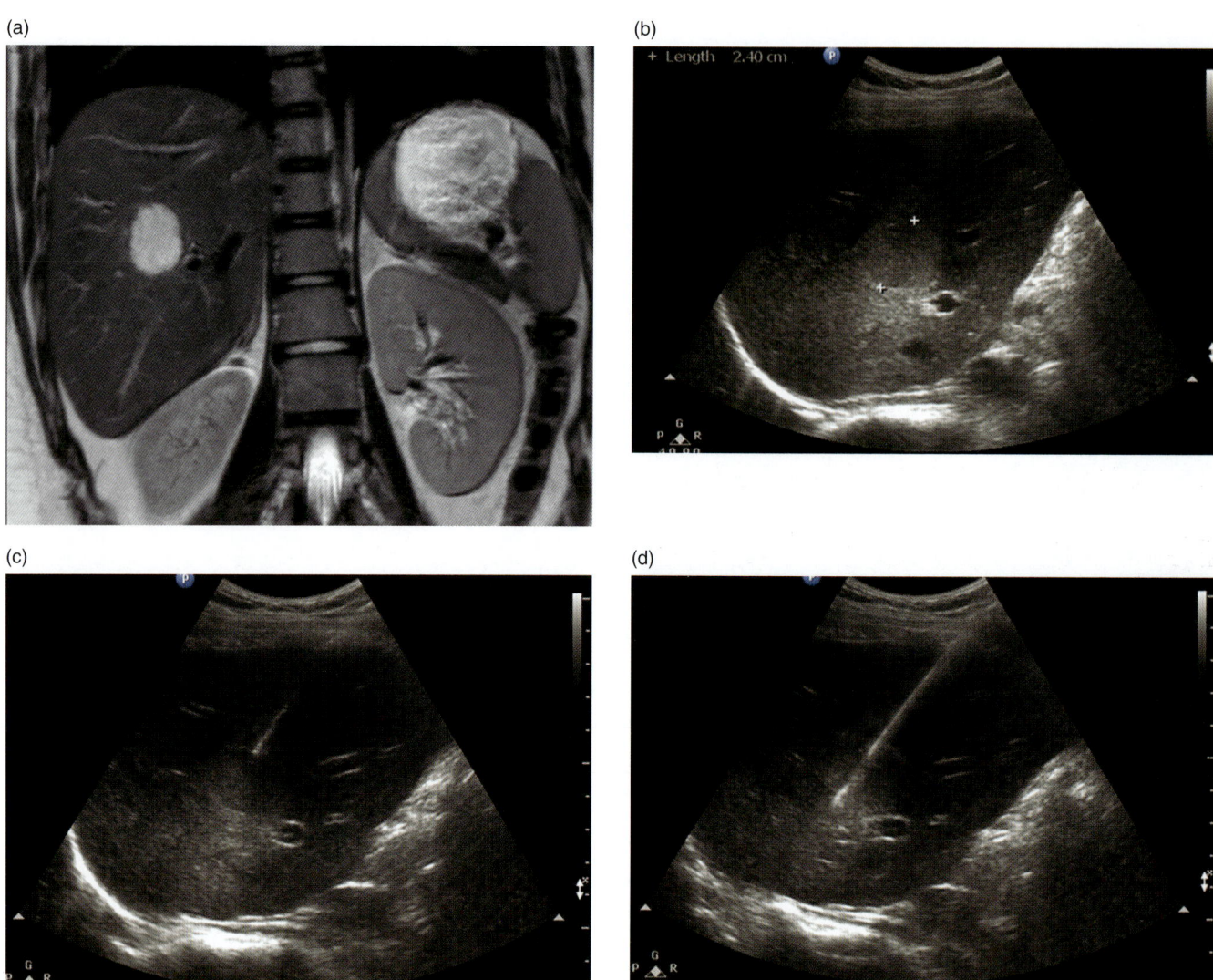

Figure 4.58 Sixteen-year-old female with incidentally discovered hepatic mass. (a) Coronal T2 MRI demonstrates a T2 hyperintense central hepatic mass. (b) Ultrasound demonstrating isoechoic mass. (c,d) Coaxial percutaneous biopsy. Pathology revealed hemangioendothelioma.

Left lobe biopsy

In some practices the left lobe is preferred for image-guided percutaneous liver biopsy (Figure 4.60). This approach is also necessary for biopsy of segmental transplants, since in these patients there is no right hepatic lobe. The preparation for the biopsy is as discussed above. A subxiphoid to subcostal midline approach is used and samples are obtained as described above for the right-lobe technique. Again, after obtaining adequate specimens the site is re-evaluated with US to look for evidence of postprocedure hemorrhage.

Hemorrhage is the major cause of morbidity in children undergoing liver biopsy, with bile peritonitis occurring less frequently. In traditional (non-image-guided) right-lobe liver biopsies the overall risk of fatal hemorrhage is around 0.1% and significant hemorrhage occurs in 0.2%. In the few studies performed, the rate of complications has been significantly lower in children undergoing US-guided biopsy, although the numbers studied have been too low to discern a difference in the frequency requiring treatment between these two groups. The risk of bleeding in children undergoing US-guided liver biopsy is increased with low-molecular-weight heparin, biopsy of focal lesions, and biopsy in children with acute liver failure, but not with aspirin and not in liver transplant patients *per se* (complication rates in the latter group are actually *lower!*).

Most complications are detectable within three to six hours after biopsy. Delayed complications are generally not detectable within 24 hours of biopsy, and may not become apparent for days to weeks following biopsy. Delayed bleeding has been reported as late as 15 days after biopsy, and hypotension and death have occurred in patients as long as nine hours after biopsy.

Tract embolization

For children in whom a history of bleeding abnormality or abnormal laboratory values suggests an increased risk of

Chapter 4 Abdominopelvic interventions

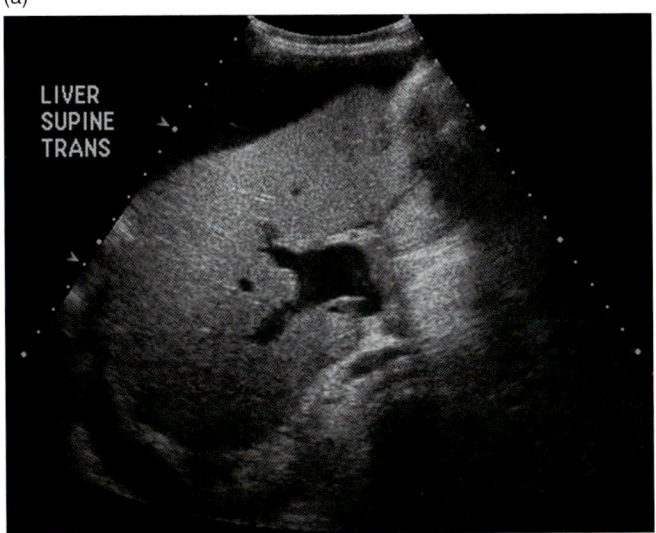

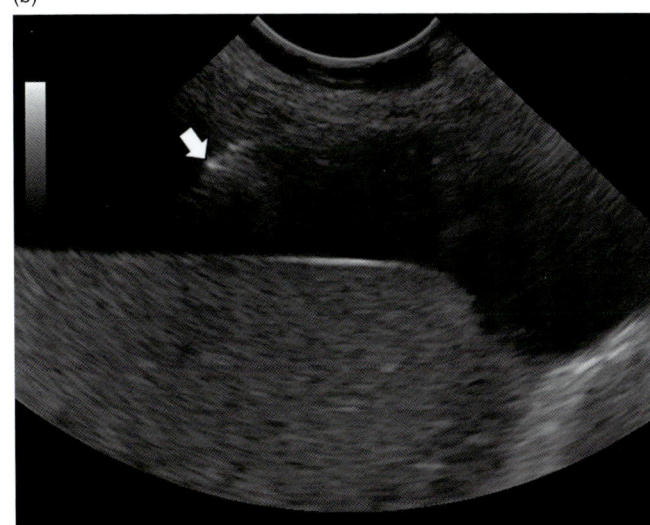

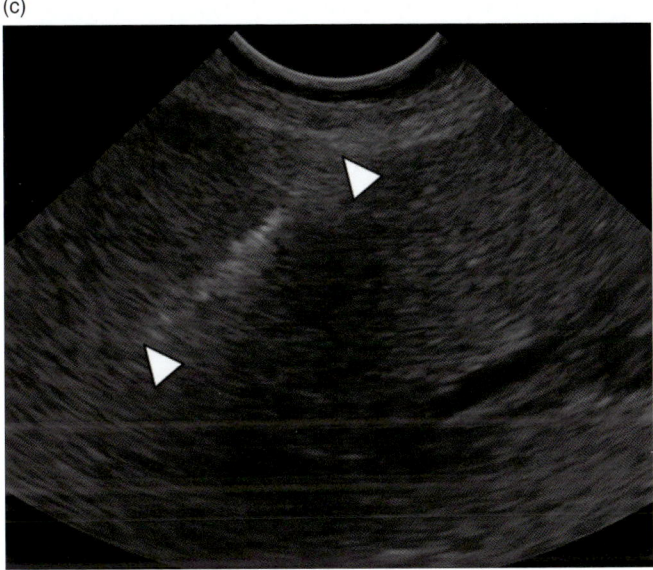

Figure 4.59 An 11-year-old male liver transplant patient requires urgent liver biopsy in the ICU. (a) Transabdominal US shows an echogenic liver and significant ascites. (b) A percutaneous transperitoneal 5-French Yueh sheathed needle (*arrow*) is introduced using US guidance at the bedside. (c) After complete evacuation of the ascitic fluid, a percutaneous 3.3 cm core biopsy of the liver is obtained with an end-cutting needle (*arrowheads*) without complication.

hemorrhage, embolization of the biopsy tract offers an effective mechanism for securing hemostasis. Because this method requires a coaxial technique, it must be planned as an adjunct prior to insertion of the biopsy needle.

Once the biopsy specimens have been obtained the core biopsy needle is removed and embolic material is injected through the coaxial needle to "plug" the biopsy tract. Although any embolic material may be used, we prefer Gelfoam® pledgets (cut from Gelfoam® sheets into 2 to 5 mm wide strips) or Avitene®. Initially we made Gelfoam® pledgets molded into "torpedoes" and pushed through the coaxial needle into the tract using the stylet. Today, we have modified the technique and place strips of Gelfoam® into a 10 ml syringe. A 1 ml syringe is connected via a three-way stopcock. About 2 ml of sterile saline is drawn into the large syringe and the material is pushed back and forth through the two syringes until a slurry is formed. At the completion of the procedure it is injected via the guide catheter as it is withdrawn from the liver while monitoring with US. If Avitene® is used it can be injected as thick slurry. In our experience this technique has been highly successful and is ideal for patients at moderate risk for hemorrhage.

Transvenous biopsy: transjugular approach

See Chapter 5.

Renal biopsy

See Chapter 6.

Splenic biopsy

Splenomegaly and the development of focal splenic lesions may occur in immune suppressed or immune deficient patients and those with such a history are at risk for metastatic disease or relapse. The nature of splenic lesions is of primary

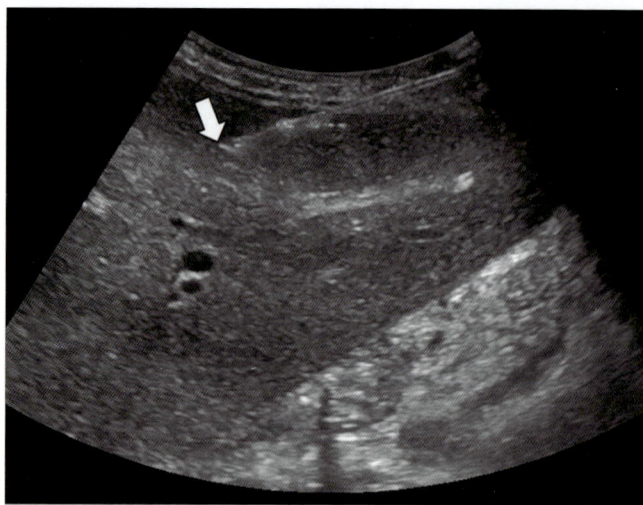

Figure 4.60 A seven-year-old male after living-donor left lobe liver transplant for liver biopsy, obtained with an automated side-cutting needle (*arrow*) from a subxiphoid approach.

diagnostic importance and defines the treatment course in these patients. In the past, FNA biopsy was the procedure of choice in these patients. Many of these patients eventually required splenectomy, with the pathological diagnosis made by sampling tissue from the excised spleen. Ultrasound-guided percutaneous core biopsy of the spleen is a relatively new procedure used to obtain core tissue samples in patients with abnormal spleens. As is the case for most percutaneous biopsies, this procedure may often be performed under deep IV sedation with local anesthetic infiltration. However, for uncooperative patients, or those with small lesions and where control of respiration is important, GA may be of benefit. An 18-gauge automated biopsy device is usually selected for this procedure. Adequate tissue is most often obtained with 18-gauge needles.

Technically, percutaneous splenic biopsy is not difficult to perform. When disease is local or unifocal, the entry site is selected at the appropriate level. With diffuse disease such as fungal infection (which is the most common presentation for splenic biopsy), the junction of the mid and distal thirds of the organ is the preferred site for biopsy in order to avoid the splenic hilum as well as inadvertent pleural transgression. If possible the entry site is planned between the left anterior and mid-axillary line.

The skin is prepared and draped in sterile fashion and buffered local anesthetic is infiltrated generously as deep as the splenic capsule. The procedure is most often performed under US guidance.

If postbiopsy tract embolization is planned (see "Tract embolization" under "Percutanueous liver biopsy," above), a coaxial system will be required. If multiple specimens are planned, a coaxial approach is useful to avoid repeated puncture of the splenic capsule. Either directly or through a coaxial guiding needle, the automated biopsy needle is advanced within the splenic parenchyma and a specimen is obtained.

More than two specimens are rarely necessary, and more than three passes at the same location may be associated with a higher rate of bleeding complication. After biopsy, and tract embolization if desired, a limited US examination is performed to evaluate for active extravasation. The patient is usually positioned in a left lateral decubitus position during the recovery period to assist hemostasis.

Pancreatic biopsy

There is seldom indication for a pancreatic biopsy in the pediatric population since primary and metastatic pancreatic tumors or other pancreatic pathology requiring biopsy for diagnosis are rare. Principles of percutaneous pancreatic biopsy are similar to those for percutaneous biopsy of any other solid organ. The decision to perform a percutaneous biopsy depends on the extent of the primary lesion, the presence of secondary pathology, and the availability of surgical alternatives (Figure 4.61). Visualization with US or CT is usually required to allow accurate placement of needles for small pancreatic lesions. Pancreatitis, bleeding and seeding of the biopsy tract, and perforation of non-target tissues are the primary risks of this procedure. A window should be sought that allows biopsy without traversing bowel or kidney. If no such window is available, a transbowel (e.g., transgastric) route of access can usually be safely employed with a 21-gauge needle.

Biopsy of nodules and masses

See Chapter 7.

Neuroblastoma

Neuroblastoma is the third most common malignancy in children and the most common extracranial solid cancer (Figure 4.62). This neural crest cell malignancy arises in the adrenal medulla or the sympathetic chain, but may metastasize. Prognosis is primarily determined by tumor genetics rather than histology alone. Although there is some controversy over this point, sufficient tissue obtained through aggressive biopsy, obtaining numerous samples from multiple quadrants within the mass with a large-bore (14- to 16-gauge) core biopsy needle can lead to determination of prognosis. A total of approximately a gram of tissue or more may be required for testing to determine the aggressiveness of the tumor, including histopathology, fluorescence in situ hybridization (FISH), image cytometry, *N-MYC*, chromosome 1p, ploidy, cytogenetics, culture and drug sensitivity, molecular biology studies, and immunohistochemistry. Electron microscopy ultrastructural studies may also be helpful. It is desirable to obtain specimens from different areas within the tumor if there is any nodular or vascular differentiation. Fine needle aspiration biopsy accompanying the core samples may be sufficient for FISH. Because core specimens may not be adequate for all potential studies, distribution and handling of the specimens should be planned carefully with the pathologist.

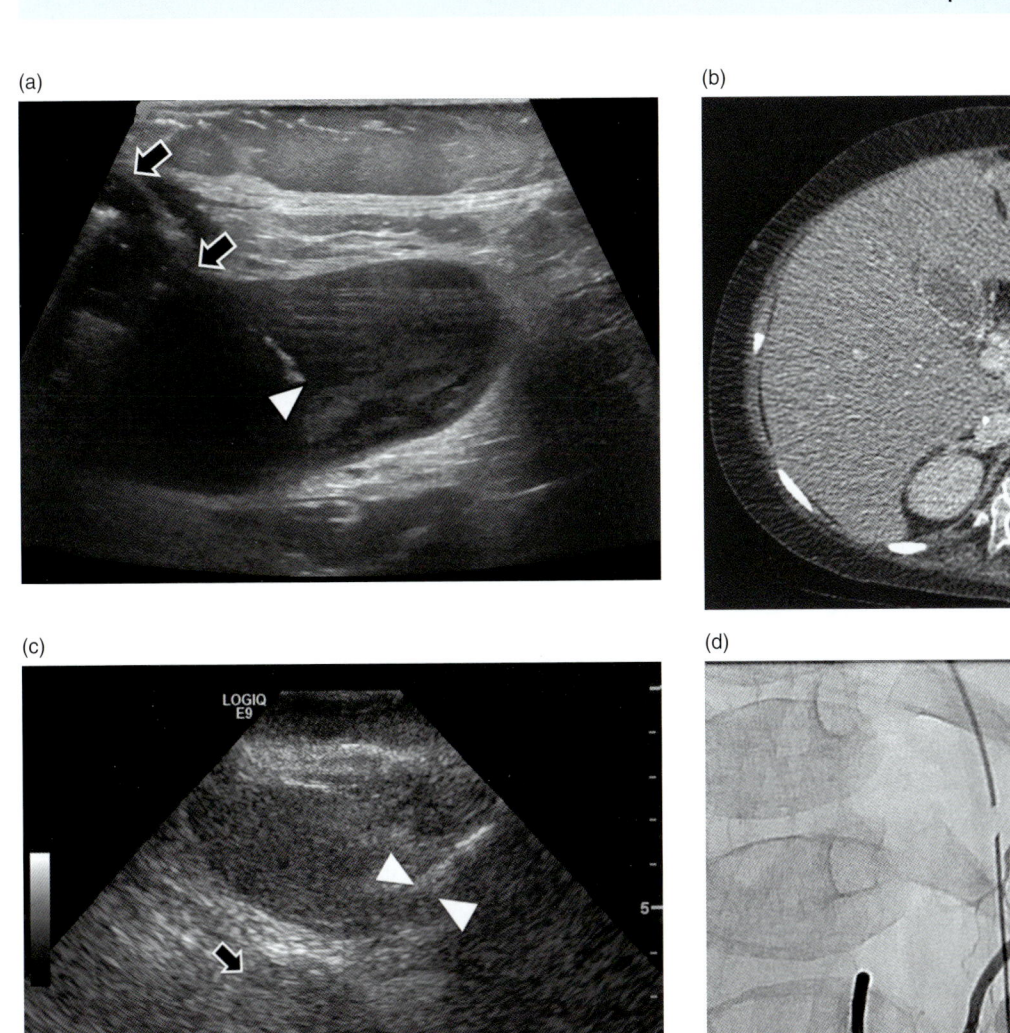
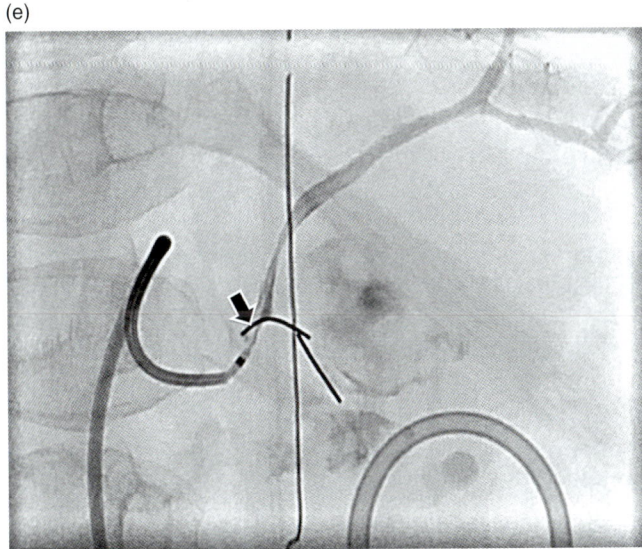

Figure 4.61 An eight-year-old male with intestinal failure developed a pancreatic pseudocyst in the lesser sac. (a) Under US guidance, through the existing gastrostomy stoma (*arrows*) transgastric access to the pseudocyst was achieved with a 22-gauge Chiba needle (*arrowhead*). (b) After successful transgastric drainage (shown in d, below) of the pseudocyst, the patient remained febrile, and a complex pancreatic tail mass (*arrow*) was noted on abdominal CT. (c) From a posterolateral percutaneous retroperitoneal approach through the space between the spleen and left kidney (*arrowheads*), US-guided biopsy of the mass (*arrow*) was obtained with an 18-gauge automated end-cutting core biopsy needle. (d) Computed tomography suggested active, contained hemorrhage in the region of the biopsy one week later. Subselective angiography shows a pseudoaneurysm of the greater pancreatic artery (*arrowhead*). The transgastric pseudocyst drain (*arrow*) projects adjacent to the gastrostomy button. (e) The pseudocyst was embolized by "sandwiching" the artery with two Hilal straight coils (*arrow*).

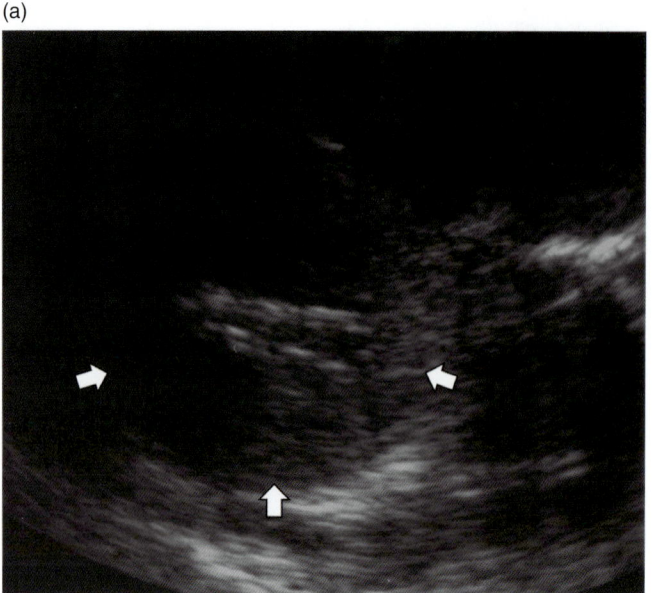 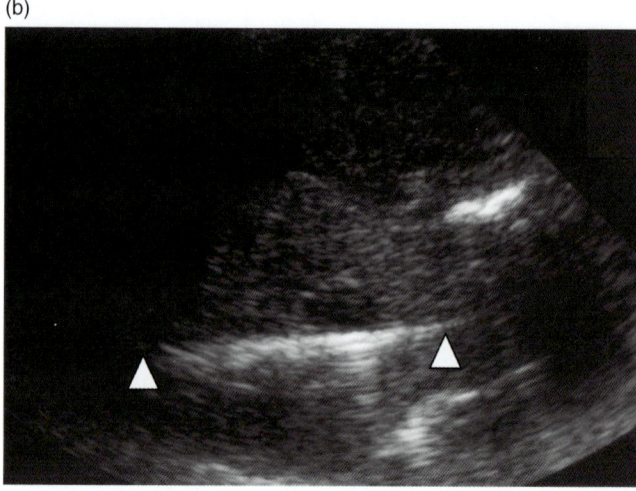

Figure 4.62 (a) An adrenal mass was identified on retroperitoneal US in this five-year-old female with fatigue and weight loss (*arrows*). (b) Multiple samples were obtained under US guidance with a 15-gauge semi-automated core biopsy needle (*arrowheads*) with a 1.2 cm throw.

Technical variations
Coaxial and tandem needle techniques

In certain cases it is helpful to either improve control or limit the number of needle passes through part or all of the prospective access pathway. The target lesion may be in close proximity to vital structures. Initial approaches to a small lesion with a large needle may provoke enough hemorrhage to obscure the target. Seeding of the biopsy tract from fragmentation or translation of pathologic (e.g., malignant or infectious) material may complicate an otherwise successful procedure. In order to increase the opportunity for a meaningful sample, and to decrease the risk of complication, coaxial or tandem needle techniques may be used alone or in combination.

For *coaxial* guidance, a larger bore calibrated guiding needle with a diamond stylet is advanced to one of two positions. For sampling a deep nodule or mass, where multiple passes through the intervening tissues are undesirable, a guiding needle may be advanced until it is near the superficial limit of the lesion. For sampling a lesion adjacent to or partially obscured by a vital structure, the guiding needle may be advanced in gradual steps to a position that, when the stylet is removed, provides safe and unobscured access to the lesion.

Once having cleared the obstacle the guiding needle may be left in this position or advanced to the perimeter of the target lesion as circumstances dictate. The caliber of the guiding needle must be sufficient to allow passage of the sampling (biopsy) needle when the stylet is removed. Additionally, the exact distance the biopsy needle can extend from the guiding needle when fully engaged must be known in order to calculate how far the biopsy needle should be advanced prior to sampling. Confirmation of these relationships before placement of the guiding needle is a necessary precaution.

Once the guiding needle is in position, it must be fixed in place in alignment with the lesion and maintained at a constant depth while the stylet is exchanged for the biopsy needle and the sample is obtained. If multiple samples are required and the lesion is sufficiently large, the angle of the guiding needle may be varied slightly between passes in order to sample different portions of the lesion. To minimize complications the stylet is usually returned to the guiding needle between passes. The same guiding cannula may of course be used to obtain FNAB and core samples from the same lesion. If brisk hemorrhage is noted during the biopsy procedure, the tract may be embolized through the guiding cannula (e.g., with Gelfoam® pledgets or Avitene®) after removal of the biopsy needle.

There are two basic principles of *tandem needle* guidance. First, it is safer to manipulate a thin (Chiba) needle than one of larger caliber. When the angle from the skin to the target lesion is difficult to gauge, passing a thin needle and confirming appropriate alignment with imaging provides a visual "pointer" to the lesion. The biopsy needle, or guiding needle if using a coaxial approach, can then be advanced in a parallel orientation alongside the thin needle. Additionally, if local anesthetic is to be infiltrated along the prospective tract, the thin needle used for this purpose may easily be detached from the hub of the anesthetic syringe and left in place during final lesion localization to provide "first pass" tandem needle guidance.

Second, it is better to pass close to (or even through!) a vital structure with a very thin needle than with one of larger caliber. A thin needle can be used as a "guard rail" to avoid

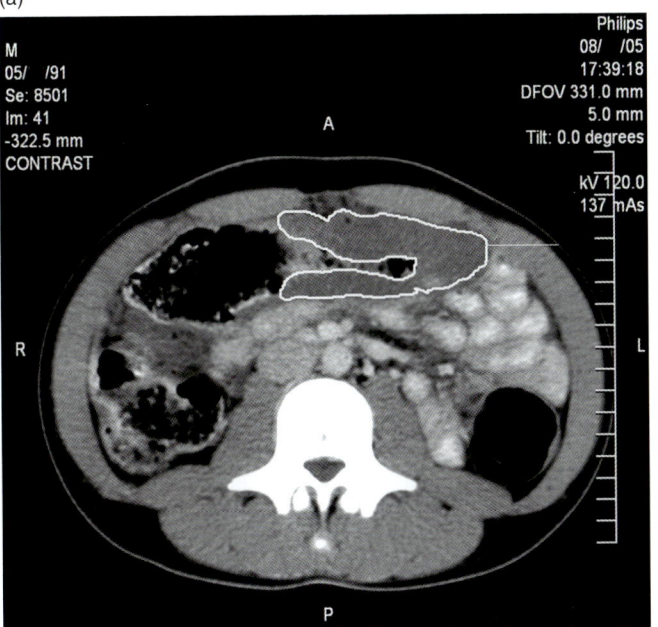 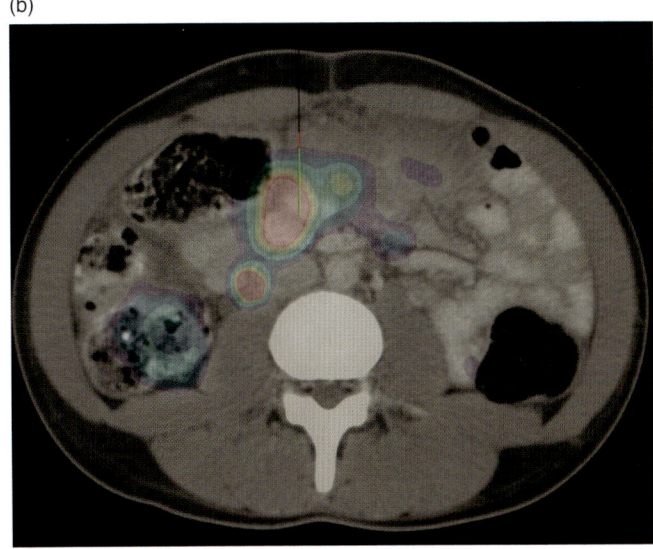

Figure 4.63 (a) Computed tomography with vascular and enteric contrast enhancement in a 14-year-old male with abdominal pain shows a soft tissue mass involving the transverse colon. (b) Stepwise reconstruction of an 18-F FDG PET-CT fusion through the same region one month later shows intense uptake although, for the purposes of guiding an intervention, co-registration might be improved with contemporaneous images on an integrated scanner.

straying from the intended pathway. By keeping to the "safe" side of the thin needle, the biopsy or coaxial needle can then be passed with less risk of complication. If there are multiple vital structures at risk, additional thin needles may be placed to "guard" them.

Molecular imaging guidance

When obtaining a tissue biopsy for suspected malignancy, the indications include an unknown tumor, metastasis from a known or unknown primary malignancy, recurrence of previously diagnosed malignancy, or secondary malignancy after prior treatment for malignancy. Conventional imaging with CT or US provides anatomic data but very little physiologic information. In any case it is difficult to differentiate vital tumor from necrosis, fibrosis, and hemorrhage. It is very difficult to avoid an unnecessary biopsy, and impossible to target the most metabolically active tissue within the target lesion. While not all malignancies are active enough to differentiate with molecular imaging, most lymphomas, sarcomas, blastomas, and carcinomas in the pediatric population will show abnormal uptake on an ^{18}F-FDG PET scan (Figures 4.56, 4.63).

Molecular imaging provides a visual representation of the metabolic activity in potential target tissues. In a large proportion of cases, PET-CT fusion will alter management compared to conventional imaging alone by avoiding a needless biopsy, enabling a percutaneous alternative to an open surgical biopsy, altering the approach to a suspicious lesion, reducing sampling error, or reducing the number of passes required to obtain diagnostic tissue.

Postprocedure and follow-up care
Specimen handling

Once the specimen is obtained it must be appropriately prepared for transit and subsequent analysis. For cytological preparations, the cells are spread onto a slide and evaluated by the pathologist to determine if an adequate sample has been obtained. Histologic samples are placed onto a Telfa® pad or suspended in normal saline or formalin depending on the specific pathologic question and the laboratory analysis that is anticipated. It is helpful to discuss the biopsy with the pathology service beforehand to determine which suspension is preferred. An adequate volume of saline should be used to avoid evaporation in transit, which may cause unintended alteration of the sample.

For the best results, there should be close cooperation between the interventionalist and pathologist. It is often preferable that the pathologist be present to receive and process the specimen. In select cases a wet reading is helpful to confirm the adequacy of the material while the patient is still under sedation or anesthesia. If needed, additional specimens can be obtained during the same session. This approach is helpful for the patient and family since it minimizes apprehension, increases efficiency, and contributes to a timely diagnosis. In select cases, a biopsy procedure may be performed on an outpatient basis.

Complications

The most important and common complication of percutaneous biopsy is bleeding. It is unusual for biopsy of even infected lesions, much less tumors and other masses, to result in infection. Pneumothorax and hemothorax may complicate any procedure that violates the thorax, whether intentionally or not. Arteriovenous fistula, pseudoaneurysm, and arterial injury are unusual complications of transhepatic or pancreatic procedures, although they may occur with virtually any abdominopelvic procedure. Similarly, bile leak and bile fistula may complicate any procedure that violates the hepatic capsule. Fistulae may also develop between hepatic arteries, hepatic veins, portal veins, and bile ducts, and hemobilia is also possible although exceedingly rare.

Hemorrhage

The entry wound should be observed frequently during the recovery period. Significant visible bleeding after percutaneous biopsy is quite rare, and easily resolved with manual compression in virtually all cases. Clinically significant bleeding in deeper tissues or potential spaces may be much more subtle, and related signs and symptoms may be delayed or misinterpreted.

Tract seeding

Tract seeding is possible but is exceedingly rare in biopsy of pediatric tumors and I have not seen a case in over 30 years of practice. Nephroblastoma and hepatocellular carcinoma are among the malignancies with an elevated risk, but use of coaxial technique with a sheathed needle significantly limits this risk.

Bile leakage and bile peritonitis

Free intraperitoneal bile is strongly inflammatory. When patients develop acute abdominal symptoms after procedures through or near the hepatic capsule or gallbladder, after excluding occult hemorrhage, presence of a free fluid collection should raise suspicion of bile leakage. Brisk leakage can precipitate liver failure and represents a surgical emergency. Symptoms are not always so prominent, and may include generalized malaise, dyspnea, shoulder pain (from diaphragmatic irritation), fatigue, fever, emesis, or irritability. If an aspirate of the fluid suggests bile leak, this should be treated as described in Chapter 5. If leakage continues undiagnosed it may result in sepsis, with progression of symptoms, or jaundice, with more obvious implications. If leakage is unrecognized and becomes walled off or encapsulated it may remain asymptomatic for months.

Controversies/issues

Outpatient liver biopsy in children

Conventional wisdom has held that pediatric liver biopsy should be performed only on an inpatient basis. However, it is our experience that under appropriate circumstances this procedure can safely be performed as an outpatient procedure. Children eligible for outpatient hepatic or renal biopsy should fulfill the following criteria, adapted for image-guided biopsy in children:

1. Patients or their legal surrogates should be given an informed choice to have the biopsy performed as an outpatient procedure.
2. Patients should be able to return to the facility where the procedure was performed within 30 minutes of any untoward symptoms.
3. Reliable observation must be available for the patient over the first 24 hours following the procedure. The designated caretaker providing observation must be able to provide transportation to an appropriate health care facility if necessary.
4. Patients should be free of identifiable and uncorrected risks for severe postbiopsy complications. Identifiable risks may include but are not limited to: cancer or bone marrow transplant, AIDS, ischemic liver disease, encephalopathy, hepatic failure with severe jaundice or evidence of significant extrahepatic obstruction, serious diseases involving other organ systems (especially cardiac or pulmonary insufficiency), and age less than one month. Potentially correctable risks include anxiety or inability to cooperate requiring sedation or anesthesia, ascites, mild coagulopathy, and use of medications (e.g., a beta-receptor antagonist) that may obscure a response to a complication.
5. The facility performing the biopsy should meet the following criteria:

   - immediately adjacent to or part of a pediatric inpatient facility to which the patient can be admitted without delay in the event of complications
   - fully approved laboratory and blood banking support
   - equipment appropriate for infants and children, for continuous monitoring of pulse, blood pressure and oxygen saturation, and for pediatric resuscitation if necessary
   - access to an inpatient bed if necessary
   - personnel experienced in providing the planned procedure and accompanying sedation, anesthesia, observation and resuscitation to pediatric patients, during the procedure and the postbiopsy period (usually, six hours) of close medical observation.

If these criteria cannot be met, children should be admitted to the pediatric inpatient facility overnight following the postbiopsy period of close medical observation. Regardless of the anticipated status of the patient, a low threshold should be maintained for continued hospitalization after biopsy if there is any evidence of bleeding, bile leak, puncture of non-target organs, or significant or prolonged postprocedure pain, until the patient's premorbid baseline has been restored.

Conclusions

When tissue is required for a pathologic diagnosis and a target can be identified with medical imaging, an image-guided biopsy using interventional techniques is the most cost-effective approach available, with the lowest rate of expected complications, the least anticipated recovery time, and the shortest requirement for hospitalization. The accuracy is equivalent to open surgical biopsy in most cases, and may exceed the capability of surgical biopsy when physiologic imaging is incorporated that enables precise targeting of the most metabolically active tissue. With a little imagination and thoughtful application of available imaging modalities and interventional techniques, there are almost no tissue targets that cannot be safely and accurately acquired.

It is essential to the success of the practice that there be strong and timely communication between the referring service, the interventionalist, and the pathology service, so that the diagnostic goal of the procedure is accomplished. It is very helpful for the interventionalist to develop the habit of examining the prepared slides with the pathologist, either intraprocedural evaluation of touch preps and frozen sections, or at least postprocedural review. This not only assures a high rate of satisfactory procedures and a valuable camaraderie with clinical colleagues, but also encourages constant process improvement and greater familiarity with diseases common to the interventionalist's patient population. Contingency planning can also allow related procedures to be performed by the interventional service, either under the same sedation or anesthesia (e.g., central venous access).

Attending tumor board and, where appropriate, seeing patients around elective procedures in the interventional radiology clinic or at the bedside will greatly enhance the interventionalist's credibility within the clinical community and more closely integrate the interventionalist into the clinical decision-making and management process.

Dilation of hollow viscera

Introduction

In 1821, Hildreth first used bougienage, a technique using a mechanical dilator, for treatment of esophageal strictures. In 1898, Russell described the first use of a pneumatic balloon dilator for treatment of lower esophageal strictures and achalasia. Over the next 50 years, numerous balloon catheters were developed for treatment of esophageal strictures. In benign disease, the results of treatment with bougies alone are comparable to surgery. In the early 1980s, modern balloon dilators were first used for the treatment of esophageal strictures. Today it is these non-surgical techniques that are the preferred approach for acquired esophageal strictures and in some cases, of congenital esophageal stenosis (CES).

Standard medical management now includes dilation with graded mechanical dilators (bougies) and inflatable balloon catheters. A variety of bougie dilators are available, including mercury-filled bougies, metal olives of different diameters (Eder–Puestow), rubber bougies, and endoscopes that are passed across strictures. Bougies are introduced transorally or retrograde via a gastrostomy and passed across the stricture to mechanically enlarge the area of narrowing. Dilation is usually accomplished without imaging and involves passing the system over a string or guide wire, although endoscopic or fluoroscopic guidance may be used concomitantly. This approach to dilation is safe and has an overall complication rate ranging between 0.4 and 8%.

In order to be effective, the bougie, a tapered dilator, must be larger than the stricture it is dilating. Thus the dilator initially exerts both transverse (perpendicular) and longitudinal (parallel) forces on the tissue just proximal to the stenosis before encountering the stricture during passage. The parallel forces create a snow-plow effect that leads to undesirable local tissue injury. In contrast, balloon dilation transmits only controlled radial forces normal to the esophageal wall at the level of the stricture. Although bougienage effectively enlarges strictures, there are disadvantages including: (1) excessive longitudinal (shearing) forces due to dilator design; (2) rigid dilator design that makes access to tortuous or angulated lumens difficult, increasing the risk of esophageal injury; (3) lack of visualization of the stricture, which makes determination of the endpoint inexact; and (4) a shorter relapse-free interval than with balloon dilation. Stark and colleagues postulate that it is the combination of decreased trauma to the esophageal wall and the larger luminal diameters that can be achieved that result in the longer symptom-free interval when dilation is performed with a balloon catheter instead of a bougie.

Since its development, there has been substantial improvement in angioplasty catheter and balloon technology, including the introduction of a large variety of catheter shaft diameters, balloon sizes, and high-pressure balloons. These technical developments have broadened the indications for angioplasty balloons, which are now routinely used to treat vascular as well as non-vascular stenoses.

Bougie-type dilators create both radial and shearing forces. With either bougienage or balloon dilation, it is the radial forces that actually dilate strictures. The shearing force is undesirable because it does not result in productive dilation of a stricture, but instead contributes to injury of the esophageal wall. The degree of shearing force developed is dependent on instrument design. McLean and colleagues evaluated different types of bougie dilators and found that the Savory–Gilliard bougie generates less shearing forces than the Maloney dilator. However, regardless of the design, it was found that bougies create more shearing force than balloon catheters. This shearing force can approach the tensile strength of the esophageal wall, putting it at greater risk for injury and perforation. However, in spite of this theoretic risk, bougienage is still used for esophageal stricture dilation and, in practice, esophageal perforation is uncommon.

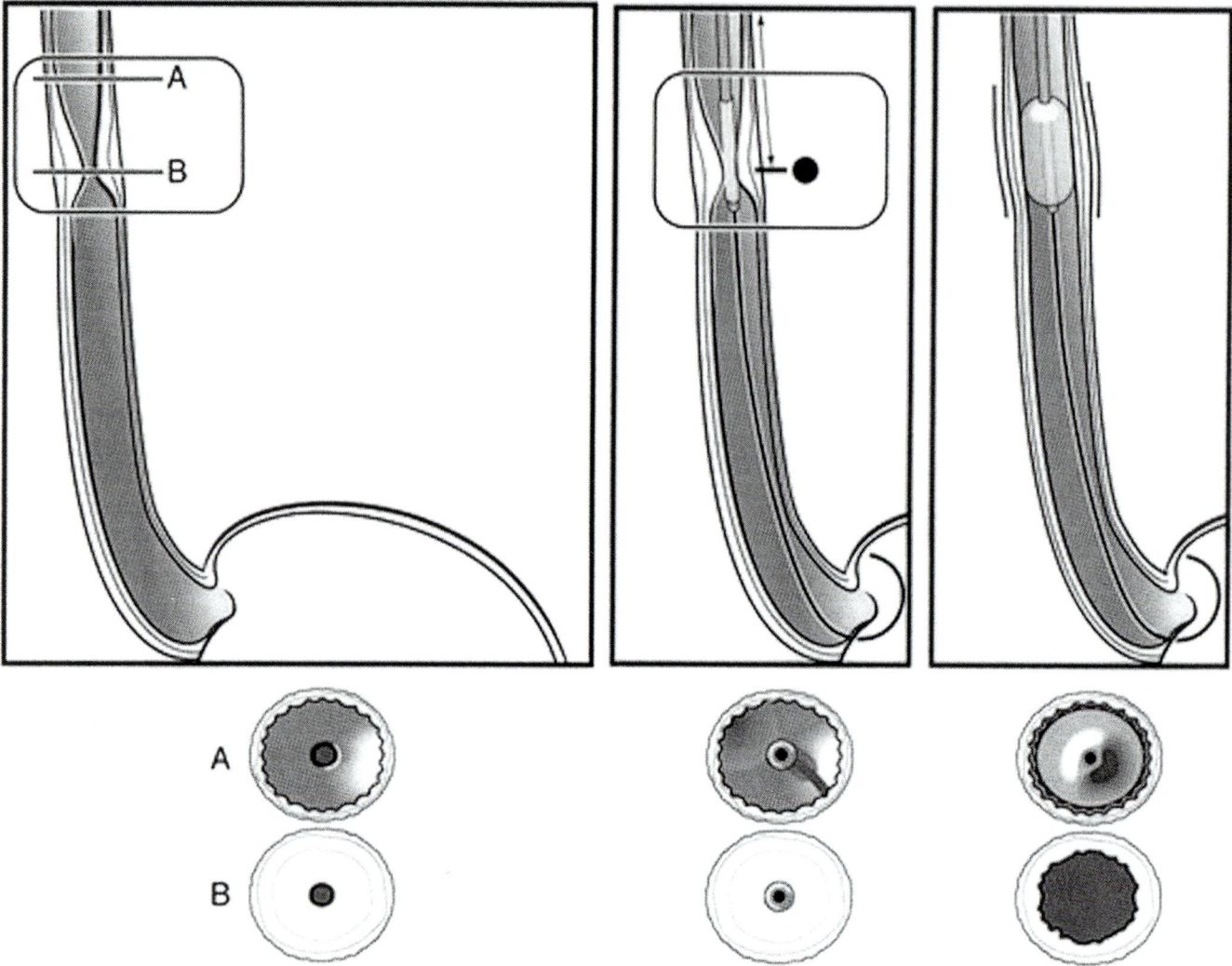

Figure 4.64 Esophageal dilation illustration. (Left) A contrast esophagram is used to measure the nearest normal caliber (A) adjacent to the esophageal stricture (B). (Middle) A directional catheter is used to navigate a guide wire across the stricture, and an initial non-compliant balloon catheter up to 2 mm smaller diameter than the "normal" diameter determined at (A) is centered on the stricture. (Right) The balloon is inflated to the intended pressure, observing the waist at the stricture. When the waist is effaced, pressure is maintained for three to five minutes as tolerated, then the balloon is deflated.

Subacute strictures respond better to dilation than do long-standing strictures that have become fibrotic. Long-term results may be judged by the symptom-free interval. Although some children remain symptom-free after one dilation, the majority of patients require serial dilations. The results of treatment are influenced by the type and extent of the stricture. Children with anastomotic strictures without ongoing inflammation have had prolonged symptom-free intervals after a single dilation. Children with anastomotic strictures and tight Nissen fundoplications on average require more than one dilation per case to achieve long-term symptom-free periods. In contrast, children with inflammatory diseases have shorter symptom-free intervals and require more than four dilations on average to achieve a long-term symptom-free period. Recurrence is most often noted in children with long-segment inflammatory strictures. Successful results using balloon catheters have been reported in adults and children by numerous authors. In collected series, success rates of approximately 90% have been achieved; however, the frequency of long-term cure or time between dilatations may vary depending upon several factors such as the etiology of the stricture, its length, and location. As a result of the success of balloon dilation as a method for treatment of esophageal strictures, we expect that this technique will continue to be utilized more frequently for treatment of these children, and will become the therapeutic method of choice (Figure 4.64).

The technique of balloon dilation can be applied to strictures involving other sites within the gastrointestinal tract. Success has been achieved with balloon dilation of achalasia, enlargement of a tight Nissen fundoplication, treatment of congenital and acquired small bowel and colonic strictures, and pyloric stenosis. Ischemic strictures develop in 3 to 36% of infants recovering from necrotizing enterocolitis. Surgical resection is still the treatment of choice. Balloon dilation is a

Table 4.18 Indications: dilation of hollow viscera

Indications for esophageal dilation
- Congenital esophageal stricture
  - fibromuscular stenosis
  - membranous web or ring
- Acquired
  - anastomotic
  - caustic
  - peptic
  - gastroesophageal reflux
  - tight Nissen fundoplication
  - retained foreign body
  - Crohn's disease
  - postinfectious (e.g., *Herpes simplex, Candida*)
  - inflammatory
  - radiation
  - syndromes (Stephens–Johnson, epidermolysis bullosa, chronic granulomatous disease)
  - secondary to sclerotherapy for esophageal varices
  - extrinsic compression

viable alternative for management of focal colonic strictures within defunctionalized bowel segments prior to re-anastomosis. To date, there have only been isolated cases reported using balloon dilation for treatment of these problems. Thus one cannot predict the utility of balloon dilation for treatment of these problems.

Indications

In adults, strictures may be associated with either malignant or benign diseases. Esophageal strictures are uncommon in the pediatric population (Table 4.18) and the vast majority of strictures are benign. Esophageal dilation procedures are indicated for children with esophageal narrowing that interferes with swallowing. Examples include primary stricture (congenital esophageal stenosis), or more often secondary stricture (e.g., postoperative or iatrogenic, anastomotic, inflammatory, caustic, radiation), webs and rings, and achalasia. Children with acquired strictures generally present with progressive symptoms, most notably dysphagia, acute obstruction secondary to lodgment of a foreign body (e.g., a piece of hot dog), or inability to take solid foods. Occasionally, malnutrition or aspiration pneumonia is the presenting symptom. When acquired causes of esophageal narrowing have been excluded, a diagnosis of congenital esophageal stenosis (CES) should be considered. In addition to the symptoms listed above, individuals with CES may also present with dysphagia for liquids with regurgitation minutes after feeding. However, these infants more frequently present with dysphagia that becomes noticeable after the introduction of semi-solid and solid foods at about six months of age. In a smaller subgroup, presentation is delayed for years and is manifest as excessive salivation, growth retardation, and recurrent respiratory tract infections.

Congenital esophageal stenosis

Congenital esophageal stenosis is a rare narrowing of the esophagus present at birth (incidence is approximately 1 in 25,000 to 50,000 live births), although it may not be symptomatic in the neonatal period. Congenital esophageal stenosis is a congenital malformation of the esophageal wall architecture. The malformation may include ectopic tracheobronchial remnants, membranous webs or diaphragms, and segmental hypertrophy of the muscularis and submucosal layers with diffuse fibrosis (fibromuscular stenosis). Stenosis secondary to tracheobronchial remnant results from sequestration of tracheobronchial tissue in the wall of the esophagus at the time of separation of the respiratory and primitive esophagus (approximately the 25th gestational day). The stenosis is usually attributed to the higher rate of growth of the esophagus compared with the tracheobronchial tree. The diagnosis may be missed by endoscopic biopsy because the heterotopic tissue lies deep beneath the normal mucosa. On radiographs, the stenosis is usually visualized in the mid-esophagus and appears irregular and very narrowed (Figure 4.65). Endoscopically, the stricture is irregular, rigid, and unyielding. Surgical excision of the stenotic segment has been the primary approach to therapy. To date, only minimal experience with balloon dilation is available; however, successful dilation is rare and is probably not the treatment of choice.

Membranous diaphragms or webs are thought to represent a form of a missed esophageal atresia similar to other Loew type 1 atresias of the digestive tract. In order to confirm this type of CES as a congenital anomaly, it is essential to exclude a web from peptic esophagitis secondary to gastroesophageal reflux. The stenosis, due to a membrane, is usually easily recognized both radiologically and endoscopically as a thin veil of tissue with regular contours. The area of narrowing is usually located in the mid-esophagus and is abrupt and sharply defined and regains its normal lumen distal to the web. Treatment may be initially undertaken with balloons or bougies. However, in most instances, surgery is indicated.

Fibromuscular stenosis has often been successfully treated with bougies and more recently balloons, but has not been studied extensively by pathologists. Pathologic proliferation of smooth muscle fibers and fibrinous connective tissue is covered by normal mucosa. Radiographs of children with fibromuscular stenosis are noted to have smooth narrowing of the distal esophagus. Endoscopically, the stenosis appeared regular and was flexible and easy to dilate. In most instances, a successful therapeutic outcome is achieved with bougienage or balloon dilation.

Congenital esophageal stenosis may be associated with other congenital anomalies. The associated anomalies may be chromosomal and involve the digestive tract, cardiovascular system, urinary tract, eye, head, face, or limbs. The most common associations include esophageal atresia with or without associated fistula, H-type esophageal fistula, duodenal

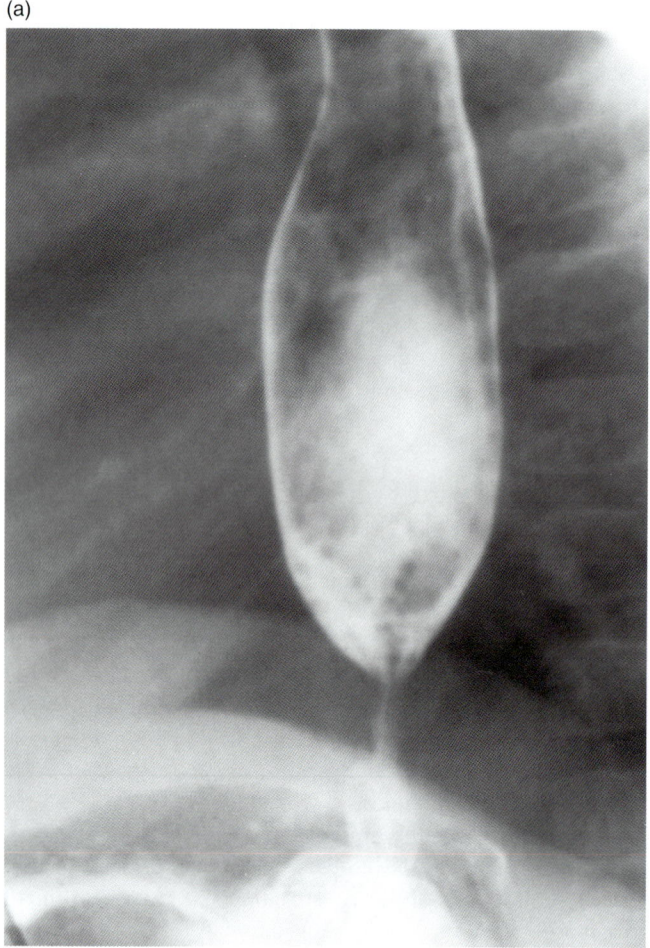 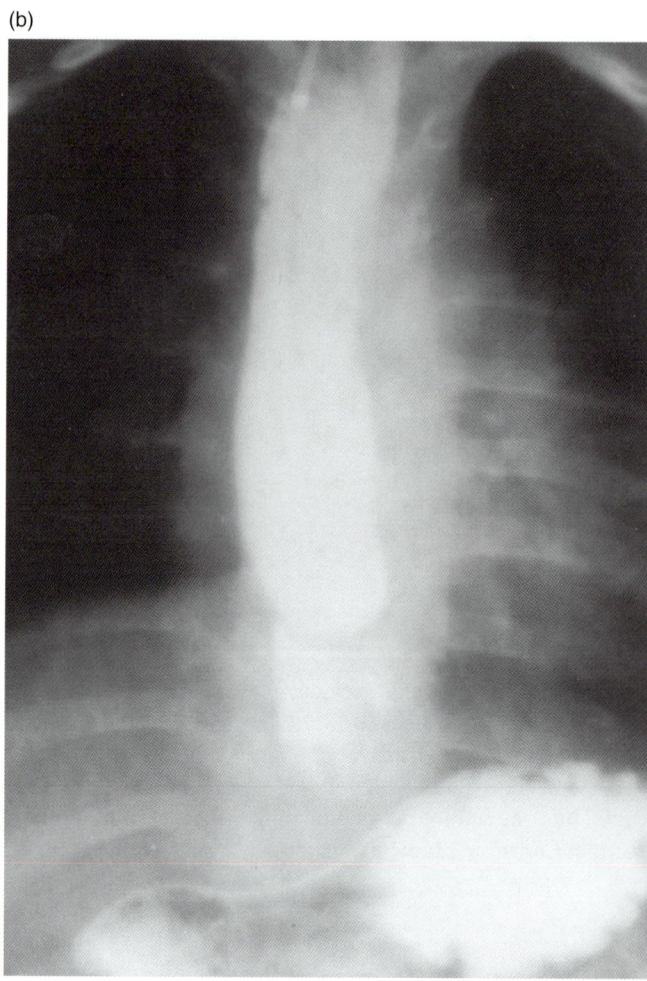

Figure 4.65 (a) A lateral distal esophagram shows a tight acquired inflammatory stricture. (b) After dilation with a 4 mm, 6 ATM non-compliant balloon, contrast is seen to pool in a contained distal perforation. A soft nasogastric tube was placed across the rupture to promote healing and the esophagus was eventually repaired surgically.

diaphragm and atresia, pulmonary valvular stenosis or left to right shunts, and Down's syndrome.

Acquired esophageal strictures

Acquired strictures occur with greater frequency than CES. An anastomotic stricture resulting from repair of esophageal atresia, with or without an associated tracheoesophageal fistula, represents the most common etiology in our experience. Strictures from a wide variety of conditions, including gastroesophageal reflux, caustic ingestion, inflammation, radiation, Stevens–Johnson and other syndromes, chronic granulomatous disease, and epidermolysis bullosa, are occasionally found.

Esophageal atresia (EA) is a rare anomaly that occurs in approximately 1 in 3,000 to 4,500 live births. The mechanism by which EA occurs is uncertain but it is postulated to be caused by fixation of the esophagus to the trachea by a fistula during its development or by failure of canalization possibly due to ischemia. Although there are several different types of EA with or without an associated tracheoesophageal fistula (TEF), the most important types are EA with distal TEF (Figure 4.66), which occurs in about 86% of cases, isolated EA in 8%, and an isolated H type fistula in 4%.

In excess of 40% of these children with EA and about 30% of those with EA and TEF have associated anomalies. The non-random association of anomalies, termed the VACTERL association, suggests a more generalized disturbance of embryogenesis. The anomalies include vertebral defects, anal atresia, cardiac abnormalities, which are the most common, TEF, esophageal atresia, renal anomalies, and radial limb dysplasia.

Treatment consists of surgical repair. A primary end-to-end anastomosis is performed whenever possible. However, if the gap between the ends is greater than 2 to 3 cm, the surgical anastomosis is more difficult and there is a greater risk for postoperative complications such as a leak or stricture. If the gap is too large for a primary anastomosis, then a cervical

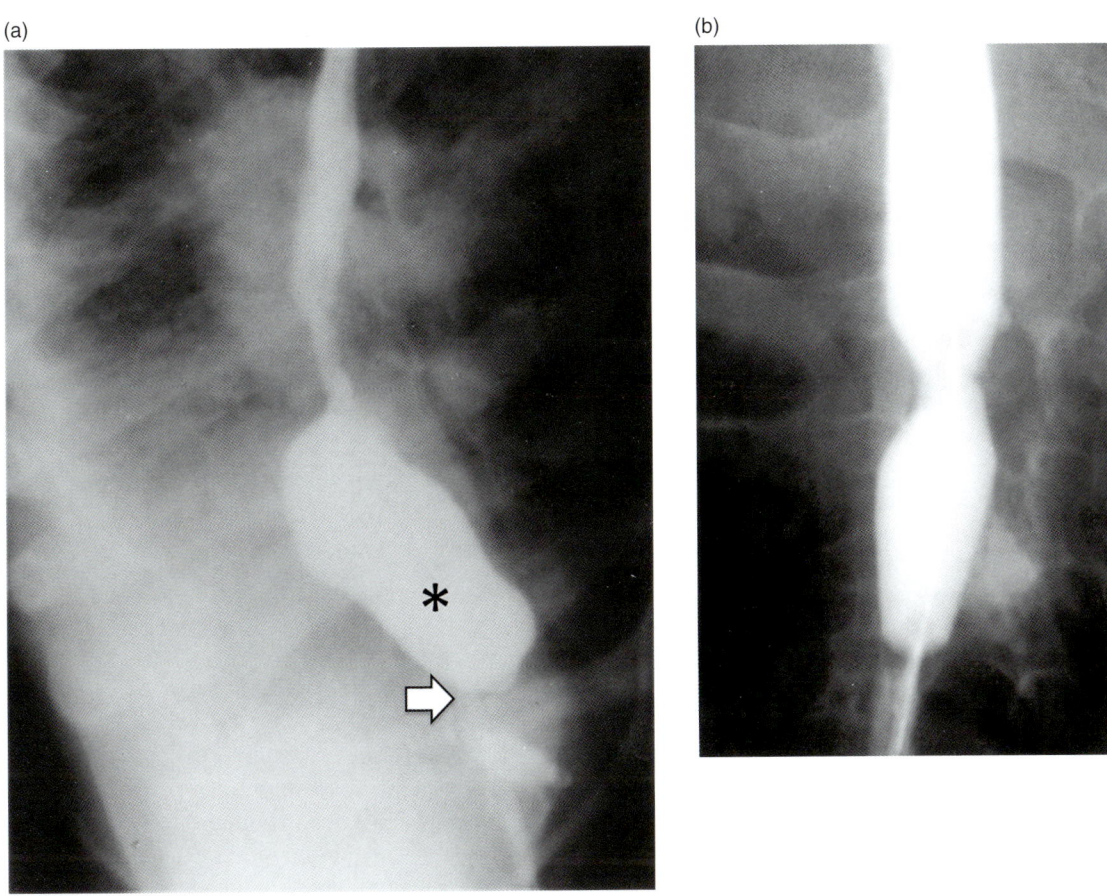
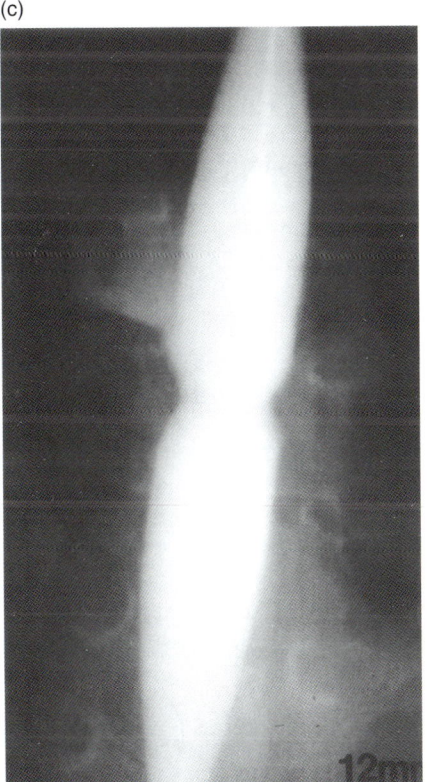

Figure 4.66 (a) An infant with surgically reconstructed esophageal atresia with distal fistula developed a postoperative anastomotic stricture (*arrow*) with proximal dilatation (*asterisk*) and dysmotility (seen in 100% of these patients). (b) A 12-mm 6 ATM balloon is partially inflated, showing a waist at the stricture. (c) The waist was almost fully effaced at 12 ATM delivered pressure. The goal of therapy is functional translation of a food bolus without dysphagia. This may require serial dilations in staged procedures.

esophagostomy can be performed in anticipation of esophageal replacement with a gastric tube or other reconstructive procedure.

Anastomotic strictures are common in the postoperative period. In addition, some children also develop strictures of the distal esophagus secondary to gastroesophageal reflux. When symptoms suggest the possibility of a stricture, endoscopy or barium esophagography is indicated for diagnosis and treatment planning.

Gastroesophageal reflux (GER) is common. In most individuals it is harmless and causes few problems. In a small subgroup of children GER may become severe and result in serious complications, including death. Complicated reflux should be considered when the patient demonstrates one or more of the following signs or symptoms: failure to thrive, hematemesis, iron deficiency anemia, intermittent wheezing, nocturnal cough, aspiration pneumonia, and apnea. Chronic GER can lead to the development of strictures and a Barrett esophagus. These strictures often will respond to balloon dilation (Figure 4.64).

Caustic ingestion is one of the most common causes of an esophageal stricture in children. Esophageal injury may result from ingestion of a variety of substances including strong alkalis, acids, ammonia, phenol, silver nitrate, and iodine. In about 80% of cases, the injured child is three years of age or younger. Historically, boys are more frequently affected. Injury is often the result of innocent negligence. Regardless of the reason for the esophageal ingestion, the result is often a severe esophageal burn. The location of the injury is somewhat dependent on the volume and type of agent ingested. Acids usually cause superficial mucosal damage primarily involving the gastric antrum with relative sparing of the esophagus. In contrast, ingestion of a strong alkali results in mucosal injury to the mouth, pharynx, and esophagus. The stomach is rarely involved. In the acute phase there is edema and ulceration. Later, there may be sloughing and denuding of the mucosa and in some cases perforation. This injury may progress to necrosis and scarring of the muscularis with resultant stricture formation. An esophageal stricture may be found as early as two weeks post caustic ingestion (Figure 4.67).

Infectious esophagitis is unusual in childhood and is most often identified in immunosuppressed patients. *Candida albicans* is the most common cause of infectious esophagitis and most often involves long esophageal segments. Other causes of esophagitis include herpes simplex type 1, AIDS, cytomegalovirus, Gram-negative bacteria, streptococcus, and mixed bacterial infections.

Rarely, non-infectious inflammatory causes of esophagitis occur. These include drugs such as antibiotics, oral potassium, anti-inflammatory agents, and cimetidine. These etiologies as well as radiation injury have all been associated with esophagitis and stricture formation.

Epidermolysis bullosa dystrophica (EBD) is a rare condition that can lead to esophageal injury with associated stricture formation. Epidermolysis bullosa dystrophica describes a

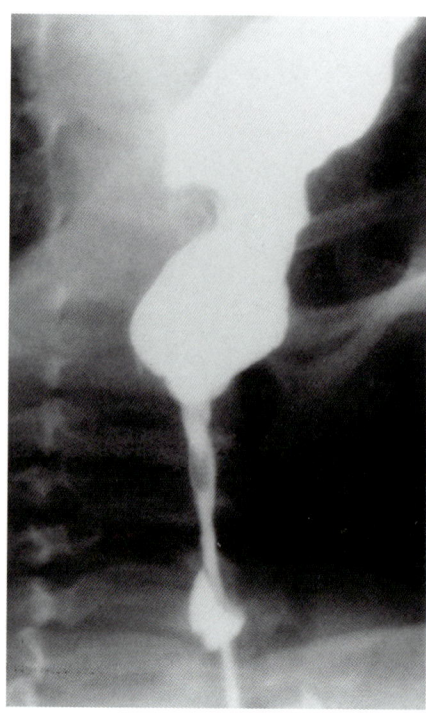

Figure 4.67 After caustic ingestion of lye, this two-year-old male developed a long esophageal stricture. This was treated with steroids acutely then referred for bougie and endoscopy, but could equally have been a suitable candidate for balloon dilation.

group of conditions that cause blistering of the skin and variable involvement of mucous membranes. The autosomal recessive type is the most severe and most often associated with esophageal disease. The esophageal lesions tend to be located in the esophagus at the level of the carina or in the extreme proximal or distal esophageal segments. When a stricture occurs, it tends to be smooth in contour, tapered, and 2 to 4 cm in length.

Stevens–Johnson syndrome is a severe form of erythema multiforme characterized by a severe systemic illness, purulent conjunctivitis, and necrotic and hemorrhagic skin and mucosal lesions. Outcome is variable but in severe cases death may occur. The esophagus is rarely involved, but when affected the lesions are characterized by vesicles, bullae, desquamation, and ulcers. Repeated episodes can result in stricture formation. Other inflammatory dermatoses, including graft-versus-host disease, mucositis secondary to chemotherapy, pemphigus, acanthosis nigricans, and lipoid proteinosis, can produce similar lesions and complications. These disorders tend to have a predilection for the proximal esophagus although any segment can be affected.

Chronic granulomatous disease (CGD) is an X-linked recessive disorder with signs and symptoms occurring before three years of age. These children have a defect in their cellular immunity because of a deficiency of neutrophil function. Due to a defect in the phagocytic function, the neutrophil can phagocytize bacteria but is unable to kill encapsulated organisms. This leads to recurrent infections, lymphadenopathy, and sepsis. Abnormalities of esophageal motility occasionally occur in these boys. In severe cases, the esophagus can be aperistaltic and thick walled, sometimes leading to long segment strictures.

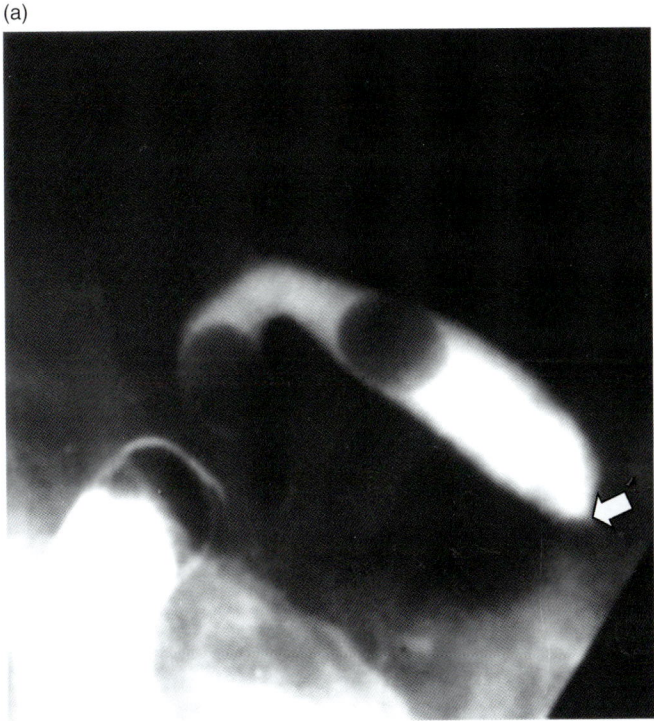 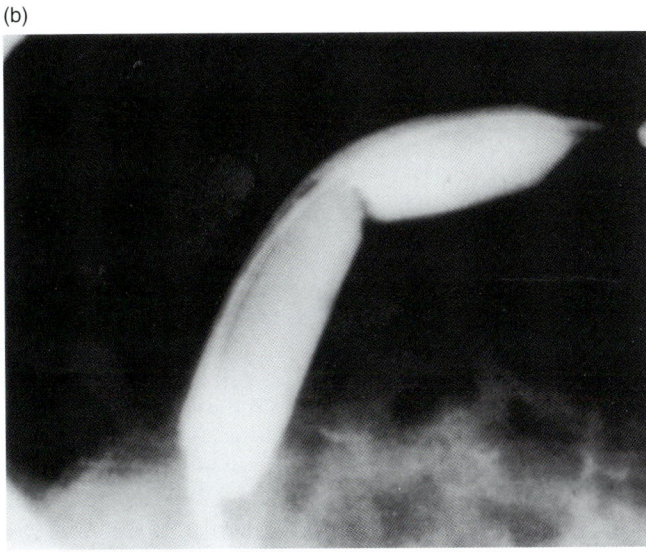

Figure 4.68 (a) A six-week-old with a history of necrotizing enterocolitis developed intermittent abdominal distention. A barium enema demonstrated a colonic stricture at the splenic flexure. (b) Measurement of nearby normal lumen resulted in selection of a 5 mm x 2 cm 8 ATM balloon, which was dilated until the stricture was effaced.

Esophageal varices result from diseases causing portal hypertension. Neonatal hepatitis, biliary atresia, complications of total parenteral nutrition, and cavernous transformation of the portal vein, are among the more common causes. Children with variceal bleeding may be treated symptomatically with endoscopic sclerotherapy. The varices are injected with a sclerosing agent such as sodium tetradecyl sulfate, in order to thrombose the offending veins. Occasionally, the esophageal wall is affected resulting in a localized stricture. Since it usually involves the distal esophageal segment, this is the site of narrowing.

Rarely, an esophageal injury may be iatrogenic. Care must be taken to avoid injury when using lasers, electrical probes, tubes, or other instruments. The young infant may be particularly prone to injury due to the relative thin wall and small luminal diameter.

Other gastrointestinal strictures

Treatable strictures in the remainder of the gastrointestinal tract include hypertrophic and much more rarely non-hypertrophic pyloric stenosis, acquired small bowel stricture from necrotizing enterocolitis (Figure 4.68), distal ileal or ileocolonic anastomotic strictures (e.g., in Crohn's disease), colonic anastomotic and more rarely inflammatory and other acquired strictures, and rectal or anorectal strictures. Generally speaking, strictures between the proximal duodenum and the distal ileum are not accessible to image-guided intervention.

Technique
Equipment

In the instance when the procedure is performed under sedation, the child must be restrained as previously described. However, in most cases, dilation is performed under GA or intubation and paralysis; therefore only light restraint is necessary. If transoral endotracheal intubation is used and a transoral route is planned for the procedure, it may be necessary to insert a bite block with a central opening in order to allow passage of the diagnostic and PTA catheters. It is our preference to use high-pressure (non-compliant) angioplasty balloons, in order to maximize the chance for a successful outcome and minimize the need for multiple balloons to enlarge the stricture to the desired diameter (Table 4.19). In these cases, the catheter shaft diameter is not important, so virtually any catheter with the appropriate balloon diameter can be used.

A variety of instruments or materials can be used to externally mark the level of the stricture. We prefer either a Beekley® spot on the skin or a hemostat clipped to the sheets, drapes, or patient gown.

Patient preparation

Anticoagulation should be discontinued prior to the procedure. The targeted lumen should be evacuated prior to the procedure. Care should be taken that the esophagus is empty

Table 4.19 Equipment: dilation of hollow viscera

Esophageal dilation
- Octostop® board (for children <2 years old or short enough to fit) or other restraining device (mummy wrap, Velcro® or other types of straps).
- 8 to 10 French feeding tube or red rubber catheter.
- 5 French JB-1 catheter.
- Guide wire (Bentson, Glidewire).
- Marker (hemostat, metallic marker, Beekley® dot).
- Percutaneous transluminal angioplasty catheter.
- Pressure gauge.

Table 4.20 Procedure summary: dilation of hollow viscera

Esophageal dilation
1. Insert an intravenous line.
2. Child is immobilized and sedated *or* under general anesthesia.
3. Limited esophagram for localization of the stricture.
4. Mark the level of the stricture using a hemostat, Beekley® dot, or other device.
5. Insert guide wire via esophageal catheter and maneuver it into the stomach.
6. Position appropriate sized balloon catheter across the stricture.
7. Under fluoroscopic guidance, inflate balloon with dilute contrast until the waist disappears. Maintain inflation for three to five minutes, or as long as the patient tolerates it.
8. Perform postprocedural esophagram prn.
9. If the procedure is performed as an outpatient, recover child until (s)he is awake and responsive, then discharge to home.
10. Soft diet and advance as tolerated.

in cases where esophageal dysfunction is accompanied by prolonged stasis. For colonic stricture, a cleansing enema may be performed if necessary. Otherwise, there is no special preparation necessary prior to dilation of a stricture except that required for general anesthesia or sedation. Initially, the decision to be made is whether to dilate the stricture under local anesthesia and sedation, sedation with intubation and paralysis, or general anesthesia. In any case, the hospital protocol for NPO preparation is followed, and the interventionalist should work closely with the other clinicians involved to make sure that the preprocedural details are in order.

When balloon dilation is considered for treatment of an esophageal stricture, it is important to examine the area of abnormality carefully prior to treatment. Both endoscopy and a diagnostic esophagram may be needed to identify and characterize the extent, location, magnitude, and number of strictures that are present. If fluoroscopically guided balloon dilation is to be performed, a barium esophagram or an examination using water-soluble contrast is always completed prior to the procedure. The esophagram should be performed on a different day than the dilation if possible. The esophagram should demonstrate the pathologic anatomy in at least two orthogonal projections so that the characteristics of the stricture are fully evaluated. In addition, it is helpful to measure the diameter of the stricture and the normal esophagus below the stenosis for treatment planning. Measurements can be made by placing a ruler over the child's chest in frontal projection or with digital technology where available. When the possibility of a CES is raised or another diagnostic issue is at question, a biopsy may be needed prior to balloon dilation or other therapy. If a biopsy is performed, it is our preference to wait one to three days before proceeding with the dilation.

Before dilation of pyloric stenosis, routine US should provide all necessary information. No bowel preparation is required prior to this procedure, although the stomach should be empty of food. Preparation for dilation of ileal, colonic, or anorectal stricture is similar to that for esophageal stricture.

Standard technique (esophageal dilation)

In our experience, the most critical aspect of dilation of an esophageal stricture is the choice of the balloon size, the type of balloon, and the endpoint of the procedure (Table 4.20). There are no controlled studies available to answer these important questions. The normal esophagus will tolerate inflation pressures up to 258 mm Hg, and can be expanded 1.6 to 2 times its resting diameter without rupture. Pressures up to 500 to 840 mm Hg have been recorded during bougienage dilation. However, neither the burst pressure of an abnormal esophagus nor the maximal diameter to which the abnormal esophagus can be stretched is known. In the case of an anastomotic stricture, the original size of the surgically created anastomosis may be known and, if so, the risk of perforation can be minimized by selecting a dilation balloon no larger than this diameter.

The choice of the balloon diameter, length, and nominal burst pressure depends on the severity, length, and location of the stricture. In order to minimize the expense of the treatment and time to complete the procedure, we try to start the procedure with the balloon diameter closest to the predicted endpoint. The actual balloon diameter selected depends on the severity of the narrowing and the type of stricture anticipated (congenital versus acquired). When the stricture is not critically narrowed, the initial esophageal dilation is with a balloon no less than 2 mm smaller than the expected endpoint (usually 8 to 12 mm). When the stricture is very tight the initial dilation will usually be more conservative at about 50 to 75% the anticipated endpoint. If, at the completion of the initial dilation, the balloon is coated with red blood the procedure is terminated. If the balloon does not "waist," a larger balloon is selected and the procedure is repeated. The maximal balloon diameter selected is approximately 10% larger than the predicted normal diameter of the esophagus.

If the procedure is performed with intravenous sedation, the patient is securely restrained. Prior to the esophageal dilation, a feeding tube or catheter is inserted through the mouth and a limited barium esophagram is performed in order to locate the stricture site, which is then marked on the chest wall. Although a variety of devices can be used to identify the level of the stricture, we prefer to use a hemostat clipped to the patient's gown. A good alternative is a Beekley® spot, a small metallic marker with an adhesive backing that can be affixed to the skin. The 8 to 10-French feeding tube or 5-French JB-1 catheter (used for contrast injection), and 0.035- to 0.038-inch Bentson guide wire, is maneuvered past the stricture and coiled in the stomach.

Although successful dilation can be achieved using either the transoral or transnasal routes, the transoral route is preferred, especially in small infants and children, because it is easier and less traumatic to pass and *remove* the large balloons at the completion of the procedure. When the esophageal narrowing is central or of moderate severity, any catheter and guide wire system will usually suffice to pass the stricture site. Tight or eccentric strictures or angulated anastomoses usually require a directional catheter and guide wire to cross the stricture. We have found the JB-1 catheter and angled Glide® wire or Bentson guide wire to be best in this situation. After the guide wire is coiled within the stomach, a standard balloon catheter is centered across the stenosis. If the stricture is tight and the angioplasty balloon will not pass, it may be useful to predilate the stricture with a low-profile catheter (van Andel catheter, other catheter/dilator), small vessel balloon, or, rarely, a microballoon.

If the transoral route is chosen, a bite block is inserted into the mouth to ease catheter placement, protect the operator's fingers, and to avoid damage to the catheter. The balloon is centered across the stricture and, under direct fluoroscopic visualization, is inflated with a water-soluble contrast medium. Balloon inflation is monitored both fluoroscopically and with a pressure gauge; balloon sizing is considered to be appropriate if an impression (waist) is identified on the inflated balloon. After disappearance of the waist, inflation is generally maintained for three to five minutes, as long as the child tolerates it. In most instances, only two or three inflations are performed. If fresh blood is noted on the balloon, the procedure is terminated since a mucosal or deeper tear has likely occurred. At the conclusion of the dilation, a water-soluble esophagram is performed to evaluate the esophagus for possible complications and the success of the dilation. The postdilation appearance of the stricture is often not predictive of outcome since luminal narrowing may result from associated edema or hemorrhage.

Technical variations

Management of eccentric stricture and pseudodiverticulum

In general, balloon dilation of esophageal strictures is a simple and straightforward procedure. In most cases, the most challenging technical aspect of the procedure is to maneuver past a tight stricture. Usually this can be easily accomplished using a JB-1 catheter and Bentson or Glidewire®. However, the operator should be aware of the eccentric stricture located in the proximal third of the esophagus, usually in children with repaired EA. In these children, the dilated proximal pouch may have an associated pseudodiverticulum, which is usually the result of previous dilations with bougies. If one is unfamiliar with this situation, it may be a source of technical difficulty and can lead to complications. A perforation can occur if rigid catheters or bougies are used for diagnosis or treatment since these instruments tend to go in a straight path often into the pseudodiverticulum. If one is uncertain of the anatomy, injection of contrast will usually quickly solve the problem.

Colonic dilation

Congenital strictures, webs, rings, and anastomotic stenoses occur throughout the small bowel and colon, albeit primarily at one end or the other. Whether a pyloric stenosis, a duodenal web, or a colonic anastomotic stricture, the principles of treatment are the same (Figure 4.69), and similar to treatment of an esophageal stricture as described above. First, pass a guide wire across the stenosis, usually assisted by a directional catheter. It is important to confirm with contrast that the catheter, and hence the guide wire, has passed through the stricture to normal bowel, as the presence of a fistula at or near the stricture is not uncommon. Next, exchange the catheter for a non-compliant balloon. The balloon must be sized according to the intended outcome. Usually, this will relate either to the known diameter of the original surgical anastomosis, or to the diameter of the nearest segment of normal caliber. The balloon should be centered on the stricture or stenosis before inflation. A blood-coated balloon should prompt termination of the procedure, understanding that serial dilations over time may be required to achieve the desired long-term outcome. Function is the ultimate measure of success.

Postprocedure and follow-up care

In most cases, esophageal and other gastrointestinal stricture dilations are performed as outpatient procedures. If the dilation is completed without difficulty or complication the child is observed in the recovery area in the radiology department for two to four hours or until the child is alert and awake. If there is suspicion of a complication or a complication has been documented, a water-soluble study of the treated segment is performed, a surgical consultation is usually called, and a hospital admission arranged. We have found significant pain and hematemesis to be good indicators of postprocedural problems after esophageal dilation. During the observation period, vital signs (pulse, temperature, blood pressure, and respiratory rate) are monitored. Initially, vital signs are recorded every 15 minutes for the first hour, then every 30 minutes for the next hour, and if all is well, every hour until discharge. Prior to discharge, the parent or guardian is reminded of the potential problems that might be encountered, and instructions for feeding and follow-up are given. If vital signs remain normal, the child is discharged with instructions to take clear liquids and, if tolerated, advanced to a soft diet by 48 to 72 hours. After esophageal dilation, children often initially prefer creamy and non-acidic foods as they are easier to tolerate.

(a)

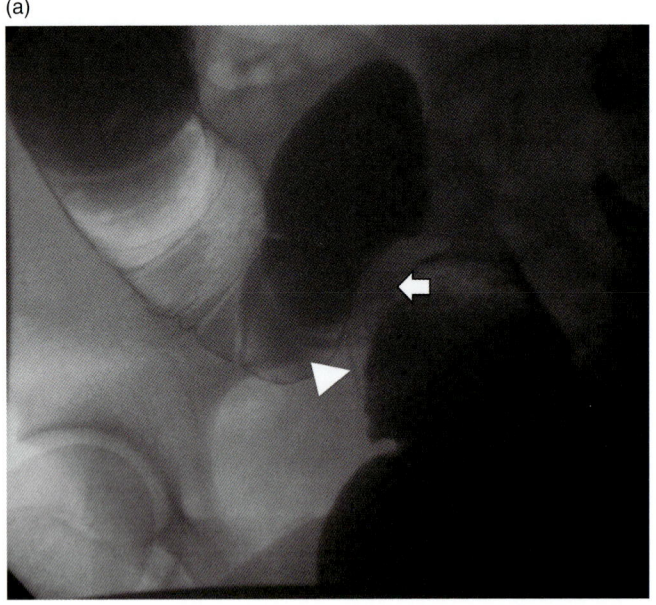

(b)

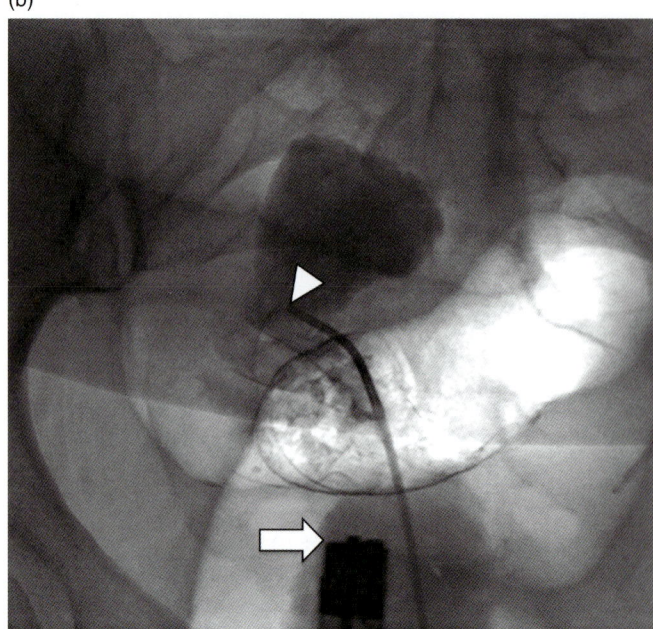

(c)

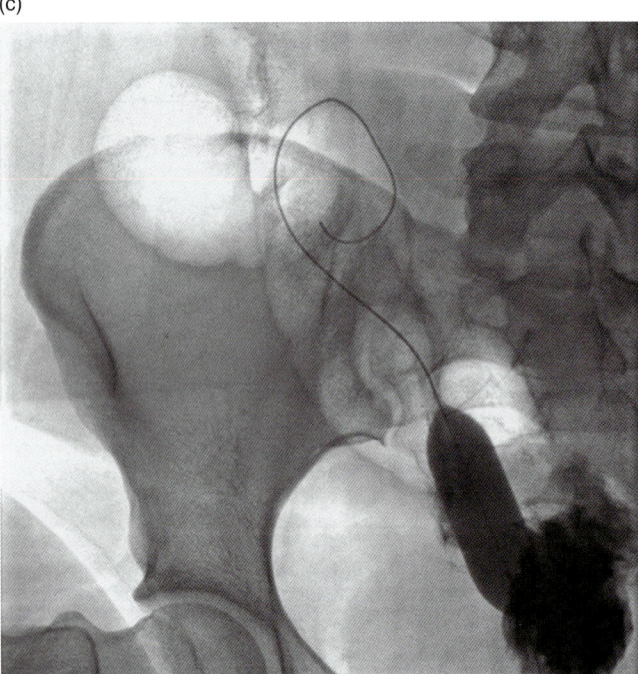

Figure 4.69 An 18-year-old female developed abdominal pain with defecation one month after total colectomy and ileorectal anastomosis. (a) A very tight stricture (*arrow*) is seen adjacent to the anastomosis suture line (*arrowhead*) on a thin barium enema. (b) Endoscopically assisted access across the ileorectal anastomosis with a directional catheter (*arrowhead*). (c) Serial dilations were performed, up to an 18 mm balloon. Discomfort resolved, and stools normalized.

The issue of when to repeat the dilation procedure must be tailored to each individual case. Strictures identified in the acute or subacute phase of development often need to be dilated one or two times per week until the diameter of the treated segment remains stable and the child is able to take solid foods or pass formed stool as appropriate. At this time the child is followed symptomatically. At this point, the stricture will often remain asymptomatic. If symptoms recur, the frequency of dilation is reduced to once per two to four weeks. As long as the child is stable, no further dilations are performed.

Technical problems and pitfalls
Balloon rupture

At times, non-compliant balloons are known to rupture during dilation. Mucosal injury may occur at the time of rupture, and after the balloon has been removed the region should be carefully evaluated for evidence of full-thickness tear. It is advisable to remove the ruptured balloon through an appropriately sized sheath, in order to avoid further injury. A sheath may be positioned by cutting the hub off the balloon catheter then passing the sheath over the catheter until the ruptured balloon is covered by the sheath, at which time both can be removed together over the guide wire.

Stiffening the balloon delivery platform

It can sometimes be difficult to navigate through loops of bowel or past redundant flexures and still have enough stiffness in the system to advance the guiding catheter and guide wire across the stricture once it is reached. We have often used an angled or curved sheath, such as a Balkin or a long straight or angled introducer, for this purpose. For example, the Check-Flo® introducer is available in lengths from 13 to 70 cm and 9 to 14 French. The sheath dilator can be advanced to the stricture, preferably engaging the stricture, and the sheath pushed forward to the tip of the dilator before the dilator is exchanged for the guiding catheter and the balloon is positioned across the stricture. In this way we have been able to treat strictures as proximal as the cecum.

Positioning for colonic dilation

Positioning the patient for balloon dilation of a colonic stricture benefits from careful preprocedure planning. It is much more convenient for the operator if the patient is reversed on the angiography table, with the perineum as close to the head-end of the table as possible. The lower extremities and feet must be supported in a lithotomy position to allow transrectal access. This is most easily managed with stirrups attached to the table rails, but a radiolucent (i.e., Plexiglas®) board, padding, and wide tape can be used to accomplish the same objective. A generous layer of absorbent padding under the patient will help avoid a messy distribution of contrast and other fluids during the procedure. Although this is a non-sterile procedure, wearing a gown, gloves, mask, and eye shield will help keep the operator and the operator's lead apron from becoming soiled.

"Kissing" balloons

During treatment of colonic strictures especially, it may be difficult to find a non-compliant balloon with a large enough diameter and an adequate nominal burst pressure to achieve satisfactory dilation. Two or three "kissing" balloons of smaller individual diameter can be substituted for a single larger balloon. When two balloons of equal diameter are used, the nominal diameter can be approximated as the diameter of an ellipse with a short axis equal to the single balloon diameter and a long axis twice the short axis. Thus the nominal diameter is approximately equivalent to the diameter of a single balloon 1.55 times the diameter of one of the two balloons.

Complications

Dilation for the treatment of esophageal and other gastrointestinal strictures has been utilized for many years. The risk of complications from bougienage and balloon dilation is well known. Perforation of the esophagus is most common and occurs in approximately 1 of 400 dilations. This is in line with numerous adult series that report complication rates of 0 to 2.2%. The most common complications are intramural laceration and transmural perforation. Laceration is contained by the esophageal wall and will usually resolve with two to three days of liquid or soft-food diet. Transmural perforation may require immediate surgical repair but, if small, will often respond to medical therapy including intravenous hydration and broad-spectrum antibiotics.

The cervical and thorocoabdominal segments were the most common sites of injury. The cervical perforations were less dangerous than the thoracic ones and usually were the result of improper introduction of the dilator through anatomic outpouchings. Thoracic perforations generally resulted from rupture of diseased segments. The use of flexible endoscopes and fluoroscopic guidance has improved dilation safety. Other complications that have been documented, but are rarely clinically significant, include bacteremia, bleeding requiring transfusion, arrhythmias, vasovagal reactions, and perforation of the stomach or small intestine with guide wires. Unfortunately, there are no large series of children treated with balloon dilation of either CES or acquired esophageal strictures. Therefore only anecdotal reports and personal experience is available describing the complications of balloon dilatation. The most significant complication reported in children is esophageal perforation with or without associated mediastinitis. As this technique gains in popularity, it is important that the range and rate of complications be more accurately documented.

Conclusions

Balloon dilation of esophageal and other gastrointestinal strictures has been shown to be safe and effective and can be a cost-effective alternative to bougienage or surgical repair or revision for treatment of gastrointestinal strictures in the pediatric population. With its many advantages, this technique should become the preferred method for treatment of acquired strictures of the esophagus and possibly other sites in the gastrointestinal tract. Congenital esophageal stenoses are often resistant to treatment with balloons and may require surgery. However, if non-operative treatment is contemplated, balloon dilation using angioplasty catheters is a reasonable alternative.

Foreign body retrieval

Introduction

Esophageal foreign bodies are common in children. Fortunately, most foreign objects (80 to 90%) pass through the gastrointestinal (GI) tract without incident. Problems can arise if a swallowed object is longer than 5 cm or thicker than 2 cm because it may not pass through the pylorus. An object retained within the stomach usually does not cause acute symptoms because it is free within the gastric lumen and does

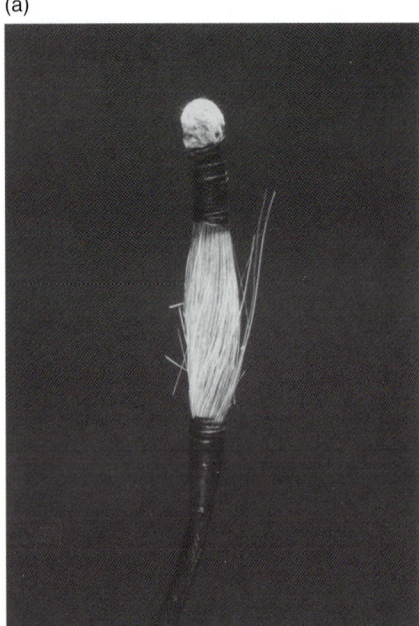
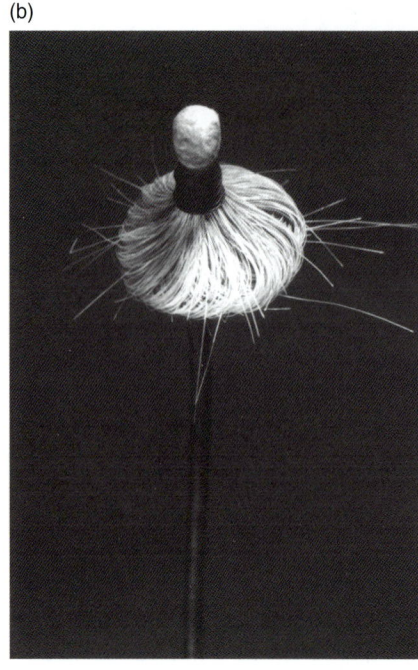

Figure 4.70 (a) This Civil War horsehair medical antique was designed for foreign body retrieval. (b) Once the device was passed beyond the esophageal foreign body, it was activated by retracting the inner core to create a soft, wide disc that assisted retrieval as it was withdrawn.

not obstruct either the gastric inlet or outlet. Thus an intragastric object may be treated conservatively and observed. If it does not pass, the retained object may be removed electively by either interventional or endoscopic techniques. However, a foreign body lodged within the esophagus can cause serious complications if untreated. For this reason, most clinicians recommend removal of an esophageal foreign body as soon as it is recognized.

Since 1937, rigid endoscopy had been the method selected for removal of esophageal foreign bodies. Today, both rigid and flexible endoscopes are used for foreign body removal. In the 1980s, the safety and effectiveness of the endoscopic approach for removal of all types of foreign bodies found within the esophagus and stomach was established. Advocates of endoscopic retrieval of esophageal and gastric foreign objects suggest that endoscopy has the advantage of: (1) direct examination of the esophagus and stomach before and after removal, (2) versatility, allowing treatment of either blunt or sharp foreign bodies, (3) increased safety, and (4) protection of the airway during foreign body removal.

The Foley catheter technique was actually introduced in the mid-1960s and has been used as an alternative to the endoscopic technique for esophageal foreign body removal. Undocumented variations of the technique could be traced to much earlier times (Figure 4.70). The Foley catheter technique is easy to learn, safe, and successful in 67 to 95% of cases. A lower rate of success has been achieved in young children with esophageal edema and tracheal compression secondary to long-standing foreign bodies. Ulceration of the esophageal mucosa is associated with the development of granulation tissue that covers the foreign body and inhibits removal with a balloon. In the absence of complicating factors, successful removal of a retained object can be expected in approximately 90% of cases. Advocates of the Foley catheter method for removal of retained esophageal foreign objects prefer this approach as the initial treatment for children who have uncomplicated esophageal foreign bodies since it: (1) is successful in over 92% of cases, (2) can be performed without general anesthesia or sedation, (3) has a very low complication rate (less than 1%), and (4) is much less costly than endoscopic removal. For example, average hospital fees associated with endoscopic removal are approximately six times greater than those of removal using the Foley catheter method.

Indications

A wide variety of objects are ingested by children of all ages. Of those objects that do not pass on their own, the majority lodge at the sites of normal anatomic narrowing, such as the hypopharynx, upper esophageal sphincter (at the level of the cricoid cartilage), aortic arch, and gastroesophageal junction. In fact, 65 to 75% of retained objects lodge in the upper third of the esophagus at the level of the cricopharyngeus muscle or thoracic inlet (Figure 4.71). If a foreign body is found at any other level, underlying esophageal pathology should be suspected (Figure 4.72). Common objects that become impacted in the esophagus include coins (found in about 80% of cases), bones, toys, disc batteries, and other found objects. If food becomes lodged it is often at the site of a stricture or anatomic narrowing.

Children with esophageal foreign bodies may present with drooling, vomiting, respiratory distress, hematemesis, airway obstruction, refusal to eat, or dysphagia. Drooling and dysphagia are among the most common presenting symptoms.

Chapter 4 Abdominopelvic interventions

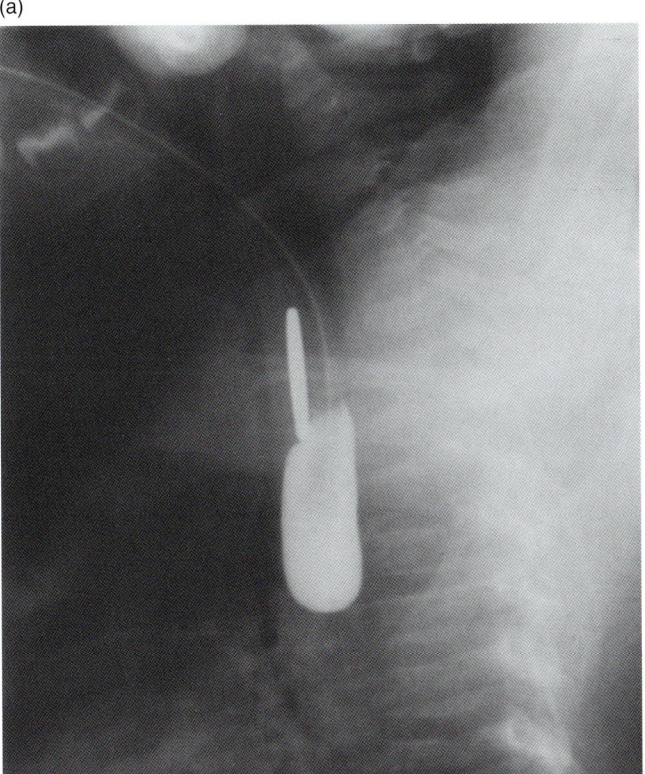
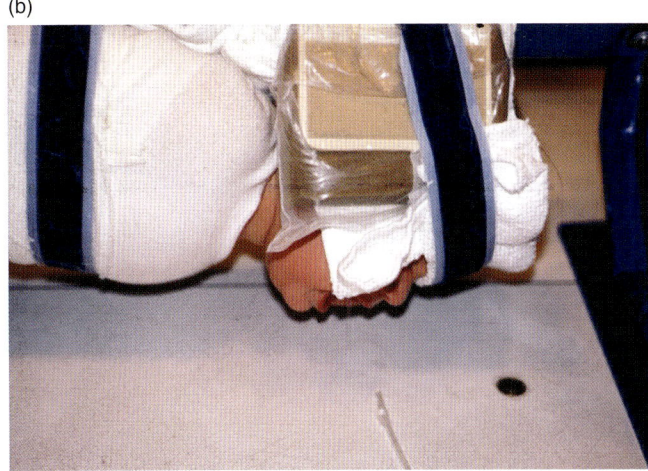

Figure 4.71 (a) A two-year-old female presented with refusal to eat and drooling. This lateral radiograph of the thoracic outlet shows a swallowed coin trapped at the level of the cricopharyngeus. A compliant Foley balloon catheter was passed beyond the coin, then the balloon was filled and withdrawn. (b) The infant, restrained on an Octostop® board in a prone Trendelenburg position, is shown as the coin (visible on the table top) has been expelled.

The presence of a foreign body lodged in the esophagus for more than 24 hours correlates most strongly with the development of major complications. When a sharp or pointed foreign body is identified, it should be removed endoscopically. However, the best treatment for blunt foreign bodies is still controversial. Current therapeutic approaches include endoscopy, blind, or fluoroscopically guided removal with a Foley catheter, passage of bougienage dilators, basket retrieval, and drug therapy.

Several authors have suggested that the time elapsed after foreign body impaction alone is an important determinant in deciding whether a child is a candidate for balloon removal. There are varying opinions as to the appropriate timing for balloon extraction. Some groups will not attempt removal after 24 hours has passed, while others will proceed after seven days or more if no contraindications are present. Our approach is to consider each case individually, based on the presence of esophageal edema or other complicating factors. If no complication or contraindication is noted, Foley catheter removal will be attempted. We suggest that any foreign object retained in the esophagus should be removed in order to resolve the child's symptoms and to prevent complications.

Absolute contraindications to non-endoscopic removal are rare but would include a retained sharp or pointed object (Figure 4.73), signs of esophageal perforation such

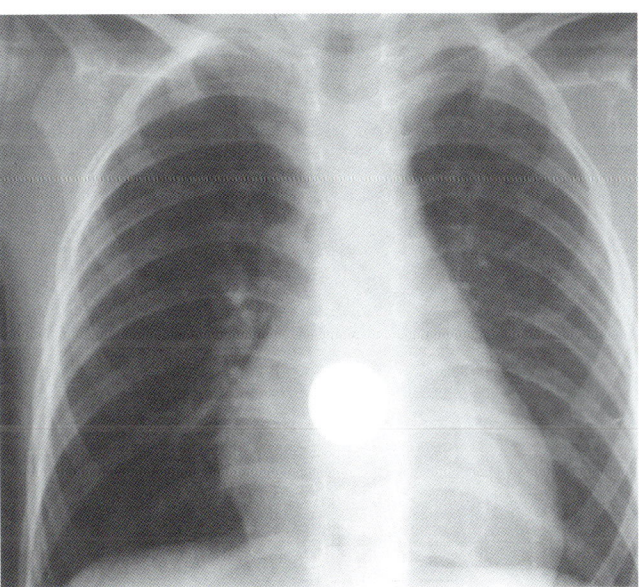

Figure 4.72 In this 33-month female a discoid foreign body projects over the distal esophagus above the gastroesophageal junction. This is an atypical position and requires a contrast study or endoscopy before a retrieval procedure is attempted, anticipating esophageal narrowing or abnormality at this point.

241

Table 4.21 Equipment: foreign body retrieval

1. Fluoroscope.
2. Octostop® board, Velcro® straps or other immobilizing devices (Figure 4.71b).
3. 12-French or larger Foley catheter with at least a 5 ml balloon.
4. Bite block or mouth gag.
5. Infant resuscitation cart.* Foley catheter end-hole punch. (Can create an end hole in a Foley catheter so that it can be passed over a guide wire).
6. JB-1 catheter and Bentson wire.
7. Tilt board should be available if it becomes necessary.
8. Foley catheter punch.

* Should be available if it becomes necessary.

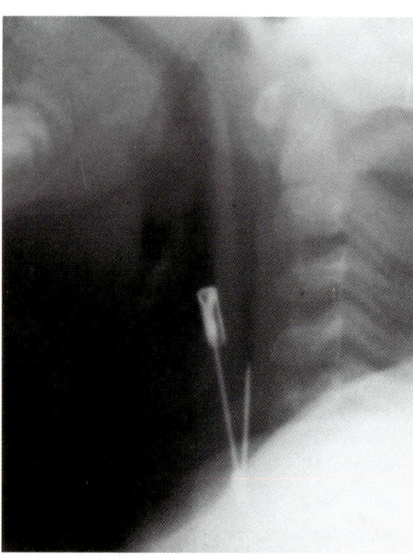

Figure 4.73 A safety pin projects outside of the esophageal soft tissues suggesting an extra-esophageal location. Removal under fluoroscopic control alone is not indicated.

as retropharyngeal gas, pneumomediastinum, pneumothorax, esophageal disruption, and recent esophageal surgery. These factors should favor endoscopic examination of the esophagus and endoscopic retrieval over Foley catheter removal. Relative contraindications to removal of esophageal foreign bodies are infrequently encountered but are important to identify prior to esophageal instrumentation. Foley catheter removal should be discouraged in the presence of esophageal or peri-esophageal edema with secondary extrinsic compression and anterior displacement of the trachea (Figure 4.74). This is associated with a high failure rate and significant potential for silent perforation due to underlying esophageal pathology such as ulceration and granulation tissue. Other relative contraindications to removal by balloon catheter include an uncorrectable coagulopathy, severe airway disease, and symptomatic lung and cardiovascular problems.

Technique

Equipment

There is no special equipment (Table 4.21) needed for removal of blunt esophageal foreign objects. Foreign body removal is usually performed in a standard fluoroscopy suite to make use of the tilt table. The procedure can be performed in an angiography suite; however, the child should be restrained on a tilt board so that a head-down position (15 to 45 degrees) can be obtained. If an Octostop®-type restraining device is not available, the procedure can still be safely and easily performed on the tabletop. In this situation, it may be helpful to restrain the child by wrapping the legs and, if

(a)

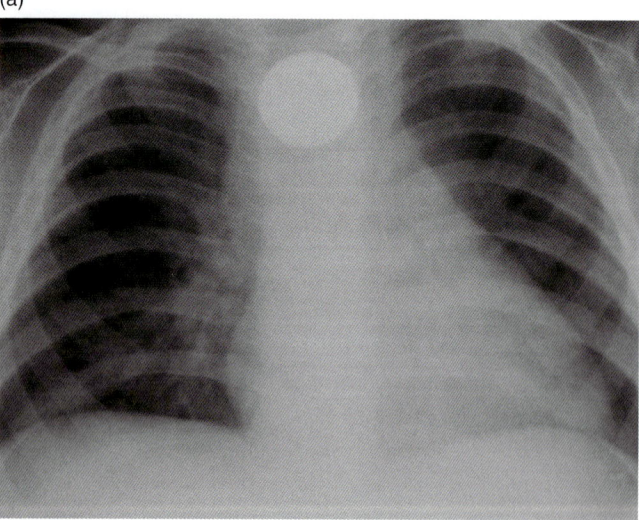

(b)

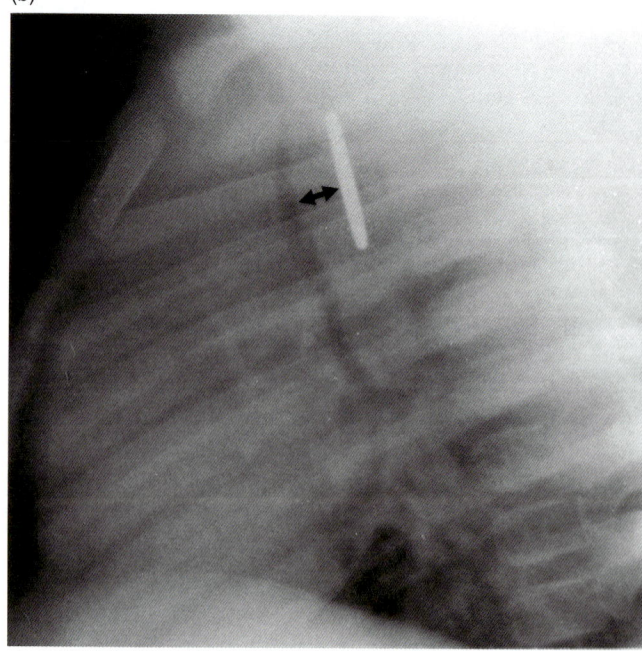

Figure 4.74 (a) In this anteroposterior view of an infant chest, the foreign body has an innocuous appearance. (b) On the lateral view, soft tissue thickening anterior to the foreign body (*double-headed arrow*) is evidence of striking edema, generally associated with esophageal erosion and development of granulation tissue.

necessary, the upper body, with elastic wrap in order to more easily maneuver and control patient motion. Any Foley catheter can be used. However, it is preferable to choose a catheter with at least a 5 ml balloon since these balloons can be routinely inflated >15 ml, which may be necessary to fully match the diameter of the esophageal lumen. Although rarely required, it is essential to have an infant resuscitation cart immediately available. This cart should include long forceps or another suitable instrument to remove an object that lodges in the supraglottic trachea. All interventional suites have a selection of directional catheters and guide wires. Remember to take catheters and guide wires to the fluoroscopy suite for use in cases where it is difficult to maneuver the Foley catheter past the lodged foreign body. In these cases, the directional catheter and guide wire will be positioned distal to the object, which can then be exchanged for a Foley catheter that has had an end hole created with a Foley catheter punch.

Patient preparation

Children suspected of having a foreign object lodged within the esophagus, stomach, or intestines, are referred for a foreign body series. This series consists of a lateral neck radiograph, frontal and lateral radiographs of the chest, and a supine abdomen. The lateral chest radiograph is omitted in some practices. However, we believe that if an object is identified within the esophagus, a lateral chest radiograph is needed to identify complications, particularly esophageal edema, and other potential contraindications to balloon removal (Figure 4.74).

In rare instances, a contrast esophagram and upper GI series may be performed if a non-radio-opaque foreign body is considered or a complication is suspected. These examinations are intended to document the presence and location of the foreign object and any associated esophageal injury, e.g., perforation. In our practice, an esophagram is not performed routinely prior to foreign body removal unless there is a known or suspected esophageal abnormality or the foreign body is lodged at an unusual location.

Standard technique

Removal of an object retained in the esophagus begins with informed consent. The fluoroscopy suite is readied and the equipment (Table 4.22) is prepared. An empty stomach is preferred to minimize the possibility of aspiration. A child less than two years of age should be restrained on an Octostop® board (Figures 4.71 and 4.75) if available, or with other methods for ease of maneuvering. Older children are wrapped in sheets, or tabletop straps may be applied if restraint is necessary. The use of topical anesthetic spray may be used in the nasopharynx but is discouraged in the oropharynx so that the gag reflex is maintained in its normal state. A Foley catheter with a balloon of at least 5 ml capacity (>12 French) is selected. Balloons with smaller diameter may not expand to fill the entire esophageal lumen. A 12-French or larger Foley catheter is chosen and tested prior to insertion by inflating the balloon with 10 to 15 ml of dilute contrast material. The Foley catheter is then inserted into the nose or mouth under fluoroscopic guidance and positioned distal to the blunt object. The child is then placed in the right anterior oblique position and the head of the table is put into Trendelenburg. The balloon is inflated with dilute contrast material until its margins are slightly flattened, indicating that the balloon has filled the entire esophageal lumen. Then, while monitoring with fluoroscopy, constant traction is applied to the balloon catheter until the object is dislodged and pulled into the mouth and expelled. Care should be taken to make sure that the object remains in contact with the balloon. If the object slips off the catheter, it will slip back into the esophagus and usually re-lodge in the esophagus at the same level. If this occurs, it is generally best to begin again and position the Foley catheter distal to the object. However, this time use the variable balloon technique as described below.

If removal has been attempted approximately three times and is unsuccessful, it is best to stop and consider referring the child for endoscopic removal. If a major complication is suspected or occurs, an esophagram should be performed. If an esophageal abnormality is confirmed, the child should be admitted to the hospital for endoscopic examination of the esophagus and removal of the object, if still present. A problem is suggested if the balloon becomes coated with blood, the child's vital signs deteriorate, or the catheter or wire appear to be extraluminal. In most instances, failed balloon removal results from an object being partly or completely covered by granulation tissue. One should avoid the use of non-compliant balloon catheters such as a Swan–Ganz or angioplasty catheter. These rigid systems may be associated with a higher risk of complications, especially esophageal laceration, due to the non-elastic nature of the catheter.

Table 4.22 Procedure summary: foreign body retrieval

Foley catheter technique

See Figure 4.75
1. Obtain informed consent.
2. Restrain child, using Octostop® board, mummy wrap in sheets, or tabletop Velcro® straps.
3. Select a Foley catheter with at least a 5 ml balloon (12 French or larger). Test inflate with dilute contrast.
4. Insert Foley catheter through the nose or mouth under fluoroscopic guidance and position it distal to the retained *blunt* foreign body.
5. Place child in right anterior oblique position and move table into Trendelenburg (head-down) position.
6. Inflate balloon until it is effaced by the esophagus and pull object into the mouth and onto the table.
7. Barium esophagram if coin not at site of normal anatomic narrowing.

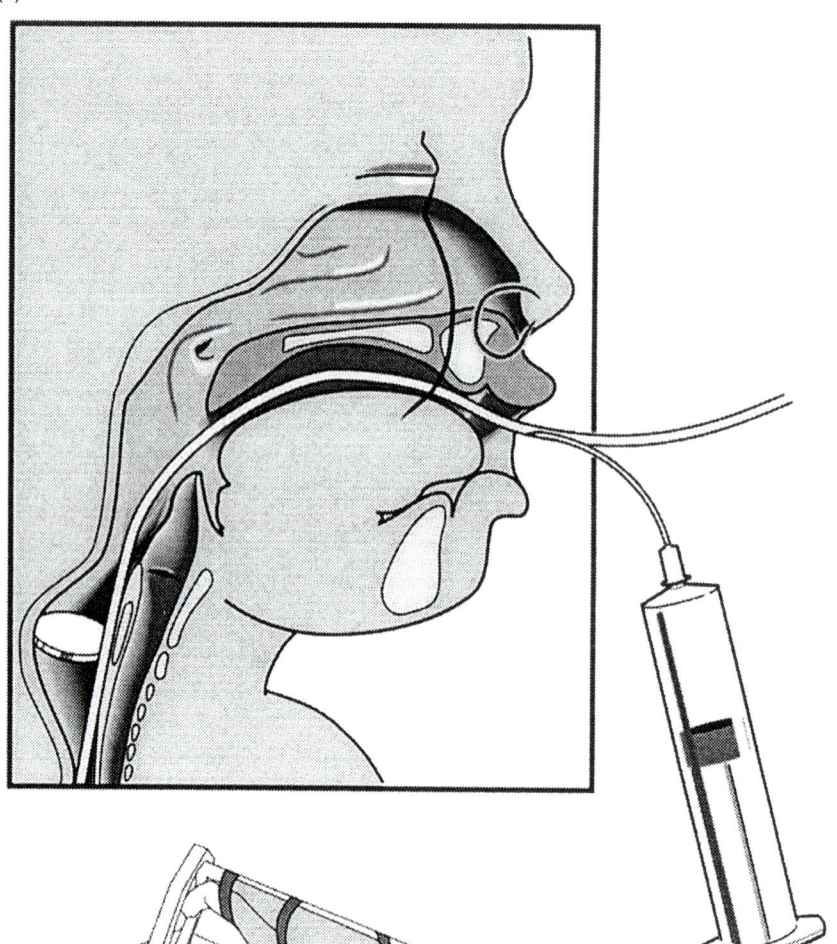

Figure 4.75 Esophageal foreign body retrieval illustration. (a) The deflated compliant balloon catheter is passed gently beyond the foreign body under lateral fluoroscopic guidance. (b) The balloon is inflated just enough to occlude the esophageal lumen, and is withdrawn so as to carry the coin toward the mouth. (c) The restrained patient should be positioned face down and in a relative Trendelenburg posture. The compliant balloon can be further inflated as it translates through the widened hypopharynx to avoid losing control of the foreign body. The foreign body is then exteriorized or retrieved.

Both the nasal and oral routes for catheter insertion work well. Operator experience and preference usually determines the approach selected. Although the nasal route allows for easier catheter insertion, there is a higher incidence of displacing the object onto the soft palate as it is removed. If this occurs, it may be difficult to remove. Reinsertion of a catheter is worth a try but usually will not dislodge the object because it adheres to the soft palate by hydrostatic pressure. We have found that the best way to remove the object in this case is either manually, by putting a finger into the mouth and over the palate and grasping it, or endoscopically. This could be a very embarrassing moment for the operator! This problem can be avoided by using the oral approach. If there is difficulty passing the Foley catheter from the mouth into the esophagus or passing the foreign body, an excellent strategy is to use a directional catheter guide wire system (JB-1 and Bentson guide wire) to maneuver past the oropharynx into the distal esophagus. Using a Foley catheter hole punch, an end hole can be created in the Foley catheter. Alternatively, other soft, end-hole catheters, such as a Council catheter or FlexiFlow® replacement gastrostomy catheter (Ross Laboratories, Columbus, OH), can be utilized. The JB-1 is then exchanged for the end-hole balloon catheter positioned distal to the object.

If the procedure was done on an outpatient basis, the child is observed briefly in the radiology department (for approximately 30 minutes) after the foreign body removal or sent back

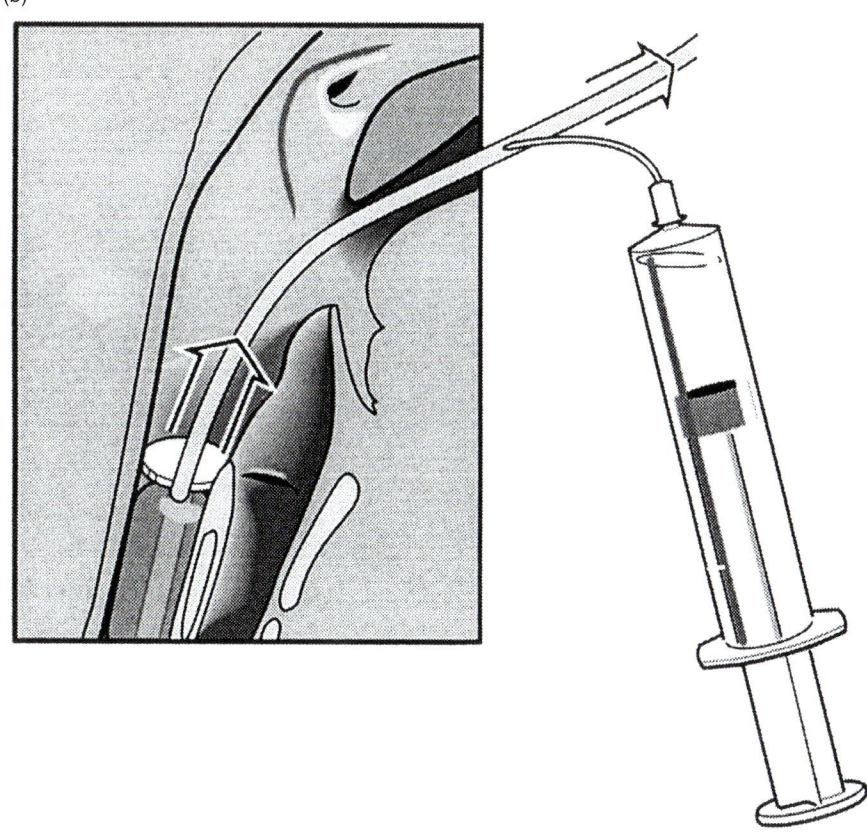

Figure 4.75 (cont.)

to the emergency room for observation. During this time, the child's vital signs are monitored and discharge instructions are reviewed. The parents are instructed to return to the hospital with the child if there is increasing or a different type of discomfort, inability to eat, or hematemesis is noted. Since there is often residual dysphagia or discomfort for 24 to 36 hours, a soft diet is recommended. Creamy, non-acidic solids and liquids are initially best tolerated. The diet can be advanced to the child's normal menu as tolerated.

During the first several hours after the procedure, blood-tinged saliva may be observed. However, significant or persistent bleeding or fever is unusual and should signal a possible complication, in which case the child should visit a physician.

Technical variations
Variable balloon inflation

In some instances, the standard approach using a fixed balloon size does not work. Problems usually result at the level of the hypopharynx where the lumen widens. This gradual enlargement allows the balloon and object to disengage and the foreign body to fall back into the esophagus. A strategy that is usually successful in this situation is to use a variable balloon inflation technique. With the standard approach, the Foley balloon is inflated and the syringe is uncoupled from the valve and removed. With the variable inflation technique, a 20 ml syringe filled with dilute contrast is left connected to the Foley catheter balloon valve. As the balloon is pulled toward the mouth, it is inflated or deflated as needed to maintain complete filling of the esophagus or hypopharynx with resultant flattening of the balloon margins until the coin is in the child's mouth or on the fluoroscopy table. (A great sound!)

Magnetic foreign body removal

Technology has produced a number of magnetic objects that may be ingested by young children, especially those less than five years of age. Ingested objects include disc (button) batteries, kitchen magnetics, toys, etc. Of these objects, the button battery poses the most risk to the child. The upper GI tract is the most common site for lodging, especially for batteries more than 2 cm in diameter.

In 1984, Jaffe and Corneli developed a magnet catheter for retrieval of magnetic foreign bodies. Although successful, the magnet used in this system was weak, therefore, a second catheter was often required for removal of the object. Since then, others have developed catheters with strong magnets, all of which appear to work well in most situations. The original Towbin catheter was modified so that the magnet catheter is directional and has an end hole allowing it to be inserted over a guide wire (Figure 4.76).

(c)

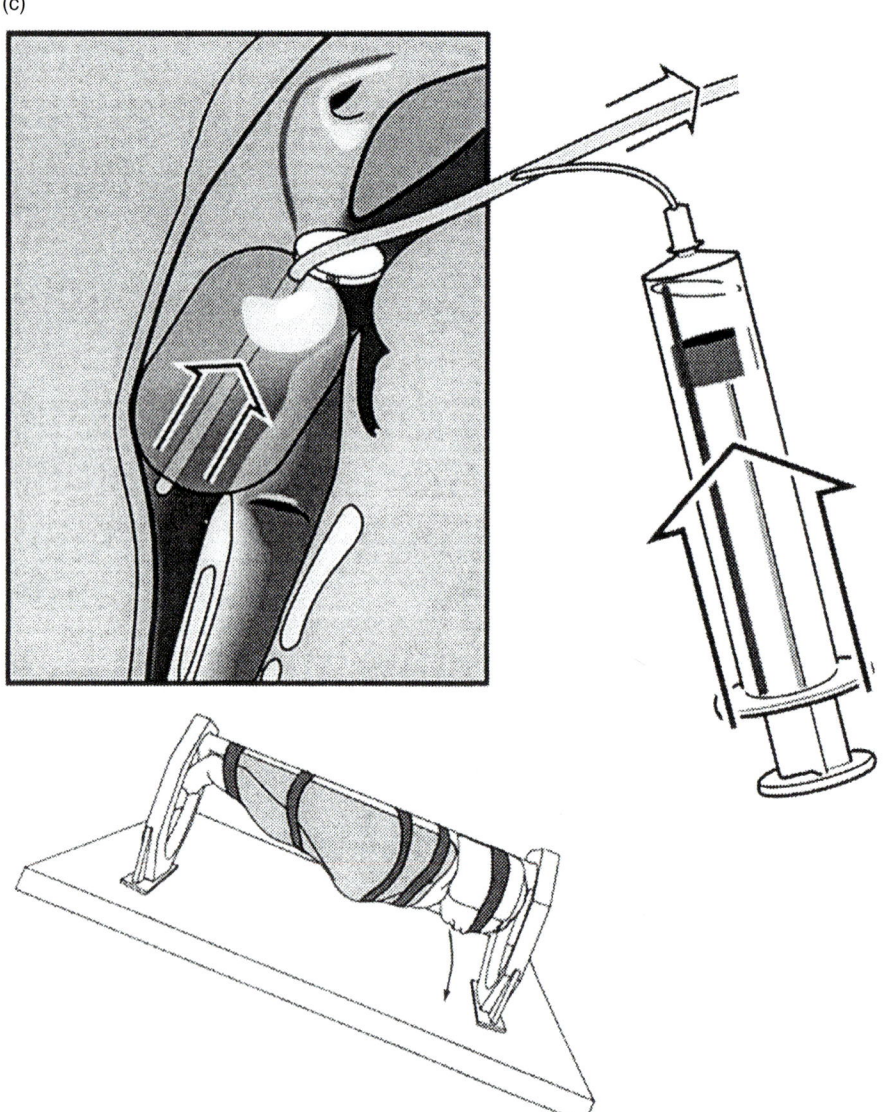

Figure 4.75 (cont.)

These magnet catheters make removal of magnetic foreign bodies easier and avoid the need for general anesthesia and endoscopic or surgical procedures (Figure 4.77). After a battery or other magnetic object is removed, an esophagram using non-ionic contrast medium is performed. Endoscopy may be necessary to evaluate the extent of injury and a follow-up esophagram is recommended in 24 to 36 hours to identify complications. Many intragastric magnetic foreign bodies are inert and cause little or no mucosal injury and do not require a postremoval contrast study. However, the decision to perform a contrast study should be made on a case-by-case basis.

Endoscopic removal of button batteries and other small objects may be difficult due to their smooth surface and mucus coating, making them slippery and difficult to grasp. Thus endoscopic removal may fail in as many as 60% of cases. In the past, if endoscopic retrieval failed, surgical removal was then performed. Today, with the availability of magnet catheters, both endoscopy and surgery can be avoided.

Removal of a magnetic object from the esophagus or GI tract is indicated whenever it is acutely lodged in the esophagus or does not pass out of the stomach. Generally, whenever an object is found within the stomach, it is allowed to pass on its own. Foreign body retrieval is considered only if the child is symptomatic or if the object can be toxic or otherwise harmful to the child.

As is the case with non-magnetic foreign objects, contraindications to removal rarely occur. Depending on the type of lodged foreign body and its location, removal might be considered in the face of a preexisting complication. This would be especially true for disc (button) batteries lodged within the esophagus. In this case, a postprocedural esophagram and

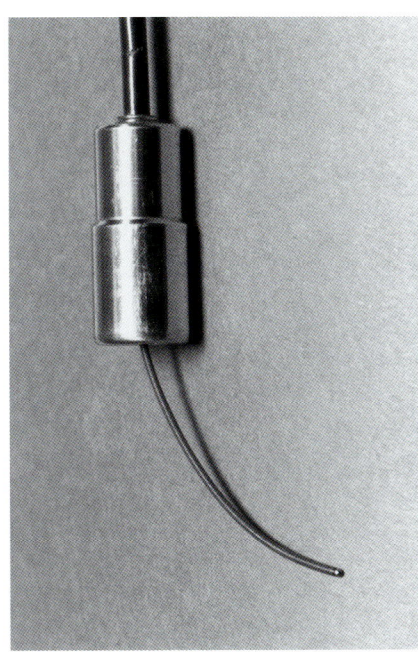

Figure 4.76 A 1 cm diameter rare earth magnet (Boston Scientific) is mounted on a catheter that can be delivered over a guide wire.

endoscopy should be performed to examine the esophageal mucosa and look for untoward effects.

The work-up of a child with a suspected magnetic foreign body is tailored to the individual situation. Whenever possible, it is best to ask the parents to bring in an example of the object ingested. If this is not possible (most cases), the identification of the object depends on experience and the history obtained from the family or referring physician. Once a magnetic foreign body is suspected, plain radiographs are all that is usually needed prior to treatment. In most cases, a foreign body series, lateral neck, frontal and lateral views of the chest, and AP abdomen, are obtained. Contrast examination of the upper GI tract is not needed and would interfere with removal of the object. Laboratory studies are not routinely obtained. Removal is otherwise identical to the Foley catheter technique.

Postprocedure and follow-up care

If the removal of the magnetic object is uncomplicated, the approach to postprocedural care is identical to that described for blunt foreign body removal. However, if an esophageal injury is suspected, the child should be admitted to the hospital and scheduled for an endoscopic examination of the esophagus or an esophagram and UGI series. If an esophageal injury has occurred, a prolonged hospital course may be required.

If a blunt object is lodged in the expected position and is removed without difficulty, no additional procedure is performed. If, however, the object is found in an atypical location, blood is present on the balloon surface, any unanticipated procedural difficulty or patient problem is encountered, or a complication is suspected, an esophagram using barium or non-ionic contrast is performed.

Complications

The main risk of foreign body removal is uncovering a preexisting injury related to the type of object ingested, the contents of the foreign body, and length of time it has been lodged in the GI tract. Most complications are minor, can be treated as an outpatient, and quickly resolve with supportive therapy alone. Major complications primarily result from the properties of the retained foreign body. The most feared complication is a result of a leaking disc battery lodged within the esophagus. Button batteries are dangerous because they contain a highly alkaline solution that can cause rapid liquefaction necrosis of the esophageal wall if leakage occurs. In addition, esophageal injury may result from a low voltage burn or pressure necrosis. Thus a button battery lodged in the esophagus must be removed emergently since injury can occur in as little as one hour, which could be fatal.

Other major complications include esophageal laceration caused by the foreign body itself or in the process of removing it, mediastinitis, and tracheoesophageal fistula (Figure 4.78). An esophagram or endoscopy is advised if a complicated esophageal injury is suspected. A follow-up esophagram may be performed 24 to 36 hours later to rule out a fistula or other complication.

Although simple, these interventional techniques are cost-effective, safe, and useful. In our experience it is worthwhile to use the Foley catheter method for removal of all uncomplicated esophageal foreign bodies. However, it may be best for this procedure to be performed by individuals experienced either in interventional techniques in general, or by pediatric radiologists who are experienced and comfortable with this procedure in children.

Major complications resulting from Foley catheter extraction of foreign bodies lodging in the esophagus occur in less than 1% of cases. Of the adverse effects that do occur, most are minor and resolve spontaneously with little or no treatment. These minor problems include blood-tinged saliva, sore throat, and a sense of a retained object secondary to esophageal irritation. These effects usually resolve without treatment in 24 to 72 hours. To maximize patient comfort, a soft diet is suggested until the symptoms subside. Major complications rarely occur but, when suspected, should be aggressively diagnosed and treated. Reported problems include esophageal perforation, mediastinitis, hemorrhage requiring transfusion, tracheoesophageal fistula, and esophagoaortic fistula formation.

Conclusions

To date, no prospective-controlled study comparing endoscopic and fluoroscopic removal techniques has been performed. Therefore one must review individual studies reporting the results of each technique separately. From this data it can be said that both techniques have merit and in

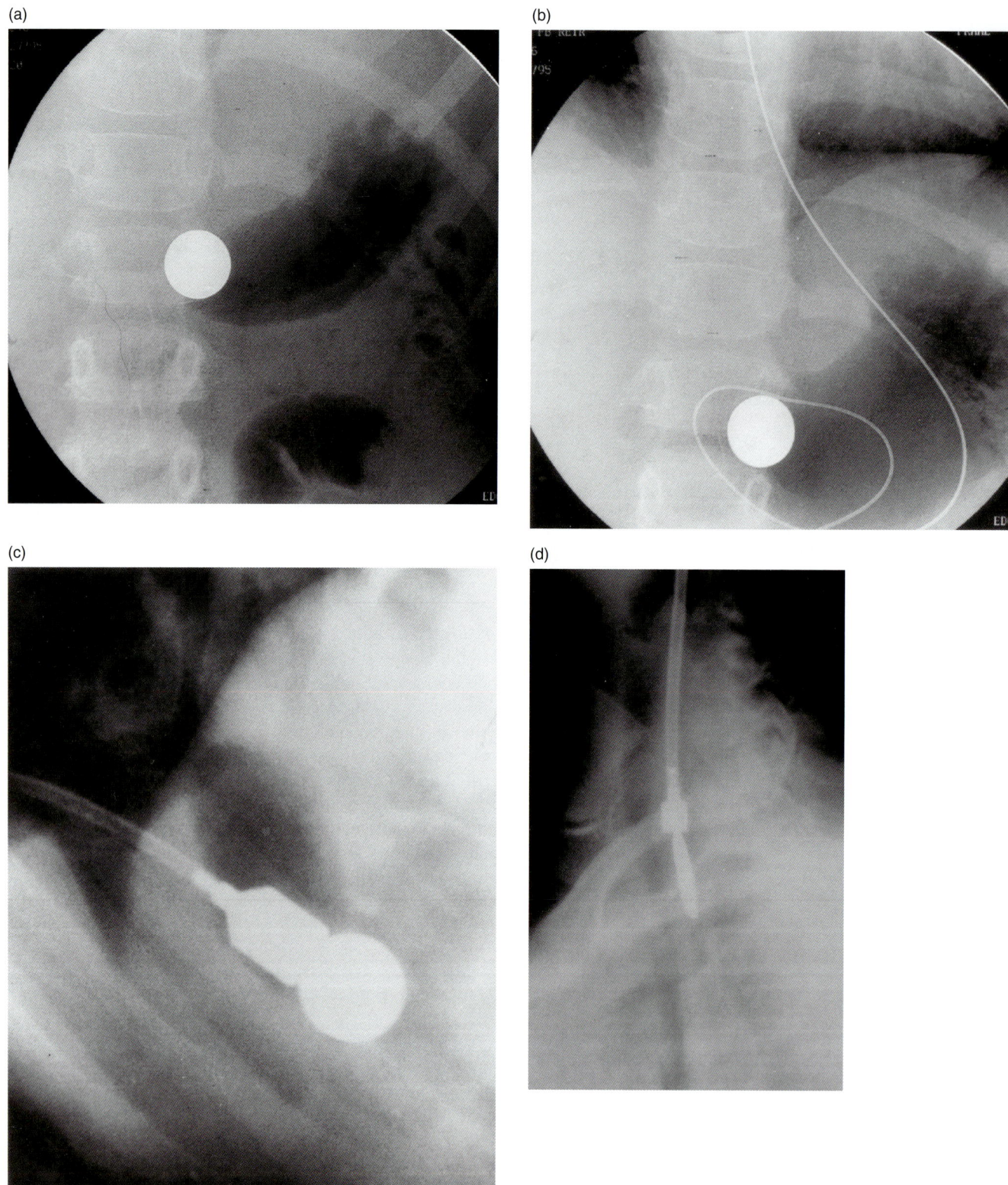

Figure 4.77 (a) A three-year-old ingested a metallic punch-out disk, seen in this fluoroscopic view of the upper abdomen projecting over the gastric antrum. (b) A 0.038-inch Bentson guide wire was advanced through a directional catheter into the stomach, and the catheter was removed. (c) The magnetic retrieval catheter was advanced over the guide wire and maneuvered until it made contact with the ferromagnetic foreign body, as seen in this lateral fluoroscopy image. (d) The magnet is withdrawn with the foreign body.

Table 4.23 Esophagoscopy versus Foley catheter method

Esophagoscopy (endoscopists)	Foley catheter method (interventionalists)
1. Can be used for removal of both blunt and sharp objects.	Lower cost: lower physician fees, no anesthesia cost, no hospitalization, or short-stay fees.
2. More often an inpatient procedure in some institutions.	Outpatient procedure, shorter procedure time.
3. Airway protected during removal of the object.	Same success rates for removal of uncomplicated blunt objects.

many situations, are interchangeable. Thus, in many institutions, the approach taken depends on the existing referral patterns, availability of the procedures, and the skills of the endoscopists and interventionalists.

In our opinion, if a radiologist with experience using the Foley catheter technique is available, children with uncomplicated blunt esophageal foreign bodies should have them removed using this method since it has a high success rate, very low complication rate, and in these days of managed care, is considerably less costly. All children with sharp or complicated foreign bodies, those at high risk for any reason, and patients who have failed Foley catheter removal should undergo endoscopic removal primarily (Table 4.23).

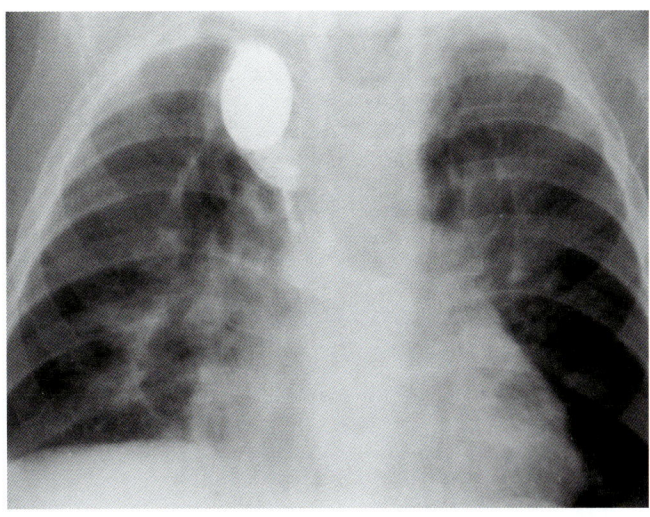

Figure 4.78 An unsuccessful attempt was made to retrieve this ingested coin by a transoral approach under fluoroscopic control. The coin is laterally displaced, indicating an extra-esophageal position likely due to esophageal perforation that may or may not have preceded the intervention.

Those who remove foreign bodies from the esophagus are occasionally tempted to hand them to the parents as souvenirs of the experience. Surprisingly often the parent will hand it back to the child, who will promptly put it in their mouth and attempt to swallow it again. Resist the temptation.

Chapter 5

Hepatobiliary interventions

Kevin M. Baskin, Richard Towbin, David Aria and Robin Kaye

Interventional radiology of the liver and gallbladder 251

Percutaneous transhepatic cholangiography (PTC) 252
Introduction 252
Indications 253
Technique 253
Equipment 253
Patient preparation 253
Standard technique 254
Ultrasound-guided access 255
Fluoroscopically guided access 255
Technical variations 257
CO_2 as a contrast agent 257
Left lateral (subxiphoid) approach 258
Postprocedure and follow-up care 258
Complications 258

Transcholecystic cholangiography (TCC) 258
Introduction 258
Indications 258
Technique 259
Equipment 259
Patient preparation 259
Standard technique 259
Postprocedure and follow-up care 259

Percutaneous cholecystostomy 259
Introduction 259
Indications 260
Technique 260
Equipment 260
Patient preparation 260
Standard technique 260
Technical variations 262

Postprocedure and follow-up care 262
Complications 262

Percutaneous transhepatic biliary drainage (PTD) 262
Introduction 262
Indications 262
Technique 263
Equipment 263
Patient preparation 263
Standard technique 264
Single-stick method 264
Double-stick method 264
Technical variations 269
Postprocedure and follow-up care 270
Complications 270

Percutaneous transhepatic biliary dilation (PTBD) 271
Introduction 271
Indications 271
Technique 272
Equipment 272
Patient preparation 272
Standard technique 272
Technical variations 273
Impassable strictures 273
Postprocedure and follow-up care 274
Complications 275

Biliary stents 275
Introduction 275

Hepatic angiography and vascular procedures 276
Hepatic venography 276
Introduction 276

Pediatric Interventional Radiology, ed. Richard Towbin and Kevin M. Baskin. Published by Cambridge University Press. © Cambridge University Press 2015.

Indications 276
Technique 276
Equipment 276
Patient preparation 276
Standard technique 277
Technical variations 277
Indirect measurement of the portosystemic gradient 277
Complications 279

Splenoportography 279
Introduction 279
Indications 279
Technique 279
Equipment 279
Patient preparation 279
Standard technique 280
Postprocedure and follow-up care 280
Technical problems and pitfalls 280
Complications 280

Transhepatic portal venography (TPV) 281
Introduction 281
Indications 281
Technique 281
Equipment 281
Standard technique 281
Postprocedure and follow-up care 282
Complications 282

Transjugular liver biopsy (TJLB) 282
Introduction 282
Indications 284
Technique 284
Equipment 284
Patient preparation 284
Standard technique 284
Technical variations 285
Needle curvature 285

Ultrasound-guided access 286
Postprocedure and follow-up care 286
Complications 286

Transjugular intrahepatic portosystemic shunt (TIPS) 286
Introduction 286
Indications 286
Technique 287
Equipment 287
Patient preparation 287
Standard technique 287
Technical variations 289
Postprocedure and follow-up care 289
Technical problems and pitfalls 289
Complications 290

Transarterial intrahepatic chemoembolization 291
Introduction 291
Indications 292
Technique 292
Equipment 292
Patient preparation 292
Standard technique 292
Technical variations 293
Postprocedure and follow-up care 293
Complications 293

Partial splenic embolization 294
Introduction 294
Indications 294
Technique 294
Equipment 294
Patient preparation 295
Standard technique 295
Postprocedure and follow-up care 295
Complications 296

Interventional radiology of the liver and gallbladder

The interventional radiologist may work with a multidisciplinary team composed of hepatologists, liver transplant surgeons, endoscopists, and pediatric surgeons in the context of a liver transplant program to provide both diagnostic services and definitive therapy for a broad variety of hepatic and biliary disorders, but may also work in a less structured setting with pediatricians, gastroenterologists, endoscopists, and pediatric surgeons to provide the same services. Percutaneous biliary procedures begin with thin-needle (Chiba) access to the biliary tree under image guidance. Access may be obtained through radicles of either the right or left main bile ducts, depending on the intended target and the optimal trajectory through the bile ducts. Manipulation of the biliary system, especially when infected, inflamed, or obstructed, may be quite painful. Simple diagnostic procedures may, in select cases, be performed under

Table 5.1 Outcome measures

To improve outcome and quality assurance analysis, it may be helpful to record the following information for each biliary procedure referral:

- Demographic information (patient name, unique identification number, date and time of procedure, age, sex, weight, date of birth, etc.)
- Primary diagnosis
- Related conditions (e.g., ascites, coagulopathy, clinical instability)
- Reason for hepatobiliary procedure; referring service and provider
- Anticipated endpoint
- Provider responsible for access (interventionalist, surgeon, nurse, etc.)
- Procedure location (interventional suite, operating room, bedside, etc.)
- Provider responsible for anesthesia/sedation (anesthesiologist, nurse, etc.)
- Preprocedural interventions (e.g., antibiotics, blood products, imaging)
- Initial access
  - entry site
  - route (e.g., transhepatic, transperitoneal, transcholecystic, femoral vein, jugular vein)
  - method (e.g., fluoroscopy, US, CT)
  - device (e.g., micropuncture needle, single wall needle)
  - number of attempts
  - reason for deferral, discontinuation or failure, if insertion not completed
- Access or drainage device and position
- Catheter manufacturer, type, lumen number and diameter, length
- Tip position
- Equipment and supplies used
- Procedure time
- Type and adequacy of anesthesia/sedation/analgesia
- Adjunctive therapies required (e.g., tract embolization)
- Complications
  - Initial access (e.g., pneumothorax, hemorrhage, extracapsular extravasation)
  - Procedural (e.g., hemobilia, bile leak, infection) and management
  - Infection (include dates)
    - type (biliary sepsis, catheter infection)
    - suspected (basis) or proven (method and results)
    - management (e.g., antibiotics, catheter removal, repeat cultures)
    - outcome
  - Catheter dysfunction (include dates)
    - type (e.g., occlusion, leak, fracture, fragment embolization)
    - management
    - outcome
  - Hemorrhagic complications (include dates)
    - method of diagnosis or documentation
    - location and extent
    - management (e.g., transfusion, blood products, fluid resuscitation)
    - outcome
  - Dislodgment or malposition (include dates)
    - method of diagnosis or documentation
    - management
    - outcome
- Other procedure-related complications or interventions?
- Removal or replacement (reason and date; endpoint achieved?)

sedation and analgesia, but more complex procedures usually require general anesthesia. The ability to control respiration is an additional advantage of general anesthesia. Liver transplant recipients, patients with bile duct reconstruction, and those with biliary ductal obstruction are often immunocompromised and are also vulnerable to biliary colonization with enteric organisms. Since manipulation of infected bile ducts may lead to serious morbidity, preprocedure antibiotics are usually given prior to initial access of the biliary tree. As has been noted elsewhere, it is vital to practice development and the process of continuous quality improvement to keep careful records of the parameters of interventional procedures and outcomes. Recommended data elements are included in Table 5.1.

Percutaneous transhepatic cholangiography (PTC)

Introduction

Percutaneous transhepatic cholangiography (PTC) was first described by Burkhardt and Muller in 1921, but it wasn't until 1974 that the modern, thin-needle technique for PTC was described by Okuda and coworkers. Prior to the introduction of this technique, surgeons in the operating room performed virtually all cholangiography using direct visualization because of the major bleeding and biliary complications that frequently occurred after multiple punctures of the liver with large-bore needles. The fine-needle technique had a significantly lower complication rate and eliminated the need for surgical intervention following cholangiography.

Ultrasound, CT, MRI, MR cholangiopancreatography (MRCP), MR with liver-specific agents (e.g., Eovist®), and nuclear medicine studies are sensitive modalities for the detection of biliary dilation and hepatobiliary pathology. Ductal anatomy, especially if intervention is anticipated, may also be imaged in real time with introduction of contrast into the biliary system. Of note, bile ducts may be normal in caliber in up to 30% of patients with biliary obstruction, especially if the obstruction is partial or intermittent or if the obstructed ducts are decompressed, such as by fistulous drainage. Percutaneous transhepatic cholangiography successfully determines the site of obstruction in 95 to 100% of cases and the etiology of the obstruction in 90 to 96% of cases in patients with dilated

Table 5.2 Indications: percutaneous transhepatic cholangiography

- Dilated ducts
- Suspected biliary calculi
- Intrahepatic obstruction
- Jaundice
- Evaluate bile leak, bile lake, biloma or biliary fistula
- As a prelude to another intervention (i.e., balloon dilation)

intrahepatic bile ducts. However, the success rate of PTC decreases as the size of the intrahepatic ducts decreases. In patients with normal or near-normal biliary ductal diameter the success rate of percutaneous cholangiography varies from 25 to 85%. The morbidity and mortality rates for PTC (3% and 0.1%, respectively) are not statistically different than those seen for endoscopic retrograde cholangiopancreatography (ERCP) (3 and 0.3%). However, ERCP is technically more difficult to perform in children, is not available in all hospitals, and is up to four times as expensive as PTC.

Indications

The indications for PTC are quite different in the pediatric population than those for adults (Table 5.2). In the adult population, stone disease and primary or metastatic tumors are the most frequent causes of biliary obstruction with secondary cholestasis. In these patients, PTC is most often performed to demonstrate the presence of intra- or extrahepatic calculi, to differentiate surgically from medically treatable jaundice, or to relieve obstruction. In children, biliary intervention is uncommon outside of the subgroup of children with liver transplantation. In children hepatobiliary obstruction due to stones or tumor is very uncommon. Instead, the most frequent indications for PTC in children are either failed magnetic resonance cholangiopancreatography (MRCP) or failed or technically unfeasible ERCP in patients in whom there is suspected biliary pathology. Percutaneous transhepatic cholangiography allows the evaluation of a biliary-enteric anastomosis after liver resection or transplantation, diagnosis of complications of liver transplantation such as bile leak or strictures, diagnosis of communication of hepatic abscess with the biliary tree, evaluation of congenital anomalies, and study of the biliary system prior to a percutaneous intervention.

Percutaneous transhepatic cholangiography may be contraindicated in the presence of an uncorrectable coagulopathy or the absence of a safe access route. Fortunately, in most instances a coagulopathy can be reversed with the administration of platelets, fresh frozen plasma, or vitamin K (see Chapter 1). If the patient's coagulopathy is not correctable, or only partially correctable, a PTC may still be attempted, if clinically indicated, with embolization of the needle tract with Gelfoam® pledgets, Avitene®, or metal coils as the guide needle is withdrawn at the end of the procedure.

Relative contraindications to PTC include ascites, a previous anaphylactic reaction to iodinated contrast, and an hepatic vascular malformation or vascular tumor in the pathway of the needle. Percutaneous transhepatic cholangiography may be more technically difficult to perform when the liver is "floating" in ascites and not apposed to the abdominal wall. In addition, the risk of hemorrhagic complications is higher when the presence of intra-abdominal fluid reduces or eliminates the tamponade effect of the liver against the abdominal wall, especially in children with coagulation abnormalities. If the ascitic fluid can be drained, PTC may be performed. If not, the procedure is generally postponed until the ascites has resolved or, at minimum, paracolic fluid abutting the liver has resolved.

When a vascular lesion or tumor is present in the liver, the inherent risk of performing a PTC depends mainly on the location of the lesion in the liver relative to the needle path and whether or not there is a coexisting coagulopathy. Imaging studies, such as CT or MRI, are of great importance in ascertaining the location and extent of the lesion and in procedure planning.

If a life-threatening contrast reaction has been documented, CO_2 may sometimes be used to outline the biliary ducts (see the discussion of CO_2 as a contrast agent in the biliary tree below).

Technique
Equipment

The equipment necessary for PTC is focused on safe and stable percutaneous transhepatic access to a bile duct peripheral to the suspected pathology. This procedure can be one of the most demanding for US guidance, especially so if a decompressed duct deep in the liver must be accessed. For this reason, the highest quality US equipment available should be used, preferably employing a high-resolution linear transducer with excellent near-field imaging as well as excellent penetration. Both US and fluoroscopic guidance have a role in these procedures, depending upon the clinical problem, the degree of biliary involvement (e.g., isolated intrahepatic ducts, lobar process, anastomotic or extrahepatic biliary stenosis), the condition of the bile ducts (e.g., ectatic, dilated, decompressed), and the nature of the liver parenchyma (e.g., firm and cirrhotic, normally compliant, partially necrotic). Recommended equipment is targeted to these parameters (Table 5.3).

Patient preparation

In adults with malignant biliary obstruction the incidence of infected bile is 25 to 36% and in those with choledocholithiasis the incidence is 71 to 90%. Stated another way, the incidence of infected bile is higher in patients with partial obstruction (64%) than in patients with complete obstruction of the common duct (10%). In patients with biliary-intestinal anastomosis the incidence of infected bile is up to 80%, although these patients may be asymptomatic. Gram-negative bacteria (*Escherichia coli*, *Enterobacter aerogenes*, *Klebsiella*, and

Table 5.3 Equipment: percutaneous transhepatic cholangiography

- High-quality US with a high-frequency linear transducer (12–18 MHz)
- Angiographic C-arm, preferably with a tilting table
- Rotational cholangiography is optional but can be useful
- Materials for sterile preparation and draping
- 22-gauge Chiba echogenic needle (0.7 mm O.D.)
- 4 French or 5 French micropuncture set with 0.018-inch stiff glide wire, mandril wire, or Roadrunner® wire and 0.035-inch stiff wire
- Additional 4 French introducer sheath with metallic or plastic cannula
- 18-gauge Chiba needle (0.018-inch approach), Yueh sheathed needle (0.035 to 0.038-inch approach)
- Connecting tubing
- 20 ml syringe filled with non-ionic contrast diluted 1:1 with normal saline
- Syringes, stopcocks, and other equipment for optional CO_2 cholangiography

Table 5.4 Procedure summary: percutaneous transhepatic cholangiography

- Administer preprocedural antibiotics
- Sedation or general anesthesia
- Position supine or partially oblique (right side up). Supine preferred for left hepatic lobe or segmental approach
- Fluoroscopic and US guidance available
- For fluoroscopically guided access, identify an entry site in the seventh to tenth intercostal space in the anterior axillary line. A subxiphoid entry point is preferred for a left hepatic lobe or segmental approach
- For US-guided access, select a dilated, relatively superficial duct in either lobe likely to be peripheral to the pathology with a long-axis relationship to the transducer
- Prepare and drape in sterile fashion
- 22-gauge Chiba needle, 5 to 20 cm in length
- Intermittent injection of dilute contrast to identify bile ducts
- When flow into biliary tree is confirmed, opacify bile ducts with contrast
- Image in multiple projections
- Maintain patient with right side down for four to six hours after procedure
- Obtain complete blood and platelet counts three to four hours after procedure

Pseudomonas) are the most common infecting organisms. In fact, *E. coli* and *Enterobacter* are implicated in almost two-thirds of cases. Gram-positive bacteria (usually *Enterococcus* spp., especially *E. faecalis*) are the causative agents in approximately 21% of cases. No information is currently available concerning the incidence of infected bile in children with biliary obstruction, but it is probably safe to assume that the major infecting organisms are similar. For that reason, prophylactic broad-spectrum antibiotics are routinely given prior to PTC. In general, intravenous ampicillin or a third- or fourth-generation cephalosporin and gentamicin are given one to two hours prior to the procedure and continued for 24 to 48 hours (see Chapter 1: "Prophylactic antibiotics").

All patients undergoing a PTC, with or without biliary drainage, have routine laboratory evaluation of coagulation (PT, PTT, and platelet count) drawn within 24 hours prior to the procedure. Patients with platelet counts between 30,000 and 50,000 are transfused with platelets, the amount depending on the patient's size and fluid status. If the platelet count is below 30,000, correction with a platelet transfusion is performed and results rechecked at least 30 minutes prior to the scheduled procedure. If the platelet count after transfusion is between 30,000 and 50,000 then it is our practice to perform the procedure with platelets infusing during and after the procedure. If the platelet count remains <30,000 the procedure is postponed until correction is established, unless diagnosis or treatment is emergent. In these situations, the decision to proceed is made by a multispecialty team after considering the relevant issues. In patients with a platelet count between 50,000 and 80,000 we may electively transfuse platelets, although this is usually decided on a case-by-case basis and in consultation with the referring service. In those patients who have a consumptive coagulopathy or who are platelet resistant, we prefer to infuse platelets during and after the procedure so that the platelet count and activity is highest as the procedure is being completed. In children with low platelet counts the total number of passes will be arbitrarily limited to a maximum of ten in most instances.

Depending on the reference values of the hospital laboratory, a PT >15 seconds and a PTT >50 seconds are usually indications for a fresh frozen plasma infusion. In addition to an infusion of fresh frozen plasma, a prolonged PT may also be treated with intravenous vitamin K. The INR (international normalized ratio) is commonly used instead of the standard PT.

Standard technique

Percutaneous transhepatic cholangiography is performed under general anesthesia. It is one of the few procedures in interventional radiology for which there is virtually no good reason to attempt under sedation (Table 5.4). The anesthesiologist should be advised if a need for suspended respiration is anticipated, so that the patient can be paralyzed in a timely fashion, as otherwise achieving this objective at the last moment can cause an untimely delay at a critical moment. The patient is placed supine with the right arm comfortably positioned above the head and properly padded and supported. The patient is secured safely in position. The sterile field should be wide, anticipating an approach from either side, which may be intercostal, subcostal, or even subxiphoid. Prior imaging should be reviewed, especially CT, MRCP, or right upper quadrant US that may demonstrate dilated bile ducts and any unexpected anatomic abnormalities. Under US or fluoroscopy the prospective tract is evaluated. The size and position of the liver are noted and the presence of intervening bowel loops assessed. The location of the lateral costophrenic angle is identified. The path of the needle is planned so as to traverse a substantial amount of liver parenchyma to optimize stability and minimize risk of transcapsular hemorrhage.

Access may be achieved under fluoroscopic or US control. In either case it is often easiest to perform the percutaneous transhepatic puncture during suspended respiration with the patient under general anesthesia and paralyzed. Once the skin is prepared and draped, local anesthesia (e.g., buffered lidocaine) is injected into the skin and subcutaneously down to the liver capsule. A 22-gauge Chiba needle is used for the PTC. In the pediatric setting needle lengths from 5 to 20 cm are available. The shortest needle possible is used as it allows the greatest degree of stability in the liver tissue.

Ultrasound-guided access

Adequate time should be taken under anesthesia to evaluate prospective routes of access with US. A long-axis approach to a relatively superficial dilated segment is preferred if one can be found (Figure 5.1). The ideal candidate segment is roughly in line with the preferred angle of needle access (approximately 30 to 45 degrees) and relatively straight in the region of expected access. The advantage of this approach is that it can be used from virtually any position, that a specific biliary duct can be targeted, that even decompressed ducts can be accessed with a high degree of precision, and that optimal geometry between the point of access and the segment to be treated can be purposefully planned. Although more superficial target ducts are preferred, deeper ducts can also be accessed in this way. Disadvantages include the fact that US access windows usually require considerable physical space, that access windows are often not optimal imaging windows in terms of image quality, and that the target duct can be obscured by nearby bone, bowel, or lung, or by a relatively tiny amount of air in the prospective tract (e.g., from prior attempts).

The patient is positioned and prepared as already described. Real-time US can be used to facilitate puncture of dilated peripheral ducts while avoiding vascular structures. It is our practice to use a freehand technique with a sterilely draped high-frequency (12 to 17 MHz) linear transducer with excellent near-field resolution and good penetration. A micropuncture kit with a 22-gauge Chiba needle is the workhorse of biliary access. Under certain conditions a 20-gauge sheathed needle with a 4 or 5 French sheath may be useful to enter a dilated biliary system, providing a larger lumen with which to aspirate thick bile avoiding multiple wire exchanges. Ultrasound can be especially helpful when no ductal dilation is present because it can direct the operator to the expected position of the duct(s) in portal triads that are readily visible on US.

In adults with dilated ducts, opacification of the biliary tree occurs in 99 to 100% of cases with four to six needle passes. The success rate in puncturing ducts that are not dilated on US examination is between 60 and 80%, and in these cases more needle passes are usually required. Similar rates are achievable in children, more so because of improved visualization using US in smaller patients. If we have not opacified bile ducts within 15 to 20 passes, we abandon the procedure. In rare instances, direct puncture of larger, more central ducts may be attempted, usually with US guidance to minimize the risk of puncturing extrahepatic ducts with the attendant higher complication rate. In selected cases direct puncture of the gallbladder (see "Transcholecystic cholangiography (TCC)," below) may be considered to opacify decompressed ducts, especially when the primary purpose is diagnostic, as in most neonatal PTC.

Fluoroscopically guided access

Fluoroscopy can be used in two ways to access bile ducts. First, if contrast, including gas or air, is already filling ducts (for example, from prior access attempts, from needle access that cannot be converted for further procedural use, or from transcholecystic injection, see below), a suitable duct can be targeted for access by triangulation. Alternatively, "blind" attempts can be made to traverse a suitable duct by inserting the needle in a statistically likely orientation, then testing with gentle puffs of contrast as the needle is withdrawn until contrast fills a tubular structure with signature biliary characteristics (i.e., slow flow toward the porta hepatis). Using this method, the needle customarily enters the liver approximately one-third of the way up from the inferior margin of the liver (usually between the seventh to tenth intercostal spaces), just anterior to the mid-axillary line, and is advanced parallel to the caudal margin of the liver and toward the ipsilateral costovertebral junction. The pleural reflection in the mid-axillary line often extends as low as the level of the tenth rib, usually well below the lung in shallow respiration. This means some punctures may be *transpleural* but not *transpulmonary*. The needle should be inserted just above the superior edge of the rib in order to avoid the neurovascular bundle. The advantage to this approach is that it usually places the trajectory of the needle in line with the right lobe biliary ducts, making catheterization of the ducts more straightforward if drainage is ultimately required.

Under fluoroscopic guidance, the needle is inserted as described in the previous paragraph until the tip of the needle is just lateral to the spine. The stylet is removed and a syringe filled with dilute non-ionic contrast is attached to clear flexible tubing, which is then connected to the hub of the needle. Dilute contrast (1:1 to 2:1 contrast to saline) is used so that the contrast can be absorbed more rapidly and persistent contrast from multiple attempts does not obscure the field.

Using fluoroscopy, preferably with magnification, the needle is slowly withdrawn as contrast is steadily but very slowly injected. The goal is to "draw" a thin, continuous line of contrast behind the retreating needle, and a persistent, thin tract of contrast in the liver parenchyma should be seen as the needle is pulled back. The needle should be pulled back to the liver periphery, but not out of the capsule, in order to minimize the number of holes in the capsule and thereby reduce the risk of bleeding. If too much contrast is injected it will form

Chapter 5 Hepatobiliary interventions

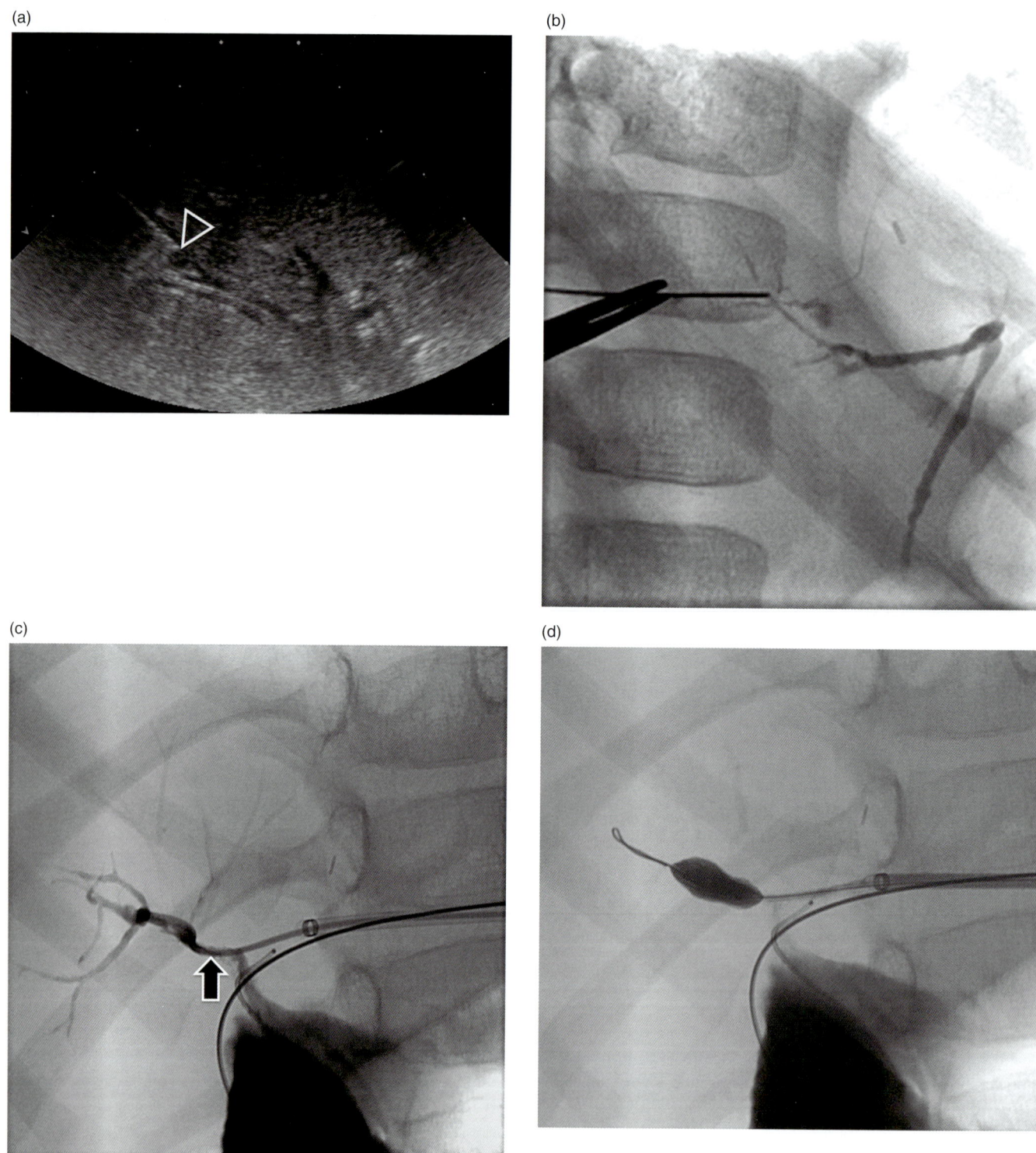

Figure 5.1 A three-year-old male cadaveric transplant recipient developed biliary sepsis. (a) A dilated duct was identified with US just superficial to a portal vein. In this image, the 22-gauge needle (*arrowhead*) is advanced into the dilated duct. (b) Initial cholangiographic injection shows only filling of irregular and severely attenuated right lobe ducts. (c) After two years treating multiple strictures in a number of intrahepatic ducts, contrast injection shows a tightly strictured right hepatic duct (*arrow*), resistant to numerous attempts at cholangioplasty. (d) A 4 mm × 2 cm cutting balloon was inflated across the right hepatic duct stricture. (e) Contrast demonstrates improved flow of contrast into right lobe ducts. (f) Two drains were left to stent-treated ducts from the left: one with the pigtail removed and extra side holes across the right hepatic duct, and a second drain across the common duct in the small bowel. The drains were subsequently removed and the patient has avoided need for retransplantation.

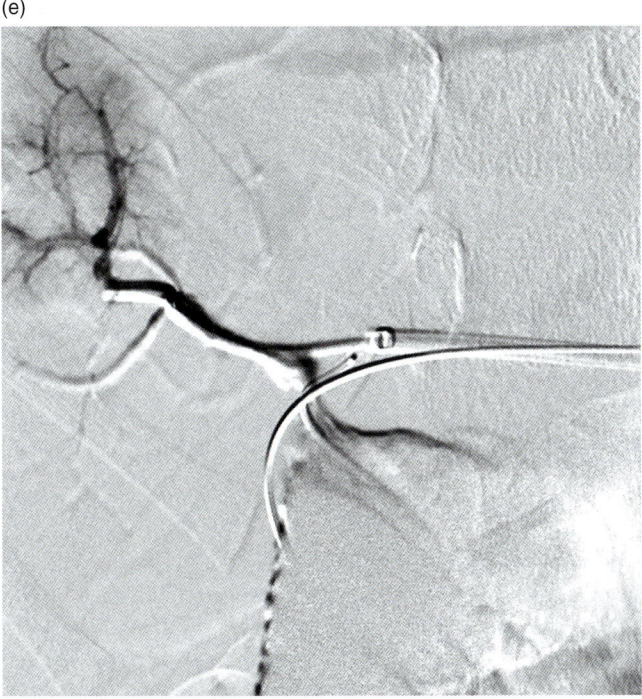
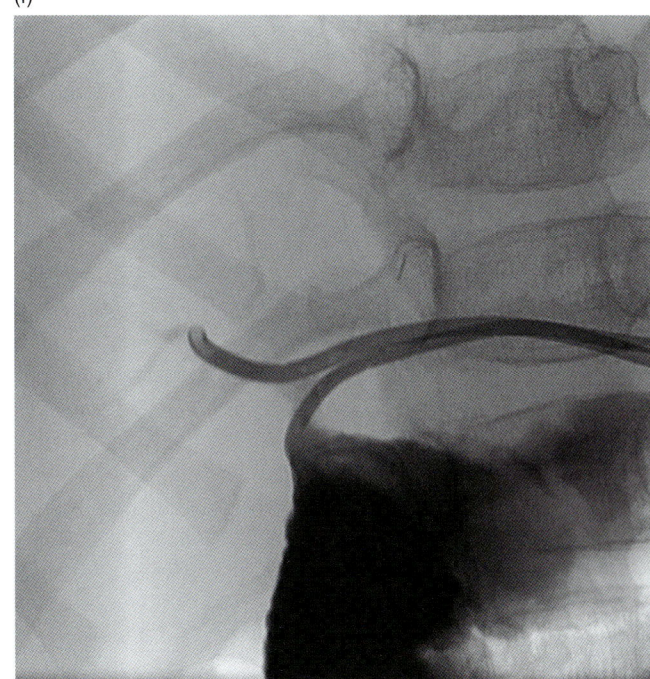

Figure 5.1 (cont.)

"puddles" in the liver parenchyma, which can hamper later attempts to opacify the biliary ducts and potentially obscure findings once the biliary ducts are opacified.

If no contrast is seen in the bile ducts on the first pass, subsequent needle passes should be made systematically, fanning out from the first tract in the cephalo-caudad direction, staying in the same coronal plane. Caudal passes should be made cautiously in order to avoid advancing the needle too far medially where inadvertent puncture of the gallbladder, porta hepatis, vena cava, or aorta might occur or where the capsule might be punctured resulting in extrahepatic, intraperitoneal injection of contrast. The latter may be quite painful and can stimulate a vasovagal response and shortness of breath. In addition, puncture of the extrahepatic ducts in an obstructed system can lead to bile peritonitis, which is a potentially serious complication. If no ducts are opacified in the original coronal plane, then the needle should be repositioned or the angle changed in the axial plane and the process repeated until ductal opacification is seen.

Whether the access needle is positioned under US or fluoroscopic guidance, location of the tip within the lumen of a bile duct must be confirmed before the biliary tree can be filled with contrast for diagnostic imaging of further procedural guidance. When injected into the liver parenchyma contrast remains near the needle tip but as soon as the needle enters a duct or vessel the contrast flows away from the tip. Hepatic veins may be recognized by the rapid flow of contrast toward the right atrium. Portal veins and hepatic arteries are recognized by rapid flow of contrast toward the liver periphery. Differentiating portal veins from hepatic arteries may be somewhat difficult, but blood flow in hepatic arteries is somewhat slower and more pulsatile than in portal veins and results in a more intense parenchymal blush. Lymphatic vessels are identified by their small size, beaded appearance, and very slow flow of contrast toward the porta hepatis. Once lymphatic channels are filled with contrast they can remain opacified for up to ten minutes.

Bile ducts are identified by the slow movement of contrast toward the hilum and by the relatively rapid appearance of a branching pattern. With a patent biliary tree, contrast will flow into the common duct and eventually into the duodenum, or into the Roux loop or jejunum in the case of liver transplant or prior surgery. Once the biliary tree is opacified it is useful to image in multiple projections including straight anteroposterior views, AP views with cranial and caudal angulation, and both anterior oblique views. Rotational biliary angiography may be useful in certain situations to clarify anatomic relationships and to reduce the number of imaging planes, and therefore time and dose, required to answer the clinical question.

Technical variations
CO_2 as a contrast agent

Because iodinated contrast has a higher specific gravity than bile, it will flow into the more dependent, posterior ducts when the patient is supine. This gravity-dependent flow may impede opacification of central ducts and almost always limits opacification of the left ducts, which are more anterior than those on the right. In order to get complete filling of the ducts several maneuvers may be used with caution. Large volumes of contrast may be injected, but this may increase the risk of septic complications. The patient may be carefully rolled onto the left side, but changing position when the patient is sedated or under general anesthesia can be challenging, and the possibility of dislodging the needle from the bile duct is high. Lowering the head of the table or tilting along the z-axis may facilitate filling of the left ducts in angiography suites outfitted with tilting tables.

Carbon dioxide (CO_2) has a lower specific gravity than bile and flows readily to the anterior ducts. It can therefore be used as a contrast agent to opacify the left ducts, which can then be selectively punctured and injected with iodinated contrast. However, injection of CO_2 has limitations and is not always effective. While the extrahepatic biliary system is well visualized with CO_2, the intrahepatic ducts are often poorly or inadequately visualized because of their small caliber and the relatively low conspicuity of CO_2. In addition, CO_2 needs to be injected cautiously because the low viscosity of the gas can cause much higher flow rates than occur with liquid contrast and, because CO_2 is compressed in the syringe, much higher volumes can be delivered with the risk of overdistending the biliary tree.

Left lateral (subxiphoid) approach

In certain situations, the left ducts cannot be visualized, despite the use of one or more of the various maneuvers described above. When there are separate right and left duct obstructions, or when a segmental obstruction of the left duct is known or suspected, or when performing a PTC in a recipient of a left lobe segmental graft, direct imaging of the left ducts is required. The right lateral approach may be used in the former two situations. This approach requires the needle to pass deeper into the liver and be directed more anteriorly and into the medial portion of the left lobe. In these cases a second puncture will usually be required, especially if intervention is necessary. However, in children with segmental transplants, because the cut surface of the liver is directed laterally and somewhat posteriorly and may have loops of bowel interposed between the cut surface and the abdominal wall, the right lateral approach is not used.

The alternative is an anterior, subxiphoid or subcostal approach. This is most easily achieved working from the patient's left side. In some rooms, this may require placing the patient feet first on the table. In almost any room this requires some preprocedure planning to position personnel, supplies, anesthesia equipment, etc., most effectively. When performed with US guidance, this approach follows naturally from the location of available US windows, and is our preference. When this technique is employed under fluoroscopic guidance, the needle is inserted in the mid-epigastrium just below the xiphoid cartilage and aimed toward the patient's right side at an angle of about 30 to 40 degrees from vertical. The needle is inserted approximately 6 to 8 cm and then is slowly withdrawn as contrast is injected, just as in the right lateral approach.

Postprocedure and follow-up care

Patients are on strict bed rest with the access site down, if possible, for four to six hours. They are observed closely in the postprocedure period, for at least four hours, for signs of septic or hypovolemic shock. Frequent vital signs are taken and a repeat hemoglobin and hematocrit are obtained four hours after the end of the procedure to look for signs of bleeding. Intravenous antibiotics are continued for at least 24 hours after the procedure.

Complications

Published series of adult patients who have undergone PTC suggest an expected rate of complication around 3 to 5% and a mortality rate of 0.1 to 0.2%. Sepsis, bile leak, and intraperitoneal hemorrhage are the most common complications, occurring in 1 to 3% of patients. Other much less frequent complications included pneumothorax, contrast reaction, vasovagal reactions, and hepatic arteriovenous fistulae. Our experience in the pediatric population has not been significantly different.

Transcholecystic cholangiography (TCC)

Introduction

If all attempts to opacify the intrahepatic bile ducts using PTC or ERCP have failed, transcholecystic cholangiography (TCC) may be attempted. Transcholecystic cholangiography has the distinction of being one of the oldest percutaneous radiologic interventions, first reported by Burkhardt and Muller in 1921. While TCC has a variable success rate in opacifying intrahepatic bile ducts in adults, in pediatric patients the intrahepatic ducts are routinely well visualized.

Indications

Besides visualization of the intrahepatic biliary tree, other indications for TCC include evaluation of the patency of the cystic duct, diagnosis of iatrogenic gallbladder or bile duct injury, evaluation of the biliary tree in patients with suspected ampullary stenosis and failed ERCP, evaluation of the distal common bile duct in cases of obstruction of the proximal common bile duct and as a prelude to gallbladder drainage (Table 5.5). In the literature most of the reported cases are in adult patients, as most of the indications for this procedure are uncommon in the pediatric population. However, TCC can be an effective way to image non-dilated biliary radicles in patients with suspected biliary disease and can be used to facilitate placement of a transhepatic biliary drainage catheter

Table 5.5 Indications: transcholecystic cholangiography

- Alternative to PTC especially when ducts are small and obstructed
- Determine patency of cystic duct to level of ampulla of Vater
- Prelude to gallbladder drainage, e.g., acalculous cholecystitis
- Opacification of biliary radicles to facilitate PTC in selected cases
- Biliary atresia

Table 5.6 Procedure summary: transcholecystic cholangiography

- Sedation or general anesthesia
- Ultrasound evaluation for route planning
- Prepare and drape in sterile fashion
- Local anesthesia at entry site
- Ultrasound-guided puncture of gallbladder
- Injection of contrast to opacify biliary tree
- Imaging obtained in multiple projections
- Rotational cholangiography may be helpful in route planning

in an obstructed but non-dilated system. It can provide a very effective means for initial opacification of non-dilated ducts in neonates, facilitating subsequent selective puncture of biliary radicles using a transhepatic route. Obviously, this procedure is not applicable to transplant patients who have no gallbladder or to patients who have had a cholecystectomy. If infection of the gallbladder, biliary tree, or soft tissues of the prospective tract is known or suspected, TCC should be deferred until the infection has been cleared.

Technique

Equipment

The equipment for this procedure is identical to that used for PTC (Table 5.3).

Patient preparation

As with PTC, the patient receives intravenous antibiotics prior to the procedure. Anemia or coagulopathy are corrected as fully as possible.

Standard technique

There are two approaches to puncture of the gallbladder. Some interventionalists prefer the shortest, most direct route to the gallbladder, which is usually transperitoneal, from a subcostal or intercostal approach. To decrease the risk of bile peritonitis, we prefer the transhepatic route when possible. With the patient supine, an intercostal approach is used (Table 5.6). Using real-time US guidance, a 22-gauge Chiba needle or sheathed needle is inserted into the gallbladder. A darting jab is usually required to puncture the gallbladder wall, but care should be taken to try to puncture only one wall to minimize the chance for bile leak. Prior to contrast injection, a small amount of bile is aspirated in order to verify the intracholecystic position of the needle and to obtain a specimen for culture or laboratory analysis if necessary. Alternatively, introduction of a small amount of air under US visualization or contrast injection under fluoroscopy can confirm proper position of the needle within the gallbladder.

Once needle position is confirmed, bile is aspirated and nonionic contrast is then slowly injected into the gallbladder in an amount sufficient to fill the bile ducts. Overdistention of the gallbladder should be avoided. If intrahepatic ducts are not well filled, patient position may be changed or the patient may be moved into the Trendelenburg position. Intravenous injection of morphine sulfate can be used to cause spasm of the sphincter of Oddi in order to facilitate filling of intrahepatic ducts. As discussed for PTC, imaging should be obtained in multiple projections. At the end of the study the gallbladder should be decompressed as much as possible before the needle is removed.

Postprocedure and follow-up care

After the procedure the patient should be kept NPO for four to six hours to prevent gallbladder contractions and decrease the risk of bile leak.

Percutaneous cholecystostomy

Introduction

Primary biliary disease is uncommon in children, but when it does occur the gallbladder is usually involved. Acute cholecystitis in children is most often idiopathic, but may be related to infectious etiologies (usually viral, bacterial, or parasitic) or, rarely, to gallstone disease. Calculous cholecystitis in the pediatric population is seen most often in girls ages 16 to 20 years, and often associated with oral contraceptives or pregnancy. In addition, gallstones may be associated with chronic hemolytic diseases, especially sickle cell anemia, congenital biliary disease, or non-hemolytic disorders such as intrahepatic cholestasis secondary to total parenteral nutrition, dehydration, pancreatitis, and cystic fibrosis. These conditions may affect either sex. Gallbladder hydrops, which is often idiopathic and not associated with cholecystitis or gallstones, may present at any age in the pediatric spectrum, and is predominately found in males. In each of the above conditions, decompression and evacuation of the gallbladder may often be curative. Traditionally, this has been accomplished by surgical drainage or cholecystectomy in those patients medically able to tolerate the operation. Currently, interventional techniques offer a minimally invasive alternative procedure for most of these patients.

Introduced around 1978, percutaneous cholecystostomy has been performed in children since the late 1980s. Catheterization of the gallbladder has been used for diagnosis, gallbladder drainage, gallstone dissolution, gallbladder ablation, and dynamic pressure and perfusion studies, as well as a route of access for other procedures, including gallstone extraction and gallbladder biopsy. Minimally invasive approaches have been shown to be a cost-effective alternative to open cholecystectomy and offer definitive therapy for young, otherwise healthy patients who require gallbladder decompression for cholecystitis.

Percutaneous cholecystostomy also offers a safe and effective method of draining the gallbladder in patients at high risk for surgery in whom gallbladder disease is known or suspected. It may be difficult to elicit clinical signs and symptoms in such patients when they are unresponsive or on a ventilator. In these patients, the need for diagnosis is paramount. Goals of therapy include defervescence, normalization of white blood cell count, or improvement in clinical symptoms and signs within 48 to 72 hours of percutaneous drainage. Failure to achieve these goals suggests either a non-biliary source of illness, or that the benefits of cholecystostomy are being masked by other medical conditions in these complex patients. Failure to respond to percutaneous cholecystostomy is also associated with a high mortality rate. Percutaneous cholecystostomy may be definitive therapy, e.g., for patients with acalculous cholecystitis, or in combination with percutaneous lithotomy, lithotripsy, or contact solvent dissolution for children with cholelithiasis. It is also an effective temporizing therapeutic maneuver until the patient is sufficiently stable for surgical cholecystectomy. At this time, cholecystostomy is considered to be the definitive therapy for children with acalculous cholecystitis (Figure 5.2).

Indications

Indications for percutaneous cholecystostomy include the need for decompression of the gallbladder (e.g., in calculous or acalculous cholecystitis, hydrops, empyema, or gallbladder perforation), cholangitis, biliary obstruction, the need for diagnostic imaging of the biliary tree, or as a route of access for additional interventions (Table 5.7). Percutaneous cholecystostomy should be regarded as the first-line intervention in critically ill patients in whom gallbladder disease is known or suspected. Because percutaneous drainage may often be definitive therapy in young and otherwise healthy patients, this is the procedure of choice in this population.

The response rate in adults is highest when clinical and radiologic signs are referable to the gallbladder and right upper quadrant, especially in the presence of a sonographic Murphy's sign or multiple radiologic signs (i.e., gallbladder wall thickening, distention, stones, and pericholecystic fluid). Clinical signs of acute cholecystitis are generally less definitive in children than in adults. Controversy remains regarding whether to drain or aspirate the gallbladder in high-risk patients who are not critically ill. This question has not been addressed in pediatric patients. Percutaneous cholecystostomy may also be useful as an alternative to percutaneous transhepatic biliary drainage (PTD, see below) in cases where biliary radicles are not sufficiently dilated or well visualized. This is an especially effective choice for diagnostic studies in neonates and small children when biliary disease is suspected.

Technique

Equipment

The equipment necessary for percutaneous cholecystostomy is similar to that used for other simple drainage procedures (Table 5.8). The smallest catheter required to achieve adequate drainage without catheter blockage should be used. A 6 to 8.5 French pigtail drainage catheter is usually satisfactory for such interventions as decompression and contact dissolution of stones. A larger tract (up to 24 French) may be necessary when secondary procedures are contemplated, such as mechanical stone removal. Only an internally locking catheter should be used, and fixation of the catheter to the skin should be secure, due to the risk of severe complications with inadvertent dislodgment.

Patient preparation

Preparation for percutaneous cholecystostomy is identical to PTC preparation, as described above. Any available preoperative imaging of the region should be reviewed, and US may be used during preparation for the procedure, to evaluate the gallbladder fossa for any abnormal vessels that may be at risk during the procedure. Vascular malformations are known to occur in this region and any large or abnormal vessels may affect the planned route of access.

Standard technique

We prefer to complete guide wire and catheter insertion under fluoroscopic control after obtaining access with US guidance (Figure 5.3). However, the entire procedure can be performed with US guidance alone if necessary (Table 5.9). Using US, the procedure can, on rare occasion, be performed at the bedside if the patient's condition is too unstable for transport to the interventional suite. In cases of difficult access, such as in obese patients or when visualization of the gallbladder is otherwise poor, CT may be used for guidance.

Following instillation of local anesthetic (if the procedure is not done under general anesthetic) either a Seldinger or a trochar technique may be used to gain initial access to the gallbladder. Specimens for bile cultures (aerobic, anaerobic, and fungal) with Gram stain should be obtained during aspiration or drainage of the gallbladder, prior to the introduction of contrast or other bacteriostatic agents. Interestingly, culture results are poorly predictive of the outcome of the intervention, and are especially insensitive in patients already receiving antibiotics. Nevertheless, if a positive culture is obtained it can be used to guide antibiotic therapy.

If a Seldinger technique is used, initial access is usually with a 21- or 22-gauge Chiba or an 18-gauge sheathed needle. The puncture site is guided by US imaging, but will usually be in the anterior axillary line in the eighth or ninth intercostal space, or, occasionally, subcostal. After passing through hepatic parenchyma (preferably through the "bare" area of the

Chapter 5 Hepatobiliary interventions

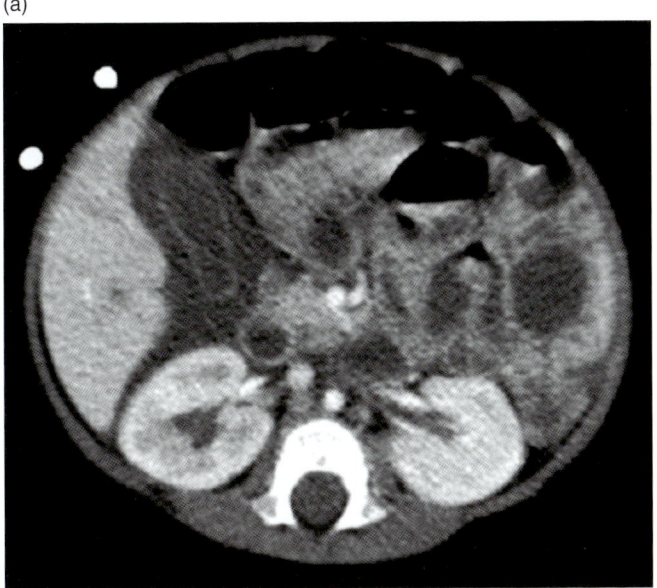

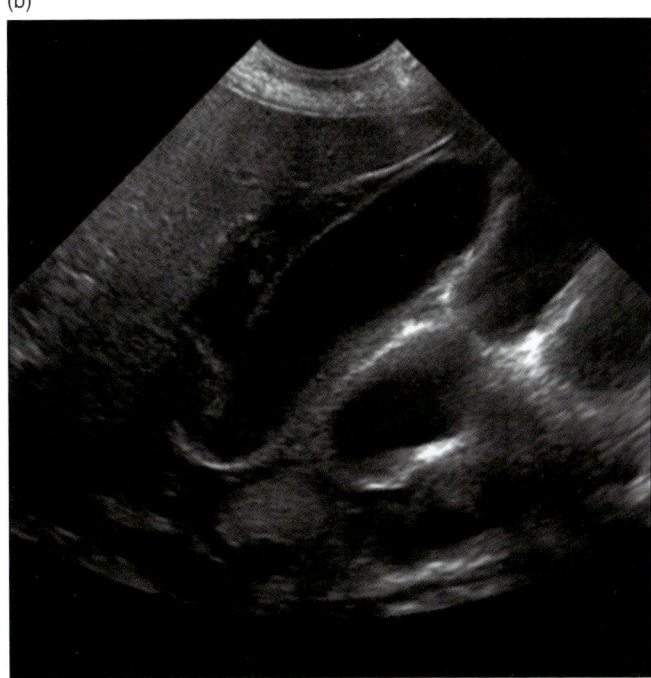

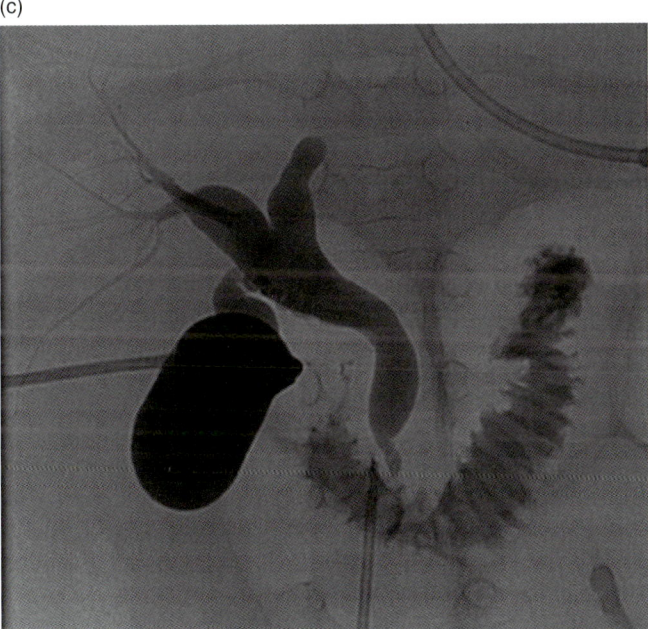

Figure 5.2 One-year-old female with severe combined immunodeficiency after bone marrow transplant with acalculous cholecystitis. (a) Axial contrast enhanced CT shows pericholecystic fluid with mild gallbladder wall enhancement and thickening. (b) Ultrasound shows gallbladder sludge prior to needle access. (c) Gallbladder drainage. Injection shows patent cystic duct.

Table 5.7 Indications: percutaneous cholecystostomy

- Gallbladder decompression
- Access route for additional interventions
- Reduction in serum bile salts, e.g., Alagille syndrome with pruritis

liver), the needle should enter the gallbladder between the fundus and the mid body. Small aliquots of bile should be obtained for cultures, leaving adequate bile within the gallbladder to keep it distended, facilitating coiling the guide wire and positioning of the drainage catheter. In an unobstructed system where infected bile is not suspected, a small amount of contrast may be instilled to opacify the gallbladder. Retrograde cholecystocholangiography may be performed through the drainage catheter after therapeutic levels of antibiotics have been achieved and the system decompressed, usually 48 to 72 hours following intubation.

A floppy-tipped mandril wire or other relatively stiff, non-kinkable wire (such as an angled Glidewire®) is advanced until

Table 5.8 Equipment: percutaneous cholecystostomy

- Materials for sterile preparation and draping
- 22-gauge Chiba needle (0.7 mm O.D.)
- 4 French or 5 French micropuncture set with 0.018-inch stiff glide wire or Roadrunner® wire and 0.035-inch stiff wire
- Additional 4 French introducer sheath with metallic or plastic cannula
- 18-gauge Chiba needle (0.018-inch approach), Yueh sheathed needle (0.035 to 0.038-inch approach)
- Connecting tubing
- 20 ml syringe filled with non-ionic contrast diluted 1:1 with normal saline
- 5 French, 6.5 French, or 8.5 French pigtail drains

the transition zone to the stiff part of the wire is intraluminal. The tract is dilated to the diameter of the drainage catheter, or may be overdilated by 1 to 2 French. Finally, a locking drainage catheter is inserted and the loop is formed and locked. The catheter is securely fixed to the skin, taking care not to kink the catheter at the skin exit site. The gallbladder is decompressed by aspiration through the drain, and the catheter is left to external gravity drainage to a drainage bag.

Technical variations

We prefer a transhepatic route for instrumentation of the gallbladder in order to decrease the risk of leakage and potentially lethal bile peritonitis. In fact, tracts formed via a transhepatic route mature more quickly than by a transperitoneal route (two versus three weeks, respectively). Cope offers an alternative approach, using a removable anchor suture to temporarily bring the gallbladder into apposition with the anterior abdominal wall, allowing a percutaneous subhepatic approach with low risk of leakage and avoiding the risks of traversing the hepatic parenchyma, in select cases. It should be noted that colon is often interposed between the anterior abdominal wall and at least a portion of the gallbladder fundus, so care should be taken to avoid a transcolonic puncture if a transperitoneal route is selected.

Postprocedure and follow-up care

The catheter is left in place for at least four to six weeks. Prior to removal of the catheter, with a guide wire in place, tract maturity should be confirmed with contrast injection. Also, cholecystocholangiography performed using the catheter can also help ensure that the cystic and common bile ducts are patent prior to removal. Prolonged drainage is rarely necessary, since the gallbladder is usually either ruled out as the origin of illness, the patient rapidly improves, or the gallbladder is surgically removed.

Complications

In the adult literature, about three quarters of percutaneous cholecystostomies are therapeutic. Interval cholecystectomy is required in only a quarter of these cases, despite the fact that stones are found in nearly half. Potential complications include gallbladder perforation with bile leakage or peritonitis, leakage of infected bile, pericholecystic abscess, chole-enteric fistula, severe vasovagal reaction with hypotension, bleeding, hemobilia, sepsis, pneumothorax, bowel perforation, accidental catheter dislodgment, and death. However, the expected complication rate is under 15%, with serious complications expected in about 5%.

Bile peritonitis is the most worrisome complication and may necessitate urgent cholecystectomy in a patient likely to be a poor surgical risk. In pediatric patients, the most commonly reported complication is asymptomatic extravasation of contrast into the gallbladder fossa without significant sequelae, although the number of reported procedures is too low to make broad generalizations about the relative risk of the procedure.

Percutaneous transhepatic biliary drainage (PTD)

Introduction

First described by Molnar and Stockum in 1974, PTD is useful to treat biliary obstruction or bile leaks. In the pediatric population these problems are most commonly seen following hepatic transplantation, especially with ischemic strictures related to hepatic artery thrombosis (Figure 5.4). Percutaneous therapy may obviate or postpone the need for retransplantation or surgical exploration, sphincterectomy, or partial hepatectomy. Percutaneous drainage plays a particularly useful role in patients with a hepaticojejunal (e.g., Roux-en-Y) anastomosis, and others in whom endoscopic drainage is difficult or contraindicated.

Indications

As a general rule, any obstructed biliary tree should be drained. Even in patients who have multifocal obstructions, in whom biliary drainage is often challenging (Figure 5.5), even when multiple catheters are used, and who are vulnerable to recurrent bouts of cholangitis and sepsis due to bile stasis in the undrained segments, the interventionalist is often called on to attempt treatment since other therapeutic options are few and costly. In cases of partial or complete biliary obstruction, PTC should not be performed unless the operator is capable of inserting a biliary drain, because of the risk of bile peritonitis is high once the diagnostic needle has been removed.

Biliary drainage is rarely needed in the pediatric population, and when needed the etiology is invariably benign (Table 5.10). Complications of liver transplantation, including anastomotic and ischemic strictures, are the most common etiologies necessitating biliary drainage. Other indications include strictures secondary to sclerosing cholangitis, postsurgical strictures

Chapter 5 Hepatobiliary interventions

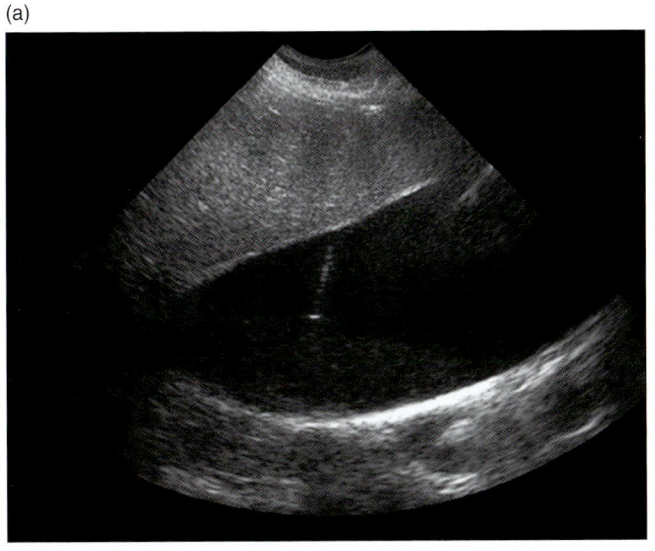

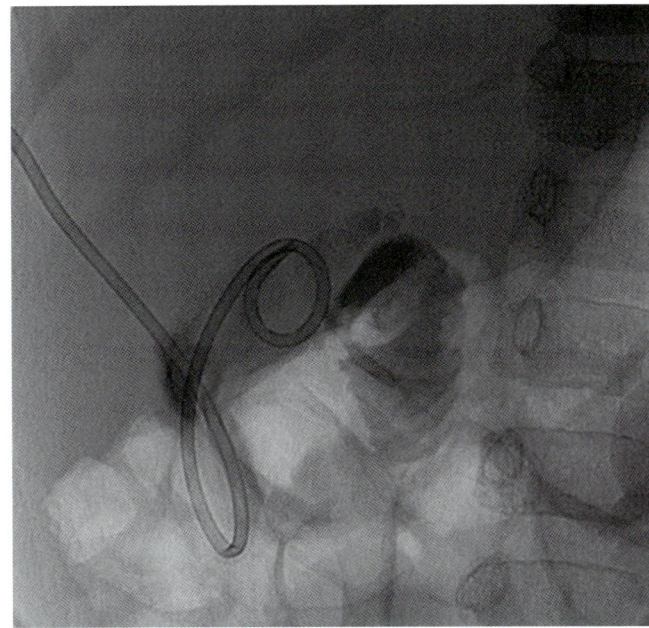

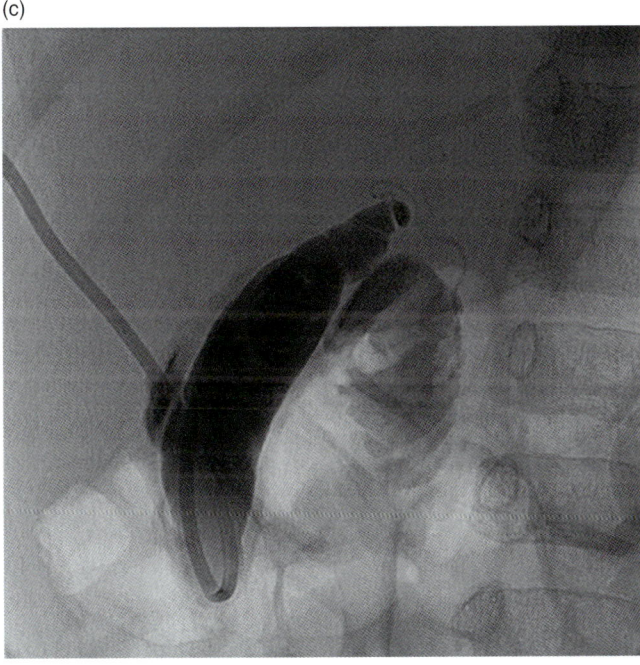

Figure 5.3 Twenty-month male with history of Alagille syndrome with refractory pruritis and hyperbilirubinemia. (a) Ultrasound-guided transhepatic needle access of the gallbladder. (b) 5 French Towbin (Duan) pigtail drainage catheter in gallbladder. (c) Contrast injection shows patency of the cystic duct. Pruritis improved.

(either at an anastomosis or due to ischemia) or trauma of the bile ducts, and congenital strictures (Figure 5.6). Patients with bile leaks (such as those associated with severe acute necrotizing pancreatitis) or large postoperative biliary defects will also benefit from percutaneous drainage (Figure 5.7).

Technique

Equipment

The PTD procedure is a modular hybrid of PTC and drainage of an abnormal fluid collection (see, for example, Chapter 4), modified for the purpose of leaving the drain in one of two places: either across the biliary–enteric connection or within the biliary tree on the access side of the stricture or obstruction. The recommended equipment requirements align with these functions (Table 5.11).

Patient preparation

Patient preparation is the same as described for PTC.

Standard technique

Single-stick method

There are two basic approaches that can be used to access the biliary tree: single stick and double stick. In the single-stick method the primary puncture of the bile duct needs to be appropriate for both opacification of the ducts and placement of a drain or stent. The biggest problem with this technique is when the primary needle puncture is within a duct that is not suitable for biliary drainage either because of its size, location, or trajectory with the common bile duct or biliary–enteric anastomosis. Often, the initial access enters a biliary radicle that is too close to the obstruction. If the guide wire cannot be maneuvered across the stenosis there may be insufficient purchase within the liver parenchyma for subsequent manipulations and placement of a drainage catheter. Also, if the biliary radicle initially entered makes an acute angle with the transhepatic tract then catheter insertion can be very difficult. In the absence of the above-mentioned technical issues, the single-stick approach is preferred. In our experience a single-needle technique is successful in most cases.

Double-stick method

In the double-stick method, opacification of the ducts is performed with the primary PTC needle puncture. The cholangiogram is used to select an appropriate duct for cannulation and a second puncture is then performed with fluoroscopic guidance. The second puncture can be done with another Chiba needle or, alternatively, if the bile duct to be entered is dilated, a larger needle (sheathed or unsheathed) that will accept a 0.035-inch or 0.038-inch guide wire can be placed. If a Chiba needle is used, a 0.018-inch flexible wire, such as an angled Glidewire® or stiff angled Glidewire® is placed into the bile duct and advanced into a stable position in the biliary tree

Table 5.9 Procedure summary: percutaneous cholecystostomy

- General anesthesia
- Intravenous antibiotics to cover enteric organisms
- Ultrasound to identify the gallbladder and mark the skin entry site
- Sterile preparation and draping of the operative field
- Ultrasound-guided, transhepatic needle puncture of the gallbladder
- Collect bile for culture and laboratory studies
- Inject contrast to illustrate pathologic anatomy
- Inserted a stiff guide wire, dilate tract, and insert drainage catheter
- Perform a transcholecystic cholangiogram. Avoid overdistention of biliary system since bile is likely infected and can cause biliary sepsis

Table 5.10 Indications: percutaneous transhepatic biliary drainage

- Obstructed biliary system
- Complication of liver transplantation
- Postoperative strictures
- Post-traumatic strictures
- Iatrogenic strictures

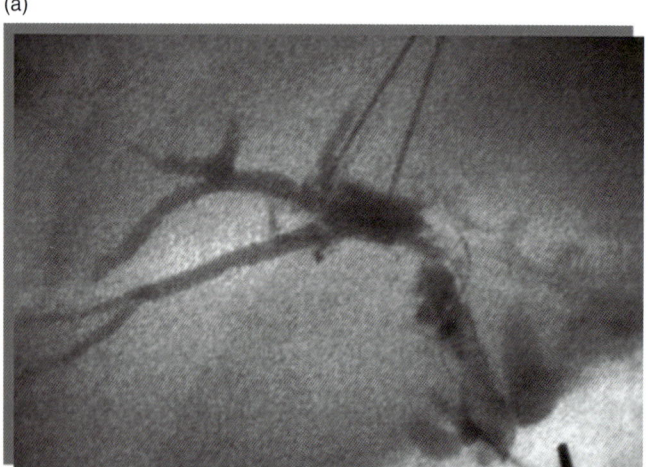
(a)

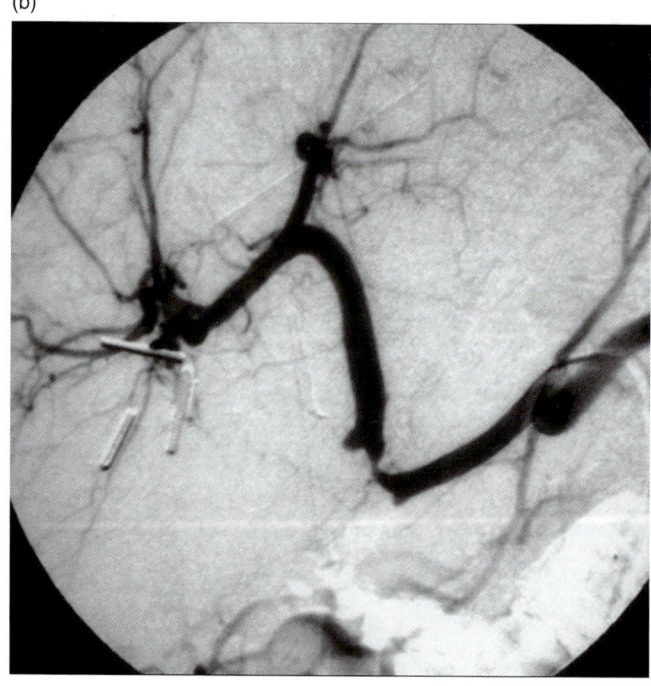
(b)

Figure 5.4 Eight-year-old female after liver transplant. (a) Percutaneous transhepatic cholangiography shows necrosis of the common bile duct. (b) Subsequent angiography revealed right hepatic artery occlusion.

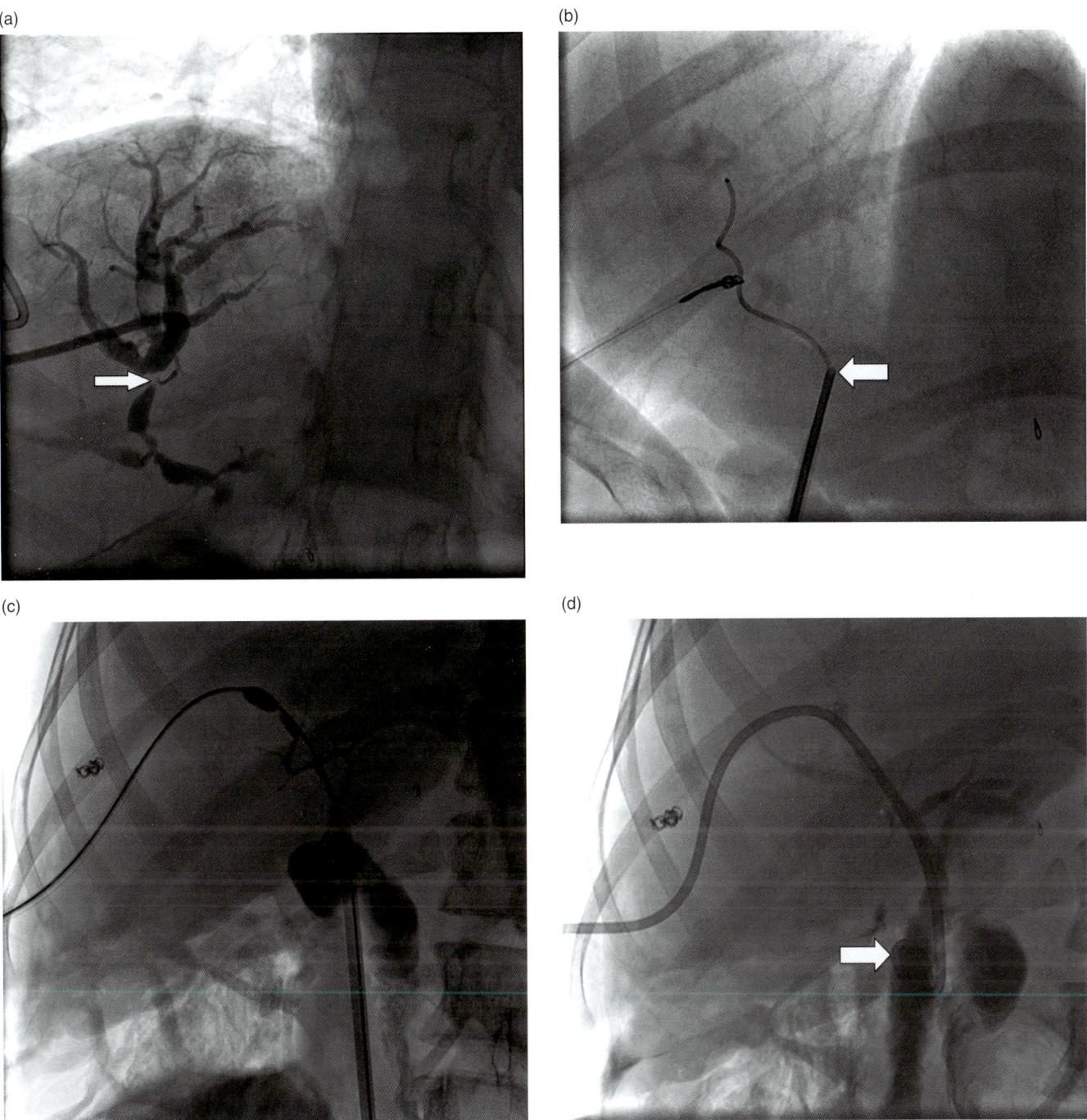

Figure 5.5 A 20-year-old female received a cadaveric whole-liver transplant in childhood. She was treated for hepatic arterial thrombosis with angioplasty by interventional radiology one month after her transplant. At age 20 she developed jaundice with an elevated gamma-glutamyl transferase (GGT) and abdominal pain. (a) Percutaneous transhepatic cholangiography shows a high-grade fixed stenosis (*arrow*) of an intrahepatic right lobe biliary duct that could not be crossed from above. (b) In a combined surgical-interventional procedure, the stenosis was crossed with a TIPS needle (*arrow*) from the small bowel through the common bile duct into the obstructed duct, and the guide wire was snared from above and exteriorized. (c) The stenosis was treated with a high-pressure PTA balloon. (d) After six months of stented drainage and serial dilations, her GGT remained normalized after removal of the catheter.

or, if possible, beyond the stricture into the duodenum or jejunal loop of a Roux-en-Y. Guide wire position distal to the stricture is preferred when possible. A 4 or 5 French coaxial, end-hole introducer system can then be used to change from the 0.018-inch wire to a 0.035-inch or 0.038-inch wire. If the guide wire is not in the distal biliary tree or duodenum, a 4 or 5 French directional catheter (JB-1 or Kumpe) can be inserted and used to direct the wire beyond the stricture. Once the 0.035-inch or 0.038-inch wire is in a stable location the tract is dilated and a 6 or 8 French catheter, often a Ring catheter, is

Chapter 5 Hepatobiliary interventions

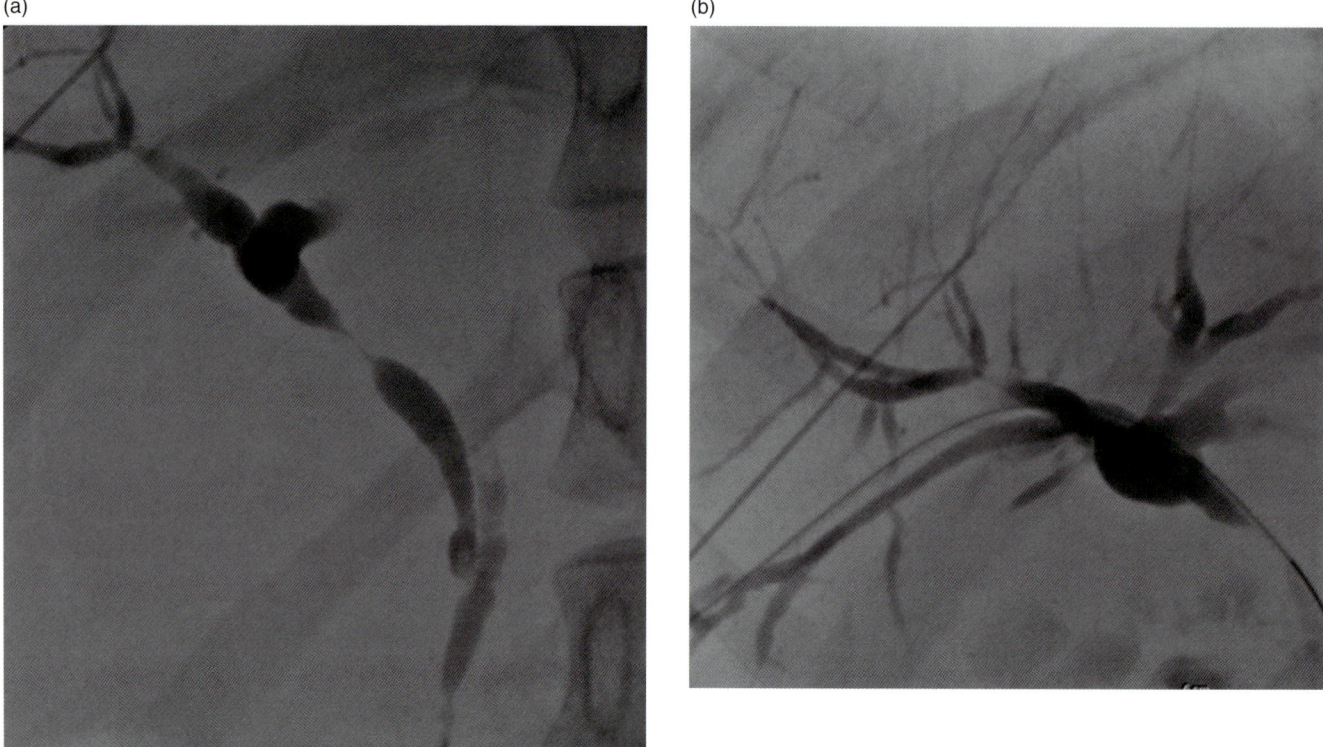

Figure 5.6 Seven-year-old female with ulcerative colitis and abdominal pain who underwent CT demonstrating central intrahepatic biliary ductal dilatation. (a) Percutaneous transhepatic cholangiography shows a high-grade short segment stricture of the common bile duct. (b) Multiple intrahepatic ductal strictures, likely sclerosing cholangitis. Note: wire in place prior to biliary dilation and drain placement.

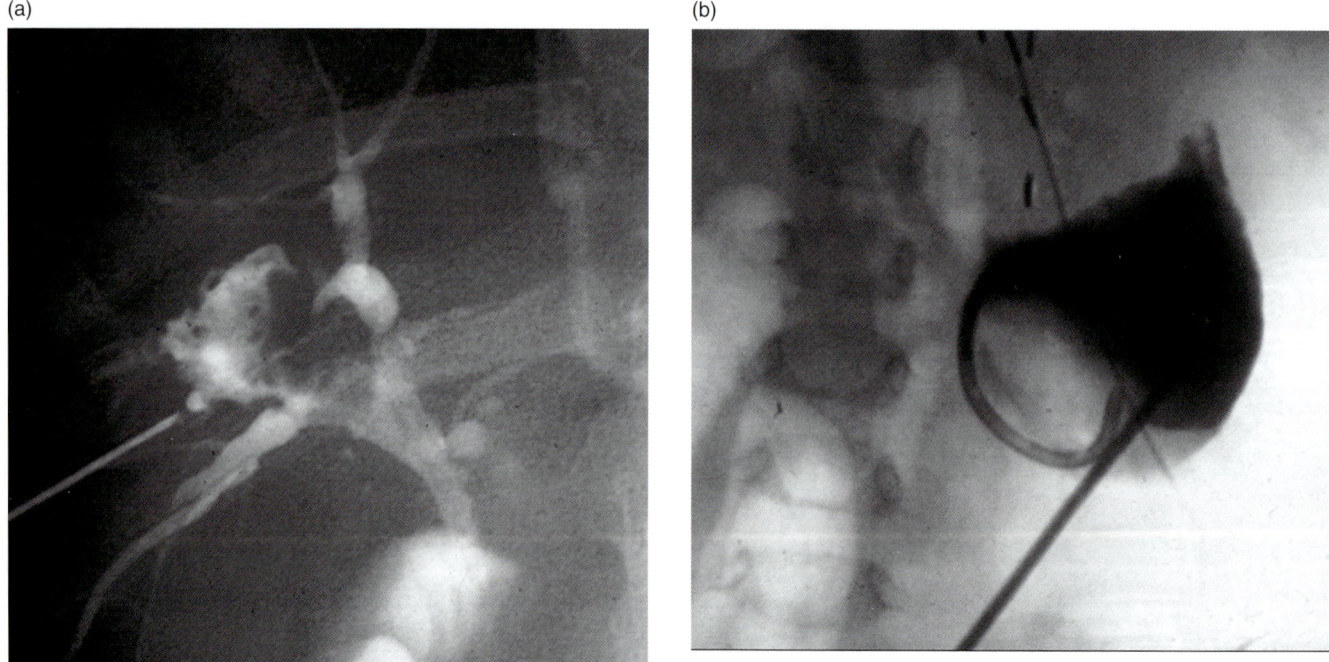

Figure 5.7 Five-year-old male post liver transplant with hepatic artery occlusion. (a) Percutaneous transhepatic cholangiography demonstrates a bile lake communicating with biliary tree. (b) Drainage of the bile lake.

Chapter 5 Hepatobiliary interventions

Table 5.11 Equipment: percutaneous transhepatic biliary drainage

- Equipment for PTC (Table 5.3)
- Guide wires: 0.018-inch glide wire, mandril, tracker; 0.035-inch angled glide wire, stiff and superstiff wires
- Dilators: 0.018-inch and 0.035-inch or 0.038-inch. 0.018-inch from 3 French – 5 French, and 0.035-inch or 0.038-inch from 4 French to 10 French
- Locking drainage catheters: 6 French to 12 French biliary and pigtail drains
- Sterile hole punch or scissors for creating side holes as needed
- Biliary drainage bag
- Retention device (SorbiView® SHIELD, Stat-Lock®, etc.)
- Suture: 2–0, 3–0 silk
- Transparent dressing

Table 5.12 Procedure summary: percutaneous transhepatic biliary drainage and dilation

- General anesthesia
- Intravenous antibiotics to cover enteric organisms
- Ultrasound to identify dilated biliary ducts and mark the skin entry site
- Sterile preparation and draping of the right lateral chest
- Fluoroscopic or US-guided, transhepatic needle passage with injection of dilute non-ionic contrast until a bile duct is entered
- Inject contrast to illustrate pathologic anatomy
- Inserted a stiff guide wire, dilate tract
- If a stricture is identified, perform angioplasty
- Measure tract length to understand where to place proximal drainage holes to maintain internal drainage
- Insert a drainage catheter
- If the child is sick one may delay performing a cholangiogram until antibiotics have a chance to sterilize the bile
- Perform cholangiogram at appropriate time. Anteroposterior, right anterior oblique, left anterior oblique, and craniocaudad views in best oblique

placed. If a stiff catheter is initially inserted, it is changed to a softer, more comfortable biliary drainage or pigtail catheter (with side holes cut into the portion of the catheter shaft that is intraductal) after five to seven days.

If in the initial drainage procedure attempts to traverse the stricture are unsuccessful, more aggressive attempts to pass the area of narrowing are not advisable. We prefer to leave a dilator, directional catheter, or straight drain carefully secured in position on the access side of the stricture. The biliary tree is drained and allowed to decompress for 48 hours or longer to allow inflammation and edema to subside. At this time, the stricture is usually more readily negotiated and a drainage catheter may be successfully placed (Table 5.12).

It may be necessary to dilate the stricture to allow passage of the drainage catheter. This can be accomplished with vessel dilators or a PTA balloon catheter (Figure 5.8). In this situation the use of a stiff wire, such as a stiff Amplatz® or ultra-stiff Glidewire®, is helpful. If the stricture is so tight that a catheter cannot be passed beyond it, a drainage catheter is positioned just proximal to the stricture.

Once the catheter is in position a cholangiogram is performed to confirm the location of the side holes and the adequacy of drainage. If the catheter has successfully crossed the stricture care must be taken to have drainage holes both proximal and distal to the stricture to promote bile drainage. The position of side holes on the catheter is easily measured in one of two ways: the bent guide wire technique or a calibrated wire. With a guide catheter in position several centimeters into the duodenum the tip of a guide wire is positioned just at the catheter tip and then bent or clamped at the catheter hub. The wire is then pulled back until the tip is proximal to the stricture but still within the duct and the wire is again bent or clamped at the catheter hub. The wire is removed and the length of wire between the bends or clamps is the length of catheter where side holes need to be made.

A second technique involves the use of a wire or catheter that has radio-opaque marks at one-centimeter intervals. The tip of the measuring device is placed several centimeters into the duodenum and the distance from the tip to a point upstream of the obstruction but within the duct can be directly measured and transferred to the drainage catheter. Once the tract length has been measured and the side holes have been cut, a guide wire is inserted into the drainage catheter until the tip is at the most proximal side hole and the wire is bent at the catheter hub. After the catheter has been inserted, the premeasured wire is placed into the catheter and advanced to the bend. The tip of the wire will then indicate the position of the most proximal side hole. The position of the drainage catheter can then be adjusted accordingly so that all side holes are intraductal. It is important that none of the side holes are within the liver parenchyma to avoid bleeding into the drain.

Separate drainage of the left biliary system is indicated in some cases. The most common indications for this include unilateral obstruction of the left biliary system, independent obstructions of both right and left systems, or unfavorable anatomy on the right from previous surgery, interventions, or disease. Other indications include ascites and uncontrollable labored respiration, as the respiratory excursion of the left lobe is less than on the right.

In cases where the left ducts are to be drained a preliminary US of the liver is often desirable, as the size and morphology of the left lobe can vary greatly. This is particularly true in the case of procedures required in patients who have received segmental liver transplants. Drainage is done from a subxiphoid approach using either the single- or double-stick method. Once the PTC has been performed and the appropriate duct chosen for placement of the drainage catheter, the technical aspects of the procedure are the same as for drainage of the right system.

In general, once the initial drainage catheter is in place the procedure is terminated. This allows the parenchymal tract to mature and the biliary tree to decompress. Decompression of

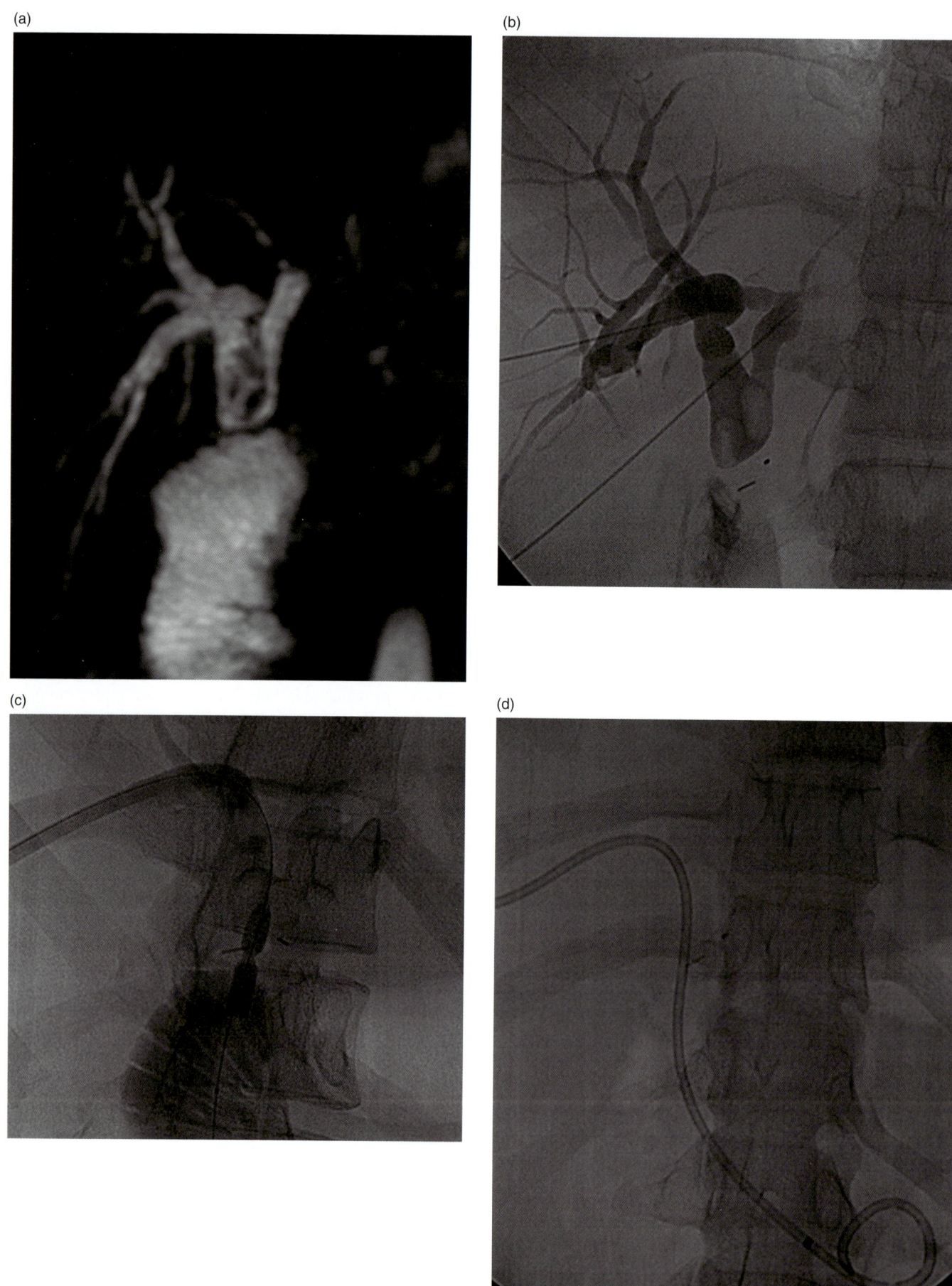

Figure 5.8 Sixteen-year-old female with history of hepaticojejunostomy and recurrent bouts of cholangitis. (a) Magnetic resonance cholangiopancreatography (MRCP) shows an anastomotic stricture and several large filling defects. (b) Percutaneous transhepatic cholangiography shows a high-grade anastomotic stricture and multiple large stones. (c) A percutaneous transluminal angioplasty balloon shows "waisting" at the stricture. (d) Biliary drain in place.

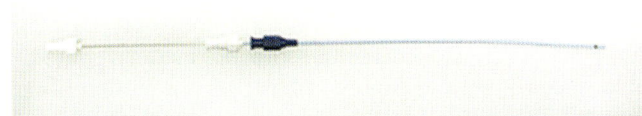

Figure 5.9 Coaxial dilator with metal stiffener.

the system allows edema and inflammation to resolve and the ducts to return to a more normal caliber. In addition, the risk of sepsis is decreased. The catheter is fixed to the skin and placed to closed gravity drainage for at least 24 hours. Depending on the patient's condition, the catheter may be clamped after 24 hours to allow internal drainage. Antibiotics are continued for at least 48 hours after the catheter has been placed. Further definitive intervention is usually postponed for two to five days, depending on the patient's condition and clinical needs.

Technical variations

We have found that the most technically demanding aspect of biliary drainage in pediatric patients is the initial entry of a dilator or catheter through the wall of the biliary radicle. It is often very difficult to dilate the intrahepatic tract, penetrate the bile duct wall, and enter the lumen over a 0.018-inch guide wire. The periductal tissue is firm and a 0.018-inch wire and 3 French dilator are not rigid enough to allow significant pushing power. As a result, the catheter can buckle just outside the duct wall, within the tract, or between the surface of the liver and abdominal wall. If one is not careful, the guide wire can inadvertently be pulled out of the biliary tree or bent.

If a micropuncture set is used, the 4 French introducer dilator is well tapered for the task. Spinning the introducer while advancing into the duct will help ease it through the transitions between tissue planes. However, if the introducer cannot be advanced smoothly into the duct, coarse and forceful effort is more likely to damage the access system than to achieve success. In this event, other techniques or devices should be considered. To facilitate entry into the bile duct an 18-gauge spinal needle can be advanced over the 0.018-inch guide wire and used to make a larger hole in the bile duct wall. Alternatively, a coaxial dilator with stiffener is available or one can be fabricated by using the metal stiffener from a 5 or 6 French nephrostomy set that can be coaxially placed within a 4 French or 5 French vascular dilator that accepts at least a 0.035-inch wire (Figure 5.9). This combination is then advanced into the biliary tree over the 0.018-inch guide wire already in position. Once the tip of the system is within the bile duct the wire and stiffener are pinned as the dilator is advanced into the biliary tree. The 0.018-inch wire and the stiffener can then be removed and exchanged for a 0.035-inch or 0.038-inch wire, which is stiff enough to maintain access during subsequent dilation of the tract and placement of the drainage catheter.

Selecting, modifying, and positioning a drainage catheter depends upon four principal factors. The first is the intended position of the catheter tip. Usually, the tip of the drainage catheter is a locking pigtail and is placed through the stricture and into the small bowel by way of the common bile duct or the biliary–enteric anastomosis, as applicable. If the stricture or the anastomosis cannot or should not be crossed during the initial procedure, and there is space in the dilated system to form a loop, then the pigtail may be left on the access side of the stricture, rather than the enteric side. Occasionally, the catheter must be advanced through the stricture in a retrograde fashion, either from the contralateral ducts or from an enteric-to-biliary approach, or left on the access side of the stricture where there may be insufficient space to form a loop (for example, when leaving a drain pulled back across a treated stricture until durable preservation of ductal diameter is proven). If the end of the drainage catheter must be left in a non-dilated duct where there is insufficient room to form a loop, the loop may be trimmed off the drainage catheter, understanding that such a modified catheter should be delivered through a sheath, to avoid traumatizing the duct with the rough-cut tip of the catheter.

The second important factor is the distance from the skin to the intended catheter endpoint. This factor will govern the necessary length of the catheter. The shortest catheter that can fulfill this requirement should be used, to minimize the external length of the catheter, and thus the opportunity for accidental dislodgment. The length of the catheter can be sized using the modified "bent guide wire" technique described in Chapter 2.

The third factor, and usually the least critical, is the optimal diameter of the drainage catheter. An 8 to 10 French catheter will suffice in most circumstances. Occasionally, a larger diameter catheter will be useful to stent a healing stricture after therapeutic interventions.

The fourth factor is the intended drainage pathway. The key to optimizing this factor is consideration of where bile is coming from and to where it should be going. If the drainage catheter is across the stricture, then side holes will be required on both sides of the stricture. If the selected catheter is not manufactured with such side holes then they must be added to the catheter shaft. This is most effectively done by creating holes no larger than the end hole of the catheter, in a spiral pattern around the shaft where it will lie on the access side of the stricture, while not extending into the hepatic parenchyma or across the capsule. If the drain is to be left on the access side of the stricture or obstruction, then side holes in the loop or end of the catheter are sufficient.

Whatever the internal configuration, the external portion of the drain should be fixed securely to the skin so as to prevent accidental dislodgment, and should be fixed in line with the access tract so as to prevent kinking of the catheter.

Postprocedure and follow-up care

The biliary drain should be flushed regularly (two to three times per day) with sterile saline. Manipulation of the catheter, including flushing, may be deferred in the initial period after accessing an obstructed system until after at least 48 hours of external drainage to reduce the risk of biliary sepsis. Daily output of any drain is monitored and recorded in the patient record. If the drain has side holes on either side of a stricture, it may be converted to a trial of internal drainage after 48 hours.

Complications

Complications of percutaneous biliary drainage may be either acute or delayed in onset. Acute complications occur in 5 to 10% of patients. Postprocedural sepsis is the most common acute complication and is due to release of bacteria and endotoxins into the lymphatic and venous circulations. The most commonly encountered bacteria are *E. coli* and *Enterobacter*, although *Klebsiella*, *Pseudomonas*, and *Enterococcus* are also relatively common. Prophylactic antibiotics are given prior to and for 48 hours after the procedure, as for PTC.

Hemorrhage is another potential acute complication. It is common to see blood-tinged bile immediately after the placement of a drainage catheter, which usually resolves within the first 24 hours. Bleeding may be intraperitoneal as a result of liver laceration, inadvertent puncture of extrahepatic vessels during PTC, or multiple punctures of the liver capsule. The most common manifestation results from inadvertent transgression of intrahepatic vessels, expressed as hemobilia, which can be seen as either bright-red blood through the drainage catheter or, less frequently, as hematochezia or melena. If bright-red blood is seen coming from the drainage catheter one easily remedied cause is the incorrect position of one or more side holes in the liver parenchyma in direct communication with a vascular channel. All that is required in that case is to reposition the catheter, confirming with a contrast injection that all the side holes are intraductal in position.

If the catheter is in good position then it must be assumed that the bleeding is a result of a biliary-arterial or biliary-venous fistula that occurred during catheter placement, seen in up to 33% of patients undergoing percutaneous biliary drainage. Clinical evidence of bleeding is seen in approximately 6% of these cases and is due to hepatic artery pseudoaneurysms (the most common cause), hepatic artery–portal vein fistulae, and varices along the transhepatic tract. One way to treat the hemobilia is to clamp the catheter and allow clotting within the biliary tree to tamponade the bleeding. Another approach is to change the catheter to a larger size to tamponade the tract, or in resistant cases to attempt direct tamponade of the bleeding vessel by gently inflating a PTA balloon catheter across the fistula.

If hemobilia persists or is severe, hepatic angiography with transcatheter embolization may be necessary to stop the bleeding. Procedurally, there are several measures that can be taken to reduce the risk of creating these vascular lesions. Patients with coagulopathy should be aggressively corrected prior to the procedure. The operator should attempt to puncture the duct peripherally so that the transhepatic tract, if at all possible, does not enter the more vascular central portion of the liver. While the number of passes through the liver with fine-gauge needles does not appear to affect the complication rate, multiple passes with larger gauge needles have been shown to increase the risk of both bleeding and bile leak.

Minor bile leak is probably present in most patients who have undergone PTD, but the vast majority of children remain asymptomatic and require no intervention. Inadvertent puncture of an extrahepatic duct or the gallbladder or multiple punctures of the liver capsule may predispose to this complication, but the same precautions that apply to reducing the risk of hemorrhage also apply here. Only rarely does bile peritonitis occur, and if it does placement of a peritoneal drainage catheter may be all that is necessary.

Pleural complications such as pneumothorax, hemothorax, and biliary–pleural fistula are uncommon. The parietal pleura often extends substantially lower than the fluoroscopically observed costophrenic sulcus, and any puncture performed along the mid-axillary line at, or cephalad to, the tenth intercostal space invariably transgresses the pleural space. Pleural complications may be avoided by choosing a puncture site closer to the anterior axillary line. However, this may make it more difficult to puncture a biliary duct.

In general, the best protection against acute complications is successful placement of a secure drainage catheter. Adequate decompression of the biliary tree decreases the risk of continued cholangitis and bile leak. Major hemorrhage and pleural complications are much less likely if an indwelling catheter tamponades the transhepatic tract. Failure to establish adequate drainage in an obstructed biliary tree, and similarly, early dislodgment of the catheter before a mature fibrous tract is formed, frequently lead to complications. Loss of the drainage catheter from an obstructed system in the immediate postprocedure period should be considered an emergency and a new catheter placed as soon as possible.

The risk of acute complications may be decreased by meticulous attention to proper technique, but delayed complications are not only much more difficult to avoid but also more likely the longer the catheter is in place. Catheter malfunction, usually due to blockage or migration, is the most common delayed complication. For the most part, if problems are recognized early they can be treated on an outpatient basis and have no significant or long-term sequelae. Early detection of these problems depends principally upon how well the patient or the patient's caretakers understand how a biliary drain works, how to properly care for the catheter, how to recognize the signs of catheter malfunction, and what to do when a problem is identified.

A blocked catheter, which is most often noticed because of bile leakage around the catheter, needs to be exchanged.

Catheters that have migrated do not drain optimally and need to be adjusted or, in most cases, exchanged. Obviously, if the catheter becomes completely dislodged it needs to be replaced. After ten to fourteen days of catheter drainage, the mature fibrous tract that forms around the catheter makes replacement relatively easy. In case of catheter dislodgment replacement should be performed as soon as possible, at least within 24 hours.

Delayed cholangitis may also result from catheter malfunction. Usually catheter exchange and antibiotic therapy will be sufficient treatment. If there are persistent or recurrent bouts of cholangitis then the possibility of independently obstructed segments, newly obstructed segments, or liver abscess should be considered and the appropriate imaging done to determine the diagnosis and direct further intervention.

Infrequently, delayed hemorrhage can occur weeks to months after the initial procedure. The etiologies of delayed bleeding include mycotic arteritis as a result of tract infection and pressure erosion of an adjacent blood vessel by the drainage catheter. Usually bleeding occurs during a routine catheter change as the old catheter is removed. The placement of a new catheter will usually tamponade the bleeding vessel and stop hemorrhage, but occasionally transcatheter embolization may be required for treatment.

Overall, the incidence of major complications in the adult population is 5 to 10% and the mortality rate is 2%. However, these statistics are derived from studies in which the majority of patients had malignant obstructions. There is a significantly lower complication rate among patients with benign disease, presumably because of the shorter duration of drainage required and because the overall health of patients with benign obstructions is better than those with malignant obstructions. In patients with benign etiologies of biliary strictures the expected rate of major complications is around 2% and the mortality rate is near zero. The complication rates in the pediatric population are generally lower in our experience; however, there are few studies available to provide objective confirmation.

Percutaneous transhepatic biliary dilation (PTBD)

Introduction

Percutaneous transhepatic biliary dilation (PTBD) became a treatment option in the late 1970s. Prior to that time surgery was the only approach available. Before liver transplantation became a viable approach to treat patients with liver failure the primary cause of biliary strictures were postoperative, primarily as a complication of a cholecystectomy. Therefore it is not surprising that biliary strictures were rarely treated in the pediatric population. This all changed in pediatric medicine when liver transplantation became a life-saving choice in the subgroup of children with liver failure. Now, in pediatric liver transplant centers, it is essential to have an interventional service that can perform these technically challenging procedures.

Table 5.13 Indications: percutaneous transhepatic biliary dilation

- Treatment of biliary strictures
- Liver transplantation
- Trauma
- Iatrogenic

Indications

In the pediatric age group virtually all biliary strictures are of benign etiology (Table 5.13), whereas in the adult population most are iatrogenic, mainly involving the extrahepatic biliary tree, or malignant, mainly involving the porta hepatis. In pediatric patients who have had liver transplantation and develop anastomotic strictures, hepatic artery thrombosis and rejection may also cause biliary strictures. Significant strictures usually cause ductal dilation visualized by invasive evaluation with ERCP or by any cross-sectional modality – US, CT, or MRCP – although early changes may be subtle. Gamma glutamyl transferase elevation (GGT more than 100 IU above the reference range), a sensitive marker of biliary injury, in conjunction with US or MRCP evidence of ductal dilation, is predictive of more than four times increased risk of stricture development after transplantation.

Other etiologies of benign strictures include congenital strictures, sclerosing cholangitis, infection, gallstones, and radiation fibrosis. Strictures need to be treated, if possible, because chronic partial obstruction predisposes the patient to repeated bouts of ascending cholangitis. Occlusion of the narrowed ducts with mucus, inspissated bile, and debris may eventually lead to cirrhosis or loss of the liver transplant.

Primary surgical repair of biliary strictures with an end-to-end anastomosis or creation of a biliary–enteric anastomosis has been the traditional management approach and generally has been effective. Surgical repair of extrahepatic biliary strictures is successful in 65 to 80% of patients, but the operative mortality rate is 2 to 13% with a stricture recurrence rate of 20 to 30%. Intrahepatic biliary strictures are not amenable to surgical repair, so retransplantation may be the only alternative to endobiliary drainage and treatment. The use of percutaneous biliary dilation is a direct and natural extension of percutaneous biliary drainage. Since Burhenne's first report in 1975, percutaneous dilation of strictures has become a feasible and successful alternative to surgery. The expected success rate for transhepatic dilation of biliary strictures may approach 85%. The morbidity rate for balloon dilation of biliary strictures ranges from 10 to 20% and the mortality rate is less than 1%. No data are available on the success rate for PTBD in the pediatric population.

Technique

Equipment

The equipment for the PTBD procedure builds on biliary access (Table 5.3) and drainage (Table 5.11). Additional equipment (Table 5.14) is necessary to either cross a stricture after temporizing drainage and antibiotic coverage have allowed normalization of inflammatory changes and evacuation of static and possibly infected bile, or to increase and maintain the diameter of the affected bile ducts sufficiently that they will conduct the volume of bile produced by the patient without generating increased intrabiliary pressure that may lead to hepatobiliary injury and cholangitis, cholestatic jaundice, bile leak, or biliary sepsis. Virtually all stents placed in pediatric patients are for temporary use (weeks to months) in patients expected to recover, although some may require retransplantation if endobiliary efforts to restore normal function fail. Metallic stents, designed for end-of-life palliation in terminal patients with biliary obstruction, are almost never used in children. When they are used, the largest deployable stent should be selected. Newer retrievable biliary stents may bridge the gap for patients with strictures unresponsive to extended efforts at conventional therapy, but too little is known about their use in children to make a recommendation at this time.

Patient preparation

Most dilations take place after transhepatic biliary drainage has been accomplished, the biliary tree has been allowed to decompress, and acute inflammation has subsided. Our practice is to allow two to five days to elapse after PTD before performing dilation. Because biliary dilation is painful we use general anesthesia. If the patient is not already on IV antibiotics, they receive a dose one to two hours prior to the procedure or at the initiation of the procedure and complete at least a 48-hour course. Empiric antibiotic selection is chosen to cover enteric Gram-negative bacteria and enterococcal species.

Table 5.14 Equipment: percutaneous transhepatic biliary dilation

- Materials for sterile preparation and draping of the field
- Guide wire: angled glidewire, stiff glidewire, Amplatz®, Roadrunner®, etc.
- Vascular sheath with side arm (5 to 7 French, sized to accommodate PTA balloons)
- PTA balloon catheters of varying sizes (2 to 12 mm)
- Inflation gauge for PTA balloon catheters
- Angioplasty catheter. High atmosphere preferred. Size equal to or 1 mm greater than normal lumen size
- Non-ionic contrast
- Stent. Usually the largest drainage catheter that will fit (6 to 12 French)
- Suture: 2–0 or 3–0
- Device to secure drain, e.g., SorbaView® shield, StatLock®, etc.
- Transparent dressing

Standard technique

A 0.035-inch or 0.038-inch guide wire is placed through the indwelling biliary drain until it is coiled securely in the biliary tree or preferably in the duodenum or jejunal limb of the Roux loop (Table 5.12). Exchanging the drain for a vascular sheath with side arm, of the same French size as the drainage catheter, facilitates both contrast injection and access to the biliary tree. The sheath is secured to the skin with Tegaderm®, Steri-Strips®, or sutures. Accidental dislodgment can result in loss of even a mature tract, so a second "safety" guide wire may be placed in order to maintain access if the sheath is lost. In addition, the second guide wire may be used to introduce a second drainage catheter or balloon, if necessary (Figure 5.10).

A cholangiogram is done via the side arm of the vascular sheath to precisely locate the stricture and to measure the diameter and length of the stricture prior to dilation. The size of the duct above and below the stricture is measured and a balloon is chosen that best approximates the "normal" ductal diameter. The balloon should be longer than the stricture but not so long that it extends into smaller caliber ducts at risk for perforation when the balloon is fully inflated. The balloon catheter is then placed over the guide wire via the vascular sheath and advanced until it is centered across the stricture. It is helpful to place a radio-opaque marker on the skin to indicate the location of the stricture so that positioning of the balloon catheter is quickly accomplished. Using a pressure gauge, the balloon is inflated with dilute contrast to the recommended pressure. Depending on the stricture either low- or high-pressure balloons may be used, although we prefer the high-pressure balloons (12 to 15 ATM) for all types of strictures. A "waist" is seen indenting the contrast-filled balloon at the site of the stricture during the early stages of the dilation, but should disappear when the balloon is fully inflated.

There are two schools of thought regarding inflation protocols. By the first approach, the balloon is inflated for five to thirty minutes. On occasion, even longer inflation times may be employed. By the second approach, concern for further injury from pressure-related ischemia of the biliary wall limits each inflation to two to five minutes, although this may not be as important a factor in strictured ducts that are already largely replaced by fibrotic tissue. Balloon inflation is maintained by frequently observing the pressure gauge to be confident that the balloon pressure is maintained. Although it may seem convenient to clamp the balloon catheter, this practice results in frequent application of subtherapeutic pressures, as the balloon pressure will drop significantly as the stricture diameter is relieved, although the clamped pressure gauge will not reflect this drop.

After PTA, an interval cholangiogram will usually be performed to evaluate ductal diameter and complications. In children with resistant strictures, up to three balloon inflations may be performed in a session. Once the dilation is finished a drainage catheter is placed. The catheter functions as a stent and is left in for a variable period of time after the dilation. It is

Chapter 5 Hepatobiliary interventions

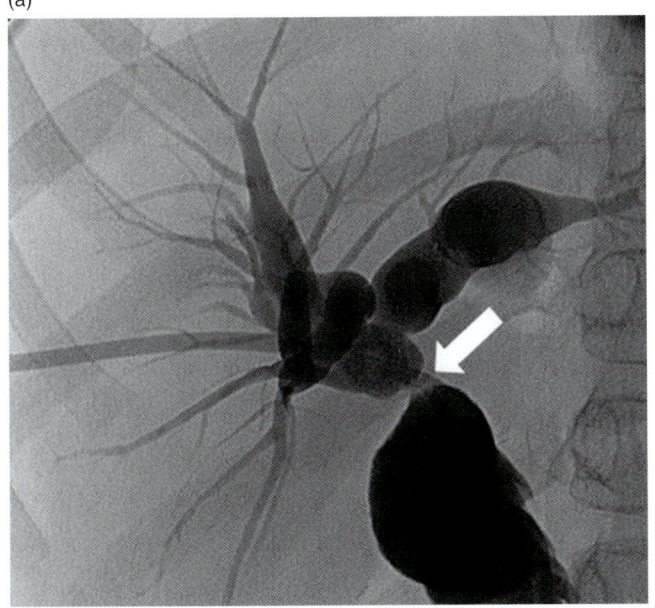
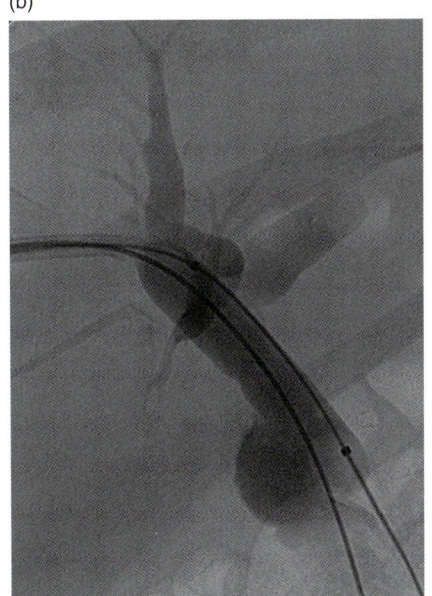
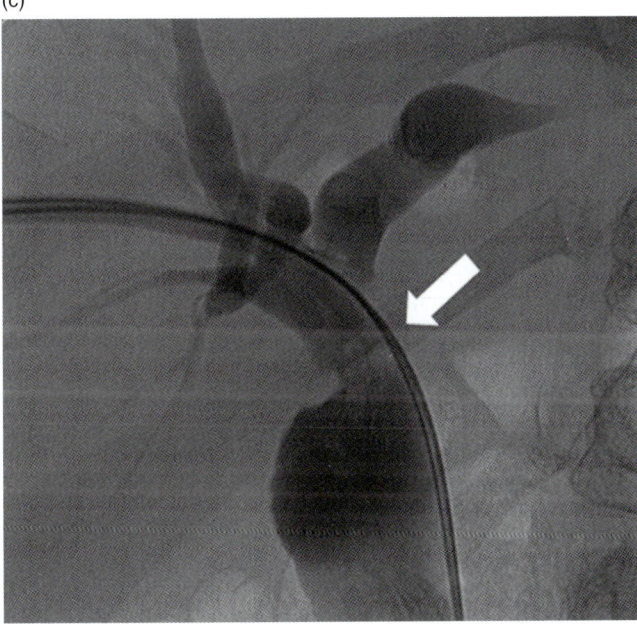

Figure 5.10 Seven-year-old female with history of resected choledochal cyst presents with recurrent cholangitis. (a) Shows stricture (*arrow*) at the choledochojejunostomy anastomosis. (b) PTA balloon dilating stricture. Note presence of second "safety" wire. (c) Successful dilation (*arrow*) of the anastomotic stricture.

not uncommon for a "stent" catheter to be left in place for three to twelve months. The frequency of balloon dilation and length of time the stent is left in place before retreatment is individualized and depends on several factors including the response of the stricture to dilation, the speed of restenosis, the number of strictures, the health of the graft, etc.

Technical variations

In general, the principles of percutaneous biliary dilation are relatively standard; however, the most effective parameters may vary. The variables include the route of approach to the stricture (Figure 5.1), the number of dilations per session, the length of time the balloon is left inflated, the size and pressure of the balloon used, the number of sessions, the amount of time between sessions, and the size of the catheter left in as a stent. In general, we maintain balloon inflation for a minimum of five minutes, and do at least two inflations per session. For more resistant strictures inflation times up to 30 minutes are used. Strictures that do not respond to PTA are considered for cutting balloon angioplasty (CBA, Figure 5.5d). Technically, the procedure and follow-up are the same.

Impassable strictures

Very rarely, a biliary stricture or obstruction proves impossible to negotiate with all conventional approaches. In our experience, if a biliary pathway was at one time patent, it will virtually

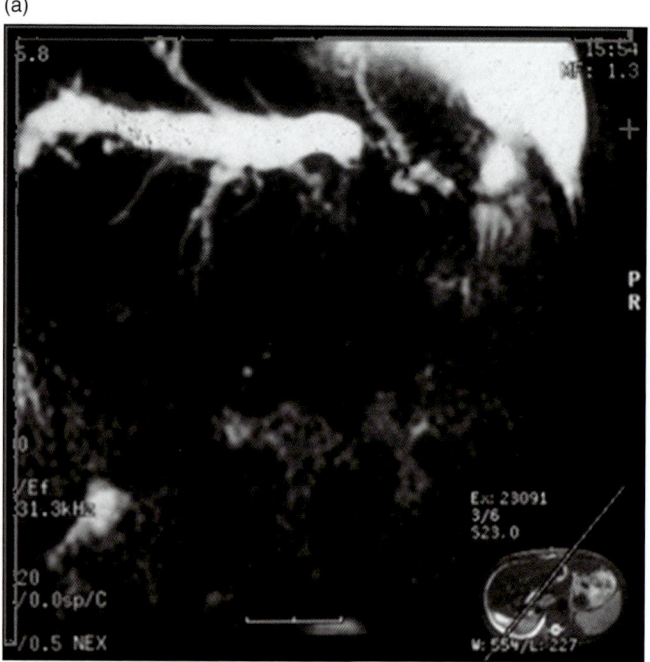 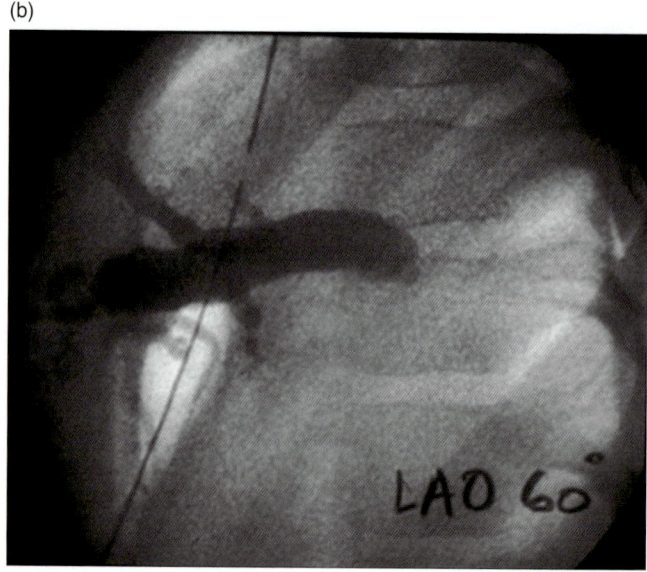

Figure 5.11 Six-year-old female with segmental liver transplant with persistent right upper quadrant pain and abnormal liver enzymes. (a) Magnetic resonance cholangiopancreatography (MRCP) shows a dilated right hepatic ductal segment. (b) Percutaneous transhepatic cholangiography confirms the abnormality. A guide wire was left in place to facilitate surgical exploration. At surgery, the common hepatic duct was found to be ligated.

always remain accessible, although it may require extraordinary effort to negotiate a wire through the probe patent connection. If passage is not possible, then this most often signifies one of two alternatives. First, the connection may have been closed by an iatrogenic event, such as inadvertent suture occlusion. Second, the connection may never have been made. For example, in approximately 10% of left-lobe living donor grafts, the plane of section (along the plane of the falciform ligament) passes to the left of the bifurcation between the segment II and segment III ducts. If both ducts are recognized at the time of graft harvest, they can both be connected at the time of graft implantation. If not, one duct may be "orphaned" and remain unconnected. This invariably results in segmental biliary dilation or bile leak within days of transplant. In the former case, surgical revision of the anastomosis may re-establish patency (Figure 5.11). In the latter case, the intrahepatic portion of the orphaned duct cannot safely be located surgically. Potential options include sclerosis of the orphaned duct, which resolves immediate symptoms but may lead to loss of half the graft, or a new interventional biliary–enteric anastomosis (neocholedochojejunostomy), which can preserve graft function and obviate retransplantation (Figure 5.12).

Postprocedure and follow-up care

Follow-up care is individualized after consultation with the referring service. If the stricture was easy to dilate repeat cholangiography should be performed after two to six weeks. Monitoring GGT levels over time (and plotting them graphically) can be very helpful in assessing response of the stricture to therapeutic interventions. If the diameter of the stricture is stable on the follow-up cholangiogram we will withdraw the catheter to a position proximal to the stricture and cap the drainage catheter. In two to four weeks we will bring the child back for contrast examination. If the stricture is stable and GGT levels have normalized, the catheter is removed. If not, the stricture is dilated and stented and follow-up is scheduled for one to three months later. The process is repeated until the catheter can be removed. There is no point removing the drain if restenosis is likely.

If the stricture were more resistant, repeat cholangiography would be in about three months. If the cholangiogram reveals residual stenosis then repeat dilation is performed and a new biliary drain is placed and left capped to allow internal drainage for at least another one to three months, to allow the tube to stent the area of stricture until complete healing has occurred. This process is repeated every eight to twelve weeks until no significant residual stenosis is seen. Once no significant stenosis remains on the follow-up cholangiogram and GGT levels have normalized, a catheter is positioned above the stricture and clamped for two to four weeks. Repeat cholangiography and GGT evaluation will then be performed. If the stricture is stable the tube may be removed.

In general, the overall recurrence rate of biliary strictures is 40 to 50% in our experience; however, percutaneous dilation can provide palliation from months to years. Because of the long potential lifespan of a young child, this is quite important as it can delay, or may even preclude, the need for retransplantation.

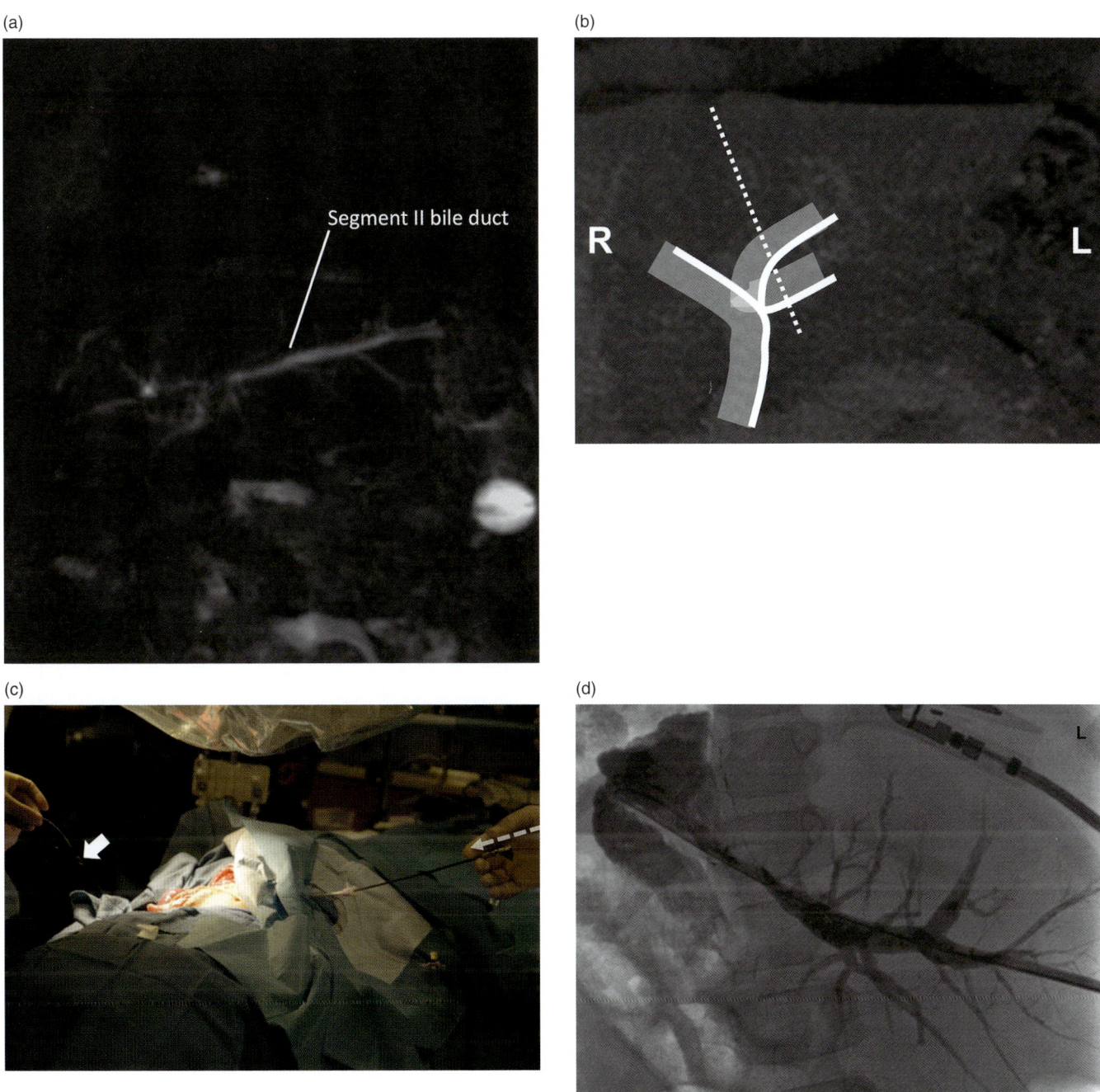

Figure 5.12 Neocholedochojejunostomy. A two-year-old with a left-lobe transplant for hepatoblastoma developed a biliary-cutaneous fistula within days of transplant. (a) MRCP showed a single dilated (segment II) duct. (b) Review of donor imaging indicated the resection plane (*dotted line*) fell to the left of the segmental bifurcation at the time of graft harvest resulting in two separate ducts for anastomosis. Only one duct was anastomosed at the time of transplant. The other duct was "orphaned". (c) Sharp canalization was performed with a Colapinto needle (Cook Medical) in a combined interventional-surgical procedure from a percutaneous transhepatic biliary access (*dashed arrow*) through the orphaned duct to a snare placed in the Roux limb of small bowel, where a guide wire was exteriorized (*solid arrow*). (d) The short transhepatic tract was serially dilated and a drain left for six months to allow the tract to epithelialize, after which the drain was removed.

Complications

The range of complications is similar to those described in the prior section on percutaneous biliary drainage. In the period after therapy, hemobilia, bile leak, bacteremia, or septicemia are most common. In the longer term, recurrent strictures, repeated episodes of cholangitis and sepsis, and drain encrustation should be looked for.

Biliary stents

Introduction

Placement of metallic biliary stents is relatively common in the adult population. The most common indication for placement of a stent is palliation of malignant biliary obstruction. Biliary

Table 5.15 Indications: hepatic venography

- Possible hepatic vein obstruction
- Measurement of portal venous pressure
- Prelude to transhepatic liver biopsy
- Anastomotic strictures secondary to liver transplantation
- Prelude to another intervention

Table 5.16 Equipment: hepatic venography

- Materials for sterile preparation and draping
- Micropuncture set, Seldinger or Potts–Cournand needle
- Connecting tubing
- Pressure transducer
- Directional catheter (4 to 5 French JB-1)
- Occlusion balloon (e.g., 3 French, 5 mm) as needed
- Vascular sheath, 4 to 5 French as needed
- Guide wires, e.g., directional guide wire (angled glidewire), mandril wire
- Non-ionic contrast (usually 300 to 320 mg% I)
- Ultrasound guidance (low-profile linear "hockey stick" transducer preferred)
- Marking pen
- Vascular sheath as needed

obstruction due to primary malignancy or metastatic disease is almost unheard of in the pediatric population. There is a case report in the literature of an endoscopically placed stent in a two-year-old girl for treatment of a congenital choledochal cyst that was placed temporarily and was removed after 16 weeks. There is a second case report of endoscopically placed biliary stents in a ten-year-old patient with Caroli's disease. To date, we have not placed a metallic biliary stent in any of our patients with treated biliary strictures. Because of the potential complications associated with stent placement, the inherent problems associated with the stents themselves, and the lack of predictable long-term results in growing children, we believe all other measures to maintain biliary patency should be exhausted before considering stent placement. Clearly, if stent placement would jeopardize a patient's chances for transplantation or retransplantation, then the procedure is contraindicated.

Hepatic angiography and vascular procedures

Hepatic venography

Introduction

Usually, imaging of the hepatic veins is performed in conjunction with other interventional procedures such as transjugular liver biopsy (TJLB) or TIPS (discussed separately in other sections of this chapter). Three different approaches are available to gain access to the hepatic veins: transjugular, transfemoral, and transhepatic. The transjugular approach is preferred when possible.

Indications

The need to image just the hepatic veins rarely arises. Ultrasound and MRI with MR angiography (MRA/MRV) can be performed initially, and may be adequate to diagnose pathology. However, if US and MRA/MRV are not adequate and additional information is necessary, hepatic venography may need to be performed (Table 5.15). The more common indications include evaluation for Budd–Chiari syndrome or venoocclusive disease, or for indirect measurement of portal venous pressure. In patients with a liver transplant, hepatic venography is performed to evaluate for suspected strictures (see Figure 8.36), either at the anastomosis or related to iatrogenic injury. In addition, hepatic vein cannulation may also be used to measure pressures when evaluating children for possible portal hypertension.

There are no absolute contraindications to hepatic venography, with the possible exception of inability to access the hepatic venous system, either due to impassable outflow obstruction or to a process that does not permit percutaneous access. Relative contraindications to venography include an uncorrectable coagulopathy, severe anemia, acute or chronic renal failure, or unstable clinical condition, and previously documented anaphylactic reaction to intravenous contrast. In the latter case, image contrast alternatives may include a gadolinium solution or CO_2 gas.

Technique

Equipment

Access to the hepatic veins is acquired by way of jugular venous access, just as for placement of a central venous catheter (see Chapter 2), if such access is not precluded by sensitivity to cardiac arrhythmia or impassable occlusion or tortuosity of the hepatic venous outflow. Otherwise, access to the hepatic veins may be achieved using percutaneous transhepatic techniques essentially identical to PTC, only directed toward an appropriate target hepatic vein instead of a bile duct. The equipment and technique for percutaneous transhepatic access is discussed in detail in Chapter 2. The required equipment follows those two procedures, with additional equipment adapted for the anatomic configuration and relationships particular to the hepatic veins (Table 5.16).

Patient preparation

Patients require little in the way of preparation for hepatic venography. Patients are kept NPO as per hospital policy prior to the procedure. All patients have an IV started and maintenance fluids are given during the procedure unless otherwise indicated. Preprocedurally, if there is any suspicion of central venous occlusion a US may be performed to assess venous

Table 5.17 Procedure summary: hepatic venography

- General anesthesia or sedation
- Imaging to define the pathologic anatomy
- Sterile preparation and draping
- Ultrasound-guided right transjugular access if possible
- Insert 5 French sheath with hemostasis valve in RIJ
- Position 5 French JB-1 or other directional catheter and 0.035-inch angled glidewire in HV
- Power or hand inject non-ionic contrast and acquire digital subtraction angiography (DSA) at one to two frames/second. Inject 3 to 10 ml/second × two seconds depending on the size of the vascular system

patency. Preprocedure labs are not routinely obtained, unless the patient has a history of liver disease or other pertinent clinical condition. If necessary, blood products are administered either prior to or during the procedure to correct laboratory abnormalities.

Standard technique

Diagnostic hepatic venography is a relatively short procedure and can be done with sedation. If there is the possibility of intervention or the clinical status of the patient or operator preference precludes sedation, then the case is done with the patient under GA. Either the transjugular or percutaneous transhepatic approach will be used (Table 5.17). For the transjugular approach, the patient is positioned with a roll under the shoulders to extend the neck, and the patient's head is turned to the side opposite the puncture site. This exposes the neck maximally and makes puncture of the internal jugular vein easier. Ultrasound of the neck is done prior to the start of the case and the skin over the internal jugular vein (IJV) is marked. The right IJV is the preferred site, followed by the left IJV and femoral veins. If all of these veins are occluded then transhepatic venography may be performed (discussed in a following section).

The skin of the neck is sterilely prepared and draped and local anesthesia using buffered 1% lidocaine is infused at the premarked insertion site. After a small dermatotomy is made, US guidance is used for direct puncture of the vein. In smaller patients a 21-gauge micropuncture needle or a 22-gauge angiocatheter is used to puncture the vein. In larger patients an 18- or 19-gauge single wall needle that accepts a 0.035-inch or 0.038-inch guide wire may be substituted for the 21-gauge micropuncture needle or 22-gauge sheathed needle. It is important to make the puncture high enough in the neck, especially in small children, ideally at least one fingerbreadth above the clavicle, to avoid inadvertently transgressing the pleural space.

Once venous blood return is obtained a wire is placed into the vein and advanced into the SVC. If a micropuncture set is used the 0.018-inch mandril or angled Glidewire® wire is exchanged through the introducer sheath for a 0.035-inch Newton wire or angled Glidewire®. The 0.035-inch wire is placed into the vein and advanced into the SVC or beyond into the IVC, if possible. The needle or micropuncture sheath is removed and exchanged for a 4 or 5 French directional catheter. If there is going to be any intervention a vascular sheath should be placed first (Figure 5.13). Depending on the suspected diagnosis either the common hepatic vein or branch veins may be injected with contrast. When hepatic vein branches are imaged a preliminary injection of contrast should be performed to make sure the tip of the catheter is not in a small venous radicle or wedged. Either a brisk hand injection or power injection of between 3 to 10 ml of contrast, depending on the patient's size, is adequate and filming is done in the frontal projection at one to two frames per second. When a complete hepatic venogram is performed the goal of contrast opacification is to visualize fifth-order branching, using the injected hepatic vein as the zero-order branch. Non-visualization of branching may signify hepatic fibrosis, from mild (loss of fifth-order branching and beyond), to moderate (loss of third- and fourth-order branching), or severe (loss of first- and second-order branching). Normal venous return to the right atrium confirms patency of the main hepatic vein, which is useful in evaluation of Budd–Chiari syndrome.

If necessary, hepatic venous wedge pressures can also be measured, as described under "Technical variations," below. The tip of the catheter is advanced until resistance is met. A gentle injection of contrast will confirm a wedged position. There will be a dense parenchymal stain in the section of parenchyma drained by the vein the catheter is wedged in and there may be opacification of portal veins.

Once the procedure is over, the catheter or sheath is removed and manual compression is applied until hemostasis is achieved. For venous punctures we hold pressure for approximately five minutes. It is sometimes helpful to elevate the patient's head. The patient should stay in bed for at least two hours after the catheter is removed.

Technical variations

Indirect measurement of the portosystemic gradient

Once the wedged position of the catheter is confirmed the catheter is attached by pressure tubing through a pressure transducer to a pressure monitor. Direct (non-wedged) pressure recordings are obtained with the catheter tip free in the right atrium, the IVC, and in an hepatic vein. Portal pressure may then be obtained indirectly by wedging an end-hole catheter tip into a branch hepatic vein or by inflating a compliant occlusion balloon catheter in a larger hepatic vein branch. The portosystemic gradient (PSG), or corrected wedge pressure, may then be calculated as the difference between the IVC and portal pressure. The normal portosystemic gradient is 2 to 4 mm Hg. A PSG > 6 mm Hg is evidence of portal hypertension, and above 15 mm Hg portal hypertension is considered to be severe.

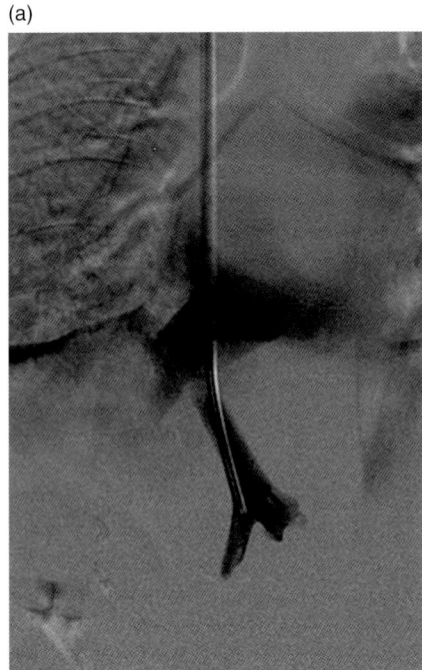
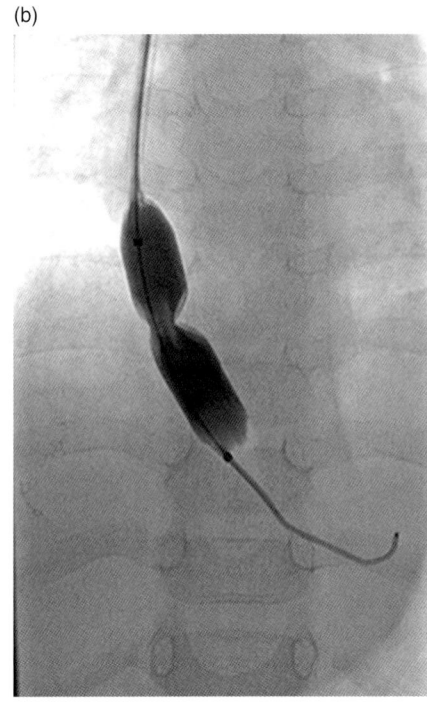
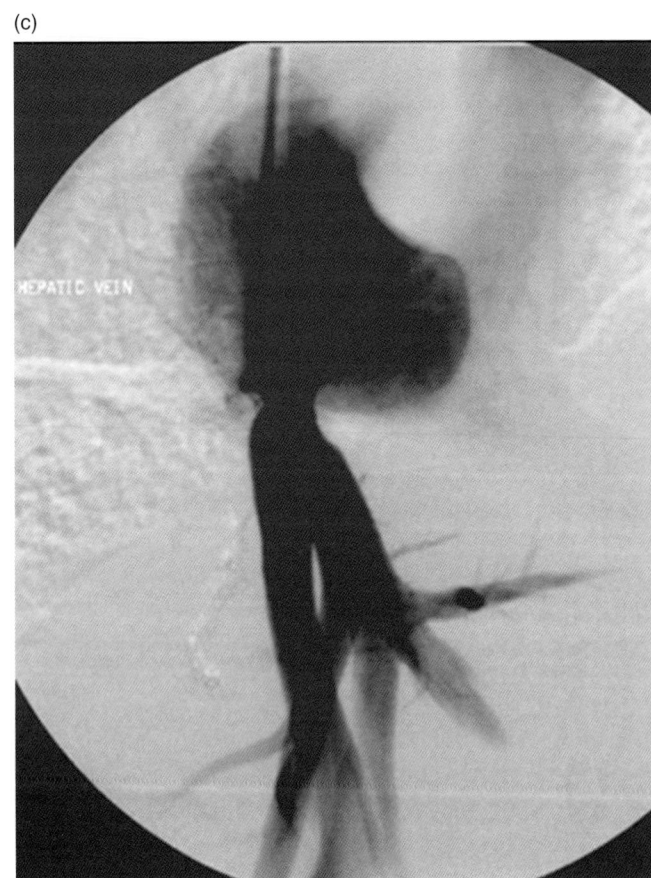

Figure 5.13 Nine-year-old female with stricture at the native hepatic venous–inferior vena cava junction. (a) Hepatic venogram with (b) waisting of PTA balloon. (c) Successful venoplasty.

Complications

Complications are extremely uncommon but can include infection, bleeding, venous thrombosis, vascular injury, capsular perforation, and cardiac arrhythmias.

Splenoportography

Introduction

Imaging of the portal vein is an important part of the work-up of patients with suspected or known portal hypertension who are being evaluated for possible liver transplantation. Currently, non-invasive, cross-sectional imaging techniques, especially US and CT, are the standard modalities used to evaluate patients with known or suspected portal hypertension. However, if the portal vein is not adequately imaged using these techniques then portal venography may be performed. There are three main angiographic methods that can be used to image the portal vein: arterial (or indirect) portography, splenoportography, and transhepatic (or direct) portal venography (discussed separately, below). In general, arterial portography is the most commonly used method in our practice. However, in those cases where arterial portography is not possible or has not provided adequate visualization of the portal and splanchnic venous anatomy, splenoportography can sometimes be useful. In patients with portal hypertension, contrast in the portal system during arterial portography is often diluted, because of inflow of non-opacified blood from an enlarged spleen. With direct injection of contrast into the splenic parenchyma, maximum contrast opacification of the splenic and portal veins can be obtained.

The technique of splenoportography was first reported in 1951 by several European authors. The technique involves puncture of the splenic parenchyma, measurement of splenic pulp pressure, and injection of contrast. Splenoportography can be a very effective method of visualizing the portal venous system with the added advantage that it allows for the direct measurement of venous pressure in the portal system. In addition, it can accurately demonstrate the site of obstruction and the presence of portal–portal collaterals, which often develop in patients with portal or splenic vein thrombosis. In addition, it allows visualization of intrahepatic portal vein radicles and evaluation of the speed and direction of flow in the portal vein and can evaluate the development of portal–systemic collateralization in patients with portal hypertension.

Indications

In our practice, virtually all splenoportography is performed in children who are being evaluated for liver transplantation and in whom cross-sectional imaging or arteriography have not provided adequate detail or information about the portal venous system. This group of children often has significant portal hypertension, splenomegaly, large collateral veins, and reversal of portal blood flow that can render arterial portography non-diagnostic even after the use of intra-arterial vasodilators.

There are several absolute contraindications to splenoportography. If the child has a tumor, cyst, or abscess in the spleen, has an uncorrectable coagulopathy, or has a condition that might predispose to splenic rupture, such as infectious mononucleosis or malaria, a splenoportogram should not be attempted. Obviously a splenoportogram is not possible in a patient who has had splenectomy. Relative contraindications would include ascites, coagulopathy, anemia, and bacteremia. In these patients once the problem is corrected the examination can be performed. Most patients with significant portal hypertension have hypersplenism with platelet sequestration and abnormal coagulation times that, in addition to hepatofugal flow in the portal vein, increase the risk of postprocedure hemorrhage. However, there are instances in which the information provided by this study is so vital to planning and patient management that we will perform it in patients with varying degrees of coagulopathy. Just as is the case for liver biopsy, tract embolization using a coaxial technique can be used to limit risk.

Technique

Equipment

The equipment used for splenoportography is similar to that used for other percutaneous procedures that access veins within a solid organ (Table 5.18). The major differences are the usual inability to visualize the target vessels in the spleen with the increased risk of non-target injection that results, and the increased instability of trans-splenic access that may easily result in accidental dislodgment or malposition from slight inadvertent manipulation or even respiratory motion.

Patient preparation

Prior to the procedure a coagulation profile is obtained and any bleeding abnormalities corrected as suggested in the guidelines provided in Chapter 1. If necessary the patient will receive blood or blood products prior to or during the procedure in order to maximally correct any abnormalities. In certain cases in which a splenoportogram is going to be performed in a patient with ascites, a peritoneal drainage catheter may be placed in advance of the procedure. Evacuating free intraperitoneal fluid brings the spleen into apposition with the body

Table 5.18 Equipment: splenoportography

- Materials for sterile preparation and draping
- Local anesthetic, 10 ml syringe and 27- or 30-gauge, 1.5-inch needle
- Scalpel (#10 blade)
- Sheathed needle
- Non-ionic contrast
- Manometer and connecting tubing
- Steri-Strips® or 2–0 or 3–0 suture

wall to help tamponade bleeding from the catheter insertion site. Prophylactic antibiotics are not routinely given.

Standard technique

The procedure is performed with the child in a supine position with the left arm raised. While it is possible to perform this procedure with the patient sedated, the vast majority of cases are performed with the patient under general anesthesia. Some interventionalists recommend that all splenoportography be performed under general anesthesia so that respirations can be completely controlled during insertion of the needle and injection of contrast. A limited US of the spleen is performed in order to choose a site for insertion of the needle. The preferred entry site is at the mid- or posterior axillary line in the lower third of the spleen. Depending on the size of the spleen, this may be intercostal or just below the costal margin. Puncture in the region of the splenic hilum is avoided to minimize the risk of hemorrhage.

After the skin has been prepared and draped in sterile fashion, local anesthesia using buffered 1% lidocaine is infused at the insertion site and a small skin nick is made (Table 5.19). Using US guidance an 18- or 20-gauge needle with a 5 French Teflon® sheath is then inserted into the spleen and advanced in the direction of the splenic hilum approximately 3 or 4 cm into the parenchyma. The needle is then withdrawn from the sheath, and if the catheter is in good position, a slow return of blood will be observed. The catheter can then be stabilized by taping or suturing it into place. At this point, the splenic pulp pressure is measured. Normal portal vein pressure is up to 15 cm H_2O, but because there is a slight gradient from the splenic pulp to the portal vein, the maximum normal pressure measured in the splenic pulp is 20 cm H_2O. Portal hypertension is diagnosed when splenic pulp pressure is greater than 25 cm H_2O.

Once the pressure has been measured, a test injection of 3 to 5 ml of contrast is performed to confirm adequate catheter position within the splenic parenchyma. Satisfactory needle position is confirmed by a relatively irregular accumulation of contrast in the parenchyma adjacent to the tip of the

Table 5.19 Procedure summary: splenoportography

- General anesthesia or sedation
- Position child in supine position with left side up
- Ultrasound spleen to select entry site in mid- to posterior axillary line in lower third of spleen
- Inject 1% lidocaine to anesthetize tract. Skin incision
- Ultrasound-guided needle puncture 3 to 4 cm into spleen (sheathed needle preferred). Secure needle in position
- Manometry or electronic measurement of splenic pressure
- Splenoportography. Hand inject 20 to 40 ml of non-ionic contrast. Film three frames/second × 2 to 3 seconds, then one frame/second × 15 to 20 seconds until venous anatomy fully identified
- Remove needle and obtain hemostasis

catheter followed by rapid filling of the splenic vein. Inadequate catheter position will most commonly show a homogeneous subcapsular accumulation of contrast that will spread slightly as the injection continues. In this case the needle can be replaced and the sheath advanced 2 to 3 cm further into the splenic parenchyma and the test injection repeated. If adequate position has not been obtained with this maneuver then the sheath should be capped and left in place, to be removed at the conclusion of the procedure, and a puncture at a new site performed. Simply withdrawing the catheter slightly to reposition is usually not adequate because injection of contrast tends to follow the tract already made by the needle and can result in a large subcapsular contrast collection. Once a new needle position is obtained, a second test injection should be done to confirm adequate position within the splenic parenchyma. A hand injection of 20 to 40 ml of contrast is then performed. Digital images are acquired at three frames per second for two to three seconds and then at one frame per second for another 15 to 20 seconds or until all the desired vessels are opacified.

Postprocedure and follow-up care

After the splenoportogram has been completed and the sheath is withdrawn, the patient is placed in the left lateral decubitus position and instructed to remain in that position for at least four to six hours. In this position the heavy spleen will tamponade the puncture against the abdominal wall. Vital signs are frequently monitored for the first four to six hours. A postprocedure hemoglobin and hematocrit may be obtained after four to six hours. A routine chest radiograph is obtained if the patient develops respiratory distress to check for the presence of a pneumothorax.

Technical problems and pitfalls

As previously mentioned, patients with significant portal hypertension often have reversal of flow in the portal venous system, so-called hepatofugal flow. Splenomegaly and formation of collateral vessels with or without spontaneous portosystemic shunts are associated with development of hepatofugal flow. As with arterial portography, if the hepatofugal flow is significant enough it can result in nonvisualization of both the extra- and intrahepatic portal veins, and often even the splenic vein, during splenoportography. It is important to not misdiagnose this as thrombosis without other confirmatory studies.

Complications

The overall expected rate of complications in splenoportography is approximately 2 to 4%. The most significant risks are splenic rupture, splenic laceration, and hemorrhage. To decrease the risk of splenic rupture, which is most often preceded by the formation of a large subcapsular or intrasplenic hematoma, the position of the needle or sheath within the splenic parenchyma must be confirmed and the needle repositioned if necessary, as described above, prior to contrast injection. Care must also be taken to avoid lacerating the splenic parenchyma and splenic capsule. We agree with the suggestion of investigators who advocate the use of sheathed needles. When using a sheathed needle only the plastic sheath is left in place, with the rigid, sharp inner needle removed, making splenic trauma with respiratory motion less likely to happen.

In order to further decrease the risk of postprocedure hemorrhage, the needle tract may be embolized, usually with Gelfoam® pledgets or slurry, as the needle is withdrawn. We suggest tract embolization be performed, especially if there is a significant risk of bleeding, such as in cases where platelet count and coagulation parameters are borderline or when there is ascites.

Other known but uncommon complications include infection, inadvertent puncture of adjacent organs such as the kidney, colon, stomach, diaphragm, or lung, injection of contrast into the peritoneal cavity, pyrogenic reactions, hemothorax, pneumothorax, and transient chemical pleuritis.

Transhepatic portal venography (TPV)

Introduction

In 1974, Lunderquist and Vang reported a new approach to examination of the portal venous system that used a modification of the technique for percutaneous transhepatic cholangiography. Transhepatic portal venography (TPV) offered several advantages over other methods for visualizing the portal venous system in that it provided direct catheterization of the portal, splenic, and superior and inferior mesenteric veins and their branches, gave the most accurate anatomic detail, and allowed direct portal venous pressure measurements. In the pediatric population, this method can also be used to do selective venous sampling in order to aid the diagnosis of infantile hypoglycemia and localize diffuse or localized pancreatic tumors.

Indications

As with splenoportography, the main indication for direct percutaneous portography is in the pretransplantation evaluation of patients with severe portal hypertension when other methods are unsuccessful or inadequate or venous sampling is needed (Table 5.20). This technique is the most accurate way to diagnose patency or occlusion of the portal, splenic, and superior mesenteric veins and to accurately measure portal venous pressure. This method can also be used for diagnosis of complications involving the portal vein after liver transplantation or splenectomy, if cross-sectional imaging has not provided enough detail or if further interventions are planned. Transhepatic portal venography is also used, along with pancreatic vein sampling, in the evaluation of infants with congenital hyperinsulinism (nesidioblastosis). Percutaneous transhepatic access to the portal vein allows several significant interventional procedures such as embolization of gastroesophageal varices or patent ductus venosus (see Figure 8.3), dilation of portal vein strictures (see Figure 8.37), infusion of chemotherapy, hepatocyte transplantation, as well as delivery of gene therapy agents.

The only absolute contraindications to transhepatic needle insertion would be a large vascular tumor or abscess within the liver parenchyma making portal vein access impossible, uncorrectable coagulopathy, or clinical instability. However, with the use of US a safe route can usually be found. Relative contraindications are the same as for PTC: coagulopathy, anemia, ascites, and previous contrast reaction. Again, postprocedural tract embolization may be useful in children with an increased risk of postprocedural bleeding.

Technique

Equipment
See Table 5.21.

Standard technique

Transhepatic portal venography is usually performed with the patient under general anesthesia. The child is positioned in a supine or slightly oblique position. The right arm is raised to a position that facilitates needle access (Table 5.22). Ultrasound of the liver is performed and the most direct route to the right portal vein is selected using a skin entry site about mid-way between the mid-axillary and anterior axillary lines. The skin

Table 5.20 Indications: transhepatic portal venography

- Pretransplant evaluation. Most imaging performed non-invasively today
- Need for imaging and venous sampling
- Confirm uncertain pathology with non-invasive imaging
- Portal venography as part of another intervention

Table 5.21 Equipment: transhepatic portal venography

- Ultrasound guidance
- 18-gauge, 4 French or 5 French sheathed needle or 22-gauge Chiba needle with a 4 French or 5 French micropuncture set
- Connecting tubing
- 0.018-inch, 0.035-inch, or 0.038-inch guide wire of choice (angled Glidewire®, Amplatz®, Rosen)
- 3 French to 5 French vascular sheath
- 3 French to 5 French directional catheter with an end-hole catheter, or a vascular dilator
- Pressure monitoring device (manometer or electronic pressure transducer)
- 3 French to 5 French pigtail catheter
- Non-ionic contrast

Table 5.22 Procedure summary: transhepatic portal venography

- General anesthesia
- Route planning
- Sterile preparation and draping
- Skin anesthesia with 1% lidocaine then skin incision
- Ultrasound sheathed needle (Yueh) placement in RPV
- Power or hand inject 3 to 6 ml/second × five seconds of non-ionic contrast and film at three frames/second × 5, then one frame/second
- Remove needle and obtain hemostasis. Consider tract embolization to reduce blood loss

overlying the proposed insertion site is marked and then sterilely prepared and draped. To facilitate insertion of the needle, a small dermatotomy is made. We prefer US to guide needle placement into the desired section of the portal vein. Ideally, a large right intrahepatic portal branch is accessed, with care being taken to not puncture the extrahepatic segment of the portal vein. Puncture of the extrahepatic segment may lead to intraperitoneal hemorrhage.

Depending on the size of the liver and the portal vein, an 18-gauge 4 or 5 French sheathed needle, which will take a 0.035 to 0.038-inch wire, is generally used. This needle and wire combination eliminates the necessity of a wire exchange and makes the procedure less time consuming. Once the tip of the needle/sheath is seen in the portal vein branch, a contrast-filled syringe with a connecting tube is attached to the sheath. Gentle suction is applied until free return of blood is obtained and then a small amount of contrast is injected to confirm satisfactory needle position within the portal vein. If the sheath is in good position within the portal vein a guide wire with a curved or angled tip (usually an angled Glidewire®) is advanced into the portal vein as far as possible and the sheath is exchanged for a vascular sheath with a hemostasis valve that is advanced into the main portal vein. However, if it appears that there will be significant difficulty in gaining initial access to the portal vein with the larger sheathed needle, then a 22-gauge Chiba needle may be used, as it is less traumatic to the liver if multiple attempts are necessary to gain access to the portal vein. The Chiba needle takes a 0.018-inch wire and, using a micropuncture set, the wire can be exchanged for a 0.035- to 0.038-inch wire followed by placement of a vascular sheath with a hemostasis valve. Then the catheter of choice can be inserted.

Once the catheter has been placed into the portal vein pressure measurements may be obtained electronically or with a manometer at the level of the mid-axillary line for reference. The mean of three readings is recorded as the portal vein pressure. A portal venogram is done with the tip of the catheter in the origin of the main portal vein, just proximal to the confluence of the superior mesenteric, inferior mesenteric, and splenic veins. Digital imaging is performed in the frontal projection injecting non-ionic contrast at a rate of 3 to 6 ml/second for a total of 15 to 30 ml (approximately 1 to 2 ml/kg over three to five seconds). Filming is done at three frames per second for three to four seconds, and one frame per second for another three to four seconds, or until the vessels being investigated are opacified. If necessary, a directional angiographic catheter can be used for selective catheterization and venograms of the splenic, superior mesenteric, and inferior mesenteric veins or their branches, as well as branches of the portal vein. From this access, percutaneous transhepatic portal procedures, including portal, splenic, or mesenteric venoplasty (see Figures 5.14 and 8.37) and portomesenteric thrombolysis (see Figure 8.43) can be performed. These procedures are discussed in greater detail in Chapter 8. In addition, investigation of gastroesophageal varices, with or without embolization, may be performed.

At the completion of the study the sheath or catheter may simply be removed. However, in cases where the patient has one or more risk factors for bleeding, the tract may be embolized with Gelfoam® slurry or pledgets, although coils can be used. To accomplish tract occlusion the sheath is withdrawn from the portal vein into the hepatic parenchymal tract and contrast injected to confirm intraparenchymal position. Once intraparenchymal position is confirmed the embolic material is deposited in the tract as the sheath is slowly withdrawn.

Postprocedure and follow-up care

Patients are kept at bed rest with their right side down for four to six hours after the procedure. A hemoglobin and hematocrit are obtained four to six hours after the procedure.

Complications

Hemorrhage, either intrahepatic hematoma or free intraperitoneal bleeding, is the main risk of this procedure. Bile leak, traumatic hepatic artery aneurysm, and arterio-portal fistula are also known, but uncommon, complications related to transhepatic needle placement. Hemo-, bilio-, or pneumothorax or inadvertent puncture of the colon or other adjacent organs are also possible complications. Infection and portal vein thrombosis have also been reported.

Transjugular liver biopsy (TJLB)

Introduction

The importance of diagnostic liver biopsy in the management of pediatric patients with severe liver disease or liver transplants is well recognized. Although the method selected may be based on the preference and experience of the operator we have developed an approach based on the presence of ascites or other complicating factors and the child's coagulation status. A conventional percutaneous US-guided core biopsy is preferred for children who have no procedure-related risk factors (see Figure 4.48). For those with mild to moderate risk factors (e.g., correctable coagulopathy with platelets 30,000 to 50,000, INR mildly abnormal) the same technique is used, but

Chapter 5 Hepatobiliary interventions

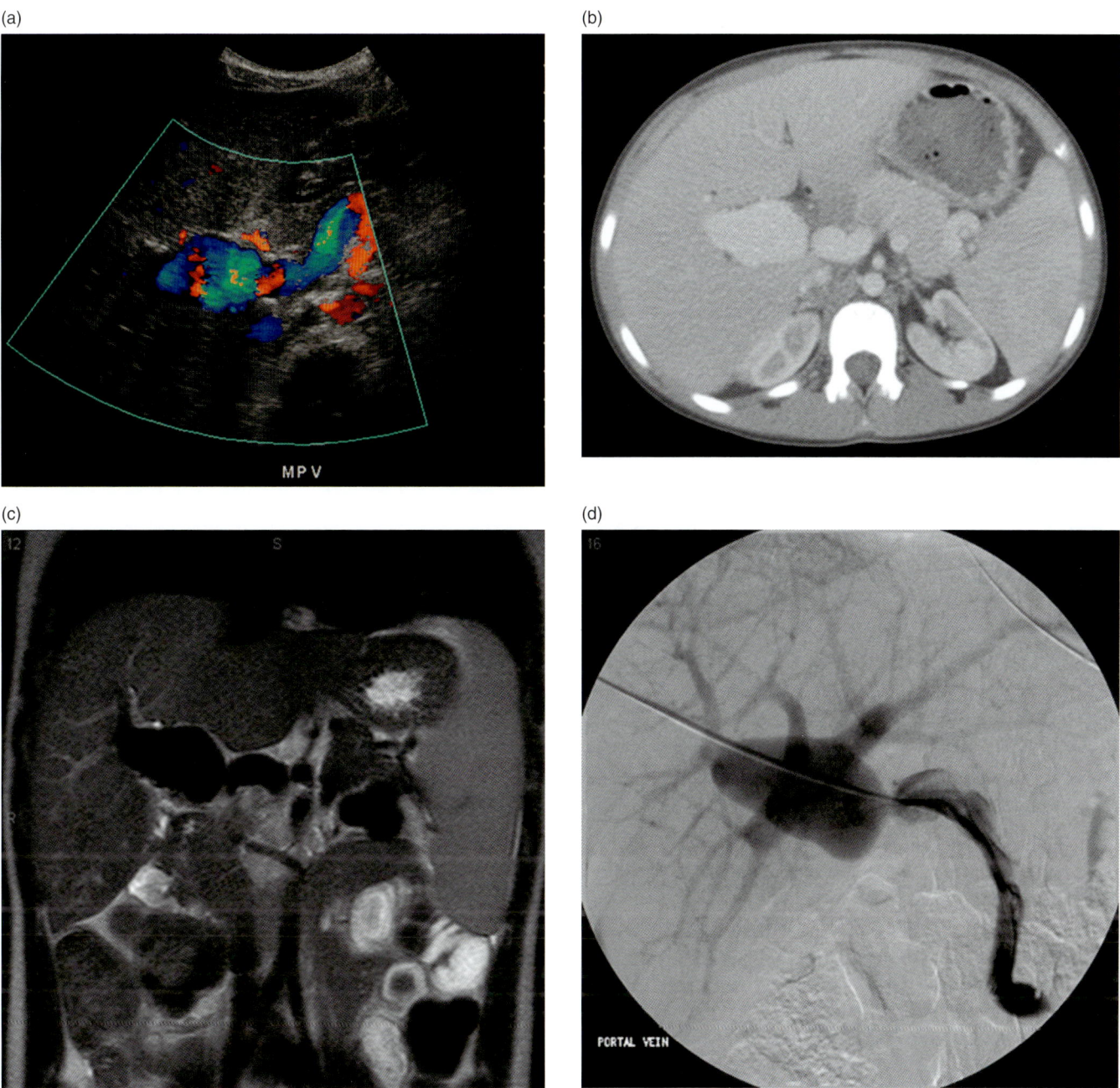

Figure 5.14 Nine-year-old female after liver transplant with a portal vein stricture. (a) Doppler US shows dilated pre-stenotic portal vein with turbulence. (b) Axial contrast enhanced CT and (c) coronal T2 MRI show anastomotic portal vein stricture with pre-stenotic dilatation. (d) Transhepatic portography with guide wire across stricture. (e) Post balloon dilation shows good response.

replacement of platelets, factors, or FFP are timed for delivery to be completed as close to the time of biopsy as possible. Some interventionalists favor coaxial embolization of the biopsy tract, usually with Gelfoam® pledgets or slurry, upon removal of the core biopsy needle. Children with an uncorrectable coagulopathy, platelets <30,000, marked ascites not amenable to drainage, those with suspected portal hypertension, or those with unfavorable anatomy are considered for a transvenous approach. The purpose of this technique is to obtain tissue for a histologic diagnosis in patients at high risk for bleeding by the standard percutaneous route. Additional advantages of the technique include the ability to obtain hepatic venous pressure measurements and to perform hepatic venography.

The first reported transjugular liver biopsy in a person was in 1967 by Hanafee and colleagues. The safety and usefulness of the transjugular approach in the adult and pediatric populations has been well established over the intervening time. The theory behind this technique is that, since the biopsy is taken via a puncture through the hepatic vein, any associated

(e)

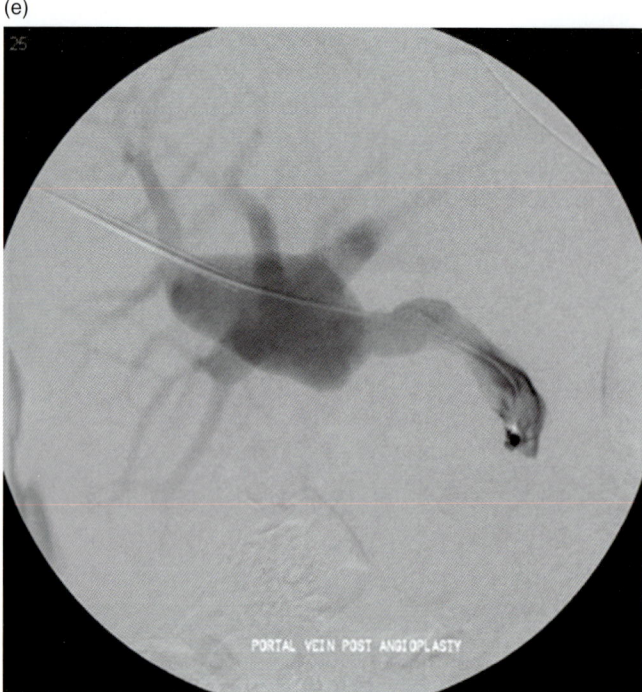

Figure 5.14 (cont.)

bleeding will be directly back into the vascular space and cause no hemodynamic problems. The disadvantages of this technique include the higher frequency of "empty" biopsy passes, the relative difficulty employing the unwieldy equipment in smaller children, and the risk of transcapsular puncture and intraperitoneal hemorrhage.

Indications

Indications for liver biopsy *per se* are discussed in detail in Chapter 4. Indications for a transjugular approach to liver biopsy include acute and chronic liver failure necessitating histologic diagnosis or grading associated with severe or uncorrectable coagulopathy, unfavorable anatomy, or ascites. Bilateral internal jugular vein thrombosis and extremely small liver size constitute contraindications. The procedure has been performed in infants as small as 12 kg. Other less common reasons to use the transjugular approach for liver biopsy include failed percutaneous liver biopsy, massive obesity, and situations in which excessive bleeding may occur as a result of percutaneous biopsy, such as suspected vascular tumor. In rare instances an alternative technique using Mansfield forceps via a femoral vein approach may be utilized.

Technique
Equipment
Several types of transjugular biopsy needles are available, including the standard Colapinto cholangiography set (9

Table 5.23 Equipment: transjugular liver biopsy

- C-arm angiographic unit
- High-resolution US with good penetration
- 3 to 10 MHz curvilinear transducer
- 18-gauge single-wall angiographic needle or sheathed needle
- 4 to 5 French directional catheter
- 7 French or 9 French transjugular biopsy set
- Non-ionic contrast
- Guide wire: Newton, angled Glidewire®, or other directional guide wire, Amplatz Super Stiff®, or Rosen
- 10 ml syringe
- Connecting tube
- Pressure tubing and transducer for pressure measurement

French catheter with 16-gauge modified Ross needle), 7 French curved catheter with 19-gauge modified Ross needle, and a biopsy gun type of needle with a 9 French catheter and metal stiffener (Table 5.23).

Patient preparation

Preprocedure labs, including PT, PTT, hemoglobin, hematocrit, and platelets, are routinely obtained. Bleeding abnormalities are corrected to the degree possible prior to the procedure, according to the guidelines described in Chapter 1. The child is also typed and cross-matched so that blood is available for transfusion if needed. Since infectious complications are very rare, prophylactic antibiotics are not routinely given.

Standard technique

In adults transjugular liver biopsy can be performed with little or no sedation, as the procedure is relatively painless. In children, the procedure may be performed with intravenous sedation but in our practice we almost always use general anesthesia.

Ultrasound examination of the liver is done to evaluate the IVC, hepatic veins, and overall hepatic size and thickness. The standard approach for this procedure is via the right internal jugular vein (Table 5.24). Use of the right external jugular vein has also been suggested as a viable alternative for access if the internal jugular vein is not available. In smaller children the angulation required to navigate the central vessels and right atrium with the angled metal stiffener from the left internal jugular vein may make this procedure difficult and even dangerous in some cases. The right internal jugular vein is punctured using real-time US guidance and the long and curved introducing catheter is inserted over a guide wire, usually an angled Glidewire®. A pre-biopsy hepatic venogram is performed to evaluate the venous anatomy. A normal free hepatic venogram confirms patency of the main hepatic vein (useful in evaluation of Budd–Chiari syndrome).

The catheter is removed and the long guide sheath is then advanced over the wire until it is in the proximal (1 to 2 cm from the origin) intrahepatic IVC. The guide wire is removed and exchanged for a stiff Amplatz® wire. A metal directional sheath, which has an arrow indicating the position of the tip of the sheath, is then advanced through the guide sheath and into the right hepatic vein. A long biopsy needle is advanced to the tip of the metal sheath. The arrow on the metal guide sheath is turned anteriorly, and the biopsy needle is advanced approximately 5 mm beyond the tip of the metal guide sheath where it is then fired to obtain a biopsy specimen (Figure 5.15). We usually obtain two or three specimens. If the right hepatic vein is not easily cannulated, then US can be used to help direct wire placement into the right hepatic vein or alternatively into the most available hepatic vein.

With the standard Colapinto or modified Ross needles, the needle is simply advanced into the liver parenchyma with syringe aspiration and the specimen is aspirated into the needle. With the automated biopsy gun, the sample is obtained as with other biopsy guns. We prefer the automated system to other approaches because it appears to obtain the most consistent and highest quality specimens. In addition, we have found that a maximum of three attempts best limits untoward effects. At the completion of the procedure an hepatic venogram may be performed to assure that there is no transcapsular hepatic bleeding. Once the biopsy and any other tests are completed the vascular sheath is removed. Direct pressure is applied to the site for a minimum of five minutes. If possible the head is elevated to 30 to 45 degrees.

Table 5.24 Procedure summary: transjugular liver biopsy

- Sedation or general anesthesia
- Ultrasound localization of right internal jugular vein. Mark skin
- Sterile preparation and draping of neck
- Infuse local anesthesia at entry site and make a skin incision
- Ultrasound-guided puncture of internal jugular vein
- Insert guide wire, dilate tract, and insert sheath
- Maneuver sheath into hepatic vein
- Insert coaxial directional metal stiffener
- Insert biopsy needle, direct sheath anteriorly or posteriorly, and obtain biopsy specimen (recommend maximum of three attempts)
- Transabdominal US may be useful for directing biopsy needle toward safest parenchymal target and to avoid vital structures, non-target organs, or liver capsule
- Hepatic venogram. If bleeding noted embolize the tract
- Remove equipment and place a dry, sterile, occlusive dressing
- Postoperative chest radiograph
- Recover with head elevated to reduce chance of bleeding
- Postprocedural hematocrit at 6 and 24 hours

Technical variations
Needle curvature

Small children, children with segmental transplants, and those with small cirrhotic livers may have horizontally positioned hepatic veins. These veins can be very difficult to catheterize

(a)
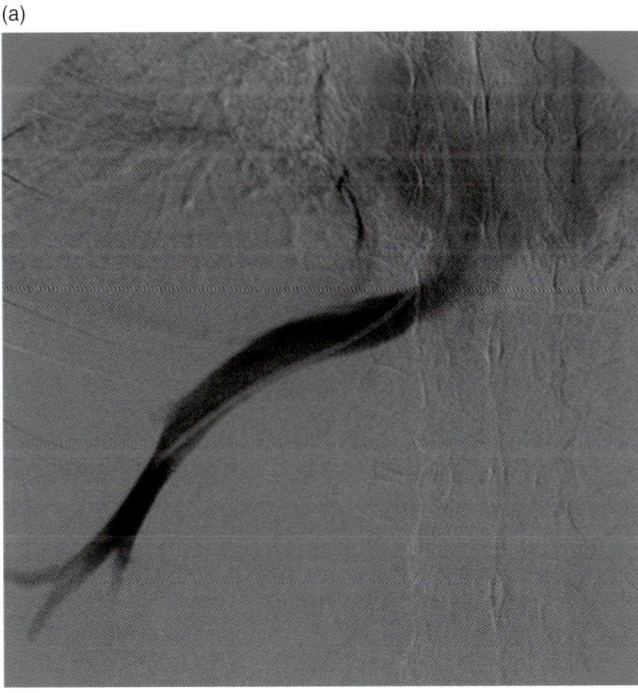

(b)
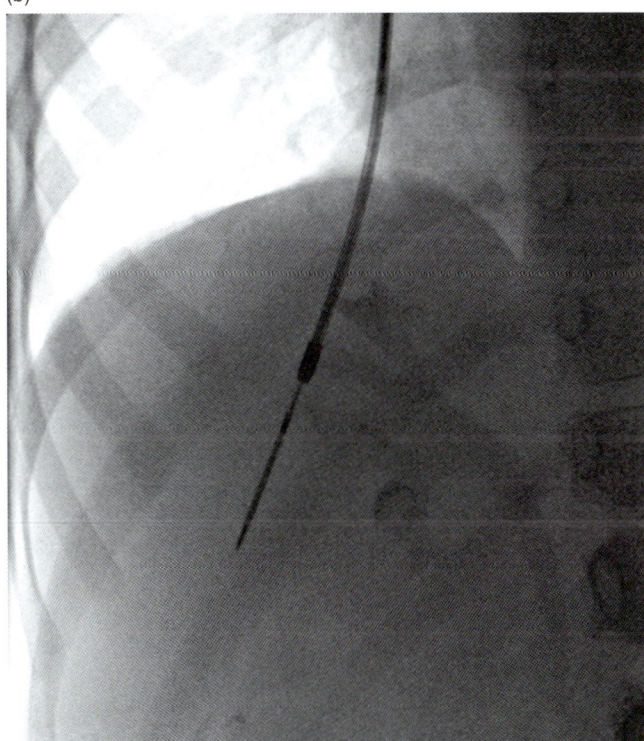

Figure 5.15 Fourteen-year-old female with autoimmune hepatitis and uncorrectable coagulopathy. (a) Right hepatic venography prior to transjugular biopsy. (b) Transjugular liver biopsy.

from the jugular approach. In some instances the use of a superstiff guide wire is all that is necessary to position the Colapinto sheath. However, increasing the distal curvature of the sheath also facilitates a successful outcome. The authors have used a prototype Colapinto sheath with distal curves of 35, 40, and 45 degrees. The sheath selected depended on the venous anatomy. The authors found that curves greater than 45 degrees interfered with the firing mechanism of the automated biopsy needle.

Ultrasound-guided access

In virtually any size child, the safety and accuracy of a transjugular approach to biopsy can be significantly improved if the intrahepatic position of the needle is guided with transabdominal US. This will require an assistant to direct the US transducer. This technique allows selection of the most convenient or accessible hepatic vein, and rotation of the angled sheath toward the greatest parenchymal mass and away from large vessels, non-target structures (e.g., gallbladder), and the liver capsule. Use of real-time US guidance of transjugular biopsy has been shown to significantly reduce complications. Alternatively, transfemoral hepatic biopsy can be performed using a flexible endocardial biopsy needle or Mansfield forceps. This technique may be indicated when the hepatic veins are not accessible from above.

Postprocedure and follow-up care

The patients are recovered with their head elevated for six hours. A hemoglobin and hematocrit may be obtained four to six hours post biopsy.

Complications

Transjugular biopsy successfully obtains adequate liver tissue in greater than 90% of patients. Failed attempts at transjugular biopsy are uncommon, but when they do occur they are usually related to difficult anatomy preventing puncture of the internal jugular vein, cannulation of the hepatic veins, or retrieval of adequate liver tissue. In patients with small, hard, cirrhotic livers not only is there a lower success rate in obtaining adequate liver tissue but, in addition, the risk of perforating the liver capsule, with its attendant bleeding complications, is higher. Subcapsular extravasation of contrast medium is relatively common after transjugular liver biopsy. Fortunately, most children remain asymptomatic. Liver capsule perforation occurs in approximately 1% of patients in large adult series and in approximately 12% of children without US assistance and can be managed, if identified, by embolization of the biopsy tract.

Minor complications, including neck hematoma, bleeding from the venipuncture, supra-ventricular tachycardia, and Horner's syndrome, can be expected in fewer than 20% of patients and major complications, including hepatic capsule perforation, cholangitis, and intraperitoneal hemorrhage, may occur in up to 3 to 5% of patients. The mortality rate of transjugular liver biopsy is very low, in the range of 0 to 0.5%. The main risk of bleeding in these patients is at the insertion site in the neck, but this is easily monitored and treated. If the venous puncture site is directly compressed for a minimum of five minutes, and the patient is kept in a semi-upright position after the biopsy is done, bleeding is very uncommon.

Transjugular intrahepatic portosystemic shunt (TIPS)

Introduction

Transjugular intrahepatic portosystemic shunt (TIPS) has been widely accepted as a treatment for adults with complications of portal hypertension, especially gastrointestinal bleeding not responsive to sclerotherapy and refractory ascites. Although a few pediatric patients are included in published reports of large series, there has been limited experience published about the applicability and feasibility of this procedure in pediatric patients. The TIPS procedure is equally applicable to pediatric patients with portal hypertension who have accessible vascular and hepatic anatomy.

Indications

The most frequent indications for TIPS in the pediatric population are severe gastrointestinal bleeding related to intrahepatic portal hypertension refractory to endoscopic sclerotherapy, especially in patients listed for liver transplantation (Table 5.25). Life-threatening gastrointestinal bleeding secondary to stomal varices in children with portal hypertension who have enterostomies and children with intractable ascites have also been shown to respond well to TIPS. The most frequent causes of pediatric cirrhosis resulting in portal hypertension include biliary atresia, congenital hepatic fibrosis, hepatitis, cystic fibrosis, alpha-1-antitrypsin deficiency, liver necrosis secondary to total parenteral nutrition, and other acquired liver disease. Several of the etiologies underlying pediatric portal hypertension, including biliary atresia with portal vein hypoplasia, congenital hepatic fibrosis with associated cavernous transformation of the portal vein, Budd–Chiari syndrome, and hepatic veno-occlusive disease, may physically preclude the performance of TIPS. Many patients with complications of portal hypertension related to these diagnoses are treated with partial or total splenectomy and surgical portosystemic shunts, usually splenorenal, if sclerotherapy of bleeding varices has been unsuccessful. The primary advantage of TIPS over repeat

Table 5.25 Indications: transjugular intrahepatic portosystemic shunt

- Severe GI bleeding secondary to portal hypertension
- Bridge to liver transplantation
- Complicated portal hypertension

sclerotherapy or surgical shunting is avoidance of potential surgical morbidity in unstable, coagulopathic patients.

The main, although only relative, contraindication to TIPS is lack of access to the right internal jugular vein, the hepatic veins, or the portal vein, from either congenital or acquired causes. Patients with biliary atresia have a high incidence of portal vein hypoplasia and other associated developmental venous anomalies, and often develop portal hypertension in the first years of life. Congenital hepatic fibrosis may be associated with cavernous transformation of the portal vein. Extrahepatic portal hypertension, almost always related to cavernous transformation of the portal vein, makes up a relatively large portion (27 to 38%) of children with variceal bleeding. These children will not benefit from a transhepatic shunt.

Technique
Equipment

Equipment necessary for TIPS is similar to that used for transjugular liver biopsy. In addition, a long 10 French sheath, angioplasty balloon catheters, and appropriate vascular stents are required (Table 5.26). A 10 mm diameter Wallstent® (Schneider USA Inc., Minneapolis, MN) has been the most commonly used endoprosthesis in the past. Alternative stents include an 8 mm Wallstent®, Palmaz® stents, Z-stents, Strecker stents and Angiomed® stents. Recently, the GORE® VIATORR® covered endoprosthesis has become an option for this procedure. The VIATORR® is 6 to 10 cm in length, with a 4 to 8 cm covered segment and a 2 cm bare metal stent component that is designed to be positioned in the portal vein. Available diameters are 8 to 12 mm, but the stent can be undersized to approximately 6 mm in the youngest patients, in order to avoid development of hepatic encephalopathy. This device has the advantages of restricting passage of mucin and bile from the parenchyma, which are common causes of failure of bare metal grafts in this location, as well as limiting stent ingrowth.

Patient preparation

Patients are prepared in a similar fashion as prior to other hepatobiliary procedures, including optimization of coagulation factors, and type and cross-match for blood products. Imaging of the jugular veins, hepatic veins, and portal veins should be reviewed prior to the procedure to insure the feasibility and determine the optimal technique for the individual patient. It is also important to assess hepatic size, especially in the anterior–posterior dimension. Ultrasound is usually very effective in this initial work-up. In some cases MR/MRA or CT/CTA may be necessary or preferred for initial evaluation. All patients receive broad-spectrum antibiotic coverage (usually with a cephalosporin) for the procedure.

Standard technique

TIPS is performed under general anesthesia. Ultrasound may be used for route planning to define an intrahepatic pathway from the hepatic vein to the portal vein, using a similar imaging plane to that used after TIPS to evaluate the endoprosthesis (Table 5.27). In this way not only can a path be selected but the length of the endoprosthesis can be estimated with fair accuracy (Figure 5.16). The overlying skin should be marked, so that the optimal location of the US transducer can be easily maintained during the procedure. Slight elevation of the shoulders with neck extension and slight rotation of the head away from the side of entry makes the internal jugular vein more accessible.

Table 5.27 Procedure summary: transjugular intrahepatic portosystemic shunt

- Preoperative testing: coagulation studies, hematocrit, type, and cross-match, etc.
- General anesthesia and intubation, consider paralysis for respiratory control
- Identify entry site over right internal jugular vein with US. Mark the skin
- Prepare and drape the skin. Make incision at the entry site
- Puncture the RIJ vein using real-time US guidance
- Insert guide wire, dilate tract, and exchange for a long sheath
- Maneuver sheath into hepatic vein
- Wedge catheter in hepatic vein branch and inject contrast or CO_2 to localize the portal vein
- Insert directional sheath and TIPS needle and puncture the portal vein
- Maneuver guide wire into portal or mesenteric vein, dilate tract, and position catheter in portal vein
- Measure pressures
- Dilate intrahepatic shunt with PTA balloon
- Position a stent in the tract between the hepatic and portal veins
- Perform a portal venogram
- Measure portal vein pressure
- Enlarge stent if necessary
- Embolize varicies if necessary
- Remove catheters, obtain a postprocedural chest radiograph
- Postoperative hematocrit three to six hours after completion of procedure

Table 5.26 Equipment: transjugular intrahepatic portosystemic shunt

- Ultrasound
- Transjugular access set (either a Ring access set (RTPS-100) or a Rosch-Uchida access set (RUPS-100), both by Cook, Bloomington, IN; Colapinto, Hawkins Angio Dynamics)
- Pressure monitoring set
- Angioplasty balloon (6 to 12 mm)
- Selection of vascular stents (6 to 12 mm)
- Connecting tube
- Catheter: Pigtail, JB-1, Cobra, or RC-1
- Guide wire: Newton, angled Glide®, Amplatz®, or Rosen
- CO_2 or non-ionic contrast

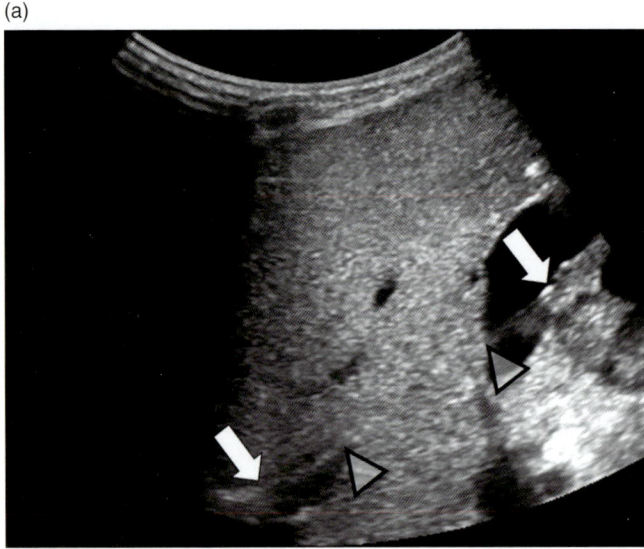 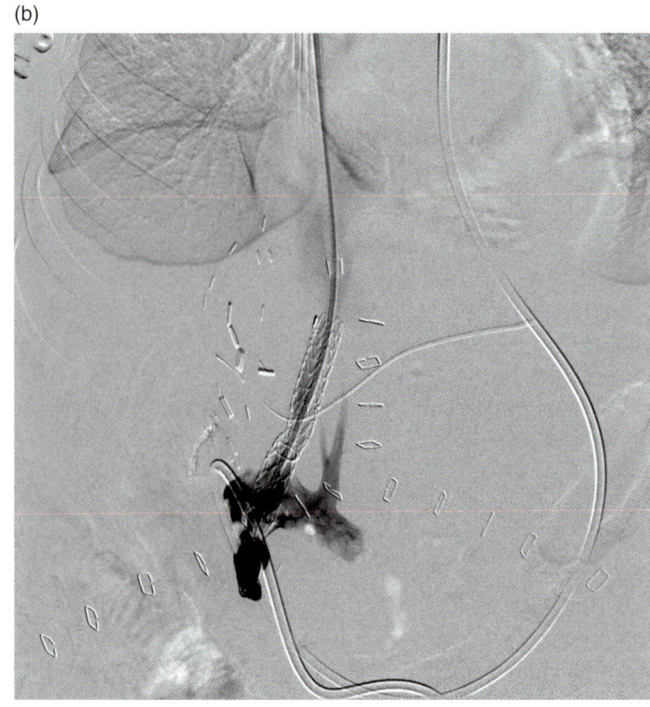

Figure 5.16 A seven-year-old male developed portal overperfusion ("small-for-size") after left-lobe living-donor liver transplantation, with profound coagulopathy, thrombocytopenia, hyperbilirubinemia, and ascites output up 13 L per day. TIPS was planned to reduce portal flow. (a) With transabdominal US, a transhepatic route (*arrowheads*) from the transplant (left) hepatic vein to the proximal portal vein was planned to match the 4 cm length of the ePTFE-covered portion of the smallest (8 mm × 6 cm) VIATORR® TIPS endoprosthesis (GORE®). A Colapinto needle (Cook Medical, *arrows*) was guided using real-time US in a single pass. (b) The TIPS graft was underinflated to 6 mm to avoid hepatic encephalopathy. Portal hypertension was reduced from 25 to <15 mm Hg. The patient recovered within a short time and the TIPS functioned as expected until he was retransplanted over two years later.

The right internal jugular vein is accessed, using the same technique as for transjugular liver biopsy (see above), and a suitable vascular sheath is placed into the vein. Via the sheath a 4 to 5 French directional catheter is advanced to the right atrium, where pressure measurements are obtained, and then into the right hepatic vein, where pressure measurements and a venogram are obtained. The right hepatic vein (RHV) tends to be the largest of the three hepatic veins, has the most optimal orientation (cephalad and posterior) to the right portal vein (RPV), and is used preferentially in the creation of the shunt. However, if the RHV is absent (e.g., left lobe segmental transplant), or too small (less than 6 to 8 mm in diameter), or if its angle with the IVC is too acute to accept the guiding cannula or access needle, then the middle or left hepatic veins may be used, remembering that their orientation to the portal vein differs.

Once position in the RHV is confirmed by venography, the sheath is advanced from the SVC into the vein. The portal vein may be identified in one of several ways, including wedged hepatic vein contrast injection (using iodinated contrast or CO_2), US-guided percutaneous transhepatic puncture of the portal vein with a small (0.018-inch) guide wire left in place, percutaneous transhepatic needle placement adjacent to the portal vein with placement of a Hilal straight coil (0.5 mm or 1.0 mm), or transarterial portography. These methods are useful if necessary to support transabdominal US route planning or if the latter method is not adequate in a given patient.

Once position of the sheath within the hepatic vein is confirmed, a metal guiding cannula with a 16-gauge Colapinto access needle is advanced through the sheath and positioned in the proximal right hepatic vein, within 3 to 4 cm of its junction with the IVC, and directed along the path previously defined, or anteriorly if only planar imaging is used. If there is a marker in the target portal vein, simultaneous biplane fluoroscopy can facilitate needle direction regardless of which hepatic vein is selected. The Colapinto access needle has a 35-degree curve over its distal 4 cm. In patients with normal hepatic and portal venous anatomy this angle greatly facilitates hepatic vein to portal vein catheterization.

If the planar fluoroscopic technique is used, the needle is advanced 3 to 5 cm through the hepatic parenchyma with short, sharp thrusts aiming somewhat peripherally in the direction of the right portal vein, which is ideally entered 2 to 3 cm from the bifurcation. If real-time transabdominal US guidance is used, the needle is advanced along the predefined route, taking care to keep both the long axis of the needle and the intended tract centered in the sound plane. In this way it is possible to achieve access and to observe the needle tip entering the portal vein.

Gentle suction is applied to the Colapinto needle with a contrast-filled syringe, withdrawing the needle slowly if necessary. Once blood has been aspirated contrast is injected to confirm needle position within the portal vein, following which a 0.038-inch stiff guide wire, usually an Amplatz Super

Stiff® wire, is advanced through the needle into the portal vein. The needle is removed and exchanged for an angiographic catheter with radio-opaque markings for measurement of the tract length. Alternatively the stiff wire can be exchanged for a calibrated guide wire that can be used to measure the tract length, or the tract length can be measured fairly accurately with US. The catheter is positioned in the proximal portion of the main portal vein, and venography and pressure measurements are performed. The patient is systemically heparinized. In older children the angiographic catheter is removed and exchanged for a 5 French 8 mm × 4 cm angioplasty balloon that is used to pre-dilate the intraparenchymal tract between the hepatic vein and the portal vein. In younger, smaller children a 6 mm balloon may be utilized.

Following dilation of the intraparenchymal tract a stent of the appropriate length and diameter is placed between the hepatic vein and portal vein, leaving at least one centimeter of stent above the parenchymal tract within the hepatic vein, and at least one centimeter of a bare metal stent below the tract, within the portal vein. The stent is then dilated with a balloon catheter to the desired diameter (Figure 5.17). If a single stent is not long enough to cross between the hepatic vein and portal vein, then an additional stent may be placed, overlapping the first. The fact that most TIPS in pediatric patients are performed pretransplant means care must be taken to place the stent(s) so that the proximal component does not protrude into the IVC nor the distal component protrude into the extrahepatic portal vein, which could compromise subsequent candidacy for liver transplantation at all and, at the minimum, would make the procedure more technically difficult.

A portal venogram is performed again, and pressure measurements are repeated in the portal vein, within the stent, and in the right atrium. The goal of the shunt procedure is to reduce the pressure gradient between the portal vein and the right atrium, ideally below 12 mm Hg, and to cause redirection of portal blood flow so that varices no longer fill. In small children the initial shunt is intentionally underinflated to 6 mm and enlarged if a gradient >15 mm Hg persists. In older children an initial shunt diameter of 8 mm is most commonly chosen. If the venogram performed after the shunt has been placed shows persistent varices then the varices should be selectively catheterized and embolized with metallic coils.

Technical variations

Technical variations in the performance of TIPS in adult patients are usually related to unusual or altered hepatic, portal, or other venous anatomy, either congenital or acquired. These variations are multiple and include the use of alternative venous approaches, methods of localizing the portal vein, type of contrast used, type of access set used to cannulate the portal vein from the hepatic vein, which stent is used, etc. While all of these variations are applicable to pediatric patients, the most common reason for technical variation is likely related to the size of the patient. This has resulted in the creation of smaller or shorter access sets and the creation of different, usually more acute, angles in the guiding sheath for the access needle. Also, distances between structures within the liver are shorter, requiring some modification in choosing the point in the hepatic vein where the needle enters the hepatic parenchyma and in the distance that the access needle is advanced toward the portal vein. In addition, the length of the intraparenchymal tract is shorter and the diameter of the involved vessels is less, which mandates choosing shorter, smaller stents.

Postprocedure and follow-up care

In the immediate post-TIPS period, liver function tests should be obtained and the patient observed for the development of hepatic encephalopathy. A baseline Doppler US examination is performed so that shunt function may be followed. Duplex US examination of the liver is performed at discharge, at three-month intervals for the first year following discharge, and at six- to twelve-month intervals after that, as long as the recipient liver is still present. Portal venography and pressure measurements can be performed electively at three-, six-, or twelve-month intervals, depending on the protocol in the institution where the TIPS was performed. Some institutions also perform elective endoscopy although this modality is usually only used in patients presenting with recurrent GI bleeding.

Patients who present with recurrent variceal bleeding or ascites are immediately evaluated. The work-up of these patients usually includes US and transjugular portal venography across the TIPS. Ultrasound is done to evaluate direction of blood flow, velocity and flow rate within the shunt, hepatic veins, and portal veins. Portal venography is performed in patients mainly to confirm shunt function, with an eye to intervention with angioplasty, revision of the existing shunt, or placement of a new shunt if necessary. Endoscopy is performed when needed, but usually not routinely. Again, the vast majority of TIPS in children are temporizing measures to get the patient to transplant and are therefore not long term. However, in those few instances where TIPS is more long term, the same approach to follow-up would apply.

Technical problems and pitfalls

Technical difficulties creating a TIPS are more common in the pediatric population. The problems causing the greatest technical difficulties most often involve difficulty achieving transhepatic access between the hepatic and portal veins that may relate to preexisting stenosis or occlusion of the right jugular vein, a small size hepatic or portal vein, a small or cirrhotic liver with secondary horizontal positioning of the hepatic veins, and the frequent occurrence of extrahepatic portal vein obstruction. Additionally, in rare cases patients with bleeding stomal varices may demonstrate low direct portal vein pressures secondary to spontaneous portosystemic shunting. In this setting normal pressure measurements do not protect against bleeding and in this situation, the size of the shunt

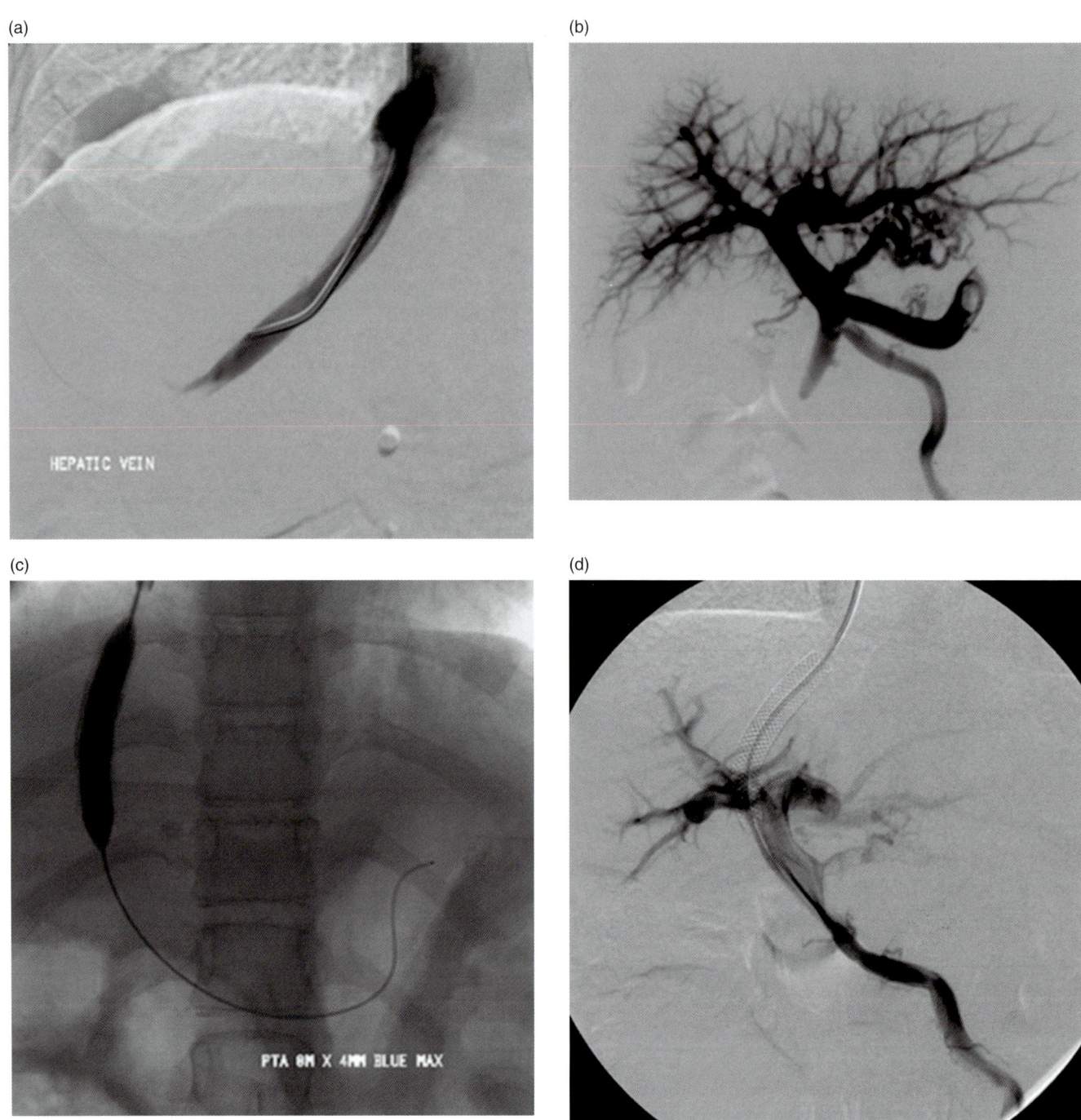

Figure 5.17 Four-year-old female with portal hypertension and upper GI bleed. (a) TIPS procedure with initial hepatic venogram (b) Portal venography shows varices. (c) Angioplasty of shunt tract. (d) Stenting of the tract with decreased varices.

should be determined by the venographic findings (reversal of hepatofugal to hepatopedal flow) rather than the pressure measurements.

Complications

In adults, excluding hepatic encephalopathy and delayed stenosis or occlusion of the shunt, serious procedural complications are reported to occur in approximately 10% of patients. Most of the procedural complications occur during the attempts to gain intrahepatic access to the portal vein and include cardiac perforation, air embolus, hepatic artery injury, portal vein rupture, splenoportal venous thrombosis, biliary duct puncture with or without hemobilia, and hemoperitoneum as a result of puncture of the extrahepatic portal vein, hepatic artery, or transgression of the hepatic capsule.

Complications also arise related to the shunt itself and include acute stent thrombosis, delayed shunt stenosis, occlusion by thrombus or ingrowth within the stent or the hepatic vein, stent shortening, and stent dislodgment or migration. Hepatic encephalopathy occurs as a result of the portocaval shunting and is related to stent diameter and degree of preexisting liver disease, among other factors. Hepatic encephalopathy is seen in 5 to 35% of patients following TIPS, some of which is *de novo* but most of which is seen in patients with a history of hepatic encephalopathy prior to TIPS. These rates compare favorably with those seen in patients after surgical portosystemic shunts, reported to be from 5 to 67%. Infants and small children, in addition to presenting a great technical challenge during transhepatic access, are at particularly high risk of hepatic encephalopathy due to the precarious balance between achieving enough flow to be therapeutic without so much flow so as to cause encephalopathy or liver failure. Staged dilation can help avoid these adverse outcomes. The direct TIPS-related procedural mortality rate in adults is low and occurs much less frequently at institutions that have performed greater than 150 TIPS procedures as compared to institutions which have performed less than 150 procedures, 1.4% vs. 3%, respectively, although virtually no pediatric practitioners have achieved anywhere near this level of experience with this procedure. The 30-day mortality rate for emergency portocaval shunts is 40 to 100%. In comparison, the 30-day mortality rate for TIPS is 7 to 45%.

Transarterial intrahepatic chemoembolization

Introduction

After neuroblastoma and Wilms tumor, primary hepatic tumors are the third most common group of intra-abdominal tumors in children. Hepatoblastoma and hepatocellular carcinoma (HCC) account for approximately 90% of the primary malignant liver tumors in childhood. The other, much rarer, types of primary malignancies include undifferentiated "embryonal" sarcoma, rhabdomyosarcoma, angiosarcoma, malignant mesenchymoma, and other sarcomas. The prognosis for children with hepatic malignancies is dismal, and the only hope for a cure is complete surgical resection of the tumor although, for a select group of patients, liver transplantation is another surgical option. Cure rates for pediatric patients undergoing complete resection of hepatoblastomas and hepatocellular carcinomas has been reported to be as high as 58% and 35%, respectively. Unfortunately, children have a resectability rate between 9.8% and 54%. Children with hepatocellular carcinoma have a poorer prognosis than adult patients with the same tumor because of this lower resectability rate, 9.8% compared to 41.6%. Ninety percent of pediatric patients diagnosed with HCC do not survive longer than one year after the onset of symptoms.

In the early 1960s, because of disappointing results with systemic chemotherapy, regional intra-arterial therapies were developed for the treatment of unresectable hepatocellular carcinoma, which worldwide is the most common primary hepatic neoplasm, as well as for other primary and secondary hepatic malignancies. Such treatments included embolization, intra-arterial infusion of chemotherapy via percutaneous or surgically implanted pumps, and chemoembolization. Chemoembolization is the infusion of chemotherapeutic agents preceded by or followed by particulate embolization with the aim of elevating tumoral chemotherapy concentration (as much as hundreds to thousands of times relative to systemic levels) potentiated by prolonged dwell time (the time the tumor is exposed to cytotoxic drug), and producing ischemia by occluding neovascularity within the tumor. Several factors permit the safe and effective use of chemoembolization in the liver. First, the liver has a dual blood supply with circulation from both the hepatic artery and the portal vein. The hepatic artery supplies approximately 20 to 40% of the circulation to the liver and the portal vein supplies 60 to 80%. In the face of occlusion of one or the other vessel, either circulation alone can support the liver. In addition, it has been shown that there is an increase in portal blood flow with a decrease in hepatic arterial flow. The liver also has the ability to increase oxygen extraction from the portal circulation in the face of decreased flow from or occlusion of the hepatic artery. Second, primary and secondary hepatic neoplasms derive their blood supply almost exclusively from the hepatic artery while the portal vein supplies normal parenchyma. Lastly, the ability to access the hepatic artery and its smaller branches has increased with the development of microcatheters and guide wires that make superselective catheter positioning into arterial branches beyond the origins of vessels to the stomach, duodenum, and gallbladder possible.

Transarterial chemoembolization (TACE) appears to prolong survival and quality of life compared to either systemic or transarterial therapy alone. We have utilized hepatic chemoembolization followed by liver transplantation in a select group of children with hepatoblastoma and hepatocellular carcinoma (HCC) who have failed systemic chemotherapy. This group of children has few options and the expectation of a near 0% survival rate over three years. We have treated children with unresectable tumors with hepatic chemoembolization that kept them free of metastasis and prepared them for liver transplant. The approach utilized was to repeat chemoembolization about every four to six weeks until the alpha-fetoprotein level was within normal limits and a liver was available for transplantation. We have found that alpha-fetoprotein is the most useful test in predicting the success or failure of the therapy. Chemoembolizations are performed until transplantation can be performed. Patients with progressive or new metastatic disease indicate failure of this approach.

Indications

Currently, transarterial chemoembolization (TACE) is not often performed in the pediatric population. However, it is an option in children who have a tumor (hepatoblastoma or hepatocellular carcinoma) that does not respond to the traditional chemotherapeutic regimens and are not candidates for complete resection. Suitability for percutaneous tumor ablation should also be considered.. There are several relative contraindications to TACE. Sepsis, hepatic encephalopathy, or complete portal occlusion should be considered absolute contraindications. When portal blood supply is significantly compromised then hepatic artery embolization could lead to hepatic necrosis with abscess formation or hepatic failure. Patients with cirrhosis and significant liver dysfunction, where the hepatic artery assumes a greater proportion of oxygen transport and nutritive function, may undergo chemoembolization if the tumor is limited to only one lobe, although the risk of hepatic infarction and abscess formation is high. If the patient has undergone previous surgery with hepatic artery ligation or has hepatic artery thrombosis, then the procedure is not feasible unless it is possible to catheterize the collateral arteries that invariably form. Post-chemotherapy bone marrow depression with leukopenia and thrombocytopenia is also a relative contraindication, although the patient is usually allowed to recover fairly completely from the effects of the previous intra-arterial chemotherapy prior to a new round. Other relative contraindications include coagulopathy, anemia, impaired renal function, and severely impaired performance status.

Technique

Equipment

The equipment and supplies necessary for transarterial chemoembolization of the liver (Table 5.28) are directed to five principal objectives: (1) providing diagnostic hepatic arteriography to define arterial supply to the tumor and to nearby anatomic structures at risk for injury from non-target embolization; (2) obtaining subselective access, as necessary, to the hepatic arterial branches supplying neovascularity to the targeted tumor(s); (3) delivery of embolic agents and chemotherapeutic agents sufficient to achieve tumor necrosis without adverse effects to non-target tissues; (4) achieving prolonged embolization of tumor neovascularity without permanent occlusion of parent hepatic arterial vessels; and (5) providing postprocedure imaging of the treatment effect.

Patient preparation

Prior to the initial procedure the patient has CT of the chest, abdomen, and pelvis to delineate the extent of the tumor and to look for metastatic disease. Prior to the first treatment, the patient has an echocardiogram and an audiogram in order to get baseline studies that are used to monitor for complications of the chemotherapy. If the patient is returning for repeat intrahepatic chemotherapy, CT is used to evaluate the effectiveness of the previously performed therapy in shrinking the tumor and in preventing metastasis. Rotational angiography can be very helpful in procedure planning as well as evaluation of prior therapy.

In our experience, we follow an extensive preprocedure protocol in collaboration with the oncologist including allopurinol, dexamethasone (4 mg/m^2), and vigorous hydration, which is started the night prior to the procedure. The morning of the procedure, prior to coming to the angiography suite, the patient receives antiemetics, a single bolus dose of dexamethasone (10 mg/m^2), and antibiotics. In the angiography suite the patient will receive mannitol 1 g/kg during the infusion of the chemotherapy. These children require at least a double lumen central line for venous access.

Standard technique

After sterile preparation and draping, arterial access is obtained. Usually a Glidewire® and a C1, RIM, or similar type catheter is used to select the celiac axis. This guide wire/catheter combination can usually be advanced into the hepatic artery without difficulty. In about 18% of patients the right hepatic artery arises from the superior mesenteric artery (SMA). If this is the case, the catheter is advanced via the SMA, into the replaced right hepatic artery. The case then proceeds in the same manner as if the origin of the hepatic artery were from the celiac axis (Table 5.29).

A single-plane DSA or rotational angiogram is then performed to assess the tumor size, feeding vessels, and tumor vascularity. If the patient is having a repeat treatment, the catheter is positioned in roughly the same position as in the original angiogram and the same contrast volume, injection rate, and filming rate are used to facilitate comparison with previous studies. In conjunction with the preprocedure CT scan, the preprocedure angiography is used to decide which hepatic artery branch will receive the chemoembolization treatment. If the catheter cannot be advanced into the hepatic

Table 5.28 Equipment: transarterial intrahepatic chemoembolization

- Diagnostic catheter: 3 to 5 French, 65 to 100 cm (JB-1, C-1, RIM, or custom-shaped with steam)
- Guide wire: 0.035-inch or 0.038-inch, 125 to 140 cm (Newton or angled Glidewire®)
- Vascular sheath: 3 French to 5 French, 8 to 15 cm
- Variable stiffness microcatheter
- Directional micro guide wire
- Gelfoam®
- Lipiodol® (optional, as selected by the interventionalist and oncologist)
- Chemotherapy agent(s) (as selected by the interventionalist and oncologist)
- Non-ionic contrast
- Connecting tubing
- Pump for chemotherapy infusion

Table 5.29 Procedure summary: transarterial intrahepatic chemoembolization

- General anesthesia
- Sterile preparation and draping of the groin
- Ultrasound femoral artery access
- Insertion of 4 to 5 French sheath with hemostasis valve
- 3 to 5 French JB-1 or visceral catheter for diagnostic angiography and procedural planning
- Consider rotational arteriography with MIP and MPR reconstructions to identify feeders and route planning, to differentiate small tumors, and for baseline to evaluate treatment outcomes
- Road mapping and selective catheterization of supplying vessel(s) to neoplasm
- Transarterial infusion of steroids, narcotics prior to treatment. If fast arterial flow, slow down (50%) with Gelfoam® embolization. Infusion of chemotherapy into neoplasm. Further decrease flow as needed
- Remove femoral artery sheath and obtain hemostasis

artery, usually because the artery is too tortuous, then a microcatheter is coaxially inserted, advanced into the desired location, and used to deliver the embolic agent and chemotherapy.

Injection of chemotherapy into both right and left hepatic artery branches in the same sitting is avoided to reduce the possibility of hepatic necrosis. Once the chosen branch has been successfully catheterized, prior to the instillation of the chemotherapeutic agent, the patient receives one-time doses of intra-arterial dexamethasone (10 mg/m^2) and morphine sulfate (0.1 to 0.2 mg/kg to a maximum of 15 mg). This is followed by partial embolization of the artery with Gelfoam® pledgets mixed in a 1:1 solution of normal saline and contrast. When slowing of arterial flow to at least 50% of normal is seen, the chemotherapy is instilled over a period of time, usually 20 to 30 minutes, followed by further embolization with Gelfoam® until hepatic arterial flow is nearly completely stopped. The goal of the embolization is to temporarily occlude peripheral arteries enough to slow flow and prolong dwell time of the chemotherapy, the effects of which may be potentiated by the ischemia that is also produced by the embolization. Since it is anticipated the patient will usually require serial procedures, proximal occlusion of the hepatic artery and permanent occlusion of the hepatic arterial bed should be avoided. Therefore the preferred embolic agent is Gelfoam®, a temporary occlusive agent. The use of permanent occlusive agents is discouraged because it can lead to proximal occlusion of the main feeding artery, which is invariably accompanied by the rapid development of collateral arteries. If the proximal artery is occluded further access to the arterial tree is prevented potentially eliminating the option of TACE.

Technical variations

Lipiodol®, an oily contrast agent, may be substituted for or combined with other agents to increase tumoral chemotherapy concentration. Although Lipiodol® is not occlusive it does have a prolonged dwell time in neovascular tumor vessels, and avoids uptake by Kupffer cells. It is not easily miscible with aqueous solutions, so compounding with the chemotherapy agent can be challenging. It also may obscure later CT evaluation of treatment response. Drug-eluting embolic spheres have proven to perform well in TACE applications, potentially reducing the time and complexity of the procedure.

Postprocedure and follow-up care

Patients are admitted to the ICU for overnight observation and continue to receive vigorous hydration. Antiemetics, including sodium thiosulfate (1.5 mg/m^2), metoclopramide (0.25 mg/kg), and diphenhydramine (0.25 mg/kg), and dexamethasone (4 mg/m^2) are given intravenously q 6 h. Morphine sulfate is given (IV/SC/IM; 0.1 to 0.2 mg/kg each two hours) as needed for pain. If the patient is afebrile, taking oral fluids, and is stable, then they are discharged to the floor the next morning. The patient is discharged from the hospital when they have recovered sufficiently from the effects of the chemotherapy.

Complications

Acute complications related specifically to hepatic chemoembolization include postembolization syndrome (pain, fever, leukocytosis), chemical hepatitis, and the inadvertent embolization of the cystic, gastroduodenal, left gastric, splenic, or superior mesenteric arteries leading to chemical cholecystitis, gastritis, gastric ulcers, duodenitis, duodenal ulcers, or pancreatitis. These complications can be avoided for the most part by careful positioning of the delivery catheter well beyond the origin of the left gastric and gastroduodenal arteries. Opacifying the fluid in which the embolic particles are delivered and using real-time subtraction during the embolization are measures taken to observe where the embolic material is deposited in order to reduce the possibility of accidental embolization of normal arteries and to monitor the progress of the vascular occlusion. However, the main risk of hepatic artery chemoembolization is hepatic necrosis leading to hepatic abscess or liver failure, even though the majority of hepatic blood supply (approximately 75%) is from the portal vein. This risk is greater if there is underlying hepatic disease or portal hypertension, and possibly if small permanent particles are used. In pediatric patients this is not as much of a concern, as chronic liver disease with cirrhosis and hepatomas arising from cirrhosis are extremely uncommon. Nevertheless, only one of the major branches of the hepatic artery is embolized at a time. If there appears to be almost equal distribution of the tumor in the right and left lobes of the liver one of the branches may be selected for the chemoembolization and chemotherapy alone may be infused in the other branch. Alternatively, chemoembolization may be alternated between the two branches every other procedure, usually scheduled four to six weeks apart.

Partial splenic embolization (see also Chapter 8)

Introduction

Although the exact functions of the spleen have yet to be fully defined, it is known that the spleen represents approximately 25% of total body lymphatic mass and that it acts as a biological filter for the clearance of bacteria, especially encapsulated bacteria. It is also essential for rapid production of antibodies after a challenge with blood-borne particulate antigens for which no preexisting antibodies exist. It serves as a reservoir for red blood cells and platelets, normally harboring approximately 4% of the body's circulating red cell mass and one-third of the body's platelets. In addition, the spleen removes senescent or damaged blood cells from the circulation.

The traditional method of treatment for hypersplenism has been surgical splenectomy. Splenectomy carries significant risks, especially in patients who are debilitated and suffering from the effects of their primary disease as well as hypersplenism, with a 30-day mortality rate as high as 14%. In addition, there is a higher incidence of life-threatening, fulminant bacterial sepsis reported in asplenic and functionally asplenic patients, and patients with congenital absence of the spleen. This increased risk of postsplenectomy sepsis is higher in children and can range from 1 to 25%, depending on the primary disease. Postsplenectomy sepsis is typically rapid in onset, is fulminant, and can have a mortality rate as high as 50%.

The first successful total splenic embolization (TSE) in humans was reported by Maddison in 1973. This procedure has been used subsequently as a preoperative adjunct in high-risk patients prior to surgical splenectomy, with the benefits of reducing splenic bulk, decreasing intraoperative blood loss, and potentially increasing peripheral platelet counts. It has also been used to treat hypersplenism, hematologic disorders, and complications of splenic trauma. However, TSE is associated with serious, often life-threatening complications including splenic abscess, splenic rupture, septicemia, pancreatitis, and pneumonia, and severe post-thrombotic syndrome. For this reason, most authors recommend the use of TSE only as an adjunct to surgical splenectomy, if at all.

In 1979, partial splenic embolization (PSE) was described as an effective but less risky alternative to TSE because it caused permanent ablation of enough splenic parenchyma to reverse and improve hematologic status while at the same time preserving enough splenic tissue to maintain its immunologic function. It has been shown both clinically and experimentally that preservation of as little as 30% of the splenic tissue is enough to provide immunologic protection against infection. Since 1979 there have been numerous reports in the literature on the safety and efficacy of PSE in children, with a reported success between 65 and 85%, similar to the results of surgical splenectomy. Recurrent hypersplenism is reported in approximately 11% of cases and appears to be related to an inadequate degree of embolization. Often these patients are re-embolized with a successful outcome.

Indications

Partial splenic embolization was developed as an alternative to surgical splenectomy to treat severe hypersplenism secondary to portal hypertension from cirrhosis, biliary atresia, portal vein thrombosis, thalassemia major, hereditary spherocytosis, Felty's syndrome, Gaucher's disease, chronic ITP, and painful splenomegaly (Table 5.30). In our practice we have used PSE for treating the thrombocytopenia caused by sequestration in hypersplenism in patients with portal hypertension, splenic lymphangiomatosis, and chronic ITP.

There are no absolute contraindications for PSE. Thrombocytopenia with or without associated coagulopathy is the most frequent relative contraindication. Patients who are candidates for PSE are usually suffering from the effects of thrombocytopenia that is refractory to platelet transfusion and need to be treated in some definitive manner. However, because of their very low platelet count surgery is a significant risk, and PSE is a less invasive way to treat the problem or temporize until the patient has regained a more normal platelet count and can more safely undergo surgical or laparoscopic splenectomy. Sepsis is also a relative contraindication to PSE. Doing this procedure while the patient is bacteremic significantly increases the risk for splenic abscess formation in the avascular/hypovascular portions of the spleen. If the patient is frankly bacteremic, then the procedure needs to be delayed until the patient has received the appropriate antibiotics and blood cultures are negative.

Technique

Equipment
See Table 5.31.

Table 5.30 Indications: partial splenic embolization

- Treatment of severe hypersplenism
- Reduce painful splenic enlargement
- Reduce portal flow
- Treat vascular malformations of the spleen

Table 5.31 Equipment: partial splenic embolization

- 4 French to 5 French vascular sheath
- 4 to 5 French catheter (JB-1, RC-1, Cobra, etc.)
- Guide wire (Newton, angled Glidewire®, etc.)
- Non-ionic contrast
- PVA particles, usually 355 to 500 or 500 to 700 microns in diameter, coils

Patient preparation

Patients who are not immune competent should receive polyvalent pneumococcal vaccine (Pneumovax®) at least two weeks prior to the procedure. Both the night before and the morning of the procedure the patient receives whole body povidone-iodine (Betadine®) or chlorhexidine baths. At least six hours before the procedure, intravenous antibiotic prophylaxis is started using gentamicin (2.5 mg/kg q 8 h) and penicillin G (250,000 U/kg/day q 6 h) or other broad-spectrum coverage of choice. *Staphylococcus epidermidis*, *Klebsiella pneumoniae*, and *Clostridium perfringens* are the pathogens most frequently isolated from splenic abscesses and are usually very effectively covered by the above antibiotic combination. If necessary, the patient is given blood or blood products, including platelets, prior to the procedure and will often receive platelets during and immediately after the procedure. If possible, a baseline nuclear medicine liver–spleen scan is obtained to evaluate splenic size and function.

Standard technique

Strict sterile conditions are observed in the angiography suite during this procedure. All personnel are required to wear at least hats, masks, and shoe covers. The angiographers also wear sterile gowns and gloves. Any visitors to the suite are required to wear surgical scrubs as well as a hat, mask, and shoe covers. Unnecessary traffic into the suite is discouraged, and often the door to the suite is locked during the procedure.

After the skin of the groin is sterilely prepared and draped, arterial access is obtained in standard fashion using the Seldinger technique. The catheter is advanced into the celiac axis, and the splenic artery is selectively catheterized (Table 5.32).

Table 5.32 Procedure summary: partial splenic embolization

- Cleansing, skin-sterilizing baths
- Pneumovax® at least two weeks prior to procedure if <12 years old
- Intravenous antibiotics at least six hours prior to procedure
- General anesthesia
- Sterile preparation and draping of the groin
- Ultrasound femoral artery access
- Insertion of 4 to 5 French sheath with hemostasis valve
- 3 to 5 French JB-1 or visceral catheter for diagnostic angiography and procedural planning
- Road mapping and selective catheterization of vessel(s) supplying spleen
- Transarterial embolization using Embospheres® or PVA particles. Prefer large particle size. Goal is embolization of approximately 60% of splenic volume.
- Postembolization angiogram to access outcome
- Remove sheath and obtain hemostasis
- Admission for treatment of postembolization pain
- CBC to look for Howell–Jolly bodies
- Cross-sectional imaging to assess splenic volume in three to six months

A single-plane DSA or rotational angiography is performed to assess splenic size, splenic artery configuration, and location of distal splenic arterial branches to the tail of the pancreas and the stomach. The catheter is then guided to the splenic artery distal to the pancreatic and gastric branches but proximal to the bifurcation of the splenic artery. This catheter position allows the particles to occlude the perimeter of the splenic vascular bed relatively homogeneously throughout the spleen. If it is not possible to exclude these distal main splenic artery branches to the pancreas and stomach from the embolization then it may be necessary to advance the catheter into the two or three main branches of the splenic artery separately. Once the catheter is in good position the embolization can proceed. We prefer to use materials that lead to permanent occlusion. The material of choice is PVA or Embospheres® with a particle size of 500 to 700 microns or larger mixed in a solution of 1,000,000 U penicillin G, 80 mg gentamicin, 10 ml contrast, and 10 ml saline until the optimal concentration of particles is achieved, which is a qualitative judgment by the interventionalist. Suspension of the embolic particles in the antibiotic solution is done to reduce the possibility of bacterial contamination, hopefully decreasing the likelihood of splenic abscess formation.

The particles are injected under real-time digital subtraction fluoroscopy until approximately 60% of the splenic vasculature has been ablated. When slowing of splenic arterial blood flow is observed a repeat planar or rotational angiogram is done to monitor the extent of embolization. If it has been necessary to position the catheter in the two or three main branches of the splenic artery this procedure is performed in each branch separately. If selective branch embolization is performed the goal is to partially ablate parenchyma supplied by all of the branches. We feel it is safer to embolize in a stepwise fashion during the procedure, doing relatively frequent angiographic checks of the amount of remaining parenchyma, in order to avoid ablating too much splenic parenchyma thereby increasing the risk of complications.

Once approximately 60% of the splenic tissue is ablated the procedure can be terminated. This is an estimation judged visually by the interventional radiologist. In order to make comparison between runs easier, the same volume of contrast, injection rate, and imaging technique are used for all of the postembolization angiograms. It appears that thrombosis can progress after the embolization has been terminated so that the end result is a greater volume of tissue being ablated than seen at the termination of the procedure, which reinforces the need to do frequent interval angiograms and be conservative with embolization. As stated earlier, there is a recurrence rate of approximately 11%. If necessary the procedure can be repeated, often successfully, if not enough parenchyma has been ablated with the first procedure.

Postprocedure and follow-up care

Patients are usually admitted to the ICU following PSE in order to monitor and control the abdominal pain that patients experience after embolization and to monitor for potential complications. Postembolization syndrome is a self-limited process, which includes mild to moderate abdominal pain, fever, leukocytosis, nausea, and vomiting, and is frequently seen after embolization of solid organs. Postembolization syndrome usually lasts for one to five days, and patients are treated with fluids, antiemetics, antipyretics, and analgesics, until the symptoms subside. The pain can be significant enough to require the use of narcotic pain medication, and "splinting" of respiratory excursion by the patient can result in significant postprocedure atelectasis or pneumonia.

We usually ask for a Pain Service consultation prior to the procedure and at their recommendation PCA pumps can be used for pain control. Beginning pain control medications prospectively and tapering them to effect is much more successful than attempting to "catch up" to the pain once it is established. Some authors advocate the use of epidural anesthesia during and after the procedure for several days and believe that this not only contributes to patient comfort and acceptance, but also leads to a lower complication rate. Bedside spirometry can also encourage deeper respirations by the patient.

The immediate postembolization period is also accompanied by an abrupt rise in WBC count, which is most likely due to the acute inflammatory reaction, with possibly a small contribution from decreased splenic capture of white cells. It can be difficult to differentiate this abrupt but transient period of reactive leukocytosis from that related to an infectious complication, especially when fever is present. Fortunately, in most cases of postembolization syndrome the temperatures usually remain below 38.5°C and the leukocytosis and left shift are not as high as would be expected if there were a splenic abscess. Very careful monitoring of the patient's clinical status is important and blood cultures are warranted if any suspicion of sepsis or splenic abscess arises. Patients continue to receive the IV antibiotics, started prior to the procedure, for at least five days after the procedure.

If the patient is stable, afebrile, and taking oral fluids, they can be discharged from the ICU to the floor, where they are observed for another one to five days prior to discharge. Some people recommend a postembolization nuclear medicine liver–spleen scan prior to discharge to evaluate the amount of residual functioning splenic tissue. If Howell–Jolly bodies are identified on blood smears in the postembolization period, it can be assumed that the spleen has been completely ablated. These children are functionally asplenic and at a higher risk for the formation of a splenic abscess. In these cases surgical removal of the spleen may be indicated.

Complications

Minor complications of this procedure, which include transient paralytic ileus, left pleural effusion, left basilar atelectasis, transient ascites, and sterile subdiaphragmatic fluid collection, are relatively frequent and predictable in the early postprocedure period. Major complications can be expected in 1 to 2.5% of cases and include splenic abscess, splenic rupture, sepsis, pancreatitis, and pneumonia. The combination of strict aseptic technique, prophylactic antibiotics, and careful postprocedure care with partial or sequential splenic embolization significantly decreases the risk of sepsis and splenic abscess formation. This is most likely due to the fact that PSE preserves enough of the splenic parenchyma to provide sufficient immunologic protection from encapsulated bacteria and preservation of the normal direction of blood flow in the splenic vein.

With TSE, when arterial flow is completely interrupted, flow in the splenic vein is reversed, potentially leading to contamination of the infarcted splenic parenchyma with bacteria from the gastrointestinal tract that can normally be present in the portal circulation. Any symptoms suggestive of infection in the postprocedure period should be rapidly and aggressively treated with IV antibiotics. Partial splenic embolization, like surgical splenectomy, may predispose the patient to splenic or portal vein thrombosis (see Figure 8.43) as a result of the almost immediate rise in platelet count combined with decreased splenic vein flow, as has been reported in TSE, although authors reporting on PSE have not cited this complication. We have not encountered this complication in children.

Chapter 6: Genitourinary interventions

Richard Towbin, Kevin M. Baskin and David Aria

History 298
Anatomic considerations 298
Interventional radiology and UPJ obstruction 300
Percutaneous renal biopsy 304
Introduction 304
Indications 304
Technique 304
Equipment 304
Patient preparation 304
Standard technique 304
Postprocedure and follow-up care 306
Complications 306
Conclusions 309
Percutaneous nephrostomy 309
Introduction 309
Indications 310
Technique 311
Equipment 311
Patient preparation 315
Standard technique 316
Access to the renal pelvis 316
Route planning 317
Catheter insertion 318
Postprocedure and follow-up care 318
Securing the catheter 318
Managing catheter exchanges and accidental dislodgment 319
Complications 319
Conclusions 320
Whitaker (pressure–flow) perfusion test 320
Introduction 320
Indications 321
Technique 321
Equipment 321

Patient preparation 321
Standard technique 321
Two-needle technique 322
One-needle technique 322
Perfusion measurement 323
Technical variations 323
Postprocedure and follow-up care 323
Technical problems and pitfalls 324
Complications 324
Conclusions 324
Percutaneous treatment of renal cysts 324
Introduction 324
Indications 325
Technique 325
Equipment 326
Patient preparation 327
Standard technique 327
Postprocedure and follow-up care 327
Complications 328
Conclusions 328
Tract dilation 328
Introduction 328
Indications 328
Technique 329
Equipment 329
Patient preparation 329
Standard technique 329
Complications 329
Conclusions 330
Percutaneous nephrolithotomy 330
Introduction 330
Indications 330

Pediatric Interventional Radiology, ed. Richard Towbin and Kevin M. Baskin. Published by Cambridge University Press. © Cambridge University Press 2015.

Technique 331
  Equipment 331
  Patient preparation 333
  Standard technique 333
  Technical variations 334
  Percutaneous management of caliceal diverticula 334
  Pelvic access with a large stone burden 334
  Postprocedure and follow-up care 335
Complications 335
Future advances 335
Conclusions 336

Balloon dilation of ureteral strictures 336
Introduction 336
Indications 336
Technique 337
  Equipment 337
  Patient preparation 337
  Standard technique 337
  Postprocedure and follow-up care 339
Complications 339
Conclusions 341

Ureteral stent insertion 341
Introduction 341
Indications 341
Technique 343
  Equipment 343
  Patient preparation 343
  Standard technique 343
  Postprocedure and follow-up care 345
Complications 347
Conclusions 348

Percutaneous endopyelotomy 348
Introduction 348
Indications 350
Technique 350
  Equipment 350
  Patient preparation 350
  Standard technique 350
  Technical variations 352
  Pediatric modifications 352
  "Stent first, hot knife" variation 354
  Postprocedure and follow-up care 354
Complications 354
Conclusions 355

History

Minimally invasive techniques are well suited for use in the child's urinary tract. As a result, the urinary tract was one of the initial systems to be treated using a percutaneous approach. In spite of the numerous percutaneous procedures that are currently available to diagnose and treat problems involving the urinary tract, it is this area of interventional practice that has grown the least in the past decade. The relatively limited involvement by interventional radiologists is likely due to a variety of factors including the preference of urologists to perform combined percutaneous and surgical procedures in the operating room.

As is the case in other systems, interventional procedures in the genitourinary system result in less pain, shorter hospital stays, and faster recovery than open surgical alternatives. In addition, in most hospitals there is a shorter time between request for and performance of the procedure with lower cost than open surgery. Despite these factors, referrals to the interventional service favor children with failed surgical procedures, after-hours procedures, or other difficult cases. A willingness to help with these cases often leads in time to more frequent referral of the many children who could benefit from image-guided therapy that are not currently being seen by the pediatric interventionalist for routine procedures.

Anatomic considerations

To successfully perform genitourinary procedures a fundamental understanding of the anatomy of the kidneys, including the peculiarities of renal vascular and morphologic anomalies and post-transplant relationships, is essential to maximize desirable outcomes while avoiding complications. While a complete review is beyond the scope of this text, the reader is encouraged to seek out some of the excellent texts and monographs that focus on this material.

With their long axis aligned with the psoas muscles, the kidneys are normally located between T12 and L2 to L3, although with ectopia they may be positioned anywhere between the thorax and the pelvis in the retroperitoneum. Their lateral borders are normally rotated 30 degrees posterior to the frontal plane. Kidneys may be malrotated, fused (horseshoe kidney), duplicated, ectopic (crossed-fused renal ectopia), dysplastic, or unilaterally absent (agenesis). Renal anomalies, surgical interventions (e.g., transplantation), or disease states (e.g., hydronephrosis) may substantially alter normal position or relationships. The patient's medical record, including prior imaging, should be consulted to clarify the anatomy of the individual patient. Additional imaging may be required to address specific issues at or before the time of the planned intervention.

The interventionalist should be mindful of the normal relationships of the kidneys when planning access and evaluating potential complications. From a posterior approach, the kidney is covered at its upper pole by the hemidiaphragm and pleurae. Below the twelfth rib, the quadratus lumborum muscle may extend almost to the lateral border of the kidney, and carries portions of the subcostal, iliohypogastric, and ilioinguinal nerves. From the more usual posterolateral approach, the transversus abdominis muscle covers the kidney. Although the liver, duodenum, and ascending colon normally lie anterior to the right kidney, any of these structures may be at risk during renal access procedures if they happen to lie more lateral or even posterior to the kidney. Similarly, the spleen, jejunum, and descending colon are subject to inadvertent injury if they lie in the trajectory of access to the left kidney. In the event the renal pelvis is perforated, incursion into the peritoneal and anterior pararenal spaces places their contents, such as the stomach and pancreatic tail, at risk for injury. Large volumes of fluid may extravasate into these compartments, and may result in significant fluid and electrolyte shifts.

While the kidneys exhibit little lateral mobility within the renal fascia, even the small amount of mobility may be enough to create challenges for a successful percutaneous renal procedure, as anyone can attest who has watched in vain as the kidney has moved away from a biopsy or access needle. Renal mobility, compounded by the resistance of the tough capsule, is particularly great in neonates and renal transplant patients, and must be considered prior to any renal intervention. The kidneys also move extensively with the diaphragm, superiorly in expiration and inferiorly with inspiration. Bolsters and body position, manipulation by the hand of the interventionalist, and respiratory control by the anesthesiologist can help stabilize the organ and bring it into a more favorable position when needed.

The renal pelvis is highly variable in its relationship to the hilum of the kidney. The pelvis may be almost completely buried within the hilum, or may protrude to such a great degree that even portions of the major calices are extrarenal. Such variation may affect the space available for and the angles that must be negotiated by instrumentation (i.e., for the manipulation of wires, sheaths, dilators, and scopes) as well as the accessibility of pelvic stones.

Contained in its tough fibrous capsule, the kidney (Figure 6.1) is normally well cushioned in perirenal fat. The increased (in obese children) or decreased (in asthenic children, neonates, and young children) abundance of this fat may affect periprocedural imaging, degrading US image quality in the former case and CT tissue differentiation in the latter. The conically shaped renal (Gerota's) fascia limits the perirenal space. The base of Gerota's fascia blends into the diaphragmatic fascia, and its apex is relatively open as it follows the ureter into the pelvis. While the anterior pararenal space is open across the midline, medial fusion of Gerota's fascia prevents extravasation to the contralateral side. Therefore blood, fluid, or pus that has extravasated tends first to distend the renal fascia, then to track inferiorly into the pelvis.

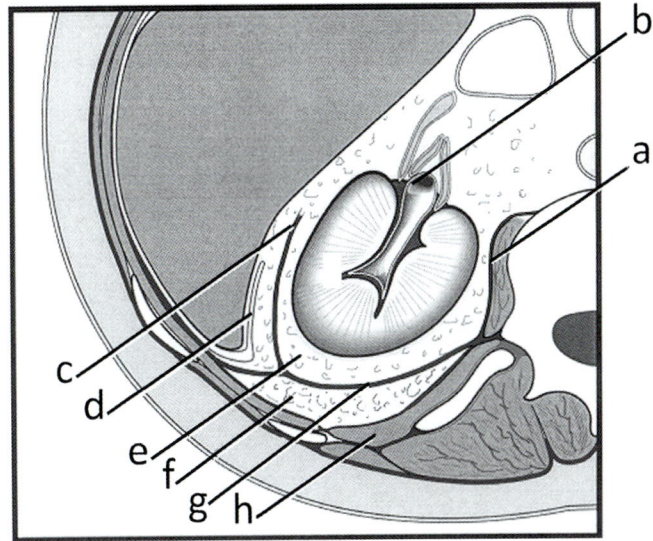

Figure 6.1 The kidney is contained in a tough, fibrous capsule. The relationships of the renal fossa and surrounding structures are illustrated. (a) psoas fascia, (b) renal hilum, (c) renal fascia (anterior layer), (d) peritoneum, (e) perirenal fat, (f) pararenal fat, (g) renal fascia (posterior layer), (h) quadratus lumborum muscle and fascia (anterior layer of thoracolumbar fascia).

Multiple renal arteries are seen in 30% of cases. When multiple renal arteries are present, there is usually a main renal artery arising normally from the aorta at the level of L1 or L2. Before reaching the hilum the main renal artery divides into anterior and posterior branches. Segmental branches of the anterior division supply anterior and polar regions of the kidney. In most cases, the posterior segmental artery is located on the posterior surface of the kidney in its middle to upper half, and supplies the remaining portion of the posterior kidney. The posterior segmental branch is particularly at risk during posterior puncture of an upper pole calyx or infundibulum medial to Brödel's line of relative avascularity.

Normal segmental vessels (or rarely, accessory or aberrant vessels) frequently cross the ureteropelvic junction (UPJ) as they course to the kidney to supply the lower pole. Specific surgical interventions were directed at these "crossing vessels" in the 1950s and 1960s, when they were considered primary candidates in the etiology of UPJ obstruction. It now appears that the likely cause of UPJ obstruction is often a dysplastic, aperistaltic segment of upper ureter, which may either happen to coexist with a crossing vessel or predispose to obstruction at that point. Because crossing vessels supply as much as 50% of the renal parenchyma, sectioning these vessels at surgery or injuring them at endopyelotomy may be a significant source of complication (e.g., new-onset hypertension or hemorrhage) or procedural failure. On the other hand, there has been no conclusive evidence yet shown that crossing vessels should be a contraindication to endourologic interventions for UPJ obstruction. If needed, CT angiography is a useful method for identifying crossing vessels, although we do not advocate this as a necessary part of preprocedural preparation at this time.

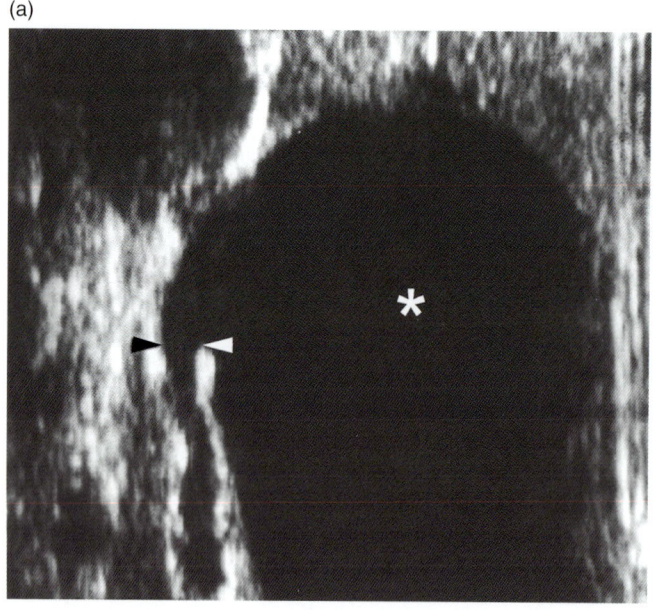
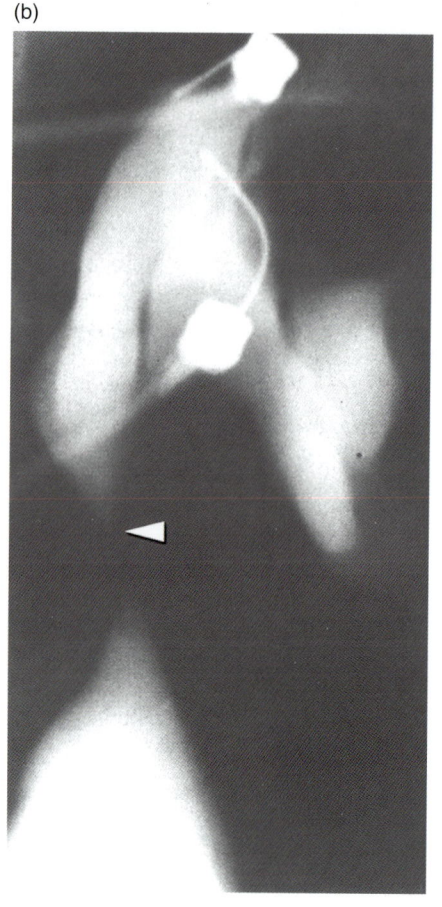
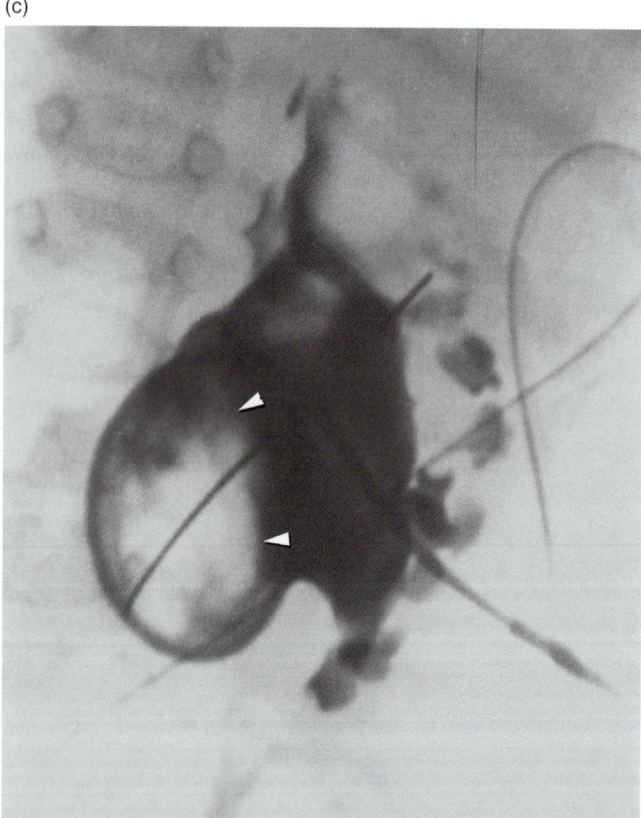

Figure 6.2 (a) A longitudinal US view using a linear transducer shows the transition point (*arrowheads*) between the grossly dilated renal pelvis (*asterisk*) and the narrowed ureter in this newborn infant with UPJ obstruction. This image illustrates the difficulty often encountered during attempts to obtain antegrade access across the UPJ obstruction, trying to go from a large cavity to a small caliber tube. On the other hand, retrograde access (e.g., via cystoscopy) in this patient would likely be effortless. (b) A fluoroscopic image obtained during provocative Whitaker testing in the same patient shows contrast medium administered at a rate of 10 ml/min through one needle into the renal pelvis. Abnormally elevated intrapelvic pressure (>35 cm H_2O) was recorded through the other needle. The fixed high-grade obstruction (*arrowhead*) characteristic of congenital UPJ obstruction is also seen in this image. (c) Initial needle access and subsequent guide wire manipulation can be impaired by retained material within the collecting system, whether by a stone or stones, hematoma, inspissated mucoid material, or as in this case by a fungus ball (*arrowheads*).

Interventional radiology and UPJ obstruction

Accurate etiologic diagnosis of UPJ obstruction, relation of apparent hydronephrosis to long-term functional impairment, and selection of an appropriate intervention remain difficult clinical problems. Compounding this difficulty is the substantial differences in prognosis after interventions in children with congenital (Figure 6.2) versus acquired (Figure 6.3) UPJ obstruction. Patients with UPJ obstruction classically present with infection (UTI is the presenting symptom in 30% of children beyond the neonatal period), pain, calculus, and hematuria, but may be identified during investigation for abdominal mass (Figure 6.4) or anomalies with a strong renal association (e.g., VACTERL). Once UPJ obstruction is diagnosed, prompt treatment is important. Without treatment, high intrapelvic pressure, intrarenal shunting, and urine stasis

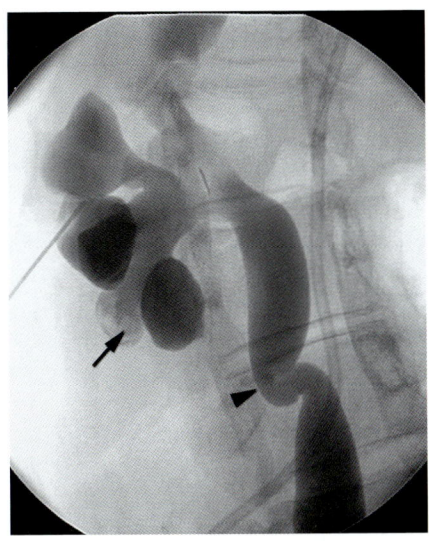

Figure 6.3 This 16-year-old girl had an open pyeloplasty performed in infancy for congenital UPJ obstruction. She now presents with caliectasis, tortuous ureter, and renal calculi (*arrow*) due to a secondary UVJ obstruction (*arrowhead*). Such acquired obstructions are often readily treated by endourologic means, with a high rate of success.

lead to progressive renal injury, deterioration in renal function, pain, increased risk of infection, development of renal calculi, and hypertension. Infection may accelerate renal injury due to obstruction, and suspicion that the two coexist should be regarded as an interventional emergency. Most renal units affected by UPJ obstruction will preserve function with treatment. Some may regain lost function.

Evaluation of UPJ obstruction for surgical intervention has historically been conducted radiologically with an intravenous urogram (IVU) or more recently by renal sonography. Today, it is more common to find hydronephrosis at antenatal ultrasonography or MRI. While upper urinary tract dilation is present in 1 of 100 pregnancies, only 20% of these represent clinically significant uropathy. With increasing frequency, the clinician must determine appropriate management for asymptomatic congenital hydronephrosis.

While hydronephrosis is not normal, it is also not synonymous with either functional obstruction or renal dysfunction in the long term. However, the implication that hydronephrosis will require surgical intervention has a significant impact on the patient and family, especially in the increasingly common situation where hydronephrosis is detected antenatally. The initial goal of medical imaging is to determine the anatomic site and functional significance of apparent obstruction. There are a number of diagnostic studies for qualitative assessment of obstructive symptoms, such as ultrasound (US), computed tomography (CT), magnetic resonance imaging (MRI), and intravenous urography (IVU), as well as for quantitative analysis of apparent obstruction, including drainage half-time by diuretic renography, resistive indices by US, and measurement of pressure–flow relationships during antegrade nephrostomy infusion (see "Whitaker (pressure–flow) perfusion test," below). Although, like any diagnostic study, each has potential sources of error or misinterpretation, used rationally these tests will yield a correct diagnosis in more than 90% of cases.

Once the diagnosis of UPJ obstruction is made, several factors influence the likely outcome of corrective interventions, including age, primary or secondary obstruction, degree of hydronephrosis, presence of a crossing vessel, and overall and differential renal function. Even though UPJ obstruction is most often congenital, diagnosis clusters around the perinatal period (predominantly due to antenatal detection) and later in life (predominantly due to symptomatic presentation). In other words, neonatal presentation tends to be asymptomatic, and the challenge is to prove that the abnormality has a functional consequence.

Although hydronephrosis in some newborns may have a different natural history from that occurring in older children and adults, intervention for all groups is unequivocally indicated when UPJ obstruction is definitively proven, or when renal function is compromised by involvement of a solitary kidney or by bilateral involvement. Secondary obstruction following open pyeloplasty should probably be treated by endourologic means in all age groups. Due to the increased risk of injury, exposure to ionizing radiation (fluoroscopy), and potential need for multiple procedures under general anesthesia, endourologic interventions for other indications may best be reserved for treatment of older children and adults, especially at facilities with less experience performing interventions in the younger age groups. Neonates and infants should be treated at centers where neonatal caregivers and interventionalists experienced with neonatal procedures are available. The goals of therapeutic intervention include improvement in hydronephrosis and stabilization or improvement in function of the affected renal unit. Open surgical pyeloplasty, although more invasive and requiring more extensive recovery than endourologic alternatives, has an 85% to 98% record of success and remains the gold standard against which alternative interventions must be measured.

While endourologic treatment of preadolescents with UPJ obstruction remains somewhat controversial, we feel it is a reasonable approach if renal function is preserved, hydronephrosis is mild to moderate, and there is no evidence of crossing vessels. For adolescents and adults, endourologic intervention is widely accepted as first-line therapy given the same parameters. Secondary UPJ obstruction is known to respond well to endopyelotomy (EP), with even better results in children (91%) than adults (73%). As interventionalists gain experience, and patient selection gets better, response of primary UPJ obstruction to this approach continues to improve. Massive hydronephrosis (i.e., high-degree obstruction), especially with a concomitant crossing vessel, significantly decreases the success rate for EP.

The coexistence of lower pole crossing vessels with UPJ obstruction may be suggested by IVU, US, retrograde ureterography, or antegrade pyelography. Computed tomography angiography (CTA), magnetic resonance angiography (MRA), and endoluminal US are all sensitive methods for identifying crossing vessels (see "Anatomic considerations," above); however, currently there is no proven ability to predict which crossing vessels are a significant factor in obstruction, or which will impact the success of EP. In the treatment of secondary UPJ obstruction, CTA may indicate the safest place

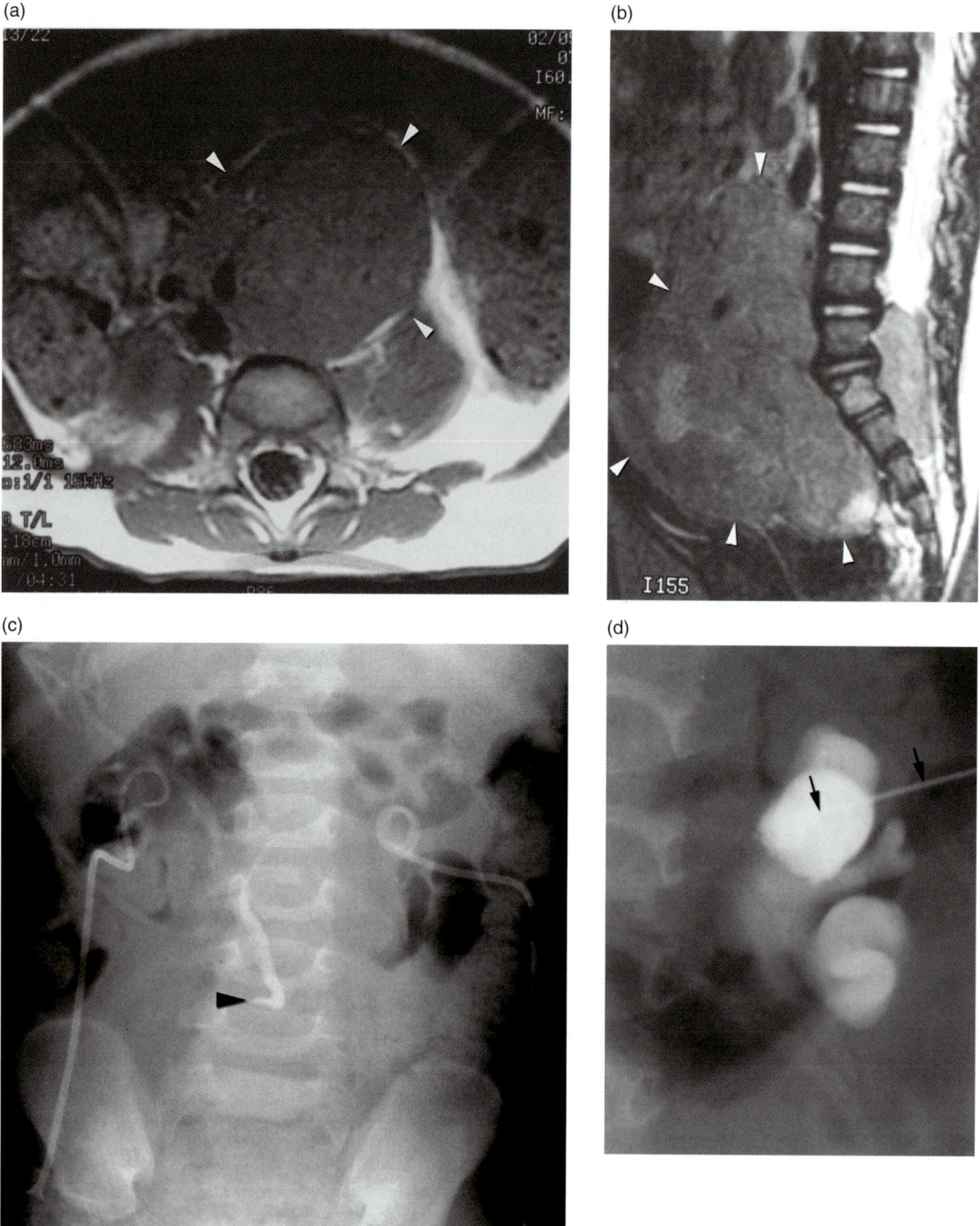

Figure 6.4 Four-year-old girl presenting with abdominal mass and bilateral hydronephrosis. Magnetic resonance imaging in the (a) axial and (b) sagittal planes shows a large abdominopelvic mass (*arrowheads*) with pre- and postsacral extension characteristic of neuroblastoma. (c) A preoperative pyelogram after insertion of bilateral percutaneous nephrostomy drainage tubes shows high-grade extrinsic mid-ureteral compression (*arrowhead*). (d) After a 21-gauge needle (*arrows*) was used to access a posterior calyx using US, dilute contrast material was injected to confirm tip location under fluoroscopy. (e) A stainless steel 0.018-inch mandril guide wire was coiled within the renal pelvis, assuring that the stiff portion of the wire (between *arrowheads*) was within the collecting system. (f) The needle is exchanged for a 4 French directional catheter (*arrowhead*) and the mandril wire is exchanged for a 0.035-inch guide wire (*arrow*). The catheter is gently advanced to the level of the obstruction, and is not advanced beyond the entry to the curve of the wire. (g) Dilute contrast medium is injected through the catheter (*arrow*) demonstrating the level of extrinsic compression (*arrowheads*) of the ureter. With the catheter tip wedged in the stricture origin, gentle probing with the directional guide wire may allow (as in this case) advancement of the catheter and wire across the stricture into the bladder. (h) With access across the narrowed ureter, an internal "double-J" stent (*arrowheads*) was deployed to relieve the obstruction. A temporary percutaneous nephrostomy drainage catheter (*arrow*) was left in place until antegrade drainage was confirmed.

Chapter 6 Genitourinary interventions

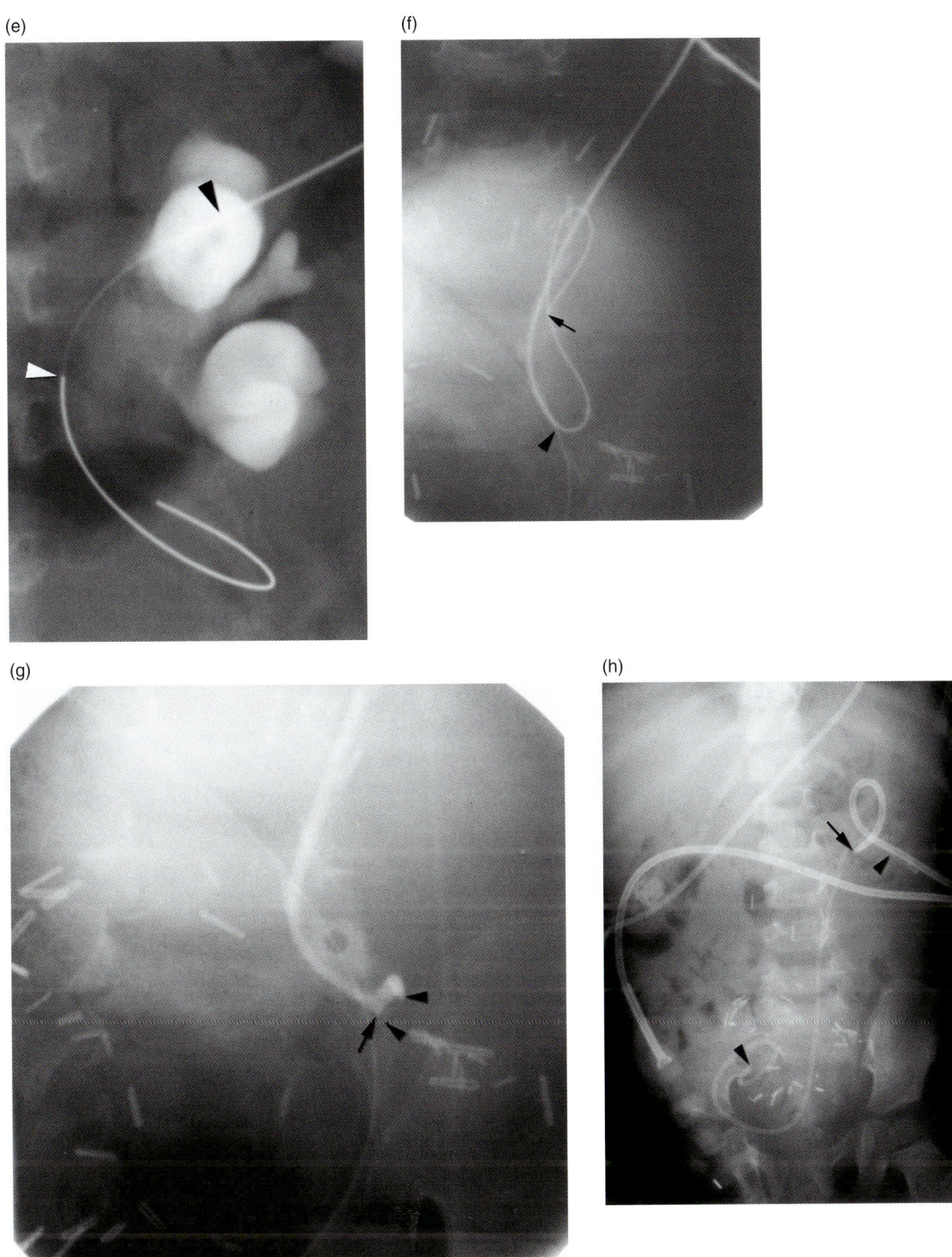

Figure 6.4 (cont.)

to make the endopyelotomy incision (usually posteromedially). Historically, infant patients with the poorest renal function preoperatively have had the greatest improvement in function following open pyeloplasty, differing from results in adults. Experience with EP in such infants is too limited to give a recommendation at this time. In rare cases where non-function of the involved renal unit is confirmed with radiographic and radionuclide studies, and non-salvageability is

303

confirmed following temporary relief of obstruction, nephrectomy may be the procedure of choice.

Percutaneous renal biopsy

Introduction

When tissue is required for the diagnosis or management of renal disease, a specimen may be obtained either by open surgery or with a needle percutaneously. In general, practitioners consider the percutaneous approach the initial procedure of choice in most cases. A percutaneous core biopsy of the kidney can be performed with or without image guidance. When image guidance is used real-time guidance, rather than marking a skin location for a blind biopsy, is the safest approach. Although all percutaneous approaches are currently considered acceptable, preference for the image-guided approach continues to grow because of the advantages of precision and safety. This section will discuss and illustrate a variety of real-time percutaneous approaches to renal biopsy.

Indications

A renal biopsy is performed in order to establish a histologic diagnosis, determine the prognosis, and clarify the therapeutic approach to a variety of renal disorders. In general, when there is a renal mass the biopsy is done using image guidance. However, when medical renal disease is suspected a biopsy may be performed with or without image guidance. Quality improvement guidelines recommend that image guidance is the key to maximize successful tissue acquisition and minimize untoward effects. In most clinical settings US guidance is all that is necessary. However, CT is an excellent alternative when it is needed in cases where a safe route cannot be visualized, for focal lesions conspicuous on CT but isoechoic on US, or in obese patients.

Technique

Equipment

There is no specialized equipment needed for a renal biopsy. The operator must decide if a biopsy guide will be used. If a guide is to be used then it needs to be fastened to the US transducer before the sterile probe cover is put on. Otherwise, all that is needed is a sterile preparation set, drape, scalpel with a #11 blade, and a biopsy needle (Table 6.1). Today, automated needles (see Figures 3.14 and 3.15) are used in most settings. It is our practice and recommendation that it is best to use the largest needle size appropriate for the size of the child and the lesion to be sampled. The needles used range in size from 14- to 18-gauge. In general, we suggest an 18-gauge needle with a 2 to 3 cm biopsy chamber for neonates and young children less than about 10 kg and any child with a greater than normal risk of bleeding. We find that a 22-gauge needle is less useful since the tissue samples obtained are often inadequate and the

Table 6.1 Equipment: renal biopsy

- Core needle
- Automated (1 or 2 cm throw), semi-automated or manual biopsy needles
- Removable core needles
- Biopsy guide for US transducer
- Sterile probe cover for transducer
- Scalpel with #11 blade
- Buffered local anesthetic
- Syringe (3 to 5 ml) with 27- to 30-gauge needle for local anesthetic
- Spinal needle (22 gauge) for deep infiltration of local anesthetic
- Formalin or sterile test tubes or containers for specimens

frequency of untoward effects is not significantly decreased compared with an 18-gauge needle. Larger children may have biopsies performed using a 16-gauge needle with a 2 to 3 cm biopsy chamber. The choice of needle size is generally based on operator preference in conjunction with pathology department needs.

One specimen may be sufficient for a parenchymal (cortical) biopsy related to a systemic disease process. The total number of specimens depends on the indication of the biopsy, the needs of the pathologist and other laboratory tests, and the quality of the sample obtained – these factors should be considered and appropriate discussions undertaken with the referring clinician and pathologist in advance of the planned procedure. We routinely get a minimum of two samples. Focal lesions are approached as in any solid organ biopsy. In order to reduce the risk for significant hemorrhage after biopsy we generally limit the maximum number of passes through one area to three, even if no tissue is obtained. Children with large renal masses (Figure 6.4) will routinely have the lesion sampled in two to four quadrants with 14- or 16-gauge needles to maximize the tissue samples for histologic examination and analysis for biological markers. The sample size will usually be discussed with the pathology service in advance to provide the specimens in the manner that is preferred.

Patient preparation

No special preparation is necessary for a renal biopsy. The procedure may be performed under sedation or general anesthesia depending on hospital/operator preference. The procedure may be performed under local anesthesia and intravenous sedation using US guidance or general anesthesia. The patient is kept NPO according to hospital anesthesia/sedation policy.

Standard technique

When a native kidney is biopsied, the child is positioned prone or with the side of the kidney to be biopsied elevated depending on the biopsy approach selected. For right-handed operators and depending upon the preferred approach, the left side is usually selected for convenience. A bolster under the abdomen may be helpful to stabilize the kidney in slender or young children. Prior to the biopsy, if cross-sectional imaging is not available, a diagnostic renal US is performed to assess *both* kidneys to exclude undiagnosed unilateral renal agenesis, to evaluate the size of the collecting systems and thickness of the cortex, and to identify renal masses or congenital anomalies, especially abnormal renal position. The procedure begins with US evaluation of the kidney to be biopsied and an entry site is marked on the skin surface with a permanent marker (Figure 6.5). Then the US probe is covered with a sterile probe cover.

Once the entry site is selected the area is prepared and draped in sterile fashion. Biopsies under intravenous sedation require local anesthetic. Procedures performed under general anesthesia do not require local anesthetic but it may be preferred for postprocedural pain control. Lidocaine 1% is infiltrated into the skin using a 30-gauge × 1.5-inch needle. A cutaneous wheal is first raised with the anesthetic, after which the remainder of the tract to the level of Gerota's fascia may be infiltrated using a 22-gauge spinal needle. Ultrasound guidance may be used to assist in the delivery of local anesthesia. The needle used for infiltration of anesthetic may also be left in place as a "tandem needle" guide to assist selection of an entry point and angle of entry with the biopsy needle (Figure 6.6). This will minimize discomfort and motion during the biopsy, as well as allow for familiarization with the desired trajectory. The biopsy is carried out using real-time US guidance using either a freehand technique or a biopsy guide. When the freehand technique is selected the probe may be positioned either posteriorly, adjacent to the needle, or on the side (see Figure 1.1). All of these approaches have been extensively utilized with successful outcomes. Regardless of the approach selected it is important to visualize the needle throughout its entire course to maximize the chance for a successful biopsy while minimizing the chance of complications (Figure 6.7).

Most parenchymal biopsies of native kidneys are obtained from the lower pole cortex of the left kidney. If possible, it is preferable to have a pathologist present or readily available to receive the specimen and confirm its adequacy. Working as a team will help keep the number of passes and procedural time to a minimum. When performing a biopsy on a transplant kidney it is especially important to understand the kidney's position in the lower abdomen and pelvis. The interventionalist's hand may be used to stabilize the more freely mobile transplant kidney during the biopsy. In these cases one may prefer to obtain a specimen from the upper pole. Since with

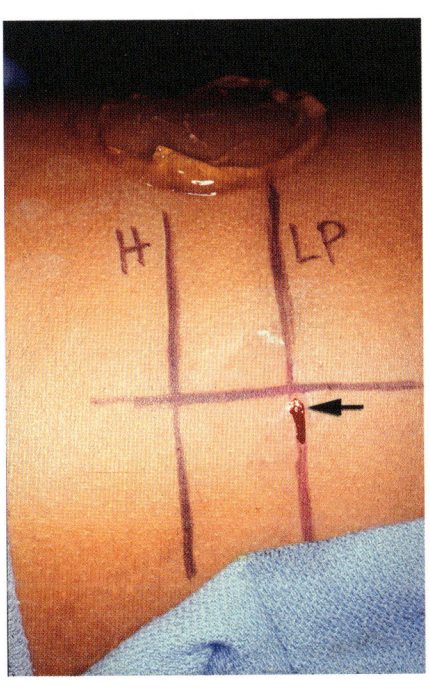

Figure 6.5 In this photograph, the patient is positioned right-side down (decubitus) with the head to the left. To obtain a core needle biopsy of renal cortex, the level of the renal hilum ("H") and lower pole cortex ("LP") were marked on the skin under US guidance with the linear transducer positioned as shown in Figure 6.7. The entry point (*arrow*) was selected in the mid-scapular line and specimens obtained using real-time US guidance.

(a)

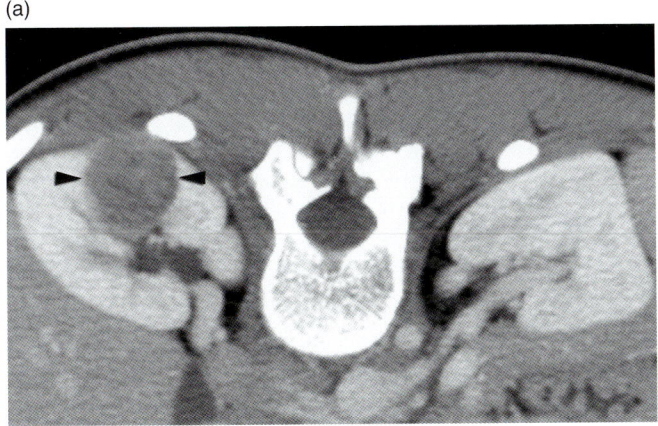

(b)

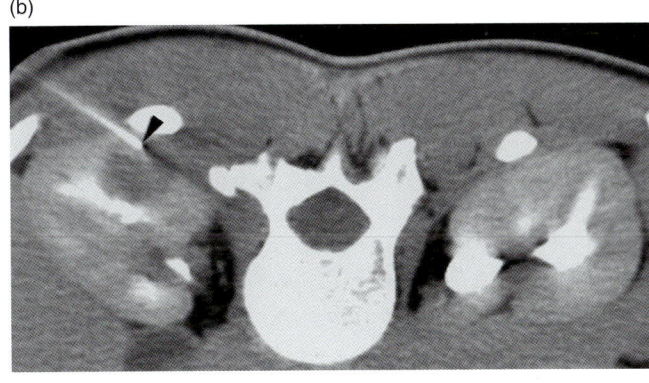

Figure 6.6 (a) Axial CT image with intravenous contrast enhancement through the hilum of the right kidney in an 18-year-old female who presented with a 3 cm × 2.5 cm × 2 cm poorly enhancing mass (*arrowheads*) in the posterior midpole. (b) With intravenous sedation, a 22-gauge Chiba needle (*arrowhead*) was used to deliver local anesthetic to the level of Gerota's fascia, then advanced to a depth of 4 cm to serve as a tandem needle guide and "guard rail". Three core specimens were then obtained from different areas within the mass with a 16-gauge automated biopsy device under CT guidance.

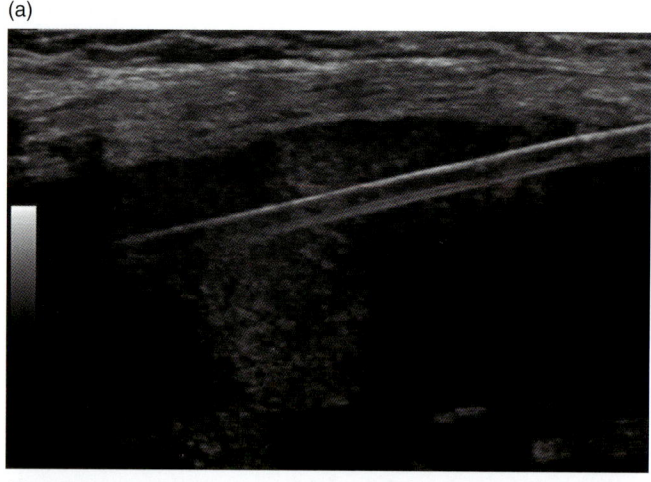
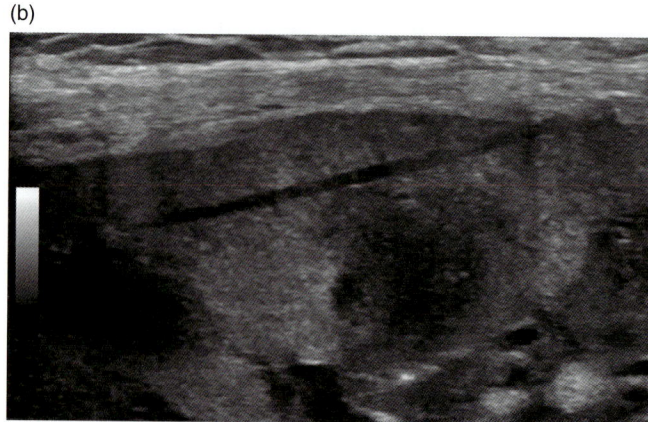
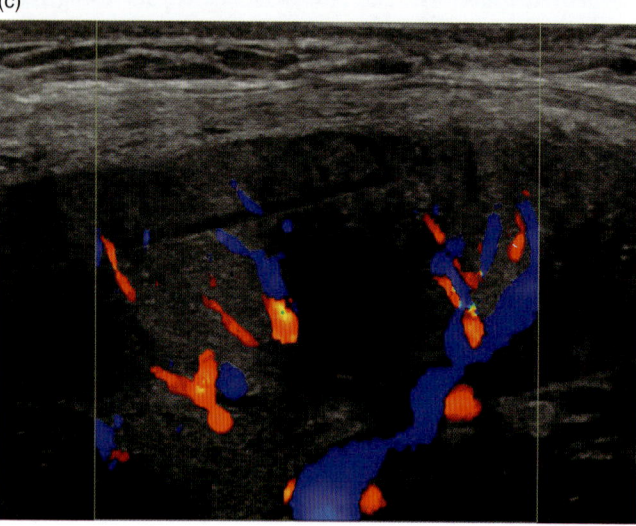

Figure 6.7 (a) A nine-year-old renal transplant recipient presents for biopsy of the renal graft. Under US guidance, a single 3.3 cm specimen is obtained from the cortex with an automated end-cutting core needle. (b) After the specimen is removed, the tissue defect is evident in the cortex. (c) Color Doppler imaging demonstrates no evidence of bleeding.

transplanted kidneys the main concerns are rejection, post-transplant lymphoproliferative disease (PTLD), and infection, a small tissue sample (i.e., 18-gauge) may suffice. However, if a lesion is larger than 2 to 3 mm, is not round, or exerts mass effect, a neoplasm should be considered (Figure 6.8). Immune-suppressed children may have a tumor secondary to transformation of PTLD or another primary tumor. In these cases it might be prudent to obtain more tissue. Be sure to discuss the diagnostic needs with the pathologist in advance since it may be necessary to split the specimen in sterile fashion at the time of the procedure to send part to pathology and part to microbiology. Regardless of the position of the kidney it is important to make certain that the selected biopsy site is not near the renal hilum, reducing the risk for severe hemorrhage or renal loss.

Postprocedure and follow-up care

Traditionally, care for patients after biopsy has consisted of bed rest, analgesia as needed, and 12 to 24 hours of observation including frequent monitoring of vital signs and urine for blood. Several studies have evaluated shorter periods of observation for patient convenience and cost. It has been demonstrated that approximately 98% of all complications were detected by 24 hours. However, only 46% of major complications were identified by four hours and 79% by eight hours after the procedure. By 12 hours all patients with major complications were known but 5% of patients with minor problems (Figure 6.9) were still not identified. However, we have found that patients who have a post-biopsy US that shows no significant bleeding or other complication, are asymptomatic, live nearby, and do not have gross hematuria by four hours after biopsy can be safely discharged to home, with clear instructions regarding when to return, confirmed contact information, and a mandatory follow-up phone call within 24 hours. For patients that do not meet these criteria, it is prudent to observe for signs or symptoms of biopsy-related complications for a minimum of 12 hours.

Complications

Although US-guided biopsy has improved the yield and safety of percutaneous renal biopsy there continues to be a high rate

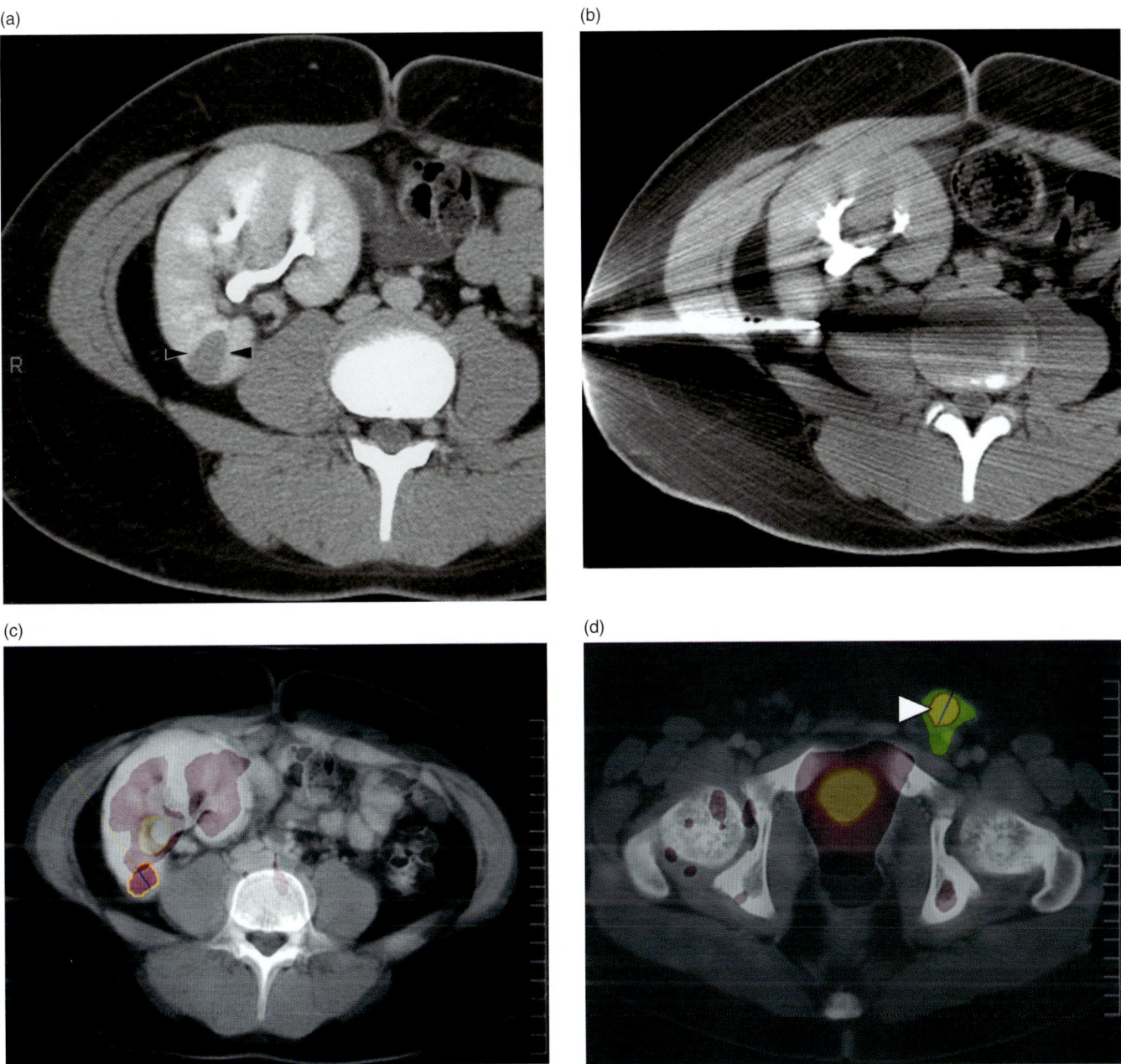

Figure 6.8 (a) An axial CT section obtained with intravenous contrast enhancement in a 14-year-old boy with a history of abdominal pain shows a new poorly enhancing pyramidal-shaped, cortical lesion (*arrowheads*) in the pelvic transplant kidney that exerts local mass effect. (b) Several core specimens obtained with a 16-gauge automated biopsy device under CT guidance resulted in the unusual diagnosis of renal cell carcinoma, undiagnosed from the donor. (c) 18-F FDG PET-CT fusion imaging obtained near the time of biopsy is shown here in the axial plane through the area corresponding to the location of the biopsied lesion (circled in yellow). There is abnormal uptake, but it is poorly distinguishable from physiologic radiotracer accumulation in the renal collecting system. (d) A PET-CT fusion performed in the same patient demonstrated much higher 18-F FDG uptake (*arrowhead*) in a left inguinal node, offering a potentially safer target for biopsy.

of complication. The literature contains experience in both adults and children, and the types and rates of complications are similar in both groups. Complication rates in reported series may vary substantially; however, clinically observable minor and major complications (Table 6.2) are observed following approximately 6 to 8% of all renal biopsies. This differs from the demonstration of asymptomatic bleeding that may be identified by imaging in up to 85% of cases. Notably, the rate of major complications is significantly lower after biopsies performed with real-time US guidance by experienced interventionalists compared to unguided biopsy with or without US marking. The use of a freehand technique for real-time US guidance is also associated with a very low rate of severe complications.

Bleeding complications are the most common after a renal biopsy. Almost all patients will have microscopic hematuria.

However, macroscopic hematuria can be expected to occur in about 6 to 8% of biopsies, and may be more prevalent after biopsy of adult-sized renal transplants in children. Care must be taken to evaluate the renal unit after biopsy for acute evidence of complication, and to monitor the patient expectantly for signs of subacute complication in the hours after biopsy (Figure 6.10). Other untoward effects include hematoma within the renal parenchymal, perinephric and retroperitoneal spaces (Figure 6.11), as well as lumbar artery aneurysms and iatrogenic arteriovenous fistulae (Figure 6.12). As is true with any biopsy, failure to obtain adequate or representative tissue is always a possibility (Figure 6.13). Although in general, diagnostic yield from percutaneous biopsies is in the range of 90 to 95%, some cases will not yield diagnostic tissue despite careful preparation and meticulous technique. Integration of evolving imaging technology with interventional techniques may help improve diagnostic yields and more effectively direct biopsy procedures in the future (Figure 6.8).

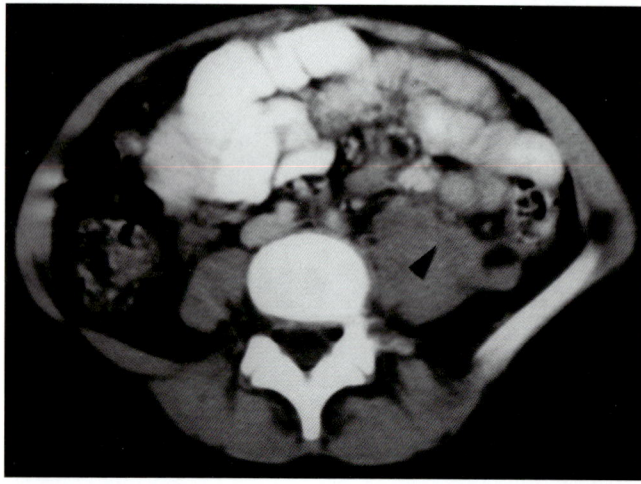

Figure 6.9 Axial CT imaging with IV contrast shows a psoas hemorrhage (*arrowhead*) after ipsilateral renal biopsy performed with image guidance. The patient complained of increasing back pain requiring IV narcotics for control approximately 12 hours after the procedure. The hemorrhage was self-limited without evidence of hypovolemia or anemia.

Table 6.2 Potential complications of renal biopsy

Minor complications
- Gross hematuria without clinical sequela
- Hematoma or perinephric hematoma not requiring intervention
- Inadvertent biopsy of the liver or other organ

Major complications
- Clinically significant hemorrhage requiring transfusion or other intervention
- Hematoma with renal compression
- Urinary outflow obstruction
- Arteriovenous fistula or pseudoaneurysm formation
- Injury to non-target organ
- Infection requiring hospitalization or specific therapy
- Peritonitis
- Pneumothorax requiring intervention

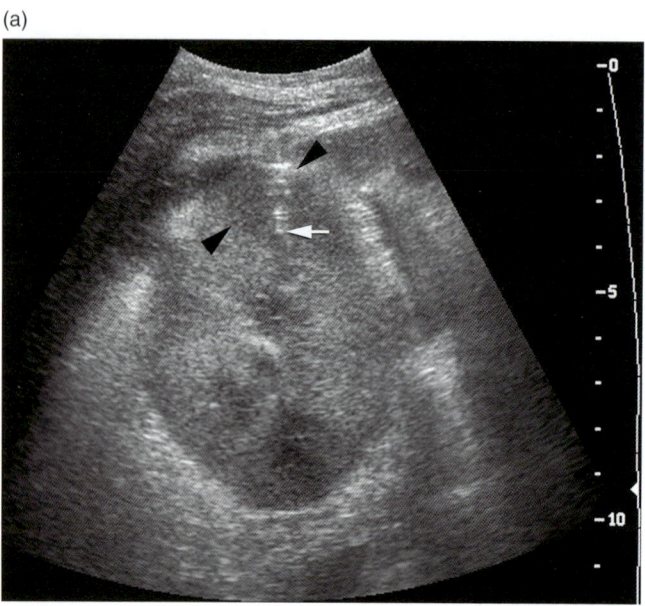
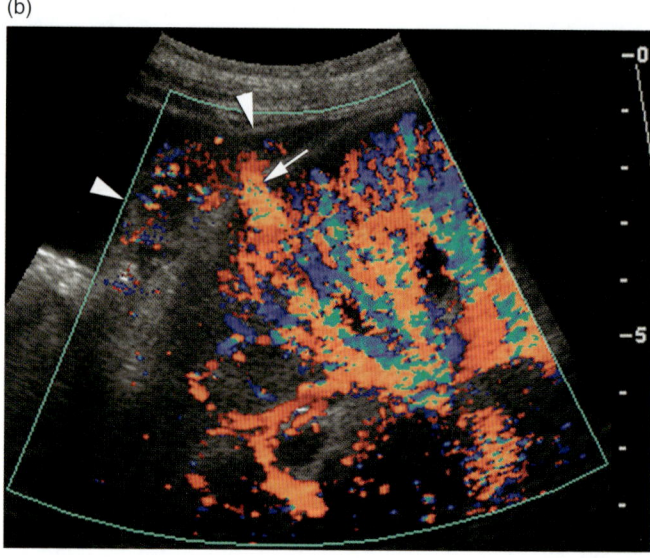

Figure 6.10 (a) A 13-year-old boy with focal sclerosing glomerular nephrosis developed fever and flank pain following renal transplantation. With the 7 to 4 MHz curvilinear transducer in a transaxial orientation, a transverse approach was used to obtain two core samples from the round cortical hypoechoic lesion (*arrowheads*) using a 14-gauge automated biopsy needle (*arrow*). (b) Immediately after the core biopsy procedure, the biopsy site was evaluated with color Doppler US in a longitudinal plane. This demonstrated active extravasation in the biopsy tract (*arrow*) with increasing subcapsular hematoma (*arrowheads*). The patient experienced persistent pain and progressive anemia requiring transfusion two days after the procedure. In similar cases direct compression with the transducer can be used to achieve cessation of transcortical color flow for five to ten minutes, usually resulting in hemostasis.

Chapter 6 Genitourinary interventions

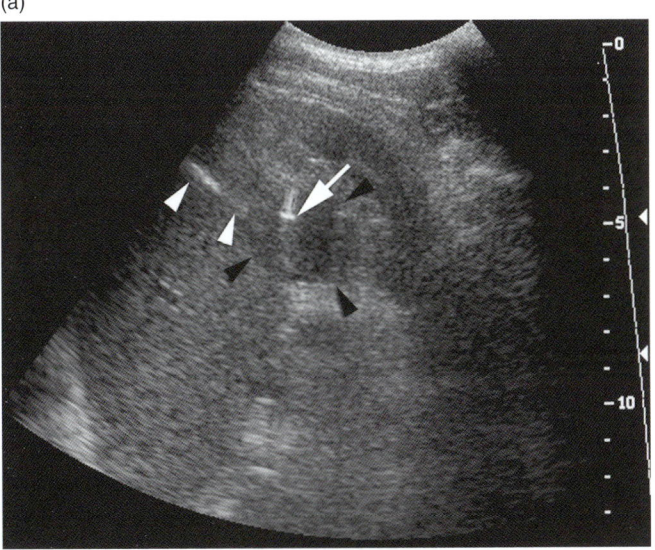
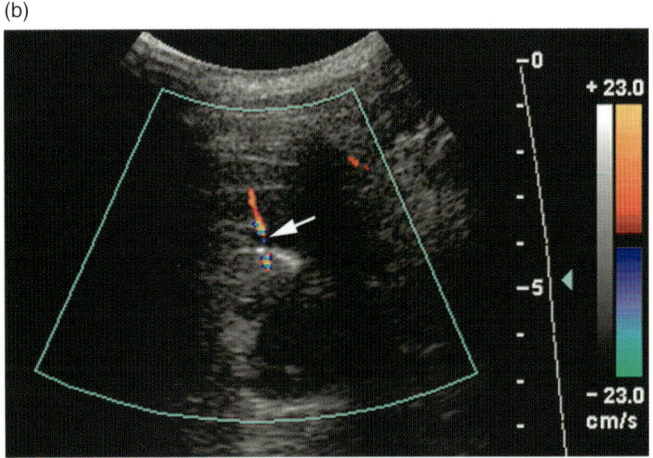
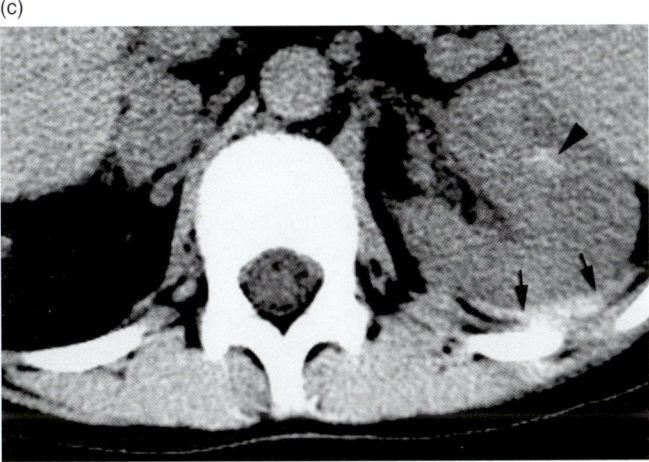

Figure 6.11 (a) A poorly compliant 18-year-old liver transplant patient with immunosuppression-induced diabetes presented with multiple abscesses. The complex mass (*black arrowheads*) in the lower pole of the left kidney was sampled using a 5 to 2 MHz curvilinear US transducer and a 21-gauge Chiba needle. The needle shaft (*white arrowheads*) and tip artifact (*arrow*) are well visualized. Aspiration produced a small amount of frank pus. A single 18-gauge core biopsy specimen was culture-positive for *Staphylococcus aureus*. (b) Color Doppler imaging obtained through the biopsy site immediately after the procedure shows a jet of extravascular blood flow (*arrow*). (c) Axial CT image with IV contrast obtained 12 hours after the biopsy shows a hematoma (*arrowhead*) within the renal parenchyma as well as a large retroperitoneal hematoma (*arrows*). The patient required a transfusion two days after the procedure.

Conclusions

Percutaneous renal biopsy is most safely achieved under US guidance in most cases. For routine parenchymal biopsies a single core specimen from the cortex is usually sufficient. Biopsy of focal lesions in the kidney is performed as any solid-organ biopsy. Hematuria is common following renal biopsy but usually clinically insignificant, although the patient should be monitored for signs of persistent bleeding or hypovolemic shock. Severe complications are uncommon. Postprocedure US surveillance and appropriate observation will identify virtually all early complications. Late complications are usually related to vascular injury, and can often be managed using interventional techniques, such as embolization of arteriovenous fistulae.

Percutaneous nephrostomy

Introduction

Percutaneous nephrostomy is one of the most frequently performed interventions for treatment of urinary tract disease and

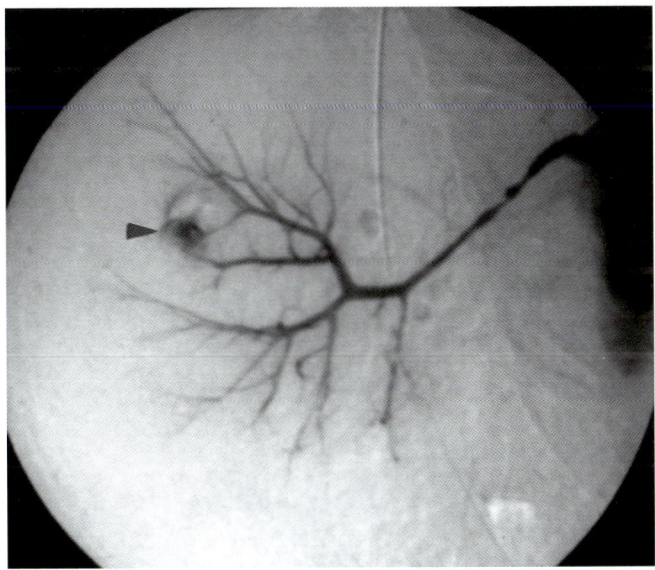

Figure 6.12 Abnormal parenchymal staining (*arrowhead*) with early venous filling is seen during this selective right renal arteriogram, characteristic of an iatrogenic arteriovenous fistula. The patient had a history of recent percutaneous renal biopsy without imaging guidance.

309

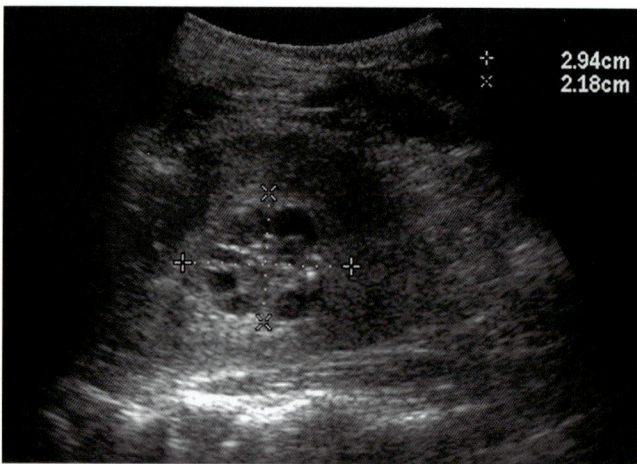

Figure 6.13 A complex cystic mass was noted in the hilum of the left kidney in this five-and-a-half-year-old boy with Henoch–Schönlein purpura-related nephritis. Under US guidance with a 7 to 4 MHz curvilinear transducer, several 16-gauge core biopsy specimens were obtained. Results were non-diagnostic, although open surgical wedge biopsy showed multicystic nephroma.

Table 6.3 Indications: percutaneous nephrostomy

- Relief of obstruction with renal insufficiency (native or transplanted kidneys)
- Drainage of pyonephrosis
- Whitaker test or antegrade pyelogram
- Drug instillation (e.g., antifungal administration)
- Treatment of renal or peri-renal collections
- Treatment of urinary tract leaks (urinary diversion)
- Access for other percutaneous endourologic procedures

is the core procedure for the development and performance of most complex interventional genitourinary procedures. The technique was first employed by Goodwin and associates in 1955 using a trochar needle for the treatment of hydronephrosis. In 1965, the translumbar catheter nephrostomy gained popularity after a report by Bartley and colleagues. In 1976, the first percutaneous stone removal was performed and eight years later endourologic technology was further extended when Clayman and colleagues showed that electrosurgical instruments could be safely used in the urinary tract. The development of these complex percutaneous endourologic techniques was made possible by the development of equipment such as progressive dilators and sheaths, the angioplasty balloon, stents, and the introduction of techniques and equipment borrowed from other specialties. These advances have led to better patient care and a closer working relationship between the nephrologist, urologist, pediatric surgeon, transplant surgeon, and pediatric interventionalist. In many instances these collaborations have led to a reduced need for open surgical procedures.

In numerous series, percutaneous nephrostomy has been successful in over 97% of pediatric patients ranging in age from one day to 18 years of age. These results compare favorably with surgical management. In most series, percutaneous nephrostomy has been performed with the entry site locally anesthetized and the child sedated with intravenous drugs.

Indications

There are several indications for placement of a nephrostomy tube in the pediatric population (Table 6.3). However, the most common indication for percutaneous nephrostomy is for relief of symptomatic urinary tract obstruction with or without renal insufficiency and pyonephrosis. The most frequent causes of ureteral obstruction were congenital ureteropelvic junction (UPJ) narrowing (Figure 6.14) and obstruction after ureteral re-implantation (Figure 6.15).

The benefits of percutaneous nephrostomy are rapidly evident in most patients and are due to improved renal function and control of infection with prompt defervescence and symptomatic improvement. Elective performance of definitive therapy can then be scheduled when necessary. Other indications for percutaneous nephrostomy include assessment of renal function (Figure 6.16), demonstration of pathologic anatomy, and differentiation between obstructed and non-obstructed dilated systems using a pressure flow study (see "Whitaker (pressure–flow) perfusion test," below).

In patients with a distended, tortuous urine-filled system, it may be difficult to demonstrate the level of obstruction at the time of initial drainage. In addition, injection of contrast may lead to bacteremia and urosepsis. Therefore in obstructed systems it may be prudent to perform a nephrostogram after the system has been decompressed and the urine sterilized. In the rare instances of obstruction caused by a fungus ball (Figures 6.2, 6.17) percutaneous nephrostomy combined with infusion of chemotherapy (e.g., amphotericin or fluconazole) has been successful.

In asymptomatic children with hydronephrosis, antegrade pyelography may be performed prior to surgical or endourologic correction to document the level and nature of the obstruction. In the child with an obstructed kidney and associated azotemia or pyonephrosis, percutaneous nephrostomy may lead to clinical improvement prior to correction of the underlying pathology. In addition, percutaneous decompression of the obstruction allows time for improvement in renal function, treatment of urinary sepsis, and a more accurate assessment of the renal unit. In some cases, such as in children with postoperative ureteral injury, leak, or obstruction from extrinsic compression or calculi, percutaneous nephrostomy may be the only intervention required. Finally, percutaneous nephrostomy may be the initial procedure required to gain access for other percutaneous endourologic procedures. Examples of these include percutaneous stone removal, percutaneous endopyelotomy, and percutaneous stricture dilation and stenting.

Few contraindications limit the performance of a percutaneous nephrostomy in a child. The primary contraindications are an uncorrectable coagulopathy and unfavorable anatomy making percutaneous access impossible or dangerous. In practice these problems rarely occur. Severe electrolyte

Chapter 6 Genitourinary interventions

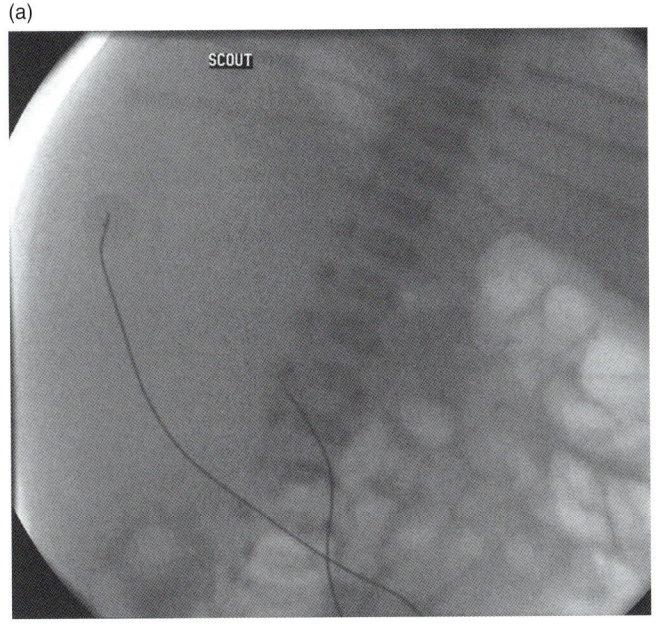

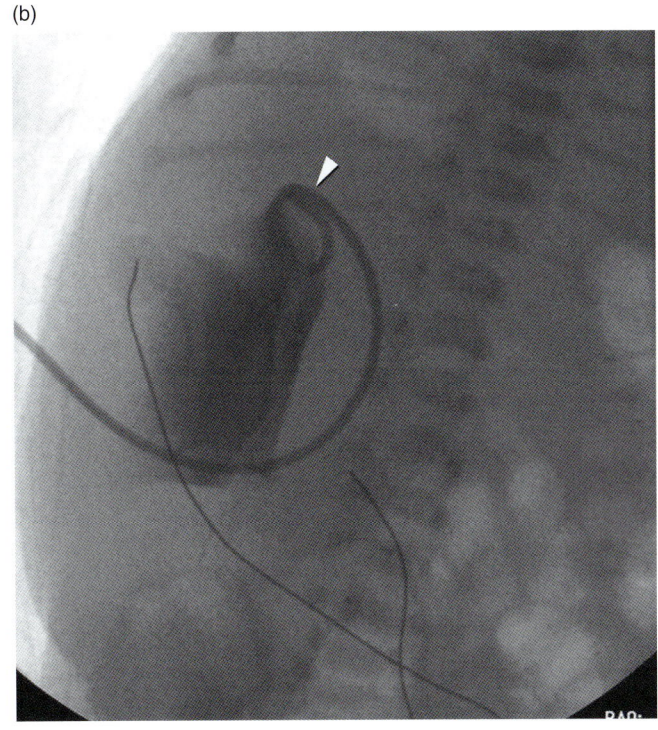

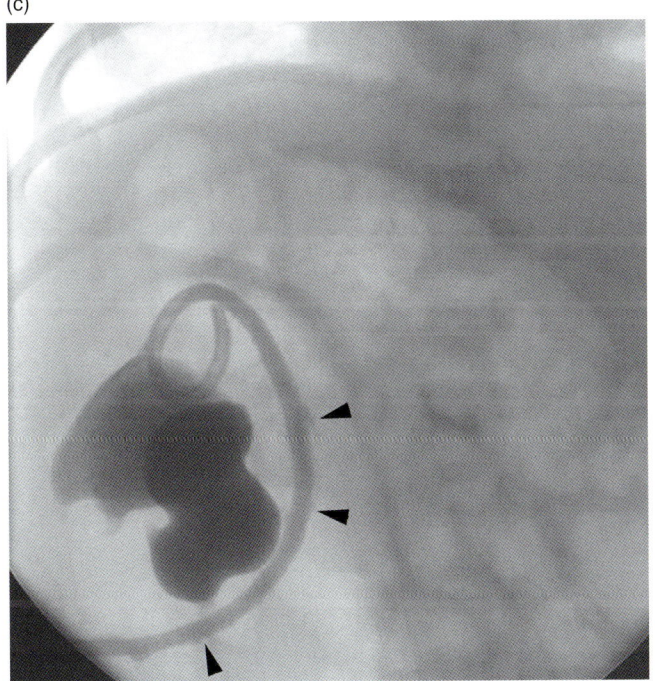

Figure 6.14 (a) Scout fluoroscopic image in a one-month-old female who presented with an abdominal mass shows displacement of the abdominal organs to the left by a large mass. Ultrasound (not shown) demonstrated hydronephrosis from UPJ obstruction. (b) An antegrade pyelogram obtained with injection of contrast material through the 6-French percutaneous nephrostomy drainage catheter (*arrowhead*) shows a grossly dilated collecting system with no antegrade flow of urine past the right UPJ. (c) An antegrade pyelogram obtained two weeks later shows interval improvement of the hydronephrosis. Reflux of contrast along the catheter tract (*arrowheads*) indicates that one of the side holes in the catheter tip has been withdrawn outside the collecting system. This can lead to leakage at the skin insertion site or formation of a urinoma, or serve as a nidus of infection.

abnormalities (i.e., hyperkalemia) should be corrected prior to percutaneous intervention.

Technique
Equipment

Performance of a percutaneous nephrostomy in the pediatric population is challenging because of the large variations in patient size (Table 6.4). Equipment routinely used in adults may be ineffective or dangerous, especially in the perinate and young infant. For example, the Cope introducer system facilitates exchange of a 0.035- or 0.038-inch guide wire for a 0.018-inch guide wire after puncture of the renal pelvis with a 22-gauge Chiba needle. While this system works well in older children and adults its use is problematic in small infants. Its side-port design (through which the 0.035- or 0.038-inch guide

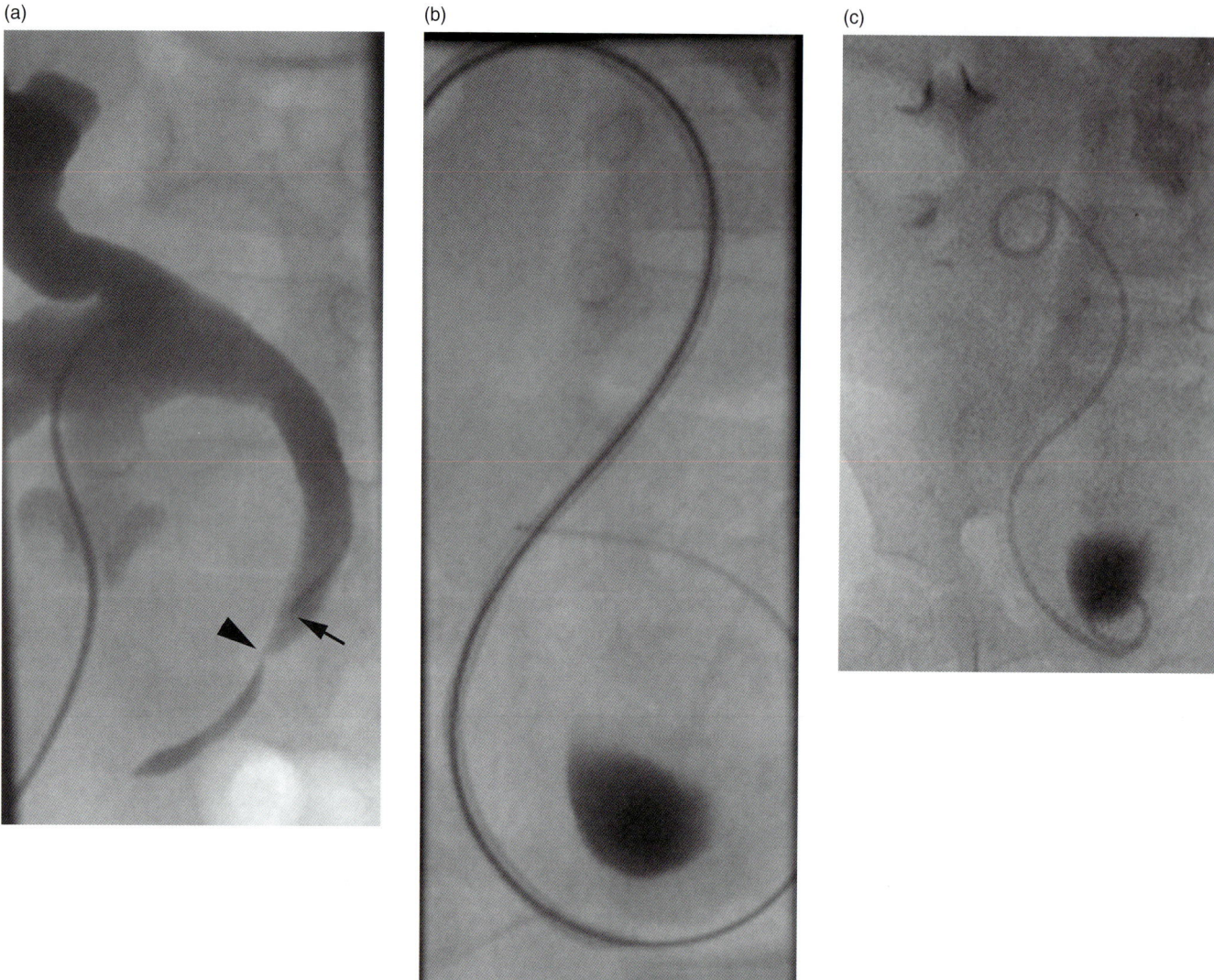

Figure 6.15 (a) Hydronephrosis with a focal ureteral stricture (*arrowhead*) is seen on this antegrade nephrostogram through a directional catheter (*arrow*) in a seven-year-old girl after renal transplant. Vascular compromise of the ureter and anastomotic complications are the most common reasons for ureteric stricture in this population. (b) After angioplasty a guide wire and catheter have been maneuvered beyond the stricture into the bladder, the length of the ureter can be measured in preparation for stent selection and deployment. (c) An adequate selection of stent lengths and sizes must be maintained. Small children, especially after transplant, may require stents that are quite short. Poorly sized stents are likely to become malpositioned and dysfunctional over time. The stent pictured here is of satisfactory length, freely coiling in the renal pelvis and bladder, without redundancy or impingement on the bladder wall.

wire will exit) will often lie outside of the renal pelvis of a small kidney, making guide wire exchange difficult or impossible, and exposing the patient to untoward effects and procedural challenges. If the outer sheath is advanced it likely will kink at the side port again making guide wire exchange problematic. Thus it is preferable to use a coaxial end-hole system (see Figure 2.14) such as the AccuStick™ system or Neff introducer, a micropuncture introducer set, or a sheathed needle to insert a 0.035- or 0.038-inch guide wire directly into the renal pelvis.

It is also important to carefully consider guide wire selection. In perinates and small infants a standard 0.035- or 0.038-inch guide wire may injure or lacerate the thin renal parenchyma. In this subgroup of patients it is helpful to avoid rigid guide wires and minimize guide wire manipulations. Thin skin, paucity of subcutaneous fat, minimal paraspinal musculature, and the short distance from the flank to the renal pelvis offers little resistance to tract dilation. The only barrier to catheter insertion is the renal capsule, which may be surprisingly tough. Thus a guide wire that does not kink such as a 0.018-inch angled Glide® wire is useful for securing initial access to the renal pelvis. Meticulous control of the needle and guide wire is important to avoid loss of access.

In the past, a 0.018-inch stainless steel mandril guide wire was used; however, on occasion the floppy tip bends, making catheter insertion difficult. If the long floppy tip is not completely within the renal pelvis, the stiff portion of the wire may be extrarenal, making passage of a dilator problematic. In

Chapter 6 Genitourinary interventions

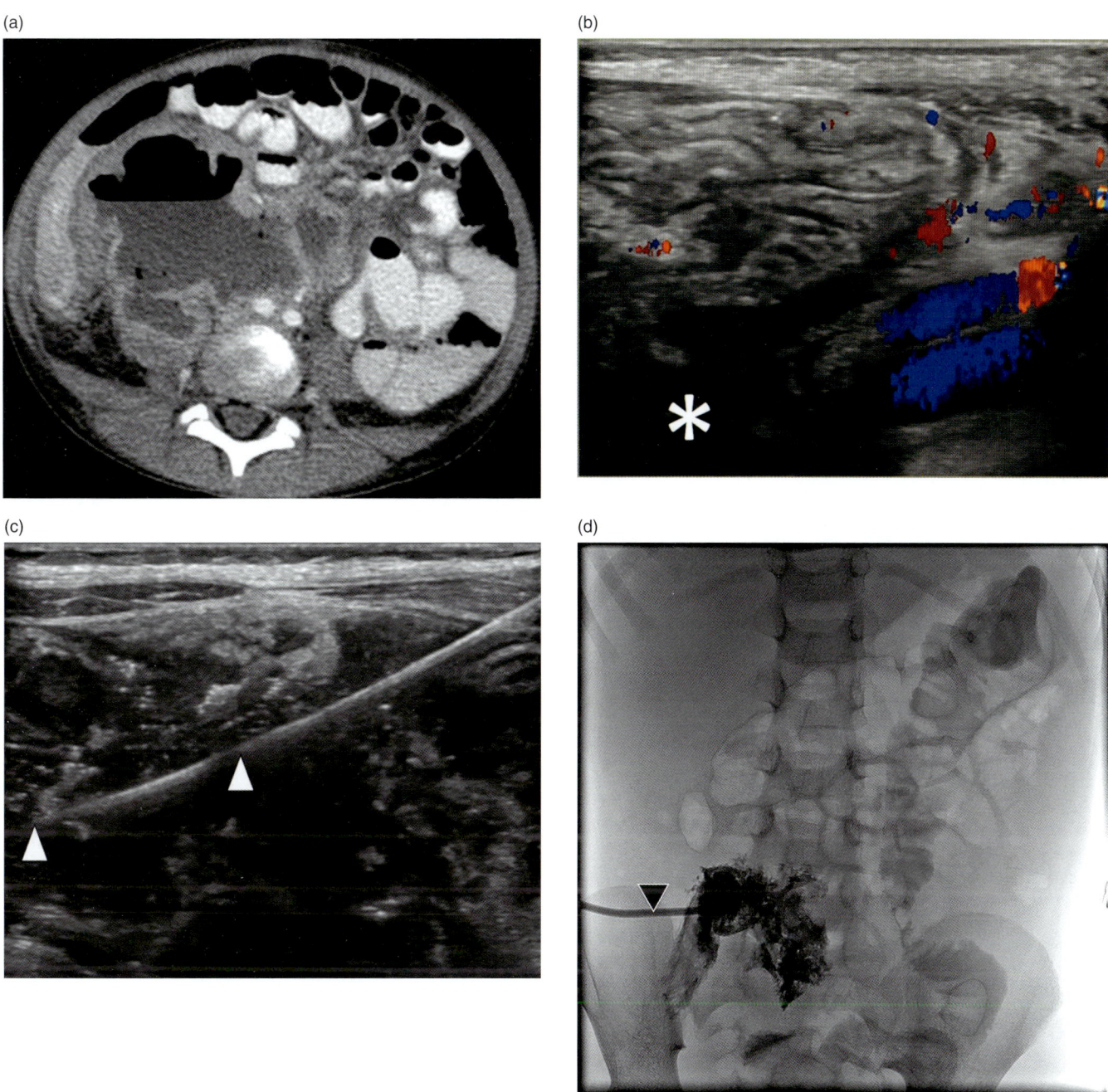

Figure 6.16 (a) Computed tomography with vascular and enteric contrast enhancement shows the right kidney with a grossly dilated collecting system with an air–fluid level, and a thin and poorly enhancing cortex in this seven-year-old male with flank pain and poor renal function. (b) Linear US with color Doppler from the right flank shows dysplastic renal parenchyma and a dilated collecting system (*asterisk*) with debris. (c) Percutaneous access was obtained with a 21-gauge Chiba needle. Ultrasound with a 6 to 18 MHz linear transducer provides high-resolution near-field guidance, with very conspicuous visualization of the needle and the 0.018-inch mandril guide wire (*arrowheads*). (d) A 10-French nephrostomy drain (*arrowhead*) is seen within the dilated collecting system. The thin cortex of this dysplastic kidney does not provide a substantial anchor for the drainage catheter, so a small amount of extravasation is not unusual. Despite decompression, this compromised renal unit did not regain significant function, and the dysplastic kidney was eventually removed.

addition, the tip may angulate as it deflects off the posterior wall of the renal pelvis making guide wire repositioning impossible. If one tries to pull the guide wire back into the Chiba needle the floppy tip can shear off (Figures 6.18, 6.19). If the guide wire cannot be withdrawn, in most cases the only choice is to remove the entire system and repuncture the renal pelvis. We have also found that the stiffness of this wire can lead to perforation of the renal pelvis. As a result this guide wire is now rarely used. Regardless of the guide wire selected it is important to maintain a straight catheter–guide-wire course during catheter insertion to avoid buckling in the retroperitoneal soft tissues.

Chapter 6 Genitourinary interventions

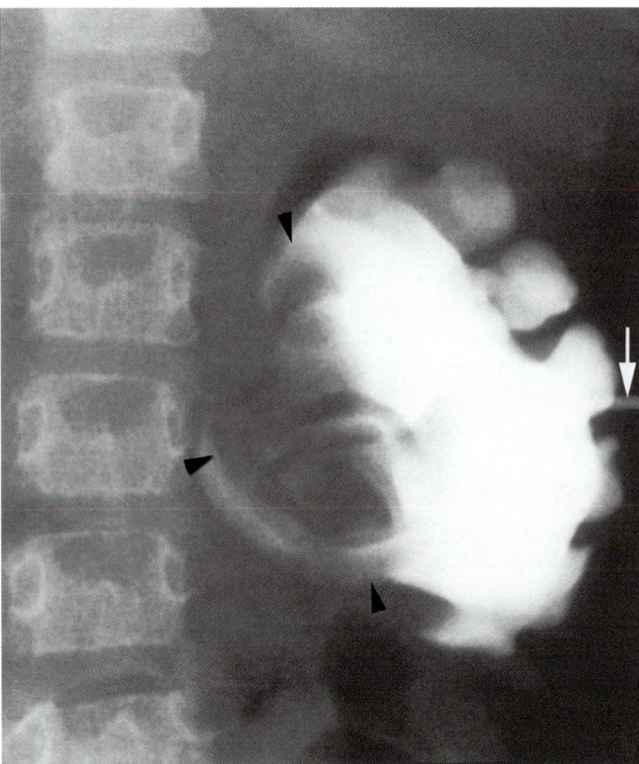

Figure 6.17 A neonate receiving IV antibiotics developed intermittent left renal outflow obstruction. A 5-French nephrostomy drainage catheter (*arrow*) was percutaneously inserted into the renal pelvis through a posterior calyx, and a sample grew *Candida albicans*. Contrast medium instilled through the catheter outlines the "fungal ball" (*arrowheads*). After transcatheter intracavitary treatment with an antifungal agent, the "fungus ball" was eradicated and the obstruction relieved.

Table 6.4 Equipment: percutaneous nephrostomy

Introducer systems
- One-step introducer system
- AccuStick™ introducer system
- Cope introducer set

Access needles
- Micro puncture system
- Sheathed needles
- TLA 19-gauge needle (accepts an 0.035- to 0.038-inch guide wire)
- Van Sonnenberg one-step needle system with removable hub
- Yueh needle (accepts an 0.038-inch guide wire)

Drainage catheters
Perinates and small children (<10 kg)
- 5-French Towbin pigtail drain
- 6-French APD
- 6-French sacks nephrostomy

Older children (>10 kg)
- VTC nephrostomy catheter systems (6-, 8-, 10-French with locking pigtail)
- APD, all purpose drain catheter (6-, 8-,10-French locking pigtail)
- Ultrathane nephrostomy catheters with Simp-Loc™ or Mac-Loc™ locking loop

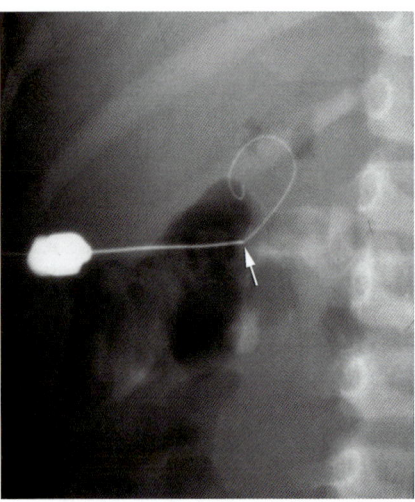

Figure 6.18 A 0.018-inch stainless steel wire through a Chiba needle angulates as it deflects off the medial wall of the renal pelvis. Attempts to pull the wire back into the needle may cause it to shear off at the sharp needle bevel (*arrow*).

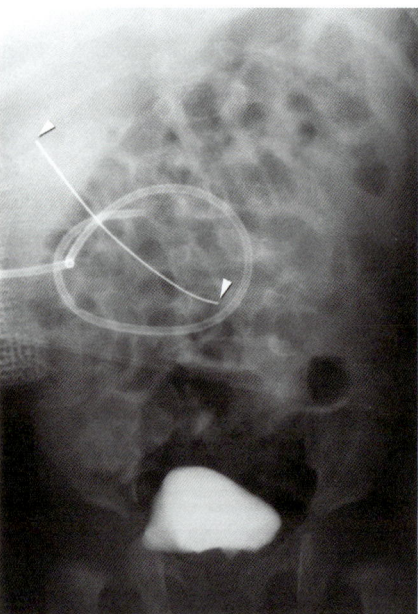

Figure 6.19 This wire fragment (*arrowheads*) was sheared off during attempts to obtain access to the renal collecting system in an infant with hydronephrosis. It was recovered using a loop snare via retrograde access using a cystoscope.

For insertion of drains ≥8-French, a variety of guide wires perform well including the Newton, angled Glide® wire, Roadrunner®, Rosen, and Amplatz® guide wires. In most cases the guide wire initially selected is the angled Glide® wire. Its hydrophilic coating and non-kinking properties facilitate catheter insertion. In those patients who are muscular or obese, or those in whom catheter insertion is difficult, a stiff guide wire such as a stiff or superstiff Glide® wire, Amplatz®, or Rosen wire is preferred.

There are a variety of nephrostomy drains available that can be used successfully in children. The choice of catheter is usually determined by physician preference. In perinates and

Chapter 6 Genitourinary interventions

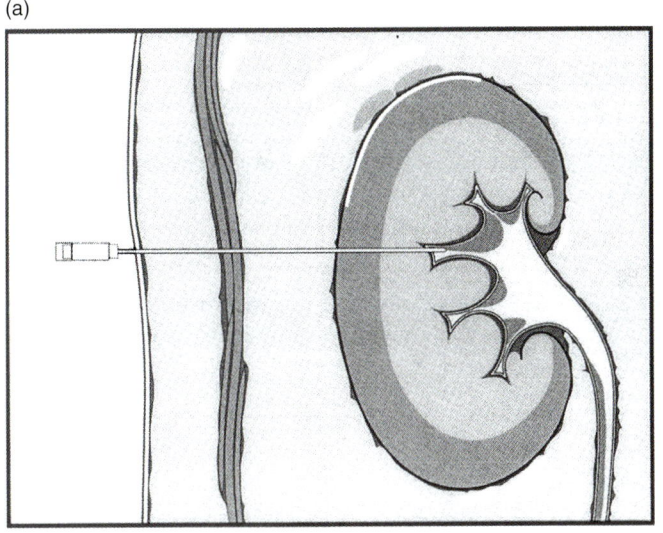

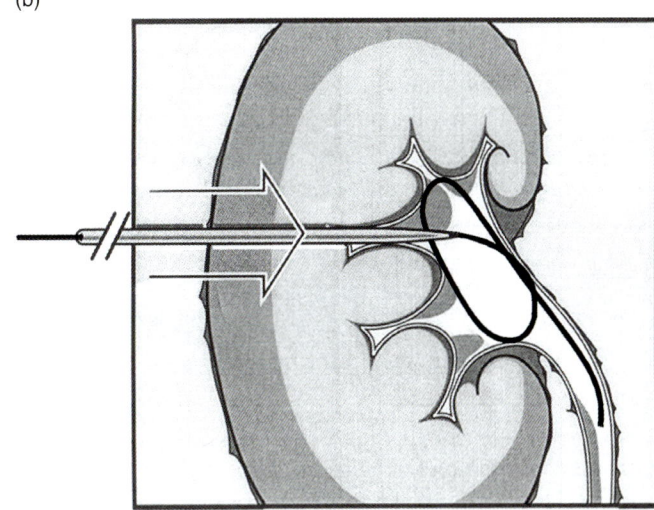

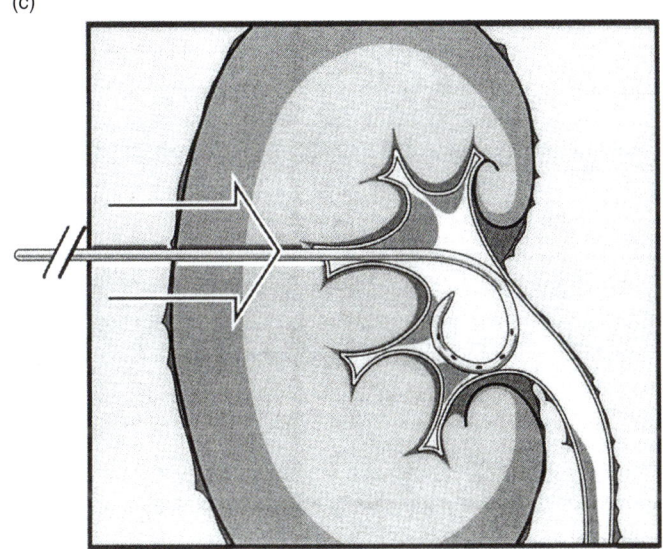

Figure 6.20 Nephrostomy illustrations. (a) Percutaneous needle access to the renal pelvis is obtained, usually with cross-sectional imaging guidance, and usually through a posterior calyx. The return of urine through the access needle confirms location of the needle tip within the renal collecting system. Contrast medium can then be administered to outline the collecting system and guide additional manipulations using fluoroscopic control. (b) Once access is secured, a directional guide wire is advanced through the needle and either the wire is coiled within the pelvis or the tip is advanced into the ureter or beyond for stability during equipment exchanges and manipulation. Hydrophilic wires must be carefully controlled, by clamping or tightly pinning at the skin surface, to prevent recoil from the collecting system and loss of access. The tract may then be developed using fascial dilators to a diameter adequate for passage of equipment or devices over the wire. (c) The nephrostomy procedure is completed by passing the pigtail catheter with its stiffener over the wire until the tip is well within the collecting system. Care is taken not to advance the stiffened catheter tip against the medial wall of the pelvis to prevent perforation or other injury. The catheter is advanced off the stiffener, and the pigtail formed, preferably within the renal pelvis. The catheter is then fixed to the patient's skin as described under "Securing the catheter."

small children a 5-French pigtail nephrostomy drainage system (Towbin drain) (Figure 6.20) or 6-French Dawson–Mueller pigtail catheter, both with a 1 cm loop, is used. The all purpose drainage (APD) catheter is available in 6-French and can be useful in the smaller patient. However, it is important to be aware that some drainage catheters require a 0.021-inch guide wire. When needed, a 0.021-inch stainless steel guide wire or Glidewire® performs well. However, the best strategy may be to avoid using these catheters so that the rarely used 0.021-inch wire does not need to be stocked.

The 5-French pigtail drain and 6-F Dawson–Mueller catheter have the advantage of a small distal loop (1 cm) and drainage holes positioned along the inner curve of the pigtail. This design prevents catheter occlusion resulting from contact with the wall of the renal pelvis and allows the pigtail to be formed within smaller cavities. The operator can be confident that all drainage holes are satisfactorily positioned within the renal pelvis once the pigtail reforms. In toddlers and older children, the standard 8-French pigtail drain works well. Locking pigtail drains may be preferred to prevent accidental dislodgment (Figure 6.21). For the rare instances where thick purulent or viscous fluid is present, larger caliber drains may be necessary.

Patient preparation

Prior abdominal imaging should be reviewed. Specifically, available cross-sectional imaging should be evaluated to confirm the location of the colon, liver, and spleen, making certain that these organs are not in vulnerable positions along the planned pathway for nephrostomy access (see "Anatomic considerations," above). For each child undergoing percutaneous nephrostomy placement or an endourologic procedure the following laboratory studies are usually obtained: CBC with platelet count, coagulation profile, and in rare cases a bleeding time. In addition, a urine culture may be obtained prior to the day of the urinary tract manipulation. Children with suspected or proven urinary tract infections are given preprocedural antibiotics. High-risk children, those with immune deficiency or other conditions predisposing to infection, children with congenital heart disease, and those in whom there are procedural difficulties or complications, are treated with antibiotics before, during, or after the procedure. The antibiotic chosen may vary with the age and underlying condition of the child. Empiric therapy guidelines are provided in Chapter 1.

Table 6.5 Procedure summary: percutaneous nephrostomy

- Select entry site in flank
- Prepare and drape skin
- Inject local anesthesia (buffered)
- Small skin incision at entry site
- Puncture renal pelvis
- Insert guide wire and coil in pelvis or direct into ureter
- Dilate tract (> catheter size)
- Insert drainage catheter
- Inject contrast
- Secure catheter

Since each child will necessarily undergo either general anesthesia (GA) or sedation the child must be NPO. Those having procedures under local anesthesia and intravenous sedation are made NPO for a minimum of one feeding in neonates and four hours in older children. Individuals requiring GA are managed by the anesthesia service and the protocol used is the same as for other patients having an operative procedure. In addition, any other routine preoperative order is obtained.

Standard technique
Access to the renal pelvis

As with many other drainage procedures a combination of US and fluoroscopic guidance is often used to achieve and secure initial access (Table 6.5). The use of US obviates the need for contrast opacification of the collecting system in most instances, reduces radiation dose, and is especially useful in patients with impaired renal function. Also, US guidance allows drainage to be performed in the fluoroscopy suite or, if needed, at the bedside. Ultrasound guidance may be used in several ways including in the selection and marking of the skin entry site for a non-guided puncture of the renal pelvis, or for real-time US guidance, either freehand or using a biopsy guide. In most situations we prefer real-time guidance with a freehand technique. A variety of retrograde fluoroscopic

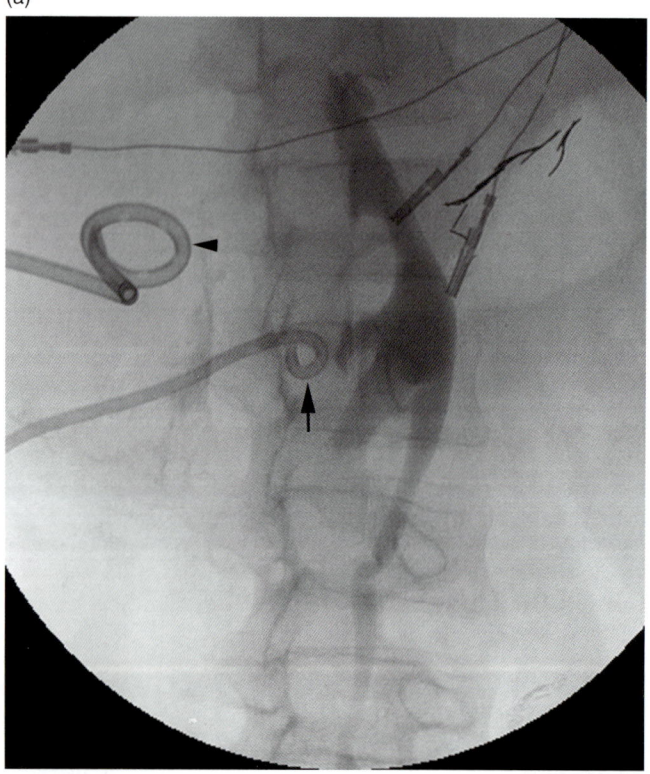

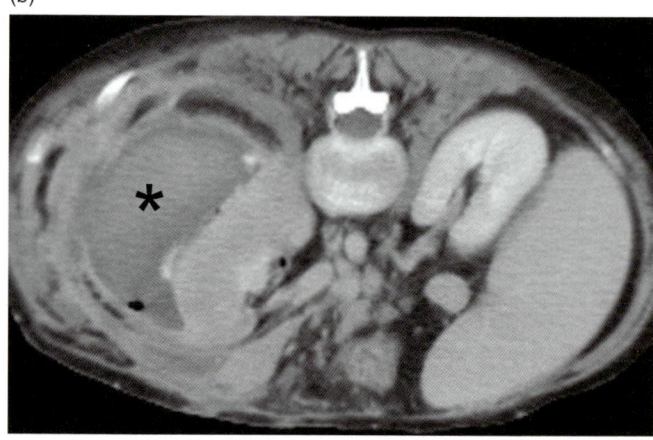

Figure 6.21 (a) In this fluoroscopic image obtained after excretory urography in this 18-year-old male trauma patient, the 8.3-French locking pigtail nephrostomy drainage catheter (*arrow*) has been accidentally dislodged from the renal collecting system. The second drainage catheter (*arrowhead*) is draining a large retroperitoneal hematoma compressing the ureter. (b) Axial CT image obtained with IV contrast through the kidneys shows a large subcapsular fluid collection (*asterisk*) related to dislodgment of the percutaneous nephrostomy catheter.

approaches are described to achieve percutaneous access to the renal collecting system, but are seldom if ever required in the pediatric population. Recently, both CT and even MRI have been suggested for use in gaining renal access. However, in the pediatric population CT is rarely necessary for guidance and is only considered for children with unusual renal anatomy, severe kyphoscoliosis or obesity, or when other guidance methods have failed.

The patient is placed either in a prone or prone-oblique position. Children are restrained on the angiography table. Children one year of age or less may be positioned on an Octostop® board or similar device while older children may be secured with Velcro® straps. Young children are usually placed on a warming device (e.g., Bair Hugger™) to maintain body temperature during the procedure. The procedure is initiated by selecting an entry site along the flank using image guidance. When anatomic landmarks are used in young children, an entry site is selected two to three fingerbreadths below the costal margin and two to three fingerbreadths lateral to the spinous processes. In older children four to five fingerbreadths are used. However, since US and fluoroscopic imaging is readily available in our practice all procedures are performed under imaging guidance. In the past renal puncture was fluoroscopically guided after injection of intravenous contrast. Currently, we have virtually replaced this approach with US guidance.

When intravenous sedation is used, skin anesthesia is initially achieved with a J-tip, then buffered local anesthesia is *slowly* injected into the skin at the entry site, after the usual sterile preparation, with a 30-gauge, 1½-inch needle to minimize discomfort. It is important to carefully and completely anesthetize the skin and deep soft tissues along the anticipated route. Inadequate local anesthesia will result in avoidable discomfort that will awaken the child and make the procedure more difficult and time consuming. The 30-gauge needle may be exchanged for a 22-gauge Chiba or spinal needle to complete anesthetizing a longer tract (to the renal capsule), when necessary. When general anesthesia is utilized this step is unnecessary. A skin incision is then made with a #11 scalpel blade and enlarged with blunt dissection.

In children, the position of the kidney in the retroperitoneum is often lower and more mobile than anticipated. In those patients in whom renal mobility is excessive, the kidney can be stabilized with a bolster positioned under the mid abdomen. In small children, manually fixing the kidney with a hand on the abdomen while the puncture is made may be helpful.

Route planning

Whenever possible an entry site is planned below the costal margin. Regardless of the approach it is important to traverse renal parenchyma and enter a middle pole calyx, if possible, especially if access to the ureter is needed. The middle and upper pole calices provide the most direct route to the ureteropelvic junction and ureter. If puncture is for decompression only, a lower pole calyx is adequate for access, and may help avoid the risk of inadvertent transpleural complications. A posterior calyx is much preferred for access, providing the most direct route for subsequent manipulations. Posterior calices are readily identified on US or using motion parallax with oblique fluoroscopic imaging, or by injecting a small amount of air or carbon dioxide gas into the collecting system.

In considering the initial approach to the kidney one should consider that any window to the pediatric kidney is likely to be narrow, and the interventionalist must work within the parameters offered by the individual patient's anatomy and body habitus. In this context, such considerations may guide the interventionalist away from the infundibulum, especially in the upper pole, where there may be an associated higher frequency of injury to the interlobar vessels (e.g., posterior segmental artery) due to their particularly large size in this region. In all cases, access through a caliceal fornix is preferred over a caliceal infundibulum, since, at worst, it exposes the child to injury of small peripheral vessels (e.g., small venous arcades) rather than large interlobar vessels (e.g., posterior segmental artery) that may supply as much as 50% of the renal parenchyma. Likewise, direct puncture of the renal pelvis is usually avoided because the renal pelvis lacks supporting parenchyma to provide tamponade against bleeding, urine leak, or premature catheter loss. Direct puncture of the renal pelvis, however, may be used for Whitaker perfusion testing or if opacification of the collecting system is required for another procedure.

Transrenal access to the renal pelvis (Figure 6.20) is achieved using a 22- or 23-gauge Chiba needle or 19-gauge sheathed needle, minimizing the risk of pneumothorax or hydrothorax. In cases with significant hydronephrosis, a Yueh sheathed needle may be used. A posterolateral approach angling the needle toward the costovertebral junction is preferred. We have found that shorter length (7.5 to 10 cm) Chiba needles are easier to control in the small infant during renal puncture and wire insertion. Caudo-cranial needle angulation is used if necessary to avoid violating the pleural space. In order to create the most direct line to the renal pelvis, especially if subsequent endourologic manipulation is planned, a posterior mid-pole calyx is entered if possible. After the kidney is punctured and a guide wire coiled within the renal pelvis, the tract is often dilated two French sizes larger than the nephrostomy catheter to ease insertion of the drain. Overdilation is especially helpful in some perinates.

In the perinate and small infant, the kidney is punctured with a 22-gauge Chiba needle and a 0.018-inch Glide® wire is positioned within the renal pelvis. The 5-French pigtail (Duan/Tobin, Cook) catheter, together with its inner (metal) cannula, is advanced over the guide wire until it reaches the first turn of the guide wire adjacent to the back wall of the renal pelvis. The inner cannula and guide wire are pinned, and the catheter is advanced until it is coiled in the renal pelvis. Although no tract dilation may be necessary, if there is any difficulty advancing the catheter system, it is best to remove it and overdilate the tract by one to two French. In most cases the cannula prevents

Table 6.6 Outcome measures

To improve outcome and quality assurance analysis, it may be helpful to record the following information for each genitourinary interventional procedure performed:

- Demographic information (patient name, unique identification number, date and time of procedure, age, sex, weight, date of birth, etc.)
- Primary diagnosis
- Reason for procedure; referring service and provider
- Anticipated endpoint
- Primary provider responsible for procedure (interventionalist, urologist, surgeon, etc.)
- Collaborating provider(s)
- Procedure location (interventional suite, operating room, bedside, etc.)
- Provider responsible for anesthesia/sedation (anesthesiologist, nurse, etc.)
- Preprocedural evaluation
  - serum creatinine
  - metabolic status (e.g., hyperkalemia, metabolic acidosis)
  - stone burden (mm^3)
- Preprocedural interventions (e.g., antibiotics, blood products, imaging)
- Initial access
  - entry method (e.g., needle nephrotomy, percutaneous nephrostomy, retrograde ureteroscopy)
  - guidance (anatomic landmarks, US, fluoroscopy, CT, nephroscopy, etc.)
  - operative site (e.g., upper pole calyx, UPJ)
  - device
  - number of attempts
  - reason for deferral, discontinuation or failure, if procedure not completed
- Access device and position
  - catheter manufacturer, type, lumen number and diameter, length
  - tip position
- Equipment and supplies used
- Procedure time
- Type and adequacy of anesthesia/sedation/analgesia
- Procedural complications (e.g., venospasm, extravasation) and management
- Adjunctive procedures
- Complications, including:
  - procedure-related infection (include dates)
    - type (septicemia, UTI, catheter tract infection, abscess)
    - suspected (basis) or proven (method and results)
    - management (e.g., antibiotics, catheter removal, repeat cultures)
    - outcome
  - bleeding and vascular injury (include dates)
    - type (e.g., hematuria, hemorrhage, AV fistula or pseudoaneurysm)
    - method of diagnosis (e.g., hemoglobin, arteriogram)
    - management (e.g., observation, transfusion, embolization)
    - outcome
  - thrombosis (include dates)
    - method of diagnosis or documentation
    - location and extent
    - management
    - outcome
  - dislodgment or malposition (include dates)
    - method of diagnosis or documentation
    - management
    - outcome
  - other procedure-related complications or interventions
- outcome at follow-up (method and date; endpoint achieved?)
  - residual stone fragments
  - change in renal function

kinking of the catheter in the subcutaneous tissue and eliminates the need for larger or stiffer guide wires.

In older children, a 19-gauge sheathed needle is used to gain access to the collecting system in most cases. Using a larger needle avoids the need to exchange a 0.018-inch guide wire for a 0.035-inch or 0.038-inch guide wire. When a Chiba needle and 0.018-inch guide wire are used, a coaxial introducer system is needed to exchange for a larger guide wire.

Catheter insertion

After successful puncture of the renal pelvis the guide wire is coiled in the renal pelvis or directed into the ureter. The tract may be overdilated (by one to two French) using standard fascial dilators, and an 8.3-French locking pigtail catheter is inserted. After insertion of the drainage catheter, contrast medium is injected to confirm satisfactory catheter position, demonstrate potential complications, and document any pathology.

In patients with renal transplants (Figure 6.15), the approach to percutaneous nephrostomy depends upon the surgical anatomy. Most transplants are extraperitoneal and located in the iliac fossa. Thus the renal pelvis usually faces posteromedially. As a result, an anterolateral approach is usually best to avoid passage through the peritoneal cavity. Real-time US is used to guide needle puncture. With intraperitoneal renal transplants CT may be necessary for preprocedural imaging or intraprocedural guidance to avoid inadvertent injury to bowel.

Postprocedure and follow-up care

Following the procedure, appropriate notes and postprocedure orders are entered into the patient's chart. It may be helpful to both patient care and ongoing quality assurance to maintain pertinent demographic and procedure-related data in an electronic database. Suggested items for data management are included in Table 6.6.

Securing the catheter

Every precaution is taken to avoid dislodgment of the nephrostomy drain. Securing the catheter begins with placement of a 3–0 suture, which is tied tightly in a criss-cross pattern over the catheter shaft. This creates a locking stitch that works like a Chinese finger torture that tightens when strain is placed upon it. In the past a retention disc was used in all children except perinates. A skin fixation device such as a SorbaView® shield or Stat-Lock® is used to protect the catheter from accidental dislodgment. In small infants an alternative method is to secure the catheter with a criss-crossing suture augmented by a tape bridge (similar to the technique used to secure umbilical artery catheters; see below). Care is taken to avoid an excessively tight skin suture, which can cause discomfort and skin necrosis.

Prior to creating a tape bridge, the skin is coated with either a liquid adhesive (e.g., Mastisol®) or a barrier film to make it sticky. After the liquid dries, the bridge is made as illustrated in Figure 3.4. Gauze is used to support the catheter at the skin exit site to avoid kinking. The catheter can then be covered with Tegaderm®, Opsite®, or a SorbaView® shield. A wooden tongue blade may be taped to the drainage catheter for added support. These precautions are successful in the majority of cases.

Managing catheter exchanges and accidental dislodgment

Occasionally a damaged or partially obstructed catheter must be replaced prior to the completion of therapy. If the original catheter has been in position for two or more weeks, the tract has probably matured and loss of access is less likely during the exchange. If the catheter has been recently placed, the danger of tract loss due to inadvertent dislodgment is much greater (Figure 6.21). The internal locking mechanism of the indwelling catheter must be released. Although some catheters are designed to easily allow unlocking, this may be accomplished by cutting off the distal end of the catheter, while pinning the proximal catheter in place at the skin. If the patient is sensitive to manipulation of the catheter, the tract should be generously anesthetized with buffered lidocaine prior to exchange.

The next priority is to secure access with a guide wire through the existing catheter, with the tip preferably positioned in the ureter, or alternatively coiled in the renal pelvis. With the wire pinned the catheter is carefully removed, pinning the wire at the skin as soon as it is uncovered. If a Glidewire is used, the wire could be pinned with a hemostat at the skin surface, to prevent the wire from slipping out inadvertently, which it is embarrassingly easy to do! The new catheter is passed with its stiffening cannula over the guide wire past the renal capsule, advanced off the cannula, locked internally, and secured to the skin as previously described.

If a wire cannot be advanced through an obstructed catheter, the catheter hub can be cut off and, if necessary, a strong suture fixed to the distal (cut) end. Using this suture to pin the catheter, a peel-away sheath may be carefully advanced over the catheter until the tip is in the renal collecting system. The old catheter remnant may then be removed through the sheath, and a guide wire advanced through the sheath, completing the exchange as described above.

If the original catheter has been inadvertently dislodged, the tract may be gently probed with a directional catheter (e.g., JB-1 or Kumpe) and an angled Glidewire after injection of a small amount of contrast under fluoroscopic guidance. If the guide wire is successfully advanced into the renal pelvis or ureter, the exchange may be completed as above. Otherwise, if catheter access for drainage or other procedures is still clinically indicated a new tract must be developed, preferably through a new skin access site.

Complications

As is true with adult patients, major complications resulting from insertion of a percutaneous nephrostomy are unusual. Microscopic hematuria, or more rarely gross hematuria, is a common minor complication and may last up to 72 hours following the procedure. In this setting the catheter should be flushed frequently to prevent blood clots from obstructing the catheter. Pain, perirenal bleeding, urine extravasation, local infection, and accidental catheter dislodgment are also potential complications. When gross hematuria occurs we often monitor the patient using an automated urine chemistry analyzer after each void and intermittent complete blood counts (CBC). The child will not be discharged to home if there is any evidence of persistent bleeding.

The most serious complications of percutaneous nephrostomy include sepsis, severe hemorrhage, and vascular injury. Sepsis is the most frequent major complication reported in pediatric series. Children with infected urine or renal calculi are at greatest risk for the development of sepsis with nephrostomy tube placement. Overdistension of the collecting system at the time of catheter placement is likely the most significant factor leading to bacteremia. Decompressing the renal pelvis prior to performing an antegrade pyelogram, especially in patients with pyonephrosis, is important to minimize this problem. In this subgroup of children it is preferable to delay a diagnostic antegrade pyelogram for 24 to 72 hours to allow decompression of the obstructed system and sterilization of urine. Patients with suspected or documented pyonephrosis require antibiotic coverage before and after the procedure. Urine Gram stain and culture should be performed so that appropriate antibiotics can be selected. Also, sepsis is more likely to occur during performance of ureteral perfusion studies due to high intrarenal pressures.

Transient mild hematuria is common after percutaneous nephrostomy and usually clears within 48 hours. This should be considered a minor complication and requires no therapeutic intervention. Severe hemorrhage requiring transfusion or other intervention is unusual and may indicate vascular injury, a clotting disorder, or an unsuspected vascular malformation. When significant bleeding occurs arteriography may be required to establish the site and cause of bleeding (e.g., vessel laceration, pseudoaneurysm, arteriovenous or arteriocaliceal fistula). If a vascular injury is identified it can be treated by selective embolization. Using a posterolateral approach for renal pelvic access along Brödel's line, and taking advantage of parenchymal tamponade, reduces the risk of vascular injury and severe bleeding. Bleeding requiring transfusion should be expected in fewer than 1% of children after image-guided renal biopsy.

Retroperitoneal hemorrhage is potentially more serious than pelvicaliceal bleeding, as it may be less evident clinically. In general, retroperitoneal hematomas are small and are asymptomatic. If a patient becomes symptomatic after unsuccessful percutaneous nephrostomy the possibility should be considered and examination with CT or US encouraged.

Leakage of urine with resultant urinoma formation has been reported in the pediatric population. This complication is more likely when the renal parenchyma is thin, as in children with chronic reflux, or when the free wall of the renal pelvis is punctured. While a small amount of urine leakage around the nephrostomy catheter can be considered normal, if the urinoma is large or becomes infected, percutaneous drainage may be required. Excessive leakage is usually due to catheter blockage especially in patients with pyonephrosis or excessive bleeding.

As noted above, surrounding anatomic structures are at risk during renal access procedures, including the liver, spleen, bowel, adrenal glands, stomach, and pancreas. Injury to these organs is usually minor and self-limited, and awareness and appropriate preprocedure imaging is usually sufficient to avoid such complications. Access to upper-pole calices, especially from an intercostal approach and more rarely from a subcostal approach, increases the risk of transpleural injuries. These may include pneumothorax, hemo- or hydrothorax, and nephro-pleural fistula. The complication rate associated with upper-pole access climbs dramatically when the route of access is above the 11th rib.

The most frequent catheter-related complication is accidental catheter dislodgment. This may be expected in 5 to 10% of patients and may happen despite suturing the catheter to the skin.

Conclusions

With the use of US for guidance, misadventures due to needle malposition are unusual. Pneumothorax is now rarely reported, as puncture above the 12th rib is usually avoided.

Considerable experience with percutaneous nephrostomy in the pediatric population has now accumulated. The results are favorable and show that with careful technique, it is a safe and effective procedure in children of all ages and sizes and is the procedure of choice in many situations.

Whitaker (pressure–flow) perfusion test

Introduction

The pressure–flow study was popularized by Whitaker in 1973. The concept was based on the observation that pressure in the renal pelvis was normal in many patients with hydronephrosis. However, with the infusion of additional fluid the intrapelvic pressure increased in the presence of obstruction. Whitaker determined that urine flow during maximum diuresis is 10 ml/min. Therefore a normal ureter should be able to tolerate this flow rate without significant dilation or increase in intrapelvic pressure. Correspondingly, the normal relative pelvic pressure (intrarenal pressure minus bladder pressure) should be ≤15 cm H_2O. When obstruction is present intrapelvic pressures of greater than 22 cm H_2O are expected. Pressures between 15 and 22 cm H_2O are considered indeterminate. The Whitaker test is best performed using fluoroscopic guidance. By using contrast medium as the perfusate (antegrade pyelogram), the normal and pathologic anatomy as well as the intrapelvic pressure can be simultaneously defined. Parenthetically, we have performed perfusion tests in the same renal pelvis using both normal saline and contrast with identical results, suggesting that the minor difference in fluid viscosity between the two is not clinically relevant.

In addition to determining the perfusion pressure at 10 ml/min, we have modified the procedure by obtaining data at a variety of flow rates. It is our preference to perfuse the renal pelvis at low (2 to 4 ml/min), intermediate (6 to 8 ml/min), high (10 ml/min), and occasionally supra-physiologic (12 ml/min) rates in order to determine the degree and perhaps significance of an obstruction. If significant pressure rises occur at low to intermediate flow rates, the significance of a partial obstruction may be greater.

Obtaining an opening pressure is an important component of the procedure. As expected, a normal or low opening pressure does not exclude a significant obstruction and perfusion through the physiologic range is important. However, opening pressures greater than 20 cm H_2O generally predict a significant obstruction. Moreover, an opening pressure greater than 35 cm H_2O indicates a high-grade obstruction and contraindicates further perfusion testing, due to risk of pyelotubular back flow with subsequent renal injury and potential sepsis. An antegrade pyelogram is performed after the opening pressure is measured. Intrarenal pressures are carefully monitored during the antegrade pyelogram to make sure that a pressure of 35 cm H_2O is not exceeded.

The Whitaker test is an objective, reproducible technique that is unaffected by glomerular filtration rate. It provides excellent definition of both the upper and lower urinary tract and permits measurement of resistance to known flow rates. The advantages of the Whitaker test over other methods include: (1) direct infusion of liquid into the renal pelvis does not require estimates of renal function to optimize the timing of images, (2) ease of performance and interpretation in most instances, and (3) results in a confident diagnosis more frequently in patients with a dilated renal pelvis of uncertain etiology. Its disadvantages are its invasiveness, the need for sedation or general anesthesia, and the potential for complications or hospital admission. At this time the popularity of the Whitaker procedure has diminished considerably due to the excellence of non-invasive imaging. However, in the proper situation the information produced is invaluable.

Indications

The primary indication for performing a perfusion study (Whitaker test) is to differentiate dilated systems that are obstructed from those that are dilated but not obstructed, and in rare cases for surgical planning. The Whitaker test is most useful for cases in which the diuretic radionuclide renogram is equivocal (with a $T_{1/2}$ between 15 and 22 min). When an antegrade pyelogram is combined with a perfusion study, one is able to define both the site and the magnitude of an obstruction. This is an advantage of performing the study with contrast using fluoroscopic guidance rather than using saline as the infusate without concomitant imaging. The Whitaker test is also the most reliable method for serial evaluation of urinary obstruction pre- and postintervention (e.g., post-endopyelotomy). Although it should be used selectively, the Whitaker test is the most reliable method available to determine the presence of obstruction.

Dilated renal grafts (e.g., postrenal transplant stenosis without evidence of rejection) are most reliably evaluated by correlating the creatinine level with findings at antegrade nephrostogram, and that in this setting a pressure–flow study contributes no additional information. Similarly, a Whitaker perfusion test is not indicated if the diagnosis can be made using non-invasive testing such as an excretory urogram or Lasix radionuclide renogram. However, as many as 10 to 15% of patients with unexplained dilation of the upper urinary tract have equivocal results on renal scanning. The Whitaker test is also contraindicated if the patient has an uncorrectable coagulopathy. In practice, non-invasive testing is successful in the majority of situations.

Technique

Equipment

The equipment selected to perform a Whitaker perfusion test and antegrade pyelogram varies with the size and age of the patient, the size and shape of the renal pelvis, the coagulation profile, and the type of fluid in the renal pelvis (Table 6.7).

Table 6.7 Equipment: Whitaker perfusion test

- Thin needles (e.g., 22-gauge Chiba)
- Can substitute sheathed needle or 5- to 8-French nephrostomy tube for Chiba
- Stopcock (three-way)
- Manometer
- Pressure transducer
- Connecting tubing
- Infusion pump capable of rates from 120 ml/h (2 ml/min) to 720 ml/h (12 ml/min)
- Multichannel pressure analyzer
- Foley catheter 6- to 12-French (use 6- to 8-French for infants and 8- to 10-French for older children)
- Contrast for infusion (ionic contrast may be used and is less expensive than non-ionic contrast)

Patient preparation

Although the Whitaker test is one of the least invasive procedures, preparation should nevertheless be completed as if for any other nephrostomy access procedure. A CBC with platelet count and a coagulation profile are usually obtained. If urine stasis or UTI are suspected, a urine culture is obtained prior to the day of the urinary tract manipulation. Children with suspected or proven urinary tract infections are given preprocedural antibiotics or possibly postponed depending upon the clinical situation. High-risk children, those with immune deficiency or other conditions predisposing to infection, children with congenital heart disease, and those in whom there are procedural difficulties or complications are treated with antibiotics before, during, or after the procedure. Since each child will necessarily undergo either general anesthesia (GA) or sedation, the child must be NPO. Those having procedures under local anesthesia and intravenous sedation are made NPO for a minimum of one feeding in neonates and four hours in older children. Individuals requiring GA are managed by the anesthesia service, and the protocol used is the same as for other patients having an operative procedure. In addition, any other routine preoperative order is obtained.

Standard technique

Interpreting the results of a perfusion test requires calculation of the differential or step-off pressure. This differential pressure is obtained by subtraction of the absolute bladder pressure from the absolute renal pressure. At a flow rate of 10 ml/min, with the bladder empty, differential pressure below 13 cm H_2O is considered normal; arbitrary values of 14 to 20 cm H_2O indicate mild obstruction; 21 to 34 cm H_2O, moderate obstruction; and above 35 cm H_2O, severe obstruction.

Technically, the first step in performing a perfusion test is to insert a Foley catheter into the urinary bladder (Table 6.8). Next, the renal pelvis is punctured using US guidance in most

Table 6.8 Procedural summary: Whitaker perfusion test

- NPO four to six hours prior to the planned procedure
- Prone position
- Sedation (GA only if unable to sedate)
- Local anesthesia injected at puncture sites
- Obtain needle access to the renal pelvis under image guidance
    - connect stopcock to needle, calibrate and zero pressure transducer
- Measure opening pressure
- Set analyzer to opening pressure level
- Begin infusion with contrast at 2 to 4 ml/min × 5 min or until measured pressure is stable
- Increase rate to 6 ml/min × 5 min or until pressure stable
- Increase to 10 ml/min × 5 min or until pressure stable
- Stop at any time if pressure reaches 35 cm H_2O
- Can repeat infusion test with filled bladder if needed
- Document normal or pathologic anatomy on spot image(s)

instances. In some cases, the puncture may be fluoroscopically guided following administration of intravenous contrast. For very large systems, a blind puncture may be performed. In general, the patient is positioned in a prone or prone-oblique position with the side to be examined elevated. Unlike access for nephrostomy placement, where a transparenchymal course is preferred, for a Whitaker test a needle may be guided directly into the renal pelvis. In infants it may be helpful to put a bolster under the abdomen to prevent the kidney from moving away from the puncture needle.

Two-needle technique

Perfusion testing may be performed using a one- or two-needle technique. We prefer the latter technique (Figure 6.22) because of the ease of simultaneous infusion and pressure

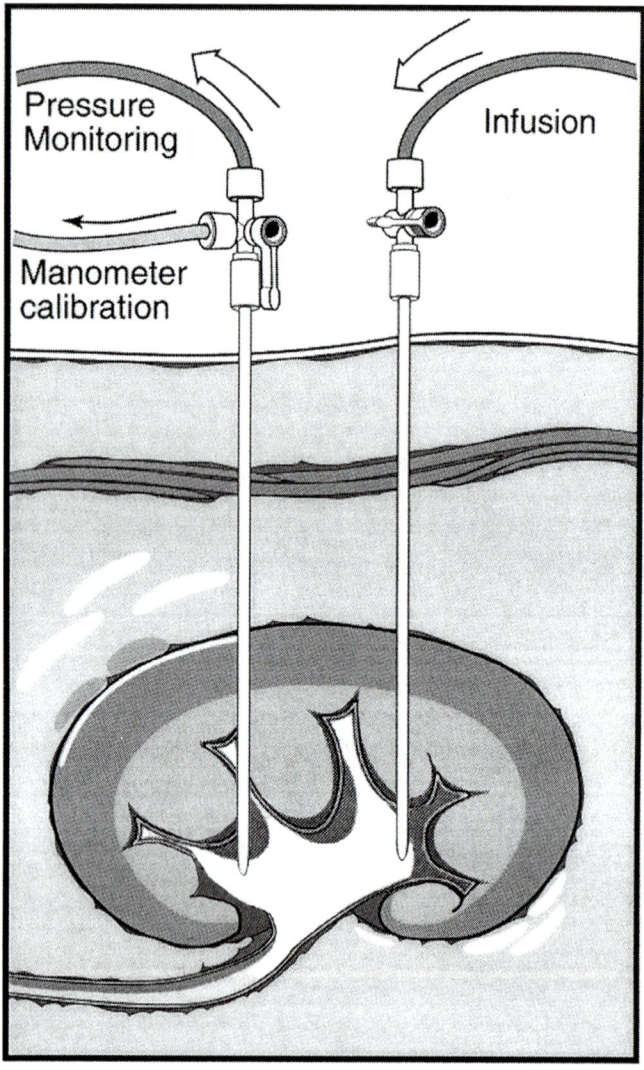

Figure 6.22 Two-needle Whitaker test illustration. Using a two-needle technique for pressure–flow monitoring, an infusion at a rate of 2 to 10 ml/min is instilled through one needle, while calibration and pressure monitoring is conducted through the second needle. Measured pressure greater than 35 cm H_2O above baseline is considered evidence of severe obstruction.

monitoring. Two 22-gauge or 23-gauge Chiba needles are inserted into the renal pelvis. In toddlers and other children with sufficiently large renal pelvises, the initial needle is positioned within the renal pelvis using a low frequency (5 MHz) transducer with a biopsy guide or using a freehand technique. Intrapelvic needle position is confirmed by aspiration of 1 to 2 ml of urine, which is sent for culture. Care is taken to replace the exact volume of urine removed with contrast so as not to distort the opening pressure. A second needle is inserted using the same technique. Once in place, the needles are secured to the skin with Steri-Strips®. In children with a larger renal pelvis, the needles can be replaced by 18- to 20-gauge sheathed needles. The inner stylets are removed and the plastic sheath is used for infusion and pressure monitoring.

Either needle can be selected for contrast infusion or pressure monitoring. However, it is helpful to use the needle with the best urine flow for pressure monitoring. The next step is to connect one needle to an infusion pump and the other to a pressure-monitoring device (manometer or multichannel analyzer). The needle selected for pressure monitoring is fitted with a connecting tube and three-way stopcock. A second connecting tube joins the stopcock to a manometer, which is filled with water until it reads >40 cm H_2O. The stopcock is closed to maintain this preset level. This maneuver will allow for a rapid determination of opening pressure once the connecting tubing is connected to a needle and the stopcock opened. One will see a rapid descent of the water level, which will come to rest at the intrarenal pressure. Alternatively, one can allow the manometer to passively fill. Once the level comes to equilibrium an opening pressure is determined. Movement of the water level with respiration is expected.

A Foley catheter is inserted and initially used to drain the urinary bladder. The Foley catheter is then allowed to continuously drain in order to keep the urinary bladder empty and maintain a baseline pressure (usually at 0 cm H_2O) that is constantly measured by the multichannel analyzer or manometer. In children who require small catheters to drain the bladder, frequent aspiration may be needed to keep the bladder empty.

Once the system is in place, an opening pressure is obtained by opening the stopcock to the manometer until its level stabilizes. If a multichannel analyzer is used, the pressure is then recorded and the stopcock opened to the multichannel analyzer, which is calibrated and set at the opening pressure just obtained.

One-needle technique

This modification can also be used but is somewhat more cumbersome (Figure 6.23). The single-needle or catheter technique is an attractive alternative in patients who already have a nephrostomy in place, are high-risk patients with a coagulopathy, and those with anatomic variations or anomalies that may have difficult renal access. Infusion and pressure movements are made by alternating the position of the three-way stopcock from infusion to pressure measurement at

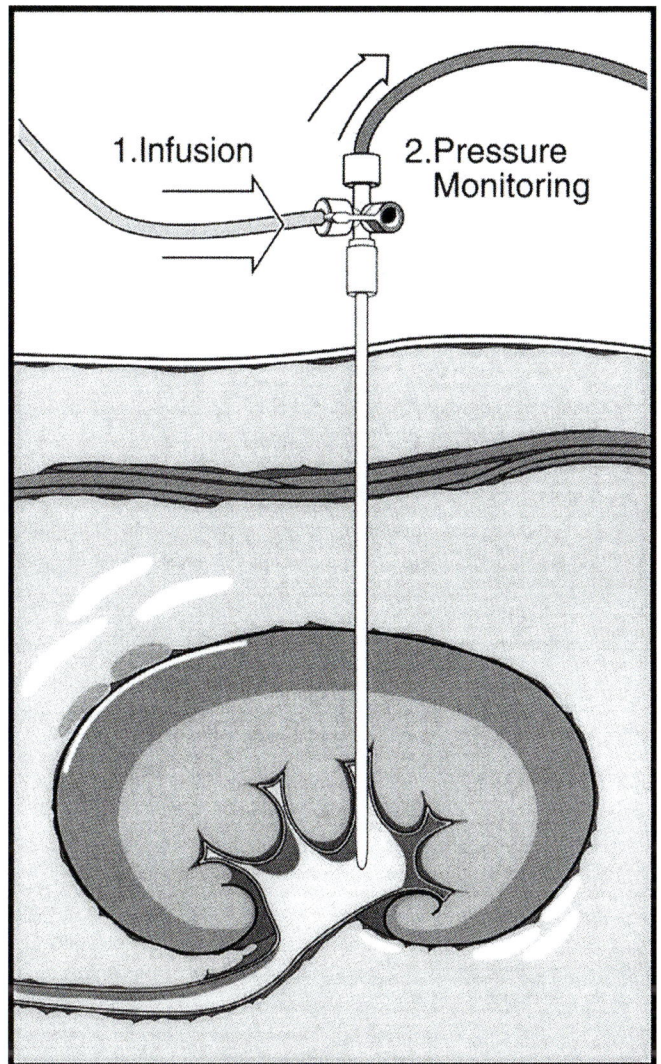

Figure 6.23 One-needle Whitaker test illustration. The one-needle variation of the Whitaker pressure–flow monitoring test may be useful in patients who already have a nephrostomy in place, or in whom more than one puncture is undesirable. The infusion can be interrupted at predetermined intervals to take pressure measurements by turning the three-way stopcock.

infusion is preferred, as is the case in our laboratory, then it is useful to begin at a low volume (2 to 4 ml/min), increase to a moderate volume (6 to 8 ml/min), and finish at a volume at the upper end of the physiologic range (10 ml/min). Using this graded technique one may be able to glean important information concerning the severity of obstruction. In some children, higher flow (supra-physiologic) rates (e.g., 12 to 20 ml/min) may be required to demonstrate obstruction.

Technical variations

The *ureteral opening pressure* is defined as the pressure at which contrast material is first seen beyond the suspected site of obstruction. With a catheter draining the bladder, contrast is instilled through a nephrostomy needle or catheter. Intrapelvic pressure is monitored as described above. Intermittent fluoroscopy is used to monitor the progress of the contrast column, and the ureteral opening pressure recorded when contrast is first detected beyond the site of suspected obstruction. Using this method, they found that a ureteral opening pressure elevated above 14 cm H_2O was 100% predictive of a positive Whitaker pressure–flow study in the same patient. Negative predictive values were not helpful. This test can easily be integrated into the conventional antegrade nephrostogram, when performed for the evaluation of suspected obstruction, and may obviate the need for more complicated studies (such as the stepped Whitaker test) when positive.

Postprocedure and follow-up care

Following the pressure–flow study, care centers around recovery of the child from sedation or GA and treatment of complications. Following the procedure, appropriate notes and postprocedure orders are entered into the patient's chart. It may be helpful to both patient care and ongoing quality assurance to maintain pertinent demographic and procedure-related data in an electronic database. Suggested items for data management are included in Table 6.6. As with other endourologic procedures under GA, children are monitored as they would be for any operative procedure. Children awakening from sedation have their vital signs continually monitored and recorded every 5 to 15 minutes for the first 30 to 60 minutes and then every 30 to 60 minutes until discharge.

When awake and alert, the child is given clear liquids to drink for the first few postprocedure hours. If liquids are tolerated the diet is advanced to solids. Discharge is considered when the child has returned to baseline neurologic status, and continued hydration is assured. In addition to monitoring vital signs, the nephrostomy site is monitored for evidence of bleeding. If no hematuria is identified, the Foley catheter is removed before the child awakens. Any complication identified is immediately treated, and the appropriate clinical service and referring physician are notified and consulted as appropriate.

predetermined time intervals. Thus in children with partial obstruction, there is a chance that the measured pressure may be falsely low due to ureteral run-off. Since renal access in most children is relatively simple, we prefer the two-needle technique whenever possible.

Perfusion measurement

Regardless of whether the one- or two-needle system is utilized, the operator may choose a single or stepped infusion rate. It is important to remember that the infusion of contrast should begin with the system at a steady state. If urine has been removed for culture or other laboratory tests the amount should be replaced volume for volume with saline before the infusion is initiated. If a single rate is selected, it is best to infuse at 10 ml/min to rule out obstruction. If a stepped

Technical problems and pitfalls

The Whitaker perfusion-flow study is customarily performed in a prone or semi-prone position. Pressure–flow relationships may be altered with changes in patient position, due to the native mobility of the kidney and its effect upon the angulation of the ureter at the UPJ. The resultant intermittent functional UPJ obstruction may be missed with conventional pressure–flow analysis. Patients who have variable results during Whitaker testing, with intermittent or unexplained symptoms, tortuous ureters, malpositioned kidneys, or previous urinary tract surgery should be considered for provocative pressure–flow testing in non-standard positions.

Failure to obtain pressure–flow measurements occur in fewer than 6% of attempted Whitaker procedures, most often during follow-up examination of a non-dilated collecting system after a successful intervention for a urinary tract lesion. Unrecognized extravasation during the pressure–flow study may confound the results, tending to yield a false-negative examination. Brief intermittent fluoroscopy allows appropriate monitoring with minimal additional radiation exposure, while ensuring that the study is completed with a full collecting system.

Complications

Complications occurring as a result of a pressure–flow study are uncommon and rarely mentioned in reports using this technique. Although no study has evaluated this point, it is likely that the use of large-bore needles or catheters and multiple puncture sites increases the risk of complications. When noted, untoward effects are usually minor and include transient hematuria, which generally clears within 24 hours. Occasionally, gross hematuria develops and can result in intrarenal clots and colicky pain. This too will usually resolve without the need for transfusion.

If bleeding is profuse and results in significant blood loss, angiography should be considered to exclude a renovascular injury. If a branch renal artery injury is noted, selective branch embolization is the treatment of choice. Other reported complications include transient flank pain with high-pressure perfusion, fluid extravasation during or after the procedure, urinary tract infection, pyelonephritis, renal abscess, peritonitis, hydrothorax, and inadvertent puncture of adjacent vessels or organs. The latter would be more likely when evaluating transplanted and ectopic kidneys. Although sepsis or bacteremia precipitated by the Whitaker procedure is seldom reported, it should be recognized that elevation of pyelocaliceal pressure during the examination may increase risk of systemic dissemination of infection from an untreated infection of an obstructed upper urinary tract.

Conclusions

Non-obstructive ureteric dilation was initially described by Shopfner in 1966. The concept that renal pelvis enlargement does not necessarily equal obstruction has since become widely accepted. Many diagnostic techniques, including excretory urography, renal US, and renal scintigraphy are able to demonstrate urinary tract dilation and, in some instances, determine the underlying etiology. When the cause of dilation is uncertain, a pressure–flow study may be a valuable tool. A Whitaker perfusion test will aid in the differentiation of non-obstructive from obstructive urinary tract dilation. As a result, endourologic or surgical intervention can be used more selectively.

Percutaneous treatment of renal cysts

Introduction

Renal cysts are common in adults but rare in children. The incidence and size of simple renal cysts increase as age advances. Approximately 5% of people have a simple renal cyst by their fourth decade of life, and by the eighth decade of life, the prevalence increases to well over 30%. In addition, cysts increase in both size and number. Cysts tend to grow more rapidly in people less than 50 years old than in those over 50 years of age. The prevalence of renal cysts in children is significantly lower. In fetuses, simple renal cysts are present in less than 0.1% of pregnancies, and most resolve prenatally. In children of all ages, there is a prevalence of 0.2% for simple cysts, and they usually range in size from 0.3 to 7.0 cm. Most cysts are found in the right upper pole. Most of these asymptomatic cysts will not change in size appreciably over time. In children, symptomatic cysts are rare. It is not known how many incidentally discovered cysts will become symptomatic. When present, associated symptoms may include pain, hematuria, ischemia, recurrent infection, obstructive uropathy, and hypertension.

The diagnosis of a benign renal cyst is usually made on the basis of the typical radiologic findings plus normal surrounding parenchyma, normal renal function, and absence of associated systemic illness or disease. In making the diagnosis of a simple renal cyst it is important to rule out a malignant or aggressive process. Although this is of concern in adults because of the risk of cystic malignancy, the risk of a misdiagnosed malignancy in childhood is small. However, to minimize the risk of a misdiagnosis the interventionalist should keep in mind the imaging features of a benign renal cyst (Table 6.9), which is defined as single and unilocular with a fibrous wall lined by a thin layer of simple cuboidal epithelium. While simple cysts are normally filled with clear fluid, they may contain blood related to trauma, or pus and debris related to superimposed infection. They do not communicate with the renal collecting system. The differential diagnosis of a cystic renal mass in a child includes common simple cysts as well as polycystic disease, acquired dysplasia, tuberous sclerosis and other syndromic diseases, glomerulocystic disease, cystic

Table 6.9 Imaging features of simple renal cysts

Ultrasonography
- Round to bulging, well circumscribed, anechoic mass
- Sharply defined posterior wall
- Surrounded by normal parenchyma
- Increased through transmission
- No central echoes (with high gain) or blood flow (with color Doppler)

Computed tomography
- Round, thin-walled mass
- Low attenuation (<15 HU)
- Non-enhancing (<10 HU increase with IV contrast administration)
- "Pseudo-enhancement" and "pseudo-thick-wall-sign" may confound interpretation

Magnetic resonance imaging
- Thin-walled, cystic lesion
- Low intensity on T_1-weighted images
- Homogeneous high intensity on T_2-weighted images

duplication, cystic Wilms tumor, previously treated malignancy, abscess, and calyceal diverticula.

Indications

Treatment is usually reserved for children with symptoms related to a renal cyst, remembering that parenchymal destruction or functional impairment are uncommon sequelae of simple renal cysts regardless of size or position. The desired endpoint of therapy is not eradication of the cyst, but resolution of the symptoms. Currently available treatment options include open surgical ablation, laparoscopic cyst ablation, retrograde marsupialization, flexible ureteroscopy and nephroscopy, and percutaneous aspiration with or without sclerotherapy (Figure 6.24).

Surgical treatment of a simple cyst may include decortication, marsupialization of the cyst, hemi-nephrectomy, or a complete nephrectomy. The advantage of the surgical approach is that it allows for direct visualization of the pathology. Thus if there is any doubt of the correct diagnosis, a biopsy can be obtained and the proper procedure performed based on the pathologic diagnosis. In addition, other pathology or problems can be addressed during the same operative procedure. Unfortunately, the perioperative complication rate is approximately 33%, making effective alternatives desirable. Perioperative complications include wound infection, problems associated with immobilization, urinary retention, atelectasis, pneumonia, and venous thrombosis. In addition, the procedure has significant postoperative pain and a relatively long convalescence.

Retrograde marsupialization and flexible ureteroscopy and nephroscopy are less invasive alternatives than open surgery. As a result, postoperative morbidity is minimized. However, there are several disadvantages to this approach including: a moderate to high degree of technical difficulty; the ability to only treat peri-pelvic cysts and not exophytic cysts; limited endoscopic visualization of the internal cyst wall; creation of a large nephrostomy tract and the need for a stent postoperatively; associated pain and discomfort; the potential for electrolyte disturbances secondary to the large volume of infusate used during the procedure; and the need for a second procedure to remove the ureteral stent.

Laparoscopic cyst ablation has the advantage of minimal postprocedural pain, no significant scarring, minimal blood loss, and a short hospital stay. This approach allows for the treatment of multiple renal cysts during the same operation including peri-pelvic and exophytic cysts, usually without the need for stents and drains at the completion of the procedure. Disadvantages of this approach include longer procedure times, need for expensive equipment and significant technical expertise, risk of injury to bowel and other organs, limited long-term results, and misdiagnosis of a benign cyst as a malignancy. Evaluation of a symptomatic cyst should include diagnostic cyst aspiration. A prospective comparison of laparoscopic de-roofing surgery and percutaneous sclerotherapy (see below) has not yet been performed, but would be helpful in more clearly defining the role of these minimally invasive approaches.

Technique

Image-guided percutaneous aspiration, with or without injection of a sclerosant, has an extremely high technical success rate and may be the least invasive alternative. With US or CT guidance, one or more cysts can be selected and accurately entered with a needle or small catheter. Once within the cyst cavity, a sterile sample of the fluid can be obtained for laboratory and microbiology analysis. If desired, contrast material can be exchanged for cyst fluid and the internal anatomy of the cyst examined.

During the same procedure, the cyst can be treated by either complete aspiration or sclerotherapy and drainage. At this time there are several sclerosing agents that can be used including absolute alcohol, hypertonic saline, doxycycline, minocycline, tetracycline, sodium tetradechol, sodium morhullate, acetic acid, talc, glue, Ethibloc® (not currently available in the United States) and recently bleomycin. Unfortunately, there are no prospective studies available to guide us as to what is the best agent. At this time, our preference is to pretreat the cyst with a local anesthetic, then sodium tetradecyl sulfate (STS) followed by either absolute alcohol or doxycycline. The reason for the use of STS is to injure the cell membranes and "cleanse" the lining of the cyst, making the subsequent treatment more likely to be successful. If necessary, a small catheter can be left in place, and the sclerotherapy can be repeated for two to three consecutive days before the catheter is removed. In general, complete cyst ablation is infrequent (approximately 10%) and reduction in size occurs in fewer than half of treated cases, although it is our experience that a significant improvement in symptoms is usually achieved. It has been our

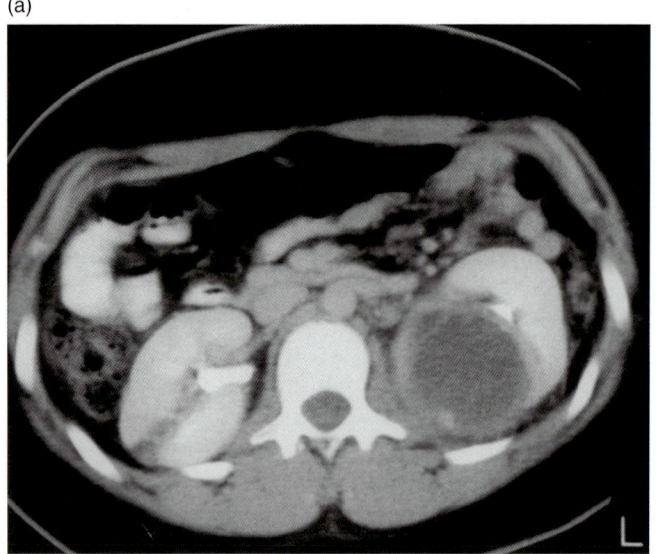
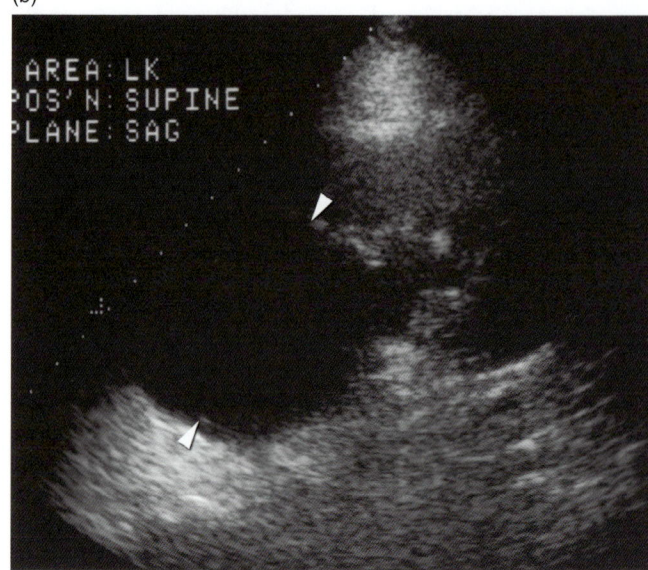
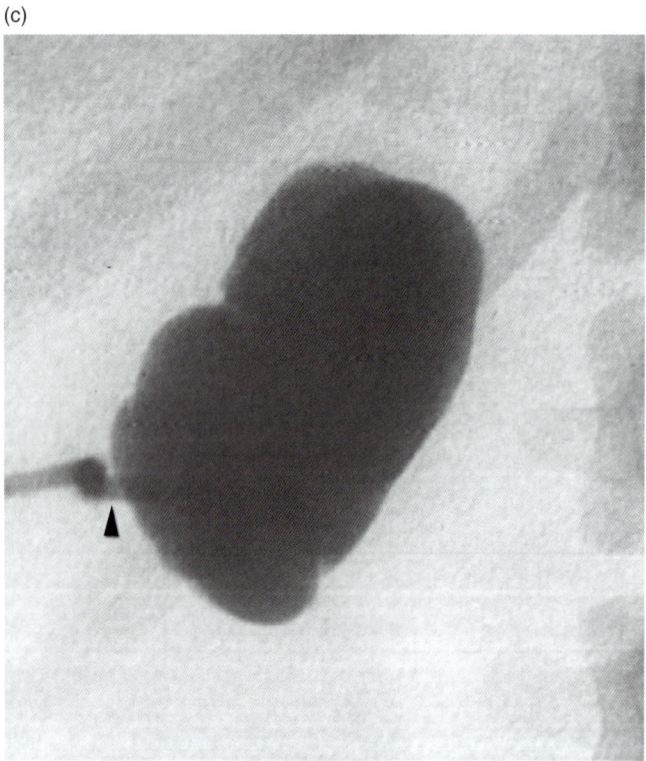

Figure 6.24 (a) An axial CT section with vascular and enteric contrast enhancement obtained through the kidneys shows bilateral renal cysts. The patient, a 15-year-old female, presented with recurring left flank pain presumed to be related to the large cyst extending from the medulla to the left renal hilum. (b) The fluid collection displayed US characteristics of a simple cyst (*arrowheads*) and was accessed with a 22-gauge Chiba needle under US guidance. (c) Under fluoroscopic control the cyst was drained with an 8.3-French APD catheter (*arrowhead*). A sample of clear fluid was obtained and the cyst evacuated before initiating sclerotherapy treatments with absolute alcohol. Although the symptoms resolved with initial drainage, ablation of the cyst required serial treatments every two weeks over a period of months. Our current practice is to repeat treatments every 24 to 72 hours.

observation that results improve with a series of treatments, but we do not have enough experience or follow-up to be certain. If the cyst is still present but the patient is asymptomatic, the therapy is considered a success, and the patient is observed and followed.

The main disadvantage of percutaneous therapy is the relatively high recurrence rate of 54%. In addition, recurrent pain in the early phase of recovery occurs in approximately 15% of patients, with an 8% rate of other complications including cyst hemorrhage. Acquired stricture of the UPJ secondary to injury by the sclerosant has been reported in as many as 2% of cases, and the overall rate of major and minor complications is reported to be 1.4% and 10%, respectively.

Equipment

The equipment needed to perform a cyst aspiration and sclerotherapy is minimal and depends upon the interventionalist's preference. If sclerotherapy is to be performed, there is little evidence to assist the selection of an appropriate agent or agents. In most cases, the cyst is punctured using US guidance and on occasion using CT guidance. The needles used most often are 22- or 23-gauge Chiba needles or a sheathed needle.

Patient preparation

Children requiring cyst drainage with or without sclerosis need no special preparation. Since either general anesthesia (GA) or intravenous sedation is needed for the procedure, the child must be NPO according to relevant hospital policies for anesthesia and sedation. In patients who are otherwise healthy, no routine laboratory tests are obtained except for a urinalysis.

A CBC with differential and platelet count and, when indicated by patient or family history, a coagulation profile are obtained preoperatively. High acuity children (ASA 3 or greater), those with immune deficiency or other conditions predisposing to infection, children with congenital heart disease, and those in whom there are procedural difficulties or complications may be treated with prophylactic antibiotics before, during, or after the procedure. The antibiotic chosen may vary with the age and underlying condition of the child. Recommendations are included in Chapter 1.

After sedation or induction with GA, the child is placed in the position that makes access to the cyst easiest. The prone or prone-oblique position with the side of interest elevated is most often chosen. The patient's position is stabilized with a combination of high-density foam sponges, rolled-up linen, or other materials, taking care to adequately protect potential pressure points. The child is secured to the tabletop with Velcro® straps and tape if necessary.

Standard technique

After sedation or anesthesia is achieved, the flank is prepared and draped in sterile fashion. Access to the cyst is achieved by US-guided needle access. An entry site is selected on the skin surface after US examination. The most direct route to the cyst is selected whenever possible. The skin is marked, and the site is prepared and draped in sterile fashion. When the procedure is performed under sedation, buffered 1% lidocaine is *slowly* infiltrated into the skin and subcutaneous tissue with a 30-gauge, 1.5-inch needle to minimize discomfort, and a small incision is made with a #11 scalpel blade. Once this step is complete, the deep soft tissue to the level of the renal capsule is anesthetized with a 22-gauge Chiba needle. Infiltration with local anesthetic may be used in conjunction with GA based on operator preference.

There is more than one approach that may be safely and successfully utilized. When the goal is simply aspiration of the cyst contents to acquire fluid for laboratory analysis, a 22- or 23-gauge Chiba needle or sheathed needle can be utilized. Using either a biopsy guide or freehand technique, the needle is advanced into the cyst. The stylet is removed, and the needle is attached to connecting tubing (small volume T-connector) and a syringe. Next, a fluid sample is obtained using sterile technique. The cyst is emptied until drainage stops, and the needle is removed.

Depending on the approach selected, the interventionalist may choose to drain the cyst before the sclerosant is injected and later, drain out the material. In these cases, either the sheath can be left in position or a drainage catheter (locking pigtail) may be inserted after the needle is exchanged for a guide wire and the tract dilated. In these cases, selection of the appropriate guide wire is most important.

If a floppy tipped guide wire is selected, one must be careful to ensure that the entire floppy segment can coil inside the cyst cavity so that the stiff portion of the guide wire is used to enlarge the tract. If the floppy segment traverses the cyst wall, it may be difficult or impossible to gain catheter access into the cyst. If the child is thickset or obese, it is helpful to use a stiffer guide wire. Thus several guide wire types should be available including an angled Glide® wire, Rosen, Roadrunner®, and stiff Glide® wire. Other guide wires can also be equally successful as long as the length of the floppy portion is minimal. The tract is dilated with fascial dilators to the size of the catheter.

Finally, the catheter chosen is usually a standard pigtail ranging in size from 5 to 8.3 French. It is important to keep in mind that the larger the drainage catheter, the larger the defect in the cyst wall will be when the catheter is removed. This may be a source of hemorrhage into the abdominal or retroperitoneal spaces or of leakage and potential injury to the tissues adjacent to the defect.

If the goal of the procedure is sclerosis of the cyst, the procedural approach is modified slightly. The procedure is performed as stated for aspiration; however, a sheathed needle (Yueh) is substituted for the Chiba needle. Once the cyst has been entered, only the minimum necessary amount of fluid is removed for culture and laboratory analysis so that the cyst does not collapse.

In the usual case, a Glide® wire is advanced and coiled within the cyst while monitoring under fluoroscopy. The needle is then exchanged for a vascular dilator and the tract enlarged to the size of the catheter to be inserted. Depending on the size of the child, a catheter is selected and inserted over the guide wire. If the patient weighs less than 10 kg, a 5- to 6-French drain with a 1 cm in diameter distal pigtail would be inserted. In children greater than 10 kg, a 6- or 8.3-French drain may be used.

Postprocedure and follow-up care

After the catheter is secured, the cyst fluid is completely drained. Dilute contrast is injected to define the limits of the cyst cavity and exclude communication with the renal collecting system (suggesting a calyceal diverticulum). The volume of contrast necessary to fill the cyst is noted, and the volume of local anesthetic or sclerosant to follow is usually approximately half this volume. Although there is no particular sclerosant that is proven to be superior to others, we have preferred the use of sodium tetradecyl sulfate (STS) followed by either doxycycline or alcohol. In selecting a volume of alcohol, we have generally used a maximum 1 ml/kg to a maximum of 50 ml.

After evacuating the contrast, a half-volume of 1% lidocaine may be instilled and allowed to remain for five to ten minutes. The lidocaine is evacuated, and a half-volume of STS is instilled. This is allowed to dwell for approximately four minutes, then it is evacuated and the primary sclerosant (usually dehydrated alcohol or doxycycline) is instilled. This is allowed to dwell from ten minutes to up to four hours, then the cyst is drained and the drainage catheter attached to a bulb suction device.

Regardless of the agent selected, the child is positioned so that the entire cyst wall is exposed to the sclerosant with the hope of destroying the cyst wall and preventing continued secretion of fluid. Hanna and Dahniya have shown that the epithelial cells lining the cyst wall become fixed and non-viable in one to three minutes after contact with the alcohol, and the cyst capsule is penetrated after four to twelve hours. In theory, the longer the contact time between the cyst wall and the alcohol, the lower the likelihood of recurrence. It is for this reason that the sclerosant may be kept in the cyst for up to four hours before being allowed to drain. Some investigators advocate a second or third injection of sclerosant to reduce the possibility of recurrence, which is similar to our recommendations for treatment of perinephric lymphoceles (see Chapter 4: "Abdominopelvic interventions"). A similar approach can be used to treat other forms of renal cystic disease, such as adult polycystic kidney disease or cysts of other solid organs such as the spleen.

At the completion of the treatment, the drain is removed and a dry sterile dressing placed. If no problems or complications have occurred, the child is discharged home after an additional 30 to 60 minutes of observation. If a second procedure is desired, the patient is scheduled to return or admitted to the hospital. In these individuals, the drain is left in place and covered to maintain sterility and reduce the chance of inadvertent removal. It is our opinion at this time that when multiple sclerosant treatments are required, they are most effectively given every day or two for the duration of therapy.

Complications

As is the case with any procedure, there is a risk of adverse effects. In addition, the recurrence of pain in the early phase of recovery is approximately 15%, and there is an 8% rate of complications including cyst hemorrhage. Acquired stricture of the UPJ secondary to injury by the sclerosant has been reported in as many as 2% of cases, and the overall rate of major and minor complications is reported to be 1.4% and 10% respectively. The potential risks of cyst puncture are similar to those seen with other percutaneous renal interventions such as renal or perirenal hemorrhage, extravasation of urine or sclerosant, injury of adjacent structures, and technical misadventures. The complications and their treatments have been discussed in prior sections. While not a complication, some patients note slight inebriation when treated with alcohol as a sclerosant. The expected effects should be explained to the patient and parents, and instructions given to older patients to avoid risky activities (such as driving or operating heavy machinery!) in the 24 hours following sclerosis with this agent.

Conclusions

Most simple renal cysts in the pediatric population are benign, although the proportion of malignant cysts is higher in children than in adults. Most solitary cysts are easily differentiated as simple or complicated on the basis of cross-sectional imaging criteria. Those that are not clearly benign must be investigated, usually via needle aspiration or biopsy, either percutaneously with image guidance or via an open surgical technique. Benign cysts usually do not impair function and are asymptomatic, characteristically discovered incidentally during investigation for other reasons. Those that are symptomatic or cause functional impairment can sometimes be safely and effectively treated via a percutaneous route with image guidance, either by aspiration alone or using a sclerosant. Where successful, this approach offers a cost-effective and minimally invasive alternative. If these approaches fail to resolve the symptoms, the patient may be better treated using a laparoscopic or even open surgical technique.

Tract dilation

Introduction

Casteneda-Zuniga and colleagues first described progressive dilation of the percutaneous tract as an adjunct to nephrostomy access in 1982. This simple technique is characteristic of transitional procedures (as described in "A modular approach to interventional radiology" in Chapter 1) in that it enables many of the complex procedures that follow below, but is not an end in itself. It is essential to enlarge a nephrostomy tract so that larger equipment can be safely and accurately inserted into the renal pelvis or distal urinary tract. As such, it is one of the fundamental modules, the bridging module, for genitourinary procedures and an essential component of the interventionalist's armamentarium.

Indications

The indication for dilation of a nephrostomy puncture site or nephrostomy tube tract is for the insertion of a stent or angioplasty balloon or for an endosurgical procedure. In the latter case, large diameter sheaths (12 to 24 French) are necessary. The contraindications to tract dilation are rare and generally are the same as those discussed for nephrostomy insertion. It is important to keep the size of the child in mind when choosing the diameter of the sheath to be left in place. In general, the sheath size recommended is two French larger

Table 6.10 Equipment: tract dilation

- Progressive dilators
- Angioplasty balloon (3 French = 1 mm)
- Non-kinking guide wire (e.g., Glide® stiff or super-stiff)

Table 6.11 Procedure summary: tract dilation

- Coil wire in cavity (e.g., renal pelvis, bladder) or stabilize in lumen (e.g., ureter)
- Dilate tract with progressive dilators or with a non-compliant balloon up to a diameter equal to or greater than the sheath or catheter diameter
- Insert sheath or catheter

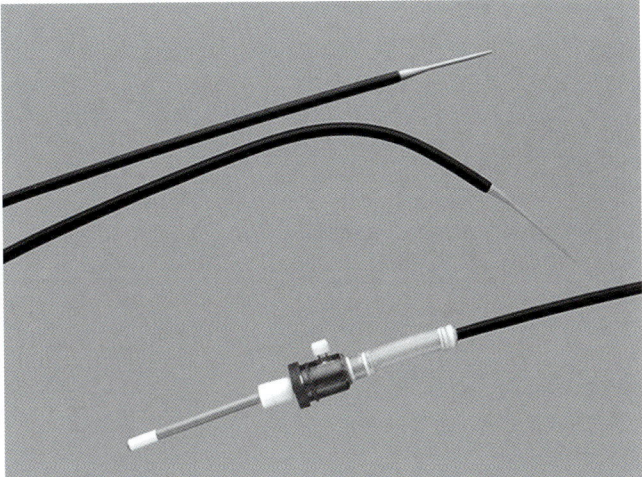

Figure 6.25 The Keller–Timmermans introducer (shown) or Rutner adapter allows balloon catheters and other instruments, such as endoscopes, to be introduced through a self-sealing port.

than the diameter of the largest instrument to be used. In small children, overdilation of a transrenal tract can lead to a fractured kidney and is performed only when necessary.

Technique

Equipment

The equipment used is usually readily available in intervention suites (Table 6.10). The only caveat in the pediatric population is the need for smaller sheaths. In the standard Amplatz® progressive dilator sets (see Figure 4.20), the dilators range from 6 to 30 French, but the smallest gray sheath is 18 French. In most children less than six years of age this is usually too large. Fascial dilators range from 4 to 36 French, and metal coaxial dilators range from 4 to 24 French. Caution must be exercised when using these dilators to avoid the risk of perforation of the renal pelvis and associated hemorrhage or fluid extravasation. If desired the tract may be dilated with a PTA balloon. This has the advantage of reduced procedure time and increased safety but has a greater expense.

Pediatric endoscopes begin at 6 French, therefore 8-French and sometimes 10-French sheaths are used. These small sheaths can be ordered. Alternatively, peel-away sheaths are also available in these sizes; however, a Rutner adapter cannot be fitted to them. A Rutner adapter is a connective device that snugly fits over the external end of a sheath, permitting an endoscope to pass through an O-ring that keeps the irrigant from leaking out and is helpful in keeping both the patient and the procedure room dry. For larger sheath sizes (18 to 24 French), the Keller–Timmermans introducer (Figure 6.25) or Rutner adapter have similar properties. As mentioned elsewhere, appropriate caution must be exercised since obstructing free egress of irrigant during these procedures may increase the risk of ureteral or pelvic perforation, fluid extravasation, and electrolyte imbalance.

Patient preparation

When nephrostomy tract dilation must be accomplished as a separate procedure from the original access, the patient record should be reviewed and current data confirmed regarding the patient's coagulation state and the absence of active infection. The appropriate NPO status should be ordered based on hospital policies. In addition, any other routine preoperative order is obtained.

Standard technique

Once access to the renal pelvis is obtained, either by direct puncture or by using an indwelling catheter, a non-kinkable guide wire is inserted and coiled within the renal pelvis or directed into the ureter or bladder (Table 6.11). Using vascular dilators, the tract is progressively enlarged at 2- to 4-French intervals to the predetermined diameter. At that point, a sheath (one French larger than the dilator) is loaded piggyback onto the dilator and positioned in the renal pelvis. If endoscopy is to be used a Rutner adapter is fitted onto the sheath to make a watertight connection. In many cases, the sheath needs to be shortened by cutting it with scissors. The shorter sheath is easier to work with and better fits the shorter pediatric endoscope.

Alternatively, once a guide wire is in position, the tract may be dilated with a percutaneous transluminal angioplasty catheter (1 mm = 3 French) instead of progressive dilators. The balloon catheter is exchanged for the appropriate-sized sheath that is necessary to provide access for percutaneous surgery. In most cases, we prefer progressive tract dilation to balloon enlargement of the tract because of the lower cost.

Complications

The two serious complications particularly associated with tract development through the renal parenchyma are renal fracture and pelvic perforation. Other complications related to tract dilation are discussed with the associated procedures (see, for example, "Percutaneous nephrolithotomy," "Percutaneous endopyelotomy," etc.).

Conclusions

With nephrostomy access, tract dilation is one of the fundamental procedures that permits more complex endourologic genitourinary interventions. The interventionalist should have more than one approach to achieve tract enlargement in a variety of situations, including small children and children with tough perirenal scar tissue. The procedure should be completed in an environment that is comfortable and familiar to the interventionalist, with high-quality imaging equipment to maximize the quality of the tract dilation or associated procedure. Although it is our preference to enlarge the tract with dilators rather than an angioplasty balloon, either approach may be used with similar safety. It is probably more important to avoid multiple renal punctures when possible and to avoid renal pelvic perforation, since these circumstances are associated with a much higher risk of significant hemorrhage and renal injury.

Percutaneous nephrolithotomy

Introduction

In industrialized countries, urinary calculi are uncommon in the pediatric population. When stones occur, they often relate to an underlying anatomic or metabolic disorder (e.g., ureteroenteric anastomic strictures, ureteropelvic junction obstruction, infundibular stenosis, stones in caliceal diverticula, horseshoe kidney, Lesch–Nyhan syndrome, hyperparathyroidism, hyperoxaluria, hypercalciuria, hypocitraturia) or may be infectious in origin. Coexisting medical problems and their treatments may also predispose to upper tract calculus formation, including relative patient immobility, chronic furosemide treatment, chronic corticosteroid treatment, and inflammatory bowel disease. Prior to the advent of percutaneous nephrostomy and extracorporeal shock wave lithotripsy (ESWL), surgical procedures were required for treatment of recurrent stone disease. Fernstrom and Johannson first described percutaneous nephrolithotomy as an alternative to surgery in adults in 1976. The technique was extended to the pediatric population by Woodside and colleagues in 1985.

Currently, management of renal calculi in both adults and children benefits from a combination of techniques. Either alone or in combination with ESWL, percutaneous nephrolithotomy and ureteroscopy may be helpful for management of calculi without surgery. The ability to treat renal calculi using a minimally invasive approach is especially important in pediatric patients with underlying anatomic or metabolic abnormalities, who may expect to require a number of stone-related procedures over their lifetimes. Both ESWL and endoscopic techniques have had a profound impact on the management of renal calculi and have limited the use of percutaneous techniques, although the realization of limitations of ESWL has led to a resurgence of interest in endourologic alternatives.

Prior to the availability of ESWL, percutaneous techniques were considered superior to open surgery because of reduced cost, decreased morbidity, shortened convalescence, and abbreviated hospital stay. In addition, the presence of a nephrostomy tract enabled subsequent removal of any residual stone fragments. Although its role has changed, the need for percutaneous stone removal persists. It is used primarily to treat individuals who are not candidates for ESWL or those with residual or complicated stone disease. Extracorporeal shock wave lithotripsy is now the treatment of choice for uncomplicated small renal calculi, while transurethral ureteroscopy is widely accepted as the method for removal of lower and mid-ureteral calculi. There has been a suggestion that single stones in the lower pole of the kidney may be more successfully treated with percutaneous nephrolithotomy rather than ESWL (due to the unfavorable angle between the lower infundibulum and the renal pelvis), albeit with a higher rate of complications, but application in the pediatric population is untested. Upper ureteral calculi are usually managed by retrograde ureteral catheterization and dislodgment back into the renal pelvis for subsequent ESWL. However, with appropriate patient stratification, percutaneous nephrolithotomy in children has shown successful results with stone-free rates at discharge of 67 to 100%.

Indications

Indications for calculus removal include pain, gross hematuria, urinary tract infection, and obstruction. Percutaneous nephrolithotomy as the initial or only therapy is preferable for patients with large stone volumes such as staghorn or branched calculi, which if fragmented are likely to cause obstruction, as well as for hard stones that are resistant to fracture by shock waves (such as cystine stones as in Figure 6.26). Additional indications include stones that are not accessible within the focus of the shock wave and with conditions that inhibit passage of stone fragments (e.g., caliceal stones or ureteral stricture). Extracorporeal shock wave lithotripsy is known to be significantly less successful with increasing stone size and multiplicity.

During the treatment of a large or staghorn calculus (Figure 6.27), percutaneous evacuation of the stone material combined with fragmentation either using ESWL or percutaneous ultrasonic lithotripsy may offer a safer and more predictable course than with ESWL alone. For these reasons, initial percutaneous nephrolithotomy has been recommended by the American Urological Association guidelines for most patients in whom staghorn calculi are likely of infectious origin, followed by ESWL as necessary. Renal calculi associated with obstruction either at the ureteropelvic junction (UPJ) or in the ureter may be better managed percutaneously. Similarly, patients with renal calculi in a horseshoe kidney, especially when the stone burden is large or complex, may benefit from

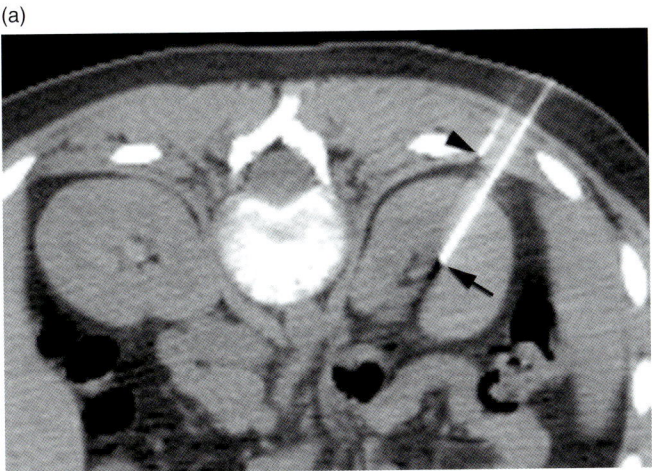
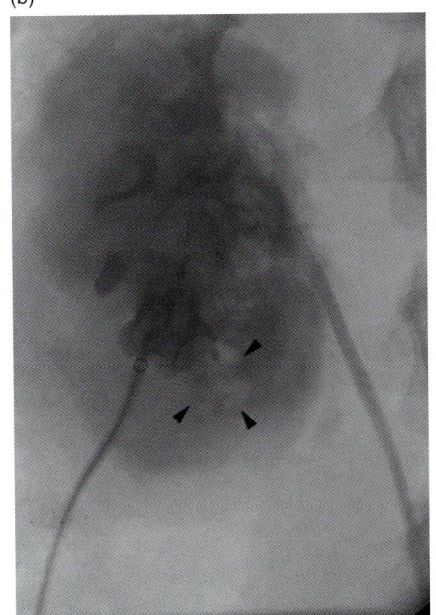
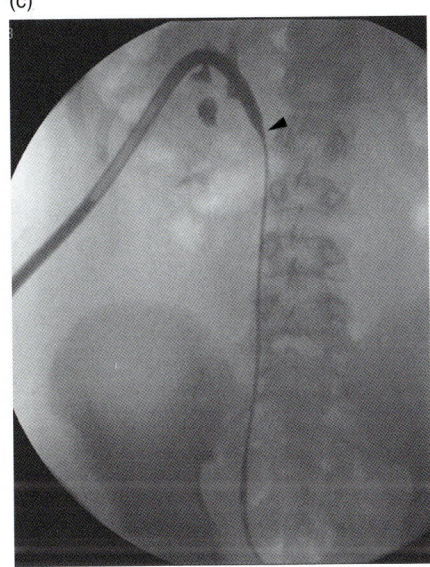

Figure 6.26 (a) Intraprocedural CT section obtained through the renal hilum with the patient in a prone position. This 15-year-old male had a history of repeated surgeries for removal of cystine stones, and now complained of pain and left ureteral obstruction. Under general anesthesia, using CT guidance, a 23-gauge Chiba needle (*arrowhead*) was used to determine a path to the kidney and using this as a tandem guide and "guard rail" an 18-gauge needle (*arrow*) was advanced through a posterior calyx into the renal pelvis. (b) After obtaining access, the patient was moved to the angiography suite where an antegrade nephrostogram was performed, showing a 1.5 cm renal calculus (*arrowheads*) too large to be retrieved through the infundibulum. (c) Over a 0.035-inch stiff wire, the percutaneous tract was dilated to 9 French, and an 8.5-French nephroureteral catheter (*arrowhead*) placed with its tip in the bladder. The patient was transferred to the urology service where holmium:YAG laser lithotripsy was performed and the stone fragments successfully retrieved with a basket.

percutaneous nephrolithotomy. Extracorporeal shock wave lithotripsy is also precluded when spinal stabilization hardware is present as in children with myelodysplasia, a group that constitutes a significant proportion of the pediatric renal calculi population. Additional relative indications for percutaneous nephrolithotomy include concomitant procedure under a single anesthesia, presence of a previously placed nephrostomy tube, inability to visualize the stone for ESWL, and prior ureterovesical surgery.

Contraindications to percutaneous nephrolithotomy are infrequent but include an uncorrectable coagulopathy and severe hyperkalemia. Limiting factors with respect to percutaneous nephrolithotomy include the degree of associated pyelocaliectasis. While older children may be successfully treated with the same instruments used in adults, smaller children warrant consideration of alternative instruments or technology appropriate for their size. Renal access may be difficult, and there may be insufficient room to maneuver instruments if the collecting system is not large enough. Also, in small children, the size of the kidney may make tract dilation to greater than 10 to 12 French dangerous for fear of long-term damage to the kidney, such as renal fracture or vascular injury.

Technique

Equipment

A wide range of instruments should be available for successful percutaneous stone removal (Table 6.12). Best results are achieved through collaboration between the interventionalist and the urologist. Stone baskets and grasping forceps are useful for removing small stones or fragments. In addition, occlusion balloon catheters and 60 ml irrigation syringes may be helpful in dislodging stones or fragments into favorable positions for retrieval. Occlusion balloon catheters may be helpful in preventing stone fragments from entering and filling the ureter. Calculi can be crushed mechanically or by using ultrasonic lithotripsy or laser fibers. These devices have

Chapter 6 Genitourinary interventions

Table 6.12 Equipment: percutaneous nephrolithotomy

Dilators
- Progressive renal dilators and sheaths 8 to 30 French

Retrieval devices
Baskets
- four wire Segura
- helical and flat wire
- loop retriever ± steerable catheter system

Grasping forceps
- with steerable catheter system
- retrieval/grasping forceps

Occlusion balloon catheter (5 to 7 French; compliant)

Ultrasonic lithotriptor

irrigation and suction ports allowing aspiration and removal of stone fragments as they are formed.

Several types of stone baskets and forceps are manufactured and some may be used through catheters. These tools may also be used through endoscopes. Different configurations of baskets, loop snares, and forceps allow selection of a device appropriate for the size and position of the stone and renal pelvis. With forceps, the stone must be identifiable on two orthogonal images (i.e., 90 degrees apart) to prevent intrarenal injury. Biplane fluoroscopy is particularly helpful to facilitate use of this equipment. If the renal pelvis is small, it may be difficult to open the basket to engage the stone. In this situation it is helpful to push the basket against the far wall of the renal pelvis.

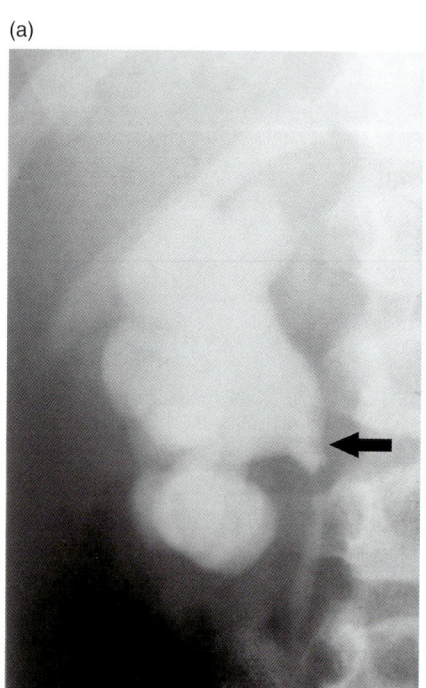
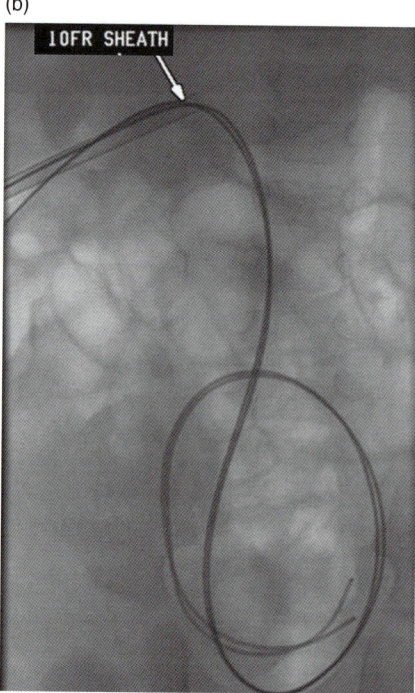
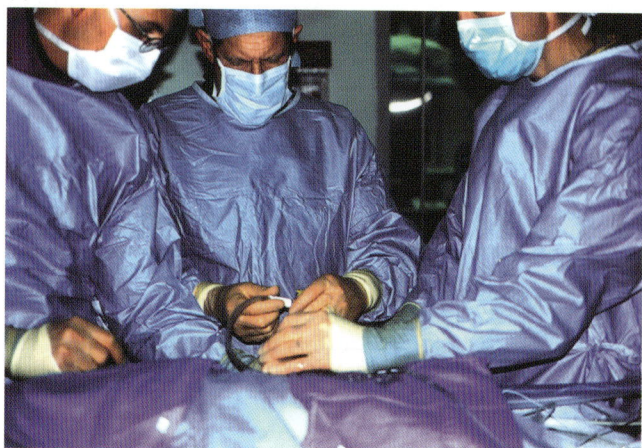

Figure 6.27 (a) Excretory urography demonstrates a renal calculus (*arrow*) lodged in the ureteropelvic junction in this 16-year-old female. (b) After obtaining percutaneous access using US guidance, the tract was dilated to 12 French with fascial dilators, and a 10-French sheath (*arrow*) was inserted, as shown on this fluoroscopic image of the abdomen and upper pelvis. Two guide wires are visualized, a safety wire alongside the sheath and a working wire through the sheath, both terminating in the urinary bladder. (c) Working together as a multidisciplinary team, the interventionalists and urologists are able to capitalize on complementary skill sets to solve difficult problems relating to access, instrumentation, manipulation, and retrieval within the urinary system. (d) In this case, having the interventionalist maneuver the sheath and endoscope (*arrowhead*) near the stone (*arrow*) under fluoroscopic guidance saved significant operative time compared to searching for the stone with the endoscope alone. (e) Once the stone is fragmented (different patient) it may be removed using stone baskets, grasping forceps, aspiration, or other similar methods.

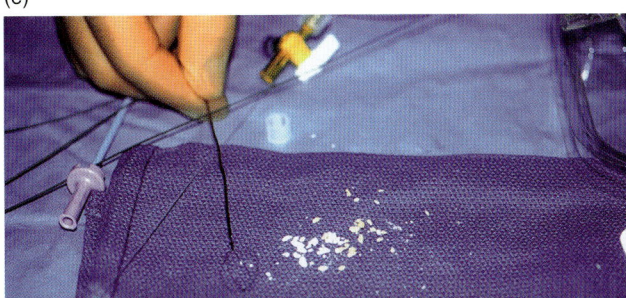

Figure 6.27 (cont.)

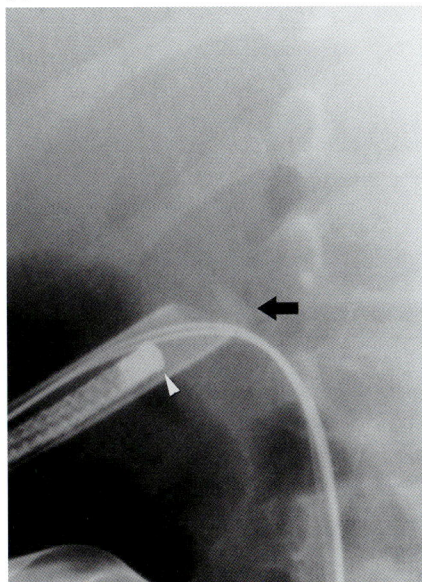

Patient preparation

Preparation for percutaneous nephrolithotomy is similar to that for percutaneous nephrostomy insertion (see above). The two procedures are often performed in sequence under the same anesthesia. From each child undergoing an endourologic procedure the following laboratory studies are usually obtained: BUN, creatinine, CBC with platelet count, coagulation profile, and in rare cases a bleeding time. A urine culture is generally obtained prior to the day of the urinary tract manipulation. Children with suspected or proven urinary tract infections are given preprocedural antibiotics. In addition, all patients should undergo a thorough metabolic evaluation due to the high rate of underlying metabolic abnormalities in children presenting with renal calculi.

Since each child will necessarily undergo either general anesthesia (GA) or intravenous sedation, the child must be NPO. As is the case for other interventions, the NPO time for sedation is according to hospital policy.

Standard technique

Percutaneous nephrolithotomy is performed under fluoroscopic guidance. In most cases, single plane C-arm fluoroscopy is adequate. However in some instances, biplane fluoroscopy is useful. In most cases, nephrostomy insertion is guided by real-time US, although fluoroscopy after contrast injection, retrograde opacification using cystoscopic guidance, or even blind puncture may be used on occasion. Securing access with a guide wire can be especially challenging when the pelvis is filled by a large stone burden (e.g., with a staghorn calculus). This problem is briefly discussed under "Technical variations," below. Cystoscopic guidance with insertion of a ureteral catheter for contrast injection may be convenient when nephrolithotomy is performed as a one-step procedure. Stone removal is performed under direct vision via a nephroscope, but fluoroscopic guidance can be time saving for localization of the stone.

Nephrolithotomy requires the establishment of a nephrostomy tract from 8 to 24 French depending on the size of the child and the nephroscope used. We prefer the use of a pediatric nephroscope (8 to 12 French) whenever possible to minimize potential complications. Stone removal can be performed in one or two stages (Table 6.13). Some interventionalists prefer the two-stage approach where on the first day a tract is established, followed by tract enlargement and stone removal at a later date. Others prefer a single-stage procedure since it can be performed under one general anesthetic. The approach that is selected will usually be based on the preferences of the treating physicians.

The location and size of the renal calculus is initially determined by US or CT examination. Excretory urography is rarely used at this time for diagnosis. Prior to the procedure, an abdominal radiograph is obtained to confirm the presence of the stone. The most important factor for successful percutaneous nephrolithotomy is appropriate placement of the nephrostomy tract. A posterolateral puncture is preferred so that a direct route to the ureter is obtained and effective tamponade achieved to limit bleeding. The target calyx depends on the location of the calculus. Pelvic and middle caliceal calculi are best approached via a middle calyx puncture. Calculi in the lower and upper pole calyces may be approached through a lower pole calyx. With multiple calculi, more than one puncture may be required.

Table 6.13 Procedure summary: percutaneous nephrolithotomy

- Select access route through posterior calyx that provides most direct approach to stone(s)
- Obtain needle access to the renal pelvis under image guidance
- Dilate tract to at least diameter of sheath
- Insert sheath (sized for nephroscope if planned) and safety wire
- If a nephroscope will be used, prevent leakage with a sealed (e.g., Rutner) adapter
- Combine fluoroscopic and endoscopic guidance to direct instruments to stone(s)
- For stones >3 cm, mechanical fragmentation (with lithotriptor or laser) is recommended
- Retrieve stones and stone fragments with grasping forceps or baskets
- Perform antegrade pyelogram to confirm absence of stones and unobstructed ureteral drainage
- A temporary nephrostomy catheter may be left for re-access if necessary or until normal antegrade drainage is confirmed

Once access to the renal pelvis has been achieved, a 0.035-inch or 0.038-inch guide wire is advanced into the ureter and preferably to the urinary bladder. The presence of a long, stiff guide wire makes later manipulations easier. If the guide wire cannot be passed into the ureter, it is initially coiled in the renal pelvis or upper pole calyx. A directional catheter (JB-1) is used if there is difficulty traversing the UPJ. In cases with a calyceal calculus, it may be challenging to get renal access and pass the calculus with a wire. In these cases, use of a 3- to 4-French coaxial sheath with a stiffener and an 0.018-inch angled Glide® wire can be helpful.

Prior to tract dilation, a generous skin incision is made. Tract enlargement is accomplished with either progressive dilators or an angioplasty balloon of appropriate size. Final tract size is dependent upon the diameter of the endoscope selected. In general, a sheath two French sizes larger than the endoscope is used. It may be helpful to cut the sheath to increase the sheath stability in the renal collecting system and make instrumentation easier. The sheath acts to tamponade the fresh tract to prevent bleeding, reduce renal injury, and maintain access to the renal pelvis for insertion of instruments and catheters.

When the tract dilation is complete and the sheath is in place, it is fitted with a sealed adapter (e.g., a Rutner adapter) through which the endoscope is inserted. This valve allows the field to remain relatively dry. Alternatively, a sheath with a rotating hemostatic valve may be used. As a precaution against loss of renal access during the procedure, a safety guide wire is inserted and coiled in the renal pelvis. However, if the primary guide wire is externalized at both the urethra and the nephrostomy tract (i.e., "body floss"), a safety guide wire is not needed.

Stone removal can be achieved using several approaches. For smaller stones, removal is accomplished under direct visualization or fluoroscopic guidance with a basket or forceps. Irrigation and aspiration with saline may be successful in removing stones or fragments smaller than the diameter of the sheath. Occlusion balloon catheters may be helpful in preventing dislodgment of fragments into the ureter. For stones greater than 1.5 cm in size, fragmentation will usually be required prior to removal. Calculi can be crushed mechanically or by ultrasonic lithotripsy. These lithotriptors have irrigation and suction ports allowing removal of fragments as they are formed.

Technical variations

Percutaneous management of caliceal diverticula

Epithelium-lined cavities protruding from the renal collecting system are termed caliceal diverticula. Although often noted incidentally on imaging obtained for unrelated reasons, stones will be found in as many as half, and almost 90% will become symptomatic within ten years of diagnosis. Multiple small, smooth, round renal calculi detected by US, CT, or KUB, or a stone in a peripheral location, may suggest the diagnosis. When patients are symptomatic, they may present with intermittent and poorly localized flank or abdominal pain, recurrent urinary tract infections, or a history of vesicoureteral reflux. Pain, infection, compromised renal function, and calculi associated with a caliceal diverticulum are indications for treatment.

Intervention should be aimed at complete evacuation of any stones and obliteration of the diverticulum. The procedure is similar to that for percutaneous stone removal from the renal pelvis, involving the same sequence of modular techniques: access, guide wire stabilization, tract dilation, and stone retrieval, as discussed above. However, the complexity of the procedure is increased by the difficulty maintaining access to the diverticulum once achieved, and by the relatively small working space available.

Access is accomplished by direct calyceal puncture under image guidance. Ultrasound is preferred for procedural guidance, if a suitable window is available. If a stone is radiographically apparent or if the diverticulum can be opacified, such maneuvers may make fluoroscopic guidance more helpful, either in lieu of or in addition to US guidance. Under certain circumstances, CT guidance may also be useful. Because a symptomatic diverticulum is often edematous or inflamed, the communication between the diverticulum and the collecting system is seldom accessible, and a retrograde approach is not recommended. Stone retrieval and obliteration of the diverticulum are accomplished in most (greater than 80%) patients treated by a direct antegrade percutaneous approach to the diverticulum.

Pelvic access with a large stone burden

While a large stone burden often simplifies localization of the renal pelvis by offering a radio-opaque target, it may reduce the room available for successfully maneuvering a guide wire to no more than a potential space, frustrating repeated attempts to secure access. However, several strategies may be employed to improve the opportunity for success. First, if urinary outflow is not completely obstructed, intravenous administration of a diuretic agent (e.g., furosemide) a few minutes prior to (re)attempting access may increase the space between the stone and the pelvic wall. This same maneuver is often helpful in gaining access to a small or undilated renal pelvis.

Second, choosing a more oblique angle relative to the stone-filled pelvis may allow the wire to slide between the stone and pelvic wall while helping to avoid driving the needle or wire tip into the substance of the stone mass.

Third, minimizing to-and-fro movement of the wire tip at the moment it exits the needle tip helps avoid kinking against the stone. With a floppy tipped wire, such as a 0.018-inch mandril wire, once the wire tip is kinked it can neither be advanced nor can it be retracted through the needle. With virtually any wire (and especially so with a Teflon®-coated Glide® wire), attempting to withdraw the tip through the sharp bevel of the access needle while the wire is under tension against the stone runs a high risk of shearing the wire tip or coating material. Once this occurs, there is little choice but to remove the wire and needle together and to reattempt access. However, slow deliberate manipulation of the guide wire in this situation may achieve success.

Postprocedure and follow-up care

At the conclusion of the procedure a plain radiograph is obtained to look for residual fragments not visible fluoroscopically. With a guide wire in place, the sheath is removed, and a Council catheter (end-hole Foley) or pigtail catheter measuring the same diameter as the tract is inserted to provide continued access to the renal pelvis if needed and to provide tamponade. Following the procedure, appropriate notes and postprocedure orders are entered into the patient's chart. It may be helpful to both patient care and ongoing quality assurance to maintain pertinent demographic and procedure-related data in an electronic database. Suggested items for data management are included in Table 6.6.

At 48 hours a repeat abdominal radiograph is obtained to look for residual stones or fragments. If none are found, a nephrostogram is performed to confirm patency of the ureter. Helical non-contrast CT is an effective alternative for identifying residual stone fragments but does not evaluate the integrity of the collecting system. If the ureter is normal, the nephrostomy tube is clamped for 24 to 48 hours, and if no problems occur, the tube is removed. It has been recommended that children be followed with a plain abdominal radiograph and either excretory urography or renal US at two to six weeks, then again at three and six months postprocedure.

Complications

The most frequent complications of percutaneous nephrolithotomy are bleeding and sepsis. In general, bleeding requiring transfusion is very uncommon. Although experience reported in the literature is limited, one may expect approximately 15 to 20% of percutaneous stone removal procedures to be associated with significant complications. Some degree of hematuria occurs in most patients, and although it is usually not of clinical significance, on occasion transfusion is needed. Delayed hemorrhage due to a leaking pseudoaneurysm or arteriovenous fistula has been reported in adult series but not in children. Infection resulting from accessing an infected urinary tract or infected calculus may occur. Preprocedural use of antibiotics, avoiding overdistention of the renal pelvis or collecting system, and adequate drainage minimize this risk.

Perforation of the renal pelvis or ureter may occur. These tears usually seal within 72 hours if adequate drainage is provided. Renal pelvic and ureteral edema requiring prolonged nephrostomy drainage is uncommon and delayed ureteral or ureteropelvic stricture has not been reported in children. Another potential complication is extravasation of irrigation fluid from the percutaneous tract producing fluid overload, pleural effusion, and retroperitoneal collections. Operators should be cautioned against preventing free fluid egress during nephroscopic procedures, especially when using small caliber endoscopes and irrigation channels in children. Careful monitoring for pulmonary compromise, or for signs of fluid extravasation into the retroperitoneum or abdomen, is important for early recognition and treatment of related complications. A postprocedural chest radiograph is important when an intercostal approach has been used to rule out hydrothorax, pneumothorax, and hydropneumothorax.

Finally, children undergoing any procedure are at risk for hypothermia. Irrigation during nephroscopic procedures may increase this risk. Using an irrigant warmed to normal body temperature, and employing techniques previously described to maintain normothermia during interventional procedures, will help avoid this complication.

Future advances

Urinary tract interventions are a good example of the aphorism that children are not small adults. Some advocate for a universal algorithm for the treatment of renal calculi, regardless of patient size. We hold the view that treatment of children should be individualized, and that stone burden, anatomic abnormalities, and patient size must be factored into the treatment algorithm. New technology, such as the "mini-perc" procedure performed through an 11-French sheath, described by Jackman and colleagues, and miniature ureteroscopes with laser lithotripsy may decrease the morbidity and increase the usefulness of percutaneous nephrolithotomy as initial or sole therapy in treatment of renal calculi in children and may reduce the need for open surgical procedures in this population. Hard stones (i.e., cystine, calcium oxalate monohydrate, and brushite) are known to be difficult to treat by ESWL, but are also difficult to identify by plain radiography. Application of newer imaging technologies may allow more accurate prediction of stone composition and thereby allow more appropriate stratification of patients.

Conclusions

Excellent historical results with nephrolithotomy has led to its application in children. While in the literature most children treated by this technique have been over five years of age, percutaneous stone removal in younger children has also been successful. In addition, percutaneous removal of ureteric stent fragments and organized clot simulating a stone has been reported in younger children with renal transplants. Indications for stone removal in pediatric series have included staghorn calculi, cystine stones, and multiple calculi.

The percutaneous approach has been especially useful in managing children who are not candidates for or have failed ESWL, and those with recurrent renal calculi who have had multiple open surgical procedures. Presenting symptoms were usually hematuria, pain, or infection. Percutaneous stone removal and ESWL have been used in combination with success. The mean procedure time can be expected to approach two hours, and the average postoperative hospitalization may be four to five days.

Today, percutaneous nephrolithotomy has been replaced in many situations by ESWL and ureteronephroscopic techniques. However, percutaneous removal of stones is still the most reliable method for certain indications. Thus an interventionalist should be familiar with the percutaneous techniques used for management of renal calculi. In addition, the modular techniques involved are nearly identical to those used for percutaneous endopyelotomy, which remains an important method for treatment of UPJ obstruction. A successful outcome is fostered by collaboration between the interventionalist and urologist. When ESWL or ureteroscopy alone are not indicated or are inadequate, percutaneous stone removal remains a viable option for the management of renal and ureteral calculi.

Balloon dilation of ureteral strictures

Introduction

Ureteral strictures in the pediatric population are often congenital or idiopathic, but may be acquired through ischemia, trauma (including penetrating injury, iatrogenic trauma with instrumentation, and trauma secondary to ureteral calculi), or, rarely, infection or malignancy. Either excretory urography or a diuretic renogram should help define the location and length of the ureteral stricture. The latter study may also quantitate differential renal function and help evaluate functional obstruction.

Although dilation of the ureter was initially reported in 1926 it was not until the development of the balloon catheter in 1979 that equipment effective for percutaneous transluminal dilation (PTA) became available. At this point, minimally invasive interventional therapies became an option. Subsequent research with animal models confirmed that ureteral strictures could be treated using a percutaneous approach. The technique of balloon dilation of ureteral strictures followed by insertion of a temporary stent was introduced in the 1980s by Banner and colleagues and Finnerty and colleagues, and has subsequently gained broad acceptance. Percutaneous treatment of ureteral strictures with balloon dilation is an attractive option given its minimally invasive nature and low risk of postprocedure hemorrhage. After the stricture is dilated, the ureter must be stented to maintain or enlarge its diameter. In adults, the overall long-term success rate is relatively low, from 50 to 76%. The success rate for ureteral angioplasty is unknown in the pediatric population. However, the predominance of benign etiologies makes this minimally invasive approach an attractive option. While serial dilations may increase the success rate substantially, such gains are partially offset by the need for multiple procedures. Certainly, shorter strictures with a good vascular supply are more amenable to transluminal balloon dilation. Longer strictures with a compromised vascular supply may be better treated with other methods, such as a transluminal incisional procedure (endoureterotomy) followed by ureteral stenting or open surgery (e.g., ureteroureterostomy) if it can be achieved without tension.

With the trend toward minimally invasive surgical therapies and cost-cutting strategies, it is likely that these as well as other interventional techniques will proliferate in the future. Certainly these endourologic interventions are safe, effective, and suited to use in children of all ages. At this time, equipment necessary to treat children is available and should not be a limiting factor in the performance of interventional procedures or the future development of interventional techniques for the pediatric population. Success of the percutaneous approach in the ureter was followed by percutaneous endourologic treatment of calculi and of ureteropelvic junction strictures first in adults then in children.

Indications

Isolated ureteral strictures are unusual in the pediatric population. However, when they are the cause of functionally significant obstruction, they are usually amenable to percutaneous therapy. As previously mentioned, ureteral narrowing may result from a variety of intrinsic or extrinsic causes (Table 6.14). The likelihood of successful percutaneous dilation of a stricture will depend upon the cause, length, and duration of the stricture. In the presence of impaired blood supply, a successful result is uncertain, but strictures present for less than three months and postoperative strictures generally respond well to balloon dilation. The location of a ureteral stricture does not appear to be of diagnostic importance. However, for successful percutaneous therapy, there must be access across the stricture so that guide wires, catheters, and

Table 6.14 Indications: balloon dilation of ureteral strictures

Intrinsic causes of ureteral narrowing
- congenital
  - intrinsic stenosis
  - anomalous insertion
  - fibrous bands
  - crossing vessels
- traumatic
- penetrating injury
- fistula
- iatrogenic
- infection (e.g., tuberculosis)

Extrinsic causes of ureteral narrowing
- retroperitoneal fibrosis
- adjacent mass

Table 6.15 Equipment: balloon dilation of ureteral stricture

- C-arm fluoroscopic unit, US with or without a biopsy guide
- Foley catheter (5 to 12 French)
- 1% lidocaine (buffered)
- Needles
  - local anesthesia
    - hypodermic needle (30 gauge)
    - spinal needle (1.5 to 3.5 inch)
  - nephrostomy
    - Chiba (22 to 23 gauge) or sheathed needle (18 to 19 gauge).
    - Yueh needle (5 French)
    - TLA (19 gauge)
- Dilators (5 to 12 French)
- Directional catheter (JB-1, Berenstein, etc.)
- Guide wire (angled Glide® wire, stiff Glide® wire, Amplatz Super Stiff®, Rosen, Newton, etc.)
- Peel-away sheath (8 to 12 French)
- Balloon dilation catheters (3 to 8 mm × 2 to 4 cm)
- Ureteral stent (6 to 10 French × 10 to 26 cm length)
- Silicone spray or liquid
- Nitinol snare (2 to 10 mm)
- End-hole Foley (use sterile punch to create end hole) or Council catheter (10 to 24 French)

other instruments can be adequately positioned. In children with tight or eccentric strictures, percutaneous techniques are often advantageous. Some advocate avoiding balloon dilation of the distal ureter in small children, where the potential for postprocedure vesicoureteral reflux has greater clinical implications than in older children and adults. In general, if the percutaneous approach seems best suited to treat the child, we will proceed especially with the availability of the Deflux procedure. Relative contraindications for percutaneous therapy include the presence of strictures longer than 2 cm, active infection, uncorrected coagulopathy, or unfavorable anatomy.

Technique
Equipment
Although ureteral strictures usually occur in older children, younger children may also be affected. Thus, it is important to maintain a variety of catheters (65 cm, 100 cm), straight and steerable guide wires (0.018-inch to 0.038-inch), stents (3 to 7 French × 6 to 26 cm), peel-away sheaths (4 to 10 French) and angioplasty balloon catheters (3 to 6 mm × 2 to 4 cm) in inventory (Table 6.15).

Patient preparation
Children requiring ureteral dilation and stenting need no special preparation. Since either GA or sedation is needed for stent insertion, the child must be NPO as per relevant hospital policies. In patients who are otherwise healthy, no routine laboratory tests are obtained except for a urinalysis.

When necessary a coagulation profile and CBC with differential and platelet count are obtained preoperatively. High-risk children, those with immune deficiency or other conditions predisposing to infection, children with congenital heart disease, and those in whom there are procedural difficulties or complications are treated with antibiotics before, during, or after the procedure. The antibiotic chosen may vary with the age and underlying condition of the child.

After the child is sedated, a Foley catheter is inserted into the urinary bladder. The child is then placed in the position that makes access to the collecting system easiest. The prone or prone-oblique position with the side of interest elevated is most often chosen. Regardless of the position, the patient is stabilized with a combination of high-density foam sponges, rolled-up linen, or other materials, taking care to adequately protect potential pressure points. The child is secured to the tabletop with Velcro® straps and tape (if necessary).

The skin entry site is selected (usually with US) and marked on the skin with a marker so that the puncture is above the level of the UPJ. This allows for an easier, more direct angle to the UPJ. This route facilitates passage of the angioplasty balloon or cutting tool and, later, stent insertion. Whenever possible, an intercostal approach is avoided to make tract dilation and catheter insertion easier and minimize the chance of hydrothorax and other thoracic complications.

Standard technique
After the induction of anesthesia or sedation, the flank is prepared and draped in sterile fashion. Local anesthesia is injected as needed with the technique described for nephrostomy insertion. Access to the renal pelvis is achieved as described under "Percutaneous nephrostomy," "Catheter insertion," above. Once the collecting system is successfully accessed, a guide wire is coiled within the renal pelvis or maneuvered into the ureter. The tract is then progressively dilated, and a peel-away sheath or valved introducer is inserted (Table 6.16). When possible, a peel-away sheath or introducer

Table 6.16 Procedure summary: balloon dilation of ureteral stricture

- Establish percutaneous renal access as discussed in Table 6.5. Access to a lower middle pole calyx allows easier access to the ureter
- Dilate the tract and insert a sheath
- Use a directional catheter and guide wire to enter the ureter. The catheter tip should be positioned above the stricture
- Inject contrast
- Mark the level of the stricture to facilitate positioning the angioplasty balloon
- Advance the guide wire distal to the stricture and coil in the bladder if convenient
- Measure the diameter of the stricture and of the normal ureter and select an appropriately sized balloon
- Center the balloon across the stricture and inflate until the stricture (waist) is effaced
- Insert a double-J or universal stent
- Maintain nephrostomy access until the procedure and follow-up imaging is complete

that is two French larger than the anticipated stent is used to facilitate later stent placement. If entry into the renal pelvis is via a lower pole calyx, a stiff guide wire (stiff Glide® wire, Rosen, Amplatz®, etc.) is helpful to avoid buckling or telescoping of the stent as it is positioned across the treated stricture.

Regardless of the location of the entry site, a directional catheter and guide wire system (JB-1, Berenstein, or cobra catheter and angled glide wire) are used to facilitate catheterization of the ureter. Once the guide wire is within the proximal ureter, contrast is injected, and the location and extent of the stricture are identified. The length and diameter of the stricture are measured, and the appropriate balloon is selected. The directional system is then maneuvered into the urinary bladder if possible.

If the stricture is difficult to pass, the directional catheter is positioned adjacent to the stricture and contrast is injected. After the level of the stricture is determined, a marker (hemostat, Beekley® dot, etc.) is placed on the patient's skin or gown to aid centering the balloon across the stricture. If necessary, a road map is created. Once the catheter is within the urinary bladder, the Glide® wire is exchanged for a stiff or superstiff guide wire. In rare cases, re-puncture of a mid-pole or upper-pole calyx will be necessary in order to successfully pass the stricture.

The approach used when a tight or eccentric stricture is present, and the guide wire cannot cross the stricture, is identical to that used when trying to catheterize a fistulous tract. The directional catheter is wedged into the proximal aspect of the stricture, which will aid passage of the guide wire (Figure 6.28). Contrast is injected and the pathologic anatomy documented with a road map or digital image. The angled Glide® wire and directional catheter are manipulated until the guide wire and catheter are across the stricture. If necessary, a 0.018-inch Glide® wire can be exchanged for a larger guide wire to initially cross the stricture. Once the catheter is distal to the stricture, a stiff guide wire is exchanged for the angled Glide® wire, and the procedure is completed as described. Additional methods for successful access across a narrowed lumen are described by Mata and colleagues.

If the stricture is extremely tight and a balloon catheter cannot be advanced across the narrow segment, several maneuvers may be attempted. Initially, advancing a straight catheter, a van Andel catheter, or a long vascular dilator across the stricture may be useful. Once the stricture is predilated, the standard PTA catheters can be used. In some cases, a small-vessel angioplasty catheter may be best. In these instances, it may be possible to dilate the stricture without exchange for additional balloon catheters. If this approach fails, the guide wire is retrieved from the urinary bladder using a loop snare and the distal end externalized through the urethra (the so-called "body floss" technique shown in Figure 6.29). A hemostat is then clamped to the proximal guide wire as it exits from the angioplasty catheter, and the low-profile angioplasty catheter and guide wire are *pulled* across the stricture in tandem. In this case a soft catheter may be passed retrograde to the point of stricture to protect the uroepithelium from a "cheese wire" laceration of the mucosa while the catheter and guide wire are pulled across the stricture. Spraying the catheters and guide wires with silicone or coating them with sterile mineral oil can enhance successful passage of the stricture. If this maneuver is unsuccessful, the catheter can be exchanged for a balloon wire, straight catheter, van Andel catheter, or tapered dilator. Alternatively, the stricture may be treated using a combination of interventional and urologic techniques. If a long introducer sheath can be positioned in the ureter, a cutting device (e.g., a cutting balloon or cutting wire) or laser may be used to incise the area of narrowing. Regardless of the method used for opening the stricture, the site must be stented. Naturally, interventionalists prefer endourologic techniques for treatment of these lesions. We have found several balloon types to be useful including low-profile balloons available in shaft sizes including: small-vessel balloons on a 3.8-French shaft, and standard balloons on shafts ranging from 5 French and up.

Initially the diameter and length of the stricture are measured. The PTA balloon selected is at least 1 cm longer than the stricture and equal to or slightly (1 to 2 mm) wider than the expected normal ureteral diameter as measured distal to the stricture. In all cases, the balloon rated for highest atmosphere inflation pressure available is selected. After the balloon is centered across the stricture, it is inflated with dilute contrast while balloon pressure is monitored with a pressure gauge. Under fluoroscopic guidance, balloon inflation progresses until the stricture (waist) disappears (Figure 6.28). If after three minutes the stricture persists, the process is repeated with a higher atmosphere (rated equal to or greater than 17 ATM) balloon or, if possible, a larger diameter balloon is utilized. If the postdilation ureterogram still shows obstruction with no significant change in the stricture diameter, a ureteral incision with a cutting device is considered if technically feasible. Once the stricture has been successfully dilated, a stent is inserted (as described in the following section) to maintain or enlarge the ureteral diameter.

Chapter 6 Genitourinary interventions

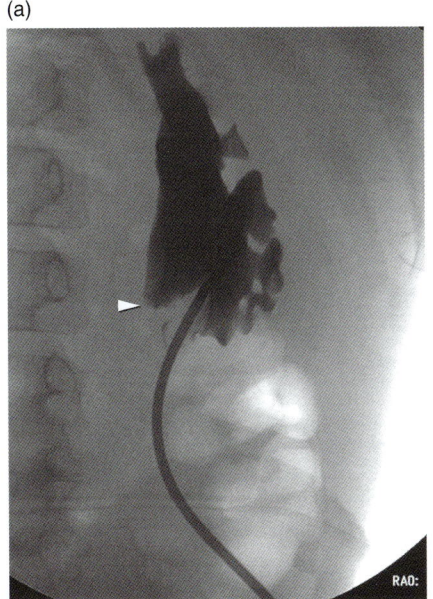
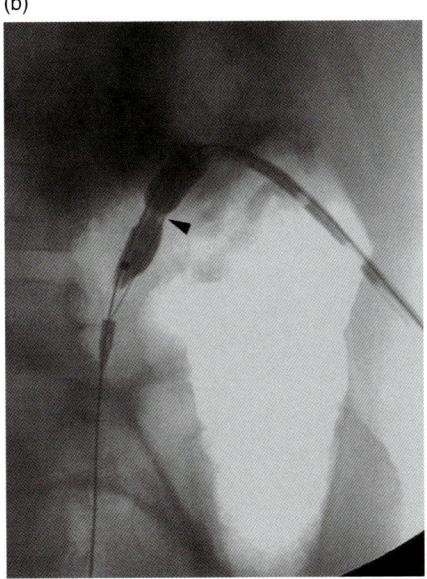
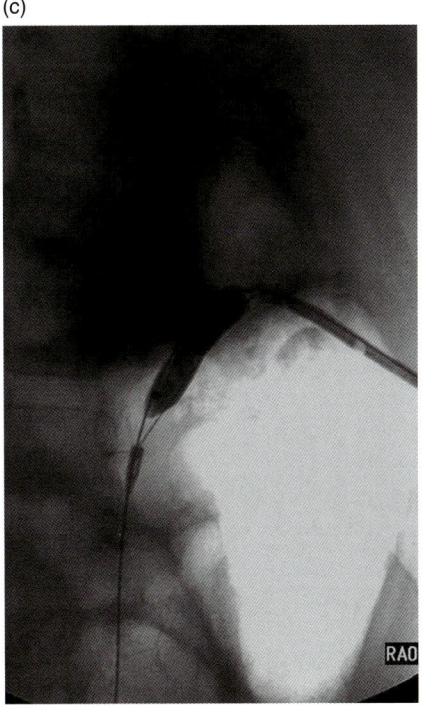
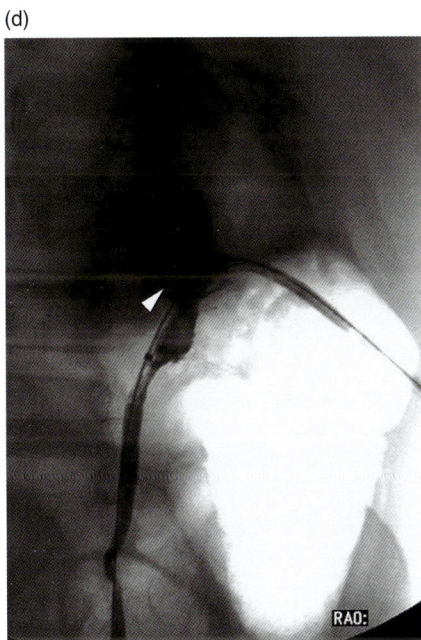

Figure 6.28 (a) An antegrade nephrostogram in this ten-year-old boy with a history of recurrent renal calculi shows a tight stricture at the ureteropelvic junction (*arrowhead*). (b) Once access to the bladder is achieved, a non-compliant angioplasty balloon 1 to 2 mm larger in diameter than nearby normal ureter is centered on the stricture (*arrowhead*) under fluoroscopic control and inflated using a pressure gauge. (c) Balloon inflation is maintained until the stricture waist is ablated or for up to three minutes. If unsuccessful the procedure may be repeated. (d) When the stricture has been successfully dilated, a stent must be placed across it to maintain or increase the diameter until healing occurs. A small amount of extravasation (*arrowhead*) is not uncommon following this procedure. With stenting and drainage it seldom requires further intervention.

Postprocedure and follow-up care

Following the procedure, appropriate notes and postprocedure orders are entered into the patient's chart. It may be helpful to both patient care and ongoing quality assurance to maintain pertinent demographic and procedure-related data in an electronic database. Suggested items for data management are included in Table 6.6. The internal stent is removed three to six weeks following balloon dilation. This requires brief sedation or anesthesia. Diuretic renal nuclear medicine scanning is performed one to two weeks after stent removal, to assess renal function and patency at the UPJ. The patient is followed with either US or diuretic renal scintigraphy at intervals of three, six, and twelve months following the procedure, then yearly thereafter.

Complications

Complication rates as high as 20% have been reported following balloon dilation of UPJ strictures, including acute postoperative obstruction (without stent placement), stent migration with or without ureterovesicular junction (UVJ) obstruction, and urinary tract infection (UTI).

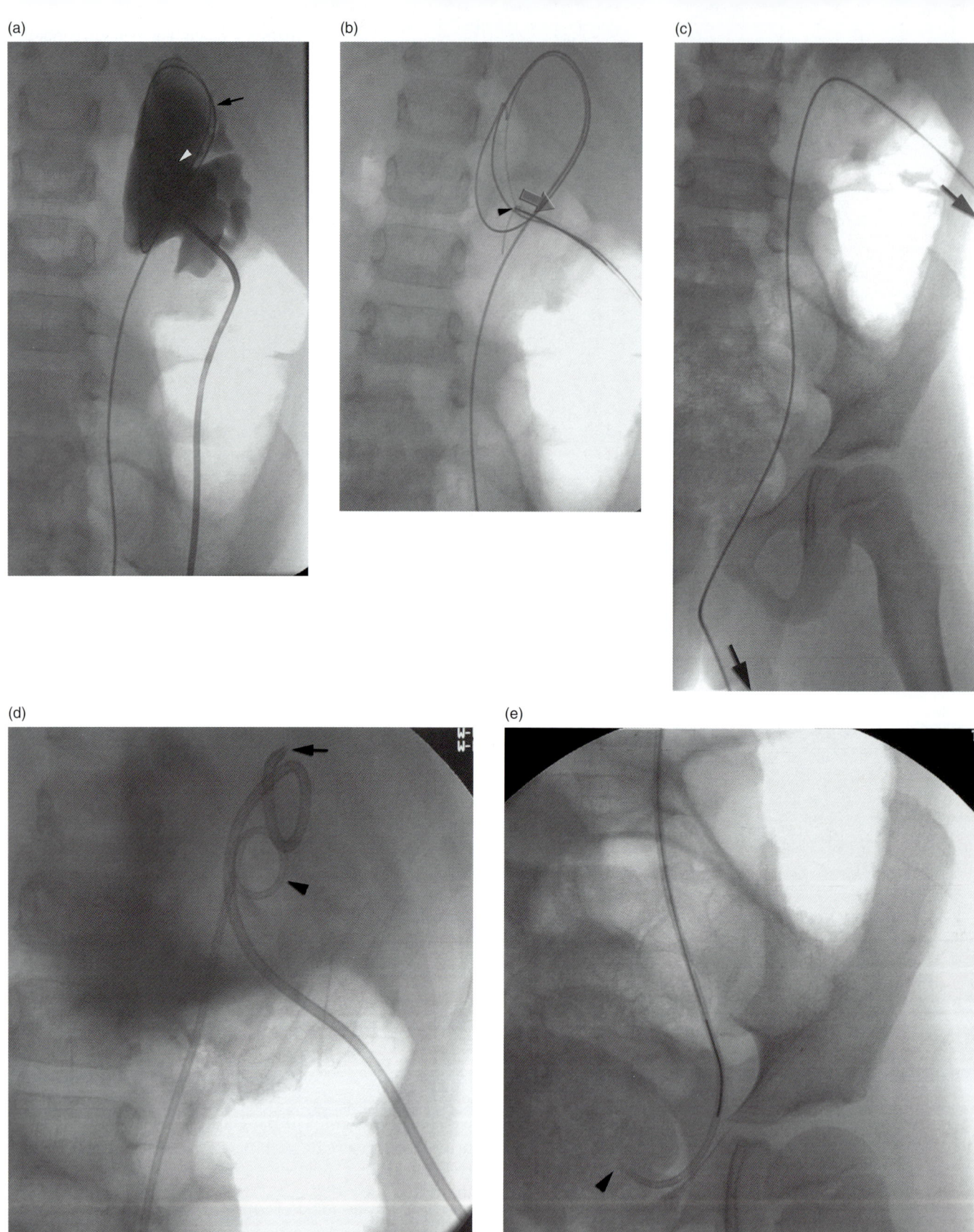

Figure 6.29 (a) This 12-year-old boy has developed a postoperative stricture following surgical ureteroureterostomy. Through the existing nephrostomy catheter (*arrowhead*) an antegrade nephrostogram is performed. Unable to pass a wire from an antegrade approach, a cystoscopic approach has been used to advance a wire from the urethra to coil in the renal pelvis (*arrow*). (b) The nephrostomy catheter has been exchanged for a sheath, through which a loop snare (*arrowhead*) has captured the transurethral wire. The superior end of the wire can now be withdrawn (*arrow*) through the sheath. (c) Having withdrawn the superior end of the wire through the existing nephrostomy access, the guide wire is now exteriorized at both ends (*arrows*), providing a stable "body floss" platform for advancing a catheter across the stricture to the bladder. (d) An internal stent (*arrowhead*) was placed across the secondary UPJ stricture, and the nephrostomy drain (*arrow*) replaced. (e) The double-J internal stent (*arrowhead*) migrated toward the kidney, interrupting antegrade flow. (f) Via a cystoscope, the lower end of the stent was snared and drawn down (*arrow*) into a satisfactory position.

(f)

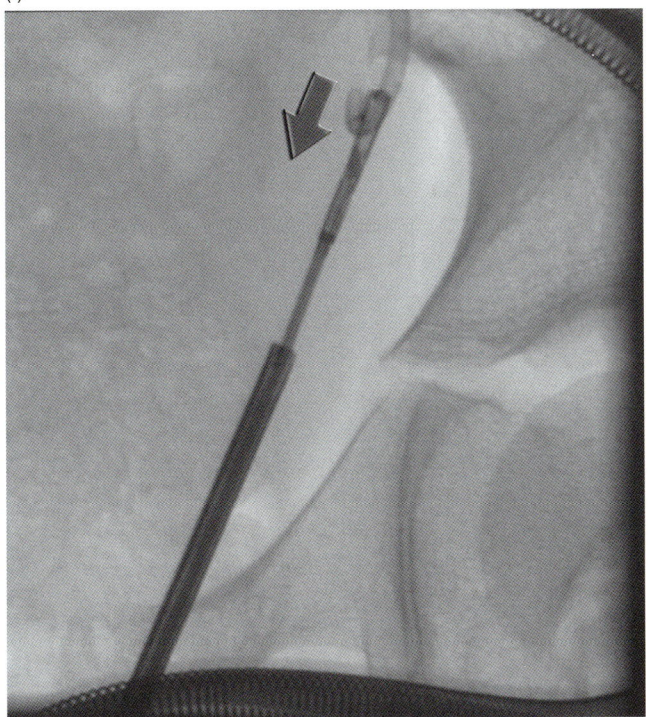

Figure 6.29 (cont.)

Conclusions

Percutaneous treatment of benign ureteral strictures begins with balloon dilation. This approach will be successful in many children, although secondary procedures may be necessary. For children with strictures that are resistant to dilation or that recur, less well tested therapies such as incision and stenting, or open surgery, may be required. To date, there is no substantial experience with stenting alone, but it is not likely to be an effective long-term therapy.

Ureteral stent insertion

Introduction

A ureteral stent is needed for the treatment of ureteral stenosis and after operative repair of the ureter, ureteropelvic junction, or ureterovesicular junction. Endourologic treatment of ureteral strictures may be accomplished by balloon dilation or incision, as discussed elsewhere in this chapter. The retrograde (cystoscopic) approach is preferred for management of a ureteral fistula or other ureteral pathology without hydronephrosis (Figure 6.29) or when cystoscopy is otherwise indicated. Percutaneous stent placement should be considered for management of ureteral obstruction in the absence of urinary tract infection and gross hematuria. Stenting can be carried out using either an internal (double-J) stent or an internal–external (universal) stent. Regardless of the stent type selected, it is best to use the largest stent possible so that the treated ureter assumes the largest diameter possible. Stent selection depends on a number of factors including personal preference, available equipment, and the anticipated duration of treatment. In most children stenting is planned as a short-term intervention (eight weeks or less) and either type of stent will do. Stenting for a prolonged period of time (greater than 12 weeks) usually requires placement of an internal stent or exchange of the universal stent to a double-J.

Each stent type has its advantages and disadvantages. Internal stents have a higher rate of patient satisfaction because they are not visible, are less apt to be inadvertently dislodged, require no maintenance, and probably have a lower infection rate – especially if long-term placement is necessary. On the other hand, they are more technically difficult to insert and special sizes (shorter lengths) must be stocked to treat children of all sizes (Figure 6.30). Internal stents are more difficult to remove and require cystoscopic or fluoroscopic guidance to guide removal. Tube mineralization, gross hematuria, and infection limit their useful life.

The universal stent is more flexible, easier to tailor to length, and easier to remove. It is a good choice when short-term use is anticipated. If the need for ureteral stenting is prolonged, the universal stent can easily be converted to an internal stent by exchange over a guide wire. Removal of the stent is performed on an outpatient basis without sedation or anesthesia in most instances. Unlike internal stents, universal stents usually have only one pigtail-shaped end (distal end). However, there are catheters with a distal locking pigtail and a proximal loop that is made to coil within the renal pelvis before exiting from the nephrostomy tract. This catheter may not be a very good choice when the catheter shaft is too long for the smaller child's ureter, as the distal end may irritate the bladder wall. Thus the catheter must be tailored to length, thereby removing its distal pigtail end and reducing the number of drainage holes. However, additional drainage holes may be created with a hole punch. In general, it is more cost effective to stock only pigtail drains (same as those used for abscess drainage) and when necessary, cut additional side holes into the catheter shaft or use pre-made ureteral catheters with side holes. In spite of its disadvantages, the double-J stent is usually preferred since it has greater stability and easier postprocedural care.

Indications

Antegrade insertion of stents into the ureter using a percutaneous technique was first performed in an attempt to palliate ureteric obstruction due to malignant disease. Since that time, stenting has become a well-established procedure for the management of ureteric obstruction of varying etiologies. Technical developments in imaging, catheters, guide wires, and stents have made percutaneous insertion easier and more effective. As a result of ongoing technical and equipment

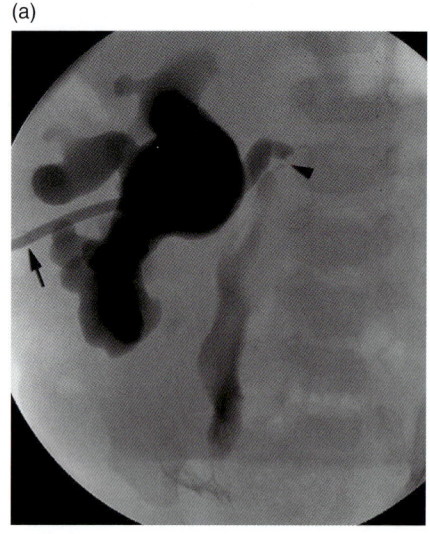
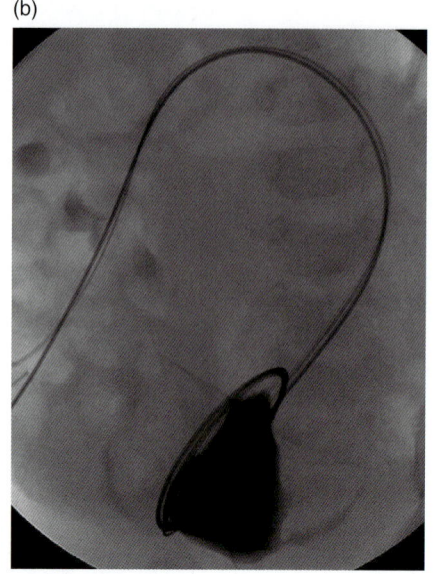
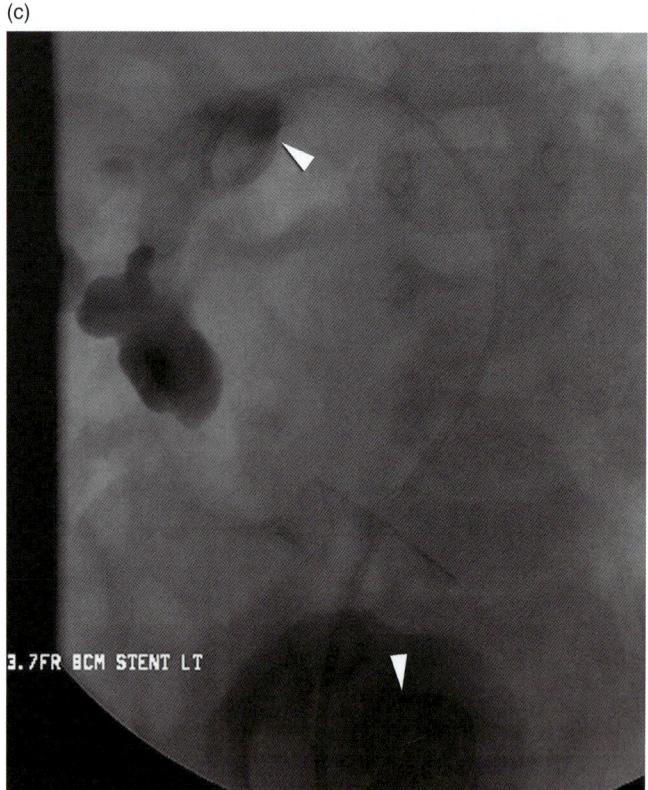

Figure 6.30 (a) Antegrade nephrostogram through the existing drainage catheter (*arrow*) in a two-year-old girl after treatment for a sacrococcygeal teratoma shows hydronephrosis and proximal ureteral stricture (*arrowhead*). (b) Through the existing nephrostomy access, two guide wires have been advanced to the urinary bladder. One is used as a safety wire, the other to deliver the internal stent. (c) At the completion of the procedure the ends of the 3.7 French, 8 cm stent (*arrowheads*) are coiled in the renal pelvis and the bladder.

improvements, the percutaneous approach is used as a primary therapy or as an adjunct to surgery, often substituting for more invasive surgical procedures.

Indications for ureteral stenting include relief of a ureteral obstruction from any cause, providing drainage while a ureteral injury heals (Figure 6.31), maintaining ureteral caliber until edema or mass effect subsides, after ureteral dilation, stone removal or surgery (Figure 6.32), and in the management of ureteral strictures. The antegrade placement of a stent may be performed after failure of the endoscopic approach due to unfavorable anatomy.

Although permanent metallic stents are now available, they are not routinely used in the child's urinary tract. Malignancy, the primary indication for insertion of a metallic stent in older patients, is rarely a problem in the pediatric population. Therefore in almost all cases of benign strictures in the child's urinary tract, temporary plastic internal (double-J) or internal–external (universal) stents are preferred for treatment.

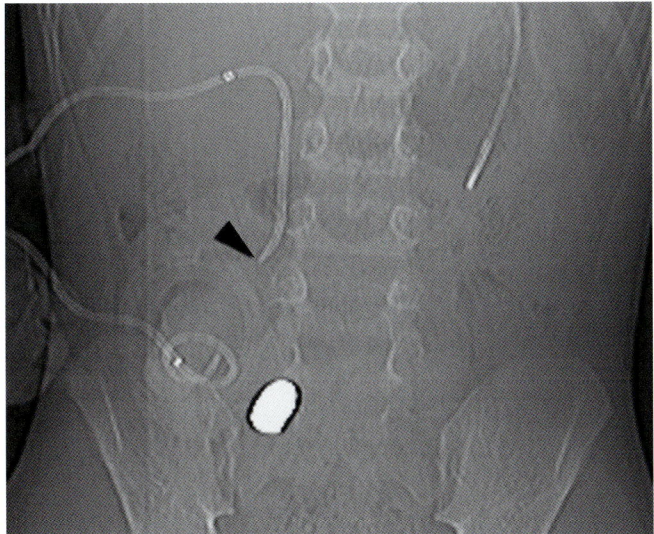

Figure 6.31 Twelve-year-old male with transection of the right ureter by gunshot. The bullet projects over the right sacral alum on this fluoroscopic view of the abdomen and upper pelvis. Under US (not shown), the mid-polar calyx was accessed with a 20-gauge needle. When urine return confirmed intrapelvic access, the initial 0.018-inch guide wire was exchanged via a 4-French micropuncture introducer for a 0.035-inch Rosen wire, which was advanced into the renal collecting system and the tract dilated to 9 French. Then an 8.5-French Cook® All-Purpose Drainage catheter was inserted, with the tip positioned in the mid-ureter (*arrowhead*).

Stents may be placed either in antegrade fashion via a nephrostomy tract or in retrograde fashion using cystoscopic guidance. The antegrade approach is advantageous in children who require other percutaneous procedures of the urinary tract, antegrade pyelography or Whitaker perfusion testing, or those who have tortuous ureters or genitourinary tract anomalies. A combined approach involving both the interventionalist and urologist may be valuable in selected cases, such as in a child who has an ileal loop with an uretero-ileal anastomotic stricture, or to treat a UPJ obstruction with an endopyelotomy. Stent insertion should be avoided or delayed whenever possible if urinary tract infection or bleeding, or a significant coagulation problem, is present.

A stent can become the nidus for infection or can be obstructed by purulent material, blood clot, or hyperplasia of irritated uroepithelium. If this occurs, attempts should be made to unclog and declot the stent by repeatedly flushing the pelvicaliceal system and ureter with sterile saline. If a more rapid result is desired, tPA infusion may be used if not otherwise contraindicated by the child's medical condition. In patients with a ureteral fistula and non-dilated upper tracts, retrograde stent insertion is the preferred route because of the ease of insertion.

Technique

Equipment

The ideal stent is non-irritating, is tailored to the child's length, resists encrustation, is readily visualized fluoroscopically, is easily inserted and removed, and is stable once in position. Although this ideal is not currently available, stents with many of these characteristics are now in use. Stents are made with a variety of materials including polyethylene, polyurethane, silicone, silastic, and other plastics (Table 6.17). Silastic stents are soft and well tolerated; unfortunately, they are more difficult to insert due to a high coefficient of friction resulting in increased resistance to advancement through the ureter. To assist placement, catheters and guide wires may be lubricated with either silicone spray or mineral oil. The preferred stent in most IR practices is stiffer and made of catheter material. A general guideline for stent length selection in children with normal kidney location is age in years plus 2 cm. Naturally, the actual length is measured using the bent guide wire technique or calibrated catheter or guide wire.

Patient preparation

Preparation for stent placement is similar to that for PCN insertion (see above); if indeed the two procedures are not performed sequentially under the same anesthesia. From each child undergoing an endourologic procedure, the following laboratory studies are usually obtained: CBC with platelet count, coagulation profile, and in rare cases, a bleeding time. In addition, BUN, creatinine, and urine culture are generally obtained prior to the day of the urinary tract manipulation. Children with suspected or proven urinary tract infections and those who are immune depressed or require procedure prophylaxis are given preprocedural antibiotics. Since each child will necessarily undergo either GA or sedation, the child must be NPO according to relevant hospital policies.

Standard technique

Placement of an internal stent is performed under fluoroscopic guidance. Prior to beginning ureteral stent placement, a second guide wire (safety guide wire) is inserted through the sheath (preferably a peel-away sheath) and coiled in the renal pelvis (Figures 6.27, 6.30). This guide wire is then secured to the drape with a hemostat and covered with a sterile towel. After a guide wire is maneuvered into the urinary bladder, a 5-French catheter is advanced over the guide wire until the tip is positioned just distal to the UVJ. The length of the ureter is measured so that the proper stent length can be selected. Ureteral length can be obtained using a calibrated catheter or guide wire, digital tools available on many angiography units, or the "bent guide wire" technique (Figure 6.33).

The bent guide wire technique is a versatile method that can be used in the GU tract as well as other systems (e.g., to measure the length of a central line; see Figure 2.39). Ureteral length is determined by positioning the tip of the guide wire under fluoroscopic guidance at a point just distal to the UVJ. The guide wire is then bent at the catheter hub. Alternatively, a hemostat may be clipped to the guide wire at this point and left in position. Next, the guide wire is pulled back so that the tip is at the UPJ and again bent or clipped with a hemostat. The

Chapter 6 Genitourinary interventions

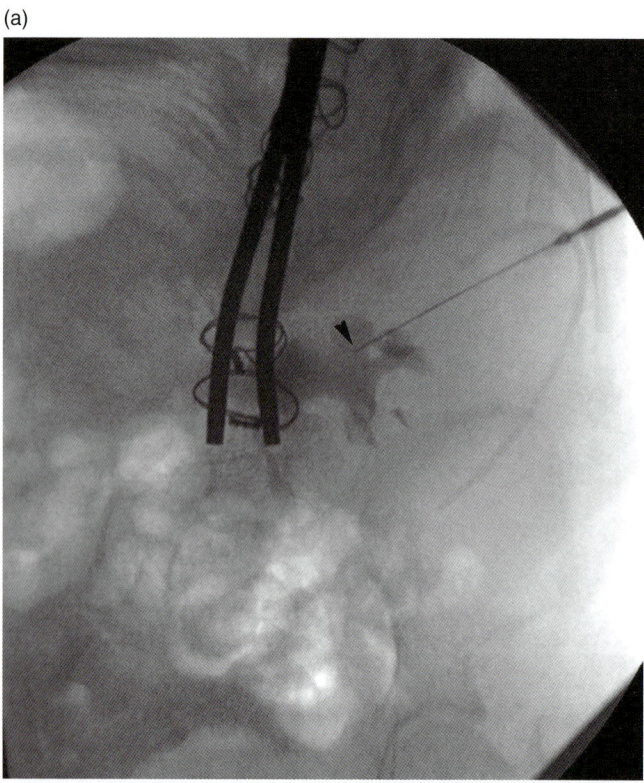

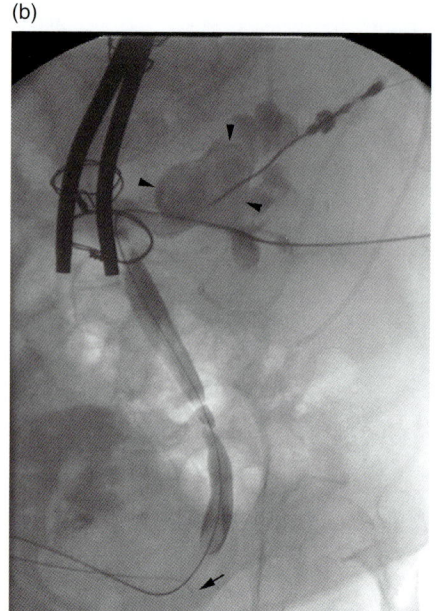

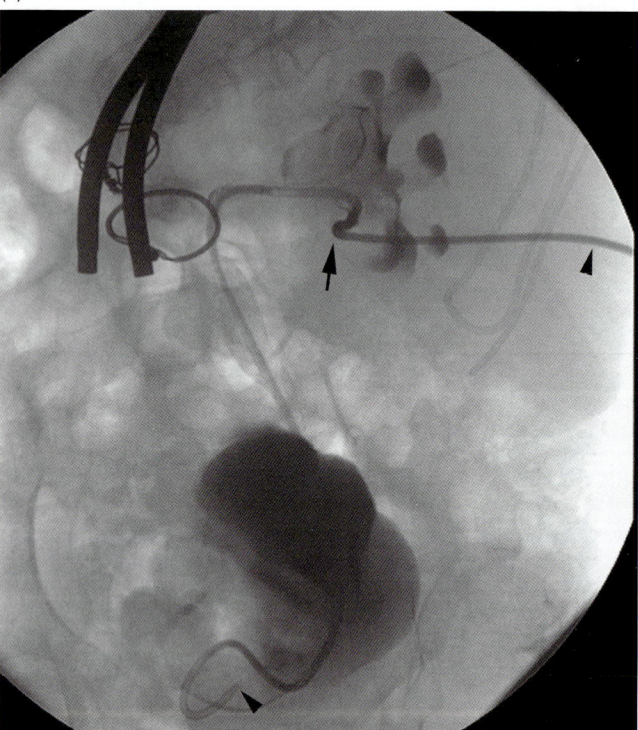

Figure 6.32 (a) This 16-year-old male with myelodysplasia has a history of multiple surgeries for removal of stones from the renal pelvis and bladder. He now presents with urosepsis and a staghorn calculus involving the renal pelvis and mid-polar calyces. A 22-gauge Chiba needle (*arrowhead*) was used to obtain access through an upper pole calyx, but a guide wire could not be advanced from this position due to the large stone burden. (b) Antegrade contrast instilled through the first needle outlined the obstructing stone (*arrowheads*) but also defined a posterior lower pole calyx through which access to the ureter and bladder was obtained with a 0.018-inch angled Glide® wire (*arrow*). (c) Using a coaxial introducer kit, the 0.018-inch wire was exchanged for a 0.035-inch Glide® wire, over which an 8-French nephroureteral (universal) catheter (*arrowheads*) was inserted. The loop (*arrow*) could not be formed in the pelvis due to the stone, but the catheter drained well. Although usually avoided in patients with spinal hardware, this patient was treated successfully with ESWL one month after this procedure.

distance between the bends or hemostats (i.e., the length of the ureter) determines the length of the internal stent. Depending on the age and height of the child, stent length usually varies from 8 to 24 cm.

Once an internal stent is chosen, a long suture looped through the distal end hole may be used to pull the stent back into the renal pelvis if it is inadvertently pushed out of the renal pelvis. The stent is fed over the guide wire and pushed via

Table 6.17 Equipment: ureteral stent insertion

- Ultrasound machine (with biopsy guide and sterile covers if needed)
- Scalpel with #11 blade
- Buffered local anesthetic
- Syringe (3 to 5 ml) with 27- to 30-gauge needle for local anesthetic
- Spinal needle (22 gauge) for deep infiltration of local anesthetic
- Puncture needle (e.g., micropuncture set, sheathed needle)
- Guide wire (e.g., mandril, glide, J, stiff)
- Dilators
- Sheath
- PTA balloon (equal to or 10% larger than the measured normal ureteral diameter)
- Stent (double-J or universal in the largest size possible for the individual patient)
- Nephrostomy tube (usually, 8 French)
- Nephrostomy drainage bag and connecting tubing
- Sterile dressing

the peel-away sheath into the renal pelvis and ureter with a pusher catheter (Table 6.18). The pusher catheter is advanced onto the guide wire and used to advance the stent into final position (Figure 6.33). Catheter positioning is intermittently monitored with fluoroscopy. Once the stent is in satisfactory position, the pusher catheter is kept abutted to the stent and counter-pressure applied while the safety suture is removed. If the stent is not in appropriate position it may be repositioned before the suture is removed.

In order to complete the procedure, the guide wire must be removed. This step is crucial to the success of the procedure and although technically straightforward often leads to problems. Again, the stent is maintained in satisfactory position by applying counter-pressure with the pusher catheter while the guide wire is slowly removed. If a safety guide wire is in position, the guide wire can be completely removed. If not, the guide wire is withdrawn until it exits the stent but is still within the renal pelvis. At this point, the guide wire is advanced and coiled in the renal pelvis to assist placement of the nephrostomy catheter. If this maneuver fails, the renal pelvis can be recatheterized via the peel-away sheath.

Next, a nephrostomy catheter (pigtail or Council) is inserted and secured to the skin. The catheter should be of similar diameter to the tract, preventing the leakage of urine. The nephrostomy tube may be left in place as long as it is clinically indicated. If another procedure is necessary, the nephrostomy is left in place for access. If no procedure is planned and no problem has occurred, the nephrostomy tube is removed after approximately 72 hours. Prior to tube removal, a nephrostogram is performed to confirm satisfactory position and functioning of the stent. If all is well, the nephrostomy is removed and the site covered with Vaseline® gauze and a dry, sterile dressing. The child is usually followed clinically, and when the stent is no longer needed, it may be removed transurethrally with a cystoscope or snared under fluoroscopic guidance. In rare cases, the stent is removed from above after a nephrostomy tract is re-established.

If a universal stent is used, it is important to be certain that the proximal drainage holes are all within the renal pelvis. If one or more side holes are in the tract or outside of the patient, urine leakage may result in significant skin irritation and a predisposition to infection. Proper catheter position can easily be confirmed with contrast injection. Unlike internal stents, guide wire removal is simple and without technical problems. In most cases, a nephrostomy tube is not needed. If the tract diameter is larger than the stent caliber (a common problem), there is usually urine drainage around the catheter for up to 24 hours until the tract closes. If leakage persists, it usually suggests catheter malfunction requiring contrast injection. If the catheter is functioning properly, one can try to seal the nephrostomy tract by covering it with an occlusive bandage. Alternatively, the tract may be tightened with a purse string suture. If unsuccessful, a nephrostomy catheter can be inserted adjacent to the stent.

Regardless of type, duration of stent placement will vary according to the underlying etiology of the stricture. Short-term placement (three to five days) is required for treatment of ureteral edema while ten to fifteen days are usually needed after ureteral surgery. Longer time periods (six to eight weeks) are usually needed to maintain ureteral caliber after endopyelotomy.

Postprocedure and follow-up care

Following the procedure, appropriate notes and postprocedure orders are entered into the patient's chart. It may be helpful to both patient care and ongoing quality assurance to maintain pertinent demographic and procedure-related data in an electronic database. Suggested items for data management are included in Table 6.6.

In the immediate postprocedural period, care centers around recovery of the child from sedation or GA and treatment of complications. Children receiving GA are observed in the recovery room, while children who have received sedation and are outpatients receive postprocedure care in the radiology department. Inpatients receiving sedation are returned to the ward for monitoring. Children having an endourologic procedure under GA are monitored in the same way as pediatric patients having any other operative procedure. Children awakening from sedation have their vital signs continually monitored and recorded every 5 to 15 min for the first 30 to 60 min and then every 30 to 60 min until discharge.

When the child is awake and alert, clear liquids are given for the first few postprocedure hours. If liquids are tolerated, the diet is advanced to solids. When children have returned to baseline neurologic status, and their continued hydration is assured (e.g., when they are tolerating liquids well), they are considered for discharge. In addition to monitoring the vital signs, the nephrostomy site and drainage area are monitored

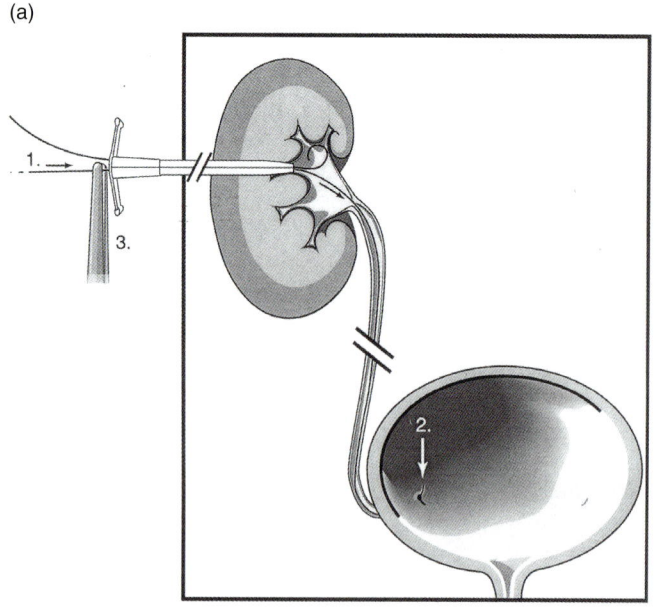

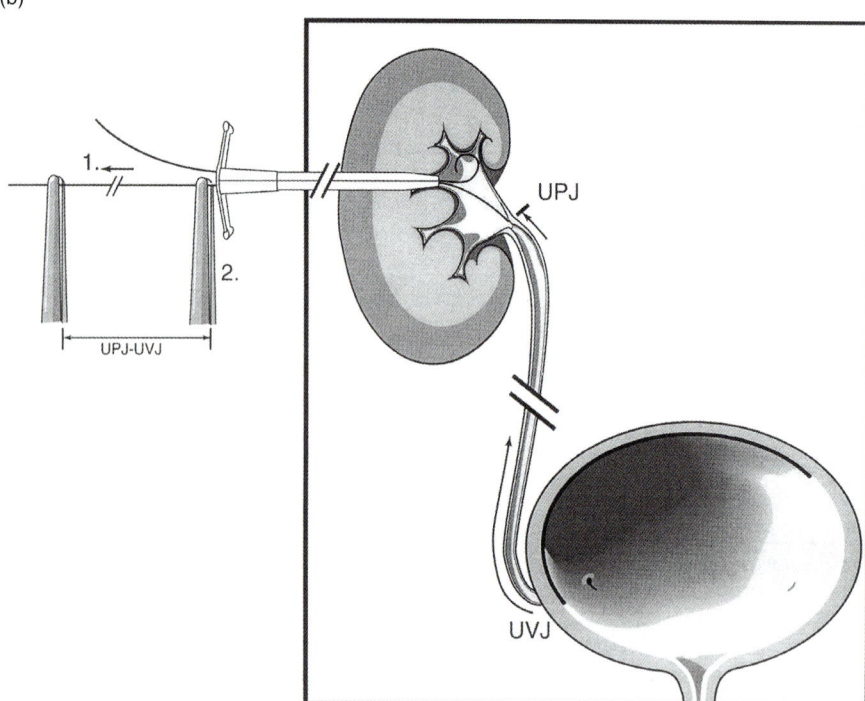

Figure 6.33 Double-J stent illustration. (a) In preparation for stent insertion two guide wires are positioned. A safety wire is inserted through the sheath and coiled in the renal pelvis. A working guide wire (*1*) is advanced until its tip is at the ureterovesicular junction (*2*). A hemostat is then clamped to the proximal end of the wire where it enters the sheath (*3*). (b) In order to measure the length of the ureter, the clamped wire is withdrawn (*1*) until the tip is visualized at the ureteropelvic junction, and a second hemostat is clamped at the sheath entrance (*2*). The distance between the two hemostats is equivalent to the length of the ureter. From this measurement the appropriate double-J stent can be selected. (c) The stent is prepared by placing a suture loop through the proximal side hole. It is then advanced over the guide wire to the sheath entrance. The pusher catheter is placed behind it, with the tips of the two catheters abutting each other (*broad arrow*). The double-J catheter can then be pushed into position until the distal end coils in the urinary bladder and the proximal end is situated in the renal pelvis. If the catheter is advanced too far it can be pulled back with the suture. (d) Once the catheter is in position, forward pressure is maintained with the pusher catheter while the suture loop is withdrawn. When properly positioned the proximal end should coil freely in the renal pelvis.

for evidence of bleeding. If no hematuria is identified, the Foley catheter is removed before the child awakens. Any complication identified is immediately treated, and the appropriate clinical service and referring physician are notified and consulted as appropriate.

When the child is discharged to home, careful and detailed verbal and written instructions are given by the interventional nurse and, if necessary, the physician. Written instructions include a list of the more common delayed complications and appropriate contact information for the interventional staff on call. If indicated, a prescription is given for antibiotics.

Analgesics are also prescribed to treat pain or discomfort. In general, we recommend mild analgesics such as acetaminophen, ibuprofen, or acetaminophen with codeine. Occasionally, an intravenous non-steroidal anti-inflammatory agent (such as Toradol®) will be necessary. If the patient's needs are not adequately managed using this approach, the child should be re-evaluated by the interventional staff or consulting services as this level of discomfort is unexpected.

Follow-up care is scheduled with the primary physician, urologist, or interventionalist and, at the appropriate time, the nephrostomy is removed. In children who have internal stents,

Figure 6.33 (cont.)

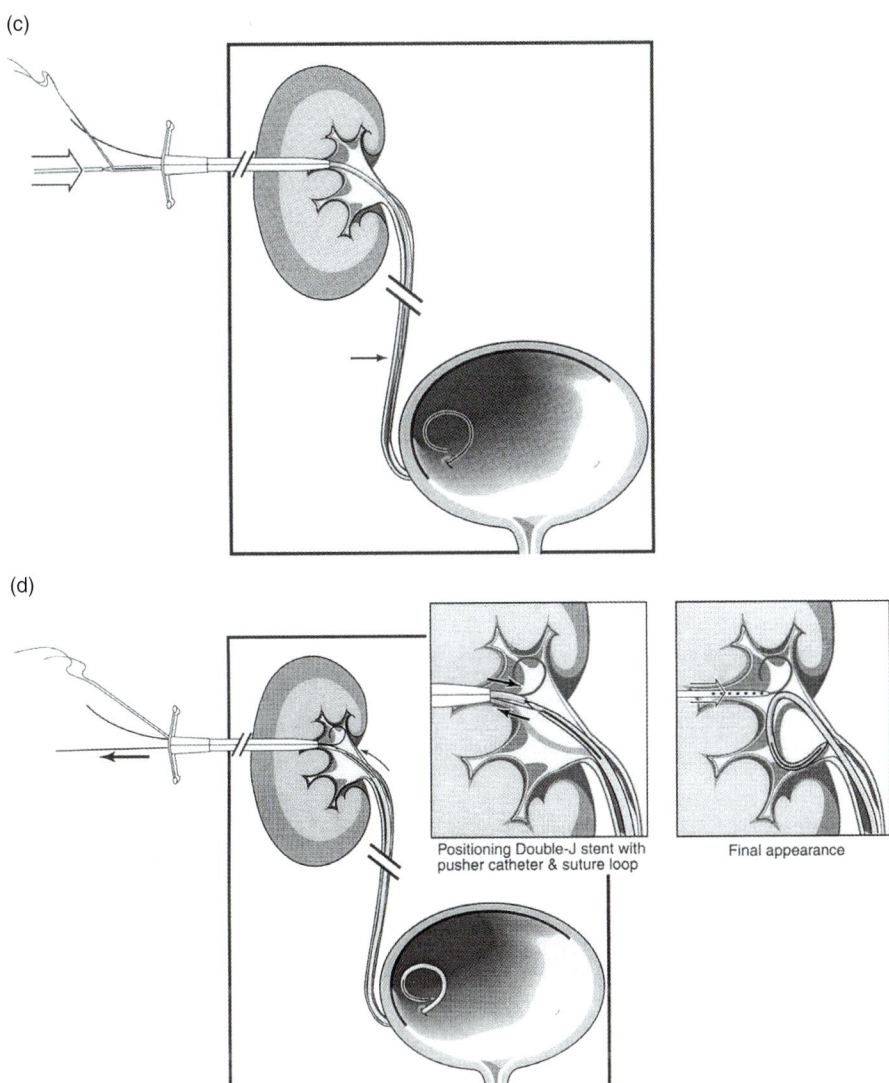

if there are no signs of ureteral obstruction or other clinical problems, the nephrostomy tube will be removed in 72 hours after stent function is confirmed by a nephrogram. If all is well, the next appointment is made in six to twelve weeks, at which time the child may be imaged to evaluate the size and drainage of the ureter. This can be accomplished with an excretory urogram, nuclear study, US, or a nephrostogram in children with universal drains. In some instances, the stent is removed without imaging based on the absence of prohibitive clinical signs or symptoms.

Complications

Any reported complication resulting from nephrostomy insertion such as bleeding, sepsis, and urine extravasation secondary to a leak or laceration may also be noted after a percutaneous surgical procedure. Complications related to stent placement are unusual in the pediatric population. Stent occlusion is probably the most common complication and occurs secondary to encrustation, bleeding, or, rarely, infection. An encrusted stent is prone to secondary infection that may lead to sepsis. Thus it is important to keep the urine dilute and sterile. Stent occlusion can be detected by cystography, antegrade pyelography, intravenous urography, or (if a PCN catheter or universal stent remains in position) nephrostomy injection. In most instances, cystography is performed. If the stent is patent, vesicoureteral reflux is seen.

Stent migration (Figure 6.34) and pain often occur if the stent is not adequately positioned or if it is not the correct length. Careful technique and accurate measurement of ureteral length and selection of a stent of appropriate diameter avoid this problem. When stents are too long, urinary bladder irritation will occur. If unavoidable, bladder spasm can be treated with urinary anesthetics or antispasmodics, such as phenazopyridine. Fistula formation between the ureter and adjacent bowel or blood vessels, and catheter erosion through

Table 6.18 Procedure summary: ureteral stent insertion

- Nephrostomy access to renal pelvis
- Dilate tract
- Insert peel-away sheath into pelvis
- Inject iodinated contrast to identify and measure stenosis
- With a directional catheter maneuver an angled hydrophilic guide wire into the bladder
- Using the bent guide wire technique or a calibrated guide wire, measure the distance from the ureteropelvic junction (UPJ) to the ureterovesicular junction (UVJ)
- Depending on the intended duration of therapy, select the universal or internal–external (shorter therapy) or an internal or double-J (longer therapy) stent of appropriate length for the measured ureter, without using a stent too short to reach from the renal pelvis to the bladder comfortably
- Place a long retention suture through a proximal end and side hole to reposition the double-J stent if necessary
- Insert the stent over a guide wire, using a pusher catheter for double-J stent insertion
- For a universal stent, secure the locking loop in the renal pelvis
- For a double-J stent, the retention suture may be removed once appropriate position is confirmed, using the pusher catheter for counter traction
- For a double-J stent, a nephrostomy catheter may be left in the renal pelvis until adequate function is confirmed

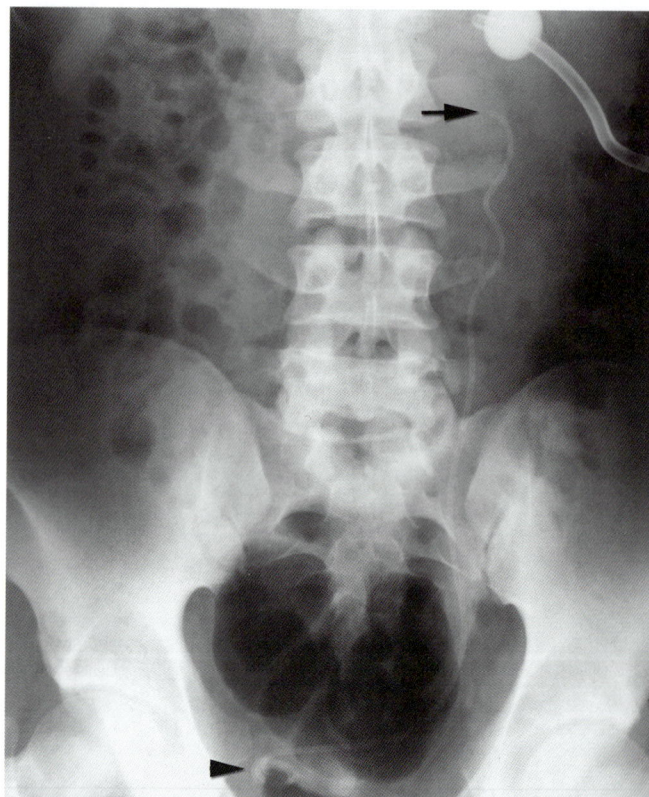

Figure 6.34 If the chosen stent is too long for the ureter, elastic recoil tends to draw the redundant catheter (*arrowhead*) into the bladder. In this case the proximal end (*arrow*) has become malpositioned too deeply in the ureter to grasp with a snare. This stent must be removed through the urethra and may be replaced either by rewiring the partially exteriorized stent from below or through the existing nephrostomy access from above.

the renal pelvis, have been reported in the adult population but as yet not in children. Once having migrated, internal stents can sometimes be snared and repositioned, either through the urethra (especially in female patients) or through an existing nephrostomy access, depending upon the direction of migration. Occasionally, they must be removed (Figure 6.35) and replaced.

The ideal timing for stent removal or replacement has not been well established. We prefer to limit the time the stent is left *in situ* to twelve weeks. With high-risk children, such as those with renal transplants on immune suppression, shorter intervals are recommended. Stents in place for long periods of time (greater than one year) have a higher incidence of mineralization and stent fracture. However, to date, this has not been reported in the pediatric population, likely due to the short duration of stenting in most patients. A stent fracture has been reported in an adult who had a stent inadvertently left in place for 17 months.

Conclusions

Dilation and stenting of the ureter are technically possible in children of all ages and sizes but require appropriate equipment. If needed, standard drains can be modified for use in children with short ureters. The ureteral diameter is usually not a limiting factor in successfully draining, dilating, or stenting an obstructed ureter. It is likely that in the future, treatment of ureteral obstruction will be the province of minimally invasive approaches.

Percutaneous endopyelotomy

Introduction

Descriptions of attempted surgical repair of the ureter appear in the literature as early as the late nineteenth century. In 1943, Davis described the intubated ureterostomy for treatment of lengthy, or multiple, ureteral and UPJ strictures. In this procedure, the ureter is incised from the outside and a stent placed to enlarge the ureteral diameter. Davis showed that the ureter would heal and maintain the larger diameter, thereby resolving the obstruction. In 1983, Wickham and Kellett and Whitfield and Mills described the endoscopic counterpart to the Davis intubated ureterostomy, using a nephroscope to treat a UPJ obstruction by incising the stricture under direct vision using a cold knife followed by stenting. In 1984, Clayman and associates showed that electrosurgical techniques could be safely applied to percutaneous therapy. The work of these and other pioneers provided the impetus and means to develop percutaneous surgical techniques in children.

Badlani and colleagues later popularized the endopyelotomy technique. Their results and those of other investigators compared favorably to results achieved by open pyeloplasty. In

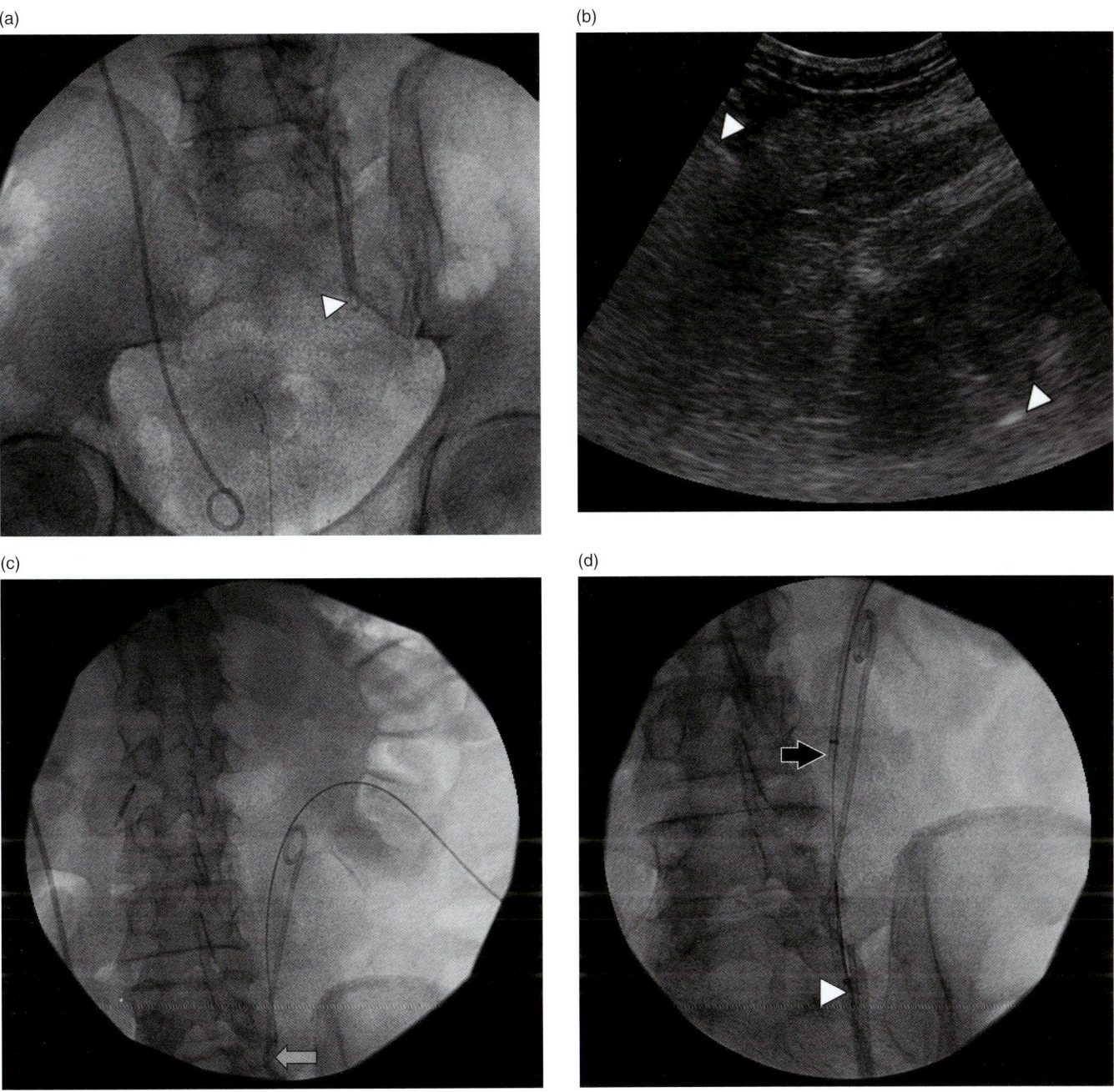

Figure 6.35 (a) The right double-J ureteral stent is in good position. The left stent (*arrowhead*) is malpositioned with the distal stent coiled in the ureter. (b) The left renal collecting system was accessed with a 21-gauge Chiba needle (*arrowheads*) using a 5 to 3 MHz curvilinear US transducer for guidance. (c) After exchanging via a 4-French Neff introducer, a 0.035-inch stiff Glide® wire (*arrow*) was advanced into the ureter. (d) A trefoil snare (*arrowhead*) through a guiding catheter (*arrow*) was used to capture the distal end of the malpositioned stent. (e) The snared stent was then withdrawn (*arrow*) through the guiding catheter (*arrowhead*). (f) A new stent was then inserted.

1987, Towbin and colleagues demonstrated that the percutaneous approach could be successfully performed on children with congenital UPJ obstruction. Since the initial report, a satisfactory long-term result has been achieved in 22 of 23 children treated.

The surgical dismembered pyeloplasty remains the mainstay for treatment of children with primary strictures of the UPJ. However, with the development of percutaneous surgical techniques, percutaneous endopyelotomy (percutaneous pyeloplasty) has become an acceptable alternative, as well as the preferred intervention for children with secondary UPJ strictures. As is the case for nephrolithotomy, percutaneous endopyelotomy (PE) can be performed as a one- or two-step procedure.

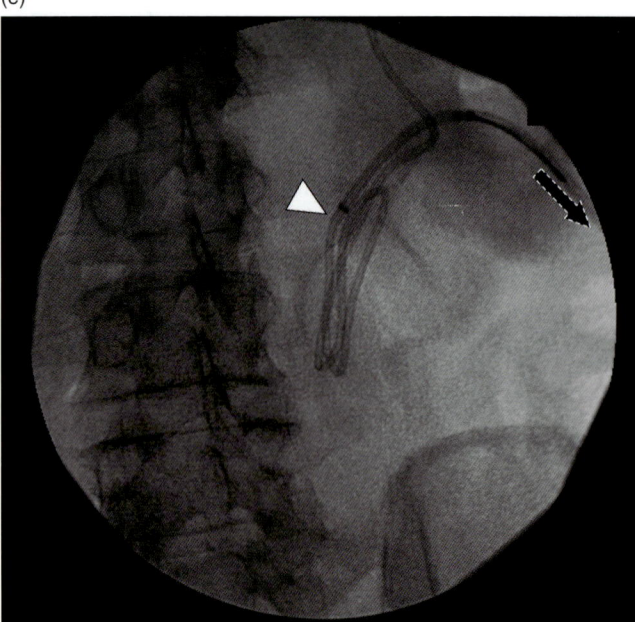
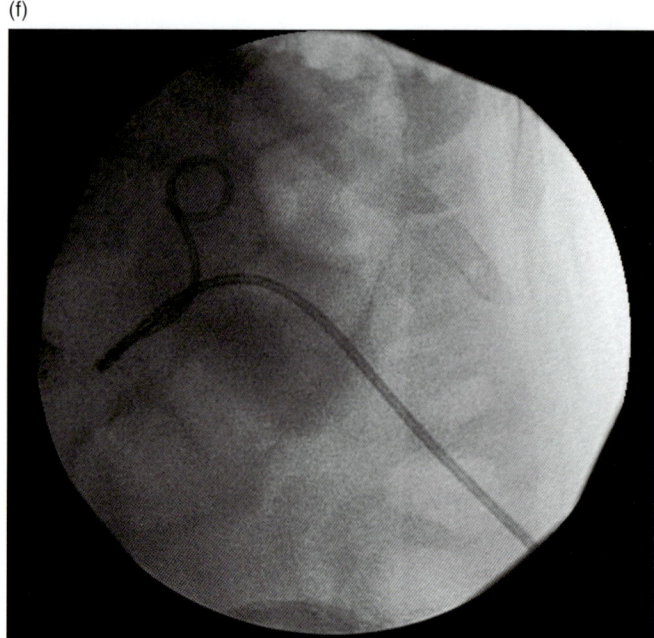

Figure 6.35 (cont.)

Indications

The indications for endopyelotomy are generally the same as those for an open surgical procedure. Children with congenital or acquired strictures of the UPJ are candidates for endopyelotomy, especially when concomitant pyelocaliceal calculi can be simultaneously treated (taking care to remove the stones prior to the endopyelotomy). In addition, these endourologic techniques are applicable to individuals with ureteral strictures. Although there are only a few absolute contraindications to either percutaneous (antegrade) or endoscopic (retrograde) approaches, children with long (greater than 2 cm) strictures respond poorly to endopyelotomy and may be best treated with an open procedure. Very small children may also benefit from open surgery; however, with the continued development of small equipment, young children have had successful minimally invasive surgical procedures. Currently, there are no studies to allow for a definitive conclusion as to the best approach. As is true for all other interventions, children with uncorrectable coagulopathy, intrarenal hemorrhage, active infection, who are medically unstable, and those with unapproachable anatomy are not candidates for minimally invasive surgery until their underlying problems are resolved. The presence of crossing vessels, especially in the face of massive hydronephrosis, may be considered a relative contraindication for a minimally invasive intervention.

Technique

Equipment

Preparation for the endopyelotomy procedure follows the modular principles previously discussed, as it is built upon the foundation of "Access to the renal pelvis," "Guide wire stabilization," and "Tract dilation" in an identical manner to other complex endourologic procedures. Therefore the bulk of the equipment required to successfully perform this procedure (Table 6.19) relates to these preparatory steps. Once a suitable tract has been developed and a sheath placed for passage of an appropriately sized nephroscope, a device must be selected for incising the ureteral or ureteropelvic junction stricture. Choices currently include a cold knife, electrocautery, laser, cutting balloon, cautery wire cutting balloon, or a "hot knife" (e.g., Bugbee electrode or Collins knife). However, once the incision is made, the enlarged tract must then be stented, and a nephrostomy catheter left in place for a short time to maintain renal access, assuring antegrade drainage and permitting re-access in the event of acute complications.

Patient preparation

Preprocedural imaging for patients with UPJ obstruction will often include renal US, diuretic renogram, excretory urogram, and perhaps abdominal (renal) CT to confirm the diagnosis and help plan treatment including identification of the safest place for incising the stricture. All patients should have sterile urine prior to the procedure. If an upper tract infection cannot be cleared due to obstruction, drainage via PCN can be used as a temporizing measure. Preprocedural IV antibiotics usually include a cephalosporin or whatever culture and sensitivity suggests. A type and screen should be obtained due to the small but real risk of bleeding requiring transfusion.

Standard technique

Percutaneous endopyelotomy may be performed by an interventionalist alone or in conjunction with a pediatric urologist

(Figure 6.36). The pediatric interventionalist establishes renal access, dilates the tract, and inserts a sheath (approximately 2 mm larger than the nephroscope) for passage of the nephroscope and other instruments. Additionally, the interventionalist positions a stable guide wire externalized at the nephrostomy site and either coiled in the urinary bladder or externalized at the urethral meatus ("body floss"). The interventionalist also provides imaging guidance for efficient positioning of the nephroscope. When necessary, the pediatric urologist, often with the assistance of the interventionalist, conducts those portions of the procedure employing nephroscopy and cystoscopy. Depending on the instrument used to incise the stricture, either the urologist or the interventionalist may conduct the maneuver.

For complex procedures it is best to work together, since together we are better able to overcome obstacles that might substantially impede the progress of either acting independently. For example, while the interventionalist may be able to pass the guide wire beyond the UPJ obstruction into the urinary bladder using conventional antegrade techniques under fluoroscopic guidance; rotation, elevation and effacement of the UPJ may result in an eccentric stricture and make

Table 6.19 Equipment: percutaneous endopyelotomy

- Directional catheter
- Exchange-length guide wire (0.035- or 0.038-inch)
- Progressive dilators with coaxial sheaths
- PTA balloon for tract dilation (3 to 8 mm)
- Nephroscope
- Electrocautery, cold knife, Acucise ureteral cutting balloon
- Internal (double-J) stent (5 to 8 French)
- End-hole Foley (use sterile punch to create end hole) or Council catheter (10 to 24 French)

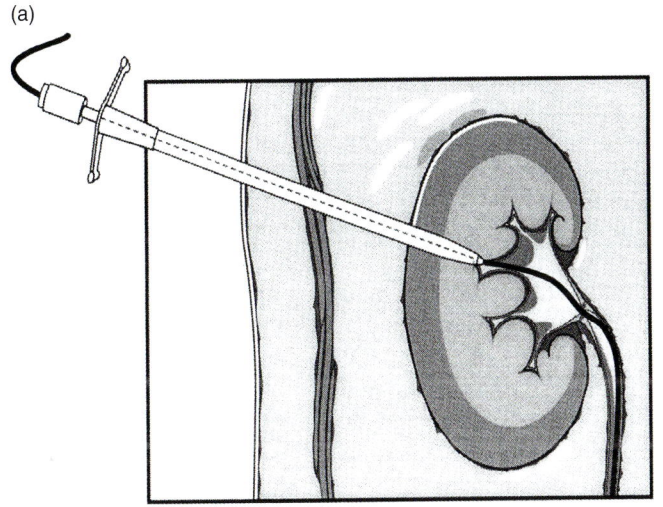

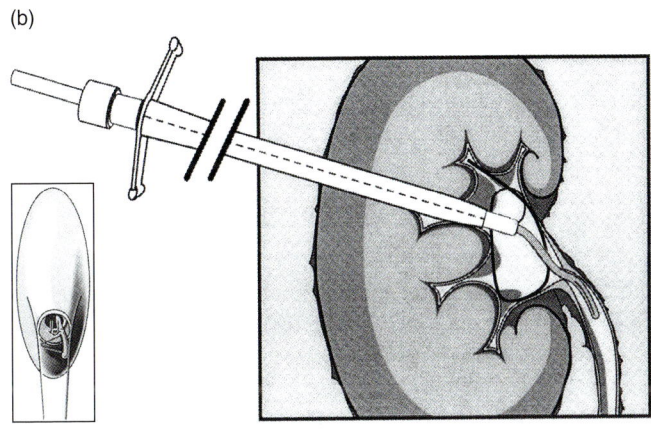

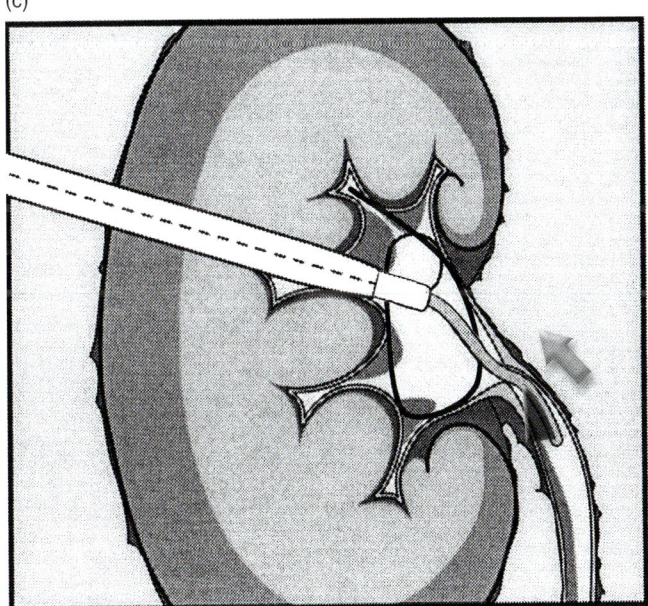

Figure 6.36 Endopyelotomy illustration. (a) Preparation for endopyelotomy is similar to other endourologic procedures: establishment of access to the renal collecting system and development of a working channel through tract dilatation and sheath insertion. A stiff guide wire is advanced to the bladder and exteriorized through the urethra if possible. (b) If the working wire is coiled in the bladder, a safety wire may be coiled in the renal pelvis or the bladder to assure access. If a nephroscope is used it is advanced to visualize the UPJ obstruction. The cutting device is then maneuvered across the stricture (*inset*). (c) Once past the obstruction, the cutting device is deployed to achieve a full-thickness incision, usually through the posterolateral wall of the UPJ, extending from the proximal ureter into the renal pelvis.

this task very time-consuming and laborious. However, retrograde (cystoscopic) passage of the guide wire by the urologist is usually accomplished rapidly and without difficulty, positioning the tip of the guide wire in the renal pelvis where it can easily be grasped and externalized by the interventionalist or urologist. Similarly, working alone the urologist will in time usually locate the UPJ with the nephroscope, at which time the incision can be made by the surgeon's method of choice. However, the interventionalist can help the urologist quickly orient the endoscope very close to the UPJ using fluoroscopy alone, following which nephroscopic location of the UPJ is greatly simplified. In both cases, substantial time under anesthesia can be saved, the rate of complications reduced, and the cumulative amount of ionizing radiation exposure decreased, taking advantage of the opportunity for beneficial collaboration.

Our approach to performing an endopyelotomy varies depending on the pathologic anatomy. For complex cases, cystoscopy is performed, and a guide wire is inserted into the renal pelvis. Retrograde guide wire placement is often easier especially in patients with severe hydronephrosis and eccentric stenosis of the UPJ. If difficulty passing the guide wire is encountered, the antegrade approach is utilized and a directional catheter and guide wire are used to probe until the guide wire is directed past the stricture into the ureter or urinary bladder.

With the child in prone or prone-oblique position, the renal pelvis is accessed via a mid-posterior or superolateral calyx using real-time US guidance (as described under "Percutaneous nephrostomy," above). Once renal access has been obtained, the tract is dilated. The tract size is determined by the size of the nephroscope or largest piece of equipment to be used (Table 6.20). After tract enlargement using a PTA balloon or progressive dilators, a sheath two French sizes larger than the nephroscope is left in place. After the stenosis has been crossed with a guide wire, it is externalized from the side opposite the site of insertion, so as to gain control of the guide wire from both ends (see "Stabilizing the guide wire," Chapter 2). A hemostat is fastened to the distal (urethral) end so that the guide wire cannot be inadvertently removed during the procedure. In this circumstance a second guide wire (safety wire) is not necessary.

A Rutner valve, or a rotating hemostatic valve, is connected to the sheath so that an endoscope can be used without the use of large volumes of water while maintaining a relatively "dry" field. Using a combination of direct vision and fluoroscopy, the endoscope is maneuvered to the UPJ, and an incision is made with a cold knife blade, electrocautery (Figure 6.37), laser, or cautery wire cutting balloon. Regardless of the instrument used, the incision is made through the full thickness of the UPJ until periureteric fat is identified. The posterolateral wall is usually selected as the site of incision, since this is an unlikely site for vessels to course. In cases where the ureter inserts into the anterior or posterior wall of the renal pelvis,

Table 6.20 Procedure summary: endopyelotomy

- Position the child on the table (prone or prone-oblique)
- Select entry site
- Inject local anesthesia (buffered)
- Obtain access to the renal pelvis, usually via a posterior mid-pole calyx
- Dilate the tract to at least the diameter of the sheath
- Position a peel-away sheath
- Catheterize the ureter
- Mark level of stricture with Beekley® dot or hemostat
- Maneuver a directional catheter and guide wire into the bladder
- Measure the diameter and length of the stricture and select the appropriate device to restore ureteral patency
- For acquired or recurrent ureteral stricture, consider a non-compliant (angioplasty) balloon
- For congenital UPJ stricture, incise stricture posterolaterally via
  - enteroscope with cautery or cutting blade, or
  - cutting balloon (e.g., Acucise®) catheter
- Place universal or internal (double-J) stent
- For double-J stent, insert temporary nephrostomy
- Perform antegrade pyelogram to confirm patency of ureter and stent function
- Remove nephrostomy when adequate function without extravasation is confirmed
- Remove stent no earlier than six weeks after incisional procedure
- Confirm function with excretory urogram prior to stent removal

the incision should extend from the proximal ureter into the renal pelvis. The procedure is completed by insertion of a 5- to 8-French internal stent and a Council (end-hole nephrostomy) or pigtail catheter.

Technical variations
Pediatric modifications

While it is possible to successfully perform percutaneous surgery with standard equipment, it is extremely helpful to use equipment modified for the pediatric population, especially in small children. The standard Teflon® (gray) sheath, which is piggybacked on the dilator, is one French larger than the dilator. In most young children, the sheath is too long. In addition, in the progressive dilator sets, the smallest Teflon sheath is 19 French, which is considerably larger than what is required in most instances. Thus modifications have been made to shorten the sheath from the standard. This can be accomplished with scissors or ordered as such from the manufacturer. The sheath is shortened after measuring the tract length and the nephroscope length. These simple changes make manipulation of the endoscope and other equipment much easier.

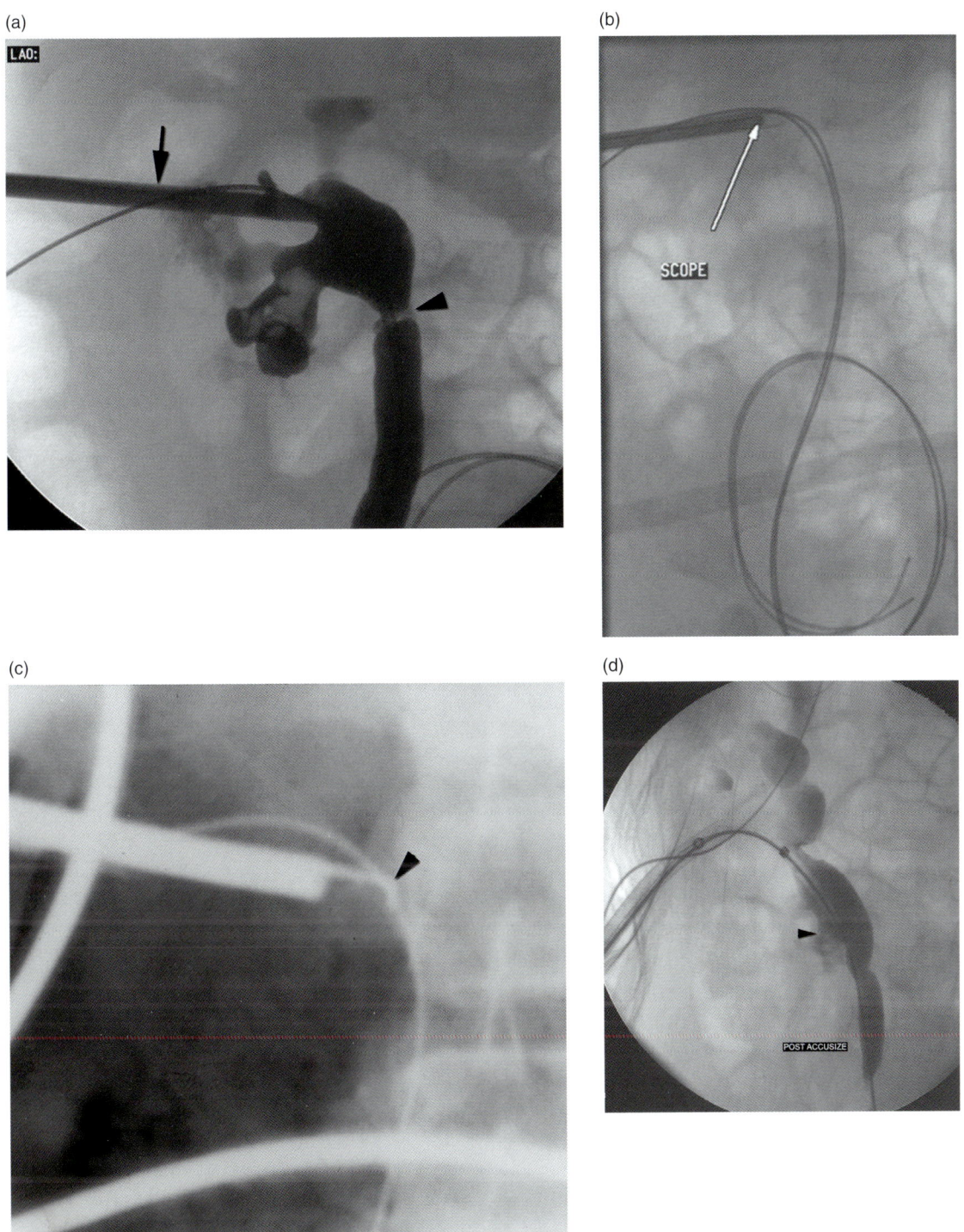

Figure 6.37 (a) With a transrenal sheath (*arrow*) providing secure access to the renal pelvis, a safety wire and a working wire are advanced past the UPJ stricture (*arrowhead*) to the bladder. (b) With combined endoscopic and fluoroscopic control, the nephroscope (*arrow*) is advanced to visualize the stricture in preparation for delivery of the cutting device. (c) In a different patient, an electrocautery device (*arrowhead*) is in position to incise the UPJ stricture. (d) After incising the stricture, it is not uncommon to observe extravasation at the site (*arrowhead*), reflecting the goal of achieving a full-thickness incision. (e) When endopyelotomy is performed, a ureteral stent must be left in place across the stricture until all leakage has resolved, the incision site has healed, and antegrade flow of urine has been confirmed with an intravenous pyelogram, usually six to eight weeks after the incision.

(e)

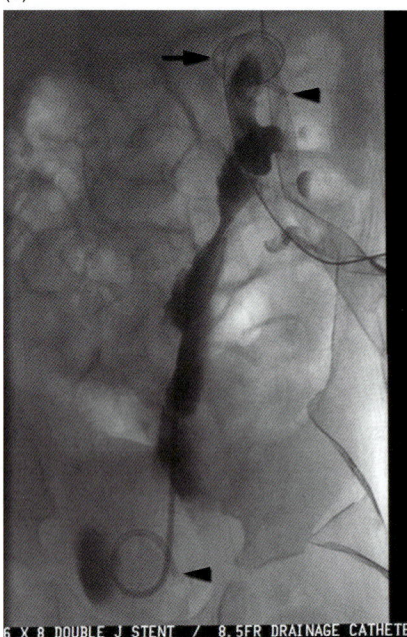

Figure 6.37 (cont.)

"Stent first, hot knife" variation

In 2000, Savage and Streem introduced a modification of the EP technique using initial placement of an internal ureteral stent to guide and simplify the ureteral incision. With the stent in place, a cutting current (through a Bugbee electrode or Collins knife) is used to incise the proximal ureter and renal pelvis. Besides better defining the UPJ, the stent provides a heat sink to protect the remainder of the ureter from thermal injury and circumvents the risk of postincision avulsion at the UPJ during stent placement. Caution must be taken to use an insulated guide wire to avoid transmitting the current in the event of contact with the active electrode.

Postprocedure and follow-up care

At the completion of the procedure, the child is admitted to the recovery room and observed for six to eight hours. Following the procedure, appropriate notes and postprocedure orders are entered into the patient's chart. It may be helpful to both patient care and ongoing quality assurance to maintain pertinent demographic and procedure-related data in an electronic database. Suggested items for data management are included in Table 6.6.

Generally, the child is admitted overnight for monitoring of vital signs and observing for untoward effects. In addition, children often require analgesia for mild to moderate discomfort. In most cases, all that is required is acetaminophen or ketorolac. In some instances, a narcotic analgesic, such as morphine or Demerol® (meperidine), is needed for a short period. After discharge, the child is instructed to resume normal activity as tolerated. Strenuous activity should be avoided for eight to ten days following the procedure.

Two weeks after endopyelotomy, the child is brought to the radiology department and the nephrostomy tube is injected with contrast. If there is prompt antegrade flow of contrast into the urinary bladder and no extravasation occurs or other complication is identified, the nephrostomy tube is removed. The internal stent is kept in place for six to eight weeks to allow the UPJ incision to heal. Prior to removal, an intravenous pyelogram is performed to evaluate the operative site. The stent is then removed through the urethra. The patient may be seen one month following stent removal for evaluation, usually with IVU or diuretic renogram. If in the asymptomatic child, renal pelvic dilation is decreased or the renogram is non-obstructive, subsequent evaluation may be planned for six months, then annually for two to three years.

Complications

In most large series, the success rate of an endopyelotomy for the treatment of strictures at the ureteropelvic junction is 85 to 90% with a range of 57 to 100%. It appears that a failed endopyelotomy does not jeopardize the success of a subsequent open surgical procedure. An endopyelotomy can be performed either percutaneously or retrograde via an endoscope. Experience has shown that the success rates achieved are similar with both techniques.

In general, the complication rate is low. The exact rate and type of complications depend somewhat upon the technical approach selected and the indication for therapy. Major complications have been reported and include hemorrhage requiring transfusion or occasionally embolization, ureteral necrosis, and ureteral avulsion. However, minor problems occur more frequently (10 to 23%) and include stent- or nephrostomy-related problems, malpositioned stent, retroperitoneal hemorrhage or urinoma, dysuria, flank pain, and infection. Stenoses of the ureter at the UVJ obstruction, or in the urethra, can occur in up to 20% of cases. This problem may result from the long duration of the procedure, local trauma, or thermal damage from the use of electrocautery to incise the stricture. The incidence and type of complications occurring using the Acucise® device appear to be similar to the other methods used to incise strictures of the UPJ and ureter, and are in the range of 11 and 9% for acute and delayed complications, respectively. It is important to realize that it is possible to lacerate adjacent blood vessels (e.g., accessory lower pole, or "crossing" vessels) and cause major hemorrhage as is true with the other devices. Although vascular injury is uncommon, it has been reported in several cases, including laceration of a common iliac artery and an ovarian vein.

Other possible untoward effects of EP include congestive heart failure, oliguria, hematuria, intrarenal clots, recurrent strictures, and hydrothorax or pneumothorax. The latter two problems can occur when the pleural space is transgressed at the time of renal access. Therefore it is imperative that the operator is aware of the likely position of the pulmonary sulcus.

Conclusions

Percutaneous endopyelotomy appears to be a safe and effective method for the treatment of both primary and secondary strictures of the ureter, UPJ, and possibly ureterovesicular junction. There are currently several methods available to incise the stricture including a cold knife, electrocautery, and the Acucise® balloon catheter. Each approach appears to result in a successful outcome with a low complication rate and good long-term patency.

The best results with percutaneous endopyelotomy have been achieved in children with a secondary stricture, occurring within a few months of an injury or surgery. In addition to postoperative strictures, congenital UPJ narrowing, strictures associated with stones, and those secondary to tumors have all been successfully managed with percutaneous therapy. Variable results have been seen with long strictures, e.g., UVJ strictures after ureteral reimplantation and ureteroenterostomy strictures. Results with balloon dilation of congenital and acquired UPJ strictures have been mixed. We have found that percutaneous endopyelotomy is an effective method of treatment in children with congenital UPJ strictures and is a good alternative for children who have contraindications to surgery or for those children and their families who elect the percutaneous approach. Balloon dilation is reserved for treatment of individuals with recurrent UPJ strictures especially those resulting from failed surgical pyeloplasty (see "Balloon dilation of ureteral strictures," above).

Open surgery still remains the gold standard for the treatment of either primary or secondary UPJ obstruction at most institutions. However, many authors now believe that the endourologic approach is superior. In general, the minimally invasive techniques described above are very well suited to treat urinary tract abnormalities in the pediatric population. Depending on the clinical (and political) situation, the interventionalist should be available to treat urinary tract disease alone or in conjunction with the pediatric urologist to provide the best outcome for the child. Proponents of endopyelotomy suggest that the reduced overall morbidity, decreased postoperative analgesic requirements, shorter hospital stay, and more rapid return to normal activity all favor the endourologic approach.

Chapter 7
Musculoskeletal and soft tissue interventions

Kevin M. Baskin, Richard Towbin, David Aria and Carrie Schaefer

History 358
Interventional radiology and musculoskeletal interventions 358
Team approach 358
Imaging guidance 358
Fluoroscopic imaging 358
Ultrasound 358
Computed tomography 358
Magnetic resonance imaging 360
Molecular imaging 360
Instruments and devices 360
Drills and other power tools 360
INTERVENTIONS IN THE SOFT TISSUES 360
Aspiration and drainage of fluid collections 360
Introduction 360
Indications 360
Technique 360
Equipment 360
Patient preparation 360
Preprocedure imaging 362
Preprocedural lab studies 362
Standard technique 362
Postprocedure and follow-up care 362
Complications 362
Conclusions 362
Biopsy of lymph nodes and soft tissue masses 362
Introduction 362
Indications 363
Technique 363
Equipment 363

Patient preparation 363
Standard technique 363
Postprocedure and follow-up care 364
Complications 364
Conclusions 364
Foreign body retrieval 365
Introduction 365
Indications 365
Technique 365
Equipment 365
Patient preparation 366
Standard technique 366
Technical variations 366
Postprocedure and follow-up care 367
Complications 367
Conclusions 367
Chemodenervation of the salivary glands 368
Introduction 368
Indications 368
Technique 368
Equipment 368
Patient preparation 368
Dosage 369
Standard technique 369
Parotid gland 369
Submandibular gland 369
Technical variations 370
Postprocedure and follow-up care 370
Complications 370
Future advances 370
Conclusions 370
Partial gland ablation and sclerotherapy of ranula 370

Pediatric Interventional Radiology, ed. Richard Towbin and Kevin M. Baskin. Published by Cambridge University Press. © Cambridge University Press 2015.

Introduction 370
Indications 371
Technique 371
Equipment 371
Patient preparation 371
Standard technique 373
Sclerotherapy 373
Partial gland ablation 373
Postprocedure and follow-up care 373
Complications 375
Future advances 375
Conclusions 375
INTERVENTIONS IN THE JOINT CAVITIES, TENDON SHEATHS, AND BURSAE 375
Arthrography and related interventions 375
Introduction 375
Indications 376
Technique 376
Equipment 376
Patient preparation 377
Standard technique 378
Postprocedure and follow-up care 379
Complications 379
ORTHOPEDIC INTERVENTIONS 380
Percutaneous treatment of cystic bone lesions 380
Introduction 380
Indications 380
Technique 381
Equipment 381
Patient preparation 383
Standard technique 383
Postprocedure and follow-up care 383
Complications 383
Issues and controversies 384
Conclusions 384
Percutaneous biopsy of solid bone lesions 385
Introduction 385
Indications 386
Equipment 388

Imaging 389
Patient preparation 389
Standard technique 389
Postprocedure and follow-up care 392
Complications 392
Bone tumor (osteoid osteoma) excision 392
Introduction 392
Indications 392
Equipment 392
Imaging 392
Drill and curettage 394
Additional equipment and supplies 394
Patient preparation 394
Standard technique 394
Technical variations 395
Postprocedure and follow-up care 396
Complications 397
Conclusions 397
Locoregional thermal ablation of bone lesions 397
Introduction 397
Indications 397
Technique 397
Equipment 397
Patient preparation 397
Standard technique 397
Postprocedure and follow-up care 398
Complications 399
Conclusions 399
Percutaneous reduction with internal fixation 399
Introduction 399
Indications 400
Technique 400
Equipment 400
Patient preparation 400
Standard technique 401
Technical variations 401
Postprocedure and follow-up care 403
Complications 403
Conclusions 403

History

In the past, the primary approach to diagnostic and therapeutic procedures involving the musculoskeletal (MSK) system has been open surgery by orthopedic surgeons, with the exceptions of joint aspiration and arthrography. Over time an increasingly broad range of these procedures are carried out using image-guided approaches, and consequently interventional radiologists are exercising a larger role, both in procedural collaboration with the orthopedic surgeons, neurosurgeons, rheumatologists, and other related proceduralists, as well as a more substantial role in clinical consultation for evaluation and management of relevant patients. It is in the MSK system that the modular approach to procedure development has worked particularly well, and this has led to an increasing diversity of patient problems that fall within the scope of practice of the pediatric interventionalist and an increasingly fertile area for innovation and collegial development of creative solutions. It is likely that this trend will continue and over time there will be fewer open procedures performed and increasing integration of interventional involvement in the care of these patients.

Interventional radiology and musculoskeletal interventions

Team approach

Interventions for problems that involve the MSK system and soft tissues can often be accomplished with improved outcomes, less surgical trauma, and a shorter recovery time if image-guided techniques are used compared to traditional open surgical approaches. For example, traumatic fracture of the pelvis with both anterior and posterior instability has traditionally been treated using a large anterior incision and plating across the reduced sacroiliac (SI) fracture. The same objective, stabilization of the posterior ring instability, can be accomplished through a small posterolateral incision with image-guided placement of one or more screws across the SI fracture after closed reduction of the dislocation. Details and advantages of this procedure are outlined below under "Orthopedic interventions." Because of the infrequency of this problem, interventionalists seldom have a depth of experience with the required hardware and delivery systems, while orthopedic surgeons usually lack training with sophisticated cross-sectional image guidance.

Collaboration allows optimal application of asymmetric skill sets to optimize high-quality outcomes not easily achieved by either subspecialty in isolation. In this domain, interventionalists can collaborate with orthopedic surgeons, trauma surgeons, neurosurgeons, rheumatologists, radiologists, oncologists, palliative care physicians, pathologists, anesthesiologists, intensivists, infectious disease physicians, and others, to derive innovative solutions to difficult problems and cost-effective solutions to common problems. A number of such innovative approaches are highlighted in this chapter. It is essential to practice development and the process of continuous quality improvement to keep careful records of the parameters of interventional procedures and outcomes. Recommended data elements are included in Table 7.1.

Imaging guidance

Fluoroscopic imaging

In the pediatric musculoskeletal system, fluoroscopic guidance is rarely used as a single modality, except for arthrography and joint injections (contrast for MR or steroids for synovitis). Rare indications include access to lytic, cystic, or blastic lesions in relatively safe locations, large (>3 cm) partially calcified soft tissue lesions, and cementoplasty procedures such as vertebroplasty. Rotational imaging with cone-beam CT reconstruction expands the use of fluoroscopy in the MSK system, allowing acquisition of volumetric images and development of route planning that can improve localization of lesions in the IR suite and ultimately reduce procedure time and radiation exposure for these complex cases. With increasing spatial resolution of these systems, the ability to visualize lesions on the angiography table rivals that in the CT suite, with potentially increased convenience and availability of interventional supplies, equipment, and supplemental imaging.

Ultrasound

Ultrasound has gained in popularity as a diagnostic modality in the MSK system over the past two decades, and has been used extensively either alone or in conjunction with fluoroscopy, for aspiration and drainage of abnormal soft tissue fluid collections, and biopsy of soft tissue masses and abnormal lymph nodes. It has also enabled retrieval of foreign bodies from the soft tissues, interventions in the salivary glands and ducts, and performance of a number of pain palliation procedures. Interventions in the soft tissues, joint cavities, tendon sheaths, and bursae can be performed with great precision and facility with US control without exposing the patient to ionizing radiation. Color Doppler adds information about the physiologic properties of target tissues, the location of vital vascular and neural structures, and pathologic hypervascularity of inflamed tissue that may be candidates for percutaneous therapy.

Additionally, there are a surprising number of procedures that can be accomplished in the bony skeleton and associated soft tissues with US guidance. For example, where the cortex has been disrupted by a malignant or inflammatory process, the abnormal bone or soft tissue mass may be readily visualized with US.

Computed tomography

Computed tomography provides exceptional bone and soft tissue resolution as well as exquisite visualization of vascular structures and nerves. In addition, CT is a precise tool for procedural guidance. For some lesions, such as osteoid

Table 7.1 Outcome measures

To improve outcome and quality assurance analysis, it may be helpful to record the following information for each musculoskeletal procedure:

- Demographic information (patient name, unique identification number, date and time of procedure, age, sex, weight, date of birth, etc.)
- Primary diagnosis (underlying disease), patient acuity, comorbid illness, ASA class, competence of patient or primary caregiver
- Any contraindicating or complicating factors
  - coagulopathy
  - infection, immunodeficiency, nutritional status, cardiorespiratory compromise
  - skin or mucosal abnormality (e.g., cellulitis, epidermolysis bullosa)
- Reason (indication) for procedure; referring service and provider; inpatient or outpatient status
- Anticipated endpoint (e.g., acquisition of fluid or tissue, resolution of symptoms, etc.)
- Primary provider responsible for procedure (interventional radiologist, orthopedic surgeon, rheumatologist, etc.)
- Collaborating provider(s)
- Procedure location (interventional suite, operating room, ICU, bedside, etc.)
- Provider(s) responsible for anesthesia/sedation (interventionalist, intensivist, anesthesiologist, nurse, etc.)
- Preprocedural evaluation (e.g., coagulation profile, creatinine, amylase, etc.)
- Preprocedure imaging (e.g., lesion localization, characterization and measurement, route planning)
- Preprocedural interventions (e.g., antibiotics, blood products, imaging,)
- Initial access
  - guidance (anatomic landmarks, US, fluoroscopy, CT, MRI, PET fusion, endoscopy, etc.)
  - operative site or pathway (e.g., percutaneous (location), transarterial, laparoscopic, open)
  - number of attempts/passes
  - reason for deferral, discontinuation or failure, if procedure not completed
- Access device and position
  - manufacturer, type, diameter, length, other pertinent characteristics
  - tip or target position
- Equipment and supplies used
- Procedure time, fluoroscopy time or estimated radiation dose
- Type and adequacy of anesthesia/sedation/analgesia
- Procedural complications (e.g., neurovascular injury, thermal injury to skin or soft tissues, bleeding) and management
- Adjunctive procedures (e.g., sclerotherapy, ablation, chemotherapy)
- Complications (major or minor), including
  - procedure-related discomfort (include dates)
    - type
    - management (e.g., NSAIDs, narcotics)
    - outcome
  - bleeding or vascular injury (include dates)
    - type (e.g., hemorrhage, AV fistula or pseudoaneurysm, thrombosis)
    - method of diagnosis (e.g., hemoglobin, US, CT scan, arteriogram)
    - management (e.g., observation, transfusion, embolization, thrombolysis)
    - outcome
  - neural injury (include dates)
    - type (e.g., thermal injury, neurolysis, impingement)
    - method of diagnosis (e.g., clinical exam, neurophysiologic testing)
    - management (e.g., observation, medication, surgical repair)
    - outcome
  - structural dysfunction (include dates)
    - type (e.g., stress riser, pathologic fracture, ligamentous injury)
    - method of diagnosis or documentation (e.g., clinical, imaging)
    - management (immobilization, stabilization, physical therapy)
    - outcome
- Other procedure-related complications (e.g., tract seeding) or interventions
- Complications, additional details
  - major
    - admission to hospital for therapy
    - unplanned increase in level of care
    - prolonged hospitalization
    - permanent adverse sequelae
    - death
  - minor
  - no sequelae
    - nominal therapy
    - short hospital stay (for observation)
  - procedurally related (within 24 hours)
  - early (within 30 days)
  - late
- For implanted devices, removal or replacement (reason and date; endpoint achieved?)
- Outcome at follow-up (method and date; endpoint achieved?)
  - postprocedural lab studies (e.g., fluid pH, culture or biopsy findings, amylase measurement)
  - response (e.g., reduction in fever, improved alignment, reduced debilitation or discomfort)
  - results (e.g., daily volume of fluid drained, radiographic evidence of resolution, hospital days)
  - treatment failure (e.g., recurrent abscess or fluid accumulation, recurrent symptoms)

osteoma, CT is best for diagnosis and procedural guidance. In order to optimize image guidance, it may be necessary to stablize the patient with appropriate padding and restraint (e.g., tape). It may also be useful to put the child in non-traditional positions to bring the target lesion and skin entry point into alignment within the image plane, and to move vital structures at risk (e.g., pleura, vessels) out of the procedural plane. Multiplanar CT reconstructions can help localize the target lesion and plan a safe and effective route. In some cases we have found it useful to localize the interventional target using CT, then complete the procedure using US guidance, thereby reducing total radiation exposure for the patient and reducing procedure time.

Magnetic resonance imaging

There has been increasing interest over time in integrating the excellent anatomic and physiologic information available with MRI with other modalities that can add fine temporal and spatial resolution for interventional procedures, especially including biopsies, spinal procedures, therapeutic injections, and loco-regional tumor ablation. Systems that combine MR with fluoroscopy, molecular imaging, and US have been explored, but to date high cost and limited utilization have restricted application of such systems in pediatric interventions.

Molecular imaging

PET-CT imaging can be very useful to obtain further physiologic information about the nature of a particular lesion, or when multiple lesions are present and there are no imaging features that distinguish one from the other. We are increasingly using PET-CT to target sites within a lesion to biopsy. We have found a subgroup of patients, i.e., osteomyelitis and neoplasia, with anatomically normal areas of the skeleton with abnormal PET activity and foci of metabolic activity within a mass. In these patients, our target is the metabolically active component of the lesion.

Instruments and devices
Drills and other power tools

There are obvious barriers to access in the bony skeleton compared to similar procedures in the soft tissues. Traditionally, interventional radiologists have used a variety of manual devices (such as trephines and biopsy needles) with tips modified to penetrate bone cortex, but these devices may take considerable force and time to gain access to the target lesion, especially when the overlying cortex is abnormally thickened due to the pathologic process. Orthopedic surgeons have been using power tools for the past three decades. These are generally available to qualified operators as a hospital resource through the operating room personnel on a first-come, first-served basis. If the use of such tools is unfamiliar to the interventional staff, thorough in-service education in proper use and safety is essential. In our experience, the use of power tools markedly shortens the procedure time and increases the accuracy and ease of the procedure. As an example, when we started to remove osteoid osteomas using trephines, it often took two hours. Now, with power tools, the case is completed in 30 to 45 minutes.

INTERVENTIONS IN THE SOFT TISSUES
Aspiration and drainage of fluid collections

Introduction

Treatment of abnormal fluid collections in the MSK system and soft tissues does not differ substantially from treatment in the abdomen, pelvis, or retroperitoneum (see Chapter 4). Management of abnormal fluid collections in the cervicofacial region (see "Partial gland ablation," below) and collections in the mediastinum and thorax (see Chapter 3) are covered in separate sections.

Indications

The purpose of aspiration and drainage of fluid collections is two-fold; to establish a microbiologic diagnosis and to drain the collection (Table 7.2). For larger collections (>3 cm), aspiration alone is unlikely to provide adequate drainage to allow successful resolution of the collection, with or without systemic therapy. Therefore, a drain 8.5 French or larger is inserted and placed to suction. There are very few anatomic limitations to successful aspiration and drainage of a fluid collection. With modern imaging, joint spaces, subperiosteal collections, and even suspected spondylodiscitis can be accessed accurately and safely.

Technique
Equipment

In general, there is no difference in the equipment used to accomplish aspiration and drainage in the musculoskeletal system and soft tissues compared to collections located elsewhere (see Table 4.13 and Figures 3.1 and 3.2).

Patient preparation

The procedure may be performed using sedation combined with generous application of local anesthesia, or with general

Table 7.2 Indications: aspiration and drainage of fluid collections

- Diagnose infection and establish antibiotic sensitivities
- Aspirate collections <3 cm
- Drain collections >3 cm

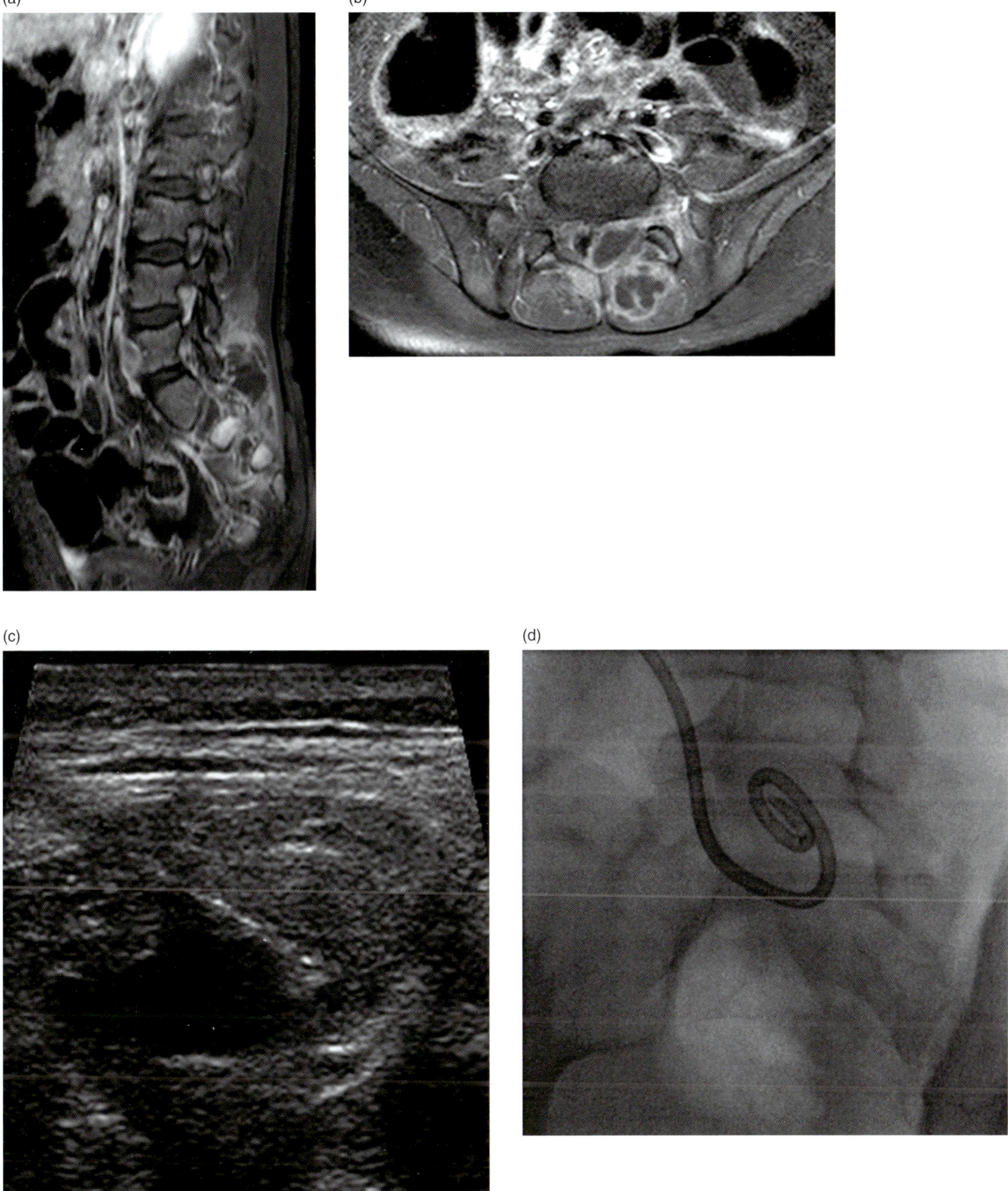

Figure 7.1 Eight-year-old female with fever and left buttock pain. (a,b) Sagittal and axial T1 FSE MRI postcontrast show abscesses involving the left paraspinal musculature with epidural extension. (c) Ultrasound-guided needle access and aspiration of purulent material. (d) 10.2-French pigtail drainage catheter placed.

Table 7.3 Procedure summary: aspiration and drainage of fluid collections

- Sedation/general anesthesia
- US (or other modality) localization of skin entry site. Mark entry site with washable ink
- Sterile preparation and draping
- US (or other modality) guided needle placement into fluid collection
- Remove fluid and send for laboratory analysis

anesthesia, depending on the patient's status and operator preference. If the periosteum is crossed, it is usually painful enough that general anesthesia is indicated.

Preprocedure imaging

In the musculoskeletal system and soft tissues, small collections may be quite difficult to localize and access. For a small collection, there is little that can be done to unequivocally differentiate fluid from phlegmon or edema. If fluid is not obtained, instillation of a small volume of non-bacteriostatic saline for irrigation and aspiration may be sufficient to obtain a sample for culture and analysis.

Preprocedural lab studies

Unless there is a history of abnormal bleeding, a known bleeding diathesis, or other condition requiring laboratory studies, preoperative laboratory studies are usually not necessary.

Standard technique

In the MSK system, small fluid collections can usually be sampled for diagnostic purposes with image-guided needle placement (Table 7.3). If fluid is not readily obtained but clearly present, a larger bore needle can be used on the premise that the collection may be too viscous for the smaller needle. If the collection is not otherwise accessible, it may be lavaged with a small volume of non-bacteriostatic saline before aspirating. If these maneuvers fail, a core biopsy specimen may be obtained for the purposes of laboratory analysis. In any case, clear goals should be set with the referring clinician and pathologist before the start of the procedure, in the event that a minimal sample is insufficient for all possible studies of interest. In the MSK system, depending on the type of infection, antibiotic coverage may be continued for six weeks or longer. For collections large enough to accommodate a formed pigtail drainage catheter leaving a catheter in place to gravity or suction (e.g, Jackson–Pratt bulb) is recommended until drainage stops (Figure 7.1). Fluid should be collected for laboratory analysis before contrast or other material is injected into the cavity.

Postprocedure and follow-up care

Following the procedure, longitudinal care of the patient should be provided as described elsewhere in this text (e.g., see Chapter 4: "Catheter fixation and drainage" and "Catheter removal"). As elsewhere, catheter management should be continued, including daily rounds under the supervision of the interventional service, until the process has resolved and the catheter has been discontinued. The interventional service may wish to schedule the patient for a follow-up visit in the outpatient IR clinic two to four weeks after catheter removal to evaluate the outcome and assure appropriate management of any complication or recurrence.

Complications

The main risks related to aspiration and drainage procedures include bleeding, infection, pain, and incomplete treatment with recurrence. Significant complications should very seldom be encountered. If a drain is placed adjacent to a bony structure, consideration should be given to the potential for catheter kinking or compression. Compression of a catheter against periosteum or within a muscle belly can be painful and should be avoided where possible.

Conclusions

The primary advantages of percutaneous aspiration and drainage with imaging guidance in the MSK system and soft tissues are less tissue trauma, shortened recovery time, and reduced cost in comparison to an open surgical procedure designed to accomplish the same objective.

Biopsy of lymph nodes and soft tissue masses

Introduction

Evaluation of the child with a soft tissue mass begins with consideration of the patient's age, the location of the mass, and the clinical history, including any known underlying predisposing conditions. The location and tissue origin of the mass can often be established with imaging. Plain radiography can be useful to examine the relationship of the mass to osseous structures and to demonstrate the presence of soft tissue calcifications. Ultrasound is perhaps most useful for characterization of soft tissue masses or nodules and to differentiate solid from cystic masses. Ultrasound offers the flexibility of a vascular study without requiring contrast administration, and can yield a great deal of physiologic information. Despite its cost and the frequent requirement for sedation or anesthesia, MRI remains the most versatile modality for analysis of a soft tissue mass. It provides excellent tissue contrast, ability to image deeply situated and large masses, can demonstrate invasion of deep tissue planes and involvement of major neurovascular bundles, and contributes significantly to the search for tumor extension and metastasis. Multiplanar reconstruction can facilitate determination of the tissue of origin, and arterial and venous imaging can help determine the vascularity of the

Table 7.4 Indications: biopsy of lymph nodes and soft tissue masses

- Possible malignancy
- Evaluate for recurrence
- Differentiate between metastasis and infection

lesion. Other modalities may offer specific advantages in limited situations, such as the evaluation of myositis ossificans with CT, and the further characterization of vascular supply, drainage, and spaces with angiography and venography.

Once a mass has been characterized to the degree possible with imaging, a few abnormal masses may be so uniquely identified that further differentiation is not necessary. For the rest, cellular or histopathologic evaluation is necessary before a final diagnosis is possible.

Indications

The differential for a palpable mass in the soft tissues includes pseudotumors, neoplastic tumors, and vascular malformations (Table 7.4). Pseudotumors in general do not require biopsy. Most can be identified by imaging characteristics in light of the patient's age, sex, location, and clinical history. Some, such as axillary breast tissue, post-traumatic lesions, and granulomata, simply need to be identified and left alone. Others, such as hematoma, cellulitis, and abscess, may require aspiration, drainage, or systemic therapy. Symptomatic periarticular cysts may benefit from aspiration and, if recurrent, steroid instillation. Vascular neoplasms and malformations, which are the most common cause of soft tissue masses in children, are considered in detail in Chapter 8.

Non-vascular neoplasms include fat-containing or adipocytic tumors (e.g., lipoma and liposarcoma), fibrous mesenchymal tumors (including such entities as nodular fasciitis and myositis ossificans, as well as infantile and adult-type fibrosarcoma), fibrohistiocytic tumors (including pigmented villonodular synovitis, giant cell tumor of the tendon sheath, dermatofibrosarcoma protuberans, and malignant fibrous histiocytoma), smooth muscle and skeletal muscle tumors (e.g., leiomyoma and rhabdomyosarcoma), a variety of soft tissue sarcomas that may be of uncertain origin, lymphoma, and tumors of neurogenic origin (e.g. schwannoma, neurofibroma, and malignant peripheral nerve sheath tumors) that may have a soft tissue presentation.

In some patients, a history of prior malignancy or predisposing factors, such as neurofibromatosis type 1, narrow the differential diagnosis. When the imaging characteristics of a previously treated malignancy are known, such as an FDG-avid lymphoma, repeat imaging with the same technique may discriminate between recurrent tumor and a benign process, and may obviate biopsy. However, the majority of abnormal nodules and soft tissue masses in children should be biopsied. Biopsy can also be useful to determine the causative organism in suspected infection or infection unresponsive to empiric therapy.

The only absolute contraindication to biopsy in the soft tissues is an arterial mass. The vascularity of each lesion should be known prior to a biopsy procedure. Biopsy should not be performed through overlying tissues that are infected, and a predisposition to bleeding should be corrected to the degree possible prior to an invasive procedure.

Technique

Equipment

The necessary equipment and standard technique for soft tissue biopsy is no different from that used in biopsies of the chest, abdomen, or pelvis (see Table 4.16).

Patient preparation

Unlike procedures in the osseous skeleton, biopsies performed in the soft tissues may be safely and comfortably completed under sedation with generous local anesthesia. There are exceptions, including (1) small lesions that are deeply situated, which may require paralysis of the uncooperative patient, (2) large masses, especially those that are hypervascular, adjacent to vital structures such as the airway, where hemorrhage may create or augment mass effect and where airway control or volume management by an anesthesiologist may be a beneficial precaution, and (3) multiple procedures planned in the same encounter, where the total procedure time is likely to exceed an hour. However, in many practices general anesthesia is preferred.

Even though US is often the most useful modality for image guidance during a biopsy procedure, it is important to review available cross-sectional imaging to localize the lesion and correlate with its US appearance, determine its suitability for biopsy, and identify any adjacent vital structures and important anatomic relationships. If there is uncertainty regarding the conspicuity of a lesion on US that has already been defined with CT, PET-CT, or MR, it is a simple matter to bring US into the CT suite so that the lesion can be localized with CT and the biopsy completed with US or CT as necessary. Regardless of which imaging modality is selected for biopsy guidance of a suspected malignancy, it is essential to sample the most representative tissue within the lesion and, where multiple lesions are present, to determine which are most metabolically active and the lesions with the safest and easiest access. We find that preprocedural PET-CT will improve target selection in >20% of cases, depending on the pathology.

Standard technique

The technique for biopsy is similar to other sites (as outlined in Chapter 4). A coaxial approach facilitates rapid acquisition of multiple specimens within each quadrant of the mass. In larger masses this can be combined with a *tandem needle* approach (see "Coaxial and tandem needle techniques," in Chapter 4), leaving the guiding tandem needles in place to

Table 7.5 Procedure summary: biopsy of lymph nodes and soft tissue masses

- Sedation/general anesthesia
- Ultrasound (or other modality) localization of skin entry site. Mark entry site with washable ink
- Sterile preparation and draping
- Ultrasound (or other modality) guided needle placement into mass lesion
- Sample all four quadrants of the lesion with >16-gauge biopsy needle if possible

assist the interventionalist in identifying which quadrants have already been sampled and which remain.

The results from percutaneous lymph node biopsy are generally not as rewarding as those from other organs. Often, several core biopsies are needed in several locations within a node in order to get an accurate diagnostic result. Otherwise, percutaneous biopsy of abdominal and pelvic nodes may be performed with imaging guidance following PET-CT. In cases of suspected lymphoma, percutaneous lymph node biopsy is usually performed with US or CT guidance. Nodes and small nodular lesions may be mobile and easily pushed away from the biopsy needle. It may be useful to stabilize the nodule: first, by introducing the tip of a semi-automated needle into the margin of the node prior to firing and, second, by "propping" the nodule opposite the needle entry site with the operator's fingertips or other suitable support. An end-cutting needle is helpful when biopsy of a small lesion is performed.

The approach to diagnosis of mass lesions in children is entirely different than in lymph nodes (Table 7.5). Percutaneous image-guided biopsy is generally the method of choice for virtually all mass lesions of childhood (Figure 7.2). Surprisingly, it is often most difficult to obtain a pathologic diagnosis in patients with very large lesions (greater than 8 to 10 cm in diameter) compared to smaller (<2 cm diameter) lesions. While the reasons for this are not entirely clear, they may include presence of extensive central necrosis, mucinoid changes, and intralesional diversity. Thus in order to maximize the diagnostic utility of the biopsy, we suggest using ≥16-gauge core biopsy needles to sample multiple quadrants within the mass, taking many samples (i.e., greater than five), and concentrating sampling in target regions where imaging suggests viability and high metabolic activity. In cystic (non-vascular) lesions, focus should be on the margin of the lesion, especially any focal nodular component, and any component that demonstrates vascularity on Doppler imaging.

Specimen handling and the usefulness of preliminary intraprocedural histopathologic evaluation (frozen section or touch-prep) have been discussed in detail in Chapter 4. It is worthwhile to repeat here that consultation, prior to the procedure, between the interventional radiologist, oncologic orthopedic surgeon, and pathologist, is extremely important to define the preferred needle route so that only the structures intended to be removed are traversed, so that the needle tract can be removed completely (if the surgeon prefers because of the risk of tract seeding), and to plan for frozen sections or other related pathology needs.

Postprocedure and follow-up care

Following the biopsy, immediate postprocedure imaging should be performed to exclude procedural complications, such as hemorrhage or injury of adjacent vital structures. If the procedure is performed with US, anatomic imaging and color Doppler of the lesion and adjacent structures may be sufficient. If the target location is in a particularly vulnerable area, CT sections through the area of interest can provide a more global assessment at the cost of a relatively small radiation dose. In most cases, the dermatotomy can be approximated with Dermabond® and covered with a transparent dressing, and no additional follow-up should be required. Postprocedural hemoglobin and hematocrit are rarely necessary, unless there is a bleeding complication. The patient and family should be informed of the possibility for postbiopsy bleeding, infection, or pain, and contact telephone numbers for the interventionalist should be given to the family. If there is a high likelihood of postprocedure discomfort, a prescription for appropriate analgesics should also be provided.

Complications

Bleeding is the most common complication of biopsy procedures in the soft tissues. When it occurs at the percutaneous entry site, it is usually readily observed and easily managed with manual compression. Hemorrhage in the deep soft tissues, the mass, or from surrounding vessels may be subtle, and in rare cases, may lead to hypovolemic shock or compression of adjacent vital structures. If there is concern for a bleed, US including color Doppler or CT of the area is recommended.

Other complications related to vascular injury during a soft tissue biopsy, such as pseudoaneurysm, arteriovenous fistula, and tract seeding are possible but rare.

Conclusions

Core biopsy of soft tissue masses, nodules, and lymph nodes should be performed to answer specific clinical questions where the answers are likely to materially affect the management of the patient. Communication between the interventionalist, clinical service, and pathologist before the biopsy should be directed to planning and executing the acquisition of sufficient representative tissue so that clinical questions are addressed in order of priority. Issues related to specimen handling, transport, and processing should be clarified with the pathology service before the procedure begins. If additional procedures are needed, such as insertion of a central venous catheter, it is ideal to perform them under the same anesthetic. Preprocedural imaging for lesion characterization and localization as well as selection of the optimal lesion to sample and the optimal level and route for sampling will help ensure a high rate of safe and successful procedures, with a low rate of

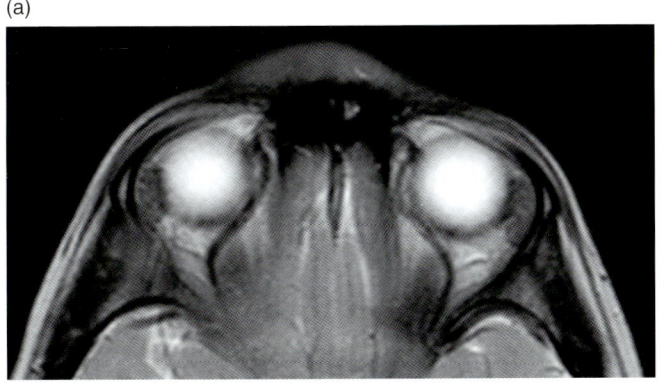
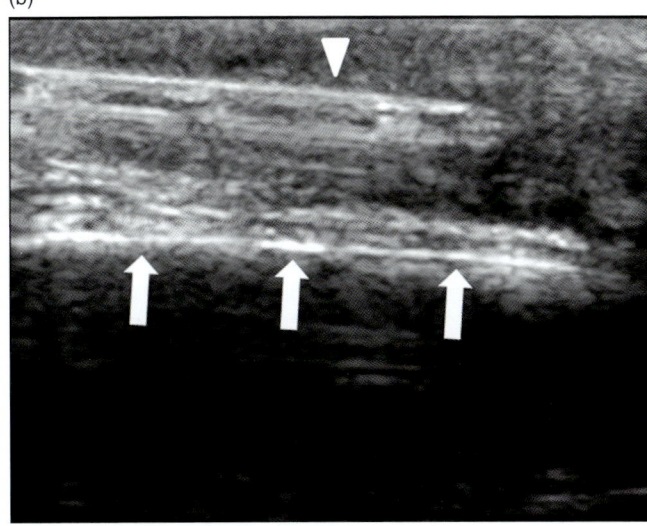

Figure 7.2 Five-year-old female with enlarging blue-colored soft tissue mass of the forehead and glabella. (a) T2 axial MRI at level of orbits showing homogeneous subcutaneous mass. (b) Ultrasound-guided 18-gauge BioPince® core needle (*arrowhead*) specimens were obtained in the mass superficial to the calvaria (*arrows*), leading to the diagnosis of lymphoblastic lymphoma.

complications and significantly lower cost than open surgical alternatives.

Foreign body retrieval

Introduction

When a potentially dangerous object is introduced into the skin or soft tissues from the outside, it places the patient at risk for injury to vital structures, infection, pain, or dysfunction. (Management of intravascular foreign bodies is described in Chapter 2, and retrieval of ingested foreign bodies is covered in Chapter 3.) These foreign bodies may be composed of a variety of materials, such as metal, glass, ceramic, plastic, mineral (e.g., rock shards and gravel), pencil graphite, or organic (e.g., bone, fish spines, teeth, wood splinters, and thorns). In addition, remnants of shoes, socks, or clothing (such as leather, cloth, or rubber) may accompany a foreign body into the wound. The entry wound and mechanism of injury may localize the foreign body in general terms, but the angle, depth of penetration, and degree of fragmentation are often uncertain. So it is that surgical removal begins with sharp and blunt exploration that may be protracted and involve considerably more trauma to tissue than originally involved in the wound.

Conventionally, foreign bodies in the soft tissues are localized with underpenetrated plain radiography first, then the radiographs are used by emergency department physicians or surgeons to guide surgical exploration and removal. For suspected objects that are difficult to identify or localize with plain radiography, US or as a last resort, CT may be used. Objects that are located near vital structures such as nerves and vessels may be left in place if they are not symptomatic or infected. Image-guided foreign body removal allows accurate localization of the foreign body and removal through a small incision with minimal additional trauma or untoward effect.

Indications

Any foreign body that causes pain should be removed if possible (Table 7.6). Removal of a foreign body in the soft tissues can be attempted for virtually any object that can be visualized with US. While objects are easiest to remove within the first 24 hours, even objects that have been embedded much longer, with accompanying inflammation, induration, suppuration, scarring, or granulation tissue, may be removed using these techniques. Many objects that are not detected on plain radiographs can be localized with US. In addition to providing information about the depth, size, and shape of the foreign object, US can also define its relationship to important anatomic structures such as nerves, vessels, tendons, ligaments, joints, and bones. Any foreign object that can be visualized should be removed under direct visualization, including objects embedded in the nose and ears. An ophthalmologist should be consulted for removal of foreign bodies in the cornea of the eye. Similarly, aspirated foreign bodies are usually removed by a pulmonologist under endoscopic visualization. Inert foreign bodies such as bullet or glass fragments that do not threaten vital structures, are not infected, and are asymptomatic may not need to be removed.

Technique

Equipment

High-quality US with good near-field resolution is very helpful for this procedure. A 10 ml or 20 ml syringe filled with sterile saline, water, or thinned US gel attached to a 16- or 18-gauge angiocatheter can be used to "float" the foreign body once it is localized. A #11 scalpel blade, splinter forceps, and a mosquito or Kelly forceps are usually sufficient to remove most foreign bodies in the soft tissues (Table 7.7).

Table 7.6 Indications: foreign body retrieval

- Painful foreign body
- Infected site of foreign body penetration
- Causing functional impairment
- Threaten adjacent tissue or organs

Table 7.7 Equipment: foreign body retrieval

- J-Tip®, 1% buffered lidocaine, 30-gauge needle
- Scalpel with #11 blade
- Sterile US gel
- Forceps, pickups
- High-frequency US transducer with small footprint
- Specimen container

(a)
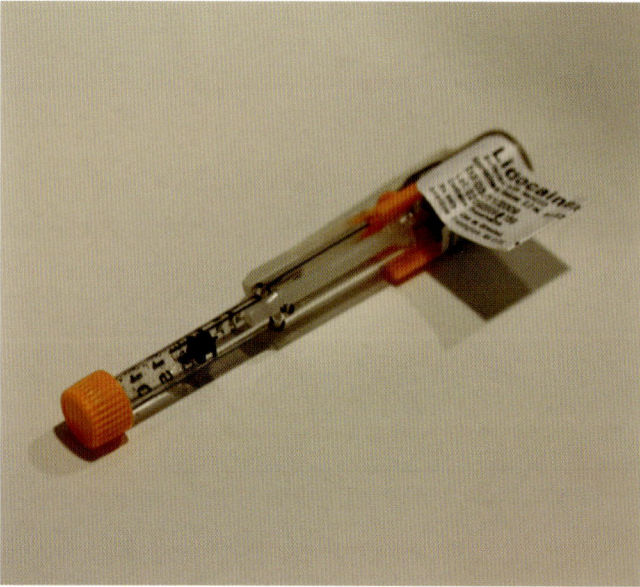

(b)
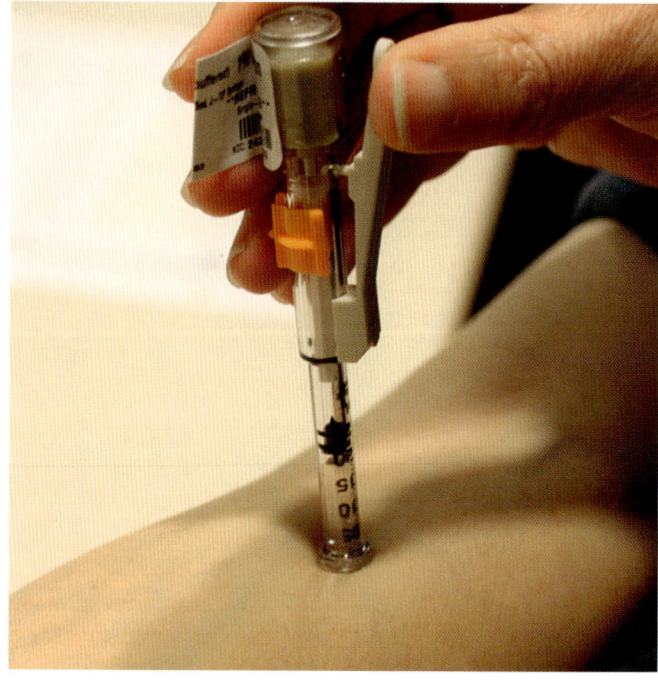

Figure 7.3 Skin anesthetic. (a,b) Use of J-Tip®.

Patient preparation

If a foreign body is suspected in a puncture wound, and cannot be removed under direct visualization, its presence should be confirmed with imaging. If the foreign body can be clearly identified with US, no other imaging is required. If US is equivocal, underpenetrated plain radiography or CT may help to confirm or further characterize the target object(s).

The puncture site may be prepared with a J-Tip® (pressurized intradermal infusion of 1% buffered lidocaine using CO_2) because of its immediate time to action (Figure 7.3). The site is then prepared and draped in sterile fashion. Infiltration with local anesthetic or regional nerve blocks may be very useful where appropriate.

Standard technique

When necessary, the child may be sedated or anesthetized. If the procedure is performed under sedation or local anesthesia only, the site is anesthetized with a J-Tip® and 1% buffered lidocaine infiltrated into the tract with a 30-gauge needle. The foreign body is visualized *en face*, to the degree possible. If the object's proximity to the skin surface makes visualization difficult, a stand-off pad or thick layer of gel may assist imaging. A stab wound is created with the scalpel blade, and carried down to the superficial margin of the foreign body (Table 7.8). The saline-filled angiocatheter or needle is advanced through the wound under US guidance, and saline is injected around the object. This has the effect of "floating" the object free from the surrounding soft tissue, and increasing its conspicuity to US imaging. Forceps are then advanced through the wound/incision, under US visualization, until they come in contact with the foreign object. The foreign body is grasped and removed (Figure 7.4).

Technical variations

In the unusual case where a foreign body is visualized on a plain radiograph or by CT but is not apparent on US, it is possible to use biplane fluoroscopy to guide forceps to the object. Failing this, a localizing needle may be placed adjacent to the foreign body to assist surgical exploration and retrieval.

Postprocedure and follow-up care

Once the foreign body, including accessible fragments, has been removed, the puncture wound is again irrigated with saline or sterile water, hemostasis is achieved, and the wound is left to heal by secondary intention. It should be dressed with a loose gauze bandage. If a skin incision has been created distant from the original puncture wound, this may be closed with suture or Dermabond® if necessary. The patient and family should be instructed to return if any signs or symptoms of infection are noted. In this case, further evaluation for a retained foreign body should be undertaken.

Tetanus toxoid prophylaxis, and tetanus immune globulin, should be considered unless the child's vaccination status is up to date. Prophylactic antibiotics are usually not necessary, but may be indicated in the case of a human bite wound, or when the foreign body involves bone or joint penetration.

Complications

Infection is the most common complication of a foreign body, although the rate of infection from non-bite wounds is small. The rate is highest in patients with a compromised immune status, or when wounds are visibly contaminated, large, jagged, or deep. Occasionally foreign bodies will be missed, or significant fragments will be left behind that may later cause infection or pain, or may migrate to a more dangerous position.

Conclusions

Wounds with a neglected foreign body are a common cause of litigation. Conventional surgical methods of removal may cause additional tissue trauma due to the difficulty of localizing the object during exploration. An image-guided approach allows detailed evaluation of the foreign body and its anatomic

Table 7.8 Procedure summary: foreign body retrieval

- Preprocedural US to identify foreign body and identify skin entry site
- Mark entry site with washable ink
- Sedation/general anesthesia as needed
- Local anesthesia with J-Tip®
- Sterile preparation and draping
- Tract anesthesia using 1% lidocaine
- Skin incision
- Identify foreign body and inject saline around it
- Forceps removal of foreign body under US guidance

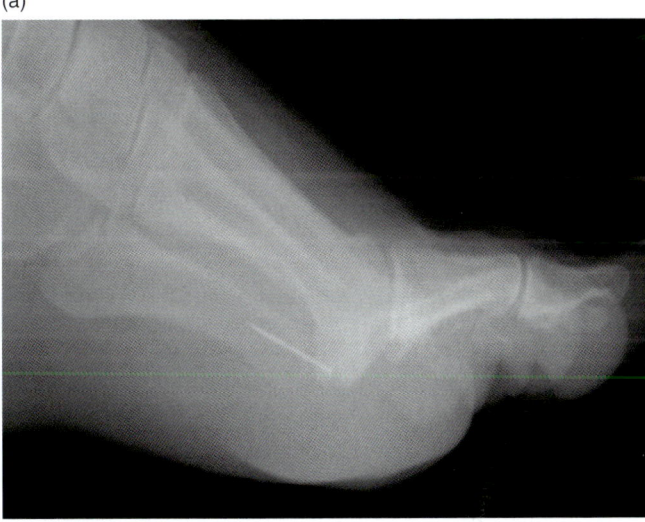

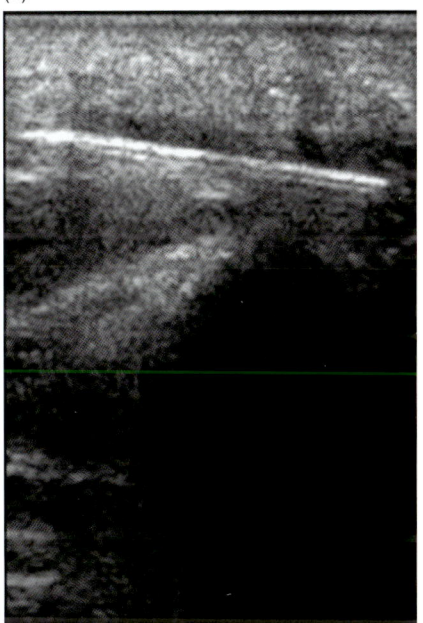

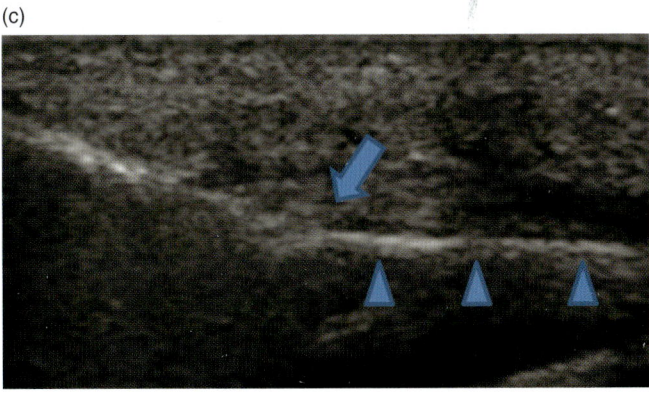

Figure 7.4 Thirteen-year-old female with sewing needle fragment in plantar soft tissues of the foot with swelling and erythema. (a,b) Lateral foot radiograph and US show needle fragment. (c) Ultrasound-guided forceps retrieval. Note: tip of forceps (*arrow*) grasping needle fragment (*arrowheads*).

context, and real-time visualization of the target object during acquisition and retrieval. This reduces the need for exploration and associated tissue injury. Although antibiotic prophylaxis is rarely necessary, there should be a low threshold for tetanus prophylaxis, as the incidence of missed tetanus prophylaxis after penetrating injuries is as high as 6%.

Chemodenervation of the salivary glands

Introduction

Excessive drooling occurs when normal swallowing is impaired, with or without elevated levels of saliva production. This occurs most frequently in the setting of cerebral palsy, but may occur due to a variety of chronic and less frequently, acute causes. Common contributing factors include inability to sense saliva pooling in the mouth and incoordination of swallowing. The inability to handle oral secretions may lead to silent aspiration, recurrent pneumonia, reactive airways disease, and other aspiration-related events. Chronically pooled secretions also lead to poor oral hygiene, gingivitis, and halitosis. Constant drooling leads to excoriation of the skin, soiled clothing, poor public acceptance, and difficulty for the caregiver. Successful control of these secretions is often life-changing for the patient and family.

For the child with excessive drooling, it is first important to establish the cause. Treatable acute causes should be identified and treated. Some patients with behavioral or neuromuscular disability may respond to behavioral modification and occupational therapy. In some circumstances, medical therapy with anticholinergic drugs such as atropine sulfate or glycopyrrolate may be beneficial in decreasing the activity of acetylcholine muscarinic receptors, and therefore decreasing saliva production. Patients who do not respond to these behavioral and medical treatments and who are at risk for aspiration-related complications may be good candidates for chemical denervation of the salivary glands.

Indications

Any child with excessive drooling who has experienced recurrent aspiration pneumonia or who has been diagnosed with other aspiration-related disorders, such as reactive airways disease with impairment of pulmonary function, is likely to benefit from this procedure. Those who have choking or severe coughing, drooling at night, poor oral hygiene or halitosis, or drooling-related skin irritation may also be reasonable candidates. Often these are children with cerebral palsy, but children with mental retardation, stroke, and degenerative neuromuscular disorders also may have chronically excessive drooling. Acute causes of excessive drooling, such as poisoning (e.g., mercury, some pesticides), infection (e.g., strep throat, tonsillitis, peritonsillar or retropharyngeal abscess) or tumors that

Table 7.9 Equipment: chemodenervation of the salivary glands

- Sterile US probe cover
- Ultrasound with high-frequency transducer
- Skin preparation liquids
- 22- to 27-gauge, 1.5-inch needles × number of glands to be injected
- Botox®: appropriate volumes and units drawn up into 1 ml syringes prior to procedure

compress the upper digestive tract are not appropriate candidates. The only contraindication to this procedure is a prior history of allergic reaction to botulinum toxin A, which may present as hives, difficulty breathing, or swelling of the face, lips, tongue, or throat. Patients with hypotonia or weakness of muscles of breathing or swallowing, may be at increased risk of life-threatening complications related to injection of botulinum toxin A. Just as with any other percutaneous procedure, injections should not be given through broken or infected skin. It is also important to inquire into the patient's surgical history, as occasionally these patients may have undergone resection of one or more glands (usually, the submandibular glands). Knowing this will save time searching for them – or worse, treating where the glands aren't.

In healthy individuals, saliva production is estimated to be between 0.75 to 1.5 liters per day. During sleep the volume drops to near zero. The submandibular glands are responsible for about 70 to 75% of the total saliva production, while the parotid produces 20 to 25%. The other salivary glands produce very little. The parotid gland production of saliva is stimulated when eating, therefore, at baseline, most saliva is from the submandibular glands.

Technique

Equipment

The only equipment required for this procedure are 1-ml syringes, 1.5-inch needles, botulinum toxin A, and a high-frequency linear transducer (15 to 7 MHz) with a small footprint, which is easiest to manipulate in this region (Table 7.9). We use Botox® A. This is an off-label use of this medication: it is not FDA approved for this purpose at the time of writing. The medication should be reconstituted with saline according to the manufacturer's directions. Other strains of *Clostridium botulinum* (e.g., B, E, and F) should NOT be substituted, as the effects of the neurotoxins produced by these other strains are not as predictable and may lead to a greater incidence of life-threatening complications. Likewise, this procedure should not, in our opinion, be performed without image guidance, due to the risk of injection of non-target structures such as vessels or facial nerve branches, with the consequently elevated risk of life-threatening complications.

Patient preparation

Due to the nature of most candidates for this procedure, they are already at risk for aspiration and do not have normal airway protective mechanisms. Therefore it does not make sense to perform this procedure with sedation, which may further compromise pulmonary integrity and function. Children tolerate this procedure well without local anesthetic or adjunct medications. However, in some practices children may undergo general anesthesia. All four glands can be safely and accurately treated in about 15 to 30 minutes.

Dosage

There are different protocols that one can use to select a starting dose of Botox®. One can calculate the dose at 0.5 U/kg/gland or use a weight-based dose of 15 U/gland for children <15 kg, 20 U/gland at 15 to 25 kg, and 25 U/gland >25 kg. We have found that the sensitivity of children to Botox® may vary and the interventionalist needs to be attentive to the effect and the child's comfort. If injection produces dry mouth, the dose should be decreased at the next treatment (usually by 5 U), and if there is still drooling or a short interval between return of symptoms, the dose can be increased so that the desired effect is titrated. The length of time Botox® has an effect varies between three and eight months in most children.

The other decision to consider is whether to inject only the submandibular glands or both submandibular and parotid glands. Some interventionalists will start with the submandibular glands, since they are responsible for the basal saliva production, and add the parotids if needed. Other practitioners inject all four at the initial visit. There is no data to tell us the best approach at this time.

Standard technique

Each gland has its own characteristic appearance, and the gland must be positively localized with US before access (Table 7.10).

Parotid gland

The *parotid gland* is wedge shaped, found in the pre-auricular space posterior to the angle of the mandible, with the base of the wedge oriented superiorly, tapering to a point inferiorly. The parotid is also divided into deep and superficial lamina by a false capsule of investing cervical fascia and the risorius muscle. Since facial nerve branches and larger vessels run deep to or through the deep lamina, the injection needle should not go deeper than the superficial lamina. To reduce the chance of facial nerve paralysis, a nerve stimulator may be used to attempt nerve activation prior to Botox® injection. If no nerve activity is observed, Botox® is injected using a standard 22- to 27-gauge, 1.5-inch needle attached to a 1 ml syringe containing botulinum toxin A mixture (usually in 0.5 to 1 ml total volume). The needle is advanced percutaneously under real-time US guidance in the long plane of the linear transducer, entering the substance of the gland and traversing its length, staying above the superficial lamina. In this way, the location of the injection in a desirable distribution is assured before the injection is begun. The syringe is then emptied as the needle is withdrawn, "lacing" the length of the gland (Figure 7.5).

Submandibular gland

The *submandibular gland* is somewhat cuboid to bilobed, located just medial to the inferior margin of the mandible,

Table 7.10 Procedure summary: chemodenervation of the salivary glands

- General anesthesia as needed
- Antiseptic preparation
- Determine dosage of Botox® per gland and prepare and label 1 ml syringes
- Ultrasound evaluation and route planning
- Ultrasound-guided needle placement within salivary gland with injection of Botox®

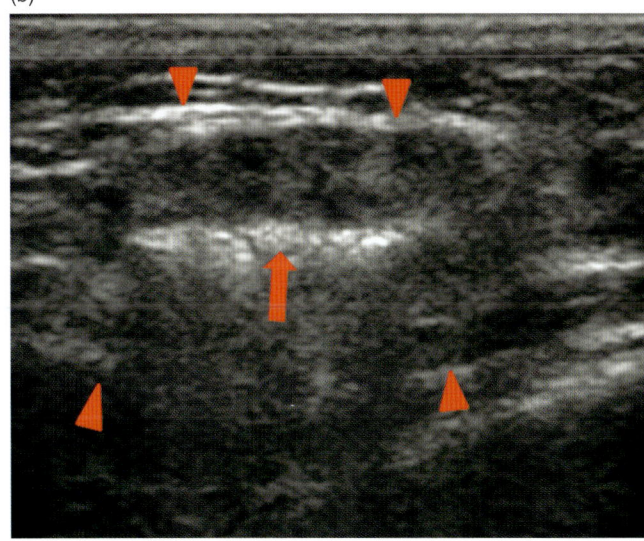

Figure 7.5 Nine-year-old male with cerebral palsy and hypersalivation with recurrent aspiration pneumonia. (a) Ultrasound-guided needle positioning (*arrow*) in parotid gland. (b) "Lacing" hyperechoic linearity (*arrow*) of gland (*arrowheads*) with Botox®.

and just anterior to the inferior aspect of the parotid gland. The deep portion of the gland is the larger portion, but also contains the gland's Wharton's duct, the glandular branch of the facial artery, and the nerve branches leading to the submandibular ganglion. The superficial portion of the gland, although the smaller part, is more accessible and is the safer target for this procedure. Using aseptic technique and US guidance a 22- to 27-gauge, 1.5-inch needle attached to a 1 ml syringe containing botulinum toxin A mixture (usually in 0.5 to 1 ml total volume) is advanced into the superficial part of the gland, and the mixture is laced across the gland as described above.

Technical variations

Some operators prefer to inject the dose into each gland as a "depot" bolus rather than "lacing" the gland as described above. There is no evidence that either technique yields different results or complications.

Postprocedure and follow-up care

No specific postprocedural care is usually needed. A dressing or bandage is unnecessary. If anesthesia was given the child is recovered. If not, the patient is discharged to home. The caregiver should be instructed to call or activate emergency medical services immediately if the patient develops difficulty breathing, fever >38°C, difficulty swallowing, facial weakness, or changes in speech in the days following the procedure.

There is usually a lag of approximately three to seven days until the therapeutic effect of the treatment is achieved. This effect persists for several weeks and the patient normally returns to baseline salivation within three to eight months after treatment. In our experience, most patients see decreasing effectiveness around three to four months after injection. The reduction in frequency of aspiration-related complications may last for a year or more. The procedure should not be repeated more often than every two to three months. The interval between treatments varies and should be tailored to the child's needs. There are unsubstantiated reports of a cumulative effect of serial treatments leading either to gland atrophy and reduced salivary output or to attenuation of the response with increased salivary output.

Complications

It is uncommon to observe complications following US-guided chemodenervation of the salivary glands. Most reported adverse effects involve injections without image guidance or after use of other *Botulinum* strains. The most severe potential complications of botulinum toxin A administration result from non-target distribution, especially when inadvertent intravascular injection occurs. This can cause severe muscle weakness in areas remote from the injection, most dangerously involving muscles of respiration. There can also be problems with vision, swallowing, heart rate, or bladder control. Local effects are also possible, including facial palsy, impairment of chewing or swallowing, as well as bruising, bleeding, swelling, or pain at the site of injection. Transient dysphagia can occur, perhaps due to changes in the viscosity of saliva. Transient xerostomia has also been reported in some patients.

Future advances

In most cases, the underlying neurologic dysfunction that results in excessive drooling and associated aspiration-related and other complications is lifelong and irreversible. The chemodenervation procedure with botulinum toxin A is temporary and self-limited. The more permanent solution currently available, gland resection, carries a high complication rate. Our experience with partial gland ablation for ranula, described below, raises the question whether this technique could be used, with appropriate neurophysiologic monitoring, to achieve a graded gland ablation, titrated to effect over a series of procedures, with the likelihood that the reduction in salivary output would last five years or more rather than five months or less.

Conclusions

Complications related to excessive drooling can be life-threatening, including aspiration-related reactive airways disease and recurrent aspiration pneumonia. These complications may result in numerous hospitalizations. In patients at highest risk, this may require more than 15 intensive care unit days per year, and may add over $100,000 per patient per year to their health care costs as well as significantly disrupting the lives of caregivers and families. Conventional pharmacologic therapy is often unsatisfactory, with undesirable side effects and uncertain benefit in many patients. Surgical gland excision is technically difficult, is not titratable or reversible, and has a high complication rate. Chemodenervation of the salivary glands with botulinum toxin A, under US guidance, is a safe and effective alternative that can be performed on an outpatient basis. It can significantly improve the lives of patients and caregivers alike, and can provide significant reduction in health care costs in patients at risk.

Partial gland ablation and sclerotherapy of ranula

Introduction

Disruption of the delicate ducts draining the salivary glands results in extravasation of serous and mucinous fluids into the periglandular soft tissues. As these fluids accumulate, they cause a local swelling, usually confined to the floor of the mouth, constituting a simple ranula. The simple sublingual ranula is usually treated by transoral surgical excision of the ipsilateral gland and evacuation of the ranula. Surgical alternatives include marsupialization with or without packing, micro-marsupialization, laser cyst, and partial gland ablation. When the accumulation dissects through the mylohyoid muscle, beyond the oral cavity, it becomes a "plunging" ranula, and may present as a swelling in the neck, submandibular, or pre-auricular region. If treated surgically, ranulas located in the neck generally require a transcervical approach with division of the mylohyoid muscle and dissection up to the floor of the mouth. While most ranulas arise from the sublingual glands, they may be related to any salivary gland, major or minor.

Swelling in the neck of a child may be solid or cystic. Since a plunging ranula should not mimic a solid mass, this can be virtually eliminated on the basis of imaging. This leaves infections (necrotic lymphadenopathy, abscess), and cystic lesions. The latter might commonly include branchial cleft cyst, thyroglossal duct cyst, lymphatic malformation, dermoid cyst, and ranula. Dermoid cysts are thin-walled cysts that contain fatty masses and may contain other differentiated ectodermal structures such as hair or nails. Branchial cleft cysts may extend any distance from the skin, usually along the margin of the sternocleidomastoid muscle, as deep as the tonsillar pillars, external auditory canal, or piriform sinus. A thyroglossal duct cyst is characteristically a midline structure between the isthmus of the thyroid and the hyoid bone. Cervicofacial lymphatic malformations are cystic lesions resulting from malformation of normal lymphatics. Most of these may enlarge with upper respiratory infections. They may also enlarge with internal hemorrhage, which may complicate the imaging appearance of these cystic structures. Solid and cystic cervicofacial masses in a child could also represent less common entities, such as teratoma or very rare malignancies such as metastatic squamous cell carcinoma or papillary cystadenocarcinoma, but are seldom confused with a ranula. Still, a fine needle aspirate from a complex fluid collection or a core biopsy of a complex cystic and solid tumor will usually provide adequate diagnostic direction to the clinical team.

An anechoic cystic neck mass can successfully be treated in almost all circumstances via drainage and sclerotherapy using the same techniques described for treatment of lymphatic malformations in Chapter 8. However, if there is any turbidity or granularity in the fluid by US, or if the diagnosis of ranula is seriously considered, then a sample of the fluid should be sent for salivary amylase analysis. Caution should be used if undifferentiated amylase analysis is substituted, as there is a possibility of confusing a foregut duplication cyst, which is a poor candidate for sclerotherapy, with a ranula, where sclerotherapy may contribute to a successful treatment plan.

Indications

Classically, a hypoechoic cystic (or pseudocystic) structure extending from the floor of the mouth, adjacent to a salivary gland, with a turbid or granular appearance on US and which contains a significant level of salivary amylase (>100 mg/dl) is a ranula. (Non-fractionated amylase may be found in other cystic foregut structures; Figure 7.6). As described above, simple ranulas are most easily and effectively treated by surgical excision of the gland and evacuation of the ranula. All other ranulas are candidates for partial ablation of the parent gland and sclerotherapy and drainage of the ranula collection. It is important to understand that testing for salivary amylase will usually require submission of the sample to an outside lab, and that a final result may not be available for one to two weeks.

There is no absolute contraindication to this approach in a properly diagnosed ranula. Relative contraindications would include inability to identify the parent gland and inability to localize and ablate the portion of the parent gland adjacent to the ranula collection without stimulating, and thus risking injury to, the facial or lingual nerve. For a suspected ranula in the midline, it is helpful to document a normal thyroid gland with appropriate imaging to avoid inadvertent ablation of an ectopic thyroid gland. In the event the skin overlying a ranula is infected, a transoral route may be considered, or the procedure can be delayed until the infection is cleared.

Technique

Equipment

The equipment and supplies for *sclerotherapy* of the ranula collection are similar to that described in the "Sclerotherapy" section in Chapter 8. This includes a 5- to 8.5-French percutaneous drainage catheter, depending upon the location and the size of the collection, suture (e.g., 3–0 Vicryl or 3–0 silk), 1% buffered lidocaine, 3% sodium tetradecyl sulfate, and dehydrated alcohol (Table 7.11). For *partial gland ablation*, supplies include a 3 ml syringe containing dehydrated alcohol connected either directly or via a short connecting tube to a 27-gauge, 1.5-inch needle. For this procedure, consideration should be given to intraprocedural neurophysiologic testing for proximity to motor branches with a nerve stimulator connected to the 27-gauge needle, especially if planning to treat the parotid gland. Consultation with a neurologist or anesthesiologist may be helpful for this aspect of the procedure.

Patient preparation

Preprocedure imaging routinely includes US, and may be supplemented by MRI in cases where the diagnosis or the gland of origin is uncertain. The procedure may be performed under general anesthesia or with procedural sedation. The anesthesia team should be advised that treatment of a lesion in the floor of the mouth may be accompanied by significant swelling that could potentially compromise the airway. If this is a concern, provision for a prolonged period of postprocedure monitoring, or even provisional admission to the intensive care unit, and delay of extubation until the airway is cleared, may be necessary.

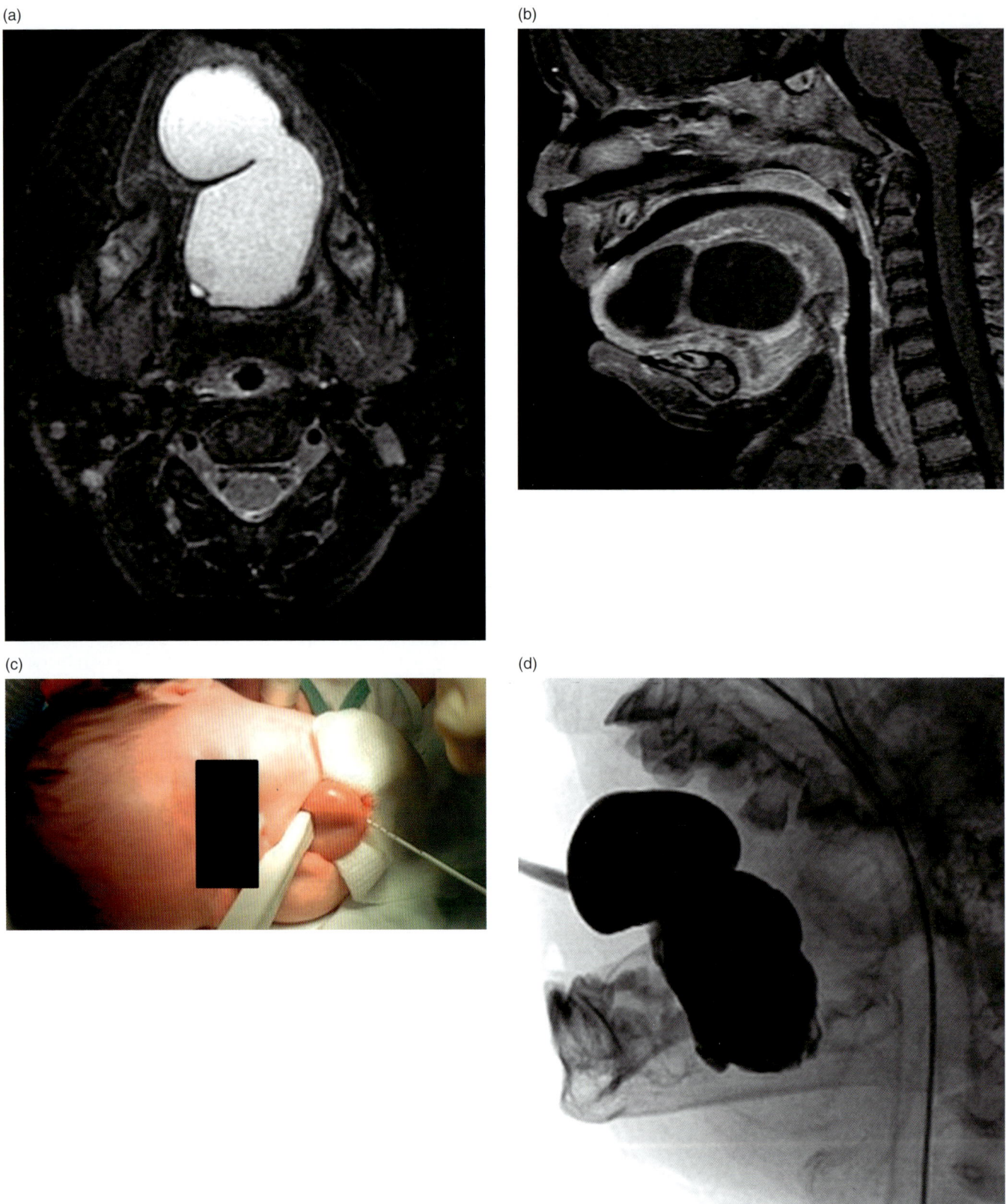

Figure 7.6 Infant presenting with painless intralingual mass and positive unfractionated amylase from aspirated fluid. (a,b) Axial T2 and sagittal T1 images show a macrolobulated cystic lesion of the tongue and floor of mouth. (c) Transglottic US-guided drain placement. (d) Cyst opacification prior to sclerotherapy and attempted partial sublingual gland ablation. After multiple interventions, salivary amylase was tested and was substantial <100 mg/dl. Pathology after surgical excision showed an intralingual foregut duplication cyst.

Table 7.11 Equipment: partial gland ablation and sclerotherapy of ranula

- Sterile US probe cover
- High-frequency US transducer with small footprint
- Skin preparation liquids
- Micropuncture or Yeuh sheathed needle
- 5- to 7-French pigtail drain
- 27-gauge, 1.5-inch needle
- Connecting tube
- Syringes, three-way stopcock
- 1% lidocaine
- Dehydrated alcohol
- Sodium tetradecyl sulfate

Table 7.12 Procedure summary: partial gland ablation and sclerotherapy of ranula

- General anesthesia
- Ultrasound examination for route planning
- Preparation and draping
- Ultrasound-guided placement of a drainage catheter
- Intralesional contrast injection to determine pathologic anatomy
- Sclerotherapy of ranula
- Connect to bulb suction device
- Partial gland ablation with dehydrated alcohol

Standard technique

Sclerotherapy

The ranula is accessed with an angiocatheter or single-wall needle sized to admit the planned guide wire, under real-time US guidance using a linear transducer with good near-field imaging capability. The pseudocyst fluid is aspirated and the volume noted. A sample is saved for laboratory analysis. A pigtail drainage catheter (5- to 6.3-French with 1 cm pigtail) is inserted into the collection using a standard technique over a 0.018-inch angled Glidewire® or stiff guide wire for 5-French drains or a 0.035-inch angled Glidewire® for 6.3-French drains.

The size and nature of the ranula is evaluated with non-ionic contrast (e.g., Optiray™ 300) injected through the drainage catheter in a volume similar to the aspirated volume. The cystic space is then anesthetized with a half volume (not exceeding 1 ml/kg) of 1% lidocaine for ten minutes, if using local anesthesia only or sedation. Next, sodium tetradecyl sulfate is instilled into the cyst (not exceeding 1 ml/kg) for three to five minutes. Finally, sclerosis is completed with a half-volume (not exceeding 1 ml/kg) of dehydrated alcohol for 15 minutes. Each agent is completely aspirated through the catheter at the end of its dwell time. At the completion of the procedure, the drainage catheter is left to bulb suction drainage. Successful end of therapy is determined by inability to easily inject an appreciable volume of contrast through a 10 ml syringe connected to the drainage catheter. The drain is removed at the end of therapy.

Partial gland ablation

Successful treatment for ranula with sclerotherapy may require several sclerotherapy sessions over several months. Partial gland ablation is usually definitive and significantly reduces the time required to achieve a successful outcome (Table 7.12). However, it makes sense to delay progression to partial gland ablation until the diagnosis is confirmed with salivary amylase determination. When partial gland ablation is performed, the gland of origin is determined by intraprocedural US as the gland adjacent to or nearest in proximity to the cystic space prior to drainage. If there is uncertainty, preprocedural MRI of the region can help to clarify relevant anatomic relationships, especially when the normal architecture of the gland is significantly altered by the ranula collection (Figure 7.7).

Usually, there will be an aspect of one gland that is directly "facing" a distinct part of the ranula collection. The purpose of partial gland ablation is to destroy the portion of the parent gland that gives rise to the disrupted duct. The prospective site for interstitial injection is first interrogated with a nerve stimulator connected to the 27-gauge needle to assure that the injection will not impinge upon motor nerves. Interstitial injection of dehydrated alcohol into the abnormal gland is then performed under real-time US guidance. In our experience, approximately 0.5 to 2 ml is sufficient to achieve a satisfactory outcome. During injection, the treated portion of the gland becomes markedly hyperechoic, at which point the injection is terminated.

Postprocedure and follow-up care

Care after *sclerotherapy* is reviewed in Chapter 8. Following *partial gland ablation*, there is often considerable swelling of the treated region. For ranula of the submandibular, sublingual, or minor salivary glands, swelling of the tongue or floor of the mouth following partial gland ablation may not peak for hours, and may threaten the airway. These patients should be treated with a controlled airway, and should be observed after the procedure until the airway is clearly safe before extubation. In some patients, this may require two to three days in the intensive care unit until extubation is safe and the patient can be discharged. This eventuality should be discussed with the patient's family during the informed consent discussion, if not earlier, so they can arrive for the procedure prepared to stay if necessary.

For ranula of the parotid gland, swelling is external to the mandible and should not threaten vital structures. Once the patient has returned to preoperative baseline status, a neurologic exam should be performed to evaluate facial and lingual nerve function and to exclude neurologic complication. The patient may then be discharged, with instructions regarding tube care, to return in five to seven days for interval assessment.

At the follow-up visit, caregivers report about the daily volume of drain output. If this has fallen to less than 5 ml per day, then the ranula bed is evaluated with physical exam

Chapter 7 MSK and soft tissue interventions

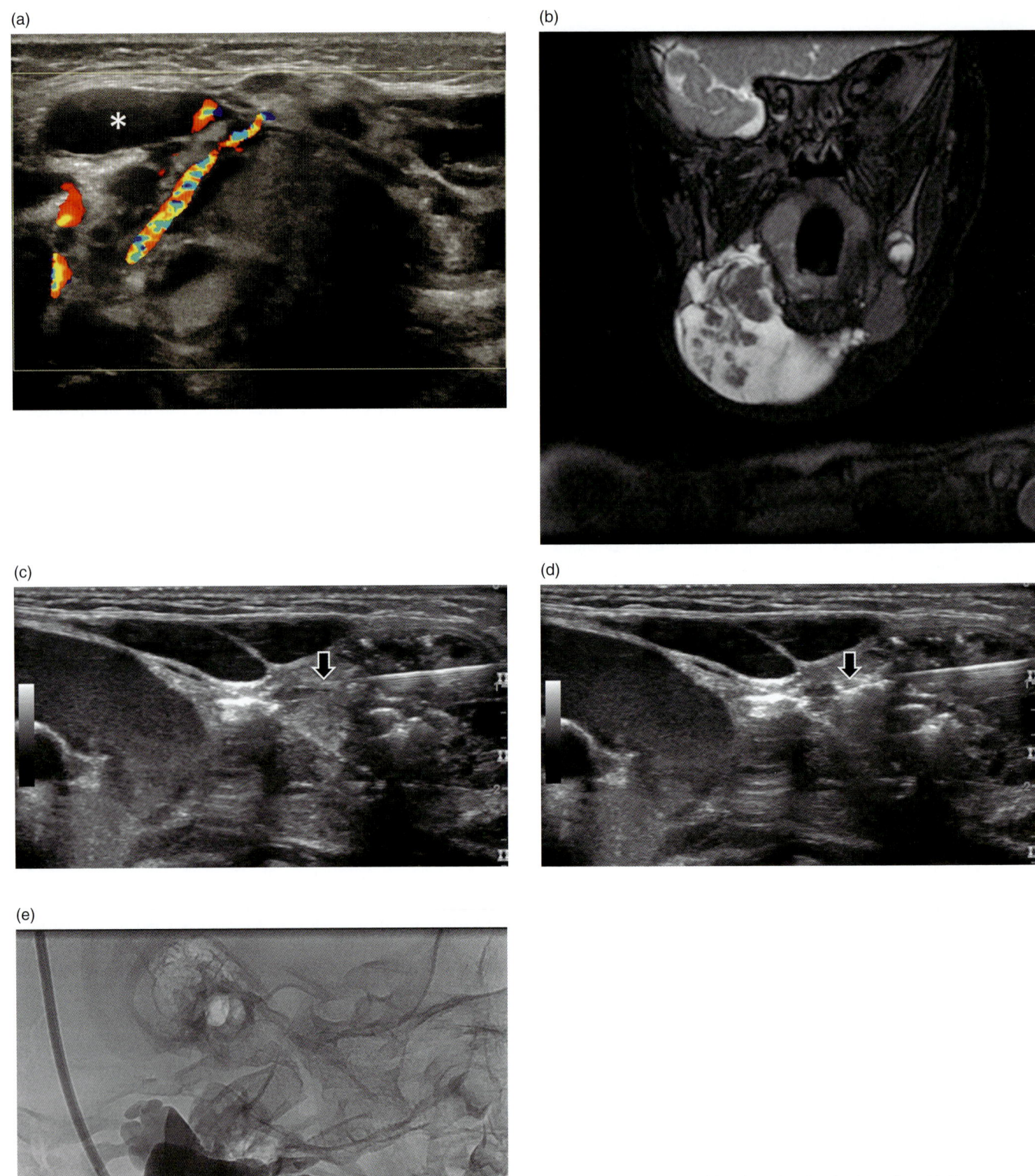

Figure 7.7 A two-year-old male with right cheek swelling. (a) Ultrasound of the submandibular region shows mixed solid and cystic components with normal vessels. A sample of the granular, turbid fluid (*asterisk*) showed an abnormal level of salivary amylase. (b) A coronal T2 fat saturation MR image shows the submandibular gland with an "exploded" appearance of the superficial lobe within the ranula fluid. (c) A 27-gauge, 1.5-inch needle is positioned under US guidance with its tip (*arrow*) within the parenchyma of one of the gland fragments adjacent to abnormal fluid. (d) With intraparenchymal injection of a small amount (0.5 to 1.0 ml) of dehydrated alcohol (*arrow*), the treated gland becomes hyperechoic. This was repeated in each of the five identifiable gland fragments adjacent to abnormal fluid. (e) A 7-French pigtail drainage catheter was placed within the fluid collection and sclerotherapy performed. The ranula completely resolved without recurrence.

and US. If the swelling has normalized and the ranula is evacuated, a gentle attempt is made to inject non-ionic contrast with a 10 ml syringe through the drainage catheter under fluoroscopy. If the collection is resistant to filling, treatment has been successful. The drain is removed, and the patient is instructed to return to the interventional radiology clinic in six weeks for a final evaluation.

If at the interval assessment after partial gland ablation, the collection remains, but tube output has diminished or stopped, it probably represents tube dysfunction, such as kinking or obstruction. The tube may need to be exchanged over a wire for a fresh tube, and the patient seen again in a few days. If instead, drainage has persisted at a substantial rate, and contrast flows relatively freely into the collection, or if the patient returns after catheter removal with recurrence of the ranula, consideration must be given to re-evaluating the gland of origin and performing another partial gland ablation procedure. If an MRI has not already been acquired, it is useful at this point to assist selection of the most likely target tissue.

Complications

Surgical approaches to ranula treatment have a relatively high rate of recurrence and other complications, especially for ranulas that do not arise from the sublingual glands. The rate of recurrence declines considerably when the parent gland is excised, but there is a compensatory rise in the rate of injury to adjacent structures. There is not a large enough cumulative experience with this procedure to estimate complication rates, although we have had no major complications in those patients we have treated. Recurrence has occurred in approximately half of the patients, but all have achieved successful treatment after one to three partial gland ablation procedures. Potential complications may include recurrence, tongue hypesthesia from lingual nerve injury during treatment of sublingual ranula, palsy of the muscles of the lower lip and chin (marginal mandibular branch of the facial nerve) during treatment of submandibular ranula, facial nerve palsy during treatment of parotid ranula, pain, bleeding or hematoma, infection, and injury to Wharton's duct (submandibular gland), Stensen's duct (parotid gland), or Rivinus' duct (sublingual gland) that may lead to obstructive sialadenitis.

Future advances

Recently, success has been reported with medical therapy of ranulas and intraoral mucoceles with an oral homotoxicological agent, Nickel Gluconate-Mercurius Heel-Potentised Swine Organ Preparation D10/D30/D200, administered over six weeks to six months, resulting in pseudocyst reabsorption and gland repair.

Conclusions

Ranulas are a relatively rare source of swelling in the oral cavity, face, or neck. They are at risk for infection and internal hemorrhage, and may cause discomfort, difficulty swallowing, and cosmetic distress. Successful medical treatment appears to be on the horizon for many cases, but is not yet part of first-line therapy. Surgical alternatives are useful in treatment of uncomplicated simple ranula, but surgical treatment in general has both a high rate of recurrence and a high rate of injury to adjacent structures, including the facial or lingual nerve. Complex cases that have failed medical or surgical therapy are good candidates for treatment with transcatheter sclerotherapy of the ranula collection combined with partial ablation of the component of the parent gland giving rise to the disrupted duct. Intraprocedural monitoring with a nerve stimulator may significantly increase safety of the procedure. Correct diagnosis of the cyst as a ranula and identification of the most likely target for ablation are critical elements of successful treatment. Patients and parents should be prepared for the likelihood of recurrence and the need for retreatment before eventual resolution of the ranula.

INTERVENTIONS IN THE JOINT CAVITIES, TENDON SHEATHS, AND BURSAE

Arthrography and related interventions

Introduction

The study of the joints and joint spaces has been performed by pediatric radiologists for several decades and arthrography is one of the oldest procedures on the pediatric interventionalist's menu. Similar techniques are useful for evaluation of the tendon sheaths and bursae. Visualization of these spaces is enhanced when they are inflamed or distended with fluid and opacified with contrast agents. Diagnostic procedures involve aspiration of fluid from these spaces or instillation of contrast through access needles, whereas therapeutic injections involve instillation of local anesthetics, steroids, and sometimes sclerosants.

With the prevalence of juvenile arthropathies, trauma, overuse syndromes, and neuromuscular diseases in the pediatric population, there is significant need for therapeutic joint, tendon sheath, and bursal injections. For example, juvenile idiopathic arthritis (JIA) effects approximate 0.5 children/1,000 with one tenth of this subgroup severely affected. In addition, the frequency of sports and other types of trauma seems to be increasing. Injection of these structures has often been performed in an office setting using palpation and topographical landmarks. Evidence from many studies indicates that a high proportion of these "blind" injections are given into non-target tissues. Simply put, they frequently miss their mark. The difficulty achieving a successful injection increases geometrically in the more anatomically complex joints, such as the temporomandibular joint (TMJ) and the subtalar joint. Since one goal of therapeutic injection is to reduce the long-term accumulation of damage to both cartilage and bone, the consequence of failed injections may be to increase chronic joint destruction and the chronic pain and dysfunction that follow. As a result, pediatric interventionalists have become considerably more involved in the treatment of children with arthritides, especially juvenile idiopathic arthritis (JIA), as well as bursitis and tendinoses (Figure 7.8).

In the next decade, it is likely that the growth of MSK procedures will be driven by treating conditions involving synovitis, bursitis, and soft tissue supporting tissues. In the majority of patients pain, snapping or clicking, and reduced range of motion are the presenting signs. The medical approaches frequently used to manage these conditions include rest, ice, elevation, NSAIDs, correction of malalignments, and stretching exercises. While these first-line methods remain useful, clinical improvement is often slow and incomplete. As a result, surgical and non-surgical treatment protocols have been developed with variable therapeutic properties. More recently, US-guided diagnostic procedures and interventions have been developed and seem to be helpful. Although in some cases MR is the preferred diagnostic method, the correct diagnosis can be made with US in most cases. In general, the US findings of tendinosis include disordered collagen fibers, variable hypervascularity, and swelling or thickening of the tendon.

A small group of drugs has become the mainstay of treatment. These injectible drugs include steroids, polidocanol, platelet rich plasma (PRP), absolute alcohol, and phenol. Steroids plus long-acting local anesthetics are used for bursal injections, polidocanol and PRP for treatment of tendons, and alcohol and phenol for the treatment of Morton's and stump neuromas.

Indications

Diagnostic arthrography is indicated for the investigation of injury to joint cartilage, ligaments, and capsule, and to assess a prosthesis for evidence of loosening (Table 7.13). The only absolute contraindication to direct arthrography is infection of the overlying tissues. The procedure may be relatively contraindicated when there is an uncorrected bleeding diathesis, although use of fresh frozen plasma and a thin needle may enable the procedure to be performed if there is an urgent indication. Diagnostic tenosynography is performed to evaluate tenosynovitis or impingement.

Aspiration is performed to decompress a joint effusion, to obtain a sample for Gram stain and culture for suspected infection, to obtain a sample for crystal analysis or blood products for suspected arthropathy or synovitis, and to evaluate fluid clarity, color, cell count, glucose, and protein. Any joint fluid present in a febrile patient, especially with sudden

Table 7.13 Indications: arthrography and related procedures

Diagnostic
- Trauma
- Evaluate pathologic synovium as a prelude to a biopsy
- Evaluate a loosened prosthesis
- Impingement syndromes
- Assess for infection
- To confirm needle tip position for an intervention, e.g., steroid injection

Therapeutic
- Synovitis
- Tendonosis
- Tenosynovitis
- Bursitis

onset of monoarticular arthritis, should be considered infected until proven otherwise, and this represents an interventional emergency (Figure 7.9). Bacteremia is the most common factor predisposing to a septic joint. Other causes are less common and include central venous catheter-related infection, IV drug use, endocarditis, and history of penetrating trauma. Immunosuppression and very young age increases the risk for developing a septic joint. Even the patient with known chronic arthropathy may have a superimposed septic arthritis. Delay in diagnosis and implementation of therapy may result in severe joint injury, including significant and irreversible loss of joint function. Conversely, timely aspiration and therapy can successfully avoid invasive joint surgery in the majority of cases. For effusions suggestive of infection that persist despite appropriate empiric therapy, a diagnosis of fungal infection, tuberculosis, or Lyme disease should be considered.

Synovial, tendon, and bursal pathology lends itself to minimally invasive treatment approaches. Inflammatory conditions involving the synovium, tendons, and bursae are now all candidates for percutaneous management along with conventional medical and surgical therapies. Oral or IV drug therapy, physical therapy, and surgery have been the mainstay for treatment of these problems. Today, a wide variety of causes of synovitis (especially JIA), tendinosis, and bursitis can be managed by image-guided injections of medication. For example, tendinoses are amenable to treatment using US guidance, including the rotator cuff, Achilles, peroneal, hip, hamstring, and ankle. In addition, we have treated teenagers and young adults with subtrochanteric, subgluteal, and iliopsoas bursitis.

Technique

Equipment

Equipment for direct arthrography and joint injections is primarily related to delivery of a contrast agent or medication into the joint space. Suitable needles should be selected based on the size of the joint and the size of the child. For example, 25- to 30-gauge needles may work well for interphalangeal

Chapter 7 MSK and soft tissue interventions

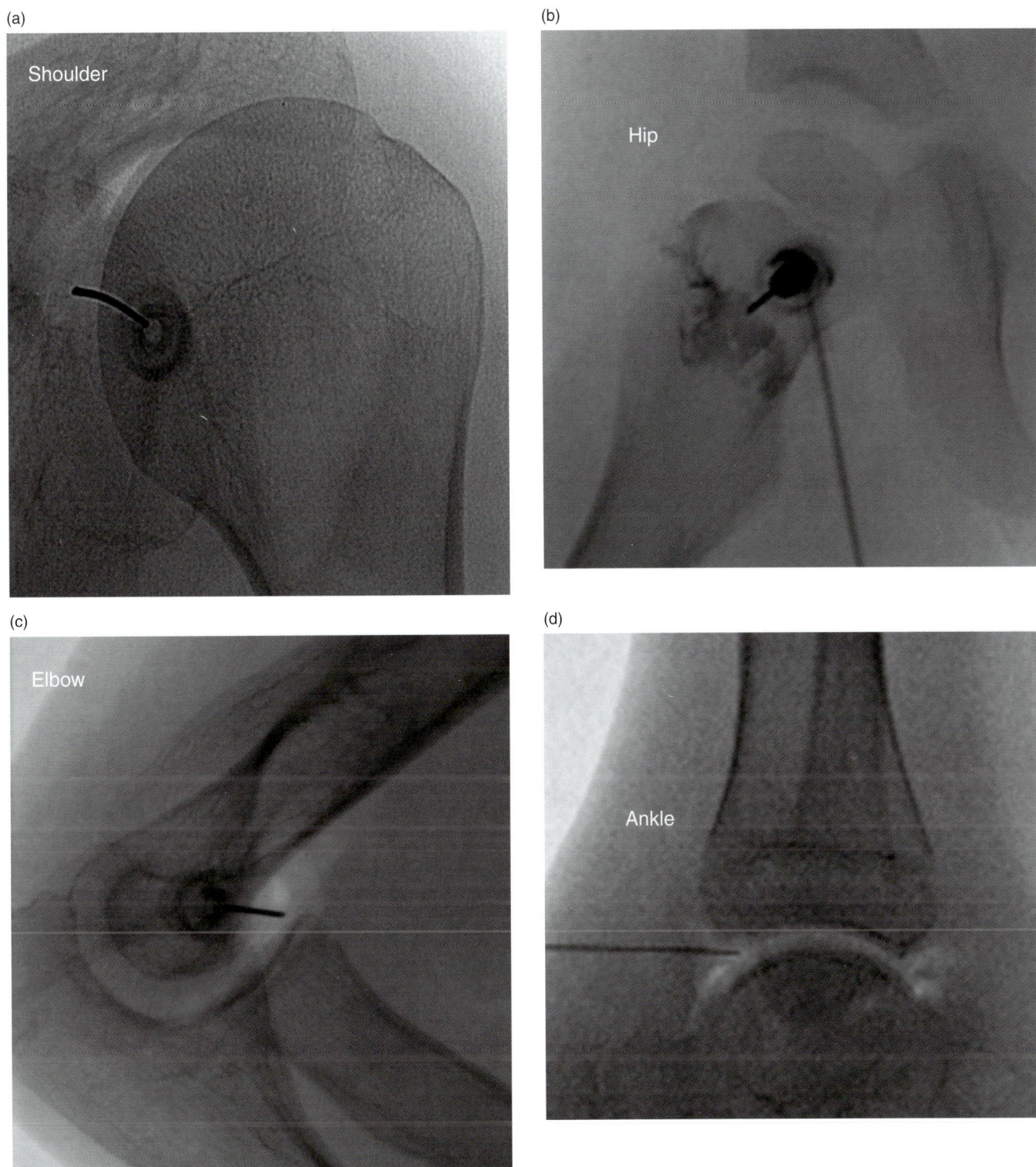

Figure 7.8 (a–g) Juvenile idiopathic arthritis potpourri. Approaches to joint access.

and wrist joints, 22- to 25-gauge 1½-inch needles for temporomandibular and subtalar joints, whereas 20- to 22-gauge 3½-inch needles will be useful in shoulder and hip joints (Table 7.14).

Patient preparation

In many cases, arthrography can be performed with local anesthesia only, others require sedation or anesthesia. If the child is not anesthetized, we would begin the procedure with a

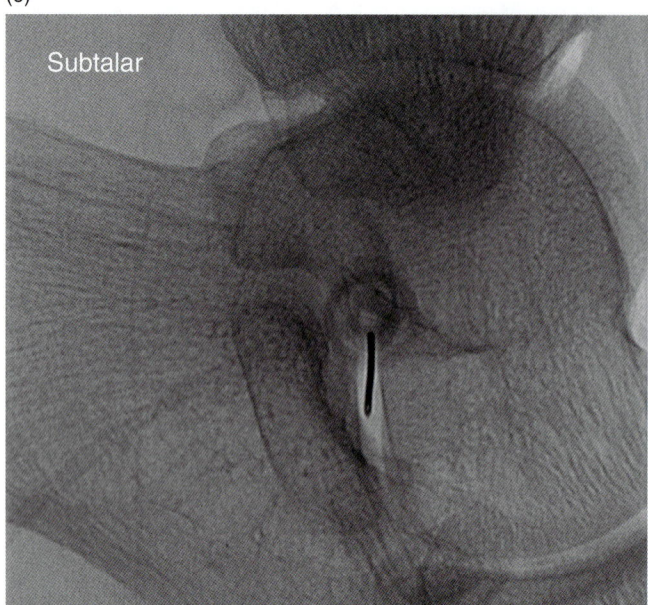

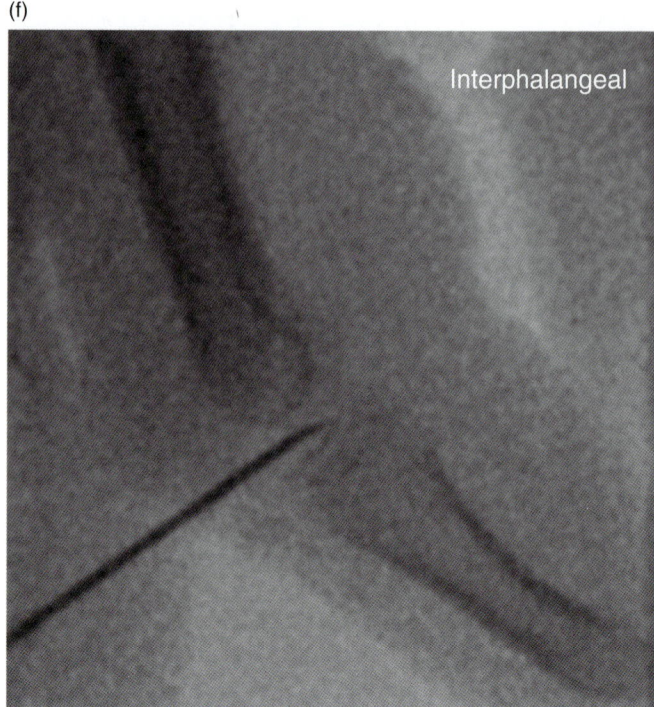

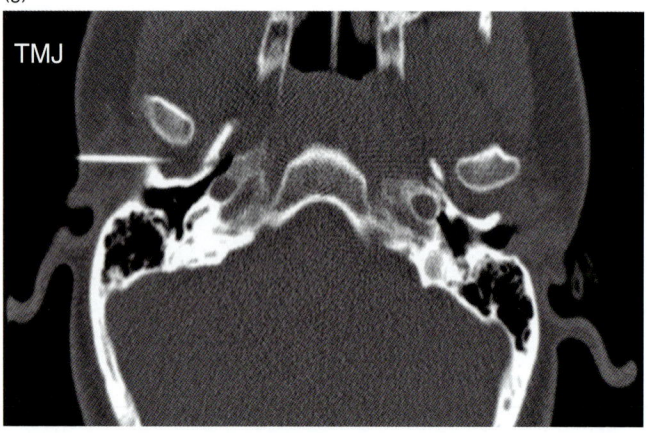

Figure 7.8 (cont.)

J-Tip® for immediate skin anesthesia followed by slow tract injection of 1% buffered lidocaine.

It is usually possible to identify a prospective access route to the joint using a radio-opaque reference object (e.g., the tip of a hemostat) under fluoroscopic guidance. The planned skin entry point is marked with a washable ink marker on the skin. Positioning the patient will depend upon the target joint.

Standard technique

The approach to each joint is unique, and a detailed discussion of positioning the patient to accommodate the features of each joint is beyond the scope of this text. The preferred approaches of the authors are summarized in Table 7.15. While these approaches may minimize common risks, they should not be interpreted as exhaustive as many successful alternative approaches may be used. The skin overlying the joint is marked, prepared, draped, and anesthetized. If fluoroscopy is used, the access needle tip is placed on the mark, perpendicular to the skin, and the needle is aligned with and centered in the beam, yielding a so-called "bullseye" appearance. The needle is then advanced toward the joint space. If firm resistance is encountered, it is probably not properly aligned. When the needle correctly enters the joint space, it should glide smoothly.

It is helpful to evaluate the progress of the needle periodically with imaging, if using fluoroscopy or CT. When the needle has advanced sufficiently, position may be confirmed in an orthogonal plane if difficulty entering the joint space is encountered. Injection of a small amount of CO_2 (except MR arthrography when non-ionic contrast is used) may be attempted. Carbon dioxide has the advantage compared to positive contrast agents that it is absorbed quickly and never obscures joint visualization (Figure 7.10). There should be minimal resistance, and the pattern of negative or positive contrast distribution should be compatible with intra-articular position. A successful injection will outline the joint cartilage and will often tend to flow into dependent recesses of the joint. Conversely, failure to outline the cartilage, and streaky, linear, or pooled contrast is not consistent with satisfactory needle placement and needle position should be revised.

Most, if not all, initial access to joint spaces, tendon sheaths, and bursae can be achieved using US guidance (Figure 7.11). This approach can, in select procedures, improve accuracy, reduce radiation exposure, and reduce overall procedure time. Successful treatment of these articular and peri-articular conditions requires substantial US guidance skills. The technical challenges to successful treatment of tendons and bursae primarily center around learning and understanding the normal and pathologic anatomy of the symptomatic area and guiding a needle into the affected area. The level of difficulty varies and usually depends on the route, diameter, and depth of the target site (Figures 7.12, 7.13).

Once needle position is confirmed within the target joint, tendon sheath, or bursa, the appropriate contrast agent or steroid mixture can be injected (Table 7.16). For arthrography, the volume of contrast mixture injected should be sufficient to completely fill the joint space; that is, until resistance to further injection is encountered. This may be as little as 0.5 ml in small joints to as much as 10 to 20 ml in larger joints. When the injection is performed as a precursor to MR arthrography, great care should be taken to maintain a continuous fluid column to avoid introduction of air bubbles into the joint space, which can easily be confused with loose bodies (Figure 7.14). The contrast mixtures and volumes used in our practice are listed in Table 7.16.

Table 7.14 Equipment: arthrography and related procedures

- Imaging for percutaneous intra-articular access: high-frequency linear transducer (7 MHz or higher), fluoroscopy, cone-beam or conventional CT
- 27- to 30-gauge needles (½-inch to 3½-inch) for injection of local anesthesia
- 1- to 20-ml syringes. Small syringes for injection of drugs. Large syringes for aspiration of joint fluid
- Sterile test tubes to send to laboratories for testing of joint fluid
- T-connector extension tubing
- Carbon dioxide gas (our preference) or non-ionic contrast for confirmation of needle position
- J-Tip® for skin anesthesia; 1% buffered lidocaine for tract anesthesia
- Contrast solution for diagnostic arthrography (see Table 7.15)
- Medications for therapeutic joint, tendon sheath, or bursa injections (see Table 7.16)

Postprocedure and follow-up care

Care following arthrography and injection therapy procedures is generally minimal and without special requirements. Some patients may need minor analgesia. Upon completion of the procedure, the patient is discharged home or to the recovery room when sedation or anesthesia has been utilized. Follow-up is tailored to the patient's condition and the clinician that is caring for them.

Complications

In this group of procedures complications are rare and are mainly related to infection and bleeding. Naturally, pain and reduced range of motion may be worsened but usually will be controlled with NSAIDs or other minor analgesics.

(a)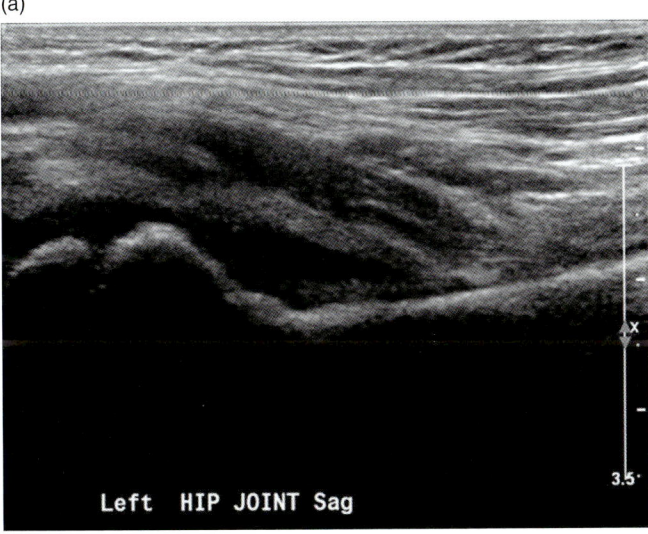

(b)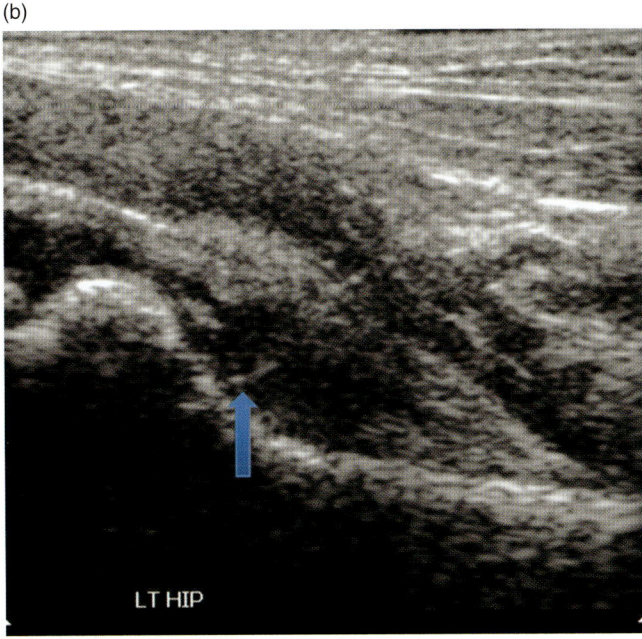

Figure 7.9 Two-year-old infant with fever and refusal to bear weight. (a) Anterior sagittal US shows moderate joint effusion. (b) Ultrasound-guided needle placement with tip (*arrow*) in hip effusion.

Table 7.15 Magnetic resonance arthrography: injected volume and positioning

Mixture for intra-articular injection:
- Optiray™ 300 5 ml
- 1% lidocaine 10 ml
- Magnevist® 0.15 ml
- Epinephrine (1:1,000) 0.1 to 0.3 ml (optional)

Shoulder arthrogram
Injection volume: 10 ml
Imaging:
- AP neutral position
- Internal rotation
- External rotation
- Abduction 90 degrees without traction
- Abduction 90 degrees with traction
- Abduction 180 degrees
- Adduction across chest

Elbow arthrogram
Injection volume: 5 ml
Imaging:
- Lateral with elbow flexed 90 degrees
- AP
- AP with medial stress
- AP with lateral stress
- Internal rotation (oblique)
- External rotation (oblique)

Hip arthrogram
Injection volume: 10 to 12 ml
Imaging:
- AP neutral position
- Frog leg lateral
- External rotation
- Abduction with internal rotation
- Abduction
- AP pull
- AP push
- Cross-table lateral as needed

Wrist arthrogram
Injection volume: 3 to 5 ml
Imaging:
- AP neutral position
- AP with radial deviation
- AP with ulnar deviation
- Lateral

ORTHOPEDIC INTERVENTIONS
Percutaneous treatment of cystic bone lesions

Introduction

The more common cystic bone lesions occurring in the pediatric population include unicameral bone cysts (UBCs) and aneurysmal bone cysts (ABCs). Up to 75% of UBCs occur in the proximal femur or humerus and are centrally located. They have a thin cortex covered by periosteum, and are lined by mesothelium. These cysts contain clear yellow fluid, unless fractured, in which case they may also contain blood. Unicameral bone cysts are susceptible to pathologic fracture. They are usually asymptomatic, but there may be associated pain or limited range of motion, especially if there is a pathologic fracture. On cross-sectional imaging, uncomplicated UBCs have the appearance of a simple bone cyst. However, when a UBC is fractured, there may be fluid–fluid levels and "fallen fragment" in the dependent portion of the bone cyst.

Aneurysmal bone cysts occur most commonly in the first and second decade of life, and are rare in children less than six years of age. More than 50% of ABCs develop in long bones and approximately 12% in the pelvis. They are expansile vascular lesions of uncertain etiology and consist of multisepated, blood-filled spaces. Patients with ABCs frequently present with pain, swelling, and if involving the vertebra, neurologic symptoms. On cross-sectional imaging, ABCs contain many fluid–fluid levels and are expansile. There may be distinct arterial feeders to the ABC, thus more of a high-flow pattern, and intralesional arteriovenous shunting may be present. Alternatively, the ABCs may have a low-flow pattern, without discernible arterial feeders, but instead slow-flow venous spaces.

Prior to therapeutic intervention of a bone cyst, percutaneous biopsy may be performed using US, CT, or fluoroscopic guidance, to obtain pathologic confirmation if the findings are atypical or the diagnosis is not already known.

Indications

The goal of treatment for a UBC is to relieve pain, prevent a pathologic fracture, and to aid in cyst healing. Symptomatic and expansile UBCs may be treated percutaneously or surgically. In the past, UBCs were treated with curettage and bone graft, but the recurrence rate was up to 40%. Today there are effective interventional options, which include percutaneous aspiration, curettage, and intralesional demineralized bone matrix injection.

Historic management of ABCs was surgical, with a high recurrence rate and significant periprocedural morbidity and mortality. Also, some ABCs are inoperable due to their location. Many effective endovascular and direct percutaneous options are now available for their treatment and management. An MRI with MRA should be obtained to assess for the presence of arterial feeders to the ABC. If arterial feeders are noted, angiography and embolization may be performed. Arterial embolization of an ABC is an effective primary treatment, but also may be performed preoperatively to reduce blood loss during surgical resection of the lesion (Figure 8.10). If the purpose of embolization is to reduce intraoperative blood loss, then surgical resection should occur the day following embolization because arterial collaterals develop quickly. Embolic agents that have been used for ABC include

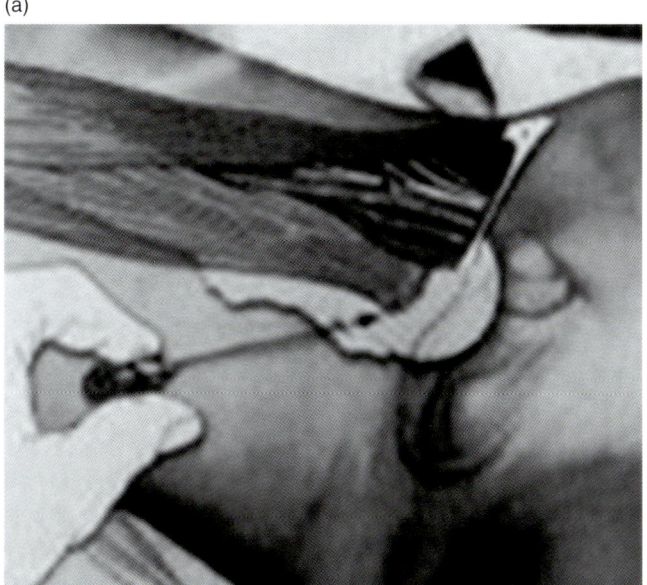
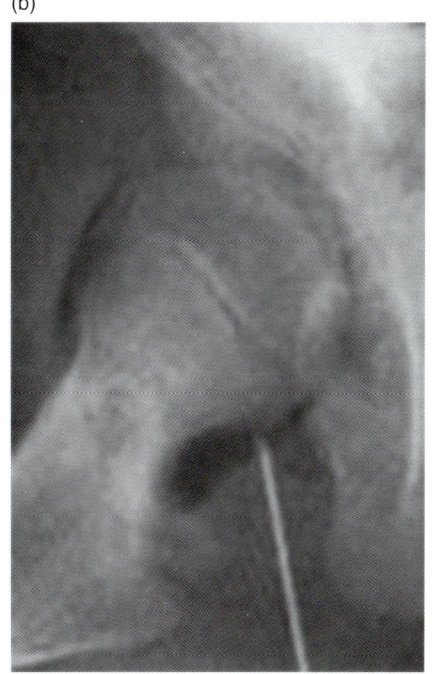
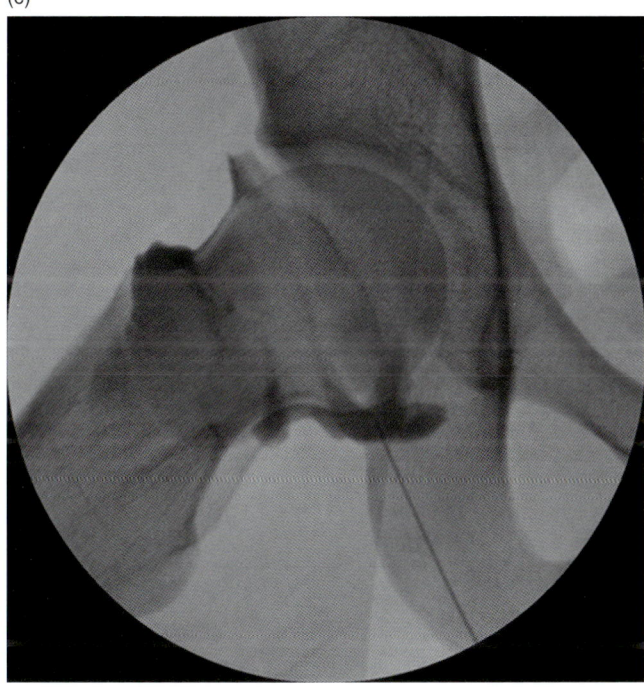

Figure 7.10 Inferior approach to hip arthrography. (a) Needle placement along inguinal crease two fingerbreadths posterior to adductor tendon. Needle parallel to the floor, directed toward the medial femoral metaphysis. (b) Carbon dioxide distends hip joint confirming intra-articular position. (c) Contrast injection of joint.

n-butyl-2-cyanacrylate (n-BCA), absorbable gelatin sponge, polyvinyl alcohol particles (PVA), ethanol, and coils. We prefer to embolize with permanent agents in case there is a delay in treatment. For low-flow ABCs, direct percutaneous puncture with intralesional injection of sclerosing agents (sodium tetradecyl sulfate (STS), dehydrated alcohol, and doxycycline) has been shown to be effective as a primary treatment. Tract embolization may reduce postprocedural oozing of blood or sclerosant. Our approach is to use a combination of STS and ethanol. Also, the percutaneous intralesional injection of n-BCA prior to surgical resection has been shown to reduce intraoperative blood loss.

Technique
Equipment
The tools utilized are variable and dependent on lesion location and goal of the procedure (Table 7.17). If an ABC is to be

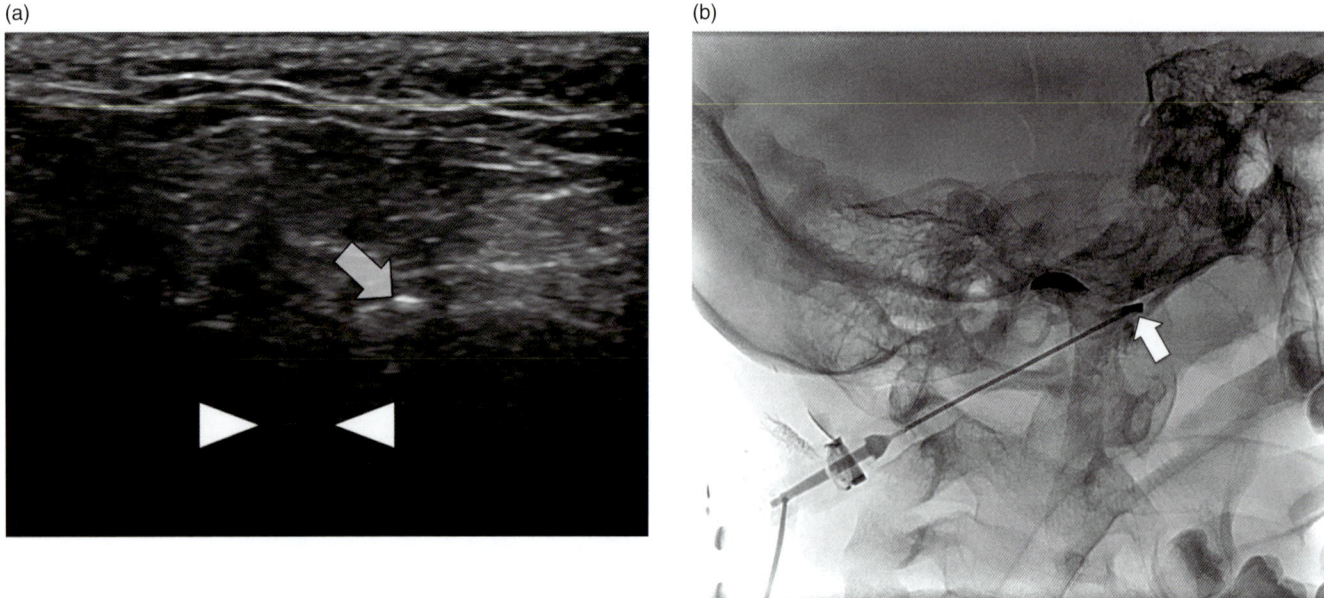

Figure 7.11 A 12-year-old female with chronic juvenile rheumatoid arthritis has decreased mandibular range of motion and acute pain, with edema and effusion in the temporomandibular joints (TMJ) by MRI. (a) Under US control, a 27-gauge, 1.5-inch needle (*arrow*) is positioned in the space (*arrowheads*) between the eminence of the squamous temporal bone and the mandibular condyle, most easily identified with real-time motion of the joint. (b) Confirmation of contrast in the superior joint space (*arrow*) requires only very brief fluoroscopy.

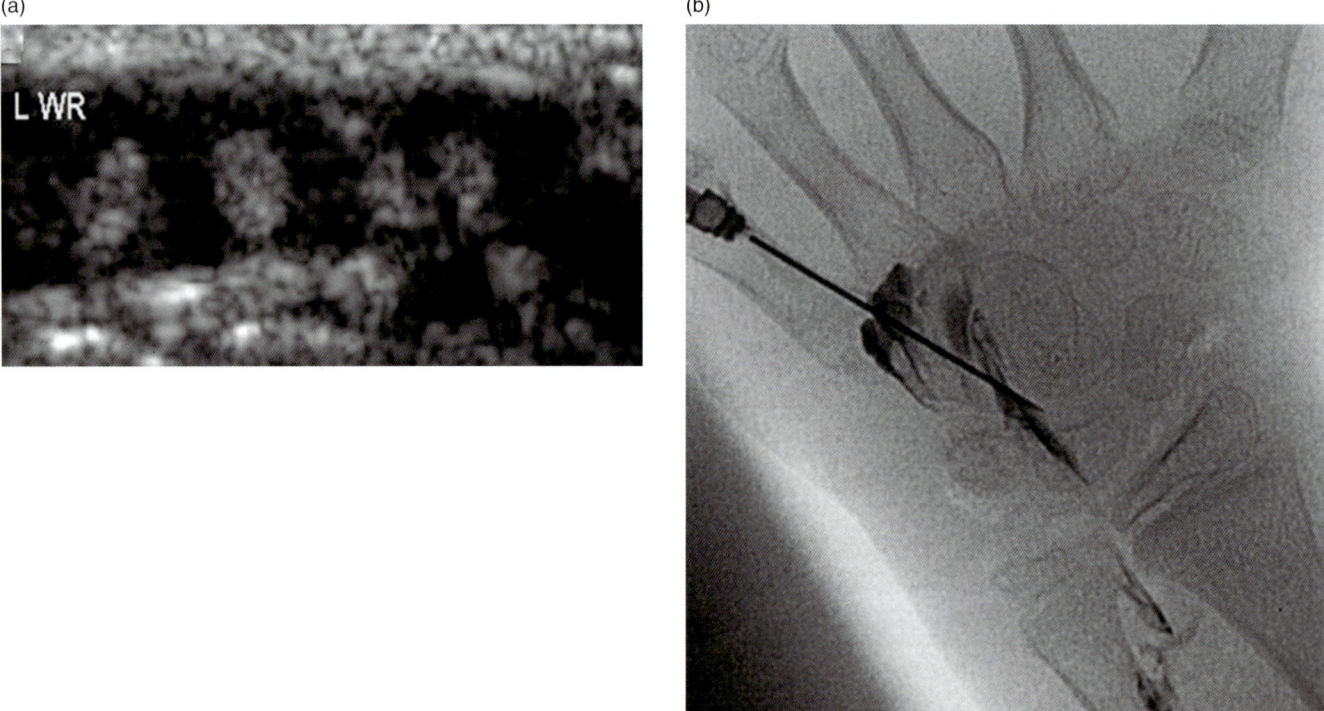

Figure 7.12 Ten-year-old male with JIA and wrist pain. (a) Ultrasound showing inflammation with fluid in the tendon sheaths (tenosynovitis). (b) Ultrasound-guided needle placement with contrast injection confirming position prior to steroid injection.

embolized, then the technique used is a standard approach to selective occlusion of feeding vessels (see Tables 8.6 and 8.7). If a direct puncture technique is planned then an 18-gauge needle, trephine or bone biopsy needle may be used in conjunction with imaging guidance to gain access into the lesion. It is important to keep in mind the technical challenges that the child presents so that the necessary equipment is available, such as power tools, pins, curettes, bone graft powder, cement, or other fillers to mechanically stabilize the lesion.

Patient preparation

Aneurysmal bone cysts are extrememly vascular and there is risk for bleeding with direct percutaneous puncture of the lesion. Thus preprocedure labs need to include a CBC to assess the hemoglobin, hematocrit, and platelets, and a coagulation profile. Any significant coagulopathy needs to be corrected prior to the procedure. We typically utilize general anesthesia for these procedures.

Standard technique

The angiogram and transarterial embolization technique is described in Chapter 8. For direct percutaneous puncture of the UBC or ABC, patient positioning depends upon the route chosen for access. Using aseptic technique, the cystic bone lesion is accessed using an 18-gauge spinal needle or bone needle (8- to 14-gauge), with imaging guidance (fluoroscopy, US, or CT). Fluid is aspirated from the UBC or ABC and non-ionic contrast injected under fluoroscopy to confirm needle tip position in the lesion (Table 7.18). For sclerotherapy of an ABC, sclerosant agents are then injected into the cyst(s) (Figure 7.15). *n*-BCA may then be injected into the cyst for preoperative intralesional injection of an ABC. For UBC, the membrane of the UBC can be stripped with a bone needle attached to a syringe through the "introducer needle," followed by intralesional injection of demineralized bone matrix.

Postprocedure and follow-up care

Most minimally invasive procedures to treat bone cysts are performed on an outpatient basis. However, the patient's clinical status, size of the cyst, and pain management needs dictate whether the patient is admitted to the hospital after the procedure. Also, limited weight-bearing or activity may be necessary, depending upon the location and size of the cystic lesion and the associated risk of a pathologic fracture. Radiographs of the cyst are obtained at two- to three-month intervals to assess for bone mineralization, healing, and reduction in the size of the cyst. Multiple sclerotherapy treatments or embolization procedures may be necessary for primary treatment of ABCs.

Complications

Because ABCs are vascular, the biggest risk of percutaneous injection of these lesions is bleeding, and given the expansile nature of ABCs and UBCs, fracture is a risk of direct percutaneous puncture.

Table 7.16 Aristospan® (triamcinolone hexacetonide intra-articular) dosage for JIA

Large joints (e.g., hip, knee, shoulder) and bursae
- 1 to 2 ml (20 mg/ml suspension) intra-articular; 1 mg/kg to 40 mg maximum

Intermediate joints (e.g., ankle, subtalar, elbow, wrist, TMJ, sacro-iliac)
- 0.5 to 1 ml (20 mg/ml suspension) intra-articular; 1 mg/kg to 40 mg maximum

Small joints (e.g., interphalangeal) and tendon sheaths
- 0.25 to 0.5 ml (20 mg/ml suspension) intra-articular; 1 mg/kg to 40 mg maximum

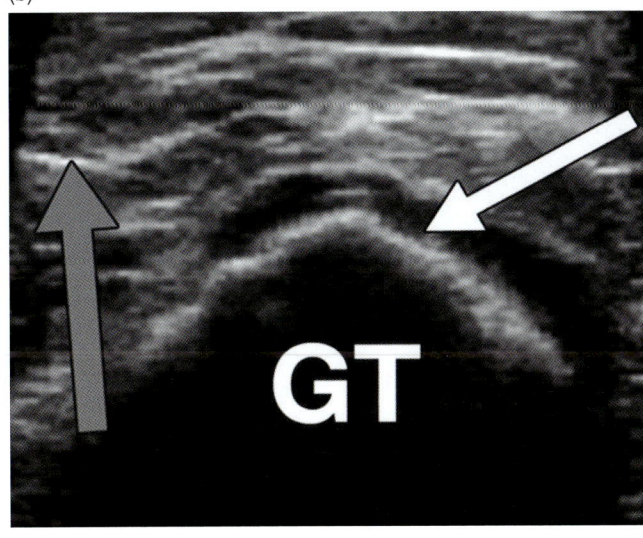

Figure 7.13 Greater trochanter bursa injection. Seventeen-year-old female athlete with lateral hip pain and point tenderness over greater trochanter. (a) Anatomic location of bursa. (b) Ultrasound-guided needle advancement (*gray arrow*) into the bursa (*white arrow*) prior to steroid injection. At three-month follow-up the patient was pain free.

Chapter 7 MSK and soft tissue interventions

(a)
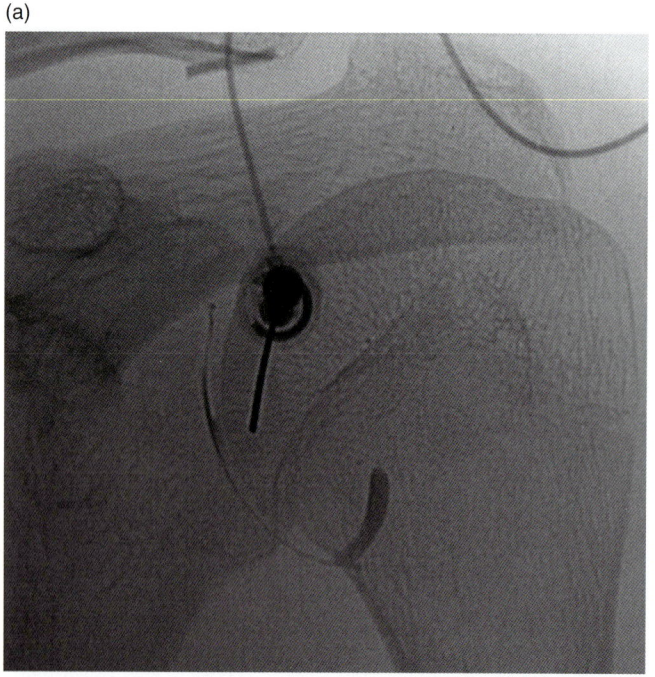

(b)
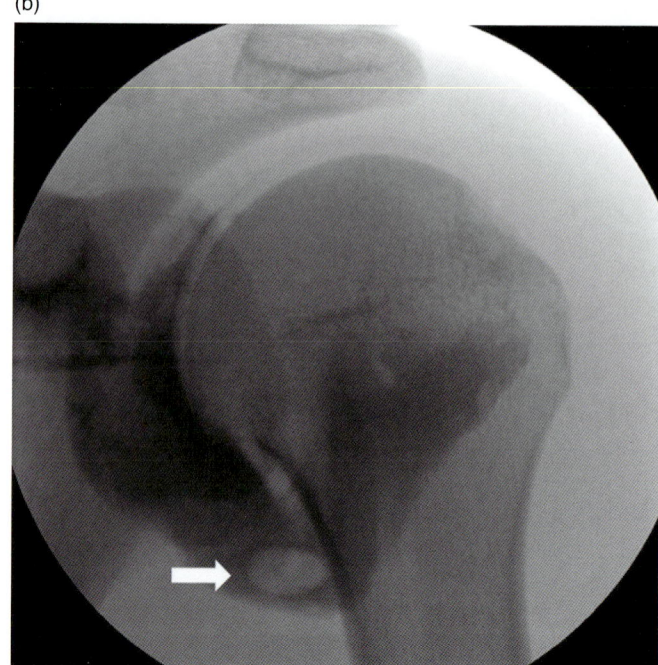

(c)
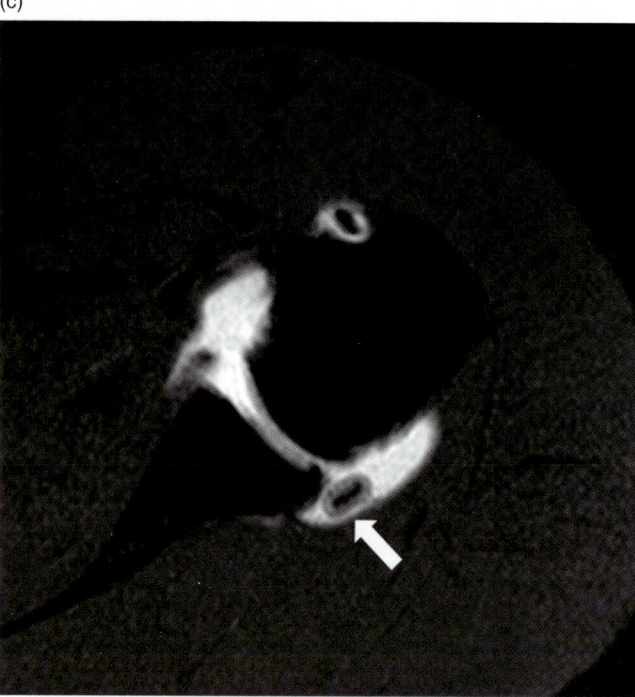

Figure 7.14 Magnetic resonance arthrography in 17-year-old male athlete with remote history of left shoulder dislocation and recurrent instability. (a) Anterior approach shoulder access with free flow of contrast from the needle tip, confirming intra-articular position. (b) Diluted Magnevist® contrast injection. Note intra-articular loose body (*arrow*) inferiorly. (c) Magnetic resonance arthrogram shows smooth, ovoid loose body (*arrow*) in the posterior recess.

Issues and controversies

There is no clear-cut consensus on the best approach to treatment. If a minimally invasive approach is selected, one cannot, at this time, know the best single agent or combination to select. Therefore operator experience and preference often determine the therapy.

Conclusions

Minimally invasive procedures have been shown to be effective and safe for the treatment of UBCs and ABCs. Unicameral bone cysts heal and pain can be relieved with the percutaneous intralesional injection of demineralized bony matrix. Arterial feeders to ABCs can be embolized as the primary treatment, or prior to surgical resection with the goal of reducing intraoperative blood loss. Also, presurgical percutaneous intralesional injection of *n*-BCA in ABCs is effective in reducing blood loss during resection, and sclerotherapy of ABCs has also been successful as a primary treatment.

Table 7.17 Equipment: percutaneous treatment of cystic lesions

- Fluoroscopy +/− CT, US
- Angiogram and embolization of ABCs (see Table 8.6)
  - hemostasis sheath and diagnostic catheters, microcatheter
  - 0.035-inch wires and microwires
  - non-ionic contrast
  - embolic material: *n*-BCA (mixed ethiodized oil), PVA, ethanol, coils
- Direct puncture of ABCs
  - Sclerotherapy
    - needles: 18-gauge, 3½-inch spinal needle or 8- to 14-gauge bone needle
    - sodium tetradecyl sulfate, dehydrated alcohol, or doxycycline
    - non-ionic contrast
- Preoperative intralesional injection of ABCs
  - 18-gauge, 3½-inch spinal needle
  - *n*-BCA mixed with ethiodized oil in 1:7 ratio, or
  - sclerosants
- UBCs
  - 18-gauge, 3½-inch spinal needle
  - 3 mm or larger bone needle (trephine)
  - demineralized bone matrix

Percutaneous biopsy of solid bone lesions

Introduction

About half of all primary bone tumors in children are benign (Table 7.19), and some of these are amenable to percutaneous therapy, such as osteoid osteoma (see below) and Langerhan's cell histiocytosis (LCH) (Figures 7.16, 7.17). Bone malignancies occur at a rate of approximately 8 to 9 per million children, and represent about 6% of all childhood malignancies. The great majority of these are sarcomas, specifically osteosarcoma and Ewing's sarcoma. There is a gradual rise in the prevalence of these tumors from age five to ten years, then a steeper rise from eleven to fifteen years of age, at which point the

Table 7.18 Procedure summary: percutaneous treatment of cystic lesions

- General anesthesia
- Route planning and access site selection
- Skin preparation and draping
- Local anesthetic and skin incision
- For embolization, see Table 8.7
- For direct puncture, image-guided percutaneous needle access
- Lesion volume assessment (contrast)
- Biopsy as needed
- Inject sclerosant, bone material, etc.

(a)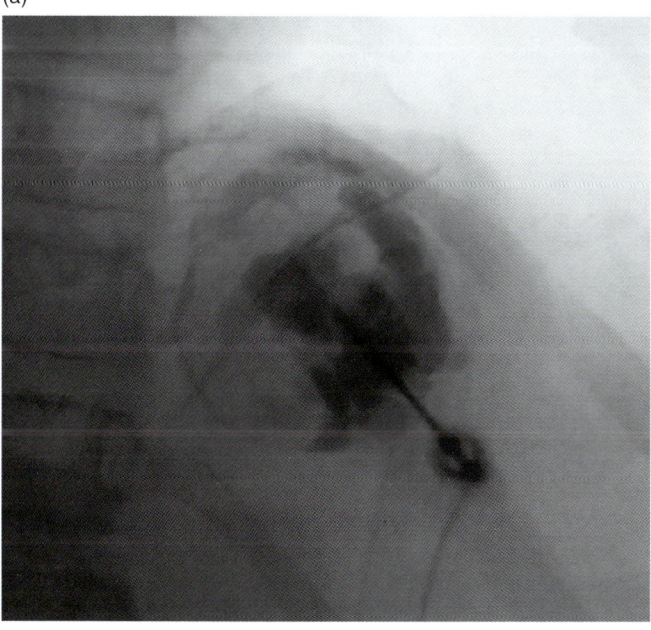

(b)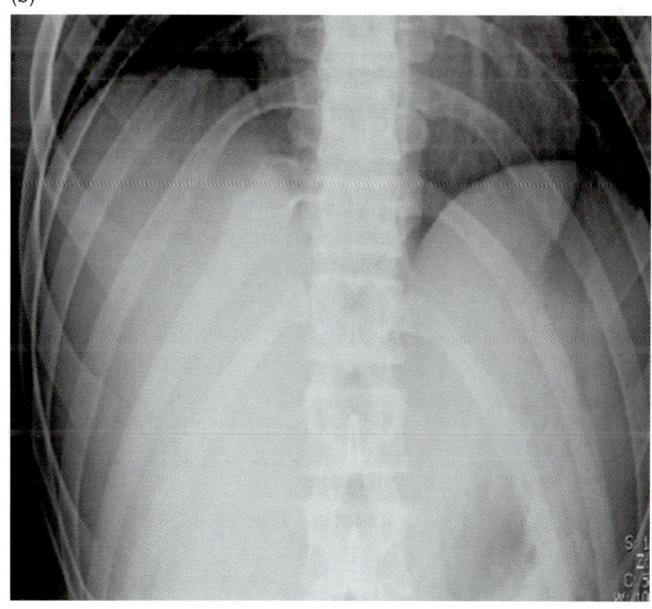

Figure 7.15 Thirteen-year-old male with aneurysmal bone cyst of right posterior 11th rib. (a) Fluoroscopic-guided needle placement and contrast injection of Ethibloc® with patient prone. (b) Four-year follow-up shows resolution of ABC with residual widening of posterior 11th rib (courtesy of J. Dubois, MD).

prevalence reaches its peak. While osteosarcoma shows a slight racial preference for African-American children, Ewing's sarcoma shows a striking preference for Caucasians. There is no other specific risk factor associated with either of these bone malignancies.

Indications

There are generally two reasons for aspirates or core biopsies from bone or surrounding soft tissue in children (Table 7.19). A bone marrow aspirate or biopsy is generally performed by staff in the department of hematology and oncology to evaluate for a systemic disease that involves bone marrow cell lines, such as the diagnosis and staging of leukemia and lymphoma, and to evaluate iron levels.

The second reason for biopsy of bone and soft tissue is to evaluate a focal bony or soft tissue abnormality suspicious for neoplasm or infection (Figures 7.18, 7.19). Classically, malignant bone and soft tissue processes progressively enlarge and are painful. The pain may be present for a considerable period of time before the diagnosis is made, intensifies over time, and may eventually become unbearable. Malignant bone tumors usually have an aggressive appearance on imaging and may be lytic, blastic, or mixed. They usually have a poorly defined margin, cortical destruction, extension into the surrounding soft tissues, and periosteal reaction variably presenting as periosteal elevation or new bone formation.

Some tumors, such as parosteal and periosteal osteosarcoma, arise at the surface of the bone. While the cortex may be intact, there is often a profound periosteal reaction and a soft tissue component that may involve part of the bone or the entire circumference. Initially the mass may be painless, but these usually become painful and tender as they progress.

One should be aware of the characteristic appearance of bone lesions that do not require biopsy (the so-called "don't touch" lesions, Table 7.20). These lesions are usually pathognomonic of a benign process, do not have malignant

Table 7.19 Indications: percutaneous treatment of bone and soft tissue tumors

Aspiration
- suspected bone marrow disease
- selected neoplasms with characteristic cytopathology (e.g., Langerhans cell)
- processes that involve or replace bone marrow (e.g., leukemia, lymphoma, neuroblastoma)
- evaluate bone marrow iron content (e.g., sickle cell disease on transfusion therapy)

Core biopsy
- evaluation of mass lesions
- evaluation of bony destructive or permeative lesions
- possible presence of metastases
- distinguish between infection and neoplasm

Management and treatment planning

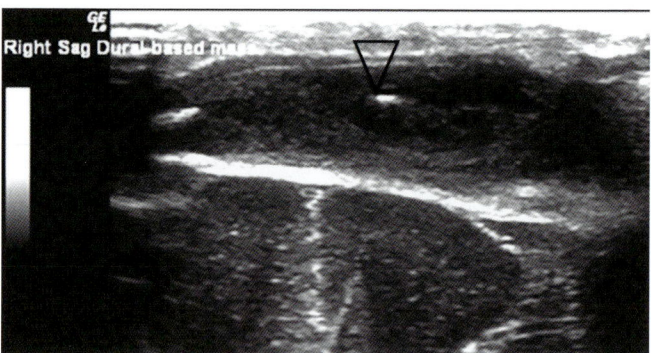

Figure 7.17 After US-guided core biopsy established the diagnosis of Langerhan's cell histiocytosis of the calvaria in this two-year-old male, steroids were laced into the substance of the tumor through a 27-gauge 1.5-inch needle (*arrowhead*). In follow-up, the tumor resolved and the skull healed.

(a)

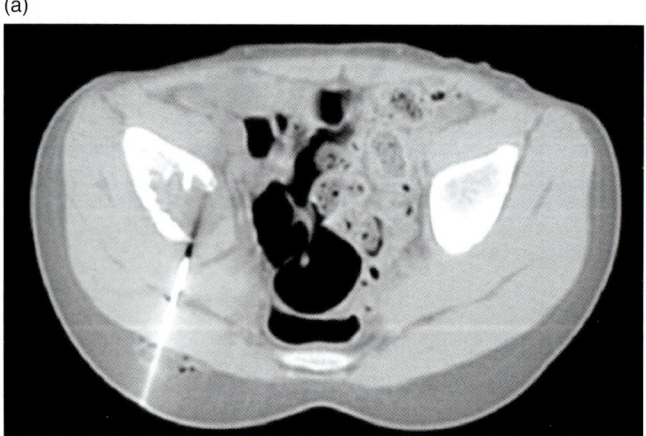

(b)

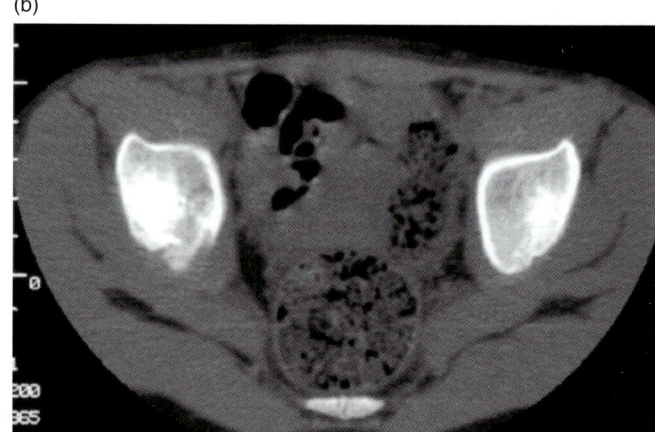

Figure 7.16 LCH right acetabulum (a) Computed tomography-guided intralesional steroid injection. (b) Two-year follow-up demonstrates bony healing (courtesy of J. Dubois, MD).

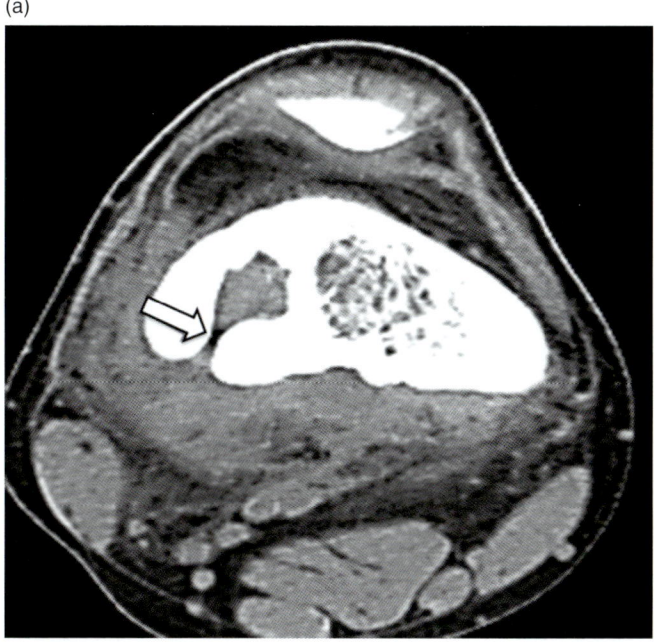
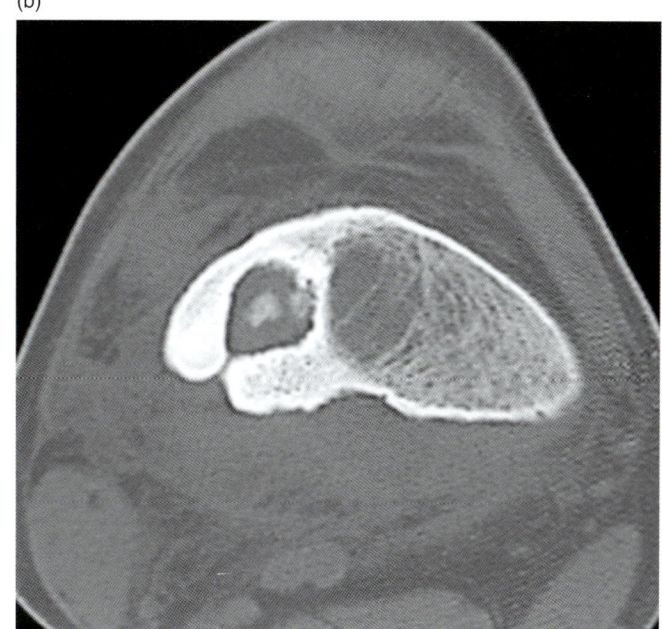
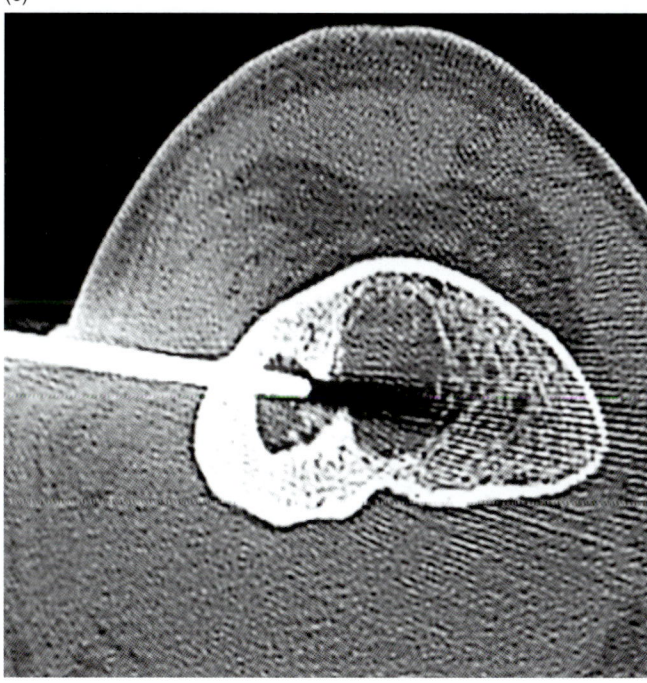

Figure 7.18 Six-year-old with chronic knee pain. (a,b) Axial soft tissue and bony window CT shows lytic lesion with associated soft tissue swelling, a central nidus, and sinus tract (*arrow*). (c) An 8-gauge Jamshidi needle was used to sample the lesion, resulting in the diagnosis of a Brodie's abscess secondary to *Staphylococcus aureus*.

potential, and often resolve over time without therapy. They are often characterized by osteolytic cortical lesions that are outlined by a thin rim of cortex that is unbroken. They may be expansile or multilobulated and may thin the cortex, but do not disrupt the cortex and do not cause a periosteal reaction. Lesions that do not meet these criteria, where malignancy cannot be excluded, may require biopsy for definitive diagnosis.

It is helpful if biopsy planning is done in close consultation with the orthopedic service, preferably with the orthopedic oncologic surgeon who will be responsible for surgical resection and reconstruction if indicated. There are circumstances under which the orthopedist will prefer to perform biopsy as part of an *en bloc* resection, and a percutaneous core biopsy may not be preferred. When a percutaneous biopsy is requested, the orthopedist may have a preference for the skin entry site and the compartments that are crossed in the needle path, and may want to have the entry site marked so that the needle tract may be excised at the time of resection to reduce the risk for remote seeding of tumor cells. This is especially true where limb sparing surgery is planned for treatment of sarcoma.

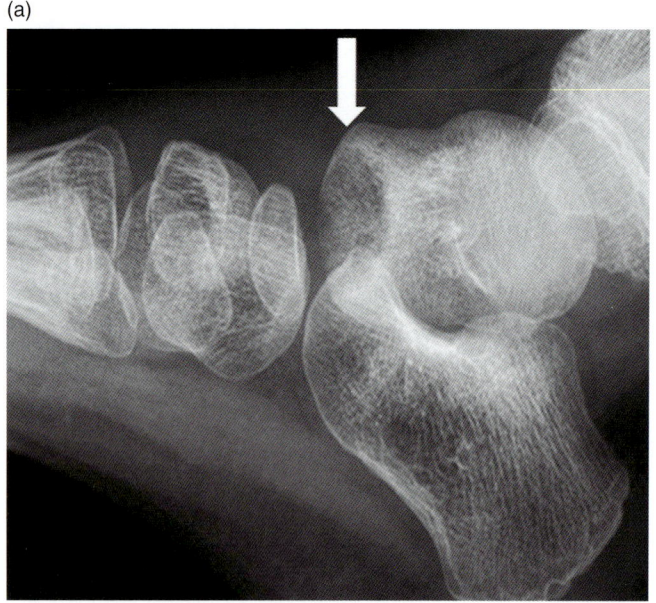
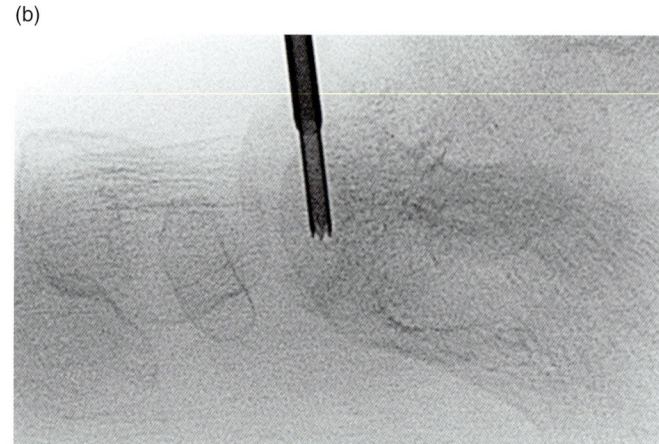
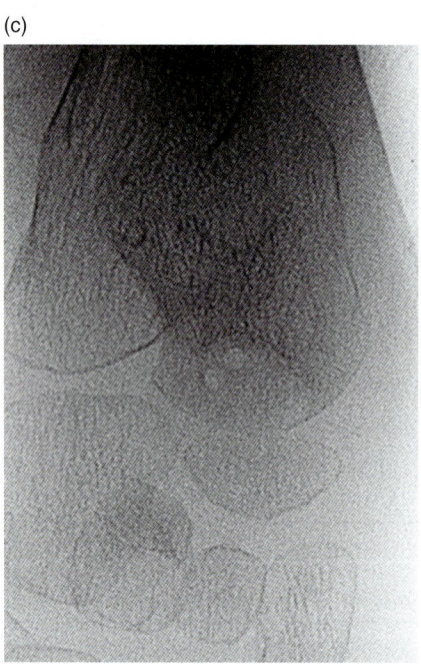

Figure 7.19 Four-year-old male with disseminated coccidioidomycosis with fever and foot pain. (a) Lateral foot radiograph shows lytic lesion in the distal talus (*arrow*). (b) Fluoroscopically guided Ackerman needle biopsy. (c) Post-biopsy frontal image shows biopsy defects within the lesion. The biopsy resulted in a diagnosis of chronic coccidioidomycosis osteomyelitis.

It is also helpful to include the pathologist and oncologist in the planning discussion, to determine what volume of tissue is required for any microbiologic, histopathologic, immunohistochemical, or genetic analysis that will be performed, and how the specimen should be transported. It may be useful to have an intraprocedural preliminary tissue evaluation performed, such as a touch preparation with Gram stain or frozen section or both, to confirm that lesional tissue has been acquired and, in some cases, to provide a provisional diagnosis. If, for example, small round blue cells are observed in the preliminary evaluation, the oncologist may wish to have a central venous access device placed under the same anesthesia. If solid bone is within the specimen, preliminary analysis may be unproductive, and a final diagnosis may await decalcification of the sample.

Equipment

A selection of bone and soft tissue sampling devices should be available (Table 7.21). The equipment and supplies used for soft tissue sampling is reviewed in other chapters. There are a variety of bone biopsy needles available, including Jamshidi®, Ackerman, T-lok™, Bierman, Conrad Crosby, Franseen, Osty-Cut® and OstyCore®, and Elson. A sterile mallet can assist initial percutaneous access to the cortex, introducing the stylet

Table 7.20 Pediatric bone and soft tissue tumors

Malignant bone tumors	Osteosarcoma (central, chondroblastic, fibroblastic, osteoblastic, parosteal, periosteal, secondary, small cell, surface, telangiectatic) Ewing sarcoma, primitive Neuroectodermal tumor Lymphoma
Malignant soft tissue tumors	Rhabdomyosarcoma (alveolar, botryoid, embryonal) Neuroblastoma Rhabdoid tumor Retinoblastoma Wilms tumor, renal clear cell sarcoma Retinoblastoma Leukemia Infantile fibrosarcoma
Cystic bone lesions	Unicameral bone cyst (UBC) Aneurysmal bone cyst (ABC)
Benign bone tumors	Osteoid osteoma, osteoblastoma Fibrous dysplasia, osteofibrous dysplasia Myofibroma Chondroblastoma, hamartoma, osteochondroma Hemangioma, Langerhans cell histiocytosis, osteomyelitis
Benign soft tissue tumors	Angiomatosis, infantile hemangioma, non-involuting congenital hemangioma, rapidly involuting congenital hemangioma, fibrolipomatous hamartoma of nerve, neurofibroma Infantile fibrous hamartoma, infantile fibromatosis, myofibroma, hyaline fibromatosis, fibromatosis coli, inflammatory myofibroblastic tumor, calcifying aponeurotic fibroma, calcifying fibrous pseudotumor Benign fibrous histiocytoma, giant cell fibroblastoma, juvenile xanthogranuloma, plexiform fibrohistiocytic tumor fetal rhabdomyoma Hibernoma, lipoblastoma, myxoma, omental-mesenteric myxoid hamartoma
"Don't touch" lesions	Non-ossifying fibroma, periosteal desmoid, fibrous dysplasia, enchondroma, bone infarct, subchondral cyst

Table 7.21 Equipment: percutaneous treatment of bone and soft tissue tumors

- Biopsy needles
  - soft tissue core biopsy needle
  - Chiba for FNA
  - bone biopsy needles
- Imaging guidance: CT, US, fluoroscopy
- Sterile transport to pathology

Imaging

Most interventional bone procedures are performed under CT guidance, as the cross-sectional images provide excellent route planning and accurate guidance. Fluoroscopy can be used to sample bone lesions, although the planar images can elevate the risk of accidental puncture of adjacent structures. ^{99m}Tc SPECT or PET images can be fused, either asynchronously or in real time, with conventional CT, cone-beam CT or even MR to help localize metabolically active lesions. Despite the oft-repeated but seldom proven rubric that US is not useful for imaging bone, there are a surprising number of bone-related lesions that can be safely and efficiently sampled under US guidance (Figure 7.20). While normally corticated bone reflects virtually all sound waves, when a malignant lesion has thinned or disrupted the cortex or has a soft tissue component, the tumor may be quite easily distinguished under US. Doppler interrogation can provide additional information about the viability of and blood flow within the lesion.

Patient preparation

There is generally no specific preparation needed in advance of a bone biopsy. As is the case for soft tissue biopsy, the laboratory tests ordered depend on the clinical situation. We do not order routine tests except for diagnostic imaging necessary to demonstrate the lesion and regional anatomy to aid in target selection and biopsy route planning. In many cases PET scanning adds information regarding the metabolically active component. This is especially useful for large masses when portions of the lesion may be necrotic. If sedation or anesthesia is planned, then the child is made NPO at the appropriate time.

Standard technique

There are several approaches that can be utilized to obtain a bone biopsy (Table 7.22). One can use an image-guided freehand technique or a guided approach (Figure 7.21). Regardless of the biopsy method used, the procedure begins with route planning and skin entry site selection. Several methods for skin site selection and marking exist. We have described our approach to site selection in prior chapters. With the freehand technique, a bone biopsy needle with a stylet is maneuvered to the target with imaging guidance. Once at the target, the stylet is removed and with substantial downward pressure the needle is rotated clockwise so that the cutting tip enters the bone and with time cuts out a tubular specimen. Depending on the

deeply enough that a coring, twisting, or drilling motion can be used to advance the hollow coaxial needle into the bone. Syringes of 5 to 20 ml can be used to aspirate tissue or fluid into the needle or to help prevent loss of the sample while withdrawing the needle. In many instances we prefer to use a trephine (Craig or Michele) and power drill to obtain bone samples especially if the cortex is intact and thick.

thickness and integrity of the cortex, this process can take considerable effort and muscle. In some cases the procedure can be facilitated by the use of a mallet (5 lbs/2.3 kg or more) to set and advance the biopsy needle or trephine into the cortex. Alternatively, power tools can be used to significantly hasten the procedure. The main downside with the freehand approach is that unless the needle is solidly within bone, needle/trephine drift can occur, potentially causing injury to adjacent structures and loss of target accuracy.

An alternative method is to use a bridging procedure to increase the ease, safety, and efficiency of the procedure. If this approach is used, a K-wire or Steinman pin is substituted for

Table 7.22 Procedure summary: percutaneous treatment of bone and soft tissue tumors

- General anesthesia
- Route planning and skin entry site selection
- Skin preparation and draping
- Local anesthetic and skin incision
- Image-guided needle access into lesion
- Specimen delivery to pathology or appropriate laboratory

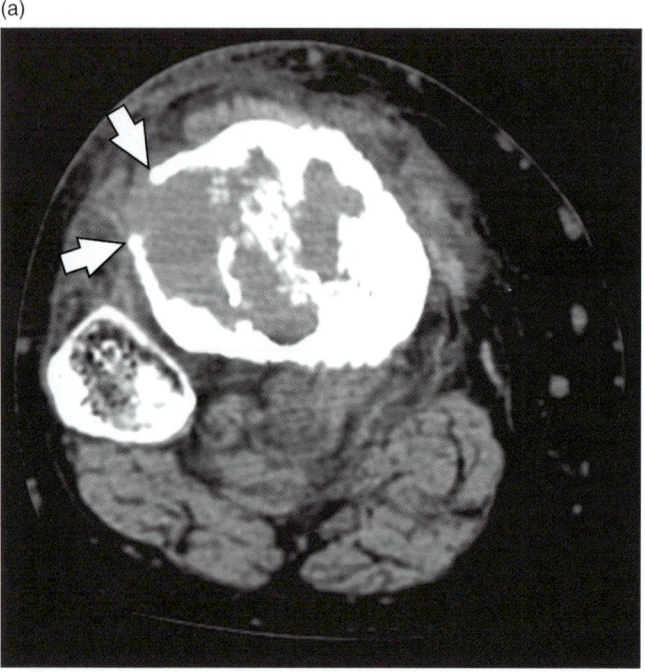

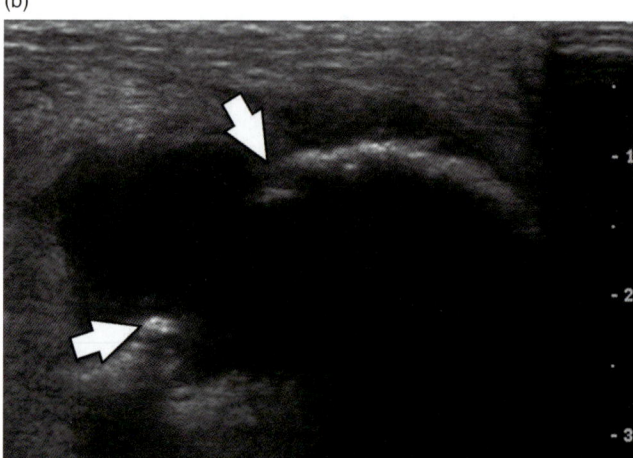

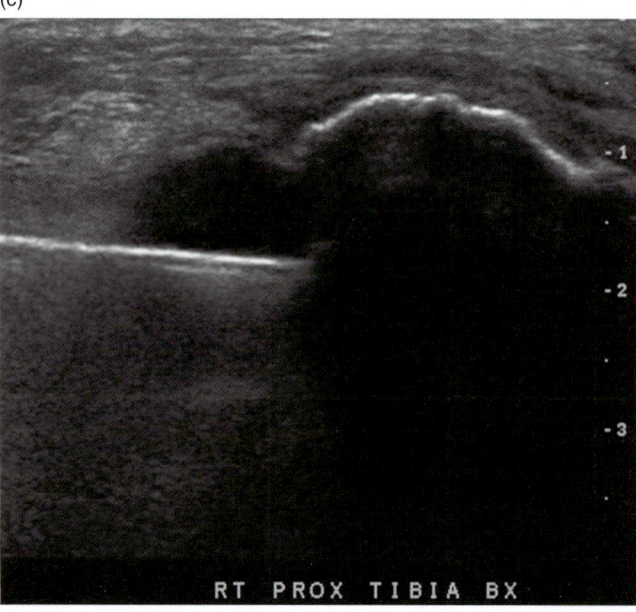

Figure 7.20 A ten-year-old female with chronic, intermittent lower extremity pain increasing in intensity, demonstrated intense radiotracer uptake in the proximal right tibia on ^{99m}Tc MDP imaging. (a) Computed tomography showed a predominately lytic lesion with disruption of the lateral tibial cortex (*arrows*). (b) Ultrasound with a linear transducer at the same location yields very similar information, except that the extent of soft tissue involvement is more clearly depicted. (c) Using US guidance, biopsy specimens were easily obtained with a conventional (soft-tissue) automated core needle.

Chapter 7 MSK and soft tissue interventions

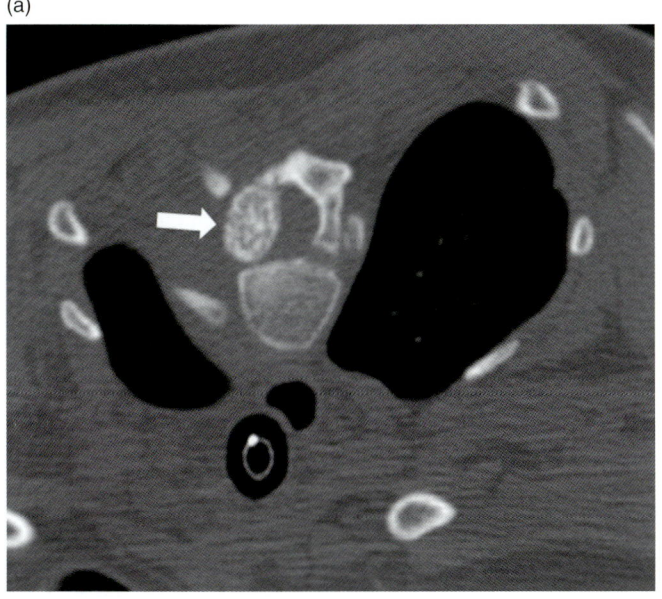

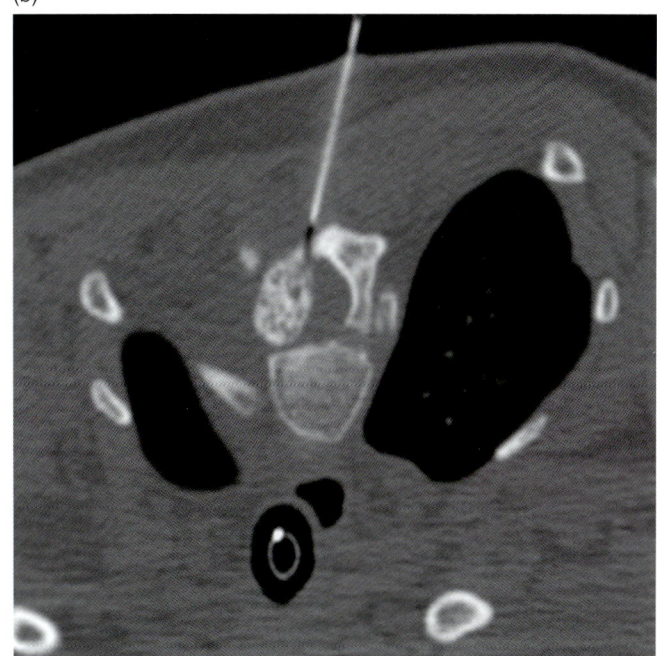

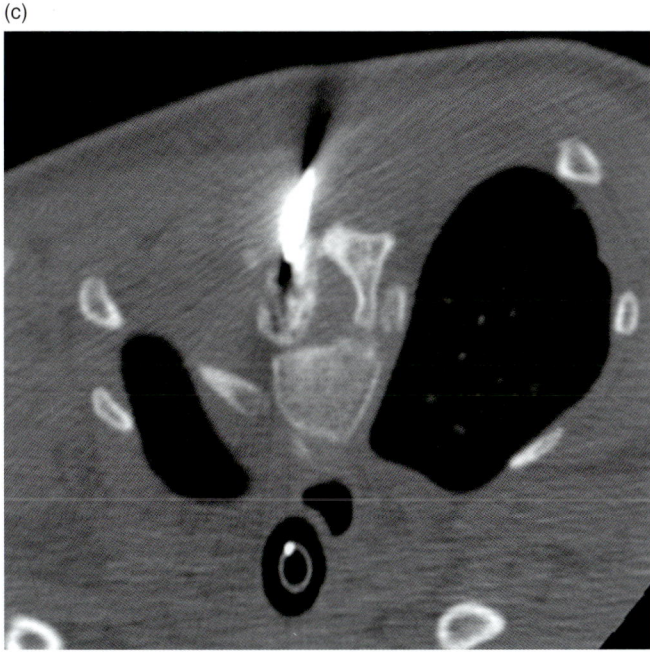

Figure 7.21 Ten-year-old female with persistent back pain. (a) Axial CT demonstrates expansile bony mass of left thoracic posterior vertebral elements (*arrow*) with narrowing of the spinal canal. (b) K-wire placement directed away from canal. (c) Coaxial biopsy needle with Ackerman needle in lesion. Diagnosis: osteoblastoma.

the needle, and using image guidance, positioned over the target and set into the cortex with a mallet. Next, the soft-tissue tract is generously dilated with forceps and a Craig needle or trephine is coaxially positioned over the pin and rotated counter-clockwise until the cutting edge is on the cortex. The length of the bone tract is measured on the CT scan and the distance transferred and marked on the bone cutting needle with a Steri-Strip®. The needle is connected to a power drill and a hole is drilled through the lesion to the prescibed length. This usually takes one to two minutes as opposed to as much as two hours if done manually.

When the drilling is completed, limited CT images are obtained to confirm needle tip position. To remove the drill and pin, the drill direction is reversed (counter-clockwise) and pulled out of the bone. The bone specimen is then removed by hammering or pushing out the pin and removing the bone specimen from around the pin. Whether using a manual or powered approach nothing needs to be done to fill the bone defect. In most cases the skin is approximated with Steri-Strips®; however, if necessary, the deeper soft tissue and skin can be approximated with sutures. A dry sterile dressing is placed over the site. If the bone defect is large or in a critical location, non-weight bearing of that extremity may be indicated. Casting is not necessary.

Postprocedure and follow-up care

In most cases, care after the procedure includes limited physical activity until the biopsy site heals (usually two to six weeks) to minimize the chance for a pathologic fracture. If the biopsy defect is in a weight-bearing location, e.g., femoral neck, non-weight bearing is preferred and crutch training is provided. Radiographs of the area are obtained four to six weeks after the procedure to assess for bone healing. In most children there is minimal postprocedural discomfort and only NSAIDs are required. If greater analgesia is needed, a narcotic analegesic is perscribed for three to five days.

Complications

The most frequent technical problem related to bone biopsy is crush artifact in the specimen that may obliterate the nature of the lesion and result in a non-diagnostic biopsy. Unfortunately, this is a difficult outcome to avoid, and does not seem particularly dependent upon the size of the sample or the method of acquisition. Multiple biopsies may improve the frequency of diagnostic tissue acquisition. In our experience, postprocedural complications are uncommon and occur in fewer than 1% of cases. When there is an untoward effect, soft tissue infection or hematoma is most likely. Osteomyelitis and pathologic fracture are known to occur, but are rare in children.

Tract seeding has been reported following core biopsy of bone malignancies. However, this is an extremely rare occurence and we have never encountered this problem. This may in part be due to our practice of performing coaxial biopsies, thereby protecting the tract from seeding.

Bone tumor (osteoid osteoma) excision

Introduction

Most focal benign bone lesions are discovered incidentally, are asymptomatic, and do not require treatment. However, some may cause intense, debilitating pain (e.g., osteoid osteoma), may cause growth disturbances like scoliosis (e.g., spinal osteoid osteoma), or angular growth deformity (e.g., physeal bar, Figure 7.22), or may weaken the bone and predispose to microarchitectural collapse (e.g., avascular necrosis). These lesions may also be associated with potentially irreversible muscle atrophy, gait and other functional disturbances, bony overgrowth, and delayed-onset osteoarthritis. Surgical options in each case include a long skin incision and *en bloc* resection of the bony lesion, often accompanied by internal fixation due to the resulting stress riser, and sometimes requiring joint replacement. Intraoperative localization of the lesion can be challenging and may lead to an incomplete removal of the lesion and the need for a second surgery. Recovery from open surgical procedures can be prolonged and generally requires intense rehabilitation and physical therapy.

Osteoid osteoma is a prototypical benign bone lesion. It is a small benign bone tumor, usually no larger than 1.5 cm in diameter although we have treated lesions over 3.0 cm (by definition, osteoblastoma). The lesion most often affects children and young adults, ranging in age from 5 to 24 years. There is a definite sex preference with reported male to female ratios of 2.6 to 3.2. The telltale symptom for this disease is local pain, which is typically more severe at night. In 30 to 75% of cases, aspirin and other non-steroidal anti-inflammatory drugs will relieve the discomfort. The time from onset of pain to diagnosis varies widely, ranging from several months to as high as nine years, as one study reported. When this lesion is seen in patients less than five years of age, it is our experience that it tends to have somewhat different properties, including a larger lesion that is less symptomatic with a higher rate of recurrence.

Interventional therapies are usually accomplished through small (1 to 2 cm) incisions, using CT guidance. The lesions can be removed by focal bone excision, either manually or using power tools, with a trephine and in some cases curettes. Today, the preferred treatment approach for osteoid osteomas is with radiofrequency ablation. When an image-guided biopsy or excision is performed a stress riser (structural weakness) is produced, and although the mechanical weakness is present, it is considerably less than that of an open surgical (wedge) resection, and recovery is much shorter and less rigorous. Alleviation of pain following percutaneous excision or ablation of the osteoid osteoma nidus is often instantaneous.

Chronic and irreversible changes related to the underlying pathology will remain present after percutaneous resection, thus a short time interval from diagnosis to definitive intervention is beneficial. Reconstructive and stabilization procedures may still be required in the event of angular or asymmetric growth disturbance or creation of a substantial stress riser.

Indications

Percutaneous bone surgery has slowly and steadily become an image-guided procedure with an expanding number of indications. The core procedure that has allowed interventionalists to grow into this complex set of procedures is the image-guided bone biopsy and the use of pins and power tools. Because of the complexity of these therapeutic and technical issues, it is essential to work as a team with orthopedic surgeons and other specialists as needed. Conditions that are amenable to percutaneous excision include osteoid osteoma, other benign bone lesions, and physeal bars.

Equipment
Imaging

Plain radiographs of an osteoid osteoma typically demonstrate a small, sharply defined, eccentric, round to oval lytic lesion

Chapter 7 MSK and soft tissue interventions

Table 7.23 Equipment: bone tumor excision

- Computed tomography guidance
- Tools: power drill, Steinman pins, K-wires, trephine/bone biopsy needle, curettes
- Dehydrated alcohol
- Suture, absorbable
- Dressing
- Crutches or wheelchair depending on age and lesion location

with reactive bone. Its characteristic feature is a lucent nidus comprised of a spongy hypervascular tissue measuring up to 1.5 cm in diameter. The nidus may contain an area of calcification. Lesions most commonly involve the long bones, including the femur, tibia, humerus, and the lumbar spine, although any bone can be affected. In 80 to 90% of cases, the lesion is located in the cortex. In general, thick laminar periosteal new bone forms adjacent to the lesion, except if the lesion is intra-articular.

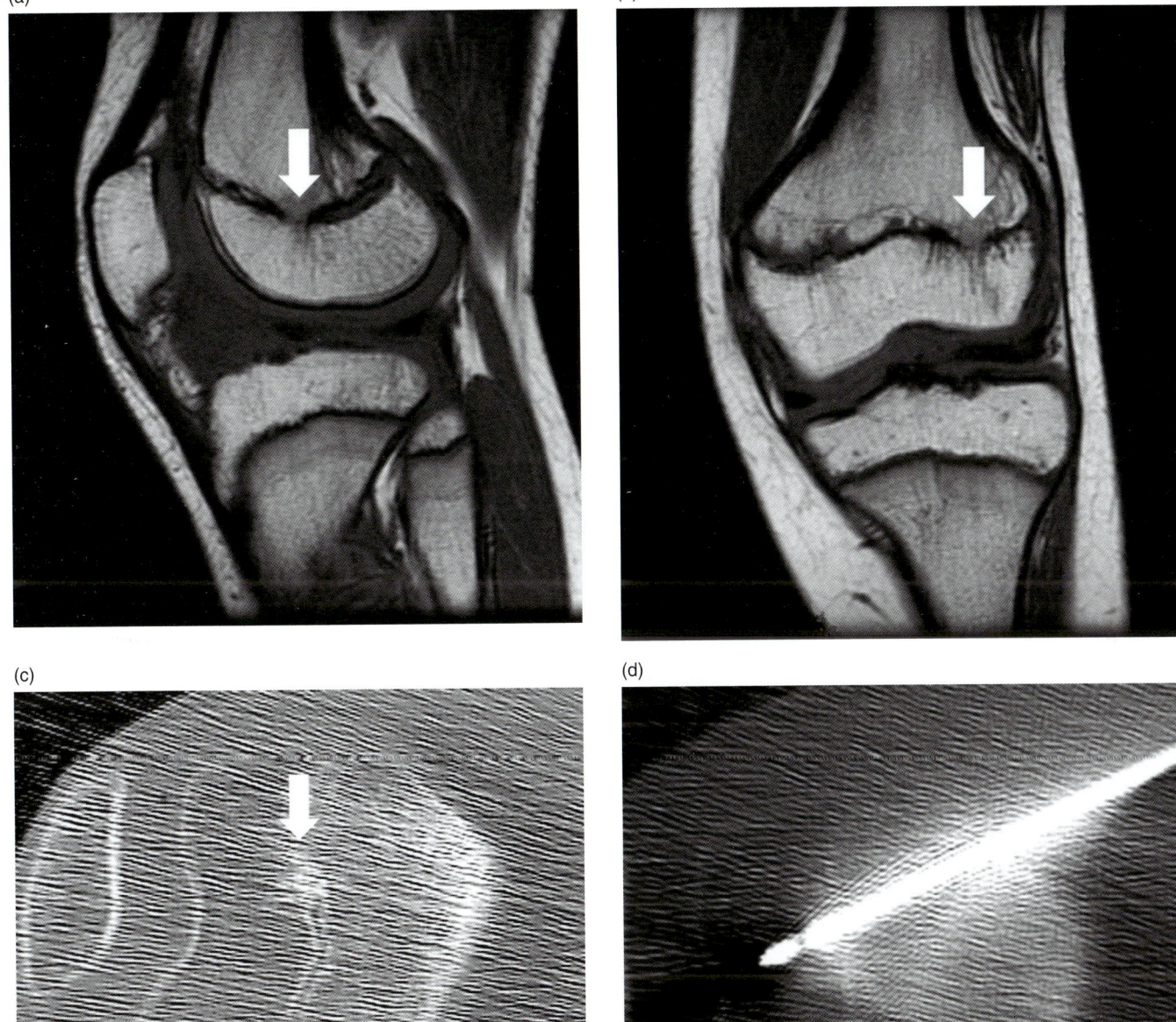

Figure 7.22 Eleven-year-old competitive ski racer suffered a displaced tibial spine fracture treated by open reduction. One year later, presented with pain, decreased range of motion, and 13 degree valgus angular deformity. (a,b) Sagittal and coronal T1 images show bony bar bridging the lateral femoral physis (*arrow*). (c) Axial preprocedural CT shows bony bar (*arrow*). (d) Pin and trephine in place through bar. (e) Post-resection of bar.

(e)

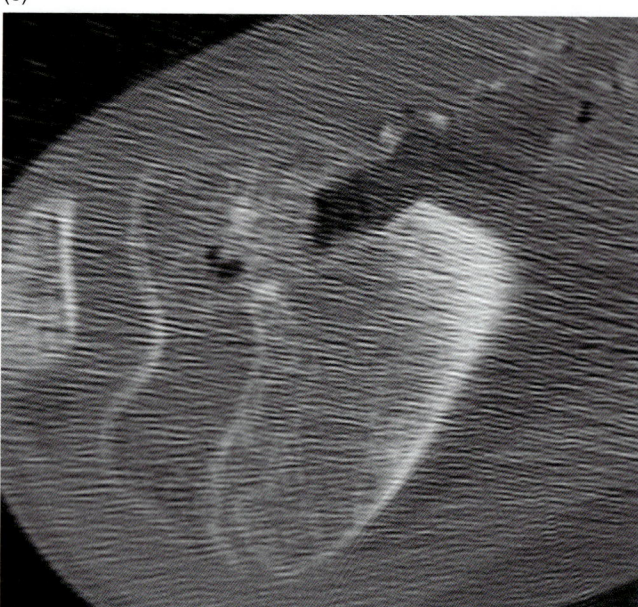

Figure 7.22 (cont.)

Imaging for diagnosis and procedural planning is usually performed on a multidetector CT, and the images are post-processed with a bone algorithm, with two objectives: first, to characterize the lesion, confirm the diagnosis of osteoid osteoma, and exclude a lesion that would require biopsy or treatment by another approach, and second, to determine a safe pathway for treatment of the lesion. If MRI has been obtained, caution must be exercised in the interpretation of the images, as osteoid osteoma is often associated with profound inflammatory changes in the surrounding soft tissues, as well as joint effusions when the lesion is near a joint, and bony overgrowth and sclerosis may be seen at some distance from the focal lesion. These findings can lead to a misdiagnosis of potential malignancy or infection. A ^{99m}Tc scan will be positive but is non-specific. The clinical history will often help improve the pre-test probability of correctly recognizing and treating the lesion.

Drill and curettage

This procedure has been successfully performed many times with a hand drill or trephine, but this method is time consuming and can be physically demanding. A power drill is a much simpler option, although this may be unfamiliar equipment to many interventional radiologists (Table 7.23). This type of equipment usually belongs to the hospital and not to a department *per se*, and can often be reserved by communicating with operating room personnel. If necessary, these colleagues can also help with in-service familiarization with operation of the equipment for the interventionalist and the interventional

Table 7.24 Procedure summary: bone tumor excision

- General anesthesia
- Route planning and skin entry site selection
- Skin preparation and draping
- Local anesthetic and skin incision
- Image-guided pin access into lesion
- Coaxial placement of trephine over pin
- Drill trephine to predetermined distance through lesion (tract length is 1.5 times the lesion diameter)
- Curettage of cavity to remove debris
- Possible instillation of dehydrated alcohol into cavity to denature residual nidus material
- Suture deep soft tissue and skin as needed
- Specimen delivery to pathology or appropriate laboratory

team. A drill motor, batteries, and a selection of Kirschner (K) wires and Steinman pins should be part of the kit, but drill bits and angled curettes may have to be requested separately (Figure 7.23). Cannulated drill bits should be available in sizes that approximate the short-axis diameter of the lesion perpendicular to the direction of approach, usually around 6 to 10 mm. It is important to assure a fit between the drill bit selected and the available K-wires or Steinman pins. Angular curettes in a similar size range can be helpful.

Additional equipment and supplies

If preferred, 95% dehydrated alcohol may be used to sterilize the excision site after lesion removal, and to denature any nidus fragments that are not removed to decrease the risk of recurrence. Since virtually all percutaneous removals result in a biopsy specimen, a sterile specimen container with formalin will also be necessary. A confirmatory diagnosis is obtained in the majority of cases.

Patient preparation

Upon review of the preprocedure scans, an approach to the lesion must be planned that best fulfills the following criteria: (1) avoid regional nerves and vessels, (2) minimize transgression of joint space or capsule, (3) provide a relatively flat cortical surface to facilitate a stable needle position that is perpendicular to the planned route of entry, and (4) allow for removal of the entire lesion with the smallest resulting stress riser possible. The best path is not always the shortest path. If neurovascular structures obscure access through the cortex nearest the skin, it is possible to approach the lesion by passing through the opposite cortical margin, or to take a perpendicular route.

Standard technique

Because manipulation of periosteum is painful, it is our preference to perform all bone procedures under general anesthesia (Table 7.24). Nevertheless, a long-acting local anesthetic (e.g., 0.25% bupivacaine) may also be administered from the

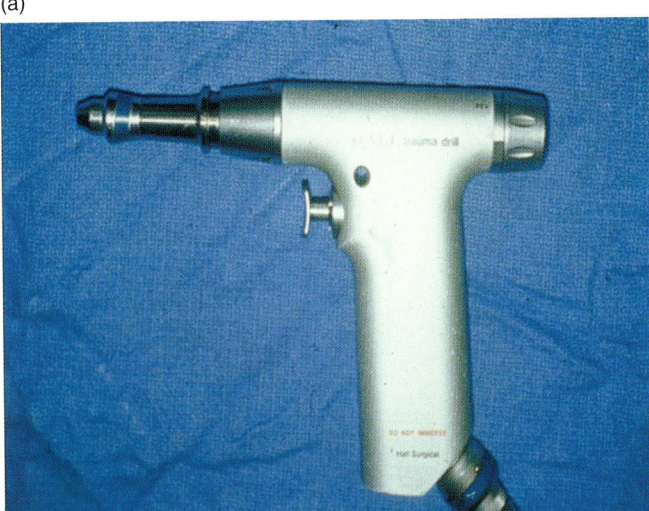 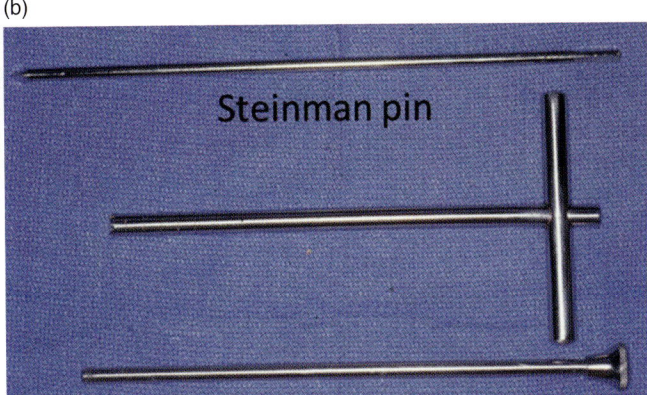

Figure 7.23 Bone biopsy equipment (a) Power drill. (b) Pin and trephine.

skin to the cortical margin to reduce postprocedure discomfort. The selection of a trephine or drill bit to remove the tumor is based on the diameter of the lesion, and should be at least 1 to 2 mm larger than the nidus so that it can be excised in a single pass (Figure 7.24). An elliptical lesion may have to be removed in two or more passes, and in such cases the device should be 1 to 2 mm larger that the short-axis diameter.

A pathway from the skin to the lesion is identified in an axial plane from preprocedure CT images. Although in many cases this will represent the shortest available path, there are important exceptions. First, selection of a pathway that avoids neurovascular structures is essential to prevent adverse complications. This may, at times, require selection of a path through the cortex *opposite* the lesion, so that the neurovascular bundle at potential risk is located well beyond the end of the planned path and, if possible, not aligned with the procedural pathway. This will, of course, create a second stress riser and increases the vulnerability of the bone to pathologic fracture, but while healing of the cortex is a temporary issue, the effect of hemorrhage or nerve injury may have much more profound implications. Second, the pathway should be planned so that there is a flat surface of cortex perpendicular to the planned path, if at all possible. This reduces the amount the drill or trephine will tend to "walk" away from the preferred path as the cortex is engaged before a substantial starter hole is formed.

Once the pathway is selected, the overlying skin is prepared and draped, and buffered local anesthetic instilled from the skin to the periosteum. A stab wound is created into the skin large enough to easily pass subsequent instruments and tools, so that devices will rotate freely without binding and potentially injuring skin. If a trephine will be used it may be advanced directly to the cortical margin (freehand technique) or a Steinman pin or similar device can be firmly seated in the cortex first to act as an orthopedic guide wire for the trephine (guided technique). Once the trephine teeth are in contact with the cortex, it is lightly embedded with a mallet, and CT images obtained to confirm or adjust the line of approach. The trephine can then be more firmly embedded with the mallet (and the guide pin withdrawn), then it is turned in clockwise fashion with forward pressure until the target depth is reached. Serial imaging can be obtained along the way to verify correct alignment and check depth and progress. The target depth is at least half-again beyond the depth (diameter) of the lesion, up to the limit of the deep cortical margin beyond the lesion.

Once the target depth is reached, the trephine is worked loose by angling it in several directions, then withdrawn completely. Sample removal is assisted with a solid pin with a flat end driven through the sample channel, e.g., using the mallet. Postbiopsy imaging is obtained to confirm that the biopsy tract contained the target lesion, and that no remnants of the nidus remain. The bony tract may be "cleaned up" with angled curettes. Optionally, the final tract may be irrigated with dehydrated alcohol to denature any unrecovered nidus fragments. The skin wound is then closed with Steri-Strips® or interrupted suture as necessary, and a sterile dressing is applied.

Technical variations

Percutaneous resection of bone can be used in a variety of conditions, from lesion biopsy to decompression of avascular necrosis to resection of a physeal bar. In each case, the procedure provides an alternative to an open surgical procedure that preserves tissue, maintains structural integrity, and reduces recovery time. These procedures follow the general principles outlined for excision of osteoid osteoma, the prototypical

Chapter 7 MSK and soft tissue interventions

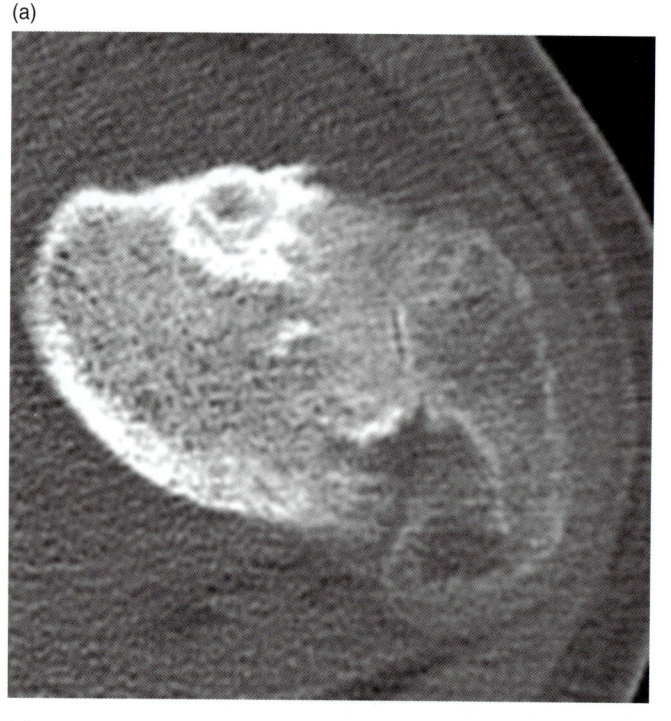

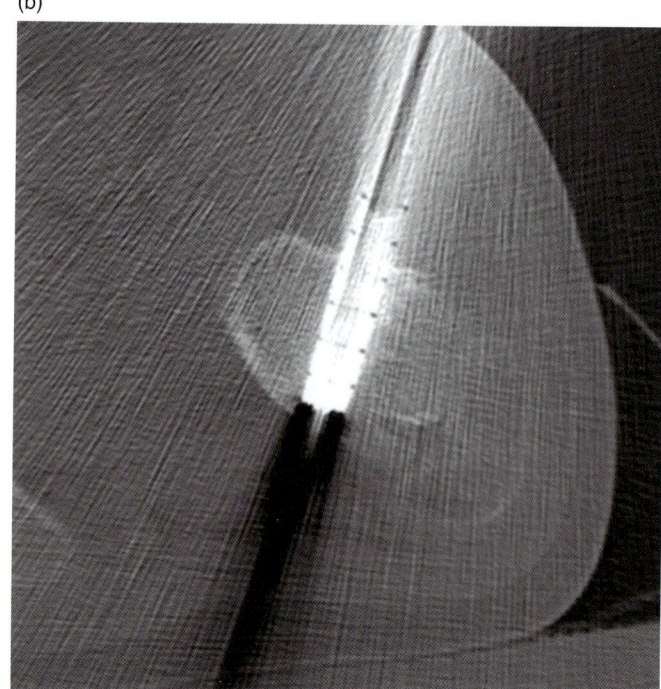

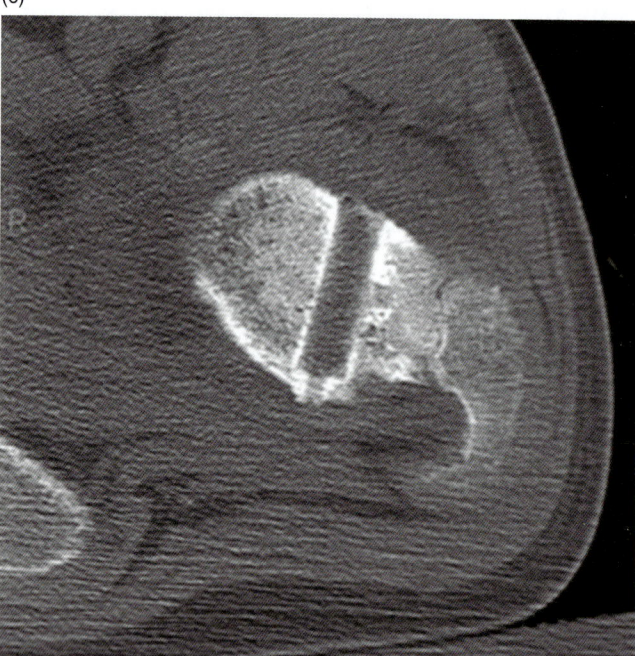

Figure 7.24 Power tool-assisted removal of femoral neck osteoid osteoma. (a) Preprocedural CT of cortical-based osteoid osteoma. Note intra-articular location of nidus, therefore no periosteal reaction. (b) Coaxial drill over K-wire. (c) Complete removal of osteoid osteoma.

benign tumor of bone in this regard. In some cases, ablation of a bone lesion can serve the same purpose even more efficiently and effectively. This option is discussed in greater detail in the following section.

Postprocedure and follow-up care

If general anesthesia or procedural sedation is used, the child will need to go to the recovery room until they awaken and vital signs are back to baseline. Minor analgesia with an NSAID is started and the family is given a prescription for a narcotic analgesic to be used if needed. Strenuous activity, physical education, and extracurricular athletics are prohibited for two to six weeks following excision of a lower extremity osteoid osteoma nidus. In addition, some children with lower extremity lesions are put on a non-weight-bearing regimen for two to six weeks. The patient is seen at two- to three-week intervals as needed in the interventional radiology clinic and a follow-up radiograph is obtained. When the tract is healed the child is able to resume normal activities.

Complications

Complications resulting from image-guided excision of an osteoid osteoma are rare, and when they occur, are generally minor. Potential complications include recurrence and pathologic fracture through the stress riser. Recurrence of symptoms may be seen in up to 10% of cases, and may either reflect incomplete excision or, less commonly, a second nidus. While fracture following percutaneous excision has been reported, it is rare. Minor complications such as cellulitis or hematoma have occurred in about 3% of cases.

Conclusions

The MSK system lends itself to percutaneous diagnostic and therapeutic procedures. We suspect that in the future a great majority of all procedures will be performed using minimally invasive techniques. If interventionalists become expert in the therapeutic options for pathology involving the bones, soft tissues, tendons, and ligaments, there is no limit to what can be accomplished. The modular approach to MSK intervention is an excellent platform to aid development of new and better solutions for soft tissue and skeletal problems.

Locoregional thermal ablation of bone lesions

Introduction

In cases of benign bone tumors, for which osteoid osteoma again serves as the prototypical lesion, it is satisfactory to devitalize the tumor in order to alleviate pain, inflammation, and associated dysfunction, since there is no known malignant potential. The characteristics of these lesions are discussed in detail in the preceding section. Thermal ablation offers the interventionalist an additional method by which to treat these benign lesions as an alternative to open or percutaneous procedures that involve removal of a larger volume of normal bone or greater potential for injury to surrounding structures. There are a variety of thermal-based therapeutic options, including laser photocoagulation, microwave ablation, and cryoablation, but radiofrequency ablation is currently the most commonly used method.

Indications

Indications for ablation of osteoid osteomas include children who have failed adequate pain management and those who do not wish to continue such therapy. Additionally, the lesion should be safely accessible by a percutaneous approach, and should be located anatomically to allow for percutaneous treatment without injuring adjacent vital structures. Radiofrequency ablation will be possible in locations adjacent to

Table 7.25 Equipment: radiofrequency ablation of bone lesions

- Computed tomography scanner
- Materials for sterile preparation and draping
- Bone biopsy needle
- Power drill, Craig needle, K-wire or Steinman pins, and drill bits
- Radiofrequency generator and related equipment
- Steri-Strips®, Dermabond®, dressings
- Crutch training, wheelchair as indicated

vulnerable structures where percutaneous excision is not advisable. Several techniques have been used to decrease this risk in vulnerable locations, such as in the spine near neural elements. Other than the usual considerations for avoiding passage through infected tissues and correction of bleeding abnormalities, there are no specific contraindications to ablation of benign bone tumors. When considering treatment of lesions that are in a vulnerable location, the experience of the operator should be weighed carefully (Figure 7.25). Adjunct neurophysiologic and temperature monitoring may be prudent when considering treatment of spinal lesions in proximity to (within 1 to 2 cm of) the spinal cord and spinal nerves. Thermal ablation may have applications in other bone-related lesions, such as in palliation of pain associated with bony metastases, that are beyond the scope of the current work.

Technique
Equipment

There are now several ablation techniques that use a variety of energies and chemicals. At this time, RF is the most commonly used device (Table 7.25). Among practitioners, there are different approaches, including freehand and coaxial techniques. Thus the equipment needed depends upon the approach selected.

Patient preparation

The planning and patient preparation for ablation of an osteoid osteoma nidus is the same as for percutaneous excision, discussed in the previous section.

Standard technique

The approach to treatment of an osteoid osteoma with radiofrequency ablation (RFA) is similar to other forms of therapy. The procedure is performed under general anesthesia. The skin entry site is selected using a preprocedural, limited CT. After sterile preparation and draping, a skin incision is made. With CT guidance, the osteoid osteoma nidus is traversed using a Steinman pin, trephine, bone biopsy needle, or drill bit, in order to create a pathway across the thickened cortex to the nidus through which the RF probe can be positioned (Table 7.26). This pathway must eventually be large enough to pass the probe; usually a 4 to 5 mm tract will suffice. The procedure may be performed manually or with power tools.

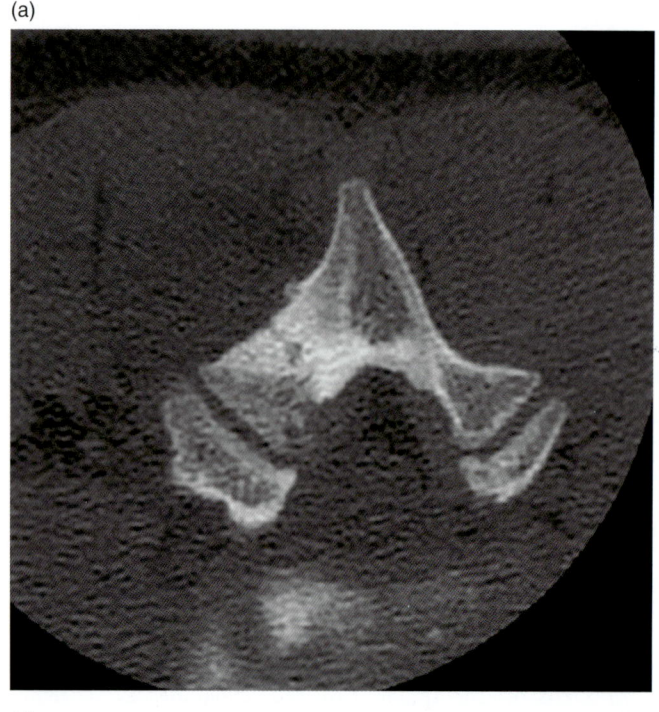
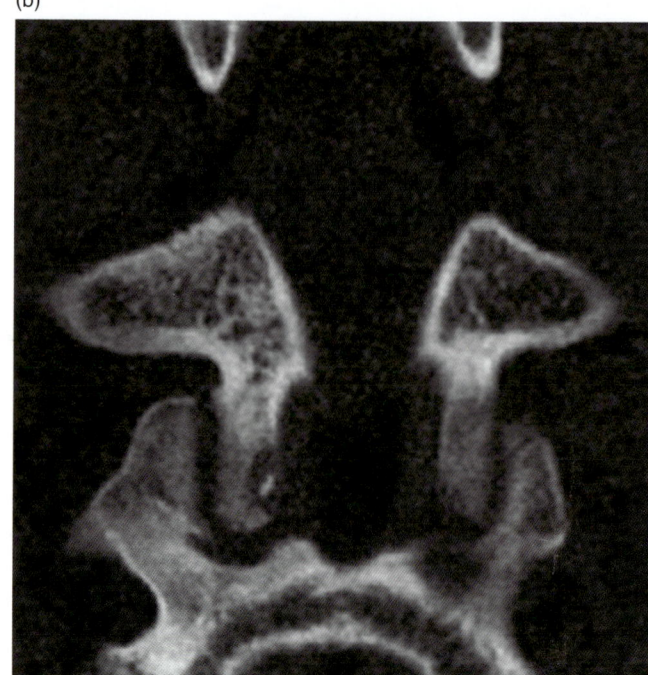
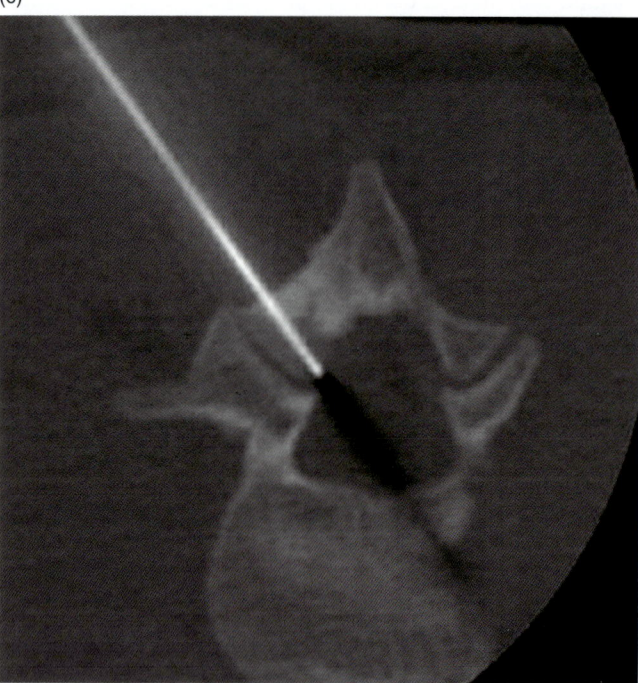

Figure 7.25 Fifteen-year-old male with low back pain, scoliosis, and intense paraspinal inflammatory changes on MRI referred for "biopsy". (a,b) Axial and coronal CT images reveal an osteoid osteoma involving a lumbar zygapophysis. (c) Radiofrequency probe traversing osteoid osteoma nidus.

A specimen may or may not be obtained, depending on the above tools used to traverse the nidus (Figure 7.26). Next, an RF probe is positioned in the defect traversing the osteoid osteoma nidus. It is preferable to position the active probe section as deep as possible to avoid skin, nerve, and adjacent tissue injury, yet still traversing the nidus. The probe is heated to approximately 90°C for five to six minutes, which allows for effective ablation of the nidus, and this may be repeated at the discretion of the interventionalist.

Postprocedure and follow-up care

The care given to these children is similar to that described for image-guided excision, above. However, because the bone defect may be smaller with percutaneous RFA of the nidus, partial or non-weight-bearing restrictions may not be necessary. The patient may therefore normally be discharged to normal activity upon recovery from the anesthesia, although participation in physical education and extracurricular sports may be limited by some practitioners until the bone defect heals. At a follow-up visit in the interventional radiology clinic, two to three weeks after the procedure, the clinical outcome can be evaluated.

Complications

The rate of symptom recurrence after RFA of osteoid osteoma is approximately the same as other percutaneous methods and is expected to be less than 10%. This includes treatment failures as well as secondary lesions. Complications have been reported in 0 to 10% in most series and include skin burns, nerve injuries, soft tissue burns, and late fractures. These untoward effects are most often the result of probe design and the length of the unshielded RF probe section that lies outside the cortex.

Conclusions

Radiofrequency ablation of osteoid osteoma is an effective treatment approach and is the most commonly used device to treat these tumors. In the future, it is likely that the use of RF and other energy sources will continue to advance minimally invasive techniques for the treatment of children with benign and malignant bone lesions.

Percutaneous reduction with internal fixation

Introduction

Severe fractures in children require reduction of the fracture fragments to a functional anatomic position, followed by fixation of the fragments to allow stable maintenance of the reduced position during healing. Fixation must be relevant to the plane or planes of instability. This is conventionally accomplished with internal or external fixators depending on the nature and location of the injury. Since the late 1950s, open reduction and internal fixation (ORIF) has been a staple for treatment of displaced and unstable fractures. Internal fixation,

Table 7.26 Procedure summary: radiofrequency ablation of bone lesions

- General anesthesia
- Route planning and skin entry site selection
- Skin preparation and draping
- Local anesthetic and skin incision
- Image-guided pin access into lesion or bone biopsy of lesion
- Radiofrequency probe placement into bone tract, confirm tip position with CT
- Heat to 90°C × six minutes per site
- Suture closure as needed
- Sterile dressing

(a)

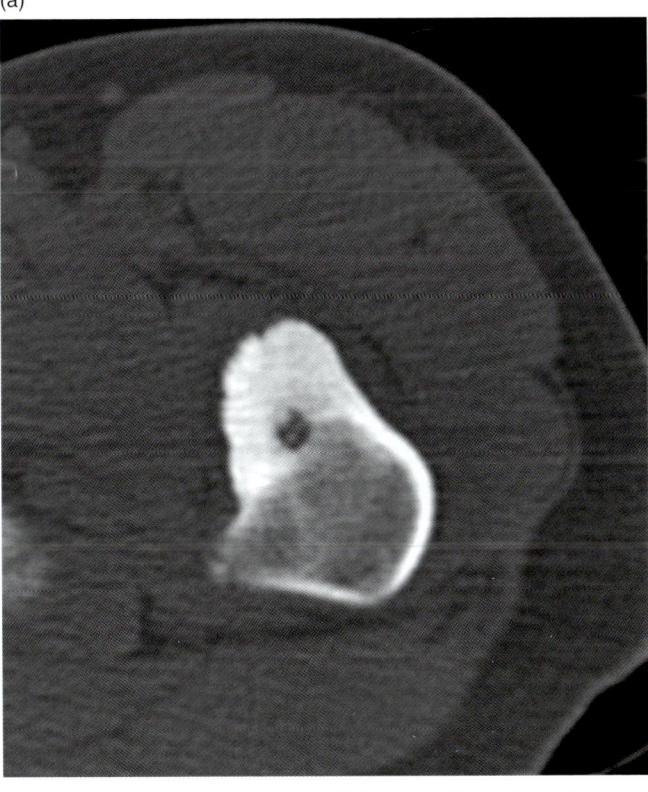

(b)

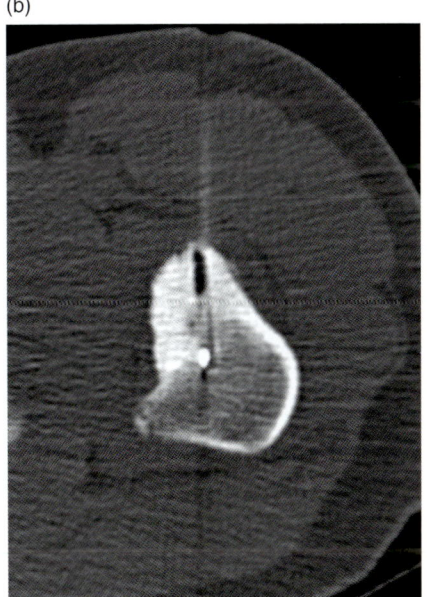

Figure 7.26 Radiofrequency ablation of left proximal femoral osteoid osteoma. (a) Preprocedural axial CT with exuberant periosteal reaction. (b) RFA probe within lesion.

with plating across the fracture plane, often requires extensive incision and exposure, which may increase risks related to accompanying tissue injury and hemorrhage. Pelvic ring fractures exemplify these risks, as they frequently involve both rotational (horizontal) and vertical instability, and may be accompanied by degloving injuries to the soft tissues as well as extensive internal hemorrhage contained by the deep pelvic fascia. Discussion of interventional approaches to these fractures highlights the opportunity for interventional radiologists to play a critical role in management of these patients, and can be extended to consideration of similar injuries elsewhere in the body.

The pelvic ring in children is more plastic than the adult pelvis, so traumatic injuries tend to include both deformation and outright fracture. Before the triradiate cartilage is closed, the pubic rami and iliac wings tend to fail before the elastic pelvic ligaments. About half of these rare fractures in children are unstable, and many are accompanied by potentially life-threatening hemorrhage. The sacroiliac (SI) joint is most commonly involved. Incomplete treatment may result in chronic debilitating pain, non-union, limb shortening, scoliosis, pelvic deformity, femoral necrosis, and degenerative disease of the hip joint. Complete treatment requires immobilization of the SI joint in a near-anatomic position.

Conventional treatment includes anterior external fixation after reduction of deformity and dislocation in the horizontal plane, for example the so-called "open book" fracture. However, anterior fixation alone cannot stabilize an unstable or displaced posterior ring injury. Placement of a plate or threaded bar across the SI joint under surgical visualization after open reduction can stabilize the vertically unstable posterior ring injury, but carries elevated risk of infection and substantial blood loss. Additionally, the highly variable and irregular morphology of the pediatric pelvis makes safe placement of iliosacral screws or pins a problematic proposition, with significant risk of neurovascular injury as well as long-term impairment of gait and function.

An image-guided percutaneous approach to closed reduction and internal fixation (CRIF), including both multiplanar imaging and volumetric reconstruction, offers substantial potential advantages over the conventional approach for treatment of this type of injury. Treating these complex problems is often best accomplished with a team of interventional radiologists and orthopedic surgeons.

Indications

Image-guided CRIF may be useful in patients subject to high-energy trauma with Tile type C (or Young–Burgess lateral compression III or vertical shear type injuries) unstable posterior pelvic fracture when external fixation alone is unlikely to adequately stabilize the posterior elements. It would not be indicated for repair of a compaction injury with significant fragmentation of the sacrum, or where there is significant soft tissue injury to the skin overlying the planned route of access, or where there is massive displacement of the fracture fragments, especially with an open fracture, after failure of closed reduction, or when the fracture is more than five days old. In these latter situations, only open reduction is likely to achieve satisfactory restoration of pelvic alignment. Inability to identify adequate bony mass for safe and effective screw placement, e.g., due to upper sacral segment dysmorphism, is also a relative contraindication to CRIF. Morbid obesity may preclude obtaining adequately penetrated images for operative planning and guidance.

Technique

Equipment

Orthopedic surgical equipment sets appropriate for this procedure, including drill motors, drill bits and taps, guides, wires, and pins can usually be ordered from the hospital's central sterile supply with the assistance of operating room personnel (Table 7.27). It is beneficial for interventional radiology personnel to have in-service training with the specialized surgical equipment and supplies related to this and other MSK, orthopedic, and trauma interventions.

Patient preparation

Due to the high-energy trauma usually required to give rise to unstable pelvic injury, the patient is at risk for hemodynamic instability either related to accompanying trauma sustained in the same event or to hemorrhage from disruption of deep pelvic tissues. Stabilization of the patient using the principles of advanced trauma life support is the first priority. Associated injuries that might threaten cardiopulmonary stability and function, neurologic function, and integrity of the urinary tract should be assessed and managed prior to interventions directed at pelvic ring injuries, although emergent compression of pelvic bony injuries may be a necessary component of the resuscitation maneuvers. Soft tissue injuries, including degloving injuries and open wounds should be documented and considered as part of preoperative planning. The preliminary evaluation, resuscitation, and management described above, as well as mechanical and imaging assessment of pelvic

Table 7.27 Equipment: closed reduction and internal fixation

- Radio-opaque marker
- 1% lidocaine
- Operative drill motor with appropriate selection of cannulated drill bits
- Kirschner smooth wire (0.62 mm)
- Narrow periosteal elevator
- Long drill guide
- 2 mm terminally threaded guide pin
- 7.3 mm cannulated partially threaded cancellous screw
- Cannulated taps
- Cannulated fully threaded cancellous screws
- Reverse ruler

injuries, and perhaps anterior external fixation of any rotational instability, will normally be accomplished by the trauma surgery team prior to referral for reduction and fixation of the posterior pelvic elements.

Standard preoperative imaging should include AP, caudal (inlet), cranial (outlet), and lateral sacral plain radiographs of the pelvis. Pelvic CT with bone windows is essential for proper assessment and planning, including localization of lumbosacral nerve roots and identification of otherwise occult fractures, such as those involving the sacral ala.

Neurodiagnostic monitoring may be useful in this and other procedures that potentially impinge upon vital neural structures in the neural foramina and spinal canal. While no substitute for informed interventional judgment, it may be helpful in this procedure during manipulation of the sacrum when foriminal structures are potentially threatened.

Standard technique

As with any similar procedure, the CT suite (or the angiographic suite when rotational angiography is substituted for CT) must be maintained to the same standard as any orthopedic surgical suite in terms of restricted access, cleanliness, air filtration, and strict adherence to sterile technique throughout the patient's exposure. Once the child has been anesthetized, (s)he can be moved to the CT gantry table and positioned to facilitate the treatment and planned imaging approach. The patient is usually placed with the injured side bolstered up approximately 20 to 30 degrees. Care must be taken to assure that the imaging equipment will not impinge on the patient and any external hardware, and that there will be sufficient space to freely maneuver drills, pins, etc., during the course of the procedure.

Once the patient is safely positioned, volumetric images are obtained through the pelvis, and the bony structures are reconstructed to assess alignment. If necessary, a closed reduction is performed, and the imaging repeated. A route is selected for placement of a compression screw perpendicular to the fracture plane that will complete anatomic reduction of the dislocation and fracture, spare neurovascular structures, and find sufficient bony purchase in the sacrum to stabilize the fracture with as few screws as possible.

The skin is prepared and draped in sterile fashion. Local anesthetic (1% lidocaine or 0.25% bupivacaine) is infiltrated from the skin to the periosteum along the defined access route. A skin incision is made, measuring approximately 1 cm in length. A smooth Kirschner (K) wire is inserted through the incision to the cortical margin of the iliac bone along the predetermined route (Table 7.28). If the trajectory is aligned with the desired route, then a sterile mallet is used to firmly set the pin in the cortex. A combination of blunt and sharp dissection is used to carry the skin incision around the wire to the iliac bone. The guide pin is inserted with a drill into the lateral iliac cortex, controlling pin direction with the drill guide. Trajectory is again confirmed with imaging as described above.

Table 7.28 Procedure summary: closed reduction and internal fixation

- General anesthesia
- Route planning and access site selection
- Skin preparation and draping
- Local anesthetic and skin incision
- Image-guided pin access across lever arm of fracture into SI joint with tip near sacrum
- Long drill guide over K-wire if exchange for a threaded pin is needed. Often using CT guidance one can directly insert a threaded pin
- Insert a cannulated screw
- Postprocedural CT scan to confirm alignment. If satisfactory, procedure finished, if not an additional screw is needed and the above steps are repeated
- Intermittant follow-up radiographs to assess healing over the next weeks to months

A long drill guide is advanced over the K-wire and the K-wire is exchanged for a 2.3 mm terminally threaded guide pin. The guide pin is advanced into the upper sacral vertebral body, caudal to the iliac cortical density and sacral alar slope, and cranial to the first sacral neural foramen. When appropriate trajectory of the guide pin has been confirmed, it is advanced as far as the midline, but not beyond, taking care not to violate the anterior cortical margin. If necessary, the prospective screw path can be prepared with a tap. A 7.3 mm partially threaded cannulated screw is then inserted coaxially after determining length with a reverse ruler, taking the thickness of the screw head and washer into account. The measurement can be confirmed with measurement software on the imaging platform. The compression screw can be tightened by hand until a perfect anatomic reduction of the SI dislocation is achieved, without overtightening. If the screw is tightened too aggressively it may compress a transforaminal fracture against the nerve root or vessels, or violate the lateral iliac cortex with the washer or screw head. The guide pin is removed by hand and the wound closed in the usual fashion (Figure 7.27).

A completely threaded cannulated screw can be used instead if a transforaminal fracture threatens the nerve root or if the SI reduction is already anatomic. If the posterior pelvic fracture is insufficiently stabilized with the first screw, additional completely threaded cannulated screws may be placed. A postprocedure pelvic CT with multiplanar reconstructions is obtained to assess position of the screw tip(s) and adequacy of the SI joint reduction.

Technical variations

The methods described can be applied to unstable fractures at other locations where the risks related to extensive dissection and tissue devitalization outweigh the benefits of an open approach. Similarly, there is a potential role for collaboration between interventional radiologists and orthopedic surgeons or neurosurgeons in percutaneous placement of

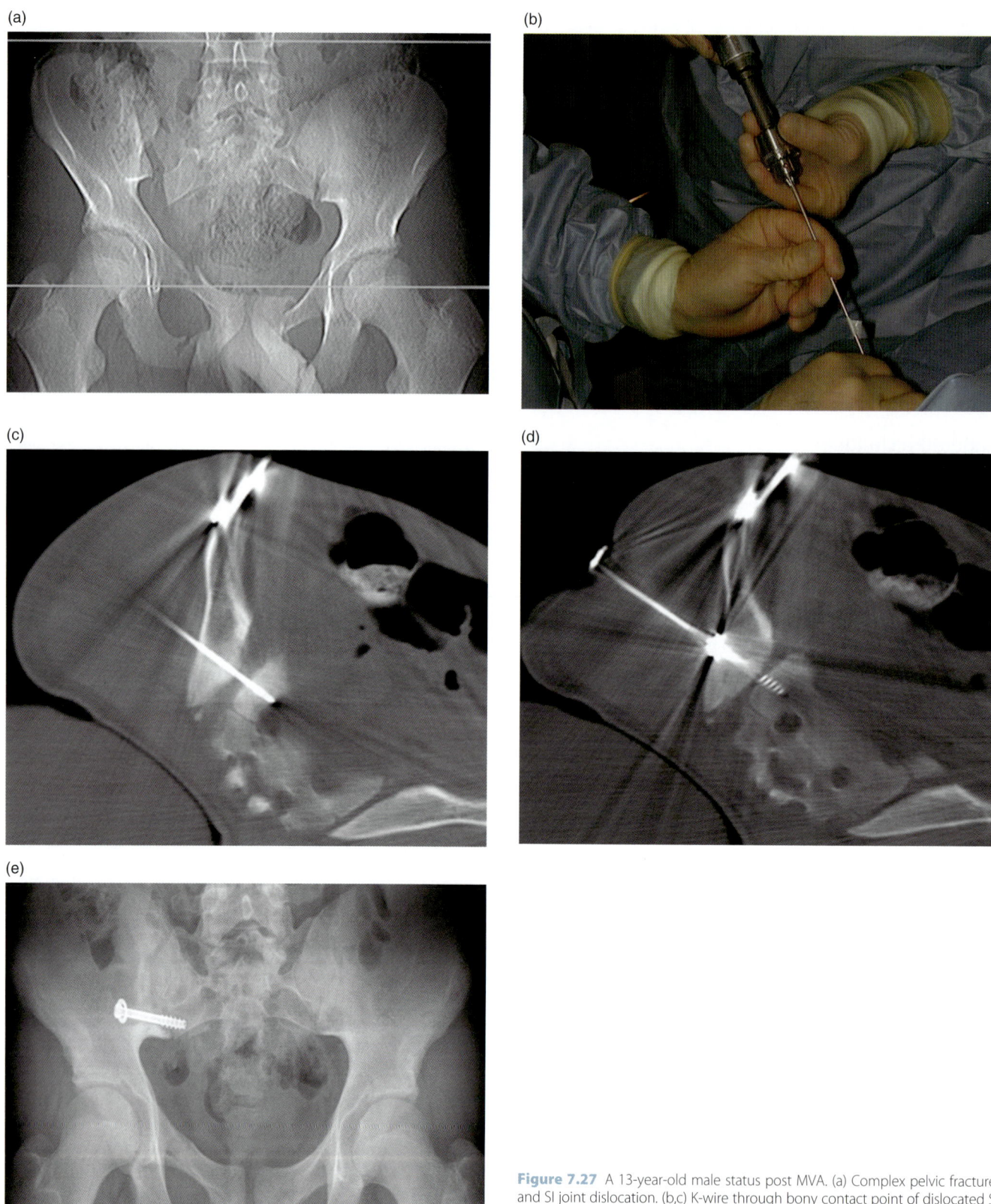

Figure 7.27 A 13-year-old male status post MVA. (a) Complex pelvic fracture and SI joint dislocation. (b,c) K-wire through bony contact point of dislocated SI joint. (d) Compression screw placed over K-wire shows repositioning and narrowing of SI joint. (e) Follow-up radiograph showing reduction with excellent result.

fixation devices where slight inaccuracies can have significant impact. For example, transpedicular screws in children may be almost as large as the pedicle diameter. Fluoroscopic guidance alone results in inaccurate placement in a large minority of cases, and such cases can occupy many hours of OR time. Preoperative CT-guided insertion of transpedicular guide pins with the use of multiplanar reconstruction for accurate route planning and trajectory confirmation can significantly improve outcomes, reduce OR time, and reduce cost.

Postprocedure and follow-up care

Intravenous antibiotics are administered for 24 hours after CRIF. Early rehabilitation with a pediatric physical therapist should be directed first to non-weight-bearing mobility as soon as is practicable, usually within one to three days after reduction and stabilization, progressing quickly to partial weight bearing with crutches for six weeks after surgery, with the goal of achieving free ambulation within three months. A return to unrestricted activity can be considered once the patient has achieved adequate strength and conditioning. Patients are usually seen at two, six, and twelve weeks following the procedure and then annually or as needed thereafter. It is important for the interventional radiologist to attend either the surgical clinic or a multidisciplinary clinic to personally follow these patients and assess their outcomes.

Complications

The use of CT guidance with accurate positioning of the screws can reduce complications and improve the outcome of these severe pelvic injuries. Complications reflected in the literature include iatrogenic neurovascular injury, especially with either concomitant transforaminal sacral fracture or violation of the neural foramen during screw insertion; malposition of the screw including violation of the lateral or anterior cortical margins; malreduction especially due to incomplete closed reduction prior to screw placement or to improper angulation of the screw relative to the fracture plane; failure of fixation especially due to inadequate stabilization or malreduction; and infection.

Conclusions

Closed reduction and internal fixation is an alternative to ORIF that may reduce procedure time, allow earlier stabilization and return to mobility, decrease tissue devitalization and neurovascular disruption, decrease intraoperative blood loss, improve bony union and soft tissue healing, and decrease risk of long-term pain and gait disturbance. Such procedures require high-quality imaging and procedural guidance, an understanding of the normal and pathologic anatomy, technical expertise related to percutaneous screw fixation and associated techniques, and close coordination and collaboration between the interventional radiologist and orthopedic surgeon.

Chapter 8
Vascular interventions

Richard Towbin, Kevin M. Baskin, David Aria and Carrie Schaefer

General angiographic considerations 405
Introduction 405
Indications 405
Technique 406
Equipment 406
Patient preparation 406
Standard technique 407
Arterial access 407
Technical variations 409
Alternative access 409
Postprocedure and follow-up care 411
Technical problems and pitfalls 411
Complications 411

Hepatic arteriography 413
Introduction 413
Indications 413
Technique 414
Standard technique 414
Technical problems and pitfalls 414
Postprocedure and follow-up care 415

Arterial embolization 415
Introduction 415
Indications 415
Technique 417
Equipment 417
Patient preparation 418
Standard technique 418
Preoperative embolization of tumors 419
Embolization of hemangiomas and high-flow vascular malformations 419
Hemangioma 423
Hepatic hemangioma (hemangioendothelioma) 423
Arteriovenous malformations 423
Arteriovenous fistulae 427

Systemic pulmonary arterial supply 429
Pulmonary arteriovenous malformations 429
Chemoembolization of hepatic tumors 429
Bronchial artery embolization 432
Arterial trauma 433
Partial splenic embolization 433
Renal ablation 433
Technical variations 435
Neonatal embolization 435
Postprocedure and follow-up care 437
Technical problems and pitfalls 437
Complications 438

Sclerotherapy 438
Introduction 438
Indications 438
Technique 442
Equipment 442
Patient preparation 442
Standard technique 442
Technical variations 444
Sodium tetradecyl sulfate 444
Bleomycin 445
Varicocele sclerotherapy 447
Postprocedure and follow-up care 448
Technical problems and pitfalls 449
Future advances 449
Complications 449

Pseudoaneurysm ablation 449
Introduction 449
Indications 451
Technique 451
Standard technique 451
Percutaneous thrombin embolization 451
Technical variations 451
Protection of the parent artery 451

Pediatric Interventional Radiology, ed. Richard Towbin and Kevin M. Baskin. Published by Cambridge University Press. © Cambridge University Press 2015.

Endovascular embolization 453
Postprocedure and follow-up care 454
Complications 454
Angioplasty and stenting 456
Introduction 456
Indications 456
Transplant vascular stenosis 456
Renal artery stenosis 458
Aortorenal syndromes 458
Venous compression syndromes 460
Technique 464
Equipment 464
Patient preparation 464
Standard technique 464
Technical variations 465
Technical problems and pitfalls 465
Complications 465
Thrombolysis 465
Introduction 465
Indications 466

Technique 466
Equipment 466
Patient preparation 469
Standard technique 470
Postprocedure and follow-up care 471
Technical problems and pitfalls 471
Complications 471
Transjugular liver biopsy 472
Transjugular intrahepatic portosystemic shunt (TIPS) 472
Vena caval filters 472
Introduction 472
Indications 472
Technique 472
Equipment 472
Patient preparation 474
Standard technique 474
Postprocedure and follow-up care 475
Complications 476

General angiographic considerations

Introduction

Most vascular interventional techniques that were initially developed for the treatment of adult vascular disease can be applied to the pediatric patient, providing appropriate technical modifications are made. There are issues specific to pediatric patients that require consideration in order to safely and successfully use vascular interventional techniques in this population. The problems that need to be overcome include the small patient size, the child's inability to cooperate, vulnerability to hypothermia and blood loss, volume limits for fluids and contrast media, the small size and fragility of access vessels, and, in the neonate, physiological differences related to fetal circulation. The wide range of patient sizes and clinical indications require that the operator be familiar with the vascular problems affecting children and techniques required to treat them. In addition, the interventionalist should be experienced with pediatric sedation and resuscitation, fluid administration, drug dosages, and contrast injection volumes for children of all ages and sizes. Catheterization supplies including needles, guide wires, sheaths, and other materials must be available in a range of sizes appropriate to the child being treated, and the operator should be familiar with the technique of custom shaping of catheters.

Indications

A large proportion of angiographic studies in the pediatric population are performed in conjunction with endovascular therapies (Table 8.1).

Current indications for diagnostic cerebral angiography include central nervous system (CNS) vasculitis, hemorrhage, cerebral ischemia, trauma, and investigation of vascular malformations, strokes, and vasospasm prior to endovascular therapy. Visceral angiography is most commonly indicated to investigate and treat hypertension, ischemia or occlusion related to organ transplantation, gastrointestinal bleeding, hemorrhage after penetrating or blunt trauma, varicoceles, and vascular malformations. Indications for extremity angiography include vascular mapping prior to surgical reconstruction of complex hand and foot anomalies, following penetrating injury and to investigate ischemic vasculopathy. In addition to the investigation of congenital heart disease, thoracic angiography is needed to study and treat hemoptysis, cyanosis (e.g., pulmonary AV malformations), and pulmonary embolism. Venography is rarely needed to investigate lower extremity venous thrombosis, but is frequently utilized to evaluate central venous catheter malfunctions, vascular malformations, and catheter-related upper extremity and central thrombosis.

Whenever possible, diagnostic catheter angiography should be avoided unless endovascular therapy is indicated, especially

Table 8.1 Indications for pediatric angiography

- Trauma
- Active bleeding (e.g., GI bleed)
- Renovascular hypertension
- Iatrogenic vascular injuries
- Vasculitides
- Collagen vascular diseases
- Prior to vascular intervention
- Surgical planning

Table 8.2 Equipment: angiography

- C-arm digital angiography unit
- Ultrasound with high-quality near-field imaging and appropriate linear transducers
- Warming device (e.g., Bair Hugger™)
- Appropriate sized puncture needles, introducer sheaths, catheters, guide wires, etc.
- Vascular sheath with side arm, as needed
- Vascular contrast (non-ionic iodinated contrast, CO_2, gadolinium, as applicable)
- Infusion pump and pressure bags
- Monitors: pulse oximeter, EKG, blood pressure
- Capnography as indicated
- Pressure transduction equipment and high-pressure tubing, as indicated
- Radiation shields
- Drugs for sedation, resuscitation, selected situations (papavarine, heparin, tPA, etc.)
- Pulse Doppler machine as indicated
- Bolsters

if less invasive imaging techniques can provide the same information. For example, ultrasound (US) may be used for the diagnosis of neonatal aortic or renal vein thrombosis. Similarly, magnetic resonance imaging (MRI) can be used to diagnose the nature of vascular masses (e.g., hemangiomas and vascular malformations), tumors, and pulmonary sequestration while magnetic resonance angiography (MRA), computed tomographic angiography (CTA), or computed tomographic venography (CTV) can be helpful to confirm the presence of central vascular occlusions such as dural sinus or inferior vena cava (IVC) thrombosis.

Technique

Equipment

Basic requirements for diagnostic angiography and vascular intervention include a modern angiography suite with a single- or biplane C-arm, high-resolution (1024 matrix) digital subtraction angiography unit with road mapping capability, variable dose acquisition and fluoroscopy, and multifield image intensifiers (e.g., 14 to 40 cm) or flat panel digital detectors (e.g., 22 to 48 cm). Rotational angiography and cone-beam CT capabilities are becoming more common with the newest generation equipment. Warming devices are necessary for infants and include warm air infusers (Bair Hugger™, Augustine Medical Inc., Eden Prairie, MN), water circulating blankets, or other methods to keep a small child normothermic. Ultrasound with Doppler capability is now standard for planning or guiding vascular access. Puncture needles, guide wires, catheters, and sheaths for children of all sizes are listed in Table 8.2. Today, the most commonly used access needle is a micropuncture needle (see Figures 2.18 and 8.1a) although we often use 22-gauge angiocatheters for access in small infants and children (Figure 8.1b). If an angiocatheter is used, the non-"safety" type (i.e., without the automated sharps retraction feature) is more suitable to this purpose. In older children, 19-gauge thin wall or 18-gauge Potts–Cournand type needles with stylets are used (Figure 8.1c,d).

Angiographic catheters should be available in sizes ranging from 3 French (usually 40 to 65 cm), to 5 or 6 French (usually 90 cm or longer). It is our preference to use 3 French catheters for children less than 10 kg, 4 French catheters for children between 10 and 30 kg, and 5 French catheters for larger children. The length and diameter of the primary and secondary curves must be proportional to the child's aorta. Therefore, a standard 4 French pre-shaped catheter may not be well suited for infants and young children in some instances. Dilute (140 to 240 mg iodine/ml) non-ionic low osmolarity contrast medium may be used with digital subtraction angiography and provides diagnostic quality images and conserves contrast, although higher concentrations may be necessary in infants and small children to compensate for the small volume of their vessels. Commonly used drugs include heparin, glucagon, dexamethasone, nitroglycerine, and papaverine (see Chapter 1). The equipment utilized to monitor children varies somewhat between interventional laboratories but should include at minimum continuous pulse oximetry and electrocardiography (EKG) and automated blood pressure cuff recorders, and preferably also intravascular pressure recording equipment and a sidestream (capnography) CO_2 monitor. Standard wall suction and medical gas outlets or appropriate substitutes are mandatory.

Patient preparation

Each child must be prepared for either deep sedation or general anesthesia. The patient is kept NPO according to relevant institutional policies regarding sedation and anesthesia. Appropriate IV fluids may be given to maintain hydration, especially in small infants. Routine blood work is usually not necessary. However, preprocedural testing is tailored to the individual patient and situation. For example, if prolonged thrombolysis is planned, baseline studies including a coagulation profile and fibrin split products are obtained. Measurements of renal and hepatic function should be obtained where appropriate. Relevant diagnostic studies should be available for guidance in tailoring the diagnostic angiogram.

For patients less than 10 kg, appropriate warming devices should be prepared before the patient is placed on the angiographic table. Physiological monitoring (pulse oximetry, blood pressure, EKG) is instituted in all cases. Side-arm (for sedation) or in-line (for general anesthesia) capnography is recommended. Intravenous access is obtained in all children prior to beginning the procedure. Restraints are applied to patients not undergoing general anesthesia. Light restraints are generally used even in children having general anesthesia. Depending on the case, other preparation may include a Foley or small rubber urinary catheter for vascular interventions and other long procedures, and placement of lead shields over the gonads and other radiation sensitive areas

Chapter 8 Vascular interventions

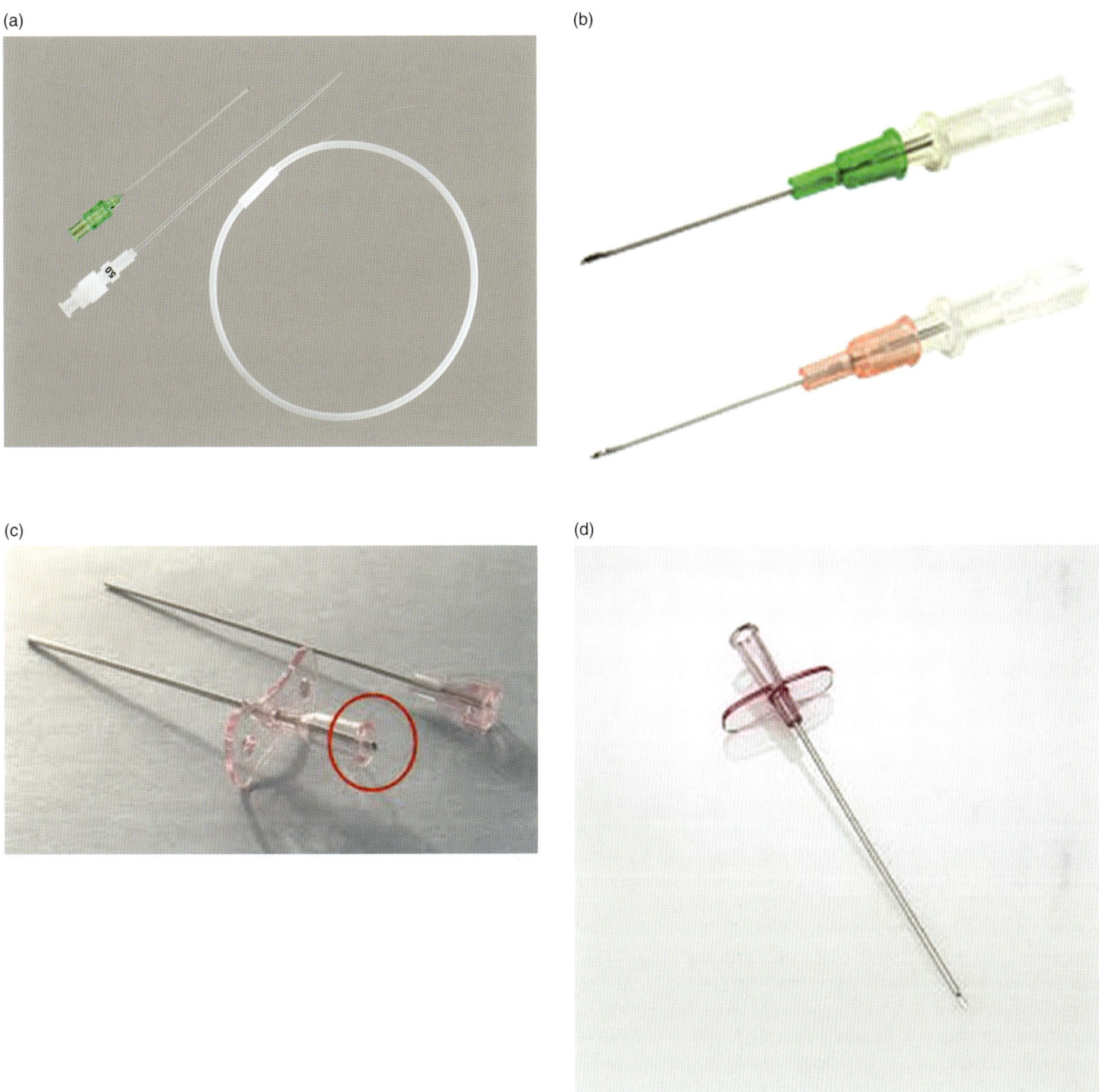

Figure 8.1 Arterial access needles. (a) Micropuncture introducer. (b) Angiocatheter. (c) Potts–Cournand needle. (d) Single-wall access needle.

whenever possible. For long cases, and for any case performed under deep sedation or anesthesia, padding of pressure points (e.g., egg crate foam, gel pads, diapers, or other cloth) to avoid neuropathy or other injury is essential, as described in Chapter 1.

Peripheral pulses (e.g., dorsalis pedis and posterior tibial) are marked on the skin so that they can be easily evaluated during or after completion of the procedure. We use a pulse Doppler or pulse oximeter to monitor lower extremity pulses during the procedure and while hemostasis is achieved after catheter and sheath removal (Figure 8.2). Standard groin preparation including shaving of pubic hair in teenagers is appropriate. In the case of femoral access both groins should be sterilely prepared and draped.

Standard technique
Arterial access

We find it helpful to place a small bolster (rolled-up towel or equivalent) under the hips to straighten the pelvic vessels somewhat by extending the pelvis, and to prevent the pelvis from moving posteriorly when the needle is advanced. In the past, initial arterial access was accomplished with a modified Seldinger technique using visible landmarks and palpation of

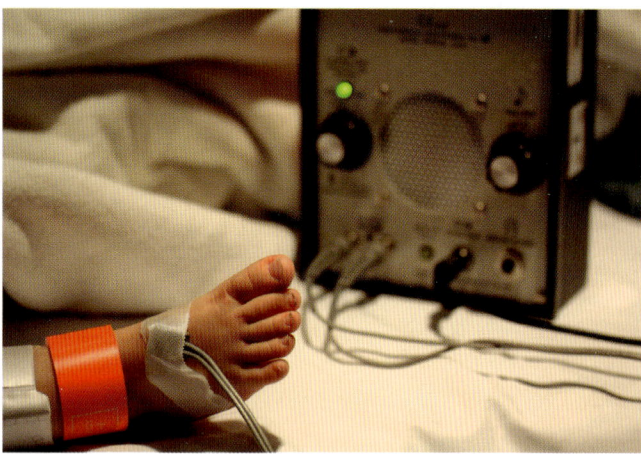

Figure 8.2 Ultrasonic Doppler flow detector. The probe is applied over the dorsalis pedis artery prior to puncture of the right common femoral artery for angiography (Parks Medical Electronics, Inc., Aloha, OR).

Table 8.3 Procedure summary: angiography

- Sedation or general anesthesia
- Puncture artery and insert a sheath (infused at 3 ml/h or greater rate, adjusted to patient size)
- Heparinize PRN (50 to 100 U/kg), may repeat every two hours during the procedure
- Selective/superselective catheterization of target vessel(s)
- Perform vascular intervention
- Remove catheter and achieve hemostasis
- Treat vasospasm or occlusion PRN
- Follow-up vascular complications with US

arterial pulses. Although this technique is still widely practiced by interventional cardiologists, it is no longer recommended for routine access, especially in infants and small children, due to the added procedure time and the relatively high prevalence of arterial injuries such as intimal dissection, pseudoaneurysm, and arteriovenous fistula associated with this technique. Real-time access guidance with US is now the preferred standard of care. The general principles of angiography in children are summarized in Table 8.3.

The *double-wall* puncture technique can be safely performed, advancing the needle tip through both walls, withdrawing the sharp stylet, and pulling back the blunt cannula until pulsatile flow is obtained, then inserting a soft-tipped guide wire into the artery. However, real-time guidance with US permits a *single-wall* technique to be performed with great accuracy and a high rate of success, advancing a single-wall needle through the superficial wall of the artery until the bevel and needle tip are securely within the arterial lumen and pulsatile flow is obtained, then advancing a soft-tipped guide wire into the artery. This may be preferable especially when lytic therapy is planned to decrease the risk of bleeding or other arterial complication. Ultrasound guidance is usually performed with a transverse view of the artery, although a long view can sometimes be useful. The ability to visualize the entire length of the needle as well as the target vessel in the long view is balanced by the difficulty overcoming partial volume artifact to keep the needle centered on the vessel in real space, not just seeing both needle and vessel in the same image plane.

If access is gained by palpation, it may be difficult to use the standard Seldinger technique for arterial puncture, especially in small infants. Instead of palpating the pulse with two fingers so that dampening can be appreciated with the distal finger, the interventionalist may use a one-finger technique. The pulse Doppler (or oximeter) is substituted for the distal finger. Using downward pressure with the needle, the artery is compressed until the pulse is no longer audible. While maintaining this downward pressure and arterial compression, the needle is thrust forward into the arterial lumen.

For patients having procedures performed under sedation, the intended puncture site is slowly and carefully injected with local anesthetic (1% buffered lidocaine), with attention to avoiding the femoral artery or vein with the infiltrating needle. It is helpful to use the smallest needle available (27- or 30-gauge) since this will minimize discomfort. A small skin incision is made approximately 1 to 1.5 cm below the site where the common femoral artery crosses anterior to the femoral head, located either by US or fluoroscopy. This assures a stable platform beneath the puncture site at the time of hemostasis at the conclusion of the procedure.

In general, it is best to puncture at or below the inguinal ligament and above the origin of the profunda femoris artery. Puncture above this level risks retroperitoneal hemorrhage as well as penetration of the hip joint and may make hemostasis more difficult. Puncture below this level may risk end-arterial injury, necrosis, and compartment syndrome. When blood return is obtained and provided no resistance is encountered the guide wire is advanced into the abdominal aorta. The operator must be careful not to "crush" the femoral artery against the guide wire or catheter while performing exchanges. Catheters or sheaths should be advanced gently over the guide wire, with as little manipulation at the groin as possible. Any vascular procedures requiring more than one catheter exchange or associated with an interventional procedure should be performed through an arterial sheath to minimize vascular trauma and to ensure vascular access in the event that a catheter becomes occluded. Some operators prefer to use a sheath in all cases. These precautions will reduce the possibility of arterial injury, arterial spasm, or occlusion.

Once the sheath is in place, Steri-Strips® or Tegaderm® are applied to secure the sheath to the drape to prevent excessive movement or inadvertent removal. The sheath may be infused with a heparinized flush solution by a pump or pressure bag. The infusion rate and volume should be limited by the use of a check flow valve (3 ml per hour for small infants) or an infusion pump, in order to avoid fluid overload. In small children, flush aortograms can be performed through a straight or pigtail catheter with multiple side holes. Pigtail catheters may cause problems as the loop may be too wide to reform in the narrow aorta. Standard injection volumes and rates for different vessels are listed for children of various ages in Table 8.4. In general, the smallest catheter that will provide

Table 8.4 Standard angiographic injection rates and volumes

Vessel	Rate, per second (total volume ml)		
	<10 kg	10 to 30 kg	>30 kg
CCA	4–5 (6–7)	6–7 (8–9)	8–9 (10–11)
ICA	2–3 (4–5)	4–5 (6–7)	6–7 (8–9)
ECA	2–3 (3–5)	3–5 (5–7)	5–7 (7–9)
vertebral	1–2 (2–3)	3–4 (4–5)	5–6 (6–7)
aortic arch	5–10 (10–20)	10–15 (20–30)	15–20 (30–40)
descending aorta	5–10 (10–20)	10–15 (20–30)	15–20 (30–40)
visceral	2–3 (4–6)	3–4 (6–8)	5–6 (10–12)
splenoportography	2–3 (10–15)	3–4 (15–20)	5–6 (25–30)
renals	2–3 (4–6)	3–4 (6–8)	5–6 (10–12)
prox extrem	2–3 (4–6)	4–5 (8–10)	6–7 (12–14)
distal extrem	1–2 (2–4)	2–3 (4–6)	4–5 (8–10)

the necessary contrast injection rate is selected. Shorter catheters are used when possible since they are able to accept higher flow rates.

The routine use of heparin for diagnostic and interventional vascular procedures is controversial. In some laboratories, children less than 10 to 15 kg are routinely heparinized immediately after insertion of a catheter or arterial sheath (50 to 100 units/kg). Heparin boluses are repeated every two hours if the procedure is still under way.

In general, contrast volume is limited to 5 ml per kg (300 mg iodine per ml) for diagnostic angiography. Complex vascular interventions may require larger volumes. In our experience, larger volumes of non-ionic contrast (10 ml or occasionally greater) are well tolerated over long procedures, if the patient is kept well hydrated and urine output remains normal. However, fluid input and output need to be carefully monitored. At the end of the procedure, pedal pulses are checked manually or with a pulse Doppler or oximeter. Hemostasis is achieved with ten minutes of manual compression. If a pulse cannot be palpated, contrast injection is made through the catheter or sheath into the access artery. If the artery is completely occluded, 2 to 3 µg/kg of nitroglycerine, diluted in 3 to 5 ml of saline, can be injected through the catheter while it is being withdrawn. Alternatively, injection of a local anesthetic around the artery may help relieve vasospasm. On occasion the response is dramatic.

At the completion of the procedure, the pulse Doppler or oximeter may again be used to monitor hemostasis at the time arterial access is withdrawn. Our approach to hemostasis is to always use manual compression, and we do not use or recommend the use of arterial occlusion devices or of sandbags or other pressure devices in the pediatric population. Initially the vessel is compressed so that there is no antegrade blood flow (no audible pulse with Doppler over the dorsalis pedis or posterior tibial artery) for one minute. Then the compressive force is reduced so that blood flow is audible but there is no bleeding from the puncture site. This lighter compression is maintained for nine minutes. After ten minutes, manual arterial compression is discontinued unless there is bleeding. This approach is intended to minimize the chance for formation of an occlusive thrombus. If rebleeding or persistent bleeding occurs, arterial compression is re-established and progress checked at five-minute intervals. In children in whom hemostasis is difficult to achieve, a hemostatic agent (such as a Surgicel® pad or StatSeal® powder) is placed over the puncture site while the vessel is compressed. The hemostatic agent is then left in place and covered by a sterile 2 × 2 gauze and a transparent dressing.

During the recovery period, the lower extremities must be kept warm. Pedal color, temperature, and pulses should be monitored frequently. If the ipsilateral foot is cool to touch and if the pedal pulses cannot be *manually* palpated, then we recommend that the patient receive another bolus of heparin intravenously. If pulses do not return within three to four hours, a heparin infusion should be started and the patient kept in the hospital for treatment and observation. Color Doppler US is useful to document the status of the femoral artery. If the femoral artery remains occluded 24 hours after the procedure, systemic thrombolysis with an intravenous infusion of tPA should be considered.

Technical variations
Alternative access
Although most transarterial procedures are performed via the femoral artery, alternate vascular access should be considered in specific situations. Since the risk of femoral artery

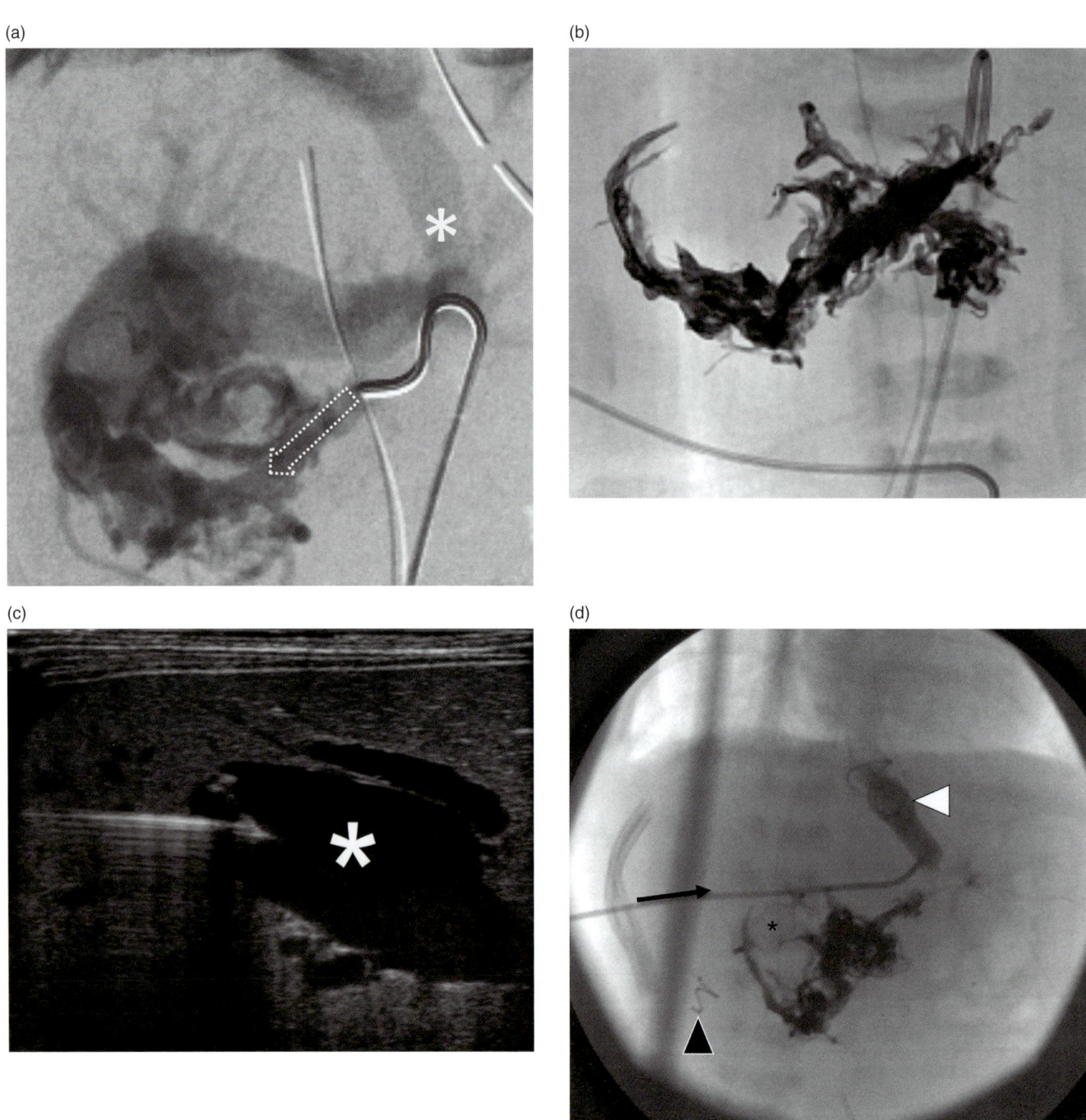

Figure 8.3 A newborn female presented with hypoxemia, congestive heart failure, and pulmonary hypertension. Initial US showed a large high-flow intrahepatic vascular abnormality. (a) A 4 French "shepherd's hook" angiographic catheter was inserted using preexisting umbilical arterial access, was formed in the aortic arch then pulled down into the replaced right hepatic artery through the SMA. Contrast injection showed hepatoportal fistulous connection (*arrow*) to a grossly enlarged right portal vein. The left portal vein drained through a patent ductus venosus (*asterisk*) to the vena cava. (b) The numerous fistulae (more than 100) could not be embolized with coils or particles. Onyx® flowable liquid was used for preliminary embolization, and resulted in dramatic, albeit temporary, clinical improvement. (c) To enable embolization of the patent ductus venosus, percutaneous transhepatic access to the portal vein (*) was obtained at the bedside in the NICU under US guidance. (d) The transhepatic access was used to deliver a 5 mm × 5 cm coil that successfully occluded the ductus (*white arrowhead*). An intrahepatic tract coil (*black arrowhead*) is visible from prior transhepatic delivery of an Amplatzer® plug to control a large residual hepatoportal fistula. Despite successful control of the abnormal vascular shunts, the child eventually succumbed to intractable pulmonary hypertension.

thrombosis is relatively high in neonates, the umbilical artery should be used for vascular access whenever possible (Figure 8.3). The main advantages of the umbilical artery approach include decreased significance of vascular occlusion since this is an artery that can be lost without concern, and the ability to use larger catheters or sheaths (4 to 5 French catheters or sheaths can be regularly utilized). The primary disadvantage of this route is difficult catheter maneuverability due to the tortuous vessel course. However, this problem can be overcome with the use of a sheath, directional guide wire, and coaxial catheter systems.

If the neonate already has an umbilical artery line in place, it can usually be easily exchanged over a guide wire for a 3 to 5 French diagnostic or delivery catheter or a 4 French arterial sheath. At the end of the procedure, the softer umbilical artery catheter can be replaced, and thus access preserved for patient monitoring or a staged endovascular procedure.

A transvenous approach can be used in neonates, by passing a catheter across the foramen ovale into the left ventricle. However, this technique may be associated with cardiac arrhythmias and requires considerable experience with neonatal cardiac catheterization. A third alternative, most useful in infants with high-flow vascular lesions in the thorax or upper abdomen, is an axillary artery puncture. Since the distal abdominal aorta and the femoral arteries are reduced in size in children with high-flow visceral lesions due to the large run-off at the level of the lesion (Figure 8.4), the axillary approach is technically easier, facilitates selective catheterization of the abnormal vessel(s), and is generally well tolerated. The main risk of this approach is the risk of brachial plexus neuropathy. For select procedures in adolescents and young adults, for example when femoral access is contraindicated, brachial access in the antecubital fossa may be helpful. It may also be useful in certain cases, such as treatment of vascular malformations, to acquire direct percutaneous access of target arteries (Figure 8.5). Finally, a translumbar approach was at one time the primary method for aortic access for angiography, although it is very seldom used in modern practice.

Postprocedure and follow-up care

Postprocedure orders include standard evaluation of the vascular access site and appropriate pulses, intravenous fluids, analgesics, and functional monitoring (e.g., neurologic status following cerebral or spinal angiography). A typical approach is to evaluate vital signs and the puncture site every 15 minutes for 30 minutes, every 30 minutes for the next hour, then every hour until the child is alert or back to neurologic baseline. Standard postprocedure recovery time for outpatient angiography is four to six hours. Whenever possible diagnostic examinations and, in certain instances, vascular interventions are performed in the outpatient setting.

Technical problems and pitfalls

The arteries and veins of infants and young children are much more reactive than those of older children and adults and are prone to vasospasm. Unintentional puncture of the femoral artery during infiltration of local anesthetic, or puncture of the femoral artery with inability to pass the guide wire, may produce spasm resulting in a non-palpable pulse. In this situation, the operator should either wait until the pulse returns to normal, which may take 30 minutes or more, or attempt to puncture the opposite femoral artery. Perivascular injection of 1% lidocaine can sometimes hasten the return of antegrade blood flow. The subintimal passage of a guide wire or catheter can easily occur with little resistance in young children. Therefore, it is important to be *gentle* and avoid probing with a guide wire. In children less than 10 kg, excessive catheter flushing can be dangerous and result in fluid overload and anemia. To avoid this issue, we recommend substitution of smaller volume syringes (e.g., 3 to 5 ml) instead of the larger syringes (e.g., 10 ml) commonly used for flushing and contrast injection. Also, maintaining and communicating a running tabulation of all fluids used is helpful. Failure to immobilize the legs and keep them warm after an arterial procedure may result in a further decrease in blood flow to the affected extremity and a hematoma. The use of oversized catheters in small arteries contributes to intimal injury, occlusion or embolization of thrombus and should be avoided.

Complications

Femoral arterial thrombosis is the most common complication following a transfemoral arterial vascular procedure in infants and young children. Factors that increase the likelihood of arterial thrombosis include small size of the patient (less than 10 kg), a hypercoaguable state or possibly the failure to heparinize, the use of large catheters, traumatic passage causing intimal injury (e.g., unsheathed balloon catheters), excessive catheter manipulation, hypothermia, and low cardiac output. The ability to detect pedal pulses by the use of Doppler monitoring does not exclude the presence of femoral artery thrombosis, as collateral pathways open quickly between the internal iliac and superficial femoral arteries to perfuse the distal extremity. In spite of the presence of collateral supply, which will usually prevent serious tissue loss, femoral artery thrombosis in infants and young children leads to leg length discrepancies in a significant number of patients. In addition, some of these children may develop claudication later in life, requiring a surgical bypass. Several strategies may be used to minimize the risk of occlusion including the use of anticoagulation (all children <10 kg), the use of a catheter size and shape appropriate for the task (the smallest catheter that will accomplish the objective is usually preferred), the use of sheaths when possible to protect the access artery, and by avoiding excessive catheter manipulation. When femoral artery thrombosis is diagnosed, patients should be treated, in the absence of contraindications, initially with full heparinization for 24 hours and then systemic thrombolysis (tPA) if needed.

Thromboembolic complications can occur in any arterial circulation but are most significant when they involve the CNS. These problems may result from wedging oversized catheters in small or spastic arteries, or from improper catheter flushing. Vessel occlusion can also be the result of subintimal dissection with a catheter or guide wire.

Pressure sores can result from long procedures and can be prevented by the use of padding at pressure points and removal of the hip bolster after femoral artery puncture.

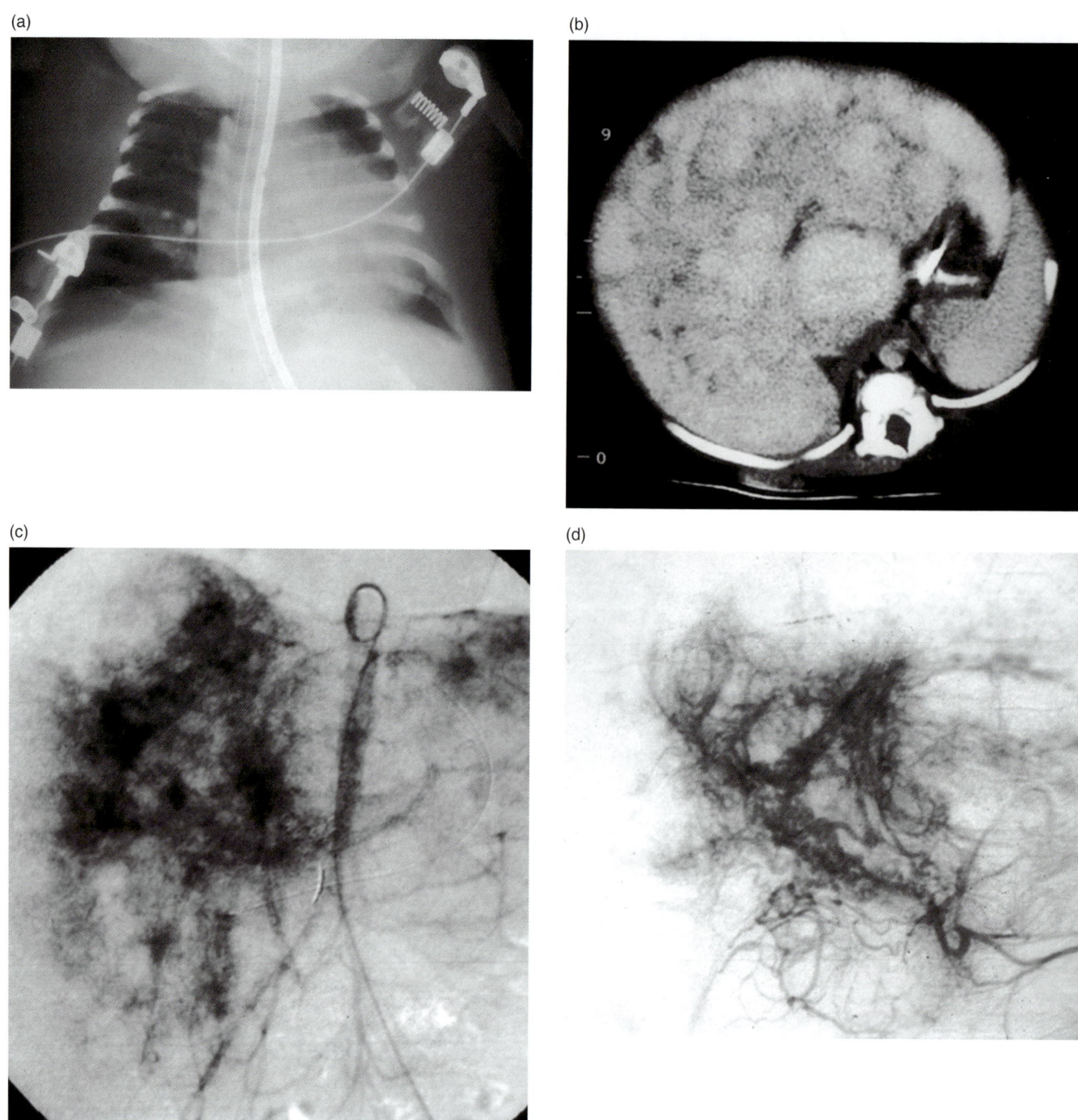

Figure 8.4 A newborn male presented with congestive heart failure and a hepatic mass. (a) Chest radiograph demonstrating cardiomegaly and mild congestive heart failure. (b) Axial contrast-enhanced abdominal CT shows hepatomegaly with marked nodular enhancement. (c) Abdominal aortogram showing marked reduction in distal aortic and common iliac diameter secondary to run-off at the celiac axis. (d) After embolization there is marked irregular contrast enhancement of the liver.

This is especially problematic in the areas of the shoulders, coccyx, iliac crest, elbows, and occiput. Padding in the axilla and careful arm, shoulder, and neck positioning will help prevent brachial plexopathy. Special attention should be paid to the position of the elbows because of the additional risk of ulnar nerve injury, and the occiput where pressure can result in hair loss. We have found the use of egg-crate foam and gel rings or pads to be effective. It is important to avoid the use of padding that is substantially radio-dense near areas likely to be included in the imaging field, since the automated detector may compensate with a significant increase in radiation dose.

(a)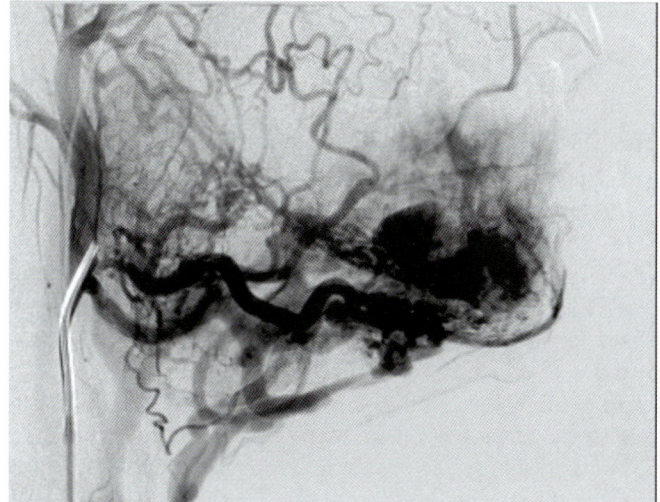

(b)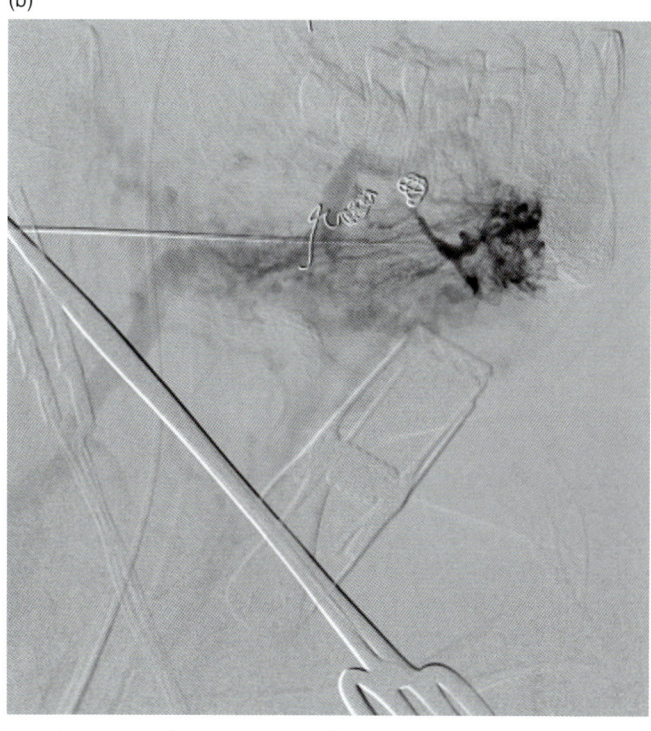

Figure 8.5 A 13-year-old male was referred by a maxillofacial surgeon for evaluation and treatment of an extensive mandibular arteriovenous malformation. (a) Arteriography from the right facial artery catheter demonstrates extensive intraosseous and soft tissue involvement of the AVM. However, due to surgical ligation of facial and lingual vessels in childhood, transfemoral access for more distal embolization was not possible. (b) Direct percutaneous US-guided puncture of a distal facial branch was obtained. Dark staining at the tip of the 21-gauge Chiba needle (stabilized by a clamp in this image) represents partial Onyx® embolization of the nidus, with contrast seen flowing through residual arteriovenous connections.

Fluid overload and anemia can result from excessive catheter flushing and may require admission to the intensive care unit for diuresis or transfusion.

Hypothermia may result in metabolic acidosis with generalized deterioration of the patient's condition and, on rare occasion, cardiac arrest. It is important to be careful when performing procedures on neonates since they are prone to hypothermia. This complication may be prevented by carefully protecting the patient with a variety of actions including warming the contrast (to approximately 27 to 32°C), covering or wrapping the infant's body with a blanket or plastic wrap, covering the head with a hat or plastic wrap since the head is the greatest source of heat loss, or using a water blanket, heater, or other method to minimize heat loss and keep the child dry.

Hepatic arteriography

Introduction

Before the introduction of US, CT, and MRI, hepatic angiography, along with the radionuclide liver–spleen scan, played a major role in the evaluation of liver masses and other types of hepatic pathology. Currently, the initial work-up of liver masses is performed with cross-sectional imaging that is safer, more sensitive, more accessible, and more cost effective than angiography. Magnetic resonance imaging with MR angiography (MRA) is usually selected for initial evaluation. If additional information is necessary US is often used. However, there are several circumstances in which angiography still plays a significant role. In the setting of a transplant center, the majority of hepatic angiography is performed on patients who will undergo or who have undergone transplantation. A smaller number of patients are referred from the neonatology, gastroenterology, oncology, and surgery services.

Indications

A common indication for hepatic angiography is in the preoperative evaluation of a patient with end-stage liver disease prior to liver transplantation. In order to evaluate whether or not a patient is a viable candidate for liver transplantation the size, patency, and anatomy of the hepatic artery, IVC, portal vein, and mesenteric veins are assessed. Initially, these vessels are evaluated with color Doppler US. If they are not well visualized because of overlying bowel gas, if the arterial or venous anatomy is distorted because of previous surgery, if the portal vein is less than 4 mm, or if there are internal echoes in the portal vein suggestive of thrombus, then angiography is usually performed. Biliary atresia is one of the major indications for liver transplantation in the pediatric age group, and it is associated with a higher frequency of vascular and visceral anomalies, including congenital absence of the intrahepatic IVC, aberrant origin of the hepatic artery, pre-duodenal portal vein, situs inversus, polysplenia, and malrotation. The other major indication for angiography in the pretransplantation evaluation is suspected congenital absence of the IVC or other congenital vascular abnormalities.

Hepatic angiography is also considered if a vascular intervention is contemplated, for example, evaluation of a neonate with a hypervascular liver mass and congestive heart failure. These masses are usually hemangioendotheliomas or cavernous hemangiomas. Cavernous hemangioma is the most common benign hepatic neoplasm in the pediatric age group. Most hemangiomas are solitary lesions and are discovered as an incidental finding in imaging studies being done for other reasons (see Figure 4.58). Children with symptomatic hepatic vascular lesions usually have large lesions and present in the prenatal period or infancy with congestive heart failure and a hepatic mass on physical or imaging examination.

Hemangioendotheliomas occur exclusively in neonates and very young infants and are more likely to be symptomatic than hemangiomas, usually presenting before six months of age. The most frequent symptoms at presentation are hepatomegaly and congestive heart failure. Hemangioendotheliomas tend to grow rapidly after initial presentation, and usually undergo slow, spontaneous regression over time. However, infants with these neoplasms are at significant risk of life-threatening congestive heart failure, ischemic damage to the heart and kidneys, portal hypertension, Kasabach–Merritt syndrome (thrombocytopenia with DIC), and tumor rupture. If the child is symptomatic the diagnosis is made with cross-sectional imaging and a plan is formulated. Cross-sectional imaging, especially MR and US, is best for discerning the extent and distribution of the lesion and is far less stressful on a sick neonate or young infant than is angiography. Angiography should be reserved for children who require vascular intervention. It is variable and somewhat controversial as to the best time to intervene in children with hemangioendotheliomas. It is our opinion that children without CHF or other life-threatening symptoms should be treated medically whenever possible. Today, propranalol has become the drug of choice in our practice since its time to action is short. Steroids and interferon remain other drug options. However, those children who fail medical therapy, or who are in CHF, or who have coagulopathy should be considered for prompt referral for angiography and embolization of the hepatic artery. Treatment of the hyperdynamic state should be accomplished before irreversible myocardial or renal injury occurs. We feel strongly that it is best to err on the side of early intervention since delayed treatment may result in a fatal outcome.

In general, there are no absolute contraindications to hepatic angiography, with the possible exception of previously documented anaphylactic reaction to intravenous contrast. Relative contraindications to angiography include an uncorrectable coagulopathy, severe anemia, hypertension, and acute or chronic renal failure.

Technique

Equipment and patient preparation are identical to that discussed above for general angiography.

Standard technique

The general elements of angiography are discussed above. For aortic injections a standard pigtail catheter with multiple side holes is used. For selective cannulation of the mesenteric vessels catheter selection is much more dependent on the preference of the operator. We most often use C-1, JB-1, Cobra, or RIM catheters. Be aware that a Simmons-type catheter may be difficult to use since the aortic diameter may be too small to allow the catheter to form. We do not routinely find this shape to be helpful in smaller pediatric patients. Once access to the desired artery is achieved, more distal access often requires the coaxial insertion of a microcatheter.

Standard injection rates and volumes for arteriography are given in Table 8.4. The exception to these suggested contrast volumes and flow rates is an SMA portogram where the injection is usually five to seven seconds with a volume of 25 to 35 ml after injection of intra-arterial papaverine or priscoline. The splenic artery may also be injected for portal venography. In children over 20 kg, we inject 45 mg of papaverine over two to three minutes prior to contrast injection. In patients less than 20 kg the dose is decreased to 22.5 mg or less, depending on the patient's weight. If the injection of vasodilator needs to be repeated, a minimum of ten minutes should pass between doses. Systemic blood pressure should be monitored. If hypotension occurs, it is easily corrected with IV infusion of normal saline in most cases.

To visualize the mesenteric arteries in neonates and young infants we film at rates of five frames per second (fps) or higher, if possible, in single plane, or 3.0 fps biplane. In larger patients we usually film at 3.0 fps single- or biplane. For studies of the portal vein we use single plane and film at 3.0 fps for the entire time in small infants and in older children at 3.0 fps for three seconds and 1 fps until the portal vein is opacified. This means that in older children the filming may last 15 to 25 seconds or longer. Filming rates in selective runs depend mainly on flow rate and can vary from 1 to 5 fps.

Technical problems and pitfalls

There are a few factors that can present problems in the interpretation of an arterial (indirect) portogram (Figures 8.37, 8.43). Splenic or superior mesenteric vein occlusion or thrombus can be simulated when there is inflow of unopacified blood from the other large tributary of the portal vein, e.g., inflow from the splenic vein during superior mesenteric artery injection and vice versa. Ultrasound or other cross-sectional imaging, evaluation of the venous phase via injection of the other artery, splenoportography, or transhepatic (direct) portography may be needed to clarify the findings. When there is significant splenomegaly there can be poor or absent

Table 8.5 Indications: embolotherapy

- Preoperative to limit blood loss
- Trauma
- Gastrointestinal bleeding
- AVMs and AVFs
- Complicated high-flow hemangiomas
- Trap aneurysms when other therapies fail or are too risky
- Iatrogenic injuries, e.g., postbiopsy bleeding

opacification of the splenic vein, suggesting splenic vein occlusion. In this case using a larger volume of contrast during splenic artery injection, splenoportography, or transhepatic portography will allow assessment of splenic vein patency. Poor visualization of the entire system may occur when there is hepatofugal flow or if there is significant spontaneous portal-systemic shunting. Finally there may be incomplete demonstration of gastro-esophageal varices if the splenic, superior mesenteric, and left gastric arteries are not all injected. Cases that require a higher total volume of contrast can be quite problematic in pediatric patients where total allowable contrast volumes are dictated by body weight or in those patients who have preexisting conditions requiring fluid restriction, such as congestive heart failure or renal disease.

Postprocedure and follow-up care

Removal of the sheath, obtaining hemostasis, monitoring the patient, recognition and treatment of complications, and conditions for discharge and follow-up are the same as those outlined above under the discussion of general angiography.

Arterial embolization

Introduction

Catheter-directed occlusion of one or more vessels (embolization) is indicated for the treatment of a wide range of pediatric conditions. Experience obtained has shown that embolotherapy can be performed safely and effectively in children of all ages and sizes. The successful outcome of catheter-directed therapy has been aided by the significant improvements in equipment and materials. The development of the variable stiffness microcatheter, coils in sizes from 0.018-inch to 0.038-inch, particulate materials ranging in size from 50 to 1,500 microns (e.g., PVA, Embospheres®, Gelfoam® powder), glue, Onyx® (Figure 8.3), and devices such as vascular plugs and locoregional ablation techniques has enabled a greater variety of vascular territories and vessel diameters to be safely catheterized and treated.

Indications

Embolotherapy may be considered for either the primary treatment of a vascular lesion or as an adjunct to another form of therapy, usually surgery (Table 8.5). The goal of the vascular intervention and the nature of the vascular supply will usually influence the materials selected, technical approach, and endpoint of therapy. There are five principal goals of therapy: control of hemorrhage, preservation of threatened vital structures, protection of organ function, alleviation of adverse effects, and cosmesis. Hemorrhage may be directly related to the lesion, such as in gastrointestinal bleeding, trauma, or rupture of an arteriovenous malformation. It may be iatrogenic, such as dehiscence of a vascular anastomosis or following tonsillectomy (Figure 8.6). It may be due to dysregulation, such as the consumptive coagulopathy of Kasabach–Merritt syndrome (Figure 8.7). Alternatively, bleeding may be anticipated, such as prior to resection of a highly vascular tumor, e.g., juvenile angiofibroma. Vital structures may be threatened by compression or obstruction, including airway, vessels, nerves, and the auditory canal. Organ and tissue function may be threatened by alterations in physiology, such as cardiac failure from high-flow peripheral arteriovenous malformations, as well as by compression or occlusion, such as obstruction of vision by tumor mass or compression of the globe by a retrobulbar hemangioma. Adverse events may include pain as well as bony or soft tissue overgrowth. Cosmesis for a child is in no way a trivial issue. Even small lesions in the central face can be disfiguring and result in serious psychological and social issues. Procedures undertaken for cosmesis should include a thorough understanding of the expectations of the patient and clear communication of the limitations of the operator and intended technique. Successful therapy does not necessarily require obliteration of the lesion or malformation. In many cases, this is not practically achievable, and efforts to reach such an outcome may result in severe complications. For example, if the goal of therapy is pain management, then the procedure is complete when pain is controlled, understanding that the pain may return and that further intervention may be required in the future.

Currently, the majority of pediatric embolization procedures are performed for the treatment of hemangiomas and high-flow vascular malformations. Today, medical therapy using propranolol has replaced surgery and embolotherapy as the initial therapy for infantile hemangiomas. In addition, there are a wide variety of other indications for embolotherapy including preoperative or primary treatment of hypervascular tumors (e.g., nasopharyngeal angiofibroma), primary or adjunctive treatment of an aneurysmal bone cyst, occlusion of a varicocele, treatment of acute or chronic bleeding from a variety of causes (e.g., hemoptysis in patients with cystic fibrosis, bleeding from an arteriovenous malformation (AVM)), and ablation of splenic or renal tissue in the treatment of hypersplenism and hypertension.

High-flow AVMs and arteriovenous fistulae (AVFs) occasionally present in the neonatal period with severe congestive heart failure. The most common of these involves the central nervous system and can take the form of galenic, pial, or dural types as well as liver involvement (hemangioendothelioma). Less commonly, diffuse AVMs of the extremity or isolated

Chapter 8 Vascular interventions

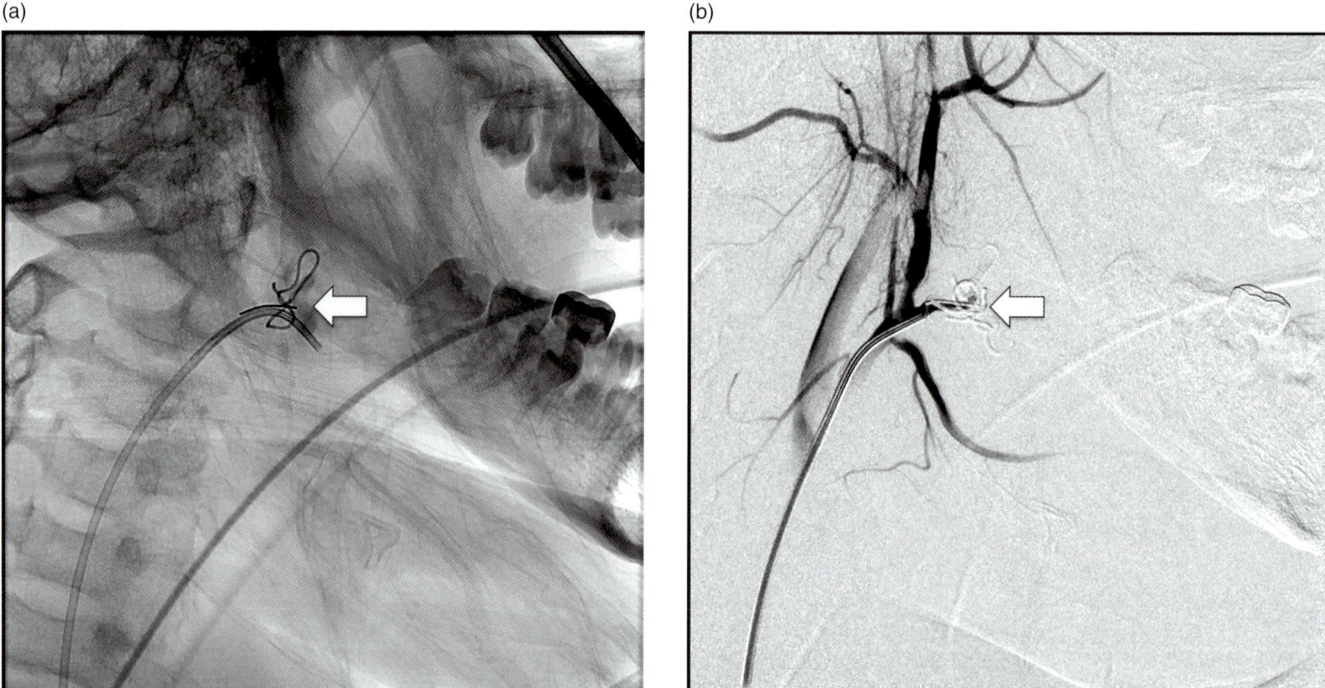

Figure 8.6 A ten-year-old female presented emergently following cardiopulmonary arrest related to massive pharyngeal hemorrhage three weeks after tonsillectomy. A suture was noted in the right tonsillar fossa associated with voluminous bleeding. Right external carotid angiography showed a defect in the proximal right facial artery. (a) Visible (*arrow*) on selective injection following initial embolization with two Hilal coils, immediately resulting in stabilization of hypotension. (b) After further embolization with a 5 mm × 3 cm tornado coil and a 5 mm × 5 cm coil through a JB-1 catheter positioned in the facial artery across the defect, complete occlusion was achieved, and the child recovered with minimal neurologic sequelae.

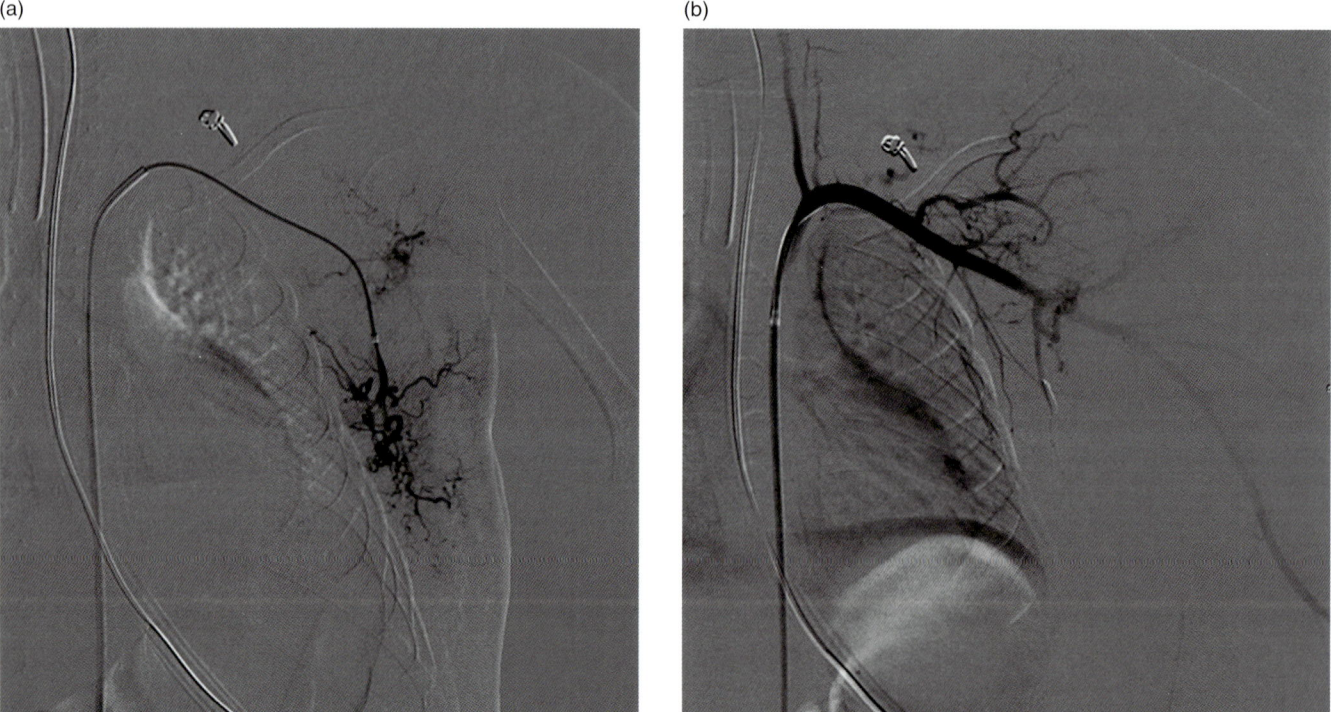

Figure 8.7 Selective catheterization of a branch of the lateral thoracic artery in a 4.8 kg, 86-day-old female with Kaposi's hemangioendothelioma and Kasabach–Merritt syndrome. (a) Microcatheter in lateral thoracic branch vessel supplying tumor. (b) After embolization using microcoils, the angiogram shows marked reduction in blood supply and tumor vascularity.

AVFs involving systemic or cardiac vessels may present with neonatal congestive heart failure. Urgent embolization, when successful, results in dramatic reversal of the cardiac failure and survival of the child. Delay in treatment often results in worsening of the congestive heart failure due to progressive myocardial ischemia and injury to other organs, e.g., kidneys and brain.

Anomalous systemic arterial supply to the lungs may be seen in isolation, in association with scimitar syndrome or pulmonary sequestration, and in patients with pulmonary atresia and ventricular septal defects. These malformations may result in severe congestive heart failure or hemoptysis. Prior to the embolization of systemic arteries, careful angiographic mapping of the pulmonary circulation should be performed.

Endangering hemangiomas (e.g., those associated with consumption coagulopathy in Kasabach–Merritt syndrome, bleeding, visual obstruction, ulceration with significant bleeding, and congestive heart failure) are generally initially treated by aggressive pharmacotherapy. Embolization may be useful in those patients failing medical management or in children who are at risk for or who present with a complication. Unfortunately, positive results are often transient and additional procedures are needed, especially in lesions with multiple arterial feeders (Figures 8.3, 8.5).

The indications for embolization of peripheral AVMs include cardiac failure, ischemic skin ulceration, bleeding, and pain. Most of these lesions are not curable by embolization alone and treatment planning should be carried out in conjunction with the appropriate surgical specialty.

Hypersplenism is an uncommon problem in childhood although a variety of etiologies may be responsible. Depending on the geographic location, the most common causes may vary. Portal hypertension, cystic fibrosis, thalassemia, and idiopathic thrombocytopenia purpura are among the more common etiologies. Total splenic embolization (TSE) is rarely indicated since it is associated with a high incidence of postprocedural abscess formation and severe postembolization syndrome. In general, TSE is only performed prior to surgical splenectomy. Instead, partial splenic embolization (PSE) is preferred to treat children with persistent severe thrombocytopenia, severe pain, or respiratory difficulty. Regardless of the etiology, the goal of PSE is to ablate 30 to 60% of the splenic parenchyma. This may be accomplished either by (1) selectively entering splenic branch arteries and systematically occluding them, or (2) positioning the catheter distal to the short gastric arteries but proximal to the bifurcation of the main splenic artery to perform particulate embolization, which we prefer. Proximal splenic artery catheter position (just distal to the short gastric arteries) allows for the injection of particulates (>300 microns) so that they will occlude the splenic parenchyma in all areas of the spleen, especially at the periphery. This has the advantage of symmetrically reducing spleen size and minimizing the time necessary to complete the procedure. Regardless of the approach selected, children will invariably develop postembolization syndrome, which consists of low grade fever (usually less than 40°C), pain, and elevated WBC count with left shift, as well as elevation of the platelet count in the first few days after treatment.

Hypertension secondary to segmental renal artery stenosis and secondary renal ischemia is a rare indication for embolotherapy. In these stenotic segmental renal artery branches not amenable to balloon angioplasty, embolization is a reasonable option and may cure or help control the child's hypertension.

Technique

Equipment

It is of paramount importance to preserve the patency of the access artery after completion of the procedure. Therefore available equipment should include the smallest possible arterial sheath, catheter, and guide wire to accomplish the procedural objective (Table 8.6). The temptation of using larger systems for easier delivery of embolic materials should be avoided since they likely expose children, especially small infants, to a higher risk of complications and are not necessary for successful occlusion of vascular lesions.

Embolization should be carried out by physicians with appropriate training and with access to pediatric anesthesia, nursing, and technical staff. High-resolution digital subtraction angiographic equipment, especially with road mapping capabilities, is essential. A selection of arterial sheaths (3 French and larger), thin-walled 3 to 5 French delivery catheters, variable stiffness microcatheters, and guide wires in short and long lengths are needed. Embolic materials include particulates, calibrated from 50 to 1,000 microns, Gelfoam®, absolute ethanol, tissue adhesives (glue and Onyx®), detachable

Table 8.6 Equipment: embolotherapy

- Arterial sheath 4 to 7 French for most indications
- Directional catheters (JB-1, Harwood-Nash, Cobra, C-1, etc.)
- Variable stiffness microcatheters (fit through a 4 French catheter with a 0.035-inch lumen)
- Guide wires (0.018- to 0.038-inch); choice depends on the vascular territory treated and operator preference
    - Bentson, hydophilic (angled Glidewire®), Newton, etc.
    - directional guide wires for microcatheters (≤0.018-inch)
- Pressure bag or infusion pump for sheath perfusion
- Embolic material
    - temporary agents
        - particles: Gelfoam®, autologous clot, Avitene® (may act as a permanent agent in some situations)
    - permanent agents
        - particles: PVA, Embospheres®, Gelfoam® powder
        - liquid: absolute alcohol, thrombin
        - tissue adhesives: glue and Onyx®
        - detachable balloons (not readily available)
    - Coils: Gianturco, platinum microcoils, Hilal, GDC, or other detachable coils, etc.

balloons, devices such as vascular plugs, ablation equipment (e.g., laser, radiofrequency, microwave, and cryoablation) and platinum/fiber and stainless steel wire/fiber coils. Unfortunately, not all of these materials are readily available and approved for use in children. Coils and particles are currently the embolic materials most often used when permanent occlusion is desired.

Patient preparation

Evaluation of a child's cardiovascular status is important in high-flow lesions. Infants in heart failure often require earlier treatment and have an increased anesthesia risk. We generally consider this an emergent indication for therapy. Assessment of the neurologic status of a patient with a facial lesion is important to exclude an existing cranial nerve abnormality. This may avoid the possibility of the finding being considered a treatment complication. Physical exam and documentation of lesion extent help to plan the likely number of treatments, especially when sclerotherapy is considered. Clinical evaluation and explanation of the treatment to the patient and parents also establishes the necessary confidence that a family must have in the treating interventionalist. Photographing lesions is important to document the baseline and subsequent improvement or need for further treatment. Routine laboratory tests are not performed unless specifically indicated. In general, children are not typed and cross-matched for either blood or platelets.

Prior to the procedure, the child should be well hydrated and have a working IV line. Corticosteroids may be given at the beginning of the procedure or 24 hours prior to the embolization, depending on the preference of the interventionalist. In most instances, it is best to prepare the child and family for a lengthy procedure. General anesthesia is usually advantageous and preferred for these procedures, since it can insure patient cooperation especially during a technically demanding, lengthy, and risky procedure. In addition respiratory and other physiologic factors may be controlled, when necessary. A urinary catheter is usually inserted because a large volume of contrast may be used. With the catheter in place, the urinary output can be monitored and bladder decompression assured. In most cases, the urinary catheter is removed before the child awakens. Systemic heparinization is suggested for infants under 15 kg, procedures involving the use of coaxial catheter systems, and procedures of the head and neck. Preoperative hematocrit, coagulation studies, and other laboratory tests are obtained on an as-needed basis.

Standard technique

In general, embolization is performed during the same session as diagnostic angiography. The angiographic approach is planned out according to the vascular territory of the lesion to be treated. Both non-invasive imaging and pre-embolization diagnostic angiography are performed to confirm the diagnosis and to finalize the interventional planning. Embolization is

Table 8.7 Procedure summary: embolotherapy

- Preoperative testing as needed
- Hydration of the child
- Puncture femoral artery and insert sheath
- Infuse sheath with heparinized saline
- Systemic heparinization (50 to 100 units/kg PRN), except children <10 kg who are routinely heparinized (50 to 75 units/kg)
- Diagnostic angiography
- Selective catheterization of pathologic vessels
- Embolize vascular pathology to complete occlusion
- Postembolization angiography

performed only after selective or superselective catheterization of the vessel(s) supplying the lesion is achieved. The precise technique utilized depends on the goal of the procedure, the nature of the lesion, and the embolic device/material being used (Table 8.7). When necessary, hypercarbia (via hypoventilation) may be helpful by producing vasodilation, thereby facilitating distal vessel catheterization.

Before deploying an embolic agent, safe catheter tip position within the abnormal vessel must be confirmed. The material utilized for vessel occlusion depends on the interventionalist's preference and experience, the type of lesion being treated, the goal of the procedure, and the availability of various materials. Particulates and coils are the most frequently used embolic agents. PVA, especially small particles (50 to 250 microns), are preferred since this material has the best chance of occluding the nidus of the lesion. In our practice, Embospheres® have replaced PVA as the particulates of choice. Embospheres® are available in a wide variety of particle sizes that generally meet the needs of the interventionalist. Recently, with the development of the liquid agent Onyx®, a third choice has become available, although it is quite costly. Coils are more often chosen for preoperative occlusions or when fluid volume excess is problematic (e.g., neonates with congestive failure secondary to arteriovenous shunting from a hemangioendothelioma). In general, coils are avoided in the proximal portions of vessels, since this approach often leads to the development of collaterals. When particles are used, we prefer to use a separate Mayo stand for any equipment containing particles. We mix the particles with contrast (1:1 ratio) via a three-way stopcock and two 6 to 10 ml syringes. One of the 6 to 10 ml syringes then acts as a reservoir for the particles while a 1 ml syringe is attached to the stopcock and eventually used for embolization (Figure 8.8). The particulate/contrast mixture is injected while observing with real-time digital subtraction fluoroscopy until blood flow becomes slow. The solution is pulsed in small boluses so that one can observe the speed of the forward flow and assess the progress of the embolization. One must be careful when flushing a catheter that has been contaminated with an embolic material since there may be residual material in the catheter. When coils or other devices are required, it may be useful to use flow-control

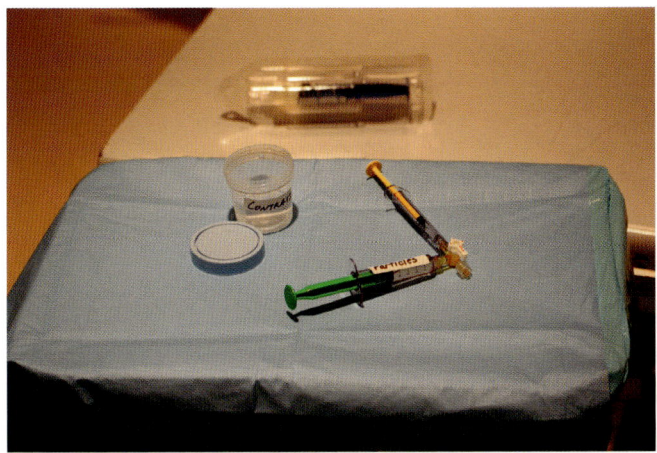

Figure 8.8 During preparation for particulate embolization, all embolic materials and related equipment are maintained on a separate sterile tray to prevent contamination of other equipment and subsequent inadvertent injection. Embolic particles are mixed using two syringes: a larger reservoir syringe and a smaller injection syringe.

techniques to assist in placing these devices in high-flow lesions. This is accomplished with proximal arterial or distal venous balloon occlusion, a tourniquet or blood pressure cuff, or glue/Onyx® control of appropriate outflow vessels.

Particles (less than 100 microns, e.g., Gelfoam® powder), tissue adhesive, Onyx®, and ethanol are extremely aggressive agents and may cause tissue necrosis when delivered to a capillary bed or end arterial circulation. In addition, these materials can pass through small collateral connections resulting in downstream embolization and untoward effects. Because of their small size, these agents have several advantages including being able to flow into the nidus of a lesion, thus increasing the chance of a cure, and may be injected through microcatheters.

Preoperative embolization of tumors

The goal of a preoperative embolization is to devascularize a lesion so that it can be excised or (in the case of bone tumors) curetted out with minimal bleeding (Figure 8.9). Embolization should be performed with the goal of occluding the vessels supplying the tumor as distally as possible while sparing normal adjacent tissue. The safest and most effective technique is selective catheterization and occlusion of the vessels feeding the lesion (Figure 8.10). The embolic agent utilized is based on the lesion type and the experience and preference of the interventionalist. In preoperative cases, "perfect is the enemy of good". Thus it is not necessary to try to completely devascularize the lesion but rather to minimize operative blood loss. It is often a good strategy to use large particles, coils, or other agents that will be the easiest and fastest to deploy. Before beginning the embolization procedure, cross-sectional imaging should be reviewed to determine the location of the mass. The vascular territory is predicted by the anatomic location of the tumor. The region of abnormality is studied angiographically to confirm and map the vascular supply, and exclude dangerous anastomotic communications with adjacent arterial territories. Once the pathologic anatomy is understood, each vascular trunk supplying the mass is selectively occluded. In general, the sequence of catheterization and embolization proceeds from distal to proximal vessels, to avoid the need to enter vessels that have already been treated and may be in spasm. For cases in which embolization is the primary therapy, it may be appropriate to utilize more aggressive embolic agents such as ethanol, small particles, or Onyx®, in an attempt to cure the patient.

Embolization of hemangiomas and high-flow vascular malformations

The management of congenital vascular lesions is challenging. In the past few years, the approach to the treatment of congenital infantile hemangiomas (CIHs) has dramatically changed. Over the past decade or two, surgery and embolotherapy were the mainstays for the treatment of CIHs. Today, medical therapy with oral propranolol is the initial therapy of choice, with both surgery and interventional solutions reserved for treatment when medical therapy fails, when there are complications, or when patients are at risk for complications. Examples of at-risk lesions are those high-flow lesions causing congestive heart failure, severe or recurrent bleeding, Kasabach–Merritt syndrome, DIC, and lesions that can lead to poor vision or unilateral blindness.

The historical lack of standardized terminology for vascular lesions resulted in confusion and interfered with data analysis and the creation of standardized therapeutic approaches. In 1982, Mulliken and Glowacki suggested a classification system based on physical examination, histology, and the natural history of the lesions. Although imperfect, this classification led to an improved categorization of lesions and a more organized approach to therapy. Presently, the accepted terminology of vascular anomalies is provided by the International Society for the Study of Vascular Anomalies (ISSVA), which classifies vascular tumors and vascular malformations. Please refer to the ISSVA classification of vascular anomalies for further reading.

Hemangiomas are the most common tumors of infancy and are noted in 1 to 2% of neonates and 10 to 12% of Caucasian children by one year of age. Interestingly, hemangiomas are three to five times more common in girls. Only 30% of hemangiomas are noted at birth, while about 70% are identified in the first month of life. Multiple lesions are found in approximately 20% of infants. The sites most often involved are the head and neck (50 to 60%), trunk (25%), and extremities (15%).

Congenital infantile hemangiomas are defined as benign vascular neoplasms that develop from the dermal capillary network and consist of masses of endothelial cells and pericytes with or without vascular lumina. Typically, a hemangioma evolves through three distinct phases: proliferative, stable, and involution. Once the lesion appears, there is rapid

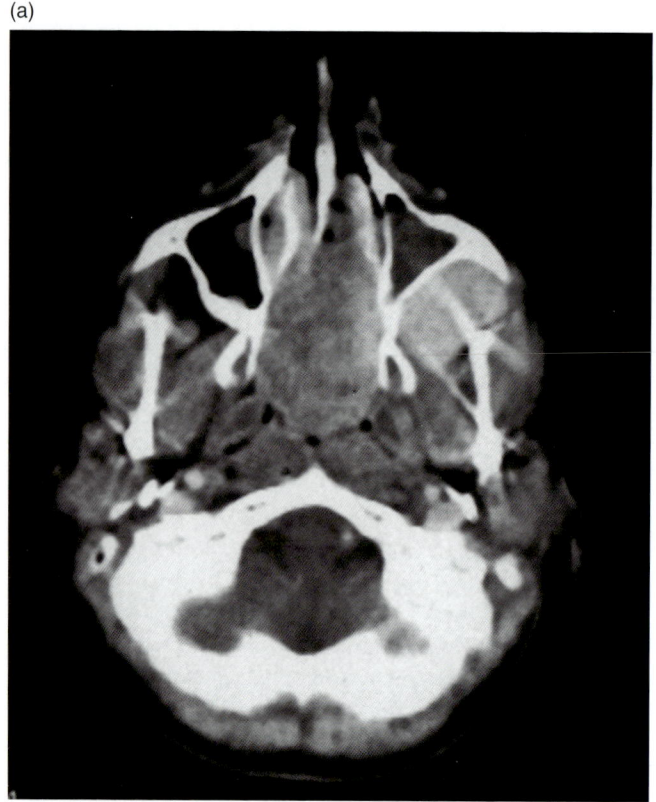

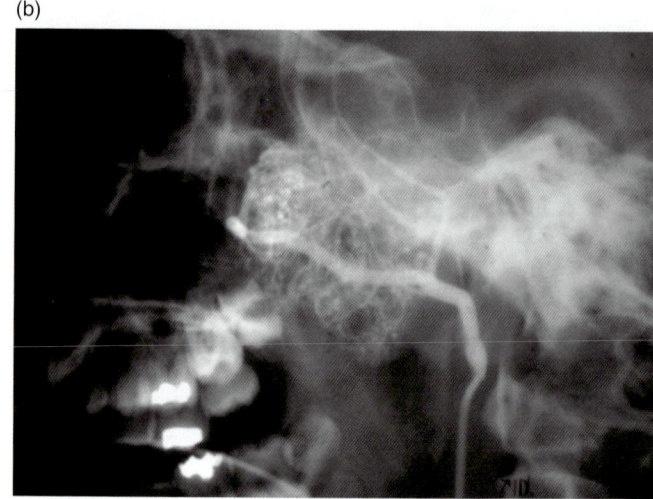

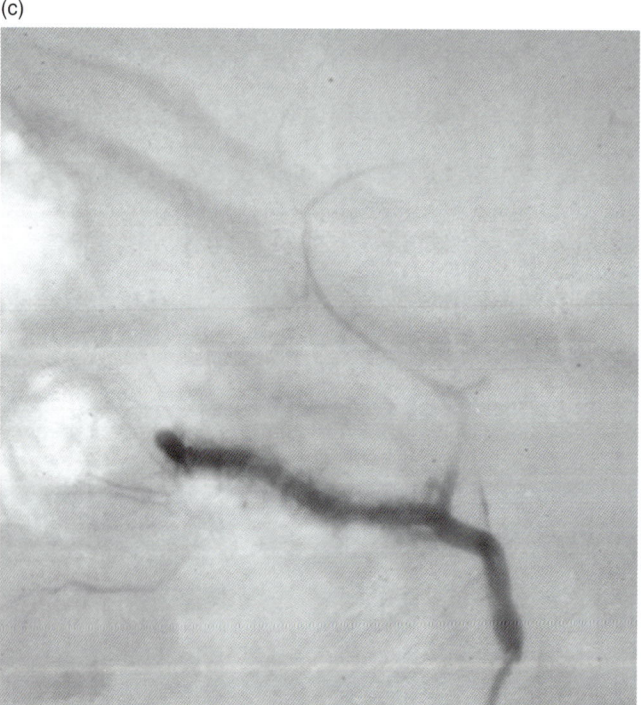

Figure 8.9 Twelve-year-old boy with epistaxis. (a) Axial CT scan demonstrates an enhancing mass originating in the left pterygo-maxillary foramen and extending into the nasal fossa and behind the maxillary sinus. Note there is widening of the pterygo-maxillary foramina with anterior bowing of the posterior sinus wall (Holman–Miller sign). (b) Selective internal maxillary artery injection shows a large enhancing mass. (c) After particle embolization, angiography demonstrates reduction in the pathologic vascularity.

growth for eight to eighteen months with maximum growth usually at one year. The rate and extent of the growth is unpredictable, but growth eventually ceases and the stable phase is then entered. During the proliferative phase, there is endothelial cell hyperplasia, 3H-thymidine uptake, and an increase in the number of mast cells. While in the involution phase, the lesions are less cellular, take up little or no 3H-thymidine, have normal mast cell counts, and have fibrosis and

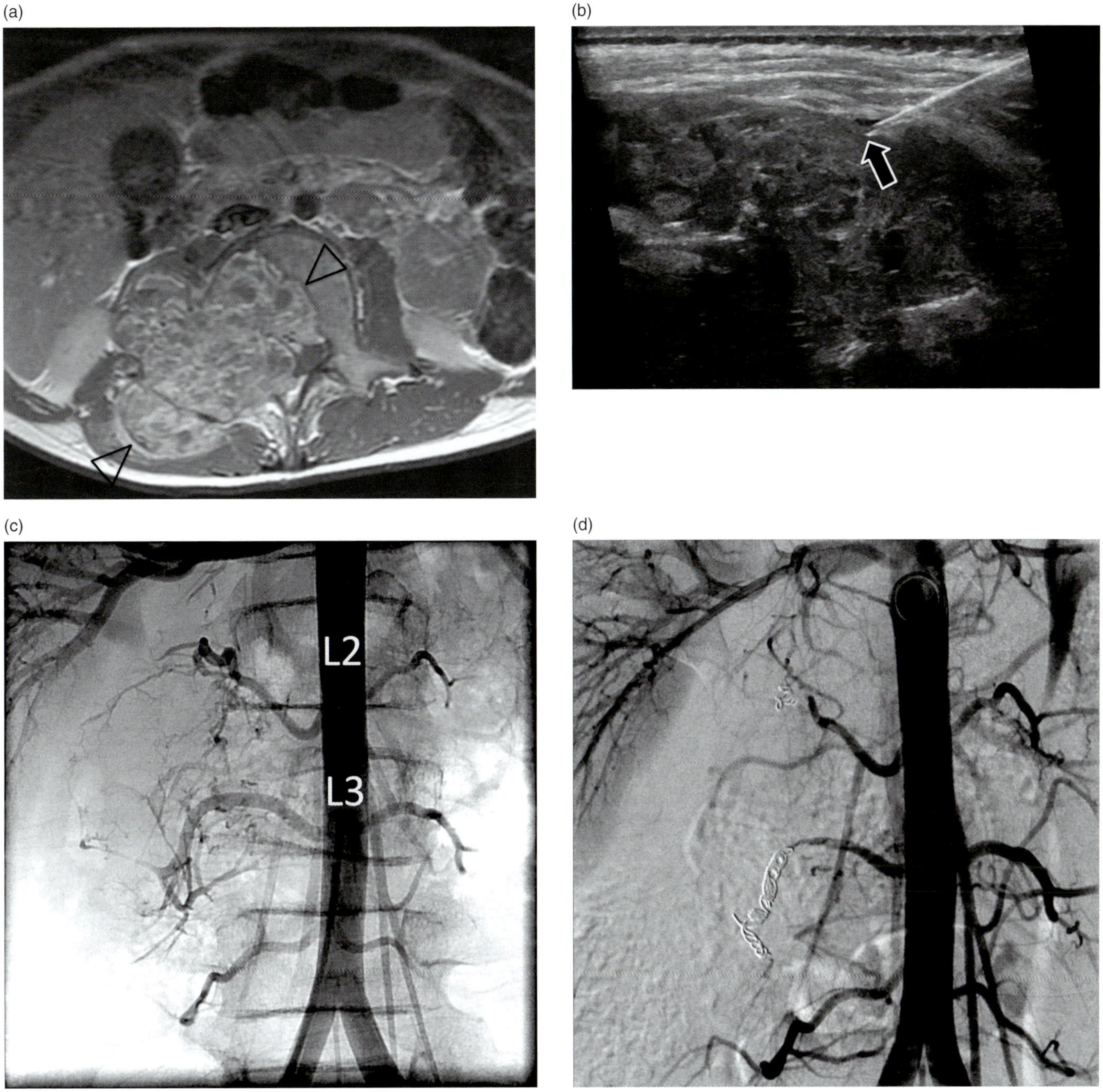

Figure 8.10 An eight-year-old female presented with back pain. (a) Axial T1 post-contrast fast spin echo MR image shows a lobulated solid and cystic 7 × 7 × 9 cm mass (*arrowheads*) centered on the L2 vertebral body that invades the spinal canal and right intervertebral foramen extending into the paraspinal tissues. (b) Under US guidance, multiple passes with a 16-gauge OstyCut® core biopsy needle obtained only blood. Several passes with an 18-gauge BioPince® core biopsy needle (*arrow*) confirmed diagnosis of aneurysmal bone cyst. (c) Abdominal aortography showed tumor vascular supply from the right second and third lumbar vertebral arteries. (d) After multiple coils were used to embolize the involved arteries, there was negligible residual tumor vascularity detectable. (e) On the following day, the tumor was completely excised surgically. The surgeons reported that the field was essentially bloodless. Spinal reconstruction was successful and the patient was asymptomatic at two-year follow-up.

fatty infiltration. The length of the stable period is unpredictable. The stable phase is followed by the involution period, when there is slow and often complete resolution of the lesion. In most series, there is a 50% chance of involution in five years, 75% chance in seven years, and 90% chance in nine years. Unfortunately, not all lesions resolve, and in about 20% of children, there are residual skin changes of cosmetic significance. All CIHs have high endothelial immunoreactivity for erythrocyte-type glucose transport protein GLUT1 (GLUT1 positive) that may be found in cells during all phases of

(e)

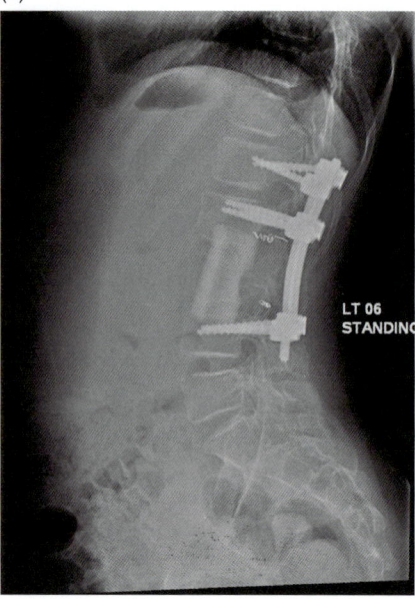

Figure 8.10 (cont.)

evolution. Interestingly, in hepatic vascular lesions, there are two types of lesions, the focal hemangioendothelioma, which is GLUT1 negative, and the multifocal hepatic infantile hemangioma, which is GLUT1 positive.

Two variants of the common juvenile hemangioma have been described: non-involuting congenital hemangioma (NICH) and rapidly involuting congenital hemangioma (RICH). The NICH is a rare, cutaneous abnormality that grows proportionately with the child but does *not* regress. There is a slight male predominance, and the lesion generally is solitary, round to oval, with the most common locations being the head and neck, extremities, and trunk. The lesions are usually pink to purple in color with an average diameter of 5 cm. Magnetic resonance imaging and angiographic findings are similar to that of congenital infantile hemangioma. However, these lesions are GLUT1 negative. Histologically, the lesion appears as a lobular collection of small, thin-walled vessels with a large and often stellate central vessel. The interlobular veins seem dysplastic, and the endothelial cells are "hobnailed" in appearance.

Rapidly involuting congenital hemangioma has similar characteristics to NICH regarding its appearance, distribution, and slight male predominance. The MR and angiographic features are similar, but RICH also have areas of inhomogeneous enhancement, larger flow voids, and arterial aneurysms on angiography. Histologically, the lesions are composed of small to large lobules of capillaries with moderately plump endothelial cells and pericytes surrounded by abundant fibrous tissue. About half of the lesions have lobular loss, fibrous tissue, and draining channels that are large and abnormal. These lesions may contain hemosiderin, calcifications, thrombus, and cyst formation. Like NICH, these lesions are also GLUT1 negative.

Vascular malformations are distinct from hemangiomas, occur much less frequently than hemangiomas, and have a significantly different natural history. These lesions are generally present at birth and tend to enlarge steadily in proportion to somatic growth throughout childhood. Males and females are affected equally. Spontaneous enlargement of lesions may result from interval problems such as thrombosis, infection, ectasia, or the development of new connections especially at puberty. Unlike hemangiomas, vascular malformations do not involute and tend to become more nodular and thickened as they age. Vascular malformations are congenital errors of morphogenesis and may involve formation of one or more vessels. Thus they can be classified as arterial, venous, capillary, lymphatic, or any combination of the above. Histologically, the lesions are not tumors and consist of abnormal clusters of vessels, have normal endothelium, normal mast cell counts, and *no non-vascular soft tissue component*.

Both hemangiomas and vascular malformations may be defined by their flow characteristics as either low-flow or high-flow. It is important to distinguish the velocity of flow through the lesion since they have different clinical behavior, prognosis, and require a different approach to therapy. Vascular abnormalities may be imaged in a variety of ways at the preference of the referring physician. In general, there is little use for plain radiography and scintigraphy in the work-up of these children. Ultrasound with Doppler can be useful in the initial evaluation and follow-up of these patients. Hemangiomas usually appear as mixed echogenic to hyperechoic soft tissue masses with internal arterial and venous flow in low-resistance vessels. Occasionally, dilated vascular spaces are identified. Distinct feeding and draining vessels may not be seen. Vascular malformations, especially high-flow types, are often distinct structures with multiple anechoic internal structures representing vessels. Spectral waveforms of feeding arteries indicate a low peripheral resistance and dilated draining veins with pulsatile flow suggesting arteriovenous communication. The exact number of supplying vessels is usually not predictable in most cases.

Magnetic resonance imaging and MRA are currently the modalities of choice for diagnosis and treatment planning in most cases. In general, T1- and T2-weighted images are performed in at least two planes (axial and coronal) prior to and after injection of contrast. Magnetic resonance angiography or MRV is obtained in cases with high-flow abnormalities. Proliferating hemangiomas usually appear as homogeneously low or intermediate signal intensity on T1-weighted images and have high signal intensity on T2 sequences. T2-weighted imaging often demonstrates flow voids in high-flow lesions. Involuting lesions are more heterogeneous in appearance. With MRA, vessels are usually identified in high-flow lesions. The appearance of vascular malformations again depends on the lesion type and blood flow characteristics. Arteriovenous malformations will generally demonstrate no significant soft tissue component, flow voids on static imaging, and distinct vessels on

MRA. Venous and lymphatic malformations are slow-flow lesions. Venous malformations can enhance homogeneously or heterogeneously if there is thrombus, or can have fluid–fluid levels if the flow is extremely slow. Lymphatic malformations consisting of macrocysts do not enhance, although there can be enhancement of tissue in microcystic lymphatic malformations. Magnetic resonance imaging is recommended to follow children after treatment. In most cases, only high-flow lesions are referred for angiography and vascular intervention. Low-flow lesions are referred for sclerotherapy without embolization.

Although angiography can accurately diagnose and define the vascular pathology, it is only recommended if it is necessary for diagnosis (e.g., a vascular neoplasm) or if vascular intervention is contemplated. Proliferating hemangiomas appear as well-circumscribed masses with intense, persistent tissue blush in a lobular pattern. Involuting hemangiomas have less intense tissue staining and lobules that are more distinctly separated by linear or patchy lucencies that represent fibrofatty septae. Hemangiomas are usually supplied by two to four slightly enlarged branches of normal feeding arteries, which often form a circumferential network around the periphery and give off numerous small feeding vessels. Arteriovenous shunting is not seen and draining veins funnel into a large vein at the base of the mass. High-flow vascular malformations are poorly circumscribed and show faint, if any, vascular blush. The AVMs are supplied by a variable number of enlarged, often ectatic, feeding arteries and have enlarged, often early-draining veins.

Hemangioma

Hemangiomas should only be embolized after failure of appropriate medical therapy (beta-blockers, usually propranolol). Exception to this approach is considered for complicated lesions, especially in young children with congestive heart failure. The technique is similar to that of treating hypervascular tumors and involves selective catheterization and occlusion of feeding arteries with small- to medium-sized particles, coils, glue, or Onyx® (Figures 8.11, 8.12). Caution should be used with coil embolization as recurrence via collaterals can occur if coils are not deployed sufficiently close to the nidus, resulting in increasing complexity of the vasculature. Because these lesions tend to recruit new vascular supplies, in most cases embolotherapy needs to be repeated several times before a stable endpoint is achieved.

Hepatic hemangioma (hemangioendothelioma)

Hepatic hemangiomas, associated with refractory congestive heart failure, should be considered for emergent treatment when the child requires respiratory support or when drug therapy fails to satisfactorily reduce the excessive blood flow. Treatment of this group of children is challenging. These infants are usually critically ill and in congestive heart failure, with possible renal insufficiency. Thus maintaining their body temperature, carefully monitoring the volume of fluids injected (via contrast and flush), and completing the treatment quickly is extremely important. Prior to treatment, the vascular pathology should be studied carefully, with MRI and US if possible, so that a thorough understanding of the problem and a treatment plan can be developed.

Although hepatic hemangiomas are always supplied by the hepatic arteries, in rare cases they may have extensive systemic collateral arterial and portal venous supply, factors that diminish the effectiveness of hepatic artery embolization. In the presence of extensive portal venous supply and poor hepatic portal perfusion, hepatic arterial embolization has resulted in extensive hepatic necrosis and death. When recognized, the portal vein–hepatic vein fistulae can be occluded with coils using a retrograde transfemoral or transhepatic portal venous approach. These small infants present technical problems in many cases. We have found that in order to minimize the risks for occlusion of the femoral artery in children less than 10 kg, a 4 French directional catheter, through which a microcatheter can be inserted, may be substituted in place of an endovascular sheath.

The type of embolic material used for embolization of the hepatic arteries varies throughout the literature. The most important factor in selecting the type of material to be used is the size of the vascular shunts within the hemangiomas. While particles and tissue adhesives are most effective in achieving distal hepatic artery branch occlusion and reducing revascularization by collaterals, these materials may result in fatal embolization to the pulmonary circulation. Proximal occlusion of the main hepatic artery, distal to the origin of the gastroduodenal artery or hepatic artery branches, using balloons or coils (our preference) has been effective in relieving cardiac failure, although glue or Onyx® are therapeutic alternatives. This approach has several additional advantages, including minimizing injected fluid volume, short time to vessel occlusion, and completion of the case with a high degree of safety. Hepatic artery branch occlusion using microcoils (0.018-inch, ≥ 5 mm length) appears to be relatively safe and effective.

It is important to keep in mind that the goal of embolization in children with symptomatic hemangioendothelioma is not to eradicate the tumor, but to control life-threatening complications, most importantly CHF, by diminishing arterial blood flow, thereby reducing the rapid AV shunting through the lesion, until the malformation involutes in the range of 12 to 18 months of age. Thus care should be taken to occlude the fewest number of vessels necessary to control the child's CHF.

Arteriovenous malformations

Arteriovenous malformations may not be cured by embolization, so this technique should be employed to treat specific symptoms or complications of the lesion, including congestive heart failure, ischemic pain and ulceration (Figure 8.13), and bleeding. In this setting, transcatheter embolization should be performed by selective catheterization of each feeding vessel

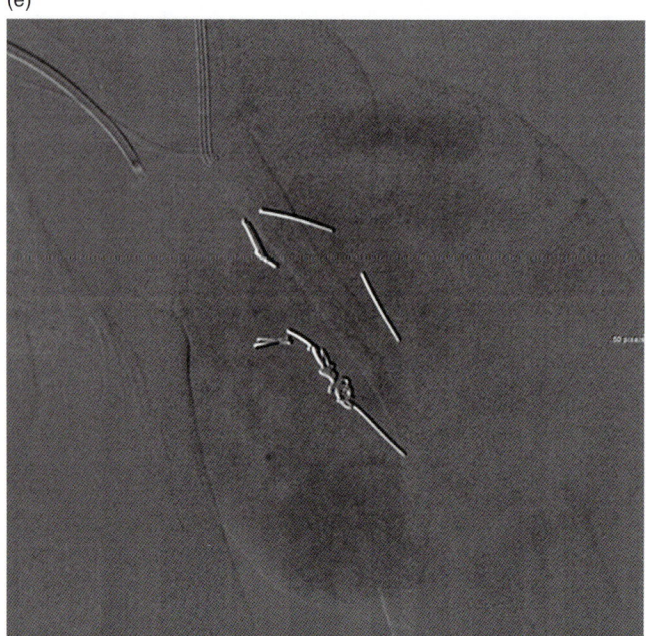

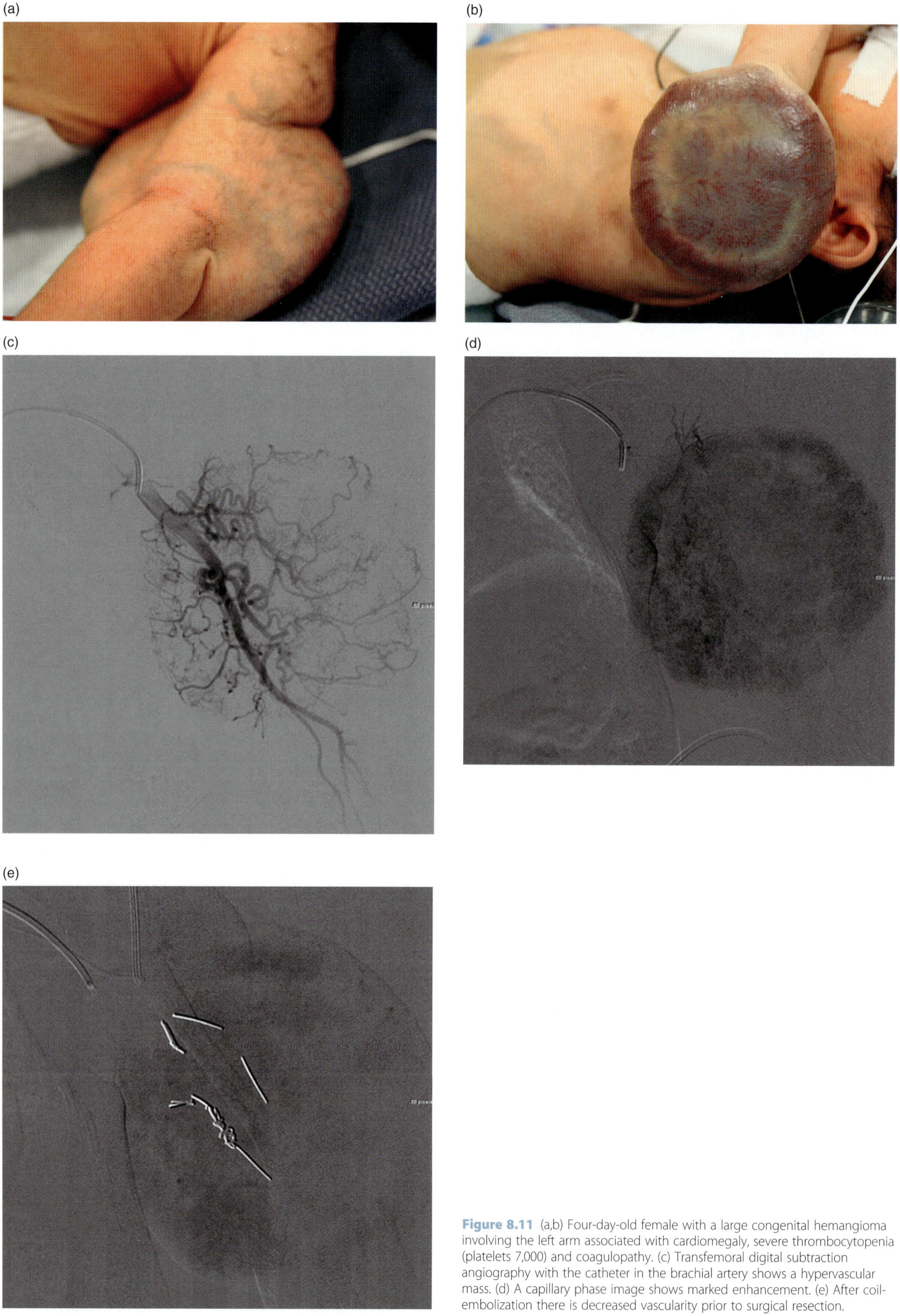

Figure 8.11 (a,b) Four-day-old female with a large congenital hemangioma involving the left arm associated with cardiomegaly, severe thrombocytopenia (platelets 7,000) and coagulopathy. (c) Transfemoral digital subtraction angiography with the catheter in the brachial artery shows a hypervascular mass. (d) A capillary phase image shows marked enhancement. (e) After coil-embolization there is decreased vascularity prior to surgical resection.

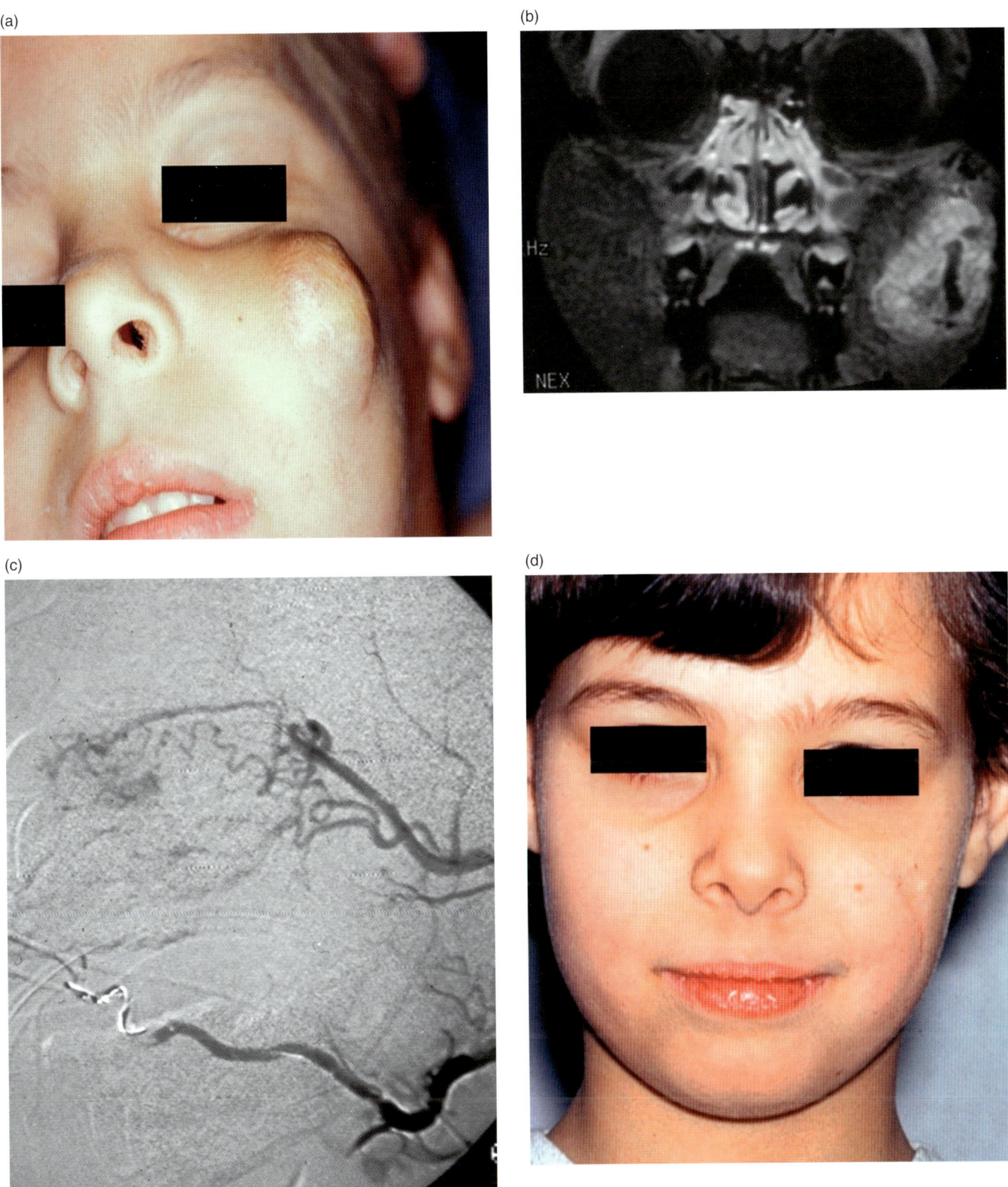

Figure 8.12 (a) A six-year-old female has a left cheek hemangioma with associated deformity. (b) Coronal T1 post-contrast MRI shows a homogeneously enhancing mass with large flow voids. (c) After coil and particle embolization the tumor vasculature is markedly reduced. (d) Photograph shows results after cosmetic repair at age eight.

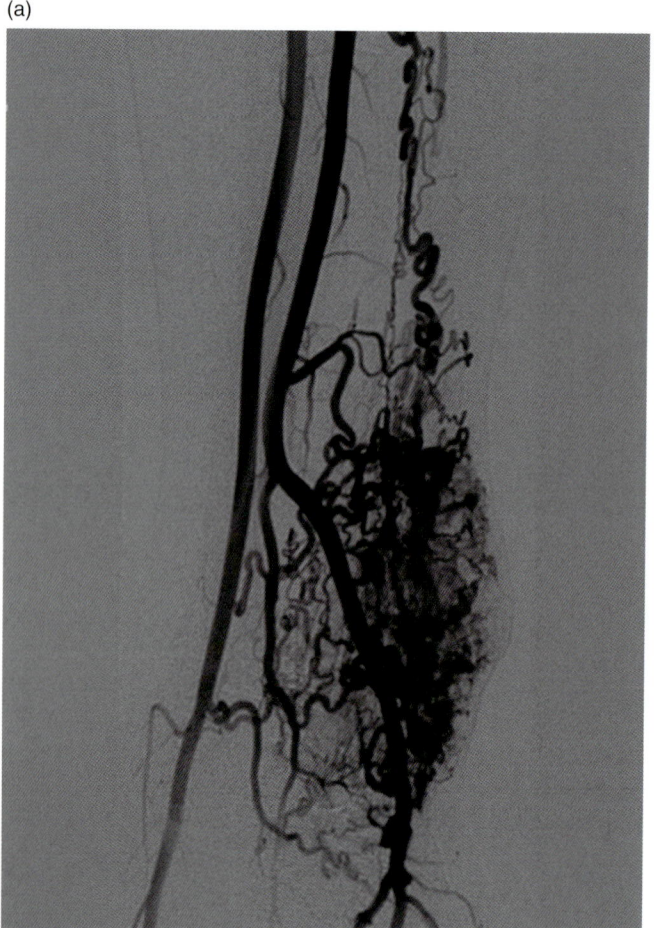
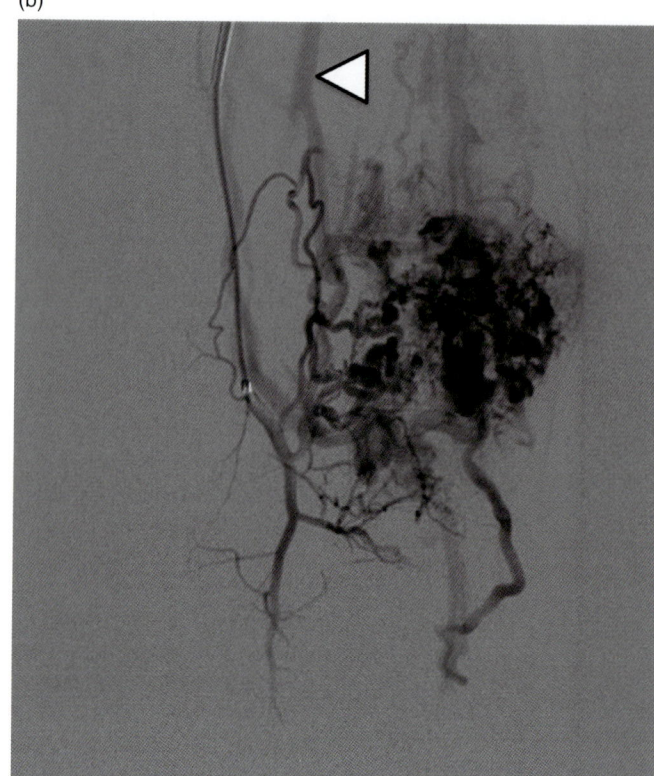
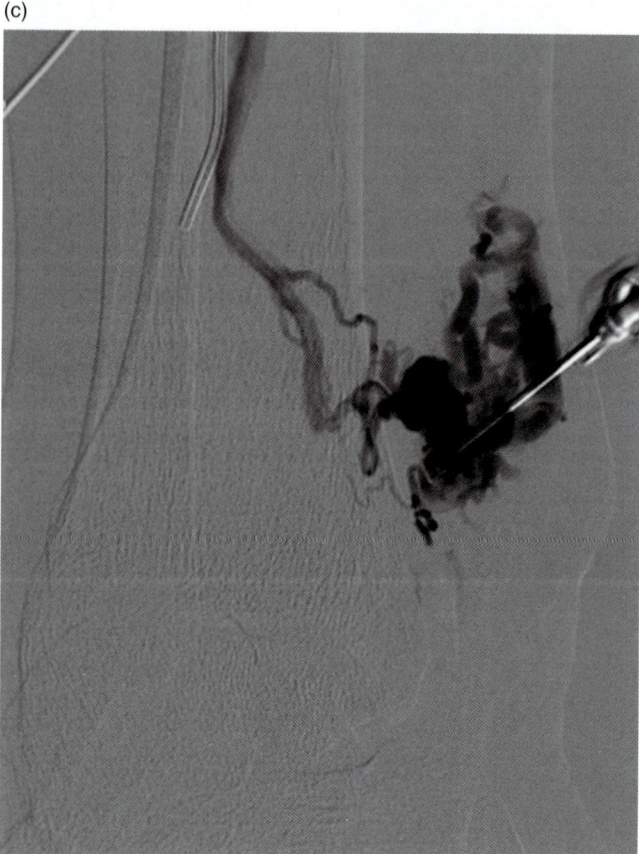

Figure 8.13 A 16-year-old female presenting with pain, ulceration, and bleeding at the right ankle. (a) A popliteal artery injection shows an AVM of the medial ankle primarily composed of arterioles with multiple arterial feeders. (b) A microcatheter positioned in the distal peroneal artery prior to ethanol injection shows arterial phase contrast with an early draining vein (*arrowhead*). (c) Contrast mixed with dehydrated alcohol is injected percutaneously directly into the nidus.

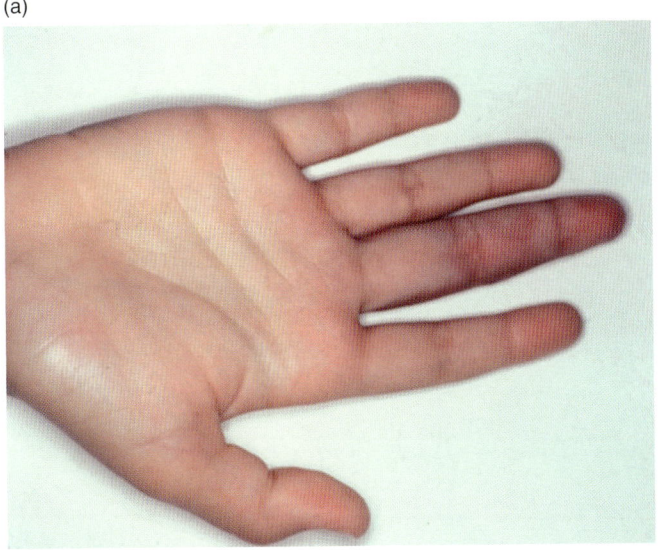
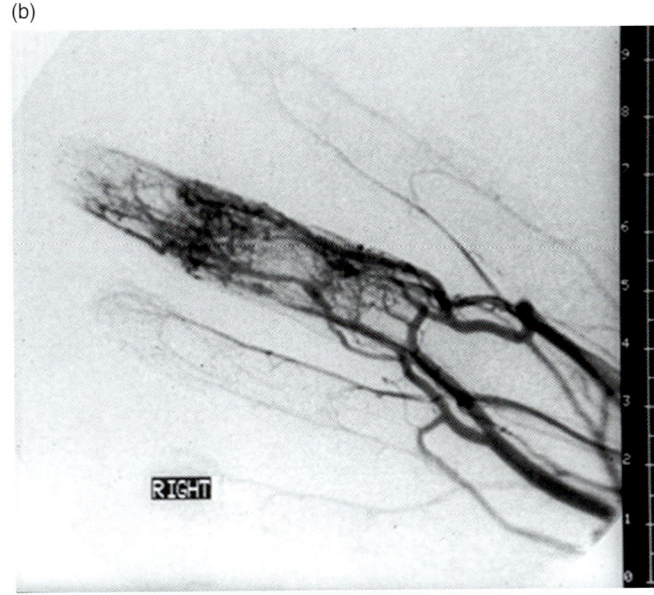
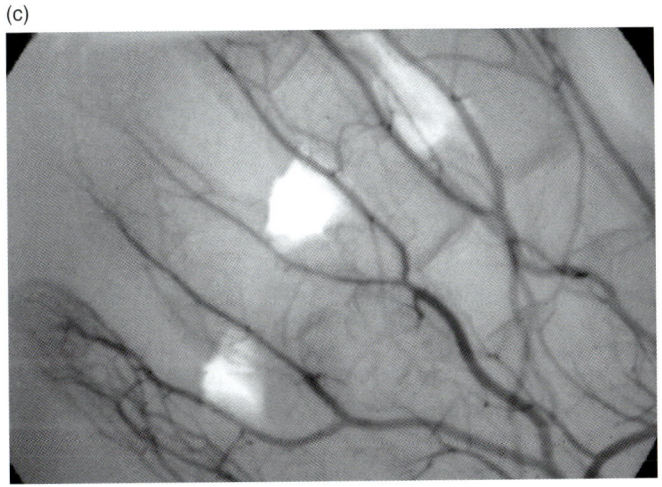

Figure 8.14 An eight-year-old male with finger claudication has had two surgical procedures for treatment of traumatic finger AVM. (a) The mildly cyanotic third finger shows fusiform enlargement. (b) Digital subtraction angiography shows enlarged medial second and lateral third common palmar arteries. Both third digit proper digital arteries are also enlarged and supply the AVM. Note segmental disruption of the lateral proper digital artery and poor supply to the tuft. (c) After direct alcohol injection into the AVM nidus no residual AVM is visualized, while the normal arterial supply is preserved.

and use of the most permanent material appropriate for the vascular territory, such as coils, glue, Onyx®, or 100% ethanol. Alternatively, in some situations, if ablation of the nidus cannot be achieved, an alternative approach is particulate embolization of feeding arteries followed by percutaneous puncture of the nidus and injection of liquid agents such as ethanol or tissue adhesive (Figure 8.14). More recently, occlusion of the proximal draining vein has also been utilized. For example, direct puncture has been shown to be highly successful in treating some endangering AVMs of the dental arcades, complicated by hemorrhage (Figure 8.5). In a few reported patients, radical intraosseous embolization with Onyx® has resulted in bony healing and apparent cure of the AVM without need for resection, considerably changing the approach to management of these lesions. Preoperative embolization prior to planned excision of the lesion should be more conservative, utilizing selective catheterization and embolization with small- or medium-sized particles. In some cases, coils may also be of use.

Arteriovenous fistulae

Arteriovenous fistulae (AVFs) may appear in isolation, in any part of the body, or in association with more complex AVMs. Because of the relative steal related to a large AVF, the concomitant presence of multiple AVFs in a complex malformation may not be revealed until the dominant fistula is occluded (Figures 8.3, 8.15). Arteriovenous fistulae occurring in isolation are usually diagnosed because of the presence of cardiac failure or cardiac overload, or following palpation of a thrill or auscultation of a bruit. Since these are curable lesions, and since they do not involute but often become larger and more symptomatic with age, it is appropriate to ablate them with transcatheter techniques, if possible, at the time of diagnosis. The goal of embolization is to occlude the fistulous connection and not simply the feeding artery. The latter approach may result in the development of collateral flow.

The delivery catheter should be placed within the fistula or within the vein immediately beyond the fistula. The most

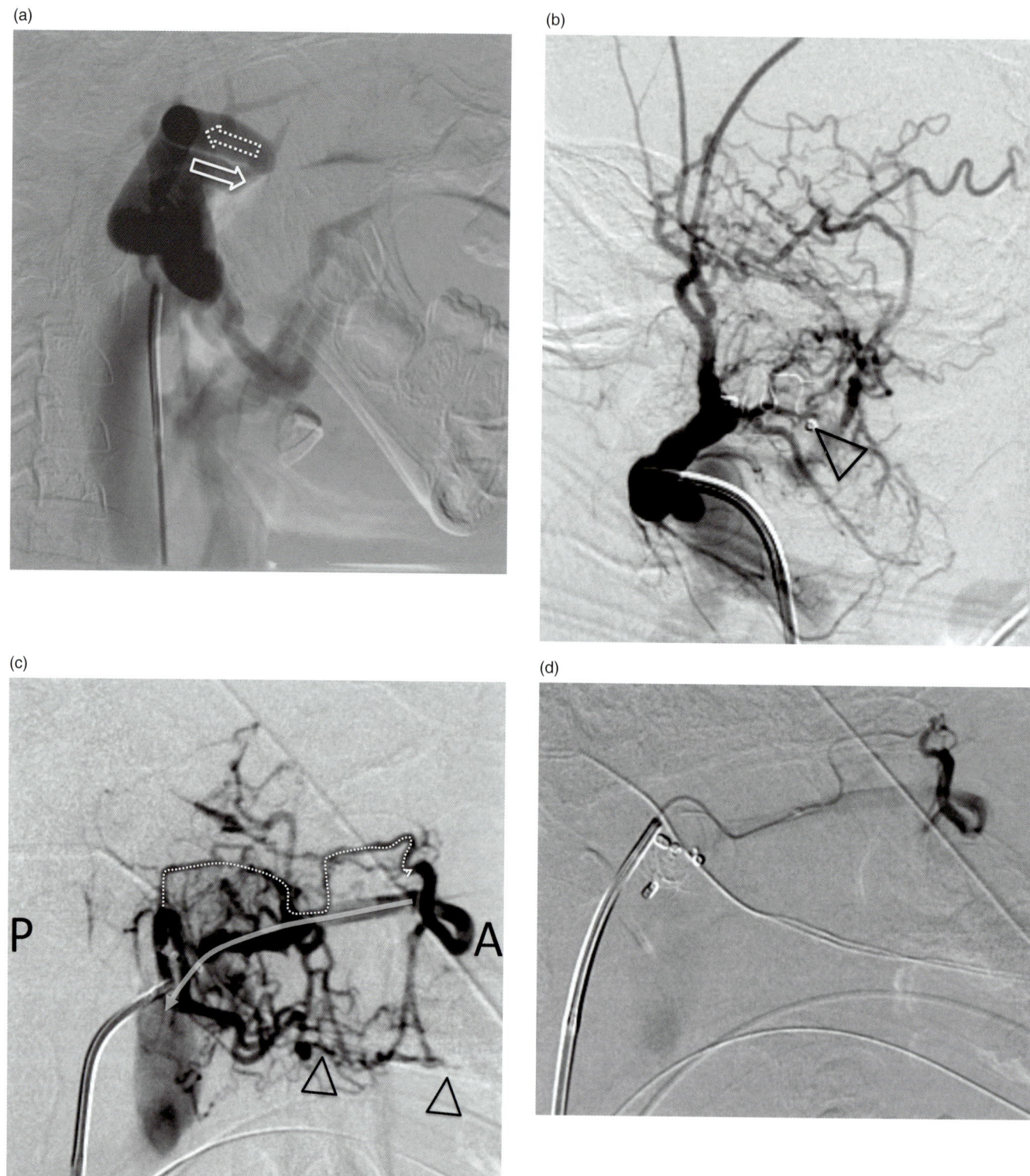

Figure 8.15 A nine-year-old male presented with an audible pulsatile mass in the right upper neck. (a) Arteriography shows a fistula between the right internal maxillary artery (*open arrow*) and the internal maxillary venous network (*dotted arrow*). (b) A 12 mm Amplatzer® vascular plug (*arrowhead*) was placed in the internal maxillary artery as close as possible to the fistula through a 6 French guide catheter by a transfemoral route. Occlusion of the low-resistance circuit revealed a complex AVM with AV fistulae. (c) After an additional plug was placed across the origin of the middle meningeal artery, a residual pterygopalatine arteriovenous fistula was visualized between a pterygoid canal arterial feeder (*dotted arrow*) and venous internal maxillary drainage (*solid arrow*) to the internal jugular vein. For orientation, the hard palate is indicated by *arrowheads*. (d) Onyx® 18 (ev3 Endovascular, Plymouth, MN) 6% ethylene vinyl alcohol copolymer liquid embolic agent was injected through a transarterial microcatheter until major palatine arterial branches were filling to the level of the hard palate, in an attempt to occlude the AV fistula. (e) After additional Onyx® administration into the proximal internal maxillary artery and feeding branches of the facial artery, the AVM was controlled to the point that palpable and (to the patient) audible pulsatility was absent.

(e)

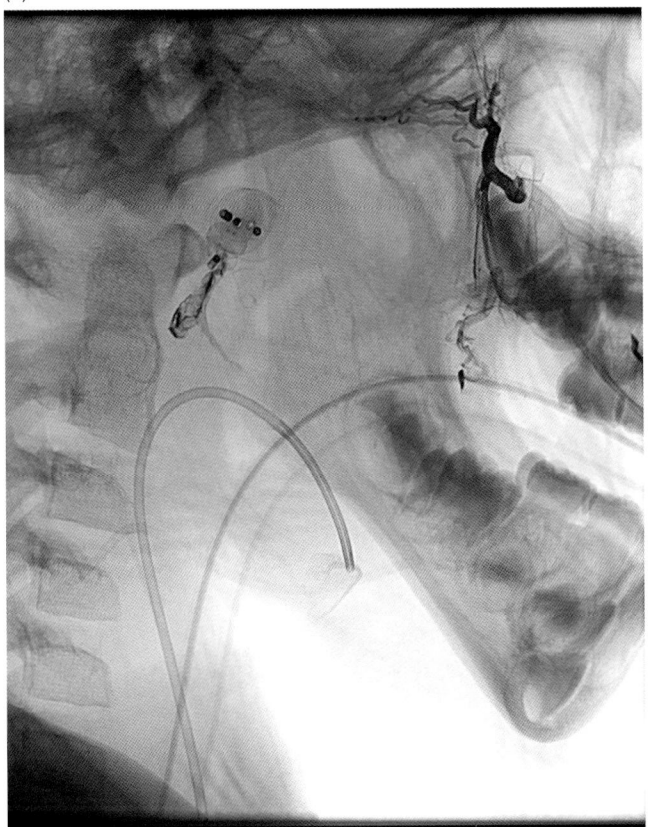

Figure 8.15 (cont.)

appropriate occlusion device will depend upon the size of the fistula and the diameter and length of the feeding artery proximal to the fistula. Vascular plugs, detachable balloons, coils, and tissue adhesive have all been used successfully. The development of vascular plugs and cardiac devices such as double clam-shell occlusion devices has provided more flexibility to treat these malformations, especially those with very large vessels (Figure 8.16). Platinum microcoils may be too soft and malleable for high-flow fistulae, thus the heavier and sturdier stainless steel and retrievable coils and vascular plugs are useful. Flow control techniques that permit accurate placement of the device and prevent migration of the material through the arteriovenous shunt include the use of a proximal occlusion balloon, a distal occlusion balloon, or a microsnare, introduced through the venous system.

Systemic pulmonary arterial supply

Systemic arterial supply to the lungs may arise from a variety of sources, including brachiocephalic arteries, coronary arteries, the ascending or descending thoracic aorta, abdominal aorta, celiac axis, or renal arteries. The central and systemic pulmonary circulation should be carefully mapped out. If possible, systemic arterial embolization should be performed in such a way as to result in all of the bronchopulmonary segmental vessels having communication with the central pulmonary arteries. Embolization of systemic arteries to lung segments that do not have dual arterial supply may result in pulmonary infarction. This outcome should be weighed against the clinical situation. Lesions such as pulmonary sequestration and scimitar syndrome usually do not have dual supply, but embolization of the systemic artery may be appropriate in order to alleviate congestive heart failure, pulmonary hypertension, hemoptysis, or other clinical symptoms. The most frequently used embolic devices for occlusion of systemic arteries to the lungs are stainless steel/fiber coils and more recently vascular plugs (Figure 8.17), although detachable balloons, Onyx®, and tissue adhesive have also been used successfully. Occlusion balloons may also be helpful in accurately deploying the embolic devices.

Pulmonary arteriovenous malformations

Pulmonary arteriovenous malformations (PAVMs) or pulmonary arteriovenous fistulae (PAVFs) may result in hemoptysis or more frequently cyanosis, CNS infection, or thromboembolism related to the loss of the pulmonary vascular filter effect of the normal capillary bed. When possible, embolotherapy is preferred to surgical resection, especially in children with multiple lesions due to the association with hereditary hemorrhagic telangiectasia (HHT). It is important to assess for additional AVMs involving the CNS and GI systems. It is particularly useful to evaluate the brain since lesions may be asymptomatic. Gastrointestinal bleeding and epistaxis are also commonly associated. In children with syndromes, and those with multiple lesions, it is possible that additional lesions will develop with time, making preservation of lung tissue important. In rare cases, the large number of lesions makes embolotherapy impossible, leaving lung transplantation as the only viable therapeutic option. Since HHT is a familial condition, it is important to evaluate family members for the condition.

Pulmonary arteriovenous malformations may be simple, consisting of a single feeding artery and draining vein, or complex, consisting of a plexiform nidus. The goal of embolization should be to ablate the arteriovenous connection, but precautions must be taken to prevent migration of the device, air, or clot through the fistula into the distal vascular bed. In general, lesions with feeding arteries >3 mm are considered for treatment. Vascular plugs, detachable balloons, and coils have been used successfully to treat these lesions. The use of a balloon occlusion catheter during coil deployment may decrease the likelihood of untoward effects. Postprocedural follow-up should consist of chest radiography and intermittent high-resolution CT scans to confirm occlusion of the treated PAVM or PAVF and to exclude the development of new lesions.

Chemoembolization of hepatic tumors

Hepatic chemoembolization (HCE) and ablative techniques have been used to treat adults with primary and metastatic

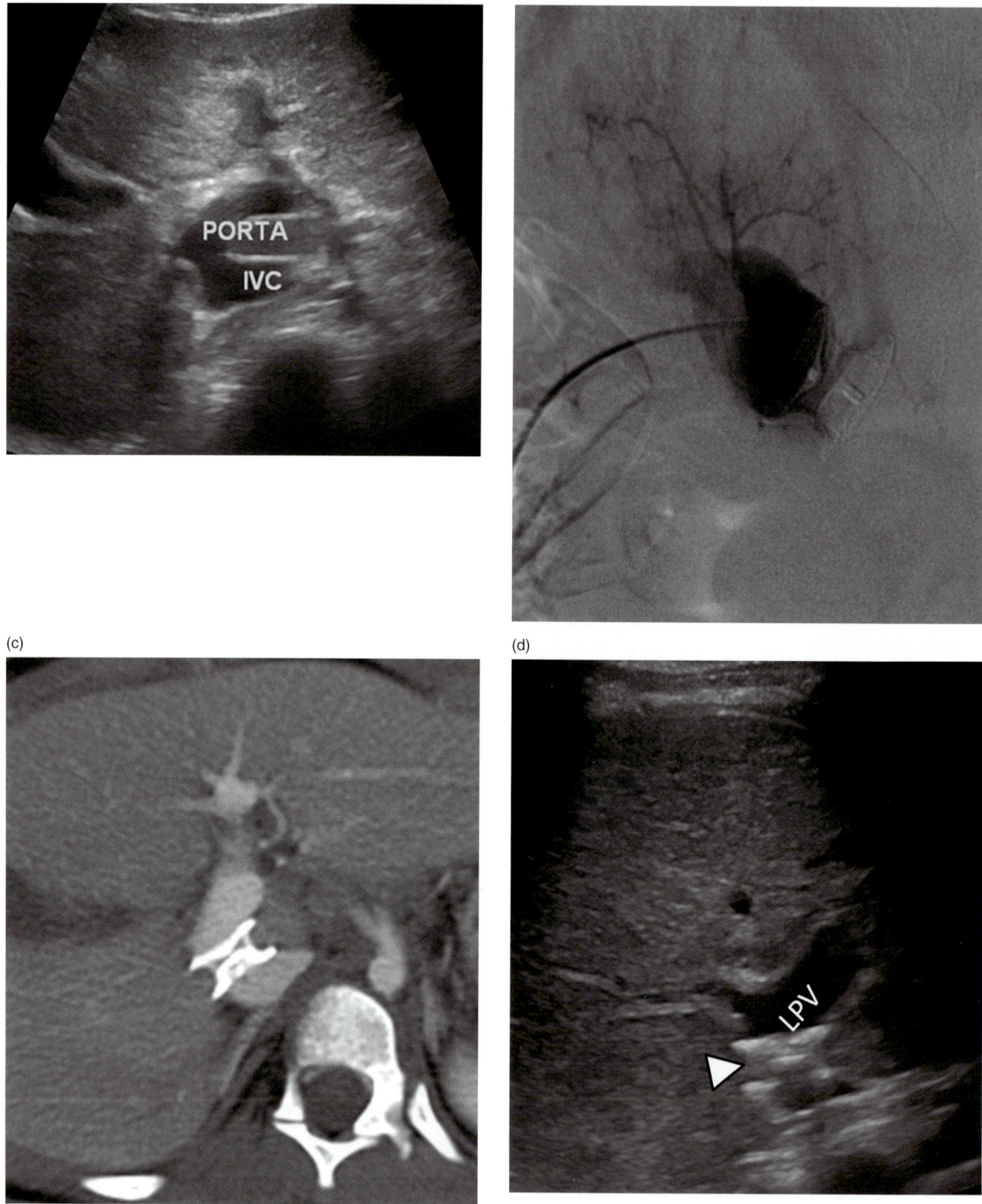

Figure 8.16 An eight-year-old female with trisomy-21 presented with digital clubbing after an episode of gastrointestinal hemorrhage. (a) Transverse US shows a type II Abernathy malformation (congenital portosystemic shunt). (b) A transhepatic portal vein catheter was used to deploy a 14 mm clam-shell ASD closure device. (c,d) Computed tomography and US imaging demonstrate fistulous closure by the clam-shell device (*arrowhead*) and intrahepatic portal vein (*LPV*) flow.

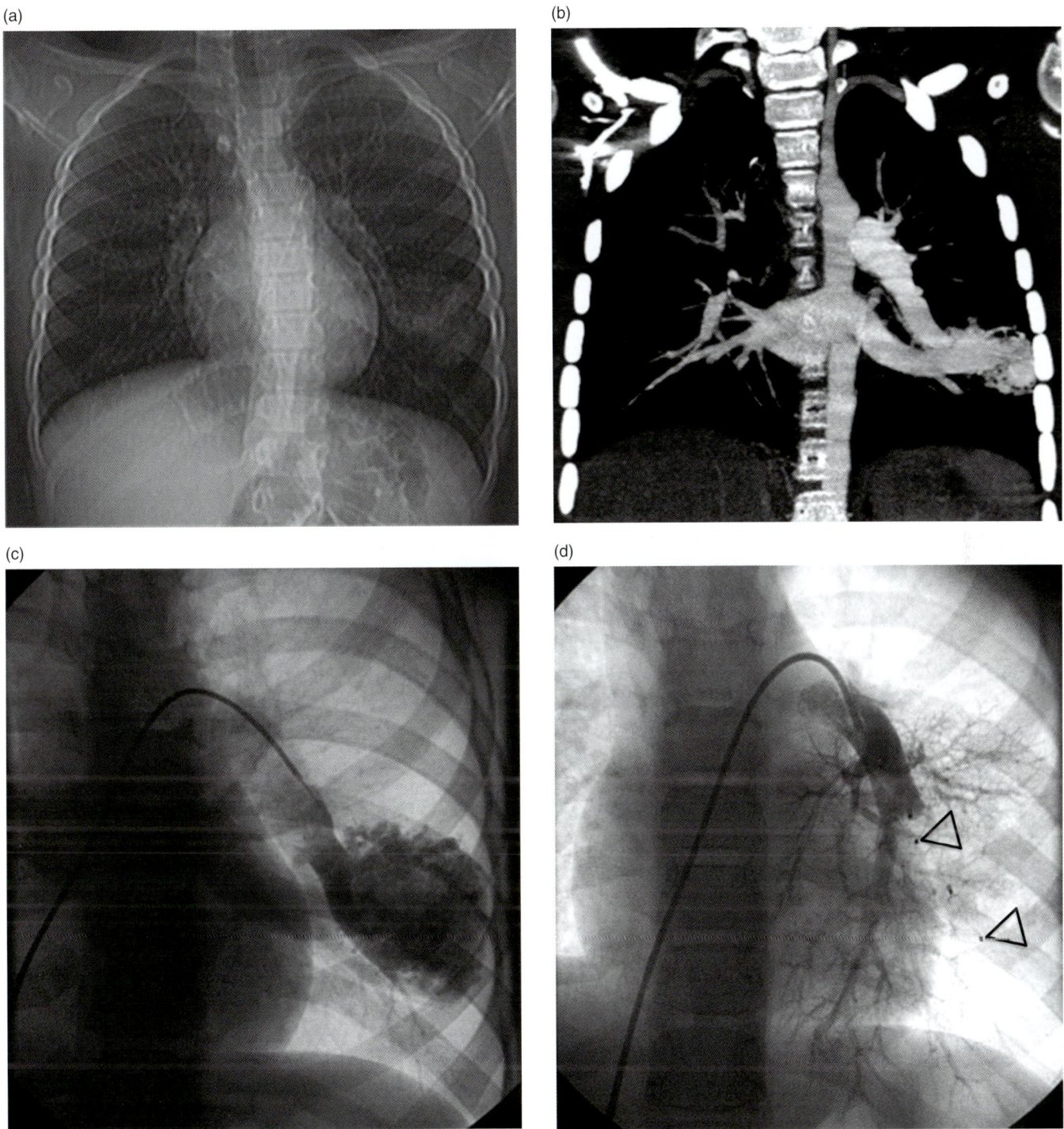

Figure 8.17 (a) A nine-year-old female had hypoxemia and "pneumonia" on a chest radiograph. (b) A coronal reconstruction from a CT angiogram shows a large left pulmonary AVM. (c) An arteriogram performed through a catheter in the left pulmonary artery shows a lower lobe pulmonary AVM with an 11 mm feeding artery. (d) Deployment of two Amplatzer® plugs (*arrowheads*) successfully occluded the AVM.

hepatic neoplasms. In children, HCE and on occasion, ablative techniques have been used for the treatment of primary neoplasms. Hepatic chemoembolization may be used as an adjunct to systemic chemotherapy in the hope that the tumor may become resectable, since the possibility of cure depends on complete resection of the neoplasm. Children with unresectable lesions and those who have failed systemic chemotherapy may be treated with a combination of HCE and liver transplantation, if the tumor responds to treatment and does not spread outside of the liver (Figure 8.18). Hepatic chemoembolization generally involves selectively infusing the hepatic arteries and, on occasion, individual portal veins, with

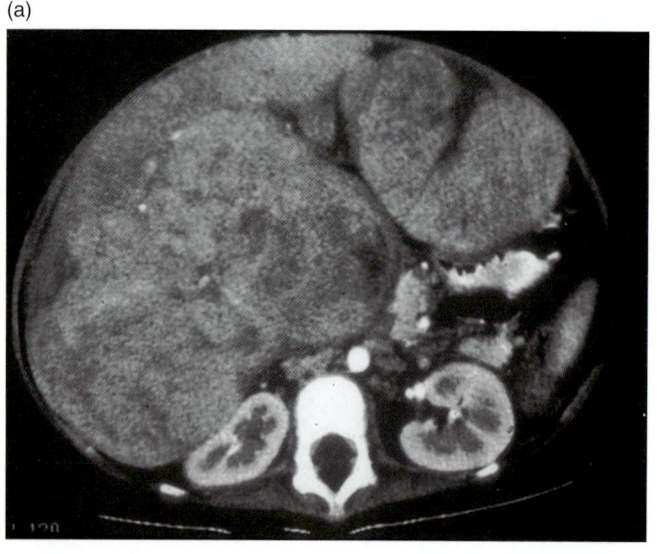
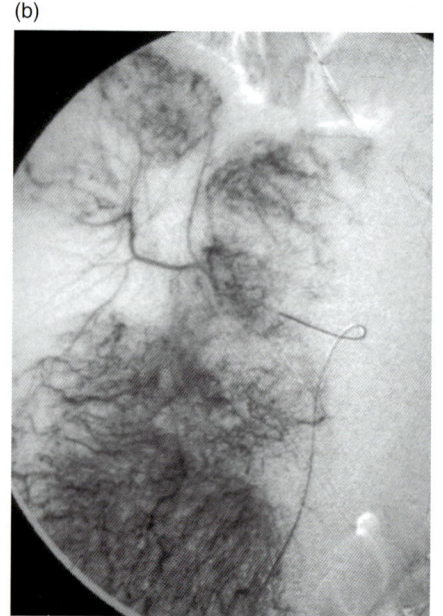
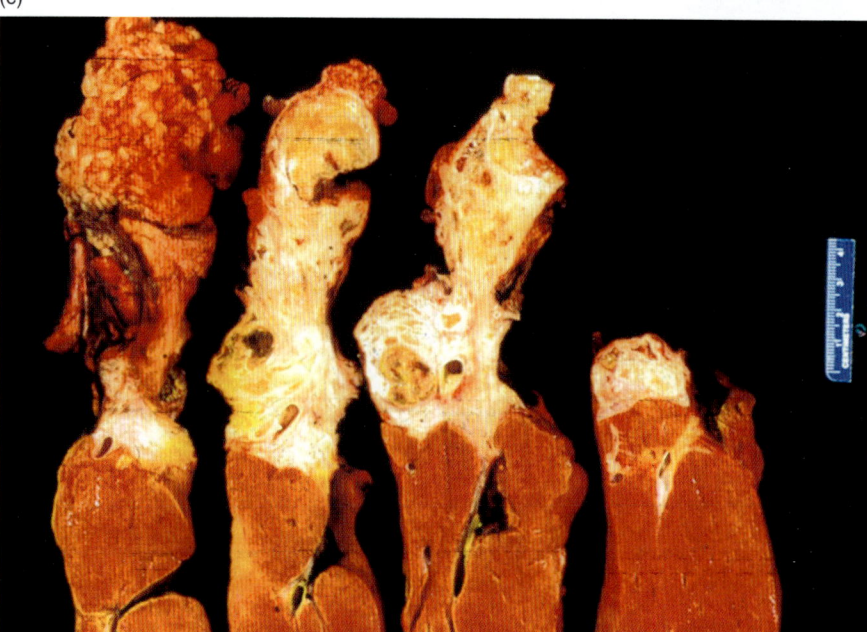

Figure 8.18 A four-year-old female presented with diffuse unresectable hepatocellular carcinoma. She required tumor reduction to qualify for transplantation. (a) Contrast-enhanced abdominal CT with diffuse nodular tumor. (b) Selective hepatic artery catheterization with multiple hypervascular hepatic lesions. (c) Explanted liver shows tumor necrosis after chemoembolization.

a chemotherapeutic agent, combined with an angiostatic agent, such as Gelfoam® or Ethiodol®. The choice of embolic agent is important. The goal of HCE is to temporarily occlude the hepatic artery in order to: (1) increase the dwell time of the chemotherapeutic drug(s) at the tumor site, (2) allow the hepatic artery to recanalize so that the treatment can be repeated at intervals dictated by the clinical protocol, imaging, and follow-up laboratory studies, especially alpha-fetoprotein, and (3) maximize the drug levels directly to the tumor, often greater than 10,000 higher tumoral concentration compared to systemic levels. The main pediatric indications for treatment are hepatocellular carcinoma and hepatoblastoma. However, the technique has also been used in patients with metastatic endocrine tumors.

Bronchial artery embolization

In the pediatric population, hemoptysis is most often secondary to pulmonary inflammation (e.g., cystic fibrosis), which may be associated with bronchial artery hypertrophy and intermittent bleeding. Alternatively, spontaneous bronchial artery to pulmonary artery fistulae, bronchial arterial hypertrophy in the presence of cyanotic congenital heart disease, or isolated systemic arterial supply to the lungs may also result in hemoptysis. In many patients, active bleeding is not identified at the time embolotherapy is considered. We have found that older children may be able to point to an area on their chest wall that corresponds to the site of pulmonary bleeding when asked. In these instances, if abnormal bronchial vessels or collaterals are identified in the predicted area in the absence of active bleeding, they are embolized. As is the case for other vascular interventions, prior to embolotherapy diagnostic angiography is performed to confirm the diagnosis and to plan therapy. In general, digital subtraction thoracic aortography is the initial study followed by selective bronchial artery injections. Selective bronchial artery injections are necessary to carefully examine the vascular territory in search for branches supplying the spinal cord. The artery of Adamkiewicz is the largest of the segmental arteries supplying the spinal cord and can be identified by its characteristic hairpin bend. The artery most often arises from the left side of the thoracic aorta at the level of T10; however, its position may vary from T7 to L4. It is right sided in 17% of patients. Regardless of the site of origin, it usually enters a single intervertebral foramen between T9 and T11. If spinal branches are identified, embolization may still be performed if the catheter can be positioned distal to the origin of the spinal branch. On occasion, it may be necessary to study other vascular territories such as the innominate artery and its branches, as they may be the source of the abnormal blood supply.

Regardless of the vascular pathology, treatment consists of selective embolization of the abnormal bronchial arteries and of any enlarged bronchial collateral arteries that can be identified. Patients with cystic fibrosis usually have multiple bronchial artery collaterals. The true bronchial arteries should be catheterized as distally as possible, and we prefer to occlude them with medium- to large-sized particles (>700 micron) or coils. Collaterals to the bronchial arteries should also be embolized if appropriate (the presence of spinal arterial supply or other CNS anastomoses should be sought for carefully prior to embolizing the bronchial artery collaterals). In patients without a history of cystic fibrosis, the technique is similar, although the lung from which the bleeding has originated may be known, and thus limit the extent of the procedure.

Arterial trauma

Embolization may be indicated to treat dissection or false aneurysms arising from major arteries or branches (Figure 8.19). In the case of dissection of major vessels, such as vertebral or carotid arteries, sacrifice of the parent artery may be appropriate in the presence of thromboembolic disease not responding to anticoagulation, or in the presence of contraindications to anticoagulation, if there is high risk of CNS complications, providing there is adequate natural or surgical collateral supply. Although there is no experience to guide therapy, in these rare circumstances, it may be appropriate to consider the alternative of placement of a vascular stent. Bleeding from peripheral arterial branches responds well to embolization. The appropriate device/material utilized depends upon the vessel involved. Coils are useful in this setting.

Children are susceptible to motor vehicle accidents, all-terrain vehicle injuries (since underage children can drive these machines in rural settings), sports injuries, and falls from heights including horses. These injuries often result in isolated or multiorgan injuries such as skeletal injuries or chest or abdominopelvic organ injuries. Erosion of vessels from mechanical abrasion or inflammation and infection may also result in significant hemorrhage (Figure 8.20). If there is significant hemorrhage with the need for repeated transfusions, threatened exsanguinating hemorrhage, or in patients who are not good candidates for surgical therapy, interventional solutions may be indicated.

Children may also sustain blunt perineal injuries from falls onto playground equipment. On occasion, this results in high-flow priapism. We have treated several children with priapism and found that it responds well to embolization of the internal pudendal or common penile artery using temporary agents, such as Gelfoam® or autologous blood clot.

Partial splenic embolization

Hypersplenism secondary to a variety of causes may be treated by subtotal embolization of the spleen. The effects of partial splenic embolization (PSE) are to improve platelet and white blood cell counts, reduce spleen size, and to decrease variceal bleeding and ascites due to portal hypertension. Partial splenic embolization involves selective catheterization of the splenic artery distal to the short gastric and pancreatic branches and embolizing 30 to 60% of the parenchymal branches. Although a variety of materials may be utilized, we prefer to use large PVA particles or Embospheres® (>700 microns) for vessel occlusion (Figure 8.21). Complications include pancreatitis, splenic abscess, and splenic vein thrombosis. The procedure is often followed by significant postembolization pain. (See Chapter 5 for a more detailed description of the procedure.)

Renal ablation

In the absence of renal carcinoma in the pediatric population, renal ablation is rarely indicated. However, ablation of part or all of the renal parenchyma by catheter embolization has been carried out in children with proteinuria, hypertension related to end-stage renal disease, or to treat hypertension secondary to segmental renal artery stenosis or occlusion, not amenable to balloon angioplasty. Total renal ablation (medical nephrectomy) is usually performed by embolization of the renal artery distal to the adrenal branches using 100% ethanol. Some interventionalists prefer to use a balloon occlusion catheter when injecting absolute alcohol to avoid reflux of the alcohol outside of the renal vascular bed. Unfortunately, the size of the balloon catheter precludes its use in many children. The volume of ethanol is best determined by contrast injection on pretreatment angiography. Renal ablation is followed by significant postembolization pain, fever (usually less than 38.9°C), and

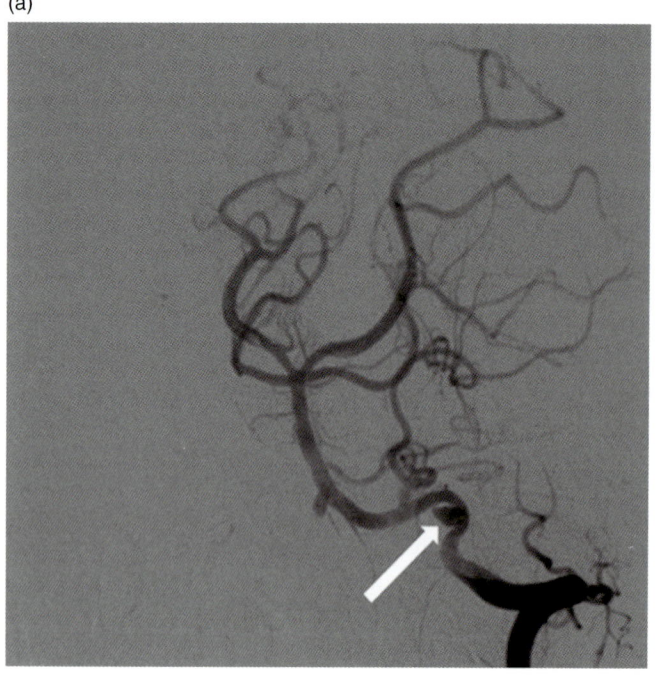
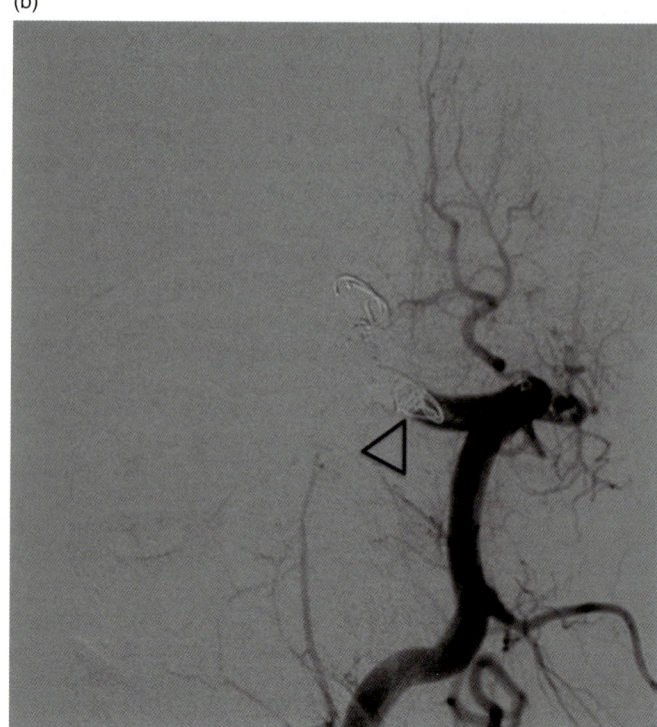
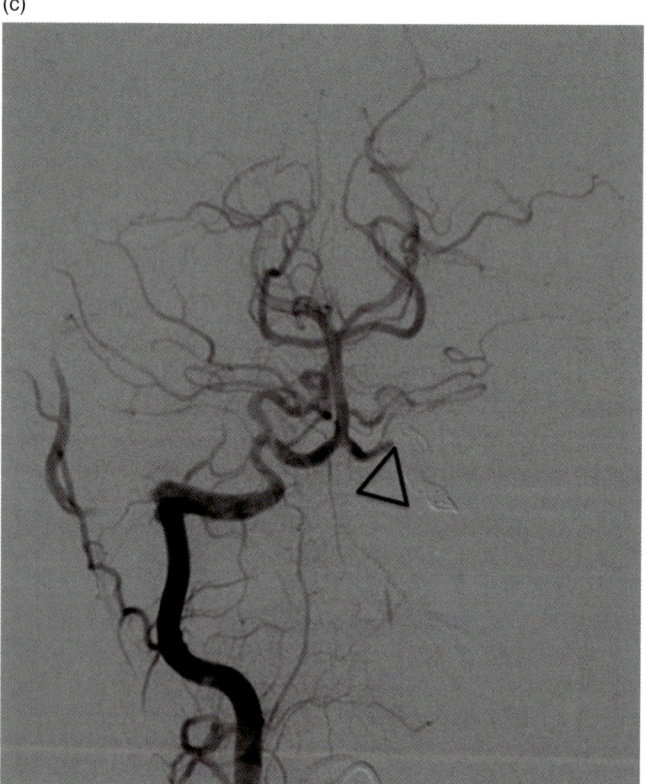

Figure 8.19 A 16-year-old male presented with loss of consciousness after head trauma. (a) A left vertebral artery injection demonstrates an aneurysm of the V4 segment (*arrow*) of the left vertebral artery. (b) Post-coil embolization (*arrowhead*) trapping aneurysm. (c) Right vertebral injection showing coiled aneurysm (*arrowhead*) without "back door" filling.

leukocytosis, and may be complicated by renal abscess. A fatal outcome has also been reported.

Segmental renal artery embolization may be performed using 100% ethanol, although microcoils may also be successful. Since the branch is generally too small to dilate with a balloon catheter, a microcatheter is generally positioned in the abnormal segmental renal artery and ethanol injected selectively.

Chapter 8 Vascular interventions

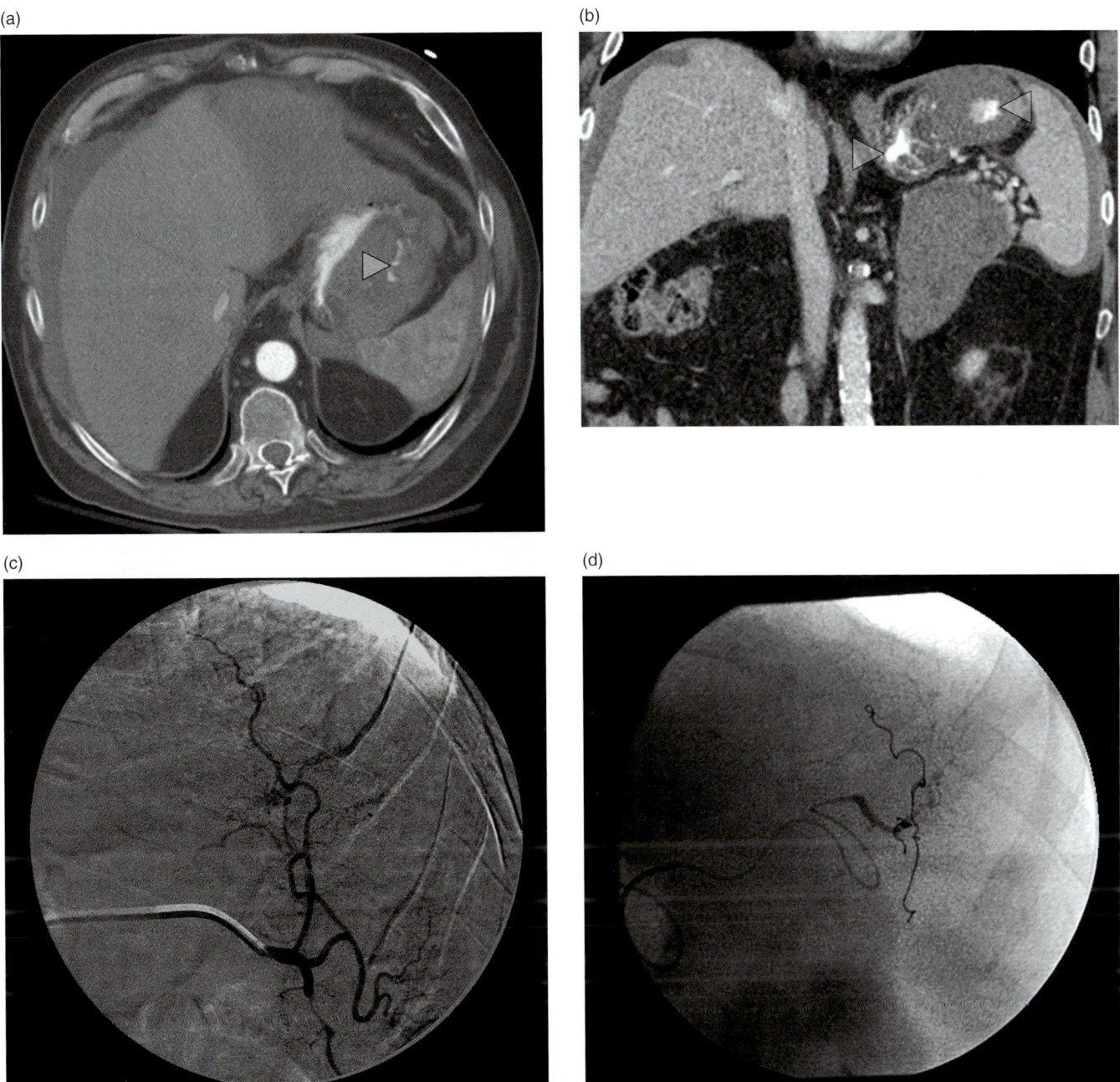

Figure 8.20 An older patient with chronic pancreatitis has become acutely anemic. (a) Axial CT of the abdomen with vascular contrast enhancement shows acute arterial-phase hemorrhage in the left upper quadrant, with extensive extracapsular hematoma. (b) Coronal reconstruction from the same CT acquisition shows acute arterial hemorrhage related to peripancreatic inflammation in a region normally supplied by splenic artery branches. (c) Splenic arteriography shows irregular vessels and hemorrhage in terminal splenic arterial branches. (d) After subselective coil embolization, no further hemorrhage was detected and the patient stabilized.

Technical variations

Neonatal embolization

Embolization in a neonate is a unique and difficult challenge that requires a more careful and measured approach when compared to that in larger children. When considering this subpopulation, it is important to keep in mind some of the issues that affect these small patients. Neonates have very little subcutaneous fat and may get hypothermic quickly. Therefore it is essential that their body temperature remains constant. To achieve this, they should be on a heating system such as the Bair Hugger™. Also, since their head sizes are relatively large relatively to their bodies, the head is a significant source of heat loss. Therefore insulating a neonate's head is a necessity. In addition, they need to remain dry throughout the procedure, and the interventionalist must be aware of fluids being infused. It may be necessary to warm fluids such as blood transfusions. Another issue is their small total blood volume. The average

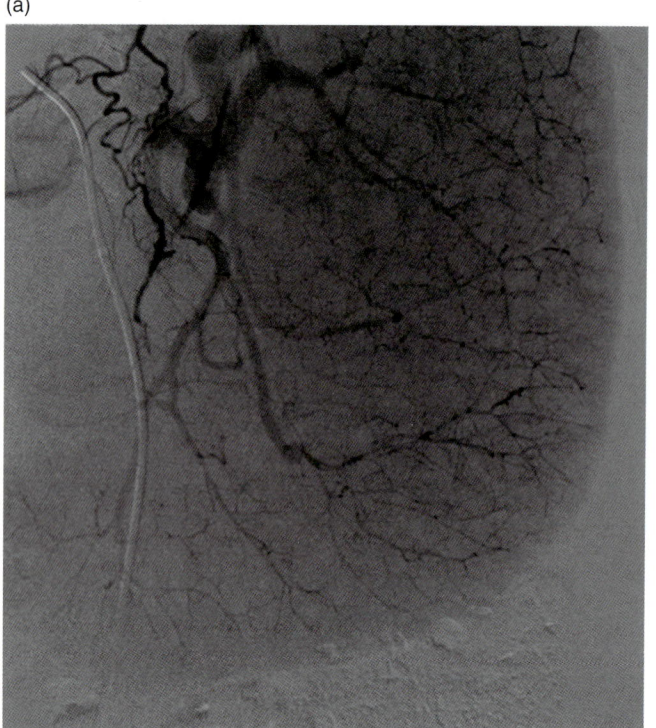
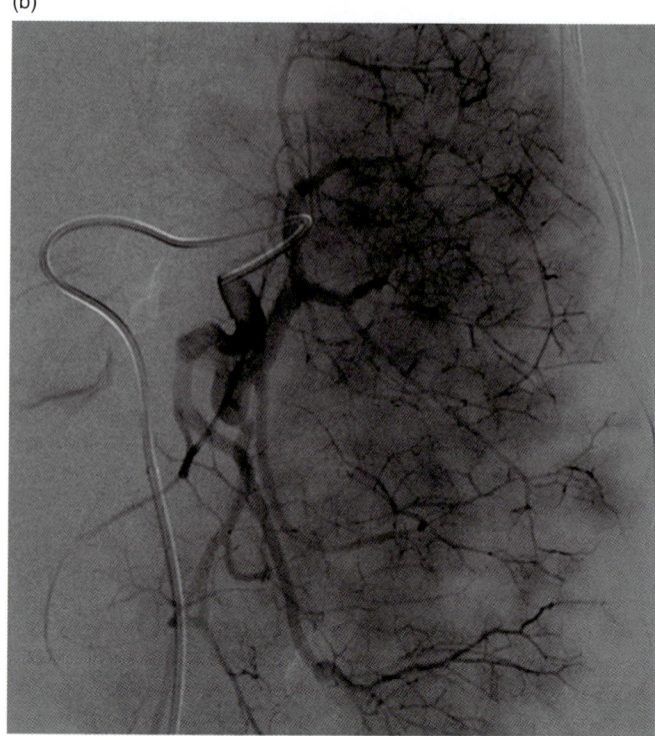
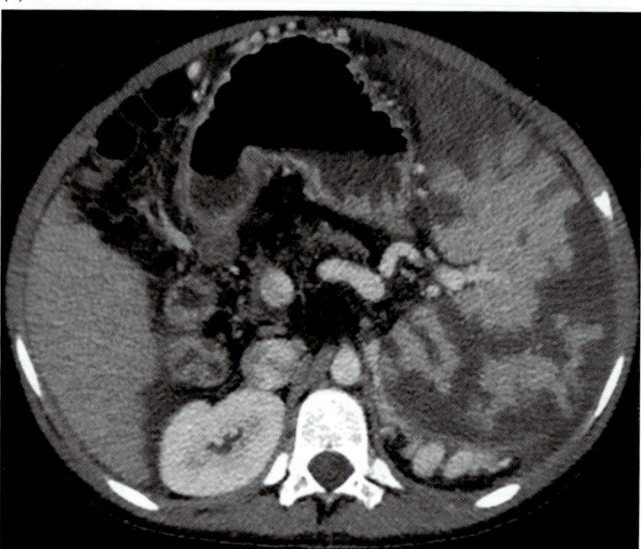

Figure 8.21 A 15-year-old female presented with cystic fibrosis, hypersplenism, and sequestration with pancytopenia for partial splenic embolization. (a,b) Pre- and post-Embosphere® (700 micron) embolization shows patchy peripheral infarctions. (c) Axial contrast-enhanced abdominal CT obtained one week later showing approximately 60% splenic embolization.

blood volume in a term infant is about 85 ml/kg. To calculate the total blood volume, you multiply (average blood volume) × (weight in kg). Therefore, as an example, a 5 kg neonate is expected to have a total blood volume of 425 ml. With this knowledge, it becomes clear that infants are at risk for fluid overload or loss. A blood loss of 15% (e.g., in this example only 64 ml) can put the child into shock. A significant increase in volume, especially if the solution is hyperosmotic, can result in acute right heart failure and pulmonary edema. To minimize these risks, we strongly recommend that when a neonatal vascular intervention is performed, all 10 ml syringes should be replaced with 3 ml or 5 ml syringes. A Foley catheter should be inserted and urine output monitored and a running total volume kept of all fluids infused. The difference between the input and output should be actively managed. In many cases, the procedure may need to be discontinued if the total volumes become too high.

Another important consideration in this subgroup is equipment selection (Table 8.8). In neonates with high-flow lesions, the distal aorta and iliac arteries are often smaller than normal because they are distal to the run-off vessels. We strongly recommend that the interventionalist uses the

Table 8.8 Equipment: neonatal arterial embolization

- Neonatal umbilical artery placement set 3.5 French to 5 French umbilical artery catheter, iris scissors, variety of specialized pick-ups, vessel finders, dilators, etc. (UAC kit)
- Umbilical tape
- 3–0 suture for counter-traction
- 4 French sheath with hemostasis valves (7 cm or longer if available)
- 4 French directional catheters (e.g., JB-1, RC, RIM, C1)
- Guide wires: 0.018-inch and 0.035-inch; angled Glidewire®, Newton
- Variable stiffness microcatheters
- 0.012-inch and 0.014-inch microwires
- 0.018-inch microcoil selection (e.g., Hilal 0.5 cm, 1.0 cm, complex coils especially 2 mm × 2 cm)
- Embospheres®
- Onyx®/glue
- Heparin 50 to 75 units/kg

smallest possible catheter or sheath in the femoral vessels and, when possible, the umbilical artery should be used for procedural access. The umbilical artery is a non-essential artery and will normally disappear shortly after birth. In sick neonates, umbilical arteries (UAs) and umbilical veins (UVs) are often catheterized by neonatologists for monitoring and drug therapy. The advantage of using the UA for intra-arterial interventions is that one may insert larger sheaths and catheters. The disadvantage is that it is a rarely used vessel and requires some special treatment to be utilized effectively. In general, we use a 4 French sheath with a hemostasis valve and a 4 French directional catheter with a 0.035-inch lumen so that microcatheters can be used coaxially. We do not routinely heparinize children with UA access. At the completion of the procedure, the UAC can be replaced. If the UA cannot be catheterized, the femoral artery is accessed. The initial arterial puncture is performed with US guidance using a micropuncture set. Once arterial access has been achieved, a 4 French directional catheter (usually a JB-1) is inserted in lieu of a sheath with hemostasis valve. The insertion of a sheath is avoided since the outer diameter of a 4 French sheath is almost 6 French and would occlude most common femoral arteries in neonates. The 4 French catheter dually serves as a sheath substitute and a guide/diagnostic catheter. Also, as a general rule, all children less than 10 kg are heparinized at 50 to 75 units/kg every two hours for the duration of the procedure.

In general, unless the interventionalist has training inserting UACs, it is probably best to ask a neonatologist to insert a UAC in any neonate that may need a vascular intervention to preserve access. In the IR suite, after the site is prepared and draped in sterile fashion, the UAC is removed over a guide wire. To assist catheter insertion, two anchor sutures are placed into the lateral margin of the umbilical stump for counter-traction when inserting the sheath. Special care needs to be taken if a 0.035-inch Glidewire® is used since the wire may unexpectedly spring out of the vessel during the exchange. An alternate strategy is to use a 0.035-inch Newton wire or 0.018-inch wire for this purpose. Selecting a sheath that will be long enough to traverse into the mid or distal aorta is helpful. Remember that the UA is a branch of the internal iliac artery, so that a UA catheter will course inferiorly from the umbilicus before curving superiorly through the iliac arteries to the abdominal aorta. This downward direction of the UA leads to added challenge in directing catheters in some instances. Once the sheath is in position, it is either sutured in place or secured with a Tegaderm® or Opsite® dressing. At this point, a selective catheter can be inserted into the aorta via the sheath, and the procedure can proceed in the usual fashion. If the UA is not available, then a standard US-guided puncture of the common femoral artery is performed.

Postprocedure and follow-up care

Following embolotherapy, children must be observed for tissue ischemia in addition to the general effects of vascular interventional procedures. Corticosteroids are routinely used in some practices and may be administered during the procedure, and also orally, in a tapering dose for approximately one week following the therapy. Steroids appear to be useful in diminishing postembolization pain. Appropriate analgesics should be ordered as needed. We have found Toradol® (ketorolac tromethamine), an NSAID, to be as effective as opioid analgesics and is worth using in cases of severe postprocedural discomfort. Toradol® may be given orally, intravenously, or intramuscularly, and oral therapy should not be used for more than five consecutive days. Intravenous administration is suggested in the immediate postprocedural period. The recommended dosage is; 0.5 mg/kg followed by bolus injection of 1.0 mg/kg q 6 h or infusion at 0.17 mg/kg/h. The maximum daily dosage is 90 mg, and maximum duration of therapy is seven days. The drug is not recommended in children younger than one year of age. Toradol® does not depress respiration, cause nausea or vomiting, urinary retention, or sedation, as do narcotic analgesics.

An increasing number of cases are being performed on an outpatient basis, especially in those children who have congenital vascular lesions but are otherwise well. These patients are observed for approximately six hours prior to discharge. In the absence of complications, they are discharged to home and followed up by telephone the next day. To date, this approach has proved to be safe and cost effective.

Technical problems and pitfalls

Arterial spasm is the most common hindrance to successful embolization. It is best avoided by using soft, small catheter systems and minimal manipulation. Calcium channel blockers, hypercarbia, and intra-arterial nitroglycerine and other vasodilators may be helpful in avoiding or reversing vasospasm.

Migration of material or devices used for embolotherapy can occur if not appropriately sized, or if flow control techniques are not used. In the case of coils, retrieval devices (e.g., snares) should be on hand to treat this complication if it occurs. Passage of excessive amounts of embolic material through AV shunts to the pulmonary circulation can result in severe pulmonary hypertension, especially in neonates, and in the presence of a patent foramen ovale, can lead to coronary artery or other systemic or cerebral artery embolization. Thus care should be taken to understand the type of malformation being treated and to minimize the use of particulate material in lesions with minimal stroma or rapid AV shunting. If uncertain about the lesion, coils or other devices may be preferred.

Complications

Tissue ischemia caused by non-target vascular occlusion is the most serious postembolization complication. Other potential problems include femoral artery thrombosis, pseudoaneurysm, vessel perforation, fluid overload with associated right heart failure and pulmonary edema, pressure sores, and radiation burns. Hemoglobinuria, cardiopulmonary complications, skin necrosis, and nerve injury may occur with the use of ethanol.

Sclerotherapy

Introduction

Vascular malformations have been classified by the International Society for the Study of Vascular Anomalies (ISSVA). The ISSVA classification divides vascular anomalies into vasoproliferative or vascular neoplasms and vascular malformations. The vasoproliferative lesions include infantile hemangiomas (IHs), congenital hemangiomas (RICH or NICH lesions), Kaposiform hemangioendotheliomas (with or without Kasabach–Merritt syndrome), spindle cell hemangioma, epitheliod hemangioendothelioma, and angiosarcoma. In general, IHs usually present between two weeks to two months of life and undergo a proliferative phase that will last months to years. Infantile hemangiomas will then begin to involute and reduce in size. In the past, many of these patients were treated with steroids or interferon and, in some patients, embolization. Today, beta-blockers are the primary medical therapy, with embolization and surgery reserved for unresponsive lesions, complicated hemangiomas, or those with persistent cosmetic issues.

In contrast, vascular malformations are subdivided into slow-flow and fast-flow vascular malformations. Slow-flow lesions consist of venous malformations (VMs), lymphatic malformations (LMs), capillary malformations (CMs), and combinations of the above. Fast-flow lesions encompass arteriovenous malformations (AVMs) and arteriovenous fistulae (AVFs). Slow-flow lesions are primarily treated with sclerotherapy, and AVMs and AVFs with embolotherapy.

Over the past five years, the number of requests for treatment of slow-flow malformations has increased substantially and this is now one of the most frequently requested vascular interventions in the pediatric population. Fortunately, the number of drugs with therapeutic effects has also increased. The result of these developments has been improved outcomes. Sclerotherapy involves the introduction of a drug into an epithelial-lined cyst or endothelial-lined vessel, with the intention of ablating the cyst or vascular lumen. Sclerosing drugs generally work by direct contact with the lining cells of the vascular malformation. In general, the longer the dwell time of the sclerosant drug, the more likely it is that the malformation will be successfully treated. Although sclerosant drugs can be very damaging to tissue when injected into a small artery or vein, they tend to be less injurious when diluted by rapidly flowing blood. Thus sclerotherapy is ideal for the treatment of lesions with slow flow such as venous malformations (VMs) (Figures 8.22, 8.23) and lymphatic malformations (LMs). It is our intention to provide an overview of sclerotherapy, since a detailed discussion is beyond the scope of this text.

Indications

Sclerotherapy is a non-specific therapy that can be utilized to treat vascular and non-vascular pathology. To be effective, it is generally best if the abnormality has relatively slow or static flow. Sclerotherapy for the treatment of non-vascular abnormalities is rare in the pediatric population. The most common non-vascular indications (Table 8.9) are for the treatment of cystic lesions, especially renal, splenic, and hepatic cysts. Vascular indications for sclerotherapy are far more frequent in childhood and include slow-flow venous and lymphatic malformations, varicoceles, and as a component of ranula treatment (see Figure 7.7). High-flow vascular malformations, such as AVMs/AVFs, are treated with transarterial embolization or direct injection into the nidus of an arteriovenous malformation. There are few absolute contraindications to sclerotherapy. However, relative contraindications, depending upon the technique and drug utilized, might include the proximity of the lesion to major nerves and skin, and the pathologic anatomy of the lesion allowing for direct outflow into major central veins or organs. It is important for the interventionalist to be familiar with techniques that control the outflow of sclerosant drugs into unwanted circulation to minimize complications. One should be aware that focal skin necrosis may result when performing sclerotherapy of vascular malformations involving the skin or that are associated with skin discoloration. When skin involvement is likely, it is important to discuss this at length with the family prior to treatment. However, good healing with minimal scarring can occur if the area does not become infected.

The choice of sclerosing agent, as is the case in many areas of intervention, is operator and case type dependent. In general, we prefer to treat VMs with absolute alcohol, although in a minority of instances sodium tetradecyl sulfate (STS) is utilized. The approach to treatment of LMs depends on whether the lesion is macrocystic or microcystic. Macrocystic lesions are usually treated with a combination of STS followed by absolute alcohol. Microcystic lesions (Figure 8.25e) do not

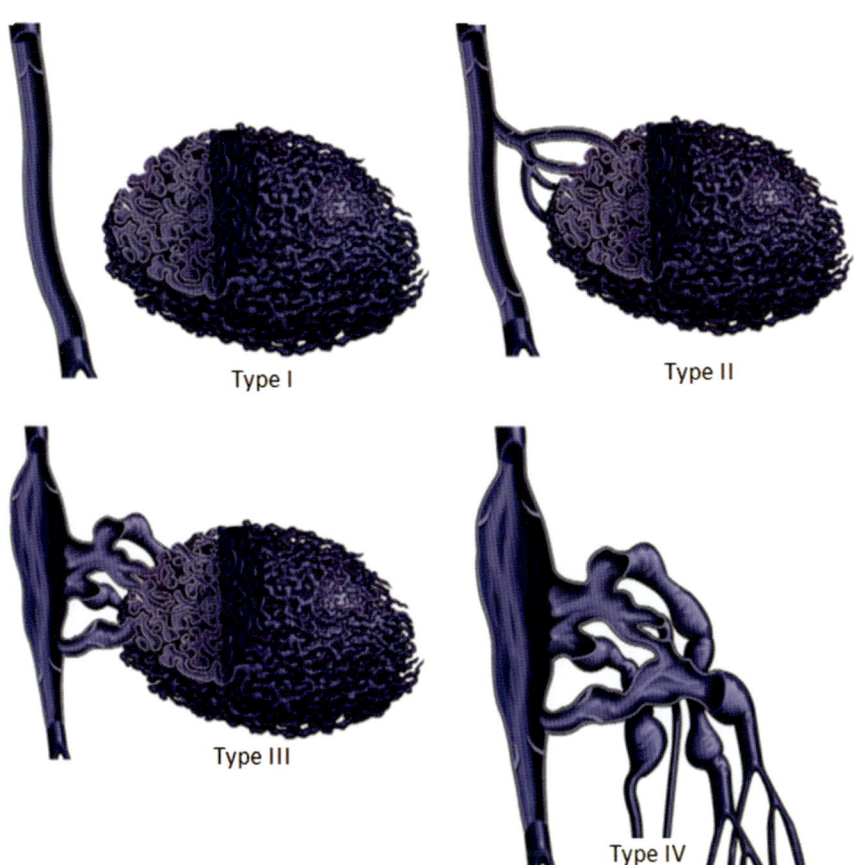

Figure 8.22 Classification of venous malformations. Diagrams of the four types of venous malformations classified by their complexity of venous drainage. Type I: Spongiform venous malformation with no direct connection to venous outflow. Type II: Similar to Type I with simple connection to venous outflow. Type III: Similar to prior types but with multiple connections to locally dilated venous outflow. Type IV: Multiple pathologic veins directly draining to locally dilated venous outflow.

tend to respond to liquid sclerotherapy with absolute alcohol or STS. Therefore foam sclerotherapy is employed, injecting the foam into each microcyst under US guidance after evacuating the cyst through a fine needle (e.g., 27-gauge, 1.5-inch hypodermic needle). The evacuation and foam instillation is performed through the same needle by way of a stopcock connected to two syringes. It is possible to treat many microcysts in each session, working through them systematically like a book: left to right, top to bottom, deep to superficial. A doxycycline foam composed of 200 mg doxycycline mixed with 2 ml normal saline, and 2 ml of 25% albumin is prepared. This mixture is combined 3:1 with air and agitated between two syringes connected by a three-way stopcock. The microbubbles increase the surface area of medication in contact with the cyst lining by approximately 40%, and are stabilized by the albumin for a longer duration of therapy. In addition, it is easy to document the treatment zone by the distributed gas pattern at the completion of the procedure. An STS foam can be prepared in similar fashion by combining 3% STS with 25% albumin in a 1:1 mixture then agitating the solution with air to create the foam. In either case, the mixture must be re-agitated before each microcyst is treated, as it tends to separate over time. Foam sclerosants should not be given if vascular run-off from the lesion is anticipated and if the patient has a right-to-left shunt, due to risk of transient ischemic neurologic events.

Over the past few years, other materials have been more frequently utilized for flow control and occlusion. This approach has primarily centered on the use of coils (both pushable and detachable) and tissue adhesives including glue and Onyx®. In some cases, a combination of materials is used.

Recently, we introduced two new therapeutic options into our vascular malformation practice: bleomycin and ablation therapy. Bleomycin has the advantage that injection produces little or no tissue edema and does not need to be intralesional to be effective. Therefore it facilitates the treatment of hemangiomas and microcystic LMs. However, bleomycin is a chemotherapeutic agent and has the risk of pulmonary fibrosis as well as minor complications such as skin hyperpigmentation, skin ulceration, and flu-like symptoms. Pulmonary fibrosis has been reported in up to 10% of patients receiving IV infusion. The incidence of pulmonary fibrosis is highest in elderly adults and in those receiving greater than 400 units total dose. Unfortunately, pulmonary toxicity has been observed in young children and those treated with lower doses. In addition, other forms of lung injury can occur such as organizing pneumonia and hypersensitivity pneumonitis. At this time, it is unclear whether the pulmonary injury will occur with percutaneous therapy since the serum drug levels achieved are small.

At this time we primarily use bleomycin for treatment of intraorbital lesions, lesions involving the tongue, floor of the mouth, soft palate, and uvula, and abnormalities that are proximate to the airway (Figure 8.24).

Ablative therapy has gained wide acceptance in the adult population for the treatment of malignancy, bone lesions, and varicose veins. Use in the pediatric population has been uncommon but is increasing. To date, our primary indication has been radiofrequency ablation (RFA) of osteoid osteomas. Lately, we have successfully used RFA for treatment of large caliber veins (>6 mm) that are associated with VMs. This approach has been especially helpful in the treatment of children with capillary-lymphaticovenous malformation with limb overgrowth, also known as Klippel–Trenaunay syndrome (Figure 8.25), varicose veins, and type 4 VMs with large outflow veins.

Table 8.9 Indications: sclerotherapy

- Slow-flow malformations, e.g., lymphatic, venous, or mixed lesions anywhere in the body
- Lymphocele
- Varicose veins
- Varicocele

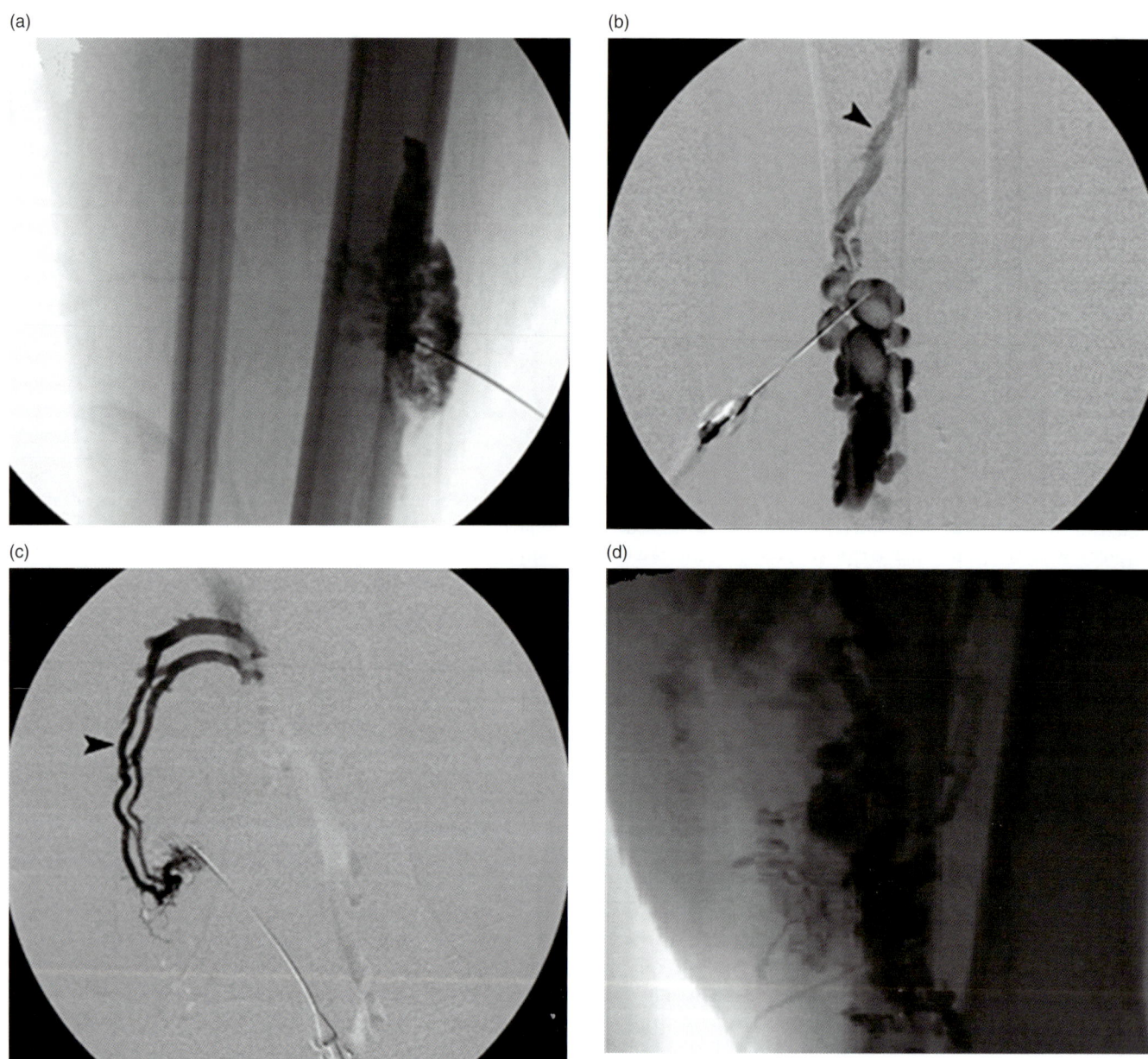

Figure 8.23 Classification of venous malformations. Images of the four types of venous malformations classified by their complexity of venous drainage. (a) Type I: Spongiform venous malformation with no direct connection to venous outflow. (b) Type II: Similar to Type I with simple connection to venous outflow. (c) Type III: Similar to prior types but with multiple connections to locally dilated venous outflow. (D) Type IV: Multiple pathologic veins directly draining to locally dilated venous outflow.

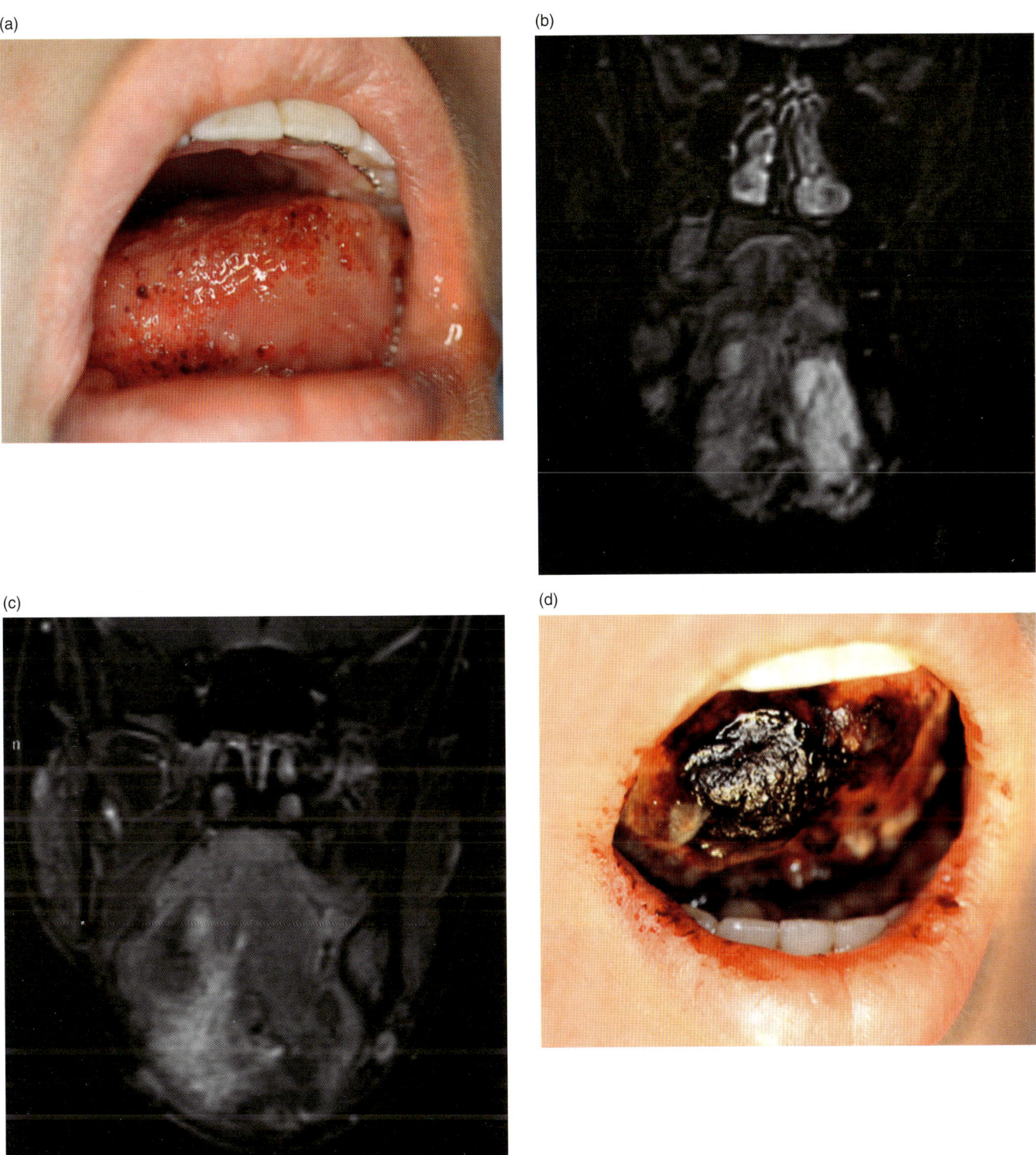

Figure 8.24 Twenty-year-old female with disfiguring venolymphatic malformation of the tongue and floor of the mouth. (a) Multiple vesicles are present on the enlarged tongue typical of microcystic venolymphatic malformation. (b,c) Coronal postcontrast T1 MRI images of the floor of the mouth and tongue show diffuse abnormality. (d) Black discoloration of the tongue from clotted blood two days after treatment will resolve over time. (e,f) One- and six-month follow-up show decreased tongue size and increased mobility.

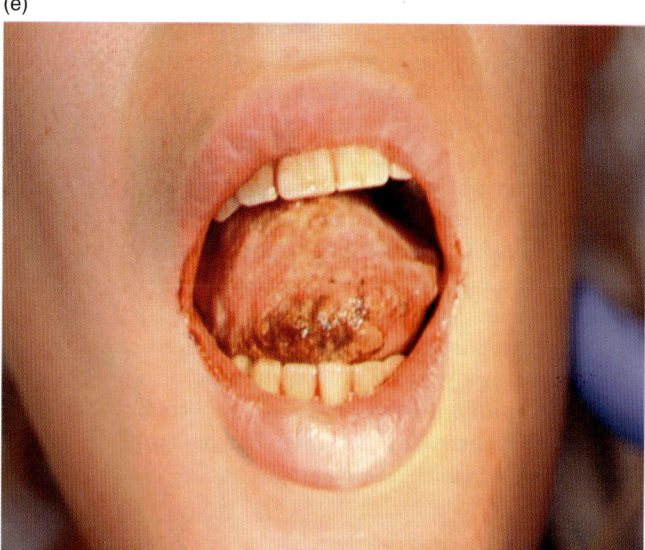
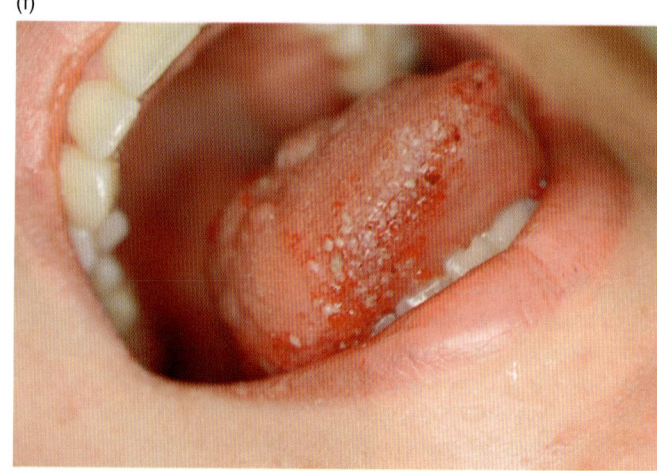

Figure 8.24 (cont.)

Technique

Equipment

Equipment needed for sclerotherapy is minimal (Table 8.10) and includes a sheathed needle of appropriate size and length for access, contrast medium and tubing for direct injection, tourniquets and compression devices, and modern imaging equipment with digital subtraction angiography and real-time digital subtraction fluoroscopy (road mapping). Platinum or steel wire coils may be useful adjuncts to the liquid agents, such as ethanol and sodium tetradecyl sulfate.

Patient preparation

Cross-sectional imaging, especially MRI of the abnormal area, is recommended prior to percutaneous therapy to diagnose and assess the extent of the abnormality, its vascular supply, route planning, and the location(s) of the direct percutaneous needle placement. In general, MRI in multiple planes prior to and after contrast injection, and MRA are performed. Ultrasound is also of use and is better able to define the internal architecture of the lesion. A focused US exam may be performed prior to or at the time of therapy. At the time of the procedure, deep sedation or general anesthesia is utilized, depending upon the patient age, sclerosant used, and preference of the interventionalist. Corticosteroids (e.g., prednisone 2 mg/kg/day) may be administered 24 hours before the procedure and maintained for seven days if needed. If a corticosteroid has not been used, it should be considered if excessive swelling occurs, if marked skin blanching during injection of the sclerosant is noted, or if excessive pain occurs. Placement of a urinary catheter is rarely utilized during sclerotherapy, which is in contrast to embolotherapy.

Standard technique

Venous malformations (Figure 8.26) are accessed percutaneously with a standard or sheathed needle (20- to 24-gauge, 1.5-inch to 2-inch in length). When free blood flow is achieved, contrast is injected and digital subtraction images are obtained. If the lesion to be treated communicates with adjacent normal veins, the contrast injection is repeated with appropriate compression or tourniquet application until the lesion can be injected with minimal or non-opacification of the draining veins. Next, the lesion is injected with sclerosant (Table 8.12). Typically, the injection of sclerosant is intermittently observed fluoroscopically to see that the intralesional residual contrast is diluted, confirming entry of sclerosant into the lesion, and to confirm filling of the VM with the sclerosant as evidenced by contrast displacement. The tourniquet or compression device is maintained in place for approximately five to ten minutes to limit outflow. Oxygen saturation, heart rate, and electrocardiographic tracing are monitored throughout the ethanol injection portion of sclerotherapy.

Patients are kept well hydrated throughout the procedure. A total dose of 1 ml/kg of 100% ethanol should not be exceeded. After sterile preparation of the overlying skin, one or more needles are inserted into the lesion and a predetermined volume of sclerosing solution is injected while venous outflow is controlled to maximize the dwell time of the agent on the endothelial surface.

Lymphatic malformations are also accessed percutaneously, with a standard or sheathed needle, or ultimately with a small caliber drain if the LM is a large macrocyst (Figures 8.25c, 8.27). The LM contents are aspirated and the volume of the cyst noted. Contrast is then injected and digital images obtained, and ultimately the contrast is aspirated to

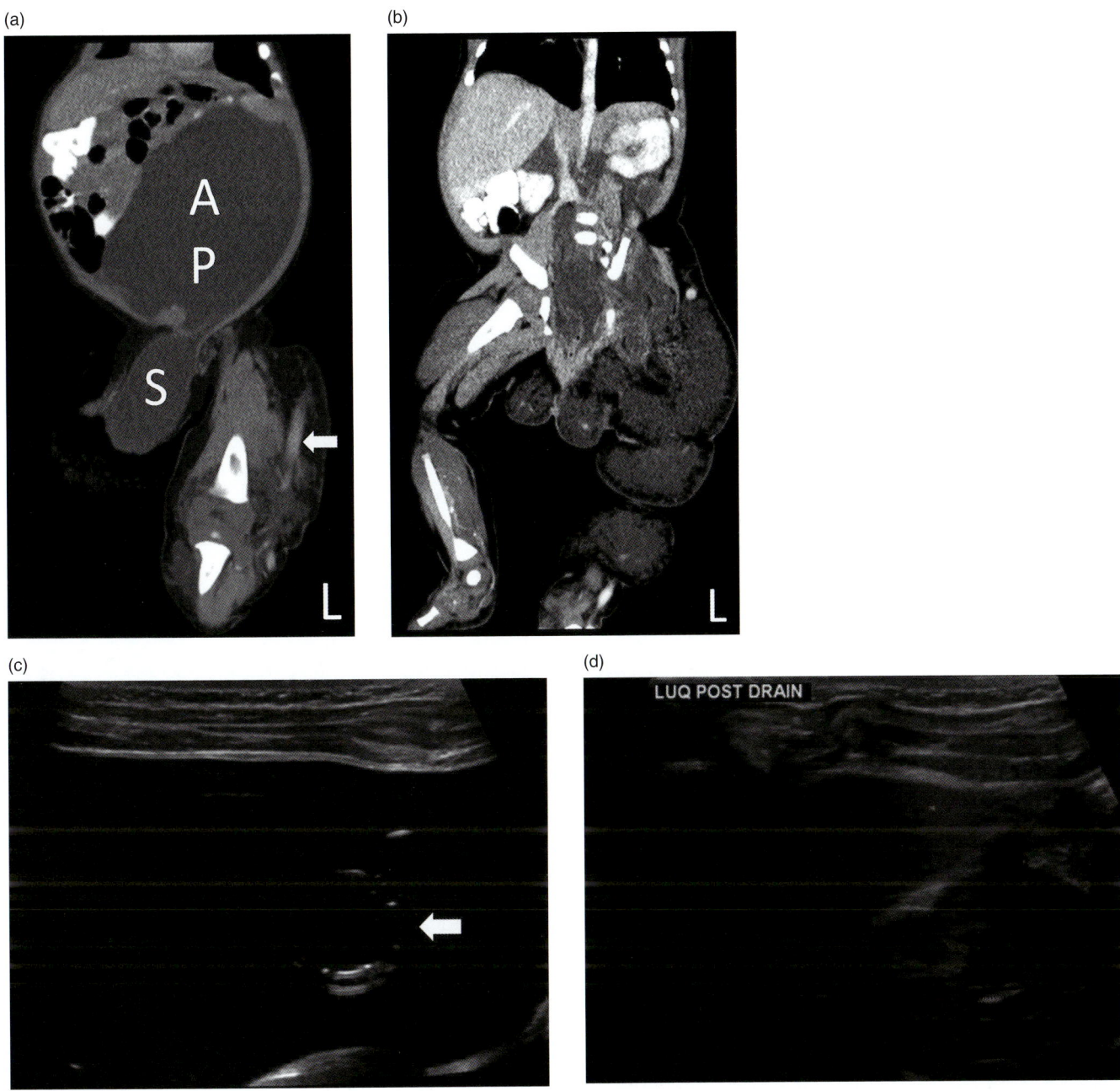

Figure 8.25 A newborn male with prenatal diagnosis of extensive vascular anomalies presents with abdominopelvic distension and left lower extremity hemihypertrophy. (a,b) Coronal CT images show extensive lymphatic malformations in the abdomen (A) and pelvis (P) extending through the inguinal canal to the left scrotum (S). A prominent vein (*arrow*) is seen in the lateral left thigh. (c) Under US guidance a 7 French drainage catheter (*arrow*) was inserted into the largest abdominopelvic LM, and 410 ml clear fluid aspirated. This was treated with combination sclerotherapy (sodium tetradecyl sulfate followed by dehydrated alcohol). (d) Ultrasound after drainage shows decompression of the LM with normalization of the position of the abdominal organs. (e) Axial T2 MR at the level of the scrotum shows innumerable LM microcysts without soft tissue mass. The larger cysts were individually treated with sodium tetradecyl sulfate foam, and the smaller microcysts were treated individually with doxycycline foam. As many microcysts as could be treated in a reasonable amount of time were treated at each session. (f) Bilateral pedal venography showed normal veins in the right lower extremity, and a persistent left embryonic sciatic vein (marginal vein of Servelle), a pathognomonic finding of Klippel–Trenaunay syndrome. (g) The urinary bladder (*asterisk*) was mistaken for a component of the LM and treated with sclerotherapy. The mucosa is thickened and irregular secondary to intense inflammation. (h) The catheter was left as a "suprapubic" catheter for several weeks until the tract matured, providing bladder drainage and allowing frequent irrigation. The bladder healed without complication and the catheter was removed without incident.

assess cyst dynamics (ability to empty the cyst of fluid/sclerosant). The sclerosant agents are then injected into the cyst and allowed to dwell per protocol, then aspirated. The approach to sclerotherapy of microcystic malformations differs in that we traverse multiple cysts with a standard needle (string of pearls), and then inject the doxycycline emulsion into the cysts as the needle is slowly withdrawn through the cysts.

(e)
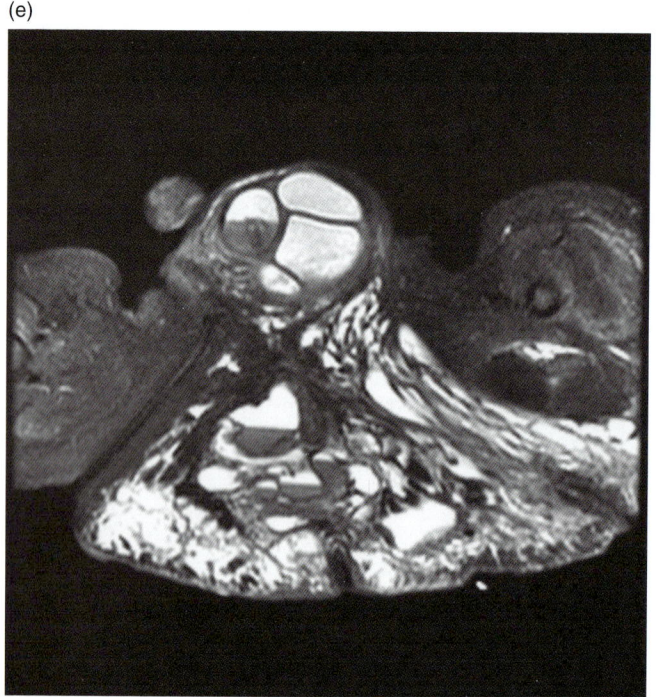

(f)
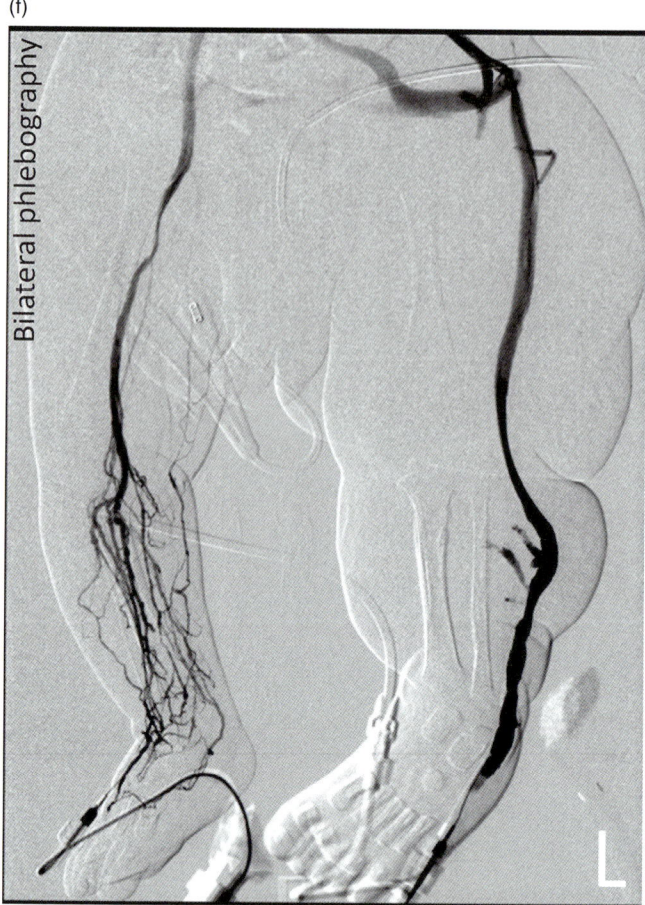

(g)
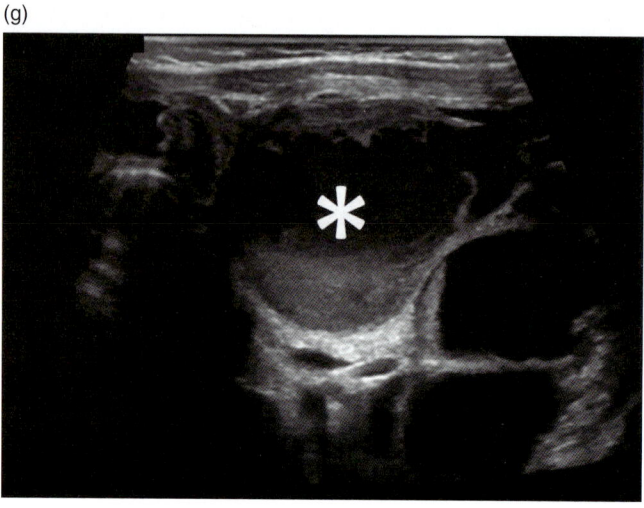

(h)
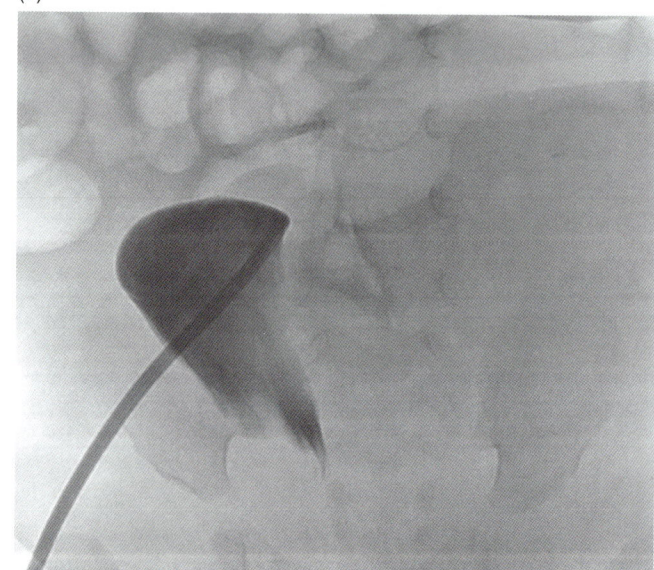

Figure 8.25 (cont.)

Technical variations
Sodium tetradecyl sulfate
Sodium tetradecyl sulfate (3%) can be used instead of ethanol, although a safe pediatric dosage range has not been published. The manufacturer's recommended limit is 10 ml (for adults). Sodium tetradecyl sulfate may have a lower incidence of nerve injury than absolute alcohol. However, this agent has not gained popularity for treatment of slow-flow lesions perhaps because of a lesser effect on vascular and lymphatic

malformations. Other sclerosants currently used in various countries include Ethibloc® (Europe and Canada) and Picibanil®, or OK-432 (Japan).

Bleomycin

Over the past five years, there has been increasing interest in and use of bleomycin, an antineoplastic agent, for treatment of hemangiomas and vascular malformations. Bleomycin is a glycopeptide antibiotic that is derived from *Streptomyces*

Table 8.10 Equipment: sclerotherapy

- Needle: angiocatheter, Chiba needle, or other needle type (20- to 24-gauge)
- Tourniquets
- Sclerosing agent: absolute alcohol, sodium tetradecyl sulfate, sodium morrhulate, doxycycline, and bleomycin (Ethibloc® and OK-432 are not available in the United States)
- Radiofrequency ablation equipment (see Table 8.11)
- Corticosteroids PRN

Table 8.11 Radiofrequency ablation settings for common procedures

- Osteoid osteoma
  - 17-gauge RFA probe with a 7 and 10 mm ablative zone
  - Six minutes at 90°C
  - Impedance: 200 to 400 Watts, preferably closer to 200
    - If impedance greater than 400 Watts, normal saline can be injected into the tract to reduce impedance
- Venous
  - ClosureFast™ catheter:
    - treatment zone: 7 cm
    - sheath with hemostasis value: 7 French
    - guide wire: 0.025-inch, 260 cm length
  - Treatment cycle: 120°C; ≤20 Watts for 20 seconds
  - To increase venous wall surface contact: tumescent anesthesia and compression (via US probe or towel roll)
  - Treatment protocol: begin 2 cm distal to saphenofemoral junction (SFJ). Initially two activations at SFJ. Then overlapping activations for length of pathologic vein. May repeat entire length or segments × 1

(a)
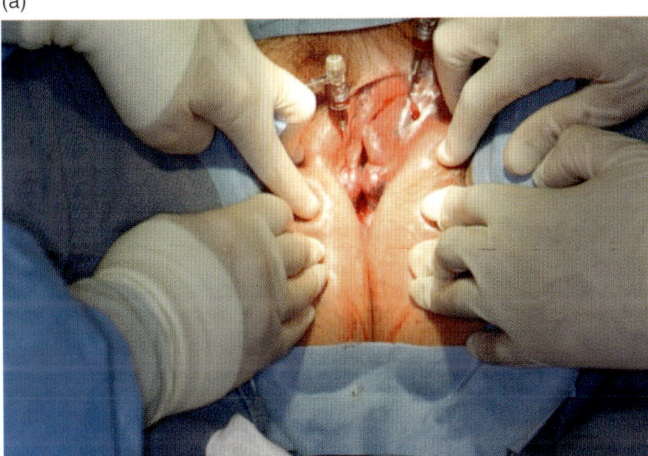

(b)
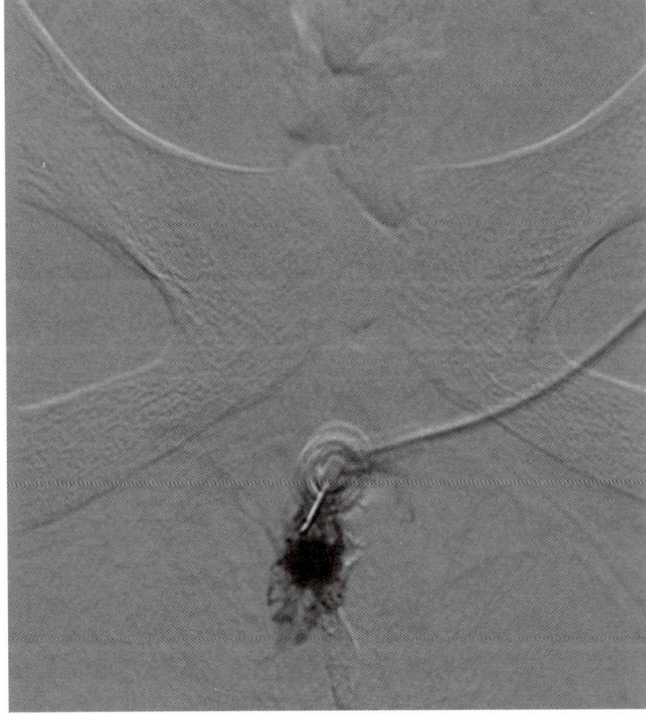

(c)
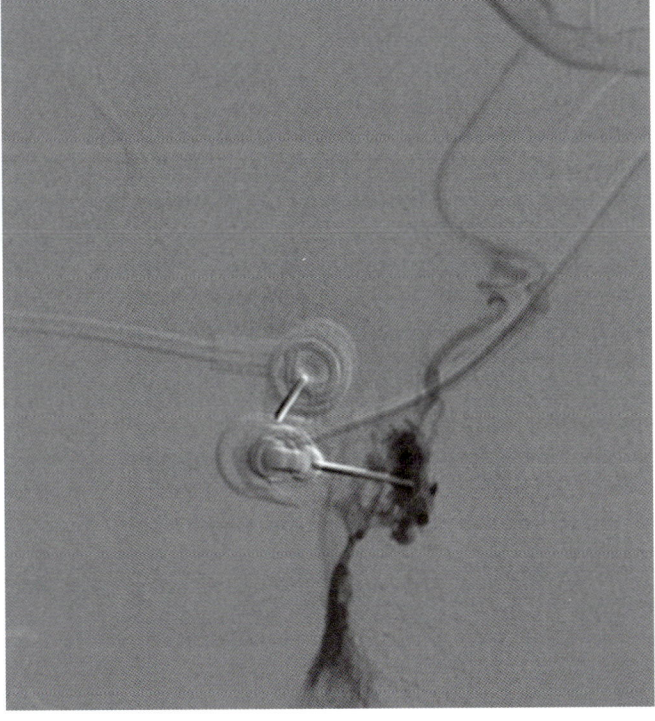

Figure 8.26 A 12-year-old female presented with bulbous venous malformations of the vulva and intense pain. (a) Bilateral adjacent vulvar lesions with needle within right VM. (b) Venogram prior to sodium tetradecyl sulfate injection of the right- and (c) left-sided lesions.

Chapter 8 Vascular interventions

Table 8.12 Procedure summary: sclerotherapy

- Preprocedural imaging to map the lesion and plan therapy
- Sedation or general anesthesia
- Sterile preparation and draping of the skin at the lesion site
- Inject local anesthesia into the entry site (if performed with sedation)
- Insert angiocather(s) into various quadrants of the lesion
- Confirm intralesional position with contrast injection
- Inject the sclerosant
- Maintain outflow obstruction if needed
- Steroids PRN

verticillus. When used as a chemotherapeutic agent, it is in the form of bleomycin A_2 and B_2 and acts by causing breaks in DNA. Bleomycin is associated with side effects ranging from fever and chills to lung problems, most notably pulmonary fibrosis. Allergic-like reactions, chest pain, shortness of breath, and oral ulcers have also been seen. The risk of pulmonary toxicity increases with cumulative dose (especially over 450,000 IU), low GFR, older age, supplemental oxygen exposure, bolus drug delivery, and prior lung disease.

(a)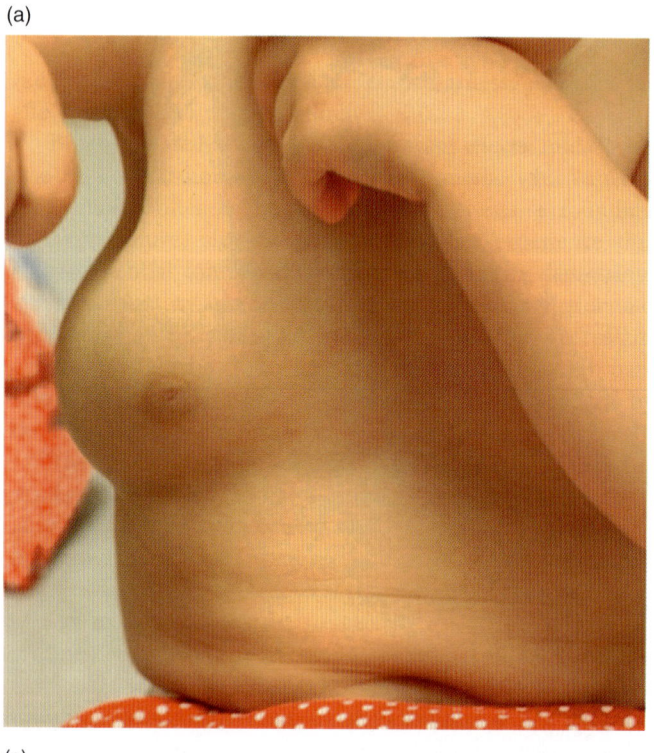

(b)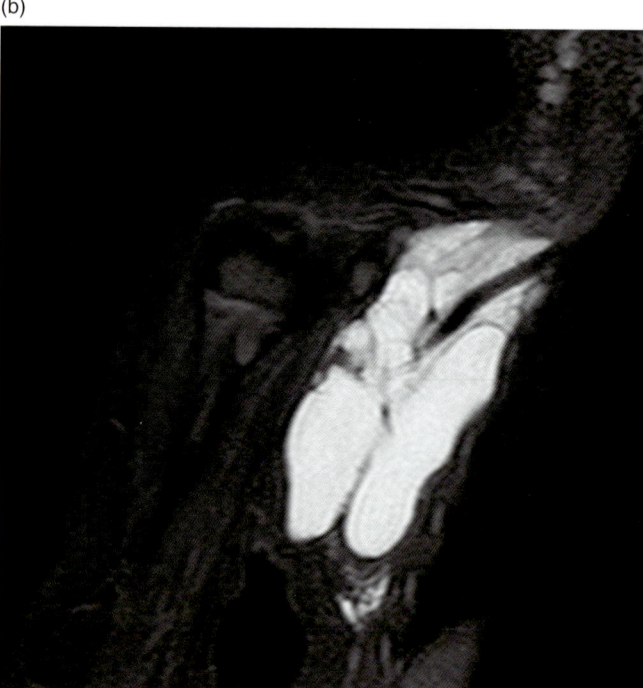

(c)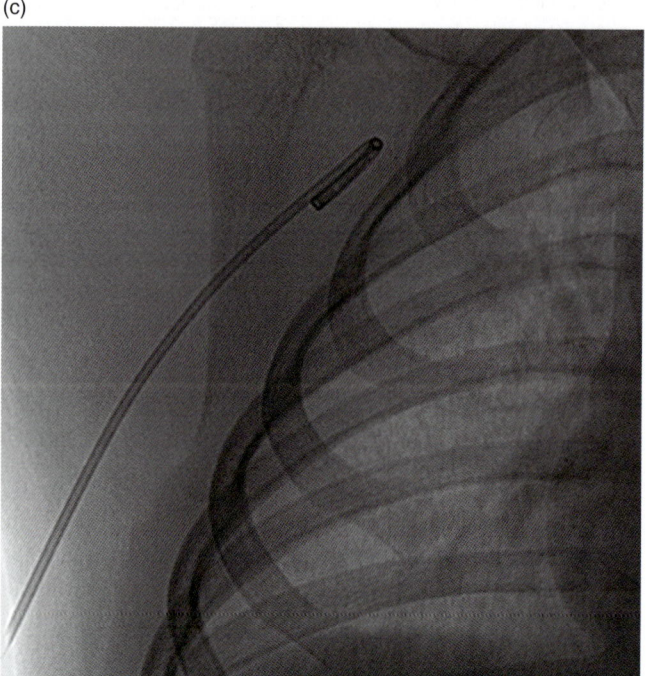

(d)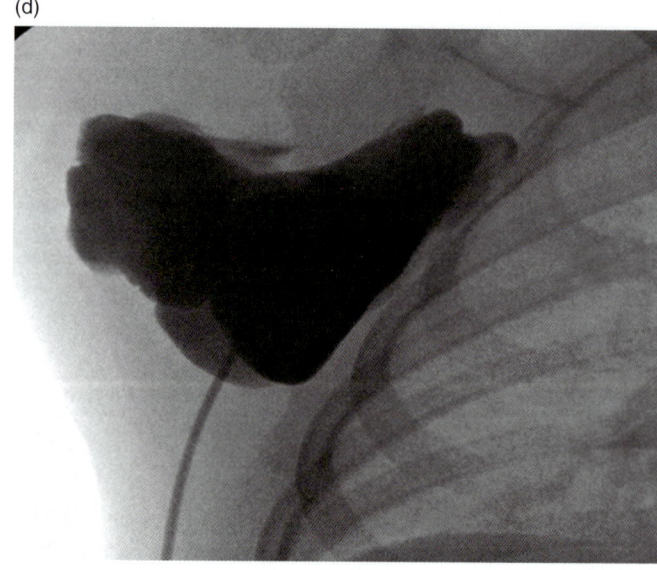

Figure 8.27 (a) A two-year-old male with right chest wall mass. (b) Coronal T2 MRI demonstrates a multiloculated macrocystic lymphatic malformation. (c) Ultrasound and fluoroscopic-guided placement of a 5 Fr Towbin (Duan) pigtail drainage catheter. (d) Contrast injection confirms placement, assures there are no draining vessels, and defines the volume of the macrocyst prior to alcohol administration.

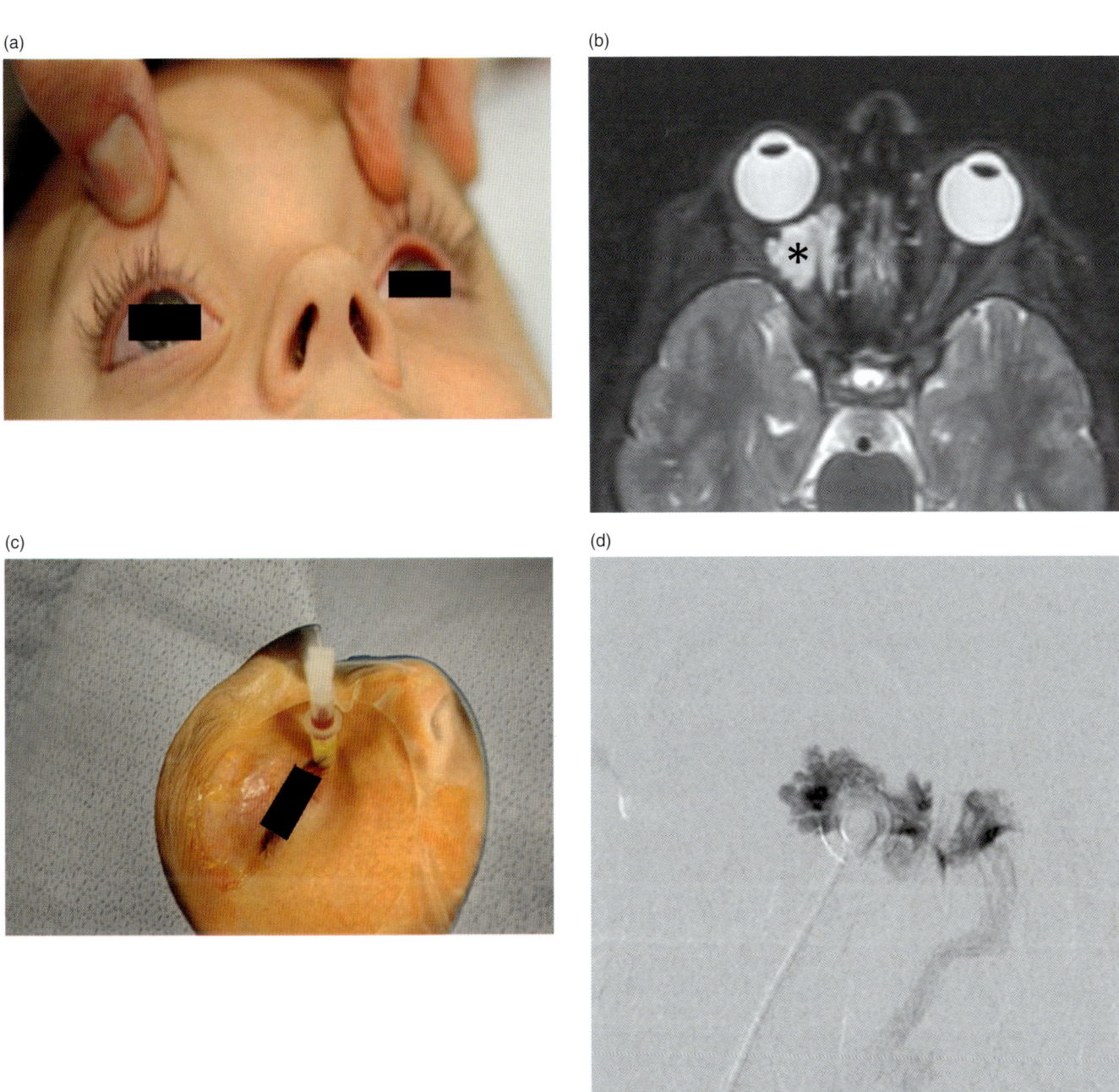

Figure 8.28 (a) Four year-old male with right exophthalmos. (b) Axial T2 MRI of the orbits shows a right postseptal, intraconal venous malformation (*asterisk*) with anterior displacement of the orbit. (c) Ultrasound-guided needle placement medial to the globe. (d) Contrast confirmation of needle location and assessment of venous drainage prior to treatment with 0.4 ml of bleomycin (20 U/ml).

Bleomycin has proven to be a useful agent for intralesional therapy of both hemangiomas and vascular malformations, with complete resolution or significant improvement of hemangiomas in over 80% of patients in both categories. Bleomycin seems to be unique in the realm of sclerosant drugs in that injection does *not* result in tissue edema. As a result, it has become our drug of choice for the treatment of lesions involving the structures around the airway, tongue and floor of mouth, and orbit (Figure 8.28).

Varicocele sclerotherapy

Sclerotherapy of varicoceles is usually indicated for teenage boys with a varicocele causing persistent inguinal pain and accompanying testicular atrophy. In this age group, reproductive functions are often not yet assessable. However, as in the adult population, varicocele embolization (usually left) is performed by catheterization of the internal spermatic vein. If the femoral vein is used for access, a Hopkins or similar broad, J-shaped catheter is directed into the spermatic vein and

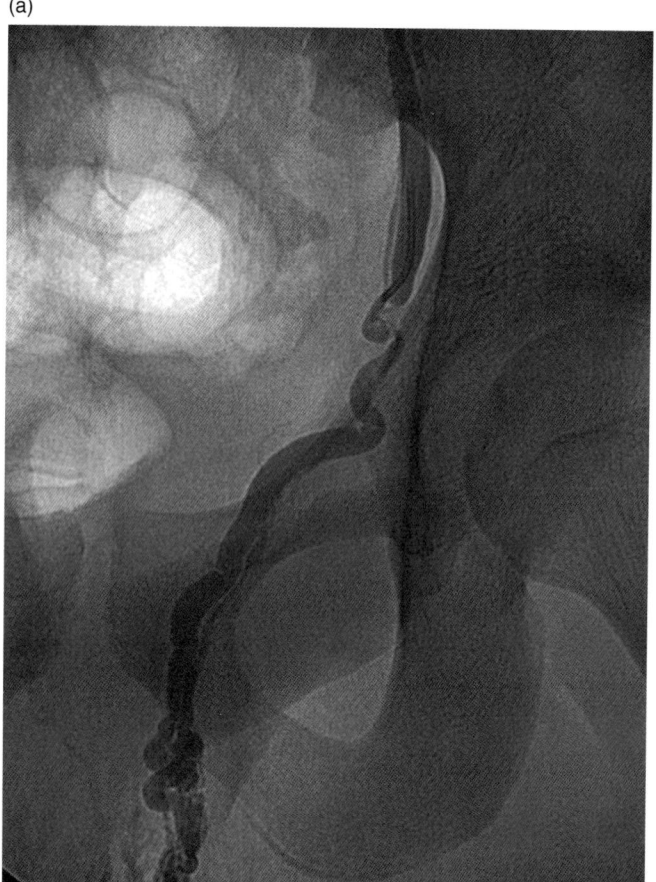 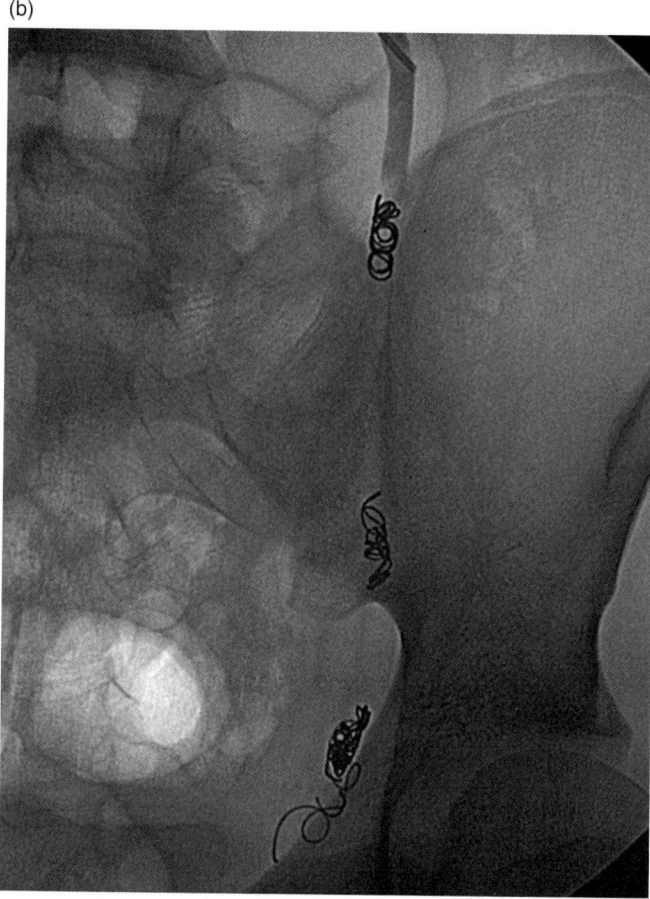

Figure 8.29 A 15-year-old male presented with left scrotal pain and testicular atrophy. (a) Venography via the left renal vein shows a prominent, tortuous left gonadal vein with dilation of the pampiniform plexus representing a varicocele. (b) Deployment of 8 cm long Gianturco vascular coils at three levels: the inguinal ligament, inferior sacroiliac joint, and superior sacroiliac joint with 3% sodium tetradecyl sulfate injected between coil groups ("sandwich" technique) relieved the patient's symptoms.

subsequently maneuvered down to the level of the inguinal ligament, over a stiff guide wire. At the current time, we prefer using the right internal jugular vein for access as it allows for easier catheterization of the left renal vein and a more stable catheter position for embolotherapy. Over the years, a variety of treatment strategies have been suggested in the literature. In general, multilevel occlusion of the spermatic vein is usually successful as long as all significant parallel channels are blocked. Today, we are using a "sandwich" technique (Figure 8.29). We usually place coils in the internal spermatic vein just above the level of the inguinal ligament, at the level of the inferior sacroiliac joint, and at the top of the iliac crest, and infuse sodium tetradecyl sulfate (agitated with air) between the coil levels. Occasionally additional coils will be placed close to the origin of the renal vein. With the advent of vascular plugs, some interventionalists have substituted them in place of coils (Figure 8.30). Although this is a fast and elegant method of occlusion, we do not prefer this approach because of the relatively high cost of plugs versus coils. As is the case for adults, the procedure is generally straightforward and good results can be expected. Unfortunately, no studies evaluating the long-term outcome are currently available in the pediatric population.

Postprocedure and follow-up care

There is no prospective study that defines the best or most effective postprocedural guidelines following sclerotherapy. Therefore there are a variety of approaches that may be used. To diminish the amount of swelling, ice may be applied, and the treated area elevated during the recovery period. Intravenous fluids are administered at double the normal maintenance rate, and urine is observed for hemoglobinuria and output volume. If output is diminished, diuretics are administered. Hydration is continued until discharge or until the hemoglobinuria clears. Some physicians prescribe appropriate analgesics (e.g., ketorolac) and oral corticosteroids in a tapering dose for one week following ethanol or tetradecyl sclerotherapy procedures. In our practice, if we observe skin blanching during the procedure, we will immediately give a single dose of IV steroid, followed by an oral steroid sequentially decreasing dose pack to be taken over the next five to seven days. These

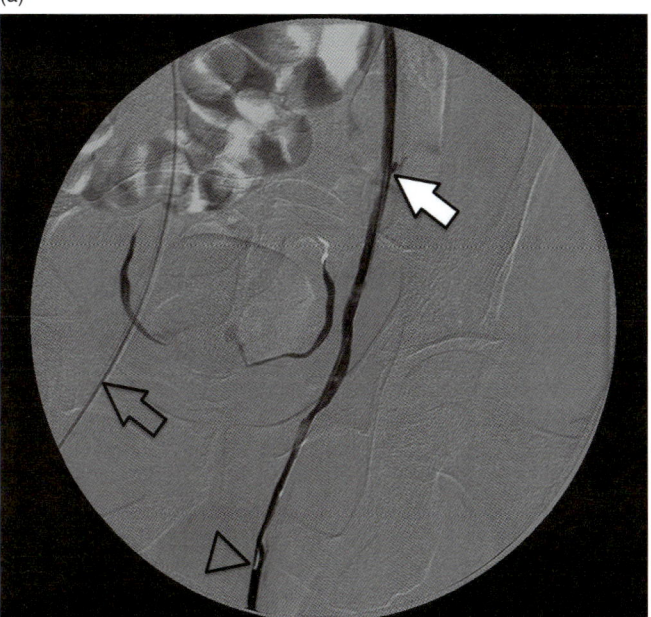 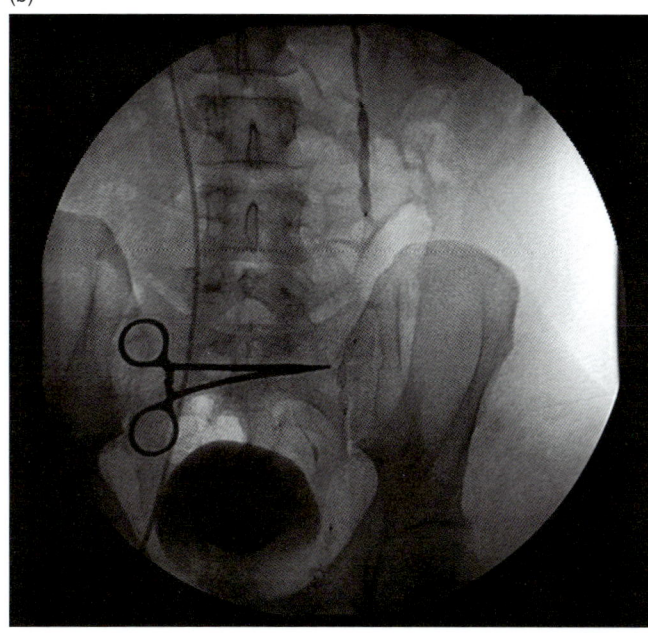

Figure 8.30 A 30-year-old male presented with testicular pain, left scrotal swelling and low sperm count. (a) A 5 French guiding catheter (*open arrow*) was advanced from the right common femoral vein through the left renal vein to the distal left testicular vein (*arrowhead*). Venography showed a branch vessel (*solid arrow*) at the upper pelvis. (b) Three Amplatzer® plugs were placed at the distal testicular vein, across the branch veins (marked with the clamp), and at the proximal vein. The pain and swelling resolved and the sperm count normalized, but the patient did complain of postembolization syndrome for several weeks after the procedure.

actions tend to limit swelling and hopefully avoid skin or other injury. At the time of therapy, the skin is observed for areas of necrosis, and if present, followed closely with appropriate antibacterial non-stick dressings, topical silver sulfadiazine (Silvadene®), and sometimes debridement. If no untoward effects occur, clinical follow-up is obtained six to eight weeks following the procedure to determine the outcome and need for further treatment.

Technical problems and pitfalls

Sclerotherapy works best in lesions with slow blood or lymphatic flow. Those lesions with large communications to adjacent veins may not respond, due to rapid wash-out of the sclerosant drug. Thus, in these situations, outflow obstruction with tourniquets, balloon catheters, or other compressive techniques are important.

Future advances

We recommend utilizing an immunohistochemical panel consisting of Prox-1, VEGFR3, CD31, and CD34 antibodies to differentiate lymphatic from venous malformations in pathologic practice.

Complications

The most frequent complications resulting from sclerotherapy include hemoglobinuria, skin necrosis, and neuropathy. Hemoglobinuria, when present, appears to be well tolerated if the child is kept well hydrated. Skin necrosis usually results from treatment of lesions involving the superficial layers of the skin but can also result from extravasation of sclerosant or inadvertent arterial injection (Figure 8.31). Any non-target instillation of sclerosant carries risk of significant complication, so verification of needle-tip location throughout the injection is essential (Figure 8.25f,g). Neuropathy, when it occurs, may be transient, presumably caused by nerve compression, stretching, or swelling (Figure 8.32), or permanent, if a direct injection occurs. Nerve injuries have been reported with the use of ethanol but apparently not with sodium tetradecyl sulfate. Cardiovascular collapse resulting in death has also been reported with the use of 100% ethanol, possibly due to pulmonary artery vasospasm resulting in acute pulmonary artery hypertension and right heart failure. Hemorrhagic pulmonary edema may also be observed. As a result, some operators perform sclerotherapy with the patient under general anesthesia while monitoring pulmonary artery pressure. This is not currently our practice for treatment of routine, uncomplicated lesions.

Pseudoaneurysm ablation

Introduction

A pseudoaneurysm is defined as a pulsating, encapsulated hematoma in communication with the lumen of a ruptured blood vessel. The pseudoaneurysm wall consists of hematoma, periarterial fibrous tissue, and adventitia. The etiology for pseudoaneurysm in the pediatric population is usually an iatrogenic arterial misadventure (see Figures 2.20, 4.61, and

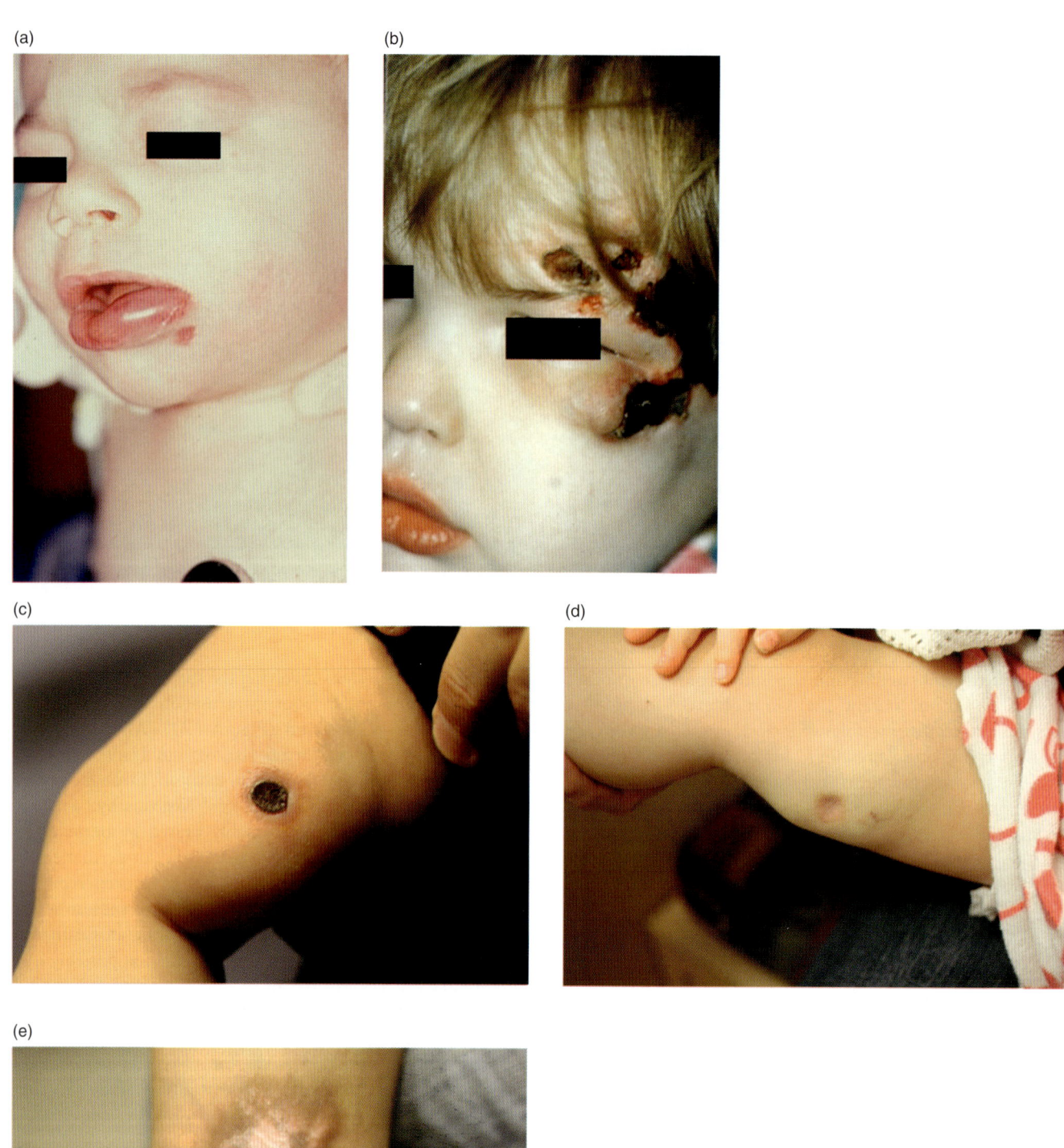

Figure 8.31 Complications of alcohol injection: a 25-year experience. (a) Acute spit fistula after direct lip injection and inferior labial branch embolization. (b) Skin necrosis after alcohol injection in distribution of the superficial temporal artery. Associated left eye blindness due to previously unknown origin of the ophthalmic artery from the superficial temporal artery. (c,d) Acute ulceration and late healing with scar formation. (e) Acute skin necrosis after direct percutaneous injection of an ankle AVM.

Chapter 8 Vascular interventions

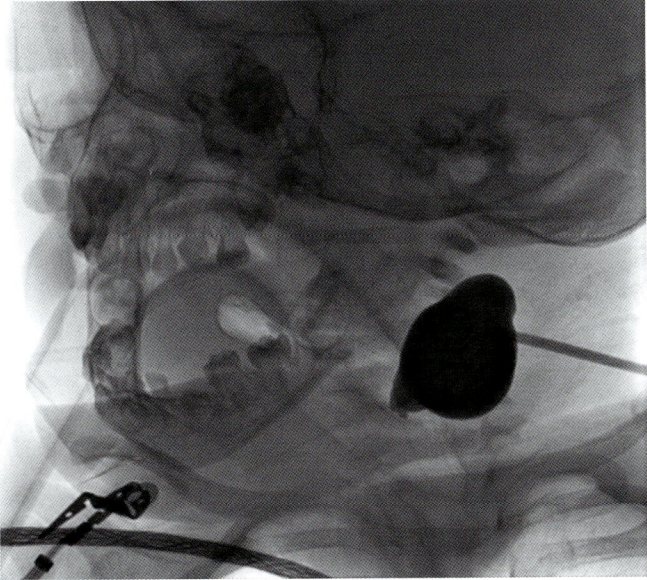

Figure 8.32 A four-year-old male was treated for a lymphatic malformation (LM) overlying the parotid gland with combination liquid sclerotherapy using sodium tetradecyl sulfate and dehydrated alcohol. Successful treatment of the LM was complicated by self-limited facial palsy, likely due to nerve stretching related to local inflammatory response.

Table 8.13 Indications: pseudoaneurysm ablation

- Interval enlargement of lesion
- Increasing pain
- Compression symptoms
- Dropping hemoglobin and hematocrit

Table 8.14 Procedure summary: pseudoaneurysm ablation

- Localize lesion with US
- Select skin entry site
- Ultrasound-guided needle insertion
- If neck is suitable, inject one drop of thrombin and wait, if not thrombosed can repeat injection
- Monitor occlusion with real-time US including Doppler
- If wide neck present may consider balloon, or covered stent to keep drug within pseudoaneurysm, or coil trapping
- Follow-up US after 24 to 48 hours if child is asymptomatic

8.33), but also includes trauma, tumor, infection, vasculitis, and inflammation. The most common etiology is iatrogenic, and a prime example of an iatrogenic pseudoaneurysm is femoral artery catheterization for cardiac catheterization or diagnostic/therapeutic angiography with inadequate hemostasis following arterial sheath or catheter removal.

Indications

Clinical diagnosis of a pseudoaneurysm is made by identification of a pulsatile mass in continuity with the lumen of the parent artery following an arterial puncture or trauma. The diagnosis is confirmed by imaging and the pathologic anatomy is demonstrated. Typically, US is the diagnostic tool of choice for superficial lesions and either CT/CTA or MR/MRA for visceral or head and neck abnormalities. Classically US shows "to and fro" flow within the aneurysmal sac on color Doppler, a communicating aneurysm neck, and, frequently, perilesional hematoma.

The presence of either a symptomatic or asymptomatic pseudoaneurysm requires treatment regardless of its location because of the risk of exsanguination (Table 8.13). Symptoms may include pain, swelling, pulsatile mass, and stable or growing hematoma.

Technique

Standard technique

Currently, the primary treatment of pseudoaneurysms is percutaneous thrombin injection utilizing US guidance (Table 8.14). Cope and Zeit first described the use of thrombin to treat pseudoaneurysms in 1986. Previously, pseudoaneurysms were treated surgically or with compression of the pseudoaneurysm neck under (US) visualization.

Percutaneous thrombin embolization

A pseudoaneurysm accessible from a percutaneous approach may be accessed using a 22-gauge thin (e.g., Chiba) needle, with the needle tip in the pseudoaneurysm but if possible directed away from the neck. Thrombin (concentration 1,000 IU/ml in a 1 ml syringe) is injected into the pseudoaneurysm in 0.1 ml increments or a drop at a time, waiting a few moments between drops to allow the clotting cascade to activate.

Under direct gray-scale US visualization, it may take as little as 200 to 300 IU up to 1,000 to 1,500 IU to thrombose the pseudoaneurysm. Thrombosis occurs rapidly and is confirmed with color-flow Doppler at the conclusion of the procedure (Figure 8.34). Care should be taken to avoid overfilling the pseudoaneurysm sac or undue compression of the pseudoaneurysm, as thrombin forced out of the sac will tend to thrombose the parent vessels. If this occurs, tPA is effective for fresh clot lysis, and should be readily available during these procedures. Although therapeutic anticoagulation should not interfere with thrombin activity, supratherapeutic anticoagulation will be more disruptive of the clotting cascade and may result in treatment failure or recurrence.

Technical variations

Protection of the parent artery

If the pseudoaneurysm has a short, broad neck, or if the parent artery is in a more hazardous location, it is possible to protect the parent artery during thrombin occlusion by carefully positioning a balloon catheter across the defect within the artery, and gently inflating it for up to several

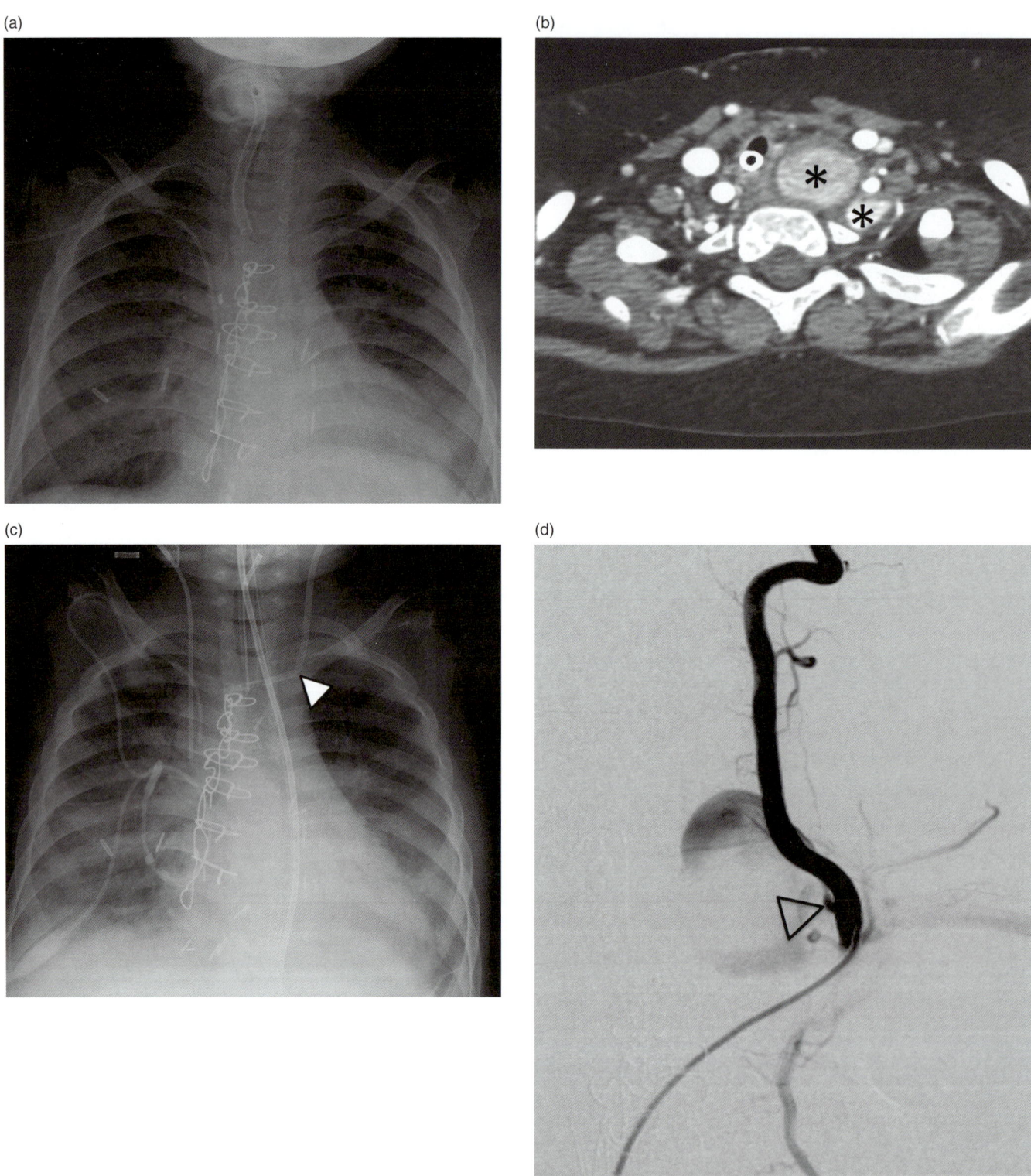

Figure 8.33 A six-year-old female heart and bilateral lung transplant recipient developed progressive respiratory distress as an outpatient, requiring progressively longer Shiley endotracheal tubes. (a) Chest radiograph shows rightward deviation of the trachea by mass effect. (b) Computed tomography with vascular contrast at the level of T1 shows a bilobed pseudoaneurysm (*asterisks*) producing extrinsic compression of the trachea. (c) Careful review of the medical record revealed attempted venous access without image guidance 11 months previously. The catheter was kinked (*arrowhead*) and removed immediately after this image was obtained. (d) Left vertebral arteriography shows an anterior wall defect (*arrowhead*) pulsing into the pseudoaneurysm sac. (e) When a percutaneous 22-gauge Chiba needle had been positioned in the pseudoaneurysm sac, a 4 mm × 2 cm PTA balloon was gently inflated across the defect to "guard" the vertebral artery during thrombin embolization. (f) Under US control, the Chiba needle was advanced percutaneously between the left carotid (*C*) and vertebral (*V*) arteries into the aneurysm sac. A wisp of thrombus is seen forming at the needle tip (*arrowhead*) as the first drop of thrombin is administered. (g) A CT with vascular contrast obtained six months later shows complete resolution of the pseudoaneurysm and normalization of the endotracheal tube position.

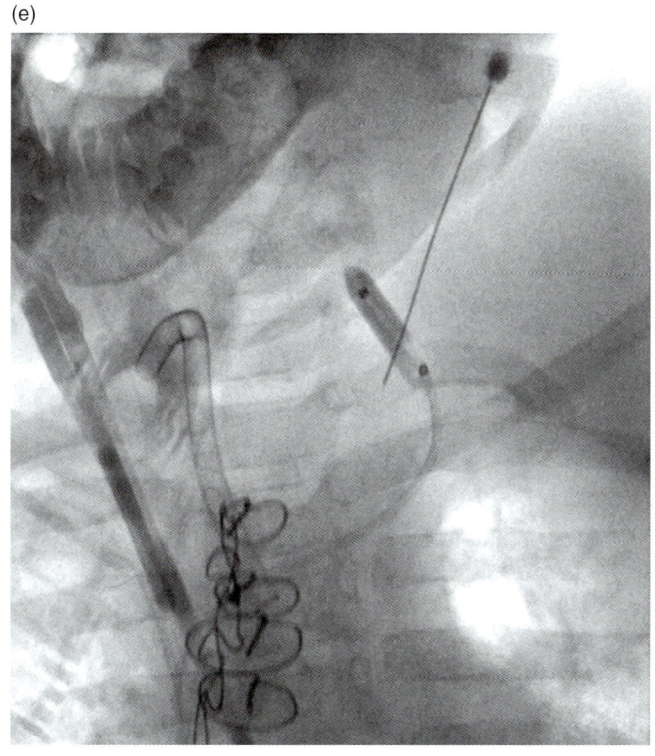
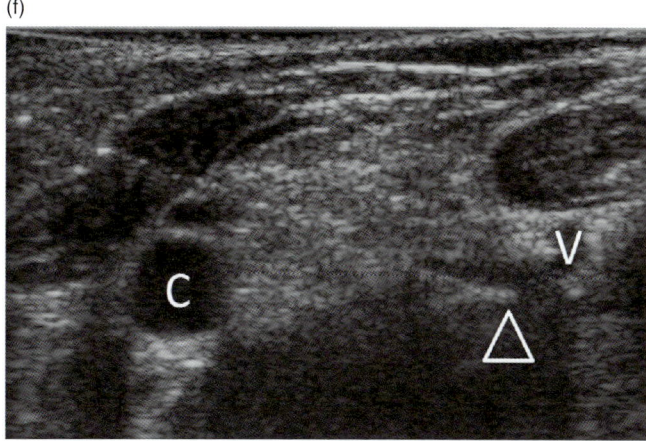
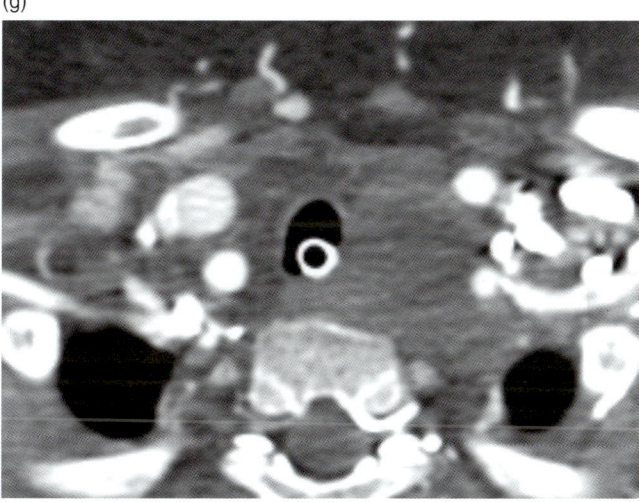

Figure 8.33 (cont.)

minutes during the time that the thrombin is percutaneously instilled into the pseudoaneurysm (Figure 8.33e). In principle, a covered stent could be used in the parent artery to exclude the pseudoaneurysm, although this technique has not been reported in children. If a safe surgical or endovascular alternative exists for treatment in such vulnerable locations, it may be preferable.

Endovascular embolization

Pseudoaneurysms involving deep arteries such as the splenic artery or neck vessels will usually require non-invasive vascular imaging e.g., US, CTA, or MRA. Once diagnosed, if direct percutaneous thrombin occlusion (Figure 8.35) is not possible, a diagnostic angiogram is performed as a prelude to therapeutic transcatheter intervention. Several approaches may be utilized to trap or occlude the pseudoaneurysm based on the pathologic anatomy and preference of the interventionalist. If trapping is the preferred approach coils or plugs are placed both distal and proximal to the lesion (Figure 4.61). Other occlusive material such as glue or Onyx® can be substituted for mechanical devices. An alternative approach is to treat the pseudoaneurysm directly by filling the aneurysmal sac. The therapeutic choices depend on the neck size and location of the pseudoaneurysm.

Chapter 8 Vascular interventions

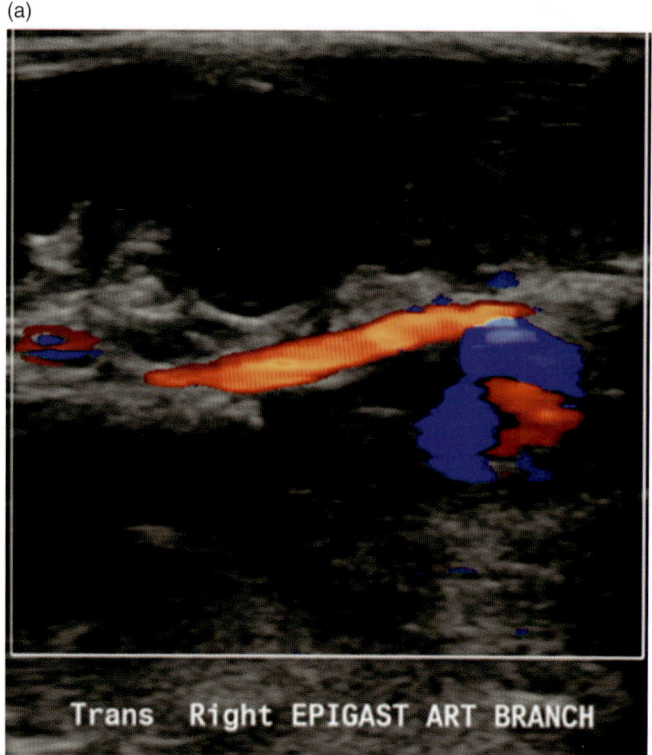

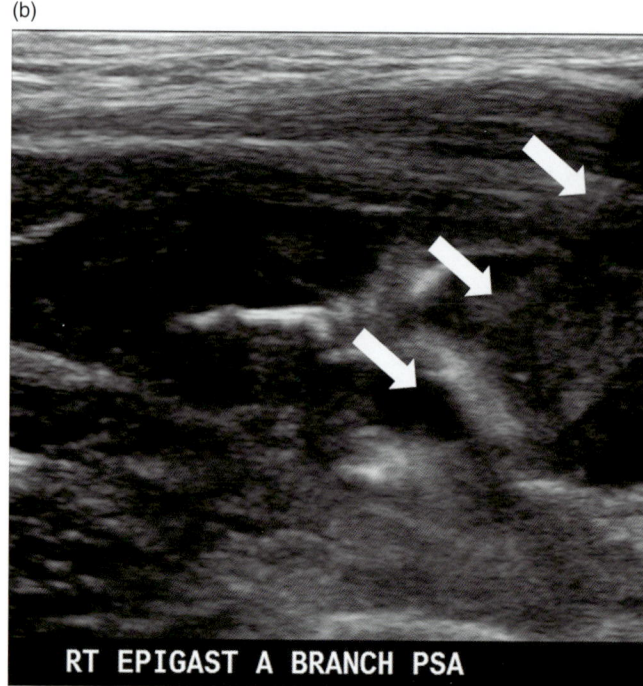

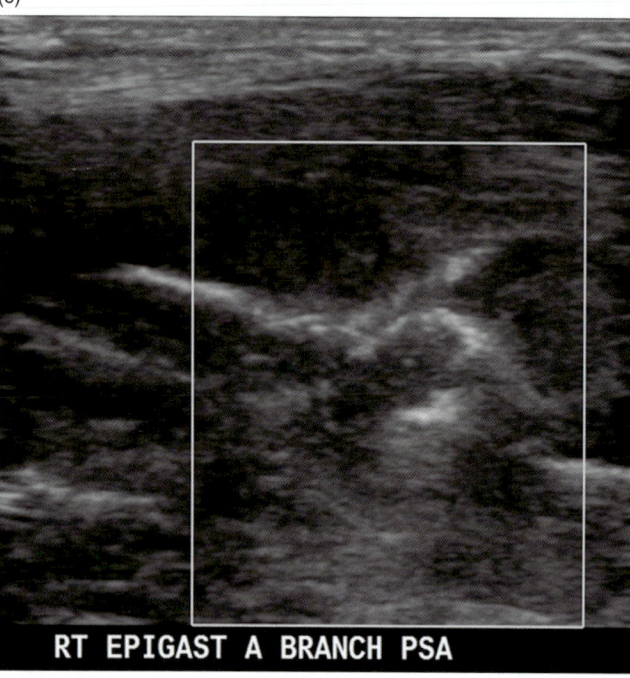

Figure 8.34 Sixteen-year-old female with a "growing" mass after paracentesis. (a) Color Doppler shows classic "ying-yang" appearance of blood flow in a saccular outpouching of a branch of the right epigastric artery characteristic of pseudoaneurysm. (b) Ultrasound-guided needle access (*arrows*) with injection of 100 IU (0.1 ml) thrombin into the sac. (c) Color Doppler US immediately after thrombin injection shows occlusion of the pseudoaneurysm.

Postprocedure and follow-up care

After completion of the procedure most children are observed in the ICU so that frequent vital signs and clinical examinations may be carried out. Special attention is paid to the circulation distal to the area treated. If there are clinical signs of abnormality, diagnostic imaging with non-invasive angiography (US, CT/CTA, MR/MRA) is obtained.

Complications

The main risk of percutaneous thrombin injection is downstream thrombin migration into the artery resulting in

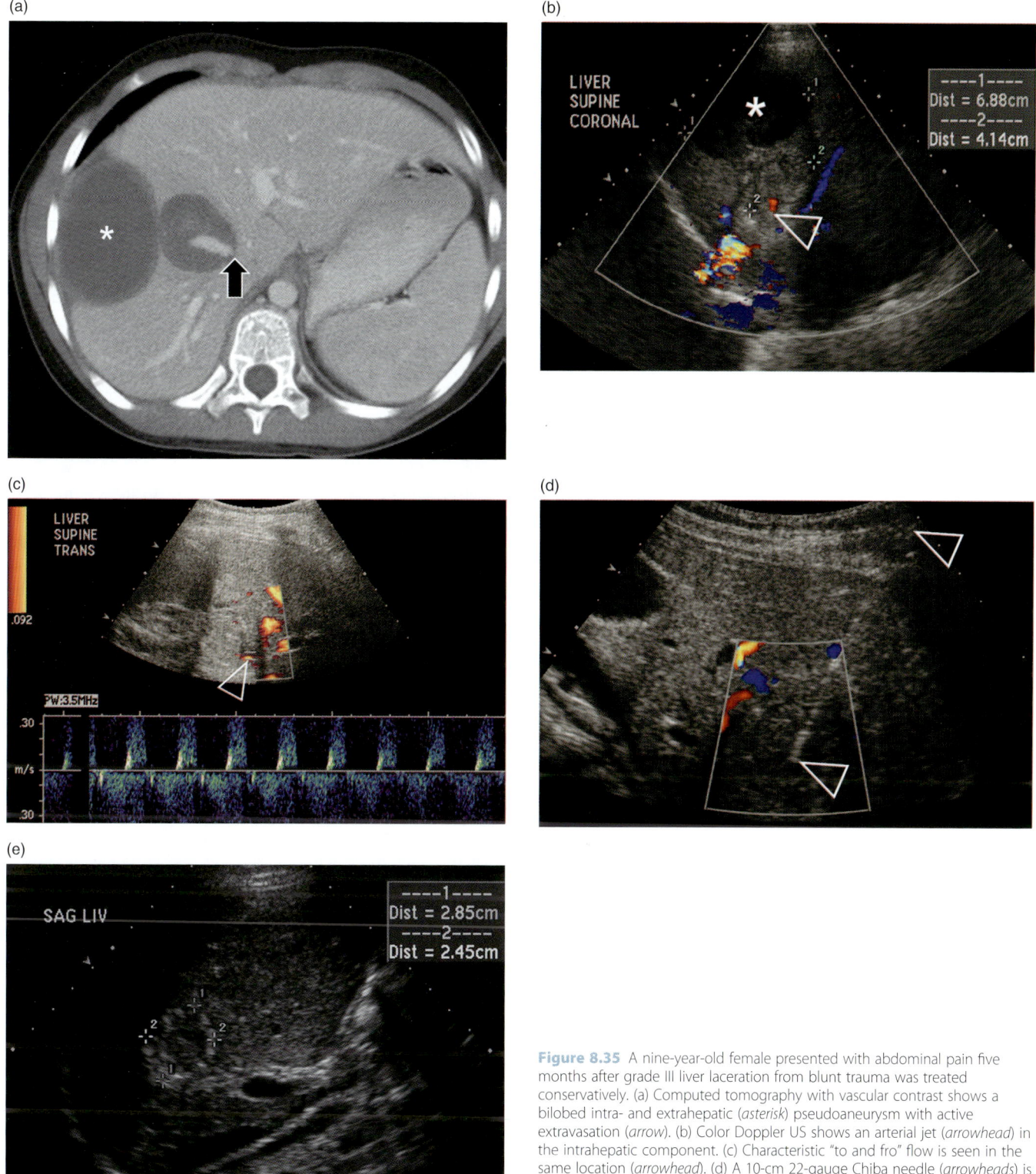

Figure 8.35 A nine-year-old female presented with abdominal pain five months after grade III liver laceration from blunt trauma was treated conservatively. (a) Computed tomography with vascular contrast shows a bilobed intra- and extrahepatic (*asterisk*) pseudoaneurysm with active extravasation (*arrow*). (b) Color Doppler US shows an arterial jet (*arrowhead*) in the intrahepatic component. (c) Characteristic "to and fro" flow is seen in the same location (*arrowhead*). (d) A 10-cm 22-gauge Chiba needle (*arrowheads*) is positioned under subxiphoid transabdominal US at the location of abnormal flow, and 250 IU thrombin injected. (e) Ultrasound 47 days later shows residual calcification but no pseudoaneurysm.

thrombosis and distal ischemia. There are techniques to reduce the embolic risk of thrombin injection, including temporary intra-arterial balloon occlusion.

Angioplasty and stenting

Introduction

The technique of percutaneous transluminal angioplasty (PTA) and vascular stenting (bare and covered) has been utilized for treatment of vascular stenoses in the adult population for over thirty years. The variety of indications and number of adult patients treated has steadily increased over the years. However, outside of the heart, PTA and stent insertion techniques have been used infrequently in the pediatric population. In recent years, the development and increasing availability of small, flexible angioplasty catheter systems and stents, designed for coronary, intracranial, and peripheral vascular use, have made it possible to treat children with vascular stenoses. As a result of these technical advances, the indications for angioplasty have increased. Placement of a stent in a young child is still avoided whenever possible since long-term patency is not known, nor is the effect on growth of the stented vessel.

Indications

The most common indications for angioplasty and on some occasions stenting in children include the treatment of portal venous and hepatic arterial and venous stenosis secondary to liver transplantation, renovascular disease, aortorenal syndromes, and venous compression syndromes (Table 8.15).

Transplant vascular stenosis

Hepatic artery thrombosis (HAT) has been reported in 5 to 11% of liver transplant recipients and in up to 25 to 30% of grafts from neonatal, infant, and small child donors. Predisposing factors include hepatic arterial kinking secondary to redundancy, reduced flow secondary to hepatic artery stenosis, allograft rejection, cold ischemia, polycythemia, use of fresh frozen plasma, and technical failure. Arterial narrowing is usually found at the site of anastomosis in the region of the porta hepatis by duplex and color Doppler US within two to three months after transplantation. In cases of complete HAT,

Table 8.15 Indications: angioplasty and stenting

- Hemodynamically significant stenosis
- Renovascular hypertension
- Anastomotic strictures usually in transplant population
- Dialysis grafts and fistulae
- Iatrogenic injuries
- Venous disease

arterial flow can sometimes be detected by Doppler in periportal collaterals, which most typically parasitize branches of the superior mesenteric artery and can result in false-negative results. However, the presence of such intra- or extrahepatic collaterals is not necessarily sufficient to protect the liver and biliary tree from ischemic injury. If left untreated, arterial stenosis may lead to complications including hepatic artery thrombosis, hepatic ischemia, biliary stricture, sepsis, and graft loss.

Hepatic artery stenosis (HAS) occurs in approximately 10% of patients after liver transplant, with 70% of the stenoses at the anastomosis. Stenosis can also occur adjacent to the anastomosis due to mechanical injury from vascular clamps. HAS usually occurs within three months of transplantation and can be clinically significant, leading to progressive deterioration of graft function. Anastomotic strictures probably result from a combination of fibrosis, reactive edema, or thrombosis at the anastomotic site while non-anastomotic strictures most often represent rejection or hepatic necrosis. While HAS may be coincidentally diagnosed during an angiographic procedure to detect the presence of HAT, it is most often diagnosed with duplex and color Doppler US examination performed in routine postoperative screening or during examination for hepatic dysfunction. If a significant HAS is detected treatment is usually indicated. Stenoses occurring in the immediate postoperative period are usually related to technical problems and require surgical intervention and anastomotic revision. Otherwise stenoses can frequently be treated with percutaneous transluminal angioplasty (PTA).

Hepatic venous outflow obstruction (Figure 8.36) is found in some 2 to 6% of liver transplant recipients. Symptomatic evidence of venous stenoses is often delayed for years after transplantation. Hepatic venous outflow obstruction may lead to portal hypertension (e.g., ascites, hepatocyte injury, splenomegaly), renal dysfunction, and lower extremity edema. Portal vein stenosis (Figure 8.37) occurs in about 1 to 8% of transplanted livers, although up to 19% of left lateral segment graft-related portal vein stenosis has been reported and may in part relate to the learning curve for transplant surgeons treating children. The incidence may be higher in children with reduced (e.g., left lobe) grafts, small portal veins, portal conduits, or significant discrepancy between donor and recipient veins.

In each of these settings, angioplasty has been shown to be effective in treatment of post-transplant vascular stenoses outside of the immediate postoperative period. Stent placement has been utilized for recurrent stenosis or suboptimal results with PTA. The outcomes after PTA and stenting have generally been excellent despite continued patient growth. Indications for PTA have not been clearly established in pediatric liver transplant recipients. Reported signs and symptoms that recommend specific angiographic evaluation include tender hepatosplenomegaly, ascites, encephalopathy, hematemesis,

Chapter 8 Vascular interventions

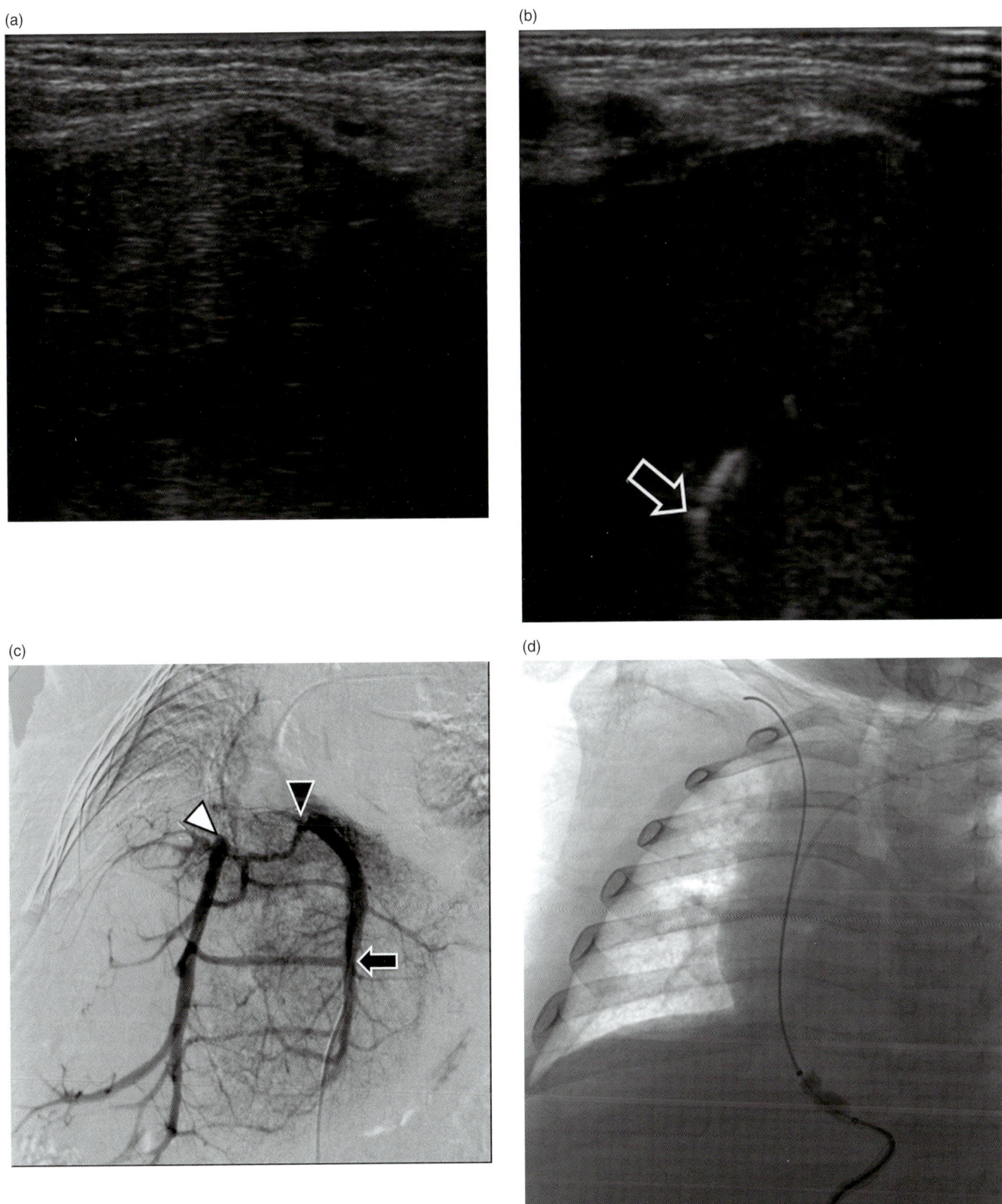

Figure 8.36 A two-month-old female with living donor left-lobe liver transplant has deteriorating liver function and evidence of venous obstruction on biopsy. (a) Because the transplant hepatic veins were not accessible from transjugular access, they were assessed with transabdominal US for percutaneous access. (b) Percutaneous transhepatic access was obtained under US control with a 22-gauge Chiba needle (*arrow*). (c) Hepatic venography from the segment 2 (*arrow*) hepatic vein shows high-grade stenosis at the anastomosis with the native IVC (*black arrowhead*). Although the segment 3 vein appears occluded (*white arrowhead*), review of donor imaging shows the graft was taken to the left of the bifurcation of the two veins. (d) A 5 mm × 2 cm 15 ATM balloon was advanced over a stiff guide wire through the 7 French endovenous sheath, and dilated, showing a tight anastomotic stenosis, (e) completely effaced at 12 ATM. (f) Postplasty venography shows good venous patency.

(e)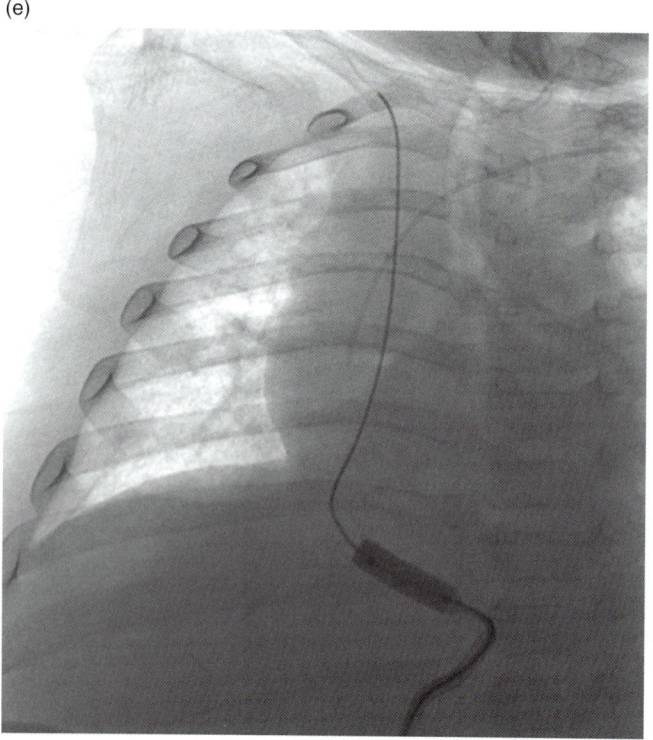

(f)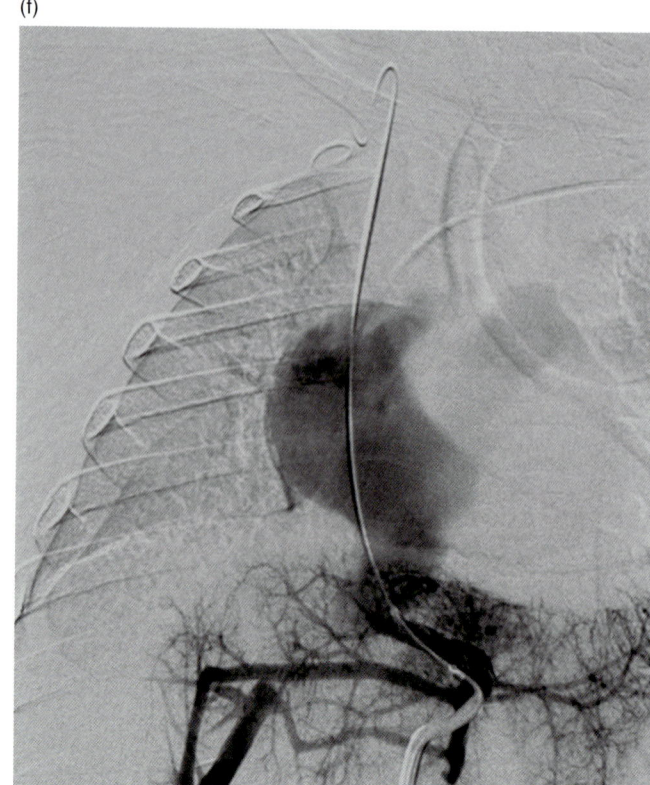

Figure 8.36 (cont.)

prolonged prothrombin time (PT), lower limb edema, stenosis of transplant vessels >50% by non-invasive imaging, evidence of elevated poststenotic flow velocity ("jet") on color Doppler US imaging, other signs of portal hypertension (including elevated liver enzymes, venous varices, and gastrointestinal bleeding), evidence of biliary stricture or biloma, pathologic evidence of hepatic venous congestion including centrilobular injury. Other causes that may not be amenable to PTA must be considered, including veno-occlusive disease such as from acute rejection, inadvertent surgical ligation, passive congestion related to elevated right atrial pressure, and extrinsic compression. Timely intervention is thought to be important in preventing ischemic allograft necrosis and resulting biliary strictures from hepatic arterial stenosis and complications related to hepatic synthetic impairment and gastrointestinal venous hypertension due to portal vein or hepatic vein stenosis.

Over the last ten years extensive research in animal models and clinical trials suggests that there may be a role for transplantation of exogenous hepatocytes in the treatment of patients in acute or chronic liver failure. However, this approach is still experimental. Hepatocyte transplantation is a relatively non-invasive endovascular technique that potentially could be used to augment liver mass with the added benefits of being relatively inexpensive and not limited by the shortage of donor organs.

Renal artery stenosis

Percutaneous transluminal angioplasty has been shown to be effective in treating stenoses of the main renal artery and proximal branch lesions. In our experience, the most common cause of narrowing requiring treatment is fibromuscular dysplasia (FMD) (Figure 8.38). The presentation of children with FMD differs from that in adults, due to a high percentage of disease involving segmental renal artery branches. Therefore, when examining patients with hypertension, it is important to study the main renal artery and segmental arteries of both kidneys to confirm the diagnosis of FMD prior to PTA. Balloon angioplasty is highly effective in the treatment of hypertension in children with FMD with success in approximately 90% of cases. In addition, vascular patency appears to be stable on follow-up. Transplant renal artery stenosis is relatively common in children undergoing cadaveric renal transplantation, and responds well to balloon angioplasty, with success rates of up to 77% reported.

Aortorenal syndromes

While FMD is the most common etiology of renal artery stenosis in some pediatric series, the aortorenal syndromes are more common in others. These aortorenal syndromes include midaortic syndrome, Takayasu arteritis, Williams syndrome, rubella syndrome, neurofibromatosis, and

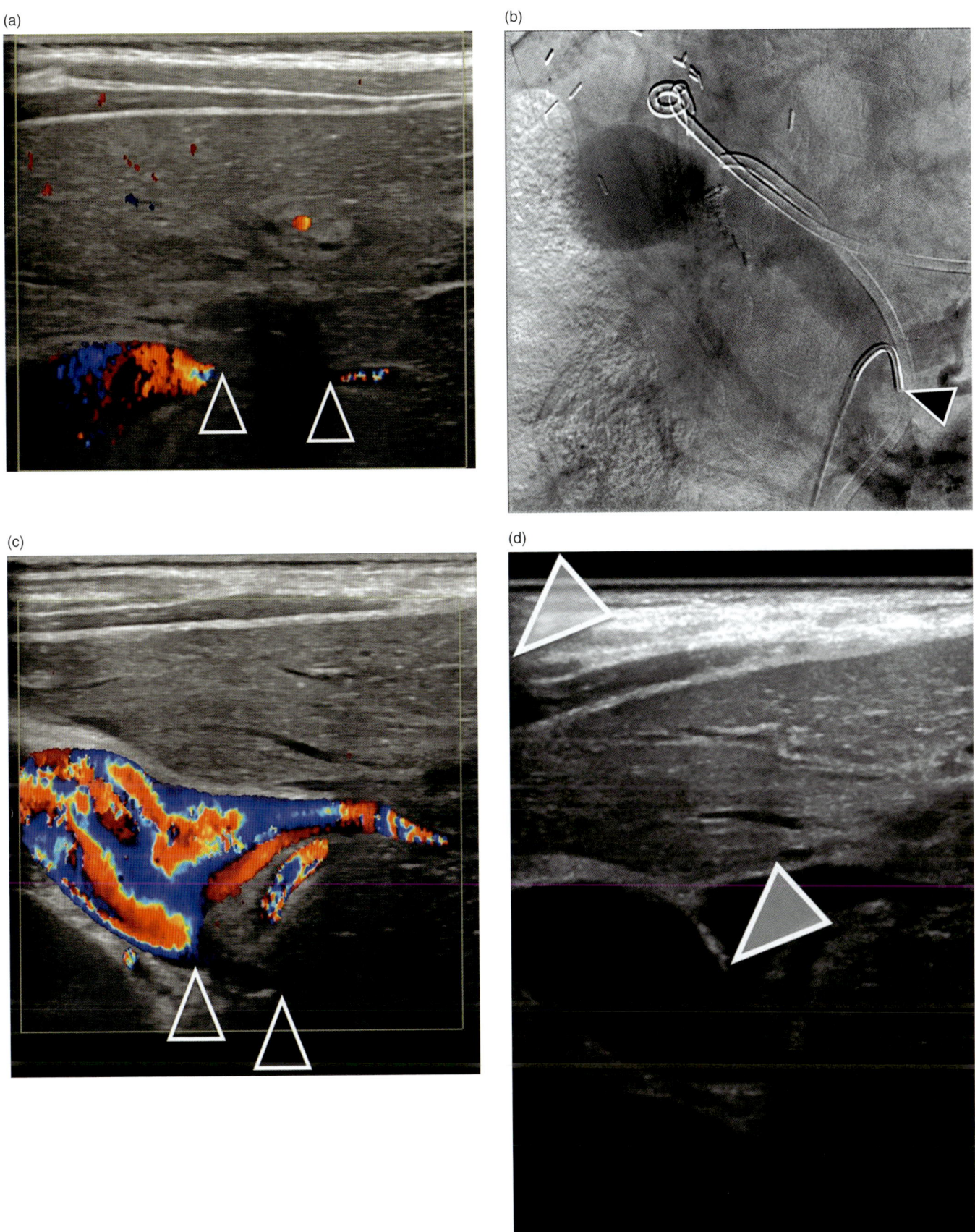

Figure 8.37 The same patient as in Figure 8.36, now 30 months of age, developed ascites and thrombocytopenia. She was also being treated for multiple intrahepatic biliary stenoses secondary to hepatic arterial thrombosis. (a) Portal narrowing (between *arrowheads*) and a "jet" on color Doppler US suggest extrahepatic portal stenosis. (b) Arterial (indirect) portography from a superior mesenteric artery (*arrowhead*) injection does not clarify the diagnosis, but rotational angiography was obtained during this injection. (c) The reconstructed images were used to orient US and plan a percutaneous transhepatic route to the extrahepatic portal vein (*arrowheads*). (d) A 22-gauge Chiba needle (*arrowheads*) was used to obtain access. Due to the favorable orientation of the access route, the needle tip could be positioned within the stenotic segment, allowing successful passage of a guide wire.

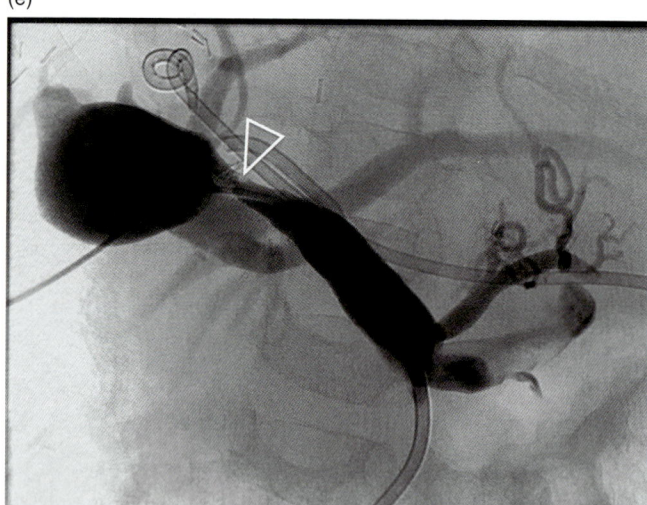
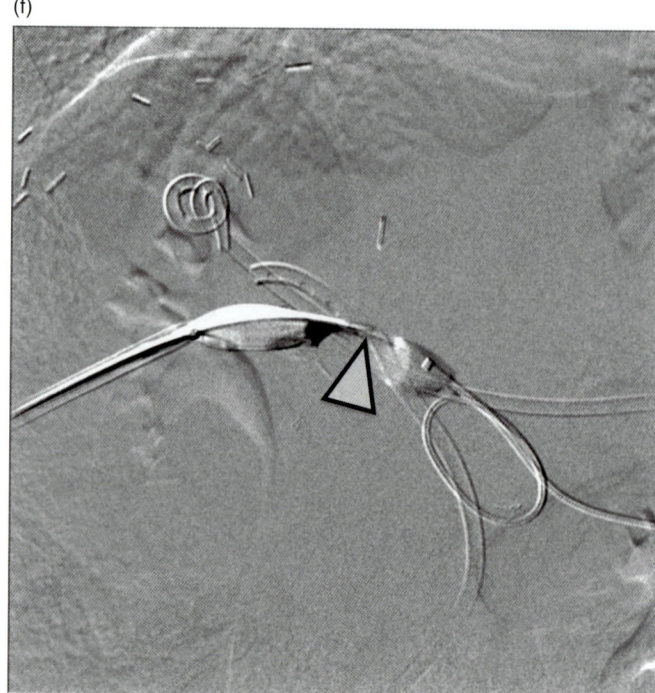
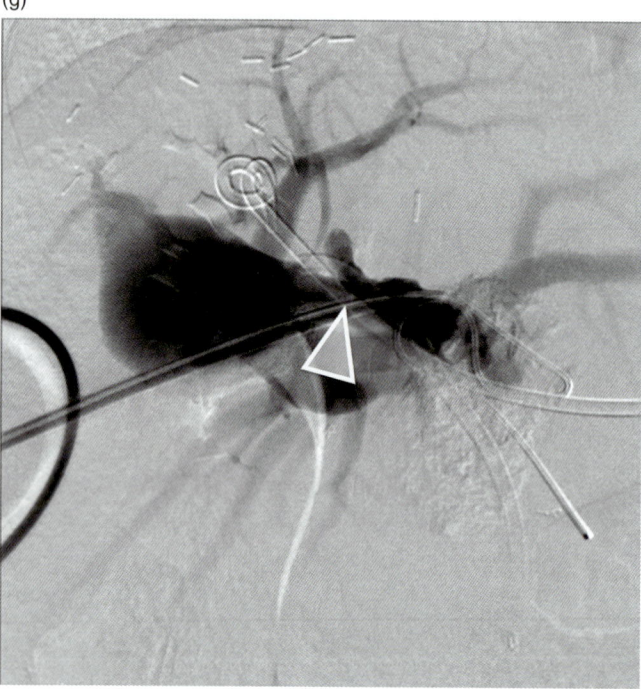

Figure 8.37 (*cont.*) (e) Direct portography clearly demonstrated the stenosis (*arrowhead*). (f) A 6 mm × 4 cm PTA balloon centered on the lesion showed a very tight stenosis (*arrowhead*), which was completely effaced with full dilation. (g) There was normal antegrade flow after venoplasty (*arrowhead*).

postradiotherapy arteritis. Unfortunately, in this group of patients with disease of the thoracic and abdominal aorta and contiguous involvement of the proximal main renal artery (Figure 8.39), PTA is usually ineffective with higher rates of treatment failure and complications. The group of syndromic renal stenosis presents a challenge to the interventionalist. In general, one should expect less than 50% of lesions to respond to conventional PTA. In this group, surgical therapy may be the best approach. However, with the advent of cutting balloon angioplasty and stents, new therapeutic possibilities are now available and being used more frequently (Figure 8.40). We have treated patients in this group successfully with cutting balloon angioplasty. We remain concerned about stenting this subgroup, although successful results have been reported.

Venous compression syndromes

Venous thrombolysis, angioplasty, and in some cases, stenting are indicated in acquired, usually central venous catheter related, venous stenosis, especially in children who need repeated venous access (see Figures 2.26 and 2.27). Other indications for treatment include venous obstructions such as in Budd–Chiari, venous compression syndromes, and intimal hyperplasia in dialysis fistulae. In our experience, the response to treatment of venous stenoses is poorer than with arterial

Chapter 8 Vascular interventions

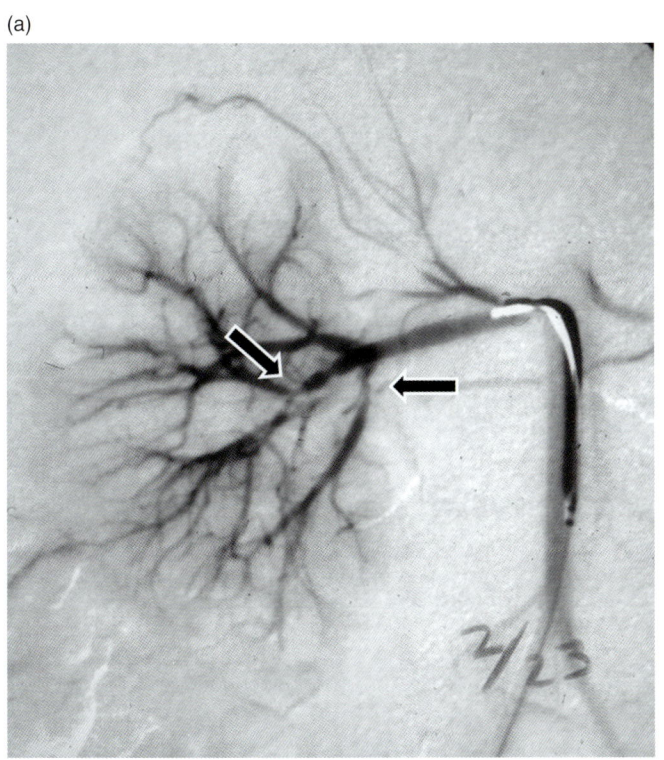
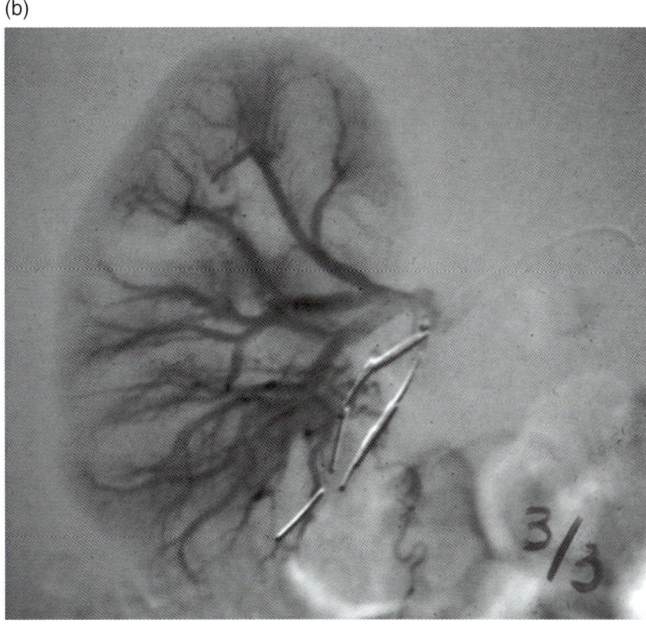

Figure 8.38 Three-year-old female with renovascular hypertension. (a) Selective right renal artery injection demonstrates fibromuscular dysplasia involving two lower pole branches vessels (*arrows*). (b) After 0.5 mm Hilal coil-embolization, the blood pressure normalized with a decreased number of antihyptertensive medications.

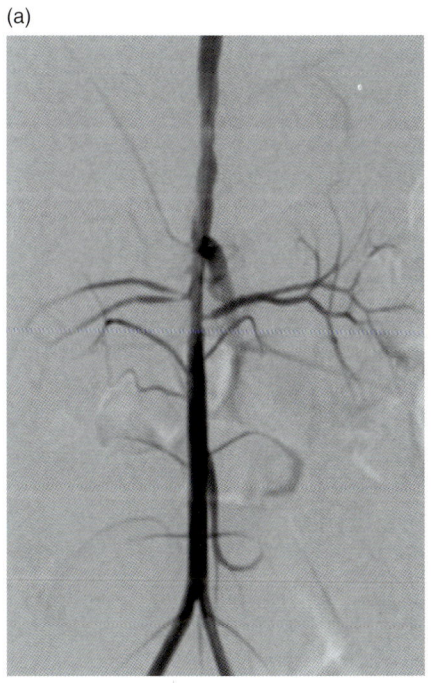
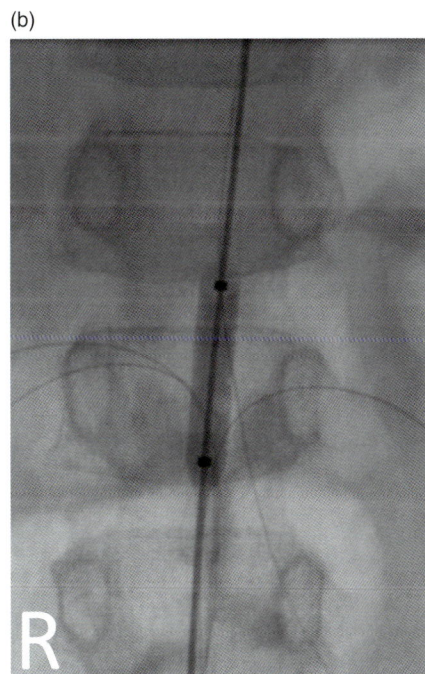

Figure 8.39 A seven-year-old male with complex congenital heart disease presented with severe hypertension despite seven antihypertensive medications. (a) Abdominal aortography showed midaortic stenosis with critical stenoses of the two right and single left renal arteries. The mean aortic pressure gradient across the aortic stenosis was 40 mm Hg. (Image courtesy of Derek Roebuck and Clare McLaren, Great Ormond Street Hospital, London). (b) With safety wires in the renal arteries and superior mesenteric artery (SMA), the aorta was dilated to 5 mm, and a 5 mm stent was placed above the SMA. The renal arteries were also dilated with 1.5 to 3.5 mm balloons. Following the procedures, the aortic gradient fell to 8 mm Hg. (Image courtesy of Derek Roebuck and Clare McLaren, Great Ormond Street Hospital, London).

lesions. In some of these patients, stent placement is an alternative and has become a primary therapy for May–Thurner syndrome (Figure 8.41) and some patients with Budd–Chiari syndrome.

Older children, usually teenagers, may present with signs and symptoms of venous compression syndromes. These include May–Thurner syndrome with compression of the left common iliac vein by the right common iliac artery,

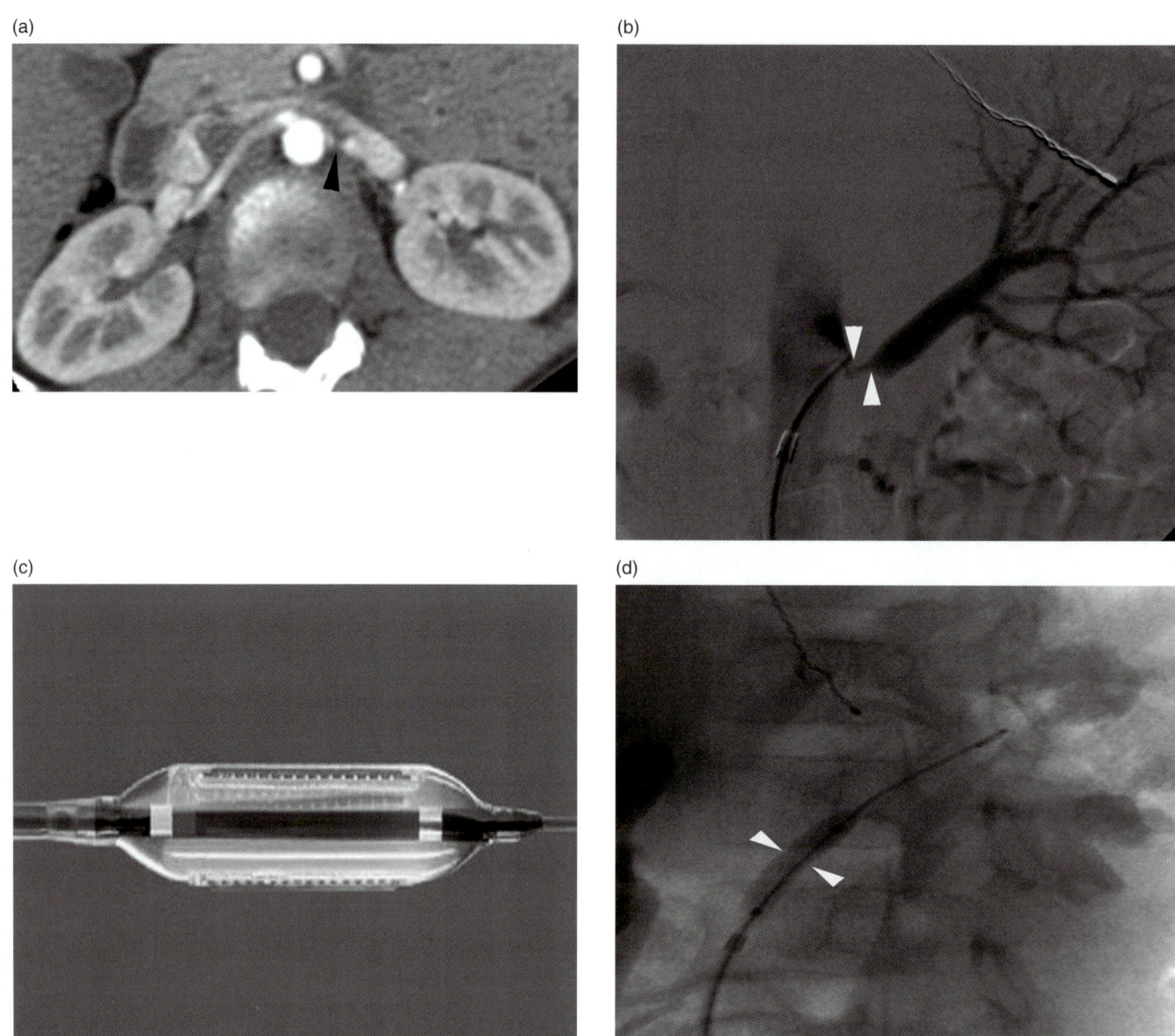

Figure 8.40 A nine-year-old, 26.6 kg male with Type 1 neurofibromatosis and hypertension with failed medical therapy and failed prior conventional renal angioplasty. (a) Computed tomography with vascular contrast enhancement shows a proximal left renal artery stenosis (*arrowhead*). (b) Selective left renal injection confirms severe proximal main renal artery stenosis with normal aorta (*arrowheads*). (c) Inflated cutting balloon. After repeated attempts to relieve the stenosis with conventional angioplasty balloons, a 45 mm Hg gradient persisted. A 4 mm × 10 mm cutting balloon (Interventional Technologies, San Diego, CA) was inflated by hand. (d) Slight residual stenosis was treated with a conventional 5 mm × 2 cm angioplasty balloon (*arrowheads*). The child was discharged the following day with significant improvement in blood pressure on a reduced dose of antihypertensive medication.

Paget–Schroetter syndrome with thrombosis of the subclavian vein usually within the costoclavicular space, and Nutcracker syndrome with compression of the left renal vein between the abdominal aorta and superior mesenteric artery.

May–Thurner syndrome is seen about three times more frequently in girls than in boys, usually in the second to fourth decade of life, with left lower extremity pain and swelling in the absence of a hypercoagulable state. As is the case with other compression syndromes, diagnosis is made with venography, US, CT, or MRI. As a result of repeated trauma or severe compression, venous thrombosis occurs with partial or complete outflow obstruction. Initial therapy usually begins with thrombolysis and is followed by stent insertion. Surgical therapy is also an alternative. In Paget–Schroetter syndrome, there is primary thrombosis of the subclavian vein as a result of forced abduction of the upper limb in young athletes, who use repetitive shoulder–arm motions. These injuries are seen in baseball pitchers, volleyball players, weight lifters, wrestlers, and even dancers. In this condition, the interventionalist is often asked to perform diagnostic studies and, if a thrombosis is identified, to perform thrombolysis. However, unlike May–Thurner syndrome, stenting is not indicated. Mild angioplasty

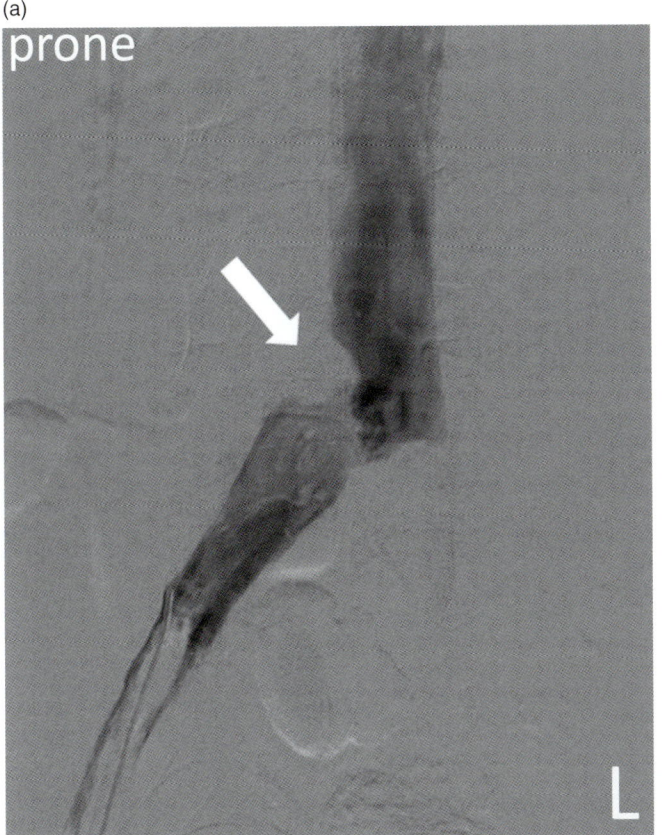
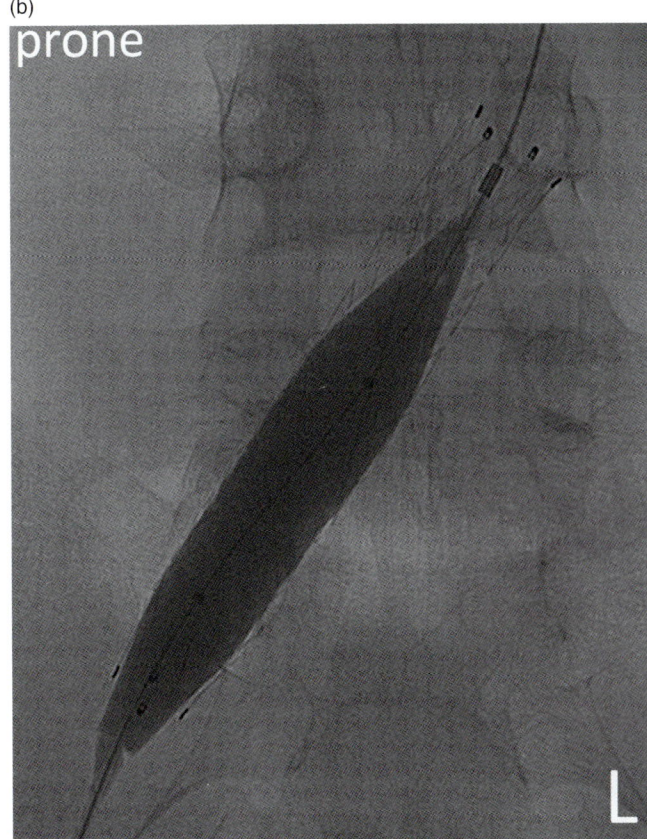
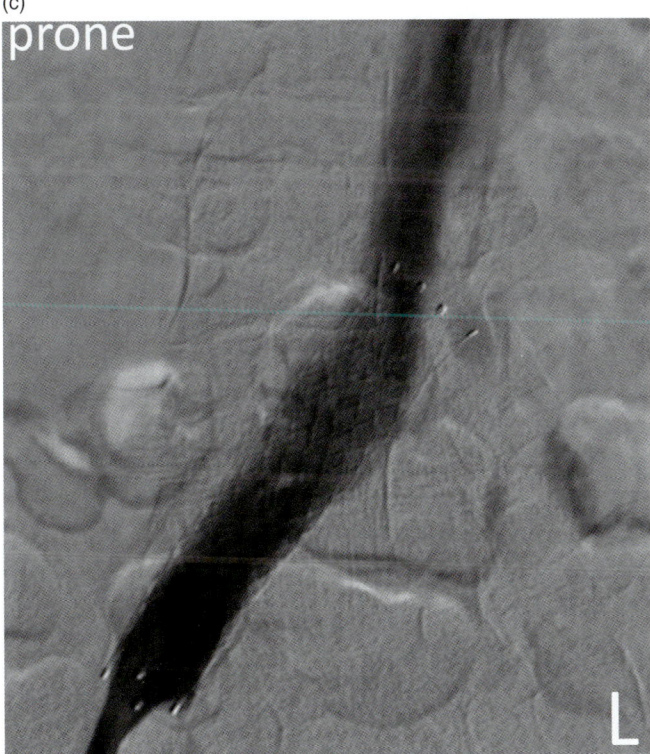

Figure 8.41 A 14-year-old male developed acute left lower extremity swelling and pain. Ultrasound demonstrated extensive DVT. Symptomatic May–Thurner syndrome recurred despite treatment with chemical and mechanical thrombolysis. (a) Digital subtraction angiography with patient prone shows left common iliac venous thrombus due to distal compression of the vein by the right common iliac artery (*arrow*). (b) A balloon-expandable 14 cm stent was deployed across the level of left iliac venous compression. (c) After deployment the vein was widely patent.

Table 8.16 Equipment: angioplasty and stenting

- Long and short sheaths with hemostasis valves (4 to 6 French)
- Directional catheters
- Directional guide wires (Glidewire®, Tracker wires, Roadrunner®, etc.)
- Variable stiffness microcatheters and 0.012-inch to 0.014-inch wires
- Angioplasty catheters (small vessel, microballoons, monorail balloons, standard)
- Intravascular pressure monitor
- Drugs:
  - vasodilators (nitroglycerine, verapamil, papavarine)
  - anticoagulants (heparin 50 to 100 U/kg to a maximum bolus of 2,000 U)
  - thrombolytic agents (tPA)
- Stents

Table 8.17 Procedure summary: angioplasty and stenting

- General anesthesia or sedation (older children)
- Skin preparation and draping
- Local anesthesia if needed
- Puncture artery, insert a sheath
- Diagnostic angiogram
- Measure pressure gradient
- Selective catheterization of stenotic vessel
- Inject heparin into the stenotic vessel
- PTA: standard or cutting balloons
- Stent for failures or complications as necessary
- Postprocedural angiogram
- Admit to ICU for overnight observation
- Maintain heparinization for 24 to 72 hours
- Convert to Coumadin® or Lovenox®
- Antiplatelet drugs (aspirin, clopidogrel bisulfate)

may be helpful preoperatively, but the treatment of choice is surgical decompression, usually by resection of the first rib. Angioplasty and stenting may have a role after surgical intervention. Renal vein Nutcracker syndrome results from entrapment of the renal vein between the abdominal aorta and superior mesenteric artery and may present with hematuria, abdominal pain (usually left flank), and on occasion testicular or left lower quadrant pain due to congestion of the gonadal vein in males or females respectively. Treatment of this entrapment is either with renal vein stenting or surgical vascular revision.

Technique
Equipment

The equipment needed for angioplasty and stenting in the pediatric population is similar to that utilized in the adult population (Table 8.16). In smaller children, catheter size is reduced proportional to patient weight. Intravascular pressure monitoring equipment, appropriately sized diagnostic and balloon angioplasty catheters from 3 to 5 French, bare-metal and covered stents, and controlled inflation devices are necessary. A vascular sheath at the vascular entry site is used to minimize vascular trauma and secondary occlusion. In small infants, the use of a sheath with hemostasis valve is occasionally not possible.

Standard PTA balloons are used in most instances since they are easiest to maneuver into position over a guide wire. In small children, it is helpful to use the balloon catheter with the smallest shaft diameter available. For children less than 20 kg, the preferred catheter is a small vessel balloon with a 3.2 French shaft diameter. If the catheter cannot be maneuvered into position across the stenosis (because the catheter is too stiff or inflexible) or it is too large (e.g., segmental renal artery) to pass through the arterial narrowing, a small vessel balloon or monorail balloon may be used. When a small vessel balloon is used, it is helpful to use a long sheath positioned as close to the stenosis as possible, maximizing the chance of positioning the balloon across the stenosis.

As is the case for other vascular interventions, the choice of guide wire is extremely important. There are a number of guide wires to choose from and the ultimate decision of which to use is often made as a result of past experience, on-site availability, and cost considerations. We find that the 0.018-inch angled Glidewire® and various 0.012-inch to 0.014-inch directional guide wires, when used with a variable stiffness microcatheter, work well especially when combined with road mapping.

Patient preparation

Routine preparation for vascular interventional procedures is discussed under "General angiographic considerations" at the beginning of this chapter. For angioplasty procedures, it may also be useful to type and cross-match the child in the event that a blood transfusion is emergently required. Long-acting anti-hypertensive medications may be changed to short-acting ones, to avoid the development of postangioplasty hypotension. Antiplatelet medication should be started 24 hours prior to the procedure. Careful attention should be paid to the fluid and electrolyte status of the child.

Standard technique

The technique used to perform renal angioplasty in a child is similar to that used in adults and involves: diagnostic angiography for mapping of the pathologic anatomy, measurement of a pressure gradient when possible, anticoagulation, and injection of vasodilators (e.g., nitroglycerine). In infants and toddlers, small femoral artery sheaths are needed to avoid arterial injury. Thus PTA is accomplished using balloon catheters with small shaft diameters (e.g., 3 to 5 French) introduced over a guide wire.

As is the case in older patients, the procedure begins with abdominal aortography and selective renal artery injections in one or more projections (Table 8.17). Superselective branch catheterization using microcatheters is sometimes necessary to delineate the anatomy of a distal branch stenosis or occlusion. Complete occlusions are often difficult to identify, but the presence of tortuous intrarenal collaterals is a reliable secondary sign of a branch occlusion. Care is taken not to cross the stenosis with a guide wire until the time for treatment. Once across the area of narrowing, the guide wire is maintained in position until treatment is completed. In addition, heparin (50–100 U/kg) is injected directly into the renal artery just prior to PTA.

Prior to angioplasty, selective renal vein renin (RVR) sampling may be helpful in confirming the source of hypertension. However, since processing the specimens is a lengthy process, one cannot use the information if PTA is planned the same day. When RVR sampling is obtained, venous access is usually obtained via a femoral vein. Although not essential, we prefer to insert a vascular sheath with hemostasis valve into the femoral vein to allow for repeated access and to protect the common femoral vein against trauma. A variety of catheters may be used to collect blood samples; however, a C-1, RC-1, or JB-1 shape is most often used although a pediatric SOS Omni® can be helpful in some cases. Approximately 3 ml of blood is collected from the infrarenal inferior vena cava (IVC) near the level of the common iliac vein confluence, suprarenal IVC near the right atrium, and from both the right and left renal veins. In selected cases, samples are collected from branch or segmental renal veins as well, depending upon the renal vascular anatomy.

Although some interventionalists confirm catheter position in the renal veins with contrast injection, others prefer to avoid contrast injection and confirm the position of the catheter by the position of the guide wire. It is controversial as to whether the injection of contrast affects the results. Regardless of the technique utilized, the blood pressure is measured at the time each blood sample is obtained.

Technical variations

In some patients, especially those with syndromic causes of renal artery stenosis (e.g., Williams syndrome, neurofibromatosis, etc.), fewer than 50% of lesions will respond to standard balloon angioplasty. In these children, cutting balloon angioplasty is a useful alternative. In our practice, we begin treatment with a standard, high atmosphere balloon about 10% larger than the native vessel diameter. If the stenosis is resistant to therapy, a cutting balloon of the same size as the adjacent normal artery is considered. Particular care must be used when treating asymmetric stenoses, as asymmetric inflation of the cutting balloon may cause one blade to cut more deeply than intended. This may result in hemorrhage or pseudoaneurysm formation. After the cutting balloon has inscribed longitudinal incisions across the stenosis, the standard non-compliant PTA balloons are then used to achieve the desired vessel diameter. As a last resort, stenting is considered if a surgical bypass is not possible. In cases in which PTA is not successful and when surgical vessel repair is not possible, or for those procedures complicated by the development of an intimal flap, arterial stenting may be considered. However, consideration must be given to the potential for growth of the patient and renal artery. It should not be assumed that implanted stents can be sufficiently enlarged by future re-angioplasty in order to accommodate growth. Also, the impact of prolonged stenting on growth and complications is unknown. For these reasons, stenting is not routinely performed in children.

Patients undergoing renal artery angioplasty should be observed in the hospital overnight in an ICU so that vital signs can be monitored frequently and heparin infused to maintain the PT at twice the normal value. Although variable, some physicians suggest the use of antiplatelet drugs, which may be continued for approximately six months.

Technical problems and pitfalls

The nature of pediatric renovascular disease may impede the success of catheter angioplasty, due to the presence of aorto-ostial or distal segment obstruction. Ischemic renal distal branch stenosis not amenable to PTA may be treated by ablation using ethanol or coils (Figure 8.38).

Complications

Complications of balloon angioplasty in children are similar to those in adults and include vessel dissection, perforation, and thrombosis.

Thrombolysis

Introduction

Systemic or catheter-directed thrombolytic therapy is infrequently required in children, although the number of children requiring treatment has steadily increased over the last five years. Over the last two decades, there has been a changing approach to clot lysis. In the 1980s, the drug of choice was streptokinase (SK), which is not fibrin-specific and has a plasma half-life of 30 minutes. This often resulted in antibody production, making retreatment difficult due to the high incidence of allergic reactions. Streptokinase was replaced by urokinase (UK), a drug that activates plasminogen directly by enzymatic action and has a shorter plasma half-life of 20 minutes. Urokinase also has the advantage of not resulting in antibody production so that allergic reactions are rare. Urokinase has now been replaced by tissue plasminogen activator (tPA), which is fibrin-specific, activates plasminogen, has a short half-life, and now is widely used for all chemical clot lysis. Interestingly, in the past several years, there has been a migration toward mechanical thrombolysis as primary therapy with catheter-directed thrombolysis as secondary therapy.

Indications

Indications for thrombolysis are varied but uncommon in the pediatric population (Table 8.18). The most common indication for tPA is to declot catheters. The more common systemic problems necessitating treatment include arterial or venous thrombosis secondary to medical catheterization (e.g., femoral artery thrombosis after cardiac catheterization or angiography), neonatal aortic thrombosis with associated renal artery involvement secondary to an indwelling umbilical arterial catheter, superior vena caval thrombosis resulting from central venous catheters, and arterial occlusions from *in situ* or embolic arterial occlusions. Early hepatic arterial thrombosis (HAT) is one of the major causes of graft failure and mortality in liver transplant recipients, and those who survive the initial event often develop ischemic biliary strictures (see Figures 5.1, 5.4, and 5.5) that if untreated may lead to need for retransplantation. When HAT is recognized, endovascular therapy (Figure 8.42) should be considered as a therapeutic option. Spontaneous thrombosis effectively treated by thrombolytic drugs also includes neonatal arterial thromboembolic occlusions (e.g., subclavian artery), dural sinus thrombosis, renal vein thrombosis, pulmonary artery thrombosis, thrombosed Blalock–Taussig shunts, hemodialysis fistulae, and other graft thrombosis. Portomesenteric thrombosis may occur from many causes, but is usually related to a provocative event, such as dehydration or sepsis, in a patient with a clotting abnormality that may have been previously undiagnosed. These patients are often treated conservatively, such as with systemic thrombolytic administration, but frequently do poorly on this regimen and may eventually progress to acute failure related to the slowly progressive occlusion of their portomesenteric veins. We advocate for early involvement of interventionalists in patient management and evaluation, and for consideration of transcatheter thrombolysis as early as possible (Figure 8.43), although this approach has not yet been widely accepted. Contraindications to thrombolytic therapy include severe coagulopathy or hypoprothrombinemia, recent surgery, and active intracranial processes. In neonates, it is important to image the brain prior to initiating thrombolytic therapy to be sure there is no intracranial hemorrhage. In premature infants, one might still consider thrombolytic therapy if there is a grade 1 or possibly grade 2 hemorrhage, in select high-risk cases. The decision algorithm is similar to that used to decide whether or not to place or continue a child on extracorporeal membrane oxygenation (ECMO).

Table 8.18 Indications: thrombolysis

- Symptomatic vascular occlusion
- Risk of pulmonary embolism
- Artery or vein recanalization
- Dialysis graft/fistula occlusion

Technique

Equipment

Thrombolysis may be achieved by pulse lysis, in conjunction with mechanical thrombolysis, by catheter-directed regional or intra-clot therapy, or by systemic intravenous

(a)

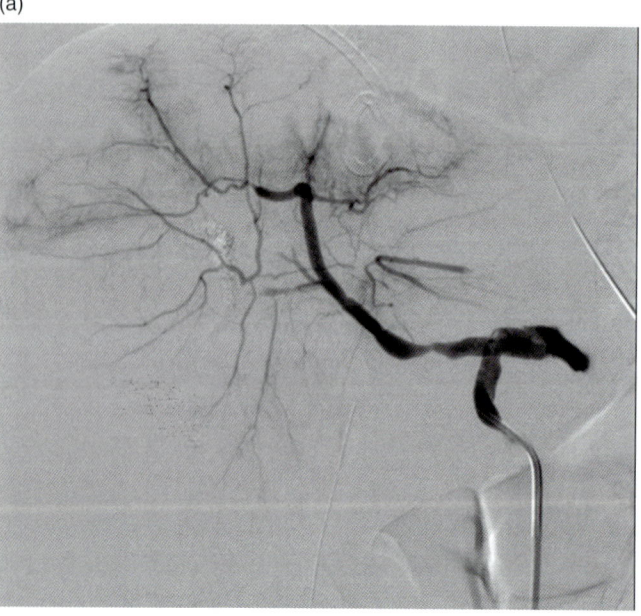

(b)

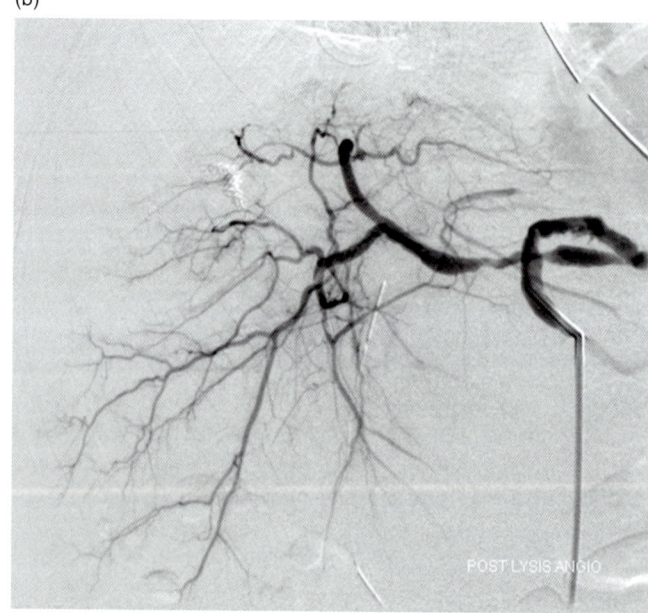

Figure 8.42 A 30-month-old male six weeks after liver transplant has patchy areas of apparent hepatic necrosis on CT, ascites, and anasarca. An initial proximal transplant hepatic arteriogram shows complete occlusion with a "meniscus" sign. (a) After pulse lysis with 2 mg alteplase, sluggish filling of irregular and attenuated transplant hepatic arteries is seen. (b) After an additional 1 mg alteplase was pulsed more distally, brisk arterial flow to the graft was restored.

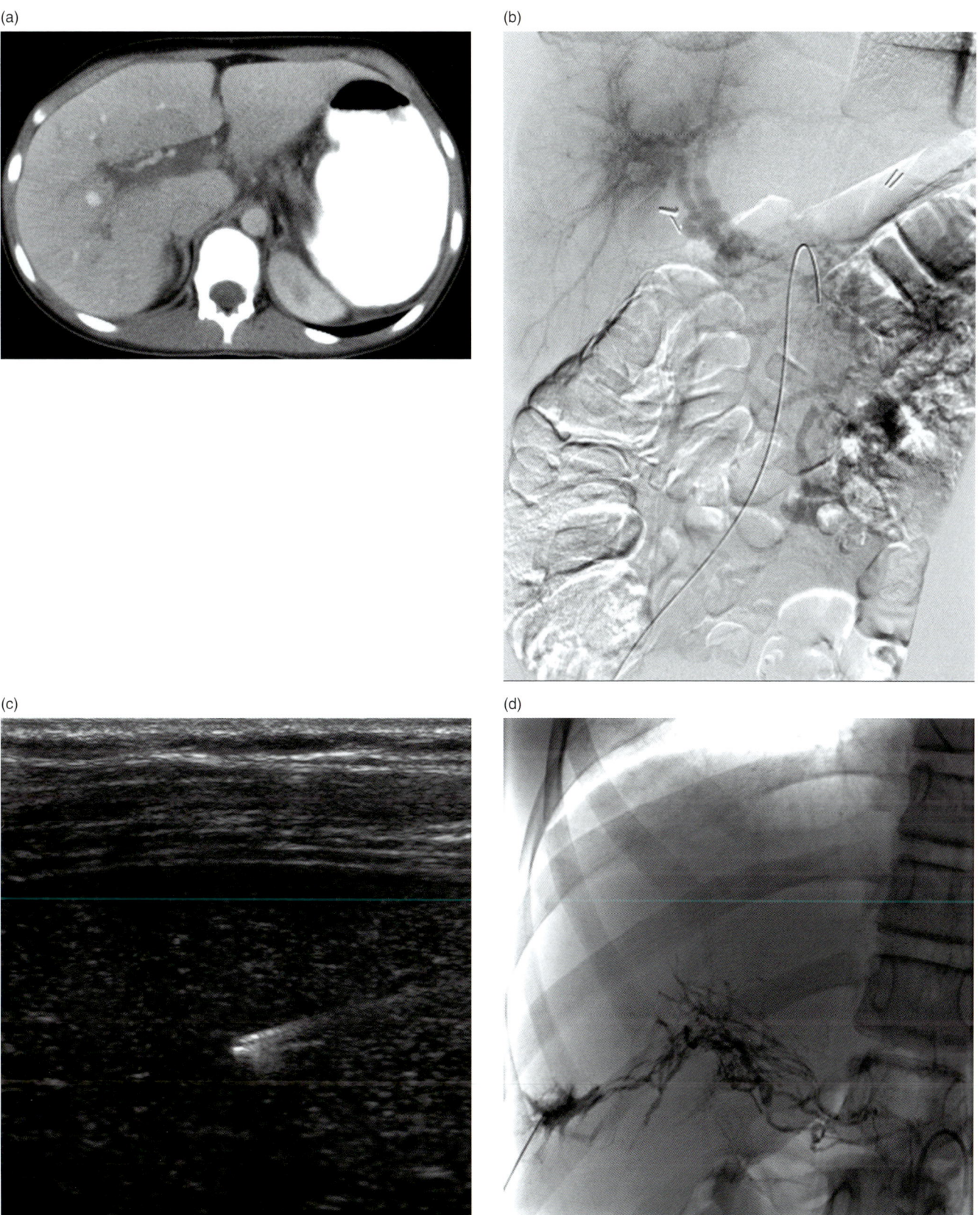

Figure 8.43 A 12-year-old female with hereditary spherocytosis was referred two weeks after splenectomy and cholecystectomy with massive portomesenteric thrombosis. (a) Computed tomography with vascular and enteric contrast shows absence of flow and clot filling intra- and extrahepatic portal veins. While this was interpreted as "old, organizing clot," its likely genesis was dated by her splenectomy. (b) Indirect portography from a superior mesenteric arteriogram shows cavernous transformation and very poor intrahepatic portal venous flow. (c) Ultrasound-guided percutaneous transhepatic portal vein access. Because no flow was visualized in the portal veins, a thick-walled structure with hyperechoic margins was targeted. (d) Contrast injection confirmed portal access by exclusion: non-pulsatile flow was directed toward the porta hepatis in a non-biliary pattern.

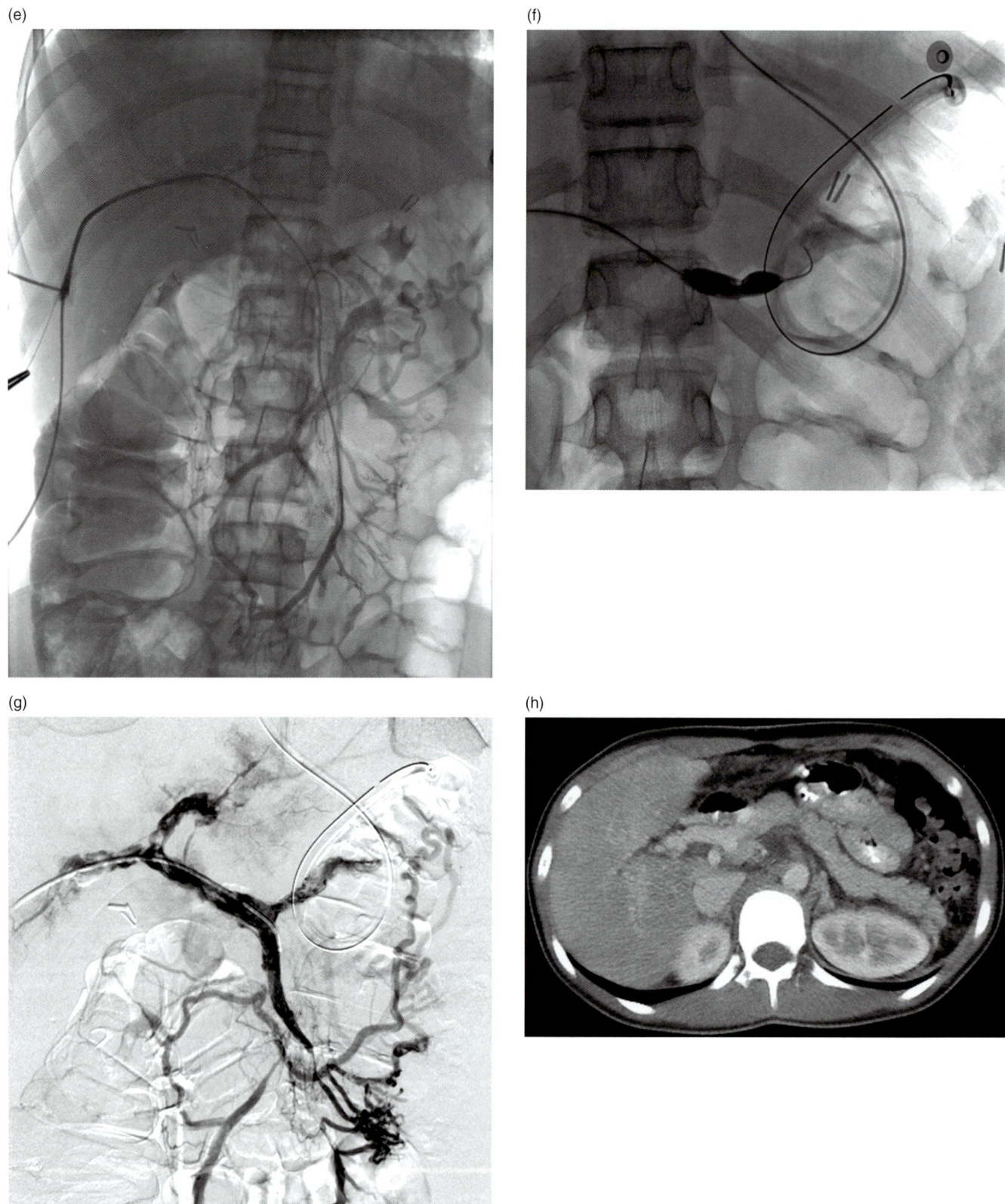

Figure 8.43 (*cont.*) (e) After 32 hours of (indirect) regional alteplase thrombolysis through a JB-1 catheter in the superior mesenteric artery, the central mesenteric veins had cleared, and the main portal vein was visualized although still filled with now non-occlusive thrombus. A 5 French pulse lysis catheter was advanced through the percutaneous transhepatic sheath across the portal veins to the mesenteric vein, and direct lytic therapy continued for 24 hours. (f) Due to persistent irregularity of the splenic vein, a 5 mm embolectomy balloon was pulled back through the splenic vein, revealing a tight stenosis, which was treated with a 7 mm × 2 cm 15 ATM PTA balloon, as shown. Additional PTA balloon maceration, spot lysis, mechanical thrombectomy, and suction removed a significant amount of remaining clot burden. (g) Completion venography shows significant improvement in portomesenteric patency. (h) Computed tomography with vascular contrast 20 months after thrombolysis shows patent portal veins with extensive mesenteric collateralization. The patient remains asymptomatic.

Table 8.19 Equipment: thrombolysis

- Sheath with hemostasis valve
- Infusion catheters (pulse spray, infusion wires, standard directional catheters)
- Drugs: tPA, heparin
- Guide wires: standard, directional, hydrophilic

Table 8.20 Preparation for rheolytic (AngioJet™) mechanical thrombolysis

- 2 × 250 ml bags of normal saline each mixed with 500 U heparin creating a 2 U/ml solution
  - First bag connected to AngioJet™ for bland mechanical thrombolysis
  - Up to 2 mg tPA (alteplase) per 100 ml may be added to this bag for combined chemical/mechanical thrombolysis
  - Second bag emptied into a reservoir to preload the AngioJet™
- Maximum run time
  - Partially occluded vessel: 220 seconds
  - Completely occluded vessel: 440 seconds
- Catheter (size/length/guide wire/recommended vessel diameter)
  - Vista: 4 French/145 cm/0.014-inch/1.5 to 3.0 mm
  - XVG: 5 French/135 cm/0.014-inch/3 to 5 mm
  - Proxi: 6 French/90 cm/0.035-inch/5 to 20 mm
  - Omni: 6 French/120 cm/0.035-inch/5 to 20 mm

infusion (Table 8.19). These patients may require frequent vascular imaging to document treatment response. Direct transcatheter therapy is performed in the angiography suite with standard vascular access techniques. The smallest possible catheter (3 French) should be used to minimize the risk of bleeding, vessel injury, or proximal vessel thrombosis. Pulse spray catheters are useful and are available in small sizes with short infusion zones and are suited for all pediatric patients including neonates and small infants. In addition, we have occasionally used pulse spray catheters to treat dural venous sinus thrombosis. Alternatively, angiographic catheters or Katzen guide wires may be used to deliver the thrombolytic agent.

A variety of devices are available for bland mechanical thrombolysis or for combined chemical and mechanical thrombolysis. Thrombus may be disrupted with a guide wire or macerated and aspirated with a combination of a compliant thrombectomy balloon and a large sheath. Partially treated clot may sometimes be macerated with a non-compliant angioplasty balloon to "shape" the recanalized lumen, to reduce turbulent flow, and to increase penetration of the clot with tPA. Automated devices include rheolytic systems, rotational or oscillating systems, and US-enhanced systems. Rheolytic thrombectomy systems (e.g., AngioJet™) use a high-pressure saline jet to macerate the thrombus and to drive thrombolytic medication into the clot substance (Table 8.20). Rotational (e.g., Trerotola™ and Amplatz®) and oscillating (e.g., Trellis™) systems macerate the clot with a high-velocity rotating helix or sinusoidal wire, and in the latter case also inject thrombolytics into the clot between terminal balloons that isolate the treated region. Ultrasound-enhanced systems (e.g., EndoWave™) improve clot penetration by thrombolytics with high-frequency US. Of these systems, we currently have the most experience with rheolytic and oscillating devices in children.

Plasminogen activators are now the agents of choice for chemical clot lysis. These include alteplase, reteplase, and tenecteplase. Alteplase has a relatively short plasma half-life (four to six minutes), and is preferred for catheter declotting. Reteplase is a second-generation agent that seems to have more rapid activity and lower systemic bleeding risk. With a longer half-life (13 to 16 minutes) and decreased fibrin binding affinity, it may have better clot penetration. Tenecteplase has higher binding affinity, the longest half-life of the three (20 to 24 minutes), greater resistance to degradation, and has shown superior outcomes for treatment of embolic stroke. Results for deep vein thrombolysis in general are satisfactory with any of these agents.

Patient preparation

Our approach to children suspected of having an arterial or venous thrombotic occlusion begins with diagnostic imaging. We prefer initial evaluation with US and sometimes MRI to define the extent and distribution of disease. In most cases, US with Doppler is sufficient to assess the vascular dynamics. Once the diagnosis is confirmed, we recommend consultation with a pediatric hematologist for a thorough clinical examination to assess for associated or predisposing conditions (including antibody to factor IV and anticardiolipin antibodies and protein S, C, and antithrombin III deficiency tests), risk factors, and discussion regarding the approach to therapy. In cases where there is non-occlusive thrombus, systemic thrombolysis may be satisfactory. However, complete or high-grade occlusion, progressive symptoms, or failed systemic therapy will usually require mechanical or catheter-directed thrombolysis. Preprocedure labs include baseline hemoglobin and hematocrit, platelets, renal function, and acid–base equilibrium markers. Coagulation studies (PT, INR, aPTT, TCT, fibrinogen level, fibrin split products, etc.) are obtained as per hospital or departmental protocol, at baseline and at minimum every four hours during therapy. These labs should be run immediately and results should be reported directly to the on-call interventional radiologist as soon as they are available. It is also sensible to consult the pediatric transplant surgical service if available to co-manage these cases in the ICU, since the skill sets are complementary and because these cases are usually so infrequent that collaborative management will reduce risk in most cases. Usually, blood is typed and crossmatched in case an emergent transfusion is needed. Preprocedure administration of unfractionated heparin in a continuous therapeutic dose is recommended. This is maintained through the course of therapy (usually administered via the endovascular sheath during continuous transcatheter therapy, but not

Table 8.21 Procedure summary: thrombolysis

- General anesthetic or sedation
- Sterile preparation and draping
- Puncture vessel, insert sheath
- Inject contrast and identify the vascular pathology
- Catheterize the occluded vessel and position the catheter within the clot
- Infuse the thrombolytic agent
- Treat the underlying stenosis PRN
- Maintain heparinization until flow has been re-established

mixed directly with tPA due to risk of precipitation) and may be continued after successful thrombolysis for a period of time at the discretion of the clinical team.

Standard technique

Currently, we prefer to start treatment with combined chemical and mechanical lysis, whenever possible, to minimize the time to recanalization and the amount of tPA that is used (Table 8.21). This approach is highly cost effective and seems to shorten infusion time and reduce the frequency and severity of bleeding complications. When mechanical thrombolysis is performed, we usually begin with a rheolytic system although oscillating devices have also been helpful. Techniques vary depending upon the age of the patient, the size of the vessel to be treated, and the technical approach selected. When mechanical thrombolysis is planned, pulsed tPA thrombolysis may be utilized if the clot seems "hard" or difficult to mechanically lyse. Standard thrombolytic dosages in children have not been established, so the following suggestions rely on extrapolation from neonatal and pediatric systemic dose recommendations, weight-based dosing in adults, and empirical experience of the authors. These suggestions assume use of alteplase, and may not be interchangeable with other plasminogen activators. If a catheter suitable for pulse lysis can be advanced across the clot, then a solution composed of 1 to 2 mg tPA in 100 ml of normal saline can be pulsed (from a 1 ml syringe) at 0.2 ml per pulse, two pulses per minute, to a maximum of 0.01 to 0.03 mg/kg. Larger doses may be used on the table, but only if continuous infusion therapy will not follow the acute treatment. If therapy is either successful or terminated due to intractable mature clot after acute treatment on the table and no further thrombolytic administration is performed, then the child should be monitored closely for at least four to six hours, but ICU admission is not mandatory.

After a dwell time of 10 to 30 minutes after pulse lysis, if clot remains mechanical thrombolysis may be initiated. In children with "soft" clots, bland mechanical thrombolysis without pulsed tPA may be adequate. If combined chemical and mechanical thrombolysis is preferred, a similar dose regimen can be used. The total run time is an important consideration when using a rheolytic system, since the main adverse effect is blood removal and significant reduction of hematocrit. Thus it is essential to monitor the fluid volume removed and obtain a hematocrit at the end of the procedure. This is particularly concerning in young children with small total blood volumes.

The advantage of these approaches is that many acute thrombotic occlusions can be completely resolved on the table without need for continuous infusion therapy. The risk of a hemorrhagic complication related to tPA therapy is significantly reduced if tPA is only given in an acute setting.

Not all thrombus will be cleared sufficiently with acute therapy, and continuous infusion durations of 40 to 60 hours are not uncommon in treatment of more chronic arterial or portal venous thromboses. More than 72 hours of continuous infusion therapy is seldom warranted, and frequently bleeding complications or coagulation factor consumption will cause therapy to be terminated before that time.

For any child in whom continuous infusion thrombolytic therapy is planned, ICU admission is mandatory. If continuous infusion is planned, a lytic catheter or Katzen wire (or both) is advanced across the thrombus. A loading dose of tPA is usually not given, although efforts at pulse lysis or mechanical lysis with adjuvant tPA may effectively represent a loading dose. In the usual case, where continuous infusion is started once the catheterized patient has returned to the ICU, the delay between on-table efforts and initiation of continuous therapy will exceed five half-lives of alteplase, although some degradation products may have residual thrombolytic activity that has a much longer half-life. The initial continuous therapy tPA dose for transcatheter infusion is 0.1 to 0.6 mg/kg/h. We usually begin at the lower end of the dosing range and, clinical conditions permitting, may double the dose rate every 12 hours until effective lysis is achieved.

When standard doses are utilized, and there are no signs of active bleeding, the tPA infusion is continued and the patient initially evaluated with angiography in 6 to 12 hours, and then every 12 hours until clot lysis is complete or until therapy is terminated. Thrombolytic therapy does not prevent clot propagation, recurrent thrombosis, or restenosis. Heparin therapy and anticoagulant therapy must always follow thrombolytic therapy.

Dural sinus thrombosis has been successfully treated by thrombolytic infusion through a microcatheter or pulse spray catheter introduced directly into the occluded sinus. The occluded sinus is accessed by transfemoral venous catheterization. A sheath is inserted, and a guiding catheter is maneuvered as close to the target area as possible. Then the infusion catheter is coaxially inserted and positioned within the clot. The infusion is often started at the most distal aspect of the thrombus and the catheter gradually withdrawn as the thrombus resolves. Complete dissolution of venous thrombosis is uncommon, although partial sinus reconstitution with collateral flow via the superficial cerebral veins may be seen.

Umbilical artery catheter-related aortic thrombosis in neonates can be treated by infusion of thrombolytic drug through the umbilical artery catheter if in place, although if directed thrombolysis is desired, a pulse spray infusion catheter is preferred. Once the umbilical catheter has been removed, isolated non-occlusive aortic as well as femoral artery thrombosis following catheterization may be treated by intravenous infusion. Keep in mind that the neonatal femoral vein is likely too small to accept a 7 French sheath, which is required for use of an AngioJet™ device or Trellis™ catheter. The results of systemic thrombolysis can be monitored by US and clinical examination. If there is aortorenal involvement or the child is symptomatic from vaso-occlusive ischemia, catheter-directed intralesional therapy is preferred.

There is little experience in thrombolytic treatment of renal vein thrombosis. Renal arterial infusion has been reported, but since this is usually a disease of newborn infants, systemic infusion is probably preferable.

Postprocedure and follow-up care

Children undergoing continuous thrombolytic therapy are *always* managed in the ICU. Bed rest is mandatory. No additional anticoagulants, aspirin, or non-steroidal anti-inflammatory medications should be administered. Frequent monitoring of vital signs, neurologic status (e.g., Glasgow Coma Scale) and whole-body evaluation of puncture sites and other regions for evidence of bleeding, and monitoring for evidence of hypoxia, hypo- or hypertension, or hypo- or hyperthermia is essential. Some precautions should be maintained in monitoring these patients with respect to their vulnerability to spontaneous bleeding. Blood pressure monitoring should be done by hand to reduce risk of bruising and petechial hemorrhage. No unnecessary venous or arterial punctures or intramuscular injections should be permitted during and for 24 hours following therapy. Unnecessary invasive procedures should be avoided, including bladder catheterization, NG insertion, and suction. All secretions and excretions should be monitored for blood.

Written orders must clearly direct that if spontaneous bleeding occurs, the infusion is discontinued immediately until the bleeding has stopped. The interventional radiologist and any other co-managing consultants must be immediately notified of any events that modify therapy, such as bleeding or consumption of fibrin or other coagulation factors, even if ICU staff are present. The thrombolytic infusion may be re-initiated on the order of the interventional radiologist if no intracranial bleeding or other major complication has occurred.

There are different approaches to following the progress of thrombolytic therapy. Some interventionalists use clinical parameters as the main criteria for continuing the drug infusion. Others also monitor laboratory values, especially fibrinogen, and continue the infusion if there are no clinical problems, and the fibrinogen level is >100, although there is no specific evidence that such monitoring is predictive of bleeding events. Some interventionalists also monitor the levels of fibrin split products and coagulation factors, and corrections are made as indicated. Fibrinogen degradation product levels are usually less than 10 mg/L, and a level greater than 40 mg/L is considered critical. Whatever regimen is selected, written orders regarding guiding parameters and mandated responses must be clearly communicated.

At the completion of the thrombolytic infusion, all patients should be effectively anticoagulated, in order to prevent re-thrombosis. Long-term administration of anticoagulants or antiplatelet medications is not well studied in children but should be considered on a case-by-case basis. Imaging evaluation is performed to evaluate the effect of therapy. Ultrasound is useful as it may be performed portably. Arteriography or venography is utilized when catheter manipulation is necessary or when management decisions mandate. The endovascular sheath may be left in place for a period of time after the conclusion of therapy and removal of treatment catheters to permit further angiography in the early post-treatment period if indicated, and to reduce the time required to achieve hemostasis after removal of the sheath by allowing the clotting cascade to normalize.

Thrombotic events often have an identifiable causative factor, and an explanation for the event should be thoroughly investigated. If vascular stenosis related to the thrombosed vessels is identified, it should be treated with angioplasty following the conclusion of thrombolytic therapy. A high rate of long-term patency can be expected in most cases.

Technical problems and pitfalls

Transcatheter thrombolysis in infants and small children is complicated by the potential for injury to the access vessels and the difficulty in maintaining the position of the catheter tip within the thrombus, due to the short length of the involved vessels, nursing issues, and lack of patient compliance. Catheter stability may be augmented by suturing catheters in place (although such suture sites are often the first to bleed during therapy), using a tape bridge, or adhering them to the skin with a large occlusive transparent dressing. In very small infants, even the shortest infusion zone lengths are too long and make it difficult to adequately position a pulse spray catheter.

Complications

Hemorrhage remote from the catheter access site is relatively infrequent in children. The most common complication is bleeding from prior arteriotomy and venotomy sites, as well as previous biopsy and surgical sites. Intracranial bleeding has been reported in a neonate. Because of this risk, neonates are examined routinely with head US prior to initiating lytic therapy. Children with an intracranial hemorrhage ≥ stage 2 are not considered candidates for treatment. The axillary artery should be avoided as an access vessel, due to the risk of brachial plexus neuropathy secondary to hemorrhage.

Children in the immediate postoperative period or those who have recently undergone open surgery, open biopsy, or other procedures (including ophthalmologic procedures) are usually not candidates for thrombolytic therapy. However, each high-risk case is considered individually.

Transjugular liver biopsy
See Chapter 5.

Transjugular intrahepatic portosystemic shunt (TIPS)
See Chapter 5.

Vena caval filters

Introduction
Pulmonary embolism (PE) is a major cause of morbidity and mortality in the adult population in the United States. Although considerably less frequent than in the adult population, the frequency, morbidity, and mortality of pulmonary emboli in children are unknown.

Inferior vena caval (IVC) filters are a well-recognized therapeutic option for adults with deep venous thrombosis (DVT) and pulmonary embolism (PE) when anticoagulation has failed or is contraindicated. Inferior vena caval filters have been used infrequently in the pediatric population because of their unknown effects on IVC growth and the frequency and severity of the long-term complications. To date, there are only a small number of reports documenting the indications and safety of IVC filter use in children. The placement of IVC filters has been limited to situations in which the medical options have been exhausted or are contraindicated. When needed, insertion of an IVC filter is technically successful in almost all cases. In view of the increasing use of retrievable filters, it seems likely that the use of filters in the pediatric population will need to be re-evaluated and will likely increase.

Indications
Interruption of the IVC for the prevention and management of DVT and PE has been well established in the adult population. Prior to 1967 and the introduction of the Mobin–Uddin filter, this was accomplished surgically. Today, insertion of a filter in the IVC is the mainstay of therapy. The current preferred treatment for DVT and PE is anticoagulation; however, there is up to a 20% recurrence rate.

In adults, there are several well-accepted indications for filter insertion, including: (1) failure of or contraindication to anticoagulation, (2) complications resulting from anticoagulation, (3) the inability to achieve adequate anticoagulation, (4) a free floating iliofemoral or caval thrombus, (5) massive PE requiring thrombolysis or embolectomy, (6) prophylaxis against PE in patients with low cardiac reserve, and (7) massive PE with residual DVT. Other indications exist but are less universally accepted. These indications include: recent surgery, poor compliance with medications, high-risk patients such as

Table 8.22 Indications: vena cava filter

- Deep vein thrombosis with contraindication to anticoagulation
- Deep vein thrombosis on anticoagulation
- Protection against PE in children with long-term immobilization at risk for PE
- Protection against PE in children undergoing risky interventions or surgeries
- Hypercoagulable states with contraindications to anticoagulation

those immobilized and in ICUs, and in some individuals prior to an operation or intervention.

Specific indications for IVC filter insertion are not well established in the pediatric population (Table 8.22). Deep vein thrombosis and PE may occur as a result of a variety of situations. Some of the more common etiologies are trauma, coagulation disorders, malignancy, heart disease, sepsis, central venous catheters (especially long-term central venous catheters), and the use of oral contraceptives in teenagers.

Although not as common as in adults, DVT does occur in children and should be considered in the child with lower extremity pain or swelling. Little has changed in the arena of clinical diagnosis; however, the approach to diagnosis has changed. Today, the diagnosis of a DVT is usually made with non-invasive imaging. Ultrasound with Doppler is now an excellent diagnostic modality to evaluate the extent of disease and follow children with DVT. Magnetic resonance imaging or CT venography may also be used in selected situations. Once DVT is considered and medical therapy fails or is contraindicated, placement of an IVC filter may be considered. In the past, even in this setting, the decision to insert a permanent filter has been a difficult one. However, with the availability of retrievable filters, the decision to protect the child with a filter has been made easier. There are no specific pediatric guidelines used to determine when it is best to insert a filter. Each child is independently evaluated and, in general, those with life-threatening conditions or those undergoing a high-risk procedure are considered as candidates for filter placement.

As is the case for other vascular interventions, contraindications are infrequent. The major reasons to delay or avoid IVC filter insertion are in a patient with an IVC that is too small to accept a filter (Figure 8.44), children with an uncorrectable coagulopathy, and when no safe or patent venous access site is available.

Technique
Equipment
When only permanent IVC filters were available, the most commonly selected filter was the 12 French Greenfield™ filter. Now with the availability of retrievable filters, the most frequently used devices are the Günther Tulip® and Celect® filters, although other filters can also be used in the pediatric

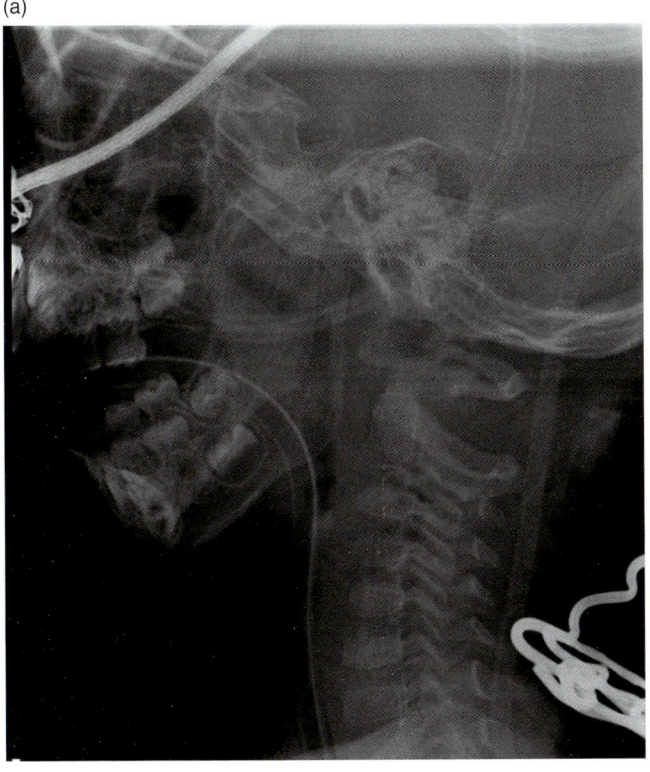

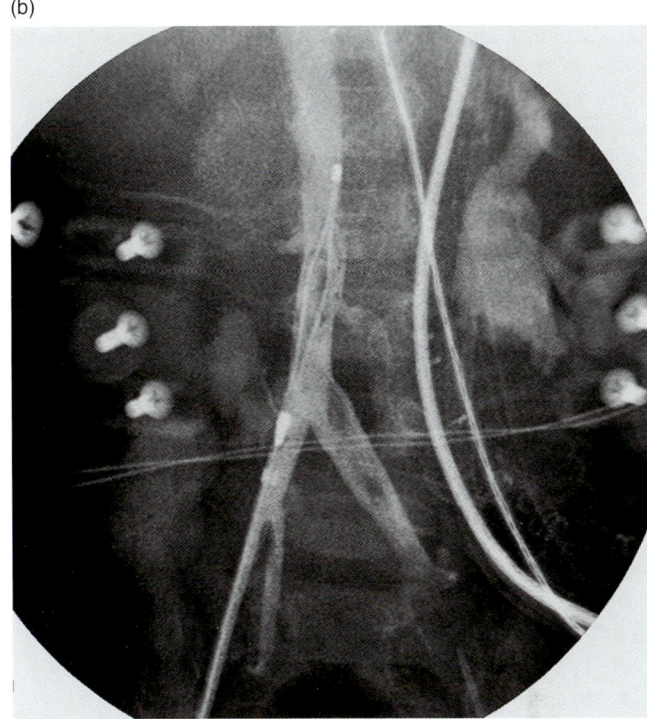

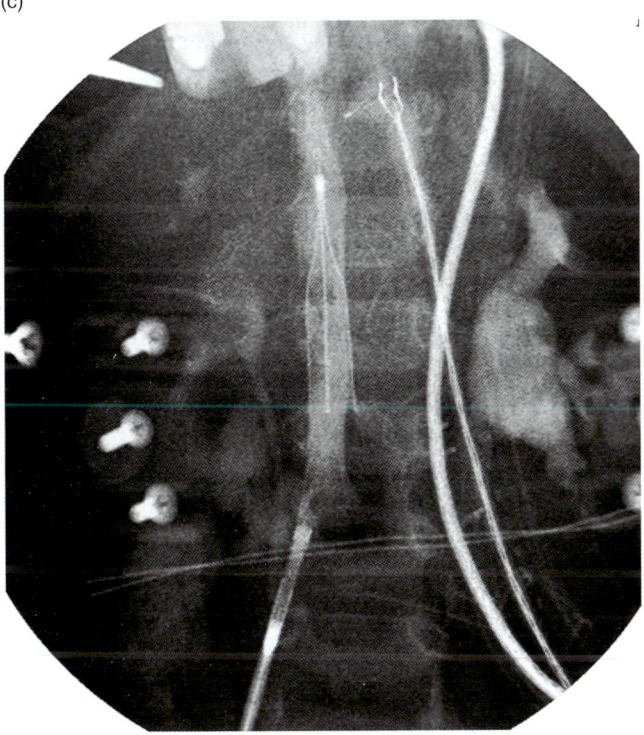

Figure 8.44 A 2.9-year-old male with central venous access-related left iliac thrombosis. (a) Head and neck trauma precluded systemic anticoagulation. (b) Preprocedure CT reconstructions indicated the infrarenal IVC had a diameter of 12 mm and was 5 mm longer that the planned Günther Tulip® IVC filter (Cook Medical). A small hand injection of contrast through the sheath assisted precise positioning of the transfemoral delivery system just prior to deployment. (c) After deployment, a small amount of contrast confirms satisfactory position with the apex in the renal venous outflow. The filter was retrieved through a transjugular sheath almost three months later when the patient's halo fixation was removed. On CT a year later, the IVC was completely occluded, but extensive collaterals visible before IVC insertion provided adequate venous return from the lower extremities and pelvis to the suprarenal IVC.

population (Table 8.23). Other filter choices include the OptEase® filter, G2 or G2 Express, or Crux® filters. These filters are suitable for children with IVC diameters that range from 17 to 30 mm. The Günther Tulip® and Celect® filters use an 8.5 French introducer while the OptEase® can be inserted via a 6 French introducer. Once the decision has been made to insert a filter into the IVC, one must consider a variety of details. Some of the important considerations are the clinical setting, the ease of filter insertion, the diameter of the IVC, the distance between the iliac bifurcation and the renal veins, the patient's age and size, the occlusion rate of the filter, the frequency of filter migration, the long-term structural integrity of the device, and potential impediments to timely retrieval. Every filter, regardless of designation, must be considered a potentially permanent implanted device, since successful retrieval is not certain.

Patient preparation

Filter insertion may be carried out using sedation or general anesthesia. The type of anesthesia selected depends on the individual child and the severity of their medical issues. Regardless of the selected method, each child is kept NPO as per institutional guidelines, and a preprocedural coagulation profile and CBC are obtained. Prior to initiating the procedure, a functioning peripheral IV should be in place.

Table 8.23 Equipment: vena cava filter

- General anesthesia or deep sedation
- Ultrasound for guided vascular access
- 7 to 8.5 French sheath with hemostasis valve
- Retrievable IVC filter
- IVC filter kit
- IVC venogram
- Vessel diameter measurements

Standard technique

Percutaneous filter insertion can be accomplished via either peripheral or central venous access. However, in the pediatric population, and especially smaller children, central venous access is almost exclusively used (Table 8.24). The right internal jugular and right femoral veins are the most commonly used entry sites. Regardless of the entry site selected, venopuncture is guided using US. Once the vein has been accessed, a sheath of appropriate size is inserted to prevent vein injury and to allow for repeated entry as needed. An injection catheter with multiple side holes is positioned in the caudal IVC, and a cavogram, using approximately 1 ml of contrast/kg, is performed over two seconds at a film rate of one to two frames/second. The length and diameter of the infrarenal segment of the IVC is determined, as is the location

Table 8.24 Procedure summary: vena cava filter

- Skin preparation, local anesthesia
- Ultrasound for venous access
- Sheath insertion
- Cavography and measurement
- Filter placement in infrarenal IVC
- Postprocedural follow-up (US, cavography)
- Filter retrieval PRN

(a)
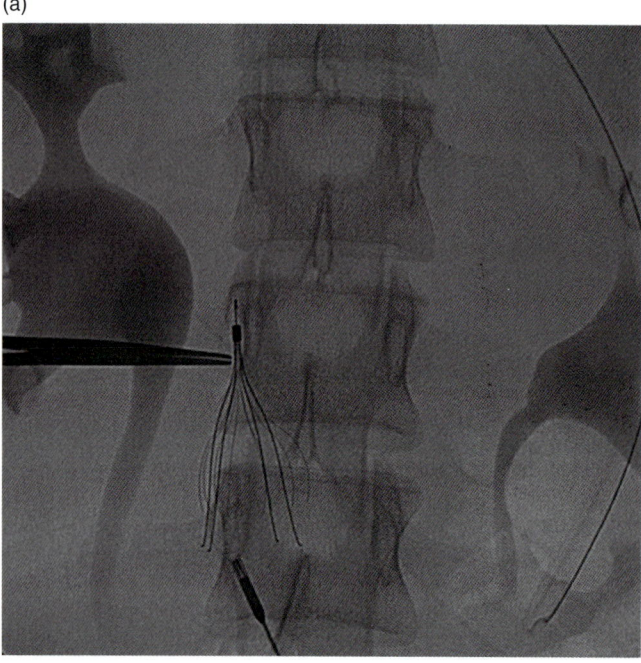

(b)
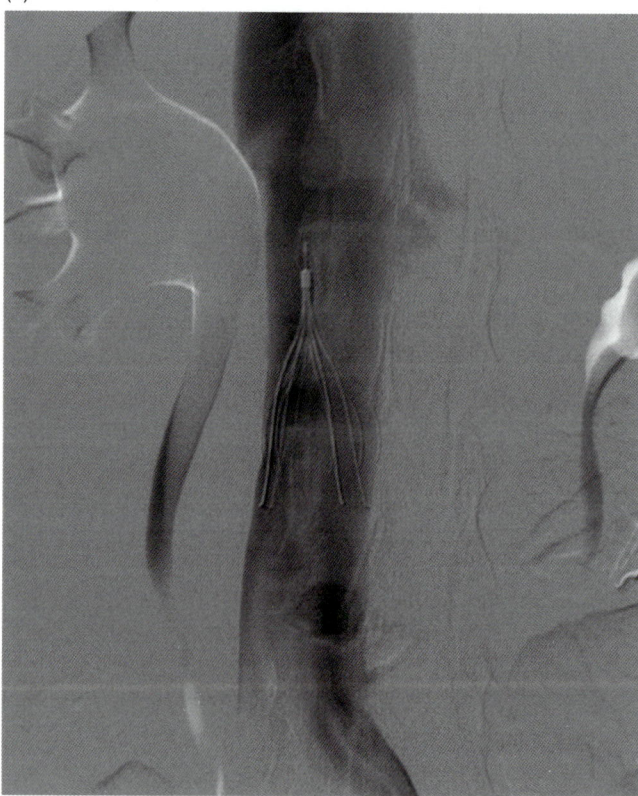

Figure 8.45 Sixteen-year-old female with right external iliac venous thrombosis at risk for pulmonary embolism. Anticoagulation is contraindicated due to recent trauma and corrective surgery. (a) A hemostat is placed at the level of the renal veins for IVC filter placement. (b) Contrast cavography shows the Celect® IVC filter (Cook Medical) positioned in the infrarenal IVC.

Chapter 8 Vascular interventions

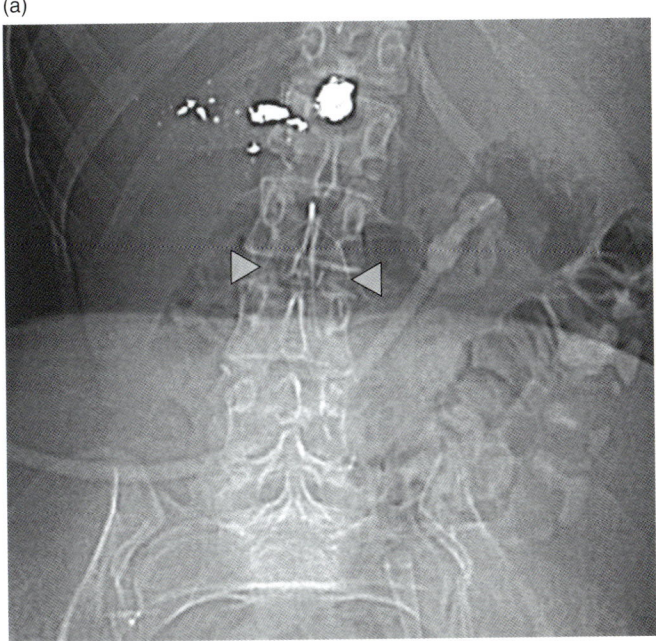
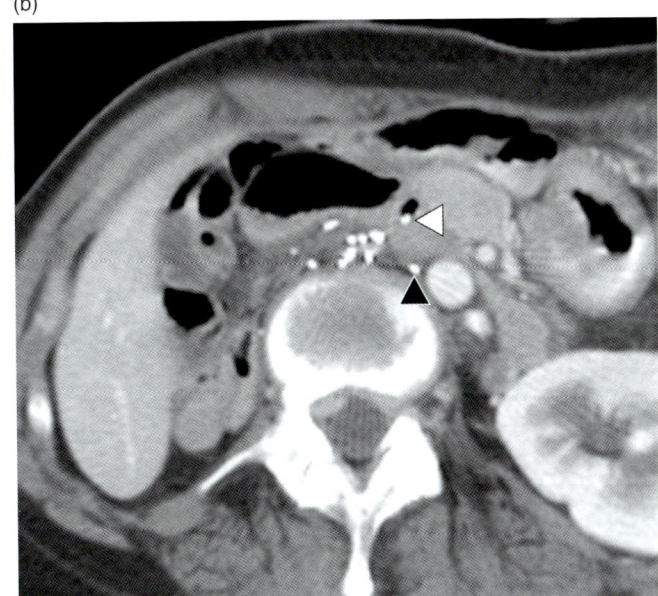
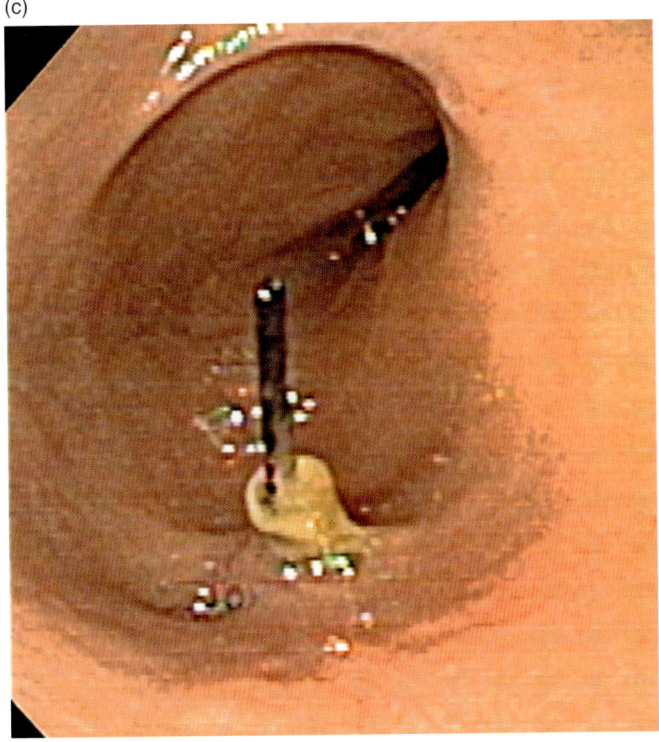

Figure 8.46 A 17-year-old female, paraplegic after a gunshot wound to the thoracolumbar spine, had an IVC filter placed at an outside hospital due to her prolonged immobility. (a) Note that the location of the filter struts (*arrowheads*) exceeds the expected diameter of her IVC. (b) Computed tomography with vascular and enteric contrast shows numerous filter struts outside the IVC, including one (*black arrowhead*) directed toward the aortic wall and one (*white arrowhead*) outlined by bowel gas. (c) The latter strut was visualized under endoscopic control and removed.

and number of renal veins, and the presence of caval anomalies. The ideal location for filter placement, in the presence of lower extremity DVT or for preprocedural protection, is in the infrarenal IVC, with the apex of the filter in the outflow of the renal veins to maximize the filter's effectiveness and to minimize venous stasis and the volume of unfiltered thrombus (Figure 8.45).

Postprocedure and follow-up care

There is no specific regimen that is followed after filter insertion. Immediately following the procedure, the child is observed for signs of complications in the ICU or other unit where vital signs can be monitored frequently. If a complication is recognized, treatment is initiated. If the child remains asymptomatic, no further scheduled follow-up is obtained. If symptoms are identified, then US, venography, or cross-sectional imaging is performed as needed. Retrievable filters should be removed when the indication for their insertion is no longer active, ideally within six months following placement, to reduce the incidence of unsuccessful IVC filter retrieval.

Complications

In the few reported series involving children, complications have been infrequently reported. However, there is limited long-term data available. Reported series demonstrate an incidence of recurrent PE and caval thrombosis of up to 4%. Unfortunately, the pediatric experience with IVC filters is limited. Therefore the low rate of complications may not be predictive of the outcome. Further experience is needed to better understand the risks and benefits of long-term IVC filtration in children. In adults, a variety of types and severity of complications have been noted. Death secondary to filter insertion has been reported in 0.12 to 3% of cases, recurrent PE in 0.5 to 34%, IVC thrombosis in 2 to 30%, IVC penetration in at least 10 to 40% (Figure 8.46), filter migration in 5 to 19%, and filter fracture in about 2% of individuals.

Index

abdominopelvic biopsy 215–29
  complications 228
    bile leakage/peritonitis 228
    hemorrhage 228
    tract seeding 228
  contraindications 215
  controversies and issues 228
  equipment 215–16
    automated systems 216
    biopsy needles 216
  image guidance 216–17, 220
    CT 217–18
    molecular imaging 217, 219
    MR 217
    ultrasound 216–17
  indications 215
  patient preparation 217–20
    pathology 218–20
    preprocedure care 218
  postprocedure and follow-up care 227
  technical variations 226–7
    coaxial and tandem needle techniques 226–7
    molecular image guidance 227
  technique 220–4
    liver biopsy 220–3
    neuroblastoma 224, 226
    pancreatic biopsy 224–5
    splenic biopsy 223–4
    tract embolization 222–3
abdominopelvic interventions 151–249
  biopsy *see* abdominopelvic biopsy
  foreign body retrieval 239–49
  gastrostomy 153–83
  hollow visceral dilation 229–39
  percutaneous aspiration and fluid drainage 191–214
  percutaneous cecostomy 183–91
ablative therapy
  bone tumors 397–9
  pseudoaneurysm ablation 449–56
  renal 208, 325, 417, 433
  salivary ranula 373

  vascular malformations 439–40, 445
abscess
  anterior abdominal wall 175
  cecostomy site 189–90
  drainage 191–214, 361
  high-risk populations 210
  interloop 203–4
  intrathoracic 112–18
  liver, amebic 204
  pelvic 199–201
  periappendiceal 201
  retropharyngeal 119
  solid organ 203–6
  splenic 204, 207
  subphrenic 203, 205
absolute alcohol 203, 208, 325–6, 328, 376
  complications of injection 450
"accordioning" of catheter body 38
AccuStick™ system 312
acetaminophen 20, 137, 185, 187, 346, 354
acetic acid 208, 325
Ackerman needle 388
acromycin 111
airway dilation 146–9
airway strictures 141–5
  see also tracheobronchial stents
Alagille syndrome 262
all purpose drainage (APD) catheter 315
allopurinol 292
alteplase 70, 469
amebic liver abscess 204
amoxicillin 12
amphotericin 110, 310
ampicillin 12, 185, 187, 254
Amplatz® dilators 172, 329
Amplatz® thrombectomy system 469
Amplatz® wire 60, 74, 116, 285, 288, 314, 338
analgesia *see* pain management
anesthesia *see* specific techniques
aneurysmal bone cysts 380, 385
  see also bone cyst therapy

angiocatheters 406–7
angiography 405–13
  complications 411–13
    femoral artery thrombosis 411
    fluid overload and anemia 413
    hypothermia 413
    pressure sores 411
    thromboembolism 411
  contraindications 405
  equipment 406–7
  hepatic 413–15
  indications 405–6
  injection rates/volumes 409
  patient preparation 406–8
  postprocedure and follow-up care 411
  technical problems and pitfalls 411
  technical variations 409–13
    transvenous approach 411
  technique 407–9
    arterial access 407
    double-wall puncture 408
    single-wall puncture 408
angiography suite 9–10
  equipment 10
  ultrasound 10
AngioJet™ thrombectomy system 469
Angiomed® Auto-Vac device 216
Angiomed® stent 287
angioplasty and stenting 456–65
  complications 465
  equipment 464
  indications 456–64
    aortorenal syndromes 458, 461–2
    renal artery stenosis 458, 461
    transplant vascular stenosis 456–8
    venous compression syndromes 460–4
  patient preparation 464
  technical problems and pitfalls 465
  technical variations 465

  technique 464–5
  see also stents; stent insertion
angiosarcoma 291, 438
angled glide wire 25, 36, 237, 312, 314, 319, 327, 334, 338, 344
antegrade colonic enema 183
antegrade (pull) gastrostomy 157, 160–5
antegrade pyelography 320–1
anterior abdominal wall abscess 175
anti-reflux procedures 157
anti-reflux valve failure 177
antibiotics
  impregnated catheters 66
  prophylactic 12
anxiolytics 17–18
aortorenal syndromes 458, 461–2
apheresis catheters 43, 47
Aristospan® *see* triamcinolone
arm port insertion 79–82
arterial embolization *see* embolization therapy
arterial spasm 437
arterial trauma 433–5
arterioportal fistula 282
arteriovenous fistula 309
  embolization therapy 415, 427–30
arteriovenous malformations 413
  embolization therapy 415, 417, 423–7
  pulmonary 429
arteritis
  postradiotherapy 458
  Takayasu 458
arthrography 375–80
  complications 379
  equipment 376, 379
  image guidance 378–9
  indications 376, 379
  patient preparation 377
  postprocedure and follow-up care 379
  technique 378–84
ASAP device 216
aspergillosis 110
aspiration and drainage 191–214

Index

aspiration and drainage (cont.)
  complications 214
  contraindications 192, 194
  equipment 193–4
  image guidance 193–8
    CT 195–8
    fluoroscopy 195
    ultrasound 195
  indications 191–3
  mediastinal fluid *see* mediastinal fluid drainage
  patient preparation 198
  postprocedure and follow-up care 210–13
    catheter fixation and drainage 212
    catheter removal 212–14
    specimen handling 212
  regional considerations 199–209
    deep pelvic collections 199–201
    pancreatic pseudocyst drainage 205, 208
    paracentesis 199
    periappendiceal abscess 201
    renal cysts 205–9
    solid organ abscess 203–6
    subphrenic and lesser sac collections 203
  soft tissue 360–2
  technical problems and pitfalls 213
  technical variations 210
    high-risk populations 210
    non-linear and curvilinear pathways 210–11
    sclerotherapy and lymphocele drainage 210
  technique 193–9
  thoracic *see* thoracic aspiration and drainage
aspirin 20
autologous blood patch 111
avascular necrosis 392
azygos arch 27–8
azygos vein 27

Bacillus spp. 67
backward reasoning 4
bacteremia 67
bacterial endocarditis 112
balloon dilation
  esophageal strictures 230–1
    balloon rupture 238
    "kissing balloons" 239
    stiffening of balloon delivery platform 239
  ureteral strictures 336–41
balloon pericardiotomy, percutaneous 121
Bard Biopty® device 216
barium 160
bent guide wire technique 35, 54, 61–2, 343, 346

Bentson guide wire 159
benzodiazepines 17–18
benzoin 160
betadine 208
Bierman needle 388
bile leak 228, 270, 272, 282
biliary tract
  obstruction 259
  sepsis 272
  stents 275
biliary-arterial fistula 270
biliary-pleural fistula 270
biliary-venous fistula 270
biliothorax 282
BioPince® device 216
biopsy
  abdominopelvic 215–29
  bone 385–92
  liver 220–2
    transjugular *see* transjugular liver biopsy
  lymph node 362–5
  pulmonary/mediastinal 123–37
    automated biopsy devices 127
    core 125–8
    FNAB 125–7
  renal 304–9
  soft tissue masses 362–5
biplane imaging 14
bleomycin 111, 439, 445, 447
"body flossing" 61, 338, 340, 351
bone biopsy 385–92
  complications 392
  "don't touch" lesions 386, 389
  equipment 388–9
  imaging 389–90
  indications 386–8
  patient preparation 389
  postprocedure and follow-up care 391
  technique 389–92
bone cyst therapy 380–5
  complications 383
  equipment 381, 385
  indications 380–1
  issues and controversies 384
  patient preparation 383
  postprocedure and follow-up care 383
  technique 383, 385
bone tumors 389
  excision 392–7
    complications 397
    equipment 392–5
    imaging 392–4
    indications 392
    patient preparation 395
    postprocedure and follow-up care 396
    technical variations 395
    technique 395–6
  locoregional thermal ablation 397–9

    complications 399
    equipment 397
    indications 397–8
    patient preparation 397
    postprocedure and follow-up care 398
    technique 397, 399
Botox *see* botulinum toxin
botulinum toxin 368
  dosage 369
  see also chemodenervation of salivary glands
bougienage 229, 231
  radial and shearing forces 229
bougies 229
bowel
  control 183
  decompression 168–9
  loops 214
  perforation 175, 181
brachial plexus neuropathy 411
brachiocephalic vein 31
branchial cleft cysts 371
Brodie's abscess 387
bronchial artery embolization 432–3
bronchopleural fistula 105
brushite stones 335
Budd–Chiari syndrome 276–7, 284, 286, 461
bullseye appearance in arthrography 378
bupivacaine 401
button batteries, removal of 246–7
  see also esophageal foreign body removal
button gastrojejunostomy 154
  complications 177
    accidental dislodgment 177
    anti-reflux valve failure 177
    loss 177
button gastrostomy 172–3
  complications 177
    accidental dislodgment 177
    anti-reflux valve failure 177
    loss 177
button jejunostomy 154, 172–4
n-butyl-2-cyanacrylate 381

calcium oxalate stones 335
calcium phosphate catheter occlusion 39–90
caliceal diverticula 334
  stones in 330
Candida spp. 67
  esophagitis 234
capnography 406
carbon dioxide, as contrast agent 257
cardiac tamponade 65, 108
catheters 10
  "accordioning" 38
  angiography 406–7
  antibiotic-impregnated 66
  apheresis 43, 47

central venous *see* central venous catheters (CVCs)
  dialysis 43, 47
  dislodgment 68
  femoral vein 39, 52–3
  fractures/tears 39
  fragmented 74, 76
  hemodialysis 31
  internal jugular vein 39, 42–51
  malposition 68–9
    catheter tip 68–71
    consequences 68
    prevention 68
    repositioning 69, 71
    unrecognized 68
  nephrostomy 345
  occlusion 39–91
    CVCs 39–91
      clot lysis 90–1
      mechanical 90
      medication precipitation 90
    mechanical 90
    peripherally inserted central *see* PICCs
  repair 89
  repositioning 69, 71
  subclavian vein 28, 39, 41, 51–2
  tip occlusion 69–73
    declotting 72
    fibrin sheath 69, 72
    follow-up 72
    heparinization 72
    thrombolysis 70–3
    thrombus 39–41
  see also aspiration and drainage; *and specific catheter types*
catheter-related bloodstream infection (CRBSI) 65–8
  diagnosis 66
  dressings 67, 93
  incidence 67
  postoperative 67
  sterile technique 66–7
  treatment 67
catheter-related thrombophlebitis 38
caustic ingestion 234
cautery wire cutting balloon 350
cavernous hemangioma 414
cavoatrial junction 25–6
cecostomy, percutaneous 183–91
  complications 187–90
    dislodgment 190
    granulation tissue 190
    occlusion and leakage 190
    peritonitis 189–90
    skin infection and abscess formation 189–90
    tube malposition 188–9
  controversies and issues 190
  equipment 184

future advances 190
indications 184–5
  latex sensitivity 185
patient support 187
postprocedure and follow-up care 187
  catheter exchange and reinsertion 187
  catheter fixation 187
preprocedure imaging 185–6
technical problems and pitfalls 187
technical variations 186
technique 185–6
central vein thrombosis 73
central venous access 22–87
  alternative pathways 27–8, 30
  blood drawing 25–88
  catheter insertion 23
  history 23
  indications 25
  indwelling venous ports 76–85
  PICCs see PICCs
  route of access 25–7
  team approach 23–5
central venous catheters (CVCs) 2, 39–76
  blood drawing 25–88
  complications 65–76
    infection 65–8
    intravascular foreign body 75–6
    malposition 68–9
    mechanical malfunction 74
    thrombosis 73–4
    tip occlusion 69–73
  contraindications 41
  conversion from indwelling venous ports 84
  difficult access 53–61
    equipment and patient preparation 54
    postprocedure and follow-up care 61
    stabilization of guide wire 60–1
    technical variations 60
    transbrachiocephalic route 54–5, 58
    transhepatic route 58–9
    translumbar route 59–61
  equipment 32
  femoral vein 52–3
  indications 41–2
  internal jugular vein 42–51
  occlusion 39–91
    clot lysis 90–1
    mechanical 90
    medication precipitation 90
    tip thrombus 39–41
  removal 92
    heparin locking 92
  repair 89
  subclavian vein 51–2
  temporary 42

venous recanalization 61–2
cephalic vein 25, 33
cephalosporins 254
cervicofacial lymphatic malformations 371
chemical cholecystitis 293
chemical pleuritis 281
chemical pleurodesis 109, 111
  pneumothorax 109
chemodenervation of salivary glands 368–70
  botulinum toxin dosage 369
  complications 370
  equipment 368
  future advances 370
  indications 368
  patient preparation 368
  postprocedure and follow-up care 370
  technical variations 370
  technique 369–70
chemoembolization
  hepatic tumors 429, 432
  transarterial intrahepatic 291–3
  see also embolization therapy
chemotherapy 41
  intracavitary 109
chest drains 105, 108
  intrathoracic abscess 112–18
  suction devices 118
Chiba needle 116, 311, 314, 327
chloral hydrate (Notec®) 18
chlorhexidine
  baths 295
  dressings 67
cholangiogram 272
cholangitis 259, 271–2
  sclerosing 271
cholecystitis 259
  chemical 293
cholecystostomy, percutaneous 259–62
  complications 261
  equipment 259, 261
  indications 259, 261
  patient preparation 260
  postprocedure and follow-up care 261
  technical variations 261
  technique 261–3
choledocholithiasis 253
cholestatic jaundice 272
chronic granulomatous disease 234
chronic lung disease 130
chylothorax 108
clinical practice development 7–11
  angiography suite 9–10
  approach 7–8
  facilities, equipment and supplies 9
  interventional radiology team 8–9

Clostridium spp.
  C. botulinum 368
  C. perfringens 295
clot lysis 72, 90–1
coagulation abnormalities 12
coagulation screen 254
coaxial biopsy guidance 134–6
coccidioidomycosis 388
codeine 346
coils, embolic 418
Colapinto needle 285, 288
Colapinto sheath 286
cold knife 350
collimation 14
colonic dilation 237–8
  positioning for 239
compartment syndrome 408
computed tomography see CT
congenital esophageal stenosis see esophageal stenosis, congenital
congenital heart disease 30
congenital infantile hemangioma 419
Conrad Crosby needle 388
contrast reactions 12–13
  subcapsular extravasation 286
contrast-enhanced dynamic fluoroscopy 38
Cope introducer 311
Cope loop catheter 189
core biopsy 125
  needles 126–8, 216
Corpak® tube 167
corticosteroids 376, 442
costoclavicular space 74
Council catheter 335, 345
Craig needle 391
CRBSI see catheter-related bloodstream infection
cross-fused renal ectopia 298
cross-sectional imaging 60
CT 1
  abdominopelvic biopsy 217–18
  and arthrography 378
  aspiration and fluid drainage 195–8
  bone tumors 393
  hydronephrosis 301
  intrathoracic abscess 115
  musculoskeletal interventions 358
  pericardiocentesis 121
  pulmonary/mediastinal biopsy 131–2, 135
  renal biopsy 307
  renal cyst aspiration 208
CT angiography 406
CT venography 406
cutting balloon
  angioplasty 465
  endopyelotomy 350
CVCs see central venous catheters

cysts
  bone 380, 385
  branchial cleft 371
  dermoid 371
  renal 205–9, 324–8
  thyroglossal duct 371
cystic bone lesions 389
cystic fibrosis 33, 145
cystine stones 330, 335

Dawson–Mueller pigtail catheter 315
declotting see clot lysis; thrombolysis
deep venous thrombosis 26, 472
  catheter-related 73–4
Demerol® see meperidine
dermatofibrosarcoma protuberans 363
dermoid cysts 371
desmopressin 12
dexamethasone 292–3, 406
dialysis catheters 43, 47
difficult access 53–61
  equipment and patient preparation 54
  postprocedure and follow-up care 61
  stabilization of guide wire 60–1
  technical variations 60
  transbrachiocephalic route 54–5, 58
  transhepatic route 58–9
  translumbar route 59–61
Dilaudid® see hydromorphone
diphenhydramine 13, 293
dislodgment of catheter 68
  see also catheters, malposition
Dolophine® see methadone
"don't touch" bone lesions 386, 389
dose-dependent radiation injury 13
doxycycline 111, 325, 381, 443
dressings
  changing 93
  chlorhexidine-impregnated 67
  occlusive 67, 105
  tape bridge 106
  thoracic aspiration and drainage 105–6
  see also individual types
drills 360
drooling 368
Dumon stent 140
duodenal ulcers 293
duodenitis 293
DuoDERM® dressing 180
dural sinus thrombosis 470
dysphagia 240

Echinococcus granulosa 203
ELA-Max® cream 17, 184, 199
electrocardiography 406
electrocautery 350
Elson needle 388

Index

embolic agents 381, 418–19
embolization therapy 415–38
   complications 438
   equipment 417–18
   indications 415–17
   neonatal 435–7
   patient preparation 418
   percutaneous thrombin embolization 451, 454
   postembolization syndrome 293, 296, 417
   postprocedure and follow-up care 437
   technical problems and pitfalls 437–8
   technical variations 435–7
   technique 418–19
      arterial trauma 433–5
      arteriovenous fistula 415, 427–30
      arteriovenous malformations 415, 417, 423–7
      bronchial artery embolization 432–3
      hemangioendothelioma 415, 423
      hemangioma 419, 423–5
      high-flow vascular malformations 415, 419, 422
      partial splenic embolization 294–6, 417, 433, 436
      preoperative embolization of tumors 419–23
      pulmonary arteriovenous malformations 429
      renal ablation 433
      systemic pulmonary arterial supply 429, 431
      tract embolization 222–3
   see also chemoembolization
Embospheres® 295
   drug-eluting 293
embryonal sarcoma, undifferentiated 291
emergence delirium 19
emergency premedication 13
EMLA® cream 17, 184, 199
empyema 99–100, 259
   management 101–5
end-cutting needles 216
endopyelotomy 2, 301, 303, 348–55
   complications 354–5
   contraindications 350
   equipment 350–1
   indications 350
   patient preparation 350
   postprocedure and follow-up care 354
   technical variations 352–4
      pediatric modifications 352
      "stent first, hot knife" 354
   technique 350–3
endoscopic retrograde cholangiopancreatography (ERCP) 253
EndoWave™ thrombectomy system 469
enoxaparin 12
Enterobacter spp. 270
   E. aerogenes 253
Enterococcus spp. 254, 270
   E. faecalis 254
enterostomy care 154
epidermolysis bullosa dystrophica 234
epidural anesthesia 296
epithelioid hemangioendothelioma 438
equipment and supplies 9–11
   catheters and wires 10
   pulse Doppler monitor 10
   safety devices 10
   warming devices 10
   see also specific items and procedures
Escherichia coli 253, 270
esophageal atresia 231–4
esophageal diameter 175
esophageal dilation 2, 229–39
   balloon dilation 230–1
   bougienage 229, 231
   complications 239
   equipment 235–6
   indications 231–5
      acquired strictures 232–5
      caustic ingestion 234
      chronic granulomatous disease 234
      congenital esophageal stenosis 231–2
      epidermolysis bullosa dystrophica 234
      esophageal atresia 231–4
      esophageal varices 235
      fibromuscular stenosis 231
      gastroesophageal reflux 234
      Stevens–Johnson syndrome 234
   patient preparation 235–6
   postprocedure and follow-up care 237–8
   technical problems and pitfalls 238–9
      balloon rupture 238
      "kissing balloons" 239
      positioning for colonic dilation 239
      stiffening balloon delivery platform 239
   technical variations 237
      colonic dilation 237–8
      eccentric stricture and pseudodiverticulum 237
   technique 236–7
esophageal foreign body removal 239–49
   complications 247, 249
   contraindications 241–2
   equipment 242
   Foley catheter technique 240, 249
   indications 240–2
   patient preparation 243
   postprocedure and follow-up care 247
   rigid endoscopy 240
   technical variations 245–7
      magnetic foreign body removal 245–8
      variable balloon inflation 245
   technique 243–5
esophageal laceration 175
esophageal stenosis, congenital 229, 231–2
esophageal strictures 229
   acquired 232–5
esophageal varices 235
esophageal webs 231
esophagitis 234
Ethibloc® 208, 325
Ewing's sarcoma 386
extracorporeal shock wave lithotripsy 330, 336

facilities 9
fecal soiling 183
femoral artery
   puncture 411
   thrombosis 411
femoral lines 20
femoral vein catheters 39, 52–3
   equipment and patient preparation 52
   postprocedure and follow-up care 53
   technical variations 53
   technique 52–5
   temporary 53
fentanyl citrate (Sublimaze®) 18–19, 21, 137
   complications 19
fibrin glue 111
fibrin sheath 69
   mechanical stripping 73
   removal 72
fibrin split products 72
fibrinolysis, intracavitary 109–11
fibrosarcoma 363
filters 14
fine needle aspiration biopsy (FNAB) 125
   needles 126–7
fistula
   arterioportal 282
   arteriovenous 309, 415, 427–30
   biliary-arterial 270
   biliary-pleural 270
   biliary-venous 270
   bronchopleural 105
   gastrocolic 175, 177
   tracheoesophageal 232–3
FlexiFlo® tube 167–8
fluconazole 310
fluid overload 413
flumazenil (Romazicon®) 20
fluoroscopy
   and arthrography 378
   aspiration and fluid drainage 195
   bone lesions 389
   gastrostomy 153–4
   musculoskeletal interventions 358
   nephrolithotomy 333
   PTC 255–7
   TIPS 288
   ureteral stent insertion 343–5
FNAB see fine needle aspiration biopsy
focal spot rating 14
foreign body
   esophageal 239–49
   in fluid collections 210
   intravascular 75–6
      localization of catheter fragment 76
      sheath size 75
   soft tissue 365–8
fracture reduction with internal fixation 399–403
   closed reduction 400
   complications 403
   equipment 400
   indications 400
   open reduction 399
   patient preparation 400–1
   postprocedure and follow-up care 403
   technical variations 401
   technique 401–2
fractured catheters 39
fragmented catheters 74
   removal of fragments see foreign body
Franseen needle 388
fungal infections 67
furosemide 335

gallbladder
   hydrops 259
   perforation 259
   radiology 251–2
gallstones 271
gastric
   herniation 175
   perforation 175
   plication, iatrogenic 180
   scintigraphy 158
   ulcers 293
gastritis 293
gastrocolic fistula 175, 177
gastroesophageal reflux 154, 157, 182

esophageal dilation 234
gastroesophageal varices 281
gastrojejunostomy 2, 153, 157
  button 154, 177
  percutaneous 2, 153, 157
  technique 167
gastrostomy 153–83
  button 154, 172–4, 177
  care of 154
  complications 175–83
    bowel perforation 175, 181
    intussusception 176, 179, 182
    malposition 176, 179–80
    occlusion and leakage 181–2
    peritonitis 175, 181
    skin irritation 177–81
    stoma ulceration 175, 179
    tract granuloma 176, 179, 181
    tube dislodgment 181
    see also specific complications
  controversies and issues 183
  equipment 157–8
    nasojejunal tube insertion 159
  indications 154–7
  laparoscopic 154
  leakage 170
  outcome measures 156
  patient preparation 157–9
  percutaneous 2, 153–4
    complications 176
    endoscopic 153
    fluoroscopic 153–4
  postprocedure and follow-up care 168–74
    catheter exchange and reinsertion 170–2
    gastrostomy/jejunostomy button 172–4
    postoperative orders and initial tube care 168–70
    replacement or exchange 173
  surgical 153, 155
  technical problems and pitfalls 174–5
    damage to deep structures 174
    difficult delivery of retention device or J-tube 175
    inability to access gastric lumen 174
    inadvertent dislodgment 175–6
    transcolonic puncture 174
  technical variations 168
    bowel decompression 168–9
    percutaneous jejunostomy 168
    push–pull gastrostomy 168
  technique 159–67
    antegrade (pull) gastrostomy 157, 160–5

nasojejunal tube insertion 159
percutaneous gastrojejunostomy 167
retrograde gastrostomy 165–7
gastrostomy tube 165–6
  balloon internal retention bumper 166
  replacement 182
gelatin sponge 381
Gelfoam® pledgets/slurry 281–3, 293, 419
general anesthesia
  bone tumor excision 395
  PICC insertion 31
  ureteral dilation 327
  ureteral stent insertion 343
genitourinary interventions 297–355
  anatomic considerations 298–9
  endopyelotomy 2, 301, 303, 348–55
  history 298
  nephrolithotomy 330–6
  nephrostomy 309–20
    tract dilation 328–30
  radiology 300–4
  renal biopsy 304–9
  renal cysts 205–9, 324–8
  ureteral balloon dilation 336–41
  ureteral stent insertion 341–8
  Whitaker (pressure–flow) perfusion test 320–4
gentamicin 185, 187, 254
Gerota's fascia 299, 305
Gianturco Z-stent 144
Glide® wire 60, 116, 261, 277, 282, 292, 319, 327, 335, 338, 373
  angled 25, 36, 237, 312, 314, 319, 327, 334, 338, 344
glucagon 406
glucose transport protein (GLUT) 1 421
glue, as sclerosant 208, 325
gooseneck snare 61
GORE VIATORR® covered endoprosthesis 287
granulation tissue
  cecostomy site 190
  gastrostomy site 176, 179, 181
grids 14
guide wires 60
  intrathoracic abscess drainage 116
  nephrolithotomy 334
  percutaneous nephrostomy 312
  stabilization 60–1
  see also individual types

Haemophilus influenzae 112
halitosis 368

hemangioendothelioma 414
  embolization therapy 415, 423
  epithelioid 438
  Kaposi's 416, 438
hemangioma 422
  cavernous *see* cavernous hemangioma
  congenital
    NICH 422, 438
    RICH 422, 438
  embolization therapy 415, 419
  endangering 417
  hepatic *see* hemangioendothelioma
  infantile 419, 438
  spindle cell 438
  variants 422
hematochezia 270
hematoma 210
hematuria 319, 324, 335, 346
hemizygos vein 27
hemobilia 270
hemodialysis catheter 31
hemoglobinuria 449
hemophiliac patients 41
hemoptysis 432–3
hemorrhage
  abdominopelvic biopsy 228
  PTD 270–1
  renal biopsy 307, 309
  retroperitoneal 309, 320, 408
  splenoportography 280
hemothorax 45, 108, 282
  PTD 270
  splenoportography 281
Hemovac® suction drain 118
heparin 12, 406
  clot lysis 72
heparin locking 92
hepatic arteriography 413–15
  contraindications 414
  indications 413–14
  postprocedure and follow-up care 415
  technical problems and pitfalls 414–15
  technique 414
hepatic artery
  aneurysm 282
  stenosis (HAS) 456
  thrombosis (HAT) 456, 466
hepatic hemangioma *see* hemangioendothelioma
hepatic necrosis 293
hepatic venography 276–9
  complications 279
  contraindications 276
  equipment 276
  indications 276
  patient preparation 276
  technical variations 277
  technique 277
hepatic venous outflow obstruction 456–7, 459

hepatic venous wedge pressure 277
hepatobiliary injury 272
hepatobiliary interventions 250–96
  hepatic venography 276–9
  outcome measures 252
  partial splenic embolization 294–6, 417, 433, 436
  percutaneous cholecystostomy 259–62
  percutaneous transhepatic biliary dilation 271–5
  percutaneous transhepatic biliary drainage 262–71
  percutaneous transhepatic cholangiography 252–8
  radiology of liver and gallbladder 251–2
  splenoportography 279–81
  transarterial intrahepatic chemoembolization 291–3
  transcholecystic cholangiography 258–9
  transhepatic portal venography (TPV) 281–2
  transjugular intrahepatic portosystemic shunt 286–91
  transjugular liver biopsy 276, 282–6
hepatoblastoma 291
hepatocellular carcinoma 228, 291
hepatofugal flow 280
hiatal hernia 162
Hickman catheter 23
high-flow vascular malformations 415, 419, 422, 438–9
history 1–2
hollow viscera, dilation 229–39
Horner's syndrome 286
horseshoe kidneys 298, 330
hot knife 350, 354
hydrocephalus shunts 76
hydrocodone plus acetaminophen (Lortab®, Vicodin®) 21
hydrocortisone 13
hydromorphone (Dilaudid®) 21
hydronephrosis 298, 301–2, 310–12, 320, 341–2
  percutaneous nephrostomy 309–20
  see also ureteropelvic junction obstruction
hydropneumothorax 335
hydrothorax 335
hypercalciuria 330
hyperoxaluria 330
hyperparathyroidism 330
hypersplenism 279
  embolization therapy *see* splenic embolization

Index

hypertonic saline 208, 325
hypnotic sedatives 18–19
hypocitraturia 330
hypothermia 335, 413

ibuprofen 20, 137, 346
imaging studies
  biplane imaging 14
  bone biopsy 389–90
  cross-sectional imaging 60
  preprocedure imaging see
    preprocedure imaging;
  see also individual modalities
indwelling venous ports 76–85
  complications 84–5
  controversies and issues 86–7
  conversion to CVC 84
  future advances 85–6
  indications 76–7
  insertion 94, 96
    arm port insertion 79–82
    documentation 95
    equipment 77–9, 94
    patient preparation 77
    procedure 95
    site closure 81
    subcutaneous tunnel 77–80
    technical problems and
      pitfalls 81
  postprocedure and follow-up
    care 81
  potential infection 96
  removal 81–4, 95
infantile hemangioma 438
infections
  CRBSI 65–8
  CVC-related 65–8
  fungal 67
  indwelling venous ports 96
  skin 177–81, 189–90
  stent-related 343
  see also abscess
inflammatory bowel disease 200–1
informed consent 10–11
infundibular stenosis 330
infusaports see indwelling venous
    ports
interloop abscess 203–4
internal jugular vein catheters 39,
    42–51
  catheter length 45–7
  catheter migration 46, 48
  equipment 42–3
  patient preparation 43
  postprocedure and follow-up
    care 50
  right internal jugular vein 41
  subcutaneous tunnel 49–50
  technical problems and pitfalls
    50–1
  technique 43–9
  ultrasound-guided access 45, 48
interventional radiology team 8–9
  interventional technologist 9
  mid-level providers 9

pediatric interventional nurse 9
  team leader 8–9
intestinal failure 27
intraperitoneal leakage 175
intrathoracic abscess drainage
    112–18
  complications 112, 118
  contraindications 115
  CT guidance 115
  equipment 115, 118
  indications 112–15
  patient preparation 115
  postprocedure and follow-up
    care 116–18
  technique 115–16
intravascular foreign body 75–6
  localization of catheter
    fragment 76
  sheath size 75
intravenous hyperalimentation
    153
intravenous urography 301
intussusception 176, 179, 182
IR see interventional radiology
    team
irrigation fluid, extravasation 335

J-tube
  buckling 175
  difficult delivery 175
Jamshidi needle 388
jejunostomy
  button 154, 172–4
  percutaneous 168
jejunostomy tube 167
jugular lines 25
jugular vein 27–8
jugular venous access 276–7, 288
juvenile idiopathic arthritis 375,
    377, 382
  triamcinolone in 383

K-wire 390, 401
Kaposi's hemangioendothelioma
    416, 438
Kasabach–Merritt syndrome
    414–15, 417, 438
Katzen wire 470
Keller–Timmermans introducer
    329
ketorolac (Toradol®) 20, 137,
    210, 346, 354, 437
kidneys 298
  agenesis 298
  capsule 299
  cross-fused renal ectopia 298
  horseshoe 298, 330
  mobility 299
  normal relationships 299
  perirenal fat 299
  stones see nephrolithotomy;
    and individual stone
    types
  see also entries under renal
Kirschner wire see K-wire

"kissing balloons" 239
Klebsiella spp. 253, 270
  K. pneumoniae 295
Klippel–Trenaunay syndrome
    443
kyphoscoliosis 179

laboratory studies 12
  preprocedure see preprocedure
    lab studies;
  see also individual procedures
Langerhans cell histiocytosis
    385–6
laparoscopic ablation of renal
    cysts 208, 325
laparoscopic gastrostomy 154
laser techniques 350
latex sensitivity 185
leaks 39
leiomyoma 363
Lesch–Nyhan syndrome 330
lesser sac fluid collections 203
leukocytosis 296
lidocaine 277, 280, 305, 319,
    327–8, 366, 401
  buffered 17
  ELA-Max® cream 17, 184, 199
  EMLA® cream 17, 184, 199
Lipiodol® 293
lipoma 363
liposarcoma 363
liver
  amebic abscess 204
  capsule perforation 286
  radiology 251–2
  see also entries under hepatic
    and hepato-
liver biopsy 220–3
  left lobe 222
  outpatient 228
  right lobe 221, 224
  transjugular see transjugular
    liver biopsy
liver transplantation
  hepatic arteriography 413
  malignant disease 291
  percutaneous drainage 203
  splenoportography 279
local anesthesia 17
  ELA-Max® cream 17, 184, 199
  EMLA® cream 17, 184, 199
  fracture reduction with
    internal fixation 401
  percutaneous nephrostomy 317
  soft tissue foreign body
    removal 366
loop snare 41
Lortab® see hydrocodone plus
    acetaminophen
lymph node biopsy 362–5
  complications 364
  contraindications 363
  equipment 363
  indications 363
  patient preparation 363

postprocedure and follow-up
    care 364
  specimen handling 364
  technique 363–5
lymphatic malformations 442
lymphocele drainage 210

magnetic foreign body removal
    245–8
magnetic resonance see MR
magnetic resonance imaging see
    MRI
malignant fibrous histiocytoma
    363
Malone antegrade colonic enema
    (MACE) 183
Maloney dilator 229
malposition of catheters see
    catheters, malposition
Manan Pro-Mag™ device 216
mandril wire 60, 116, 261, 277,
    312, 335
mannitol 292
Mastisol® 160
May–Thurner syndrome 62,
    461–2
mechanical malfunction 74
  fragmentation 74
  "pinch off" 74–5
  radiographic grading 75
mechanical occlusion 90
mechanical thrombolysis 71
mediastinal fluid drainage
    118–23
  complications 123
  equipment 119
  indications 119
  patient preparation 120
  postprocedure and follow-up
    care 123
  technical variations 121–3
    mediastinal window
      creation 121, 124
    percutaneous balloon
      pericardiotomy 121
  technique 120–1
  see also aspiration and drainage
medication precipitation 90
melena 270
meperidine (Demerol®) 19, 137,
    354
mesenchymoma, malignant 291
metallic stents 140–1
methadone (Dolophine®) 21
methylprednisolone 13
metochlopromide 293
metronidazole 185, 187
micropuncture introducer sets
    42, 406–7
midaortic syndrome 458, 461
midazolam (Versed®) 18
minocycline 66, 208, 325
modular approach 4–7
  completion module 5
  core module 4

transitional module 5
molecular imaging
   abdominopelvic biopsy 217, 219, 227
   musculoskeletal interventions 360
   pulmonary/mediastinal biopsy 133
Monopty® device 216
morphine 21, 210, 293, 354
MR angiography 26, 406, 413
   embolization therapy 422–3
   see also angiography
MR cholangiopancreatography (MRCP) 252–3
MRI 1
   abdominopelvic biopsy 217
   arthrography see arthrography
   bone tumors 394
   embolization therapy 422–3
   hydronephrosis 301
   musculoskeletal interventions 360
   pulmonary/mediastinal biopsy 133
   sclerotherapy of vascular malformations 442
   vascular interventions 406
MRSA 99
mucormycosis 110
multicystic dysplastic kidneys 28
musculoskeletal interventions 356–403
   history 358
   imaging guidance 358–60
      CT 358
      fluoroscopy 358
      molecular imaging 360
      MRI 360
      ultrasound 358
   instruments and devices 360
   interventional radiology 358
   outcome measures 359
myelodysplasia 344
myositis ossificans 363

naloxone (Narcan®) 19–20
Narcan® see naloxone
nasogastric tube feeding 153
nasojejunal tube insertion 2, 153, 159–60
   equipment 159
necrotic tumor 210
necrotizing enterocolitis 235
needles
   abdominopelvic biopsy 216
   bone biopsy 388
   end-cutting 216
   gauge 216
   pulmonary/mediastinal biopsy 126–8
   side-cutting 216
   thoracic aspiration/drainage 102
   see also specific types
Neff introducer 312

neocholedochojejunostomy 275
neonates
   analgesia 21
   atrial clots 73
   catheter-related thrombosis 73
   embolization therapy 435–7
   esophageal stenosis 231–2
   imaging studies 14
   local anesthesia 17
   naloxone 19–20
   renal mobility 299
   renal outflow obstruction 314
   sedation 18
   ureteropelvic junction obstruction 301
nephroblastoma 228
nephrolithotomy 330–6
   complications 335
   contraindications 331
   equipment 331–2
   future advances 335
   indications 330–2
   patient preparation 333
   postprocedure and follow-up care 335
   technical variations 334–5
      caliceal diverticula 334
      pelvic access with large stone burden 334–5
   technique 333–4
nephrostomy catheter 345
nephrostomy drains 314–15
   insertion 2
nephrostomy, percutaneous 309–20
   complications 319–20
   contraindications 310
   equipment 311–16
   indications 310–14
   outcome measures 318
   patient preparation 315–16
   postprocedure and follow-up care 318–19
      catheter exchange and accidental dislodgment 319
      catheter security 318
   technique 316–18
      access to renal pelvis 316–17
      anesthesia 317
      catheter insertion 318
      infants 317
      route planning 317–18
      transrenal access 317
nephrostomy tract dilation 328–30
   complications 329
   equipment 329
   indications 328
   patient preparation 329
   technique 329
nephrotic syndrome 44
nesidioblastosis 281
neuroblastoma 224, 226, 302
neurofibromatosis 363, 458, 461

neuropathy 449
Newton wire 116, 314
NICH see non-involuting congenital hemangioma
Nissen fundoplication 230
nitinol snare 160–1
nitinol stent 144
nitinol wire 60, 116
nitrogen washout 108
nitroglycerine 406, 409, 437
nodular fasciitis 363
non-involuting congenital hemangioma (NICH) 422, 438
non-steroidal anti-inflammatory drugs see NSAIDs
Notec® see chloral hydrate
NSAIDs 12
nutcracker syndrome of renal vein 464

occlusion of catheters see catheters, occlusion; catheters, tip occlusion
occlusive dressings 67, 105
occult transfixation of small bowel/colon 174–5
OK-432 111
olive oil 111
Onyx® 419
"open book" pelvic fractures 400
open surgical pleurodesis 111
opioid analgesics 19
   morphine 21, 210, 293, 354
Opsite® dressing 105, 167, 319, 437
orthopedic interventions 380–403
   bone biopsy 385–92
   bone tumors
      excision 392–7
      locoregional thermal ablation 397–9
   cystic lesions 380–5
   percutaneous reduction with internal fixation 399–403
oscillating thrombectomy systems 469
osteoblastoma 391
osteoid osteoma 4
   excision 392–7
osteomyelitis 388
osteosarcoma 68, 386
   parosteal 386
   periosteal 386
OstyCore® needle 388
OstyCut® needle 388
outpatient liver biopsy 228
oximeter 408–9
oxycodone (Percocet®) 21

padding 15
pain management 20–1
   patient-controlled analgesia (PCA) 296
   see also individual drugs

Palmaz® stent 144, 287
pancreatic biopsy 224–5
pancreatic pseudocyst 205, 208
pancreatitis 203, 293
papaverine 406, 414
paracentesis 199
parapneumonic effusion 101–5
paravertebral vein 27
parotid gland 369
partial splenic embolization 294–6, 417, 433, 436
partial thromboplastin time 254
particulate embolic agents 381, 418–19
patent ductus arteriosus 281
patient positioning 15
patient preparation 10–12
   general principles 10
   informed consent 10–11
   laboratory studies 12
   NPO status 11
   pregnancy testing 12
   preprocedure medications 12
   prophylactic antibiotics 12
   see also individual procedures
patient safety 12–15
   contrast reactions 12–13
   general principles 10
   premedication 12–13
      emergency 13
   radiation dose management see radiation safety
patient-controlled analgesia (PCA) 296
Pedialyte® 169
pediatric interventional nurse 9
pelvic abscess 199–201
   inflammatory bowel disease 200–1
   transgluteal drainage 199–201
   transrectal drainage 199–200, 202
pelvic pressure 320
pelvic ring fractures 400
   "open book" 400
   see also fracture reduction with internal fixation
pentobarbital sodium (Nembutal®) 18–19
Percocet® see oxycodone
percutaneous thrombin embolization 451, 454
percutaneous transluminal angioplasty 456–64
   see also angioplasty and stenting
percutaneous transluminal dilation 336
periappendiceal abscess 201
pericardiocentesis 118–23
   complications 123
   CT guidance 121
   equipment 119
   indications 119
   patient preparation 120

Index

pericardiocentesis (cont.)
  postprocedure and follow-up care 123
  technical variations 121–3
    mediastinal window creation 121, 124
    percutaneous balloon pericardiotomy 121
  technique 120–1
perineal injuries 433
peripheral nerve sheath tumors 363
peripheral pulses 407
peripherally accessed system ports 77
peripherally inserted central catheters *see* PICCs
perirenal fat 299
peritonitis
  abdominopelvic biopsy 228
  gastrostomy 175, 181
  percutaneous cecostomy 189–90
PET 1
PET-CT 198
  soft tissue biopsy 363
PICCs 27–39
  blood drawing 25–88
  catheter measurement 36
  complications 38–9
    accidental dislodgment 86
    catheter dysfunction 38–9
    catheter-related thrombophlebitis 38
  equipment 32
  indications 27–9, 32
  patient preparation 30–3
  postprocedure and follow-up care 36–7
  removal 36–7
  technical problems and pitfalls 37–8
  technical variations 36
  technique 33–6
    angled glide wire 36
    modified bent guide wire technique 35
    ultrasound-guided access 34–5
pigmented villonodular synovitis 363
pigtail catheter 315–16, 318
"pinch off" 74–5
plasmapheresis 42
platelet count 254
platelet dysfunction 12
platelet-rich plasma 376
Pleur-evac® drain 105
pleural effusion 98–9
pleural fluid collections *see* thoracic aspiration and drainage
pleurodesis
  chemical 109, 111
  open surgical 111

pneumatocele 114
pneumonia 99, 110
  parapneumonic effusion 101–5
pneumonostomy 112
pneumopericardium 108
pneumoperitoneum 176
pneumothorax 105, 108, 282, 335
  biopsy-related 137
  chemical pleurodesis 109
  PTD 270
  splenoportography 281
polidocanol 376
polyvalent pneumococcal vaccine (Pneumovax®) 295
polyvinyl alcohol particles 381, 418
portal hypertension 280, 286, 290, 414
portal overperfusion 288
portosystemic gradient 277
ports 2, 25
positron emission tomography *see* PET
postembolization syndrome 293, 296, 417
postprocedure lab studies 107
postradiotherapy arteritis 458
post-transplant lymphoproliferative disease 306
Potts–Cournand type needles 406–7
povidone–iodine (Betadine®) 295
power tools 360
prednisone 13, 442
pregnancy testing 12
premedication 12–13
  emergency 13
preprocedure imaging
  percutaneous cecostomy 185–6
  thoracic aspiration/drainage 101, 104
preprocedure lab studies
  pericardial/mediastinal fluid drainage 120
  thoracic aspiration/drainage 101
preprocedure medications 12
pressure sores 411
prilocaine 17
priscoline 414
prothrombin time 254
pseudoaneurysm ablation 449–56
  complications 454
  indications 451
  postprocedure and follow-up care 454
  technique 451–3
    endovascular embolization 453, 455
    percutaneous thrombin embolization 451, 454

  protection of parent artery 451–3
pseudodiverticulum 237
Pseudomonas spp. 67, 253, 270
  P. aeruginosa 114
psoas hemorrhage 308
PTC *see* transhepatic cholangiography, percutaneous
PTD *see* transhepatic biliary drainage, percutaneous
pulmonary arteriovenous malformations 429
pulmonary artery stenosis 63
pulmonary embolism 472
pulmonary nodules 130
  marking for resection 137–40
    complications 140
    equipment 138
    indications 138
    patient preparation 138
    postprocedure and follow-up care 139
    technical variations 139
    technique 138–9
pulmonary sequestration 417
pulmonary/mediastinal biopsy 123–37
  complications 137
  contraindications 126
  equipment 126–8
    core biopsy needles 126–8
    FNAB needles 126–7
  imaging modalities 130–3
    CT 131–2, 135
    molecular imaging 133
    MR 133
    ultrasound 133
  indications 125–6
  patient preparation 128–9
  postprocedure and follow-up care 136–7
  specimen handling 134
  technical variations 134–6
  technique 130, 133
    chronic lung disease 130
    pulmonary nodules 130
pulse Doppler monitor 10, 408–9
pulse oximetry 406
push–pull gastrostomy 168
pyeloplasty 301
pyloric stenosis 235–6
pyonephrosis 319

Quick-Core® semi-automated needle 216

radiation fibrosis 271
radiation safety 13–15
  alternative modalities 13
  appropriate focal spot rating 14
  biplane imaging 14
  collimation 14
  dose-dependent radiation injury 13

  effective use 13
  filters 14
  grids 14
  limiting image number 14
  limiting redundant imaging 14
  optimization of hardware and imaging configuration 14
  prompt "stand down" 14
  shielding 14–15
ranula treatment 370–5
  complications 375
  contraindications 371
  equipment 371, 373
  future advances 375
  indications 371–2
  patient preparation 371
  postprocedure and follow-up care 373–5
  technique 373–4
    partial gland ablation 373
    sclerotherapy 373
rapidly involuting congenital hemangioma (RICH) 422, 438
reflux 39
regional anesthesia 17
  soft tissue foreign body removal 366
renal arteries 299
  ablation 417, 433
  stenosis 458, 461
renal biopsy 304–9
  complications 306–10
  equipment 304
  indications 304
  patient preparation 304
  postprocedure and follow-up care 306, 308
  technique 304, 305–7
renal cysts 205–9, 324–8
  complications 328
  diagnosis 206
  imaging features 325
  indications for therapy 325–6
  percutaneous treatment 325–6
    disadvantages 326
    equipment 326
    image-guided aspiration 208
    laparoscopic ablation 208, 325
    patient preparation 327
    postprocedure and follow-up care 327–8
    retrograde marsupialization 208, 325
    sclerotherapy 208, 325
    standard protocol 327
    surgical 207
renal failure 31
renal pelvis 299
  perforation 335
  transrenal access 317
renal transplantation, percutaneous nephrostomy 318

renal vein
  nutcracker syndrome 464
  renin sampling 465
Replicare® dressing 180
repositioning of catheters 69, 71
restraints 406
reteplase 469
retrograde gastrostomy 165–7
retrograde marsupialization of renal cysts 208, 325
retroperitoneal hemorrhage 309, 320, 408
retropharyngeal abscess 119
rhabdomyosarcoma 291, 363
rheolytic thrombectomy systems 469
RICH see rapidly involuting congenital hemangioma
rifampin 66
Roadrunner® wire 116, 314, 327
Romazicon® see flumazenil
Rosen wire 116, 314, 327, 338
Ross needle 285
rotating hemostatic valve 60, 352
rotational thrombectomy systems 469
rubella syndrome 458
Rutner adapter 329
Rutner valve 352

safety devices 10
salivary glands
  chemodenervation 368–70
  parotid gland 369
  partial ablation 370–5
  ranula 370–5
  submandibular gland 369–70
Savory–Gilliard bougie 229
schwannoma 363
scimitar syndrome 417, 429
scintigraphy, gastric 158
sclerosing agents 325, 328, 381, 438
  see also individual agents
sclerosing cholangitis 271
sclerotherapy of renal cysts 208, 210, 325
  disadvantages 209
  equipment 209
  treatment approach 209
sclerotherapy of salivary ranula 370–5
  contraindications 371
  equipment 371, 373
  patient preparation 371
  technique 373
sclerotherapy of vascular malformations 438–49
  complications 449–50
  equipment 442, 445
  future advances 449
  indications 438–41, 443
  patient preparation 442
  postprocedure and follow-up care 448–9

technical problems and pitfalls 449
technical variations 444–8
  bleomycin 445, 447
  sodium tetradecyl sulfate 444
  varicocele sclerotherapy 447–9
technique 442–3, 445–6
scoliosis 392
sedation 15–21
  complications 19
  emergence delirium 19
  risk index classification 16
  see also individual drugs
sedation formulary 16–19
  anxiolytics 17–18
  hypnotic sedatives 18–19
  opioid analgesics 19
  postprocedure pain management 20–1
  reversal agents 19–21
  topical, local, tumescent and regional anesthesia 17
sepsis 67
  percutaneous nephrostomy 319
septic arthritis 37
septic thrombophlebitis 67
septicemia 67
shielding 14–15
side-cutting needles 216
silastic catheters 47
silastic stents 345
silicone catheters 47
silicone stents 140
silver nitrate 111, 203
single wire method 36
skin irritation/infection
  cecostomy site 189–90
  gastrostomy site 177–81
skin necrosis 449
slow-flow vascular malformations 438–9
snares
  embolization therapy 437
  gooseneck 61
  loop 41
  nitinol 160–1
  transfemoral 39
sodium morrhuate 208, 325
sodium tetradechol 325
sodium tetradecyl sulfate 208, 325, 328, 381, 438, 444
sodium thiosulphate 293
soft tissue aspiration and drainage 360–2
  complications 362
  equipment 360
  indications 360
  patient preparation 360
  postprocedure and follow-up care 362
  technique 361–2
soft tissue biopsy 362–5

complications 364
contraindications 363
equipment 363
indications 363
patient preparation 363
postprocedure and follow-up care 364
specimen handling 364
technique 363–5
soft tissue foreign body removal 365–8
  complications 367
  equipment 365–6
  indications 365–6
  patient preparation 366
  postprocedure and follow-up care 367
  technical variations 366
  technique 366–7
soft tissue tumors 389
solid organ abscess 203–6
SorbaView® dressing 105, 319
specimen handling
  abdominopelvic biopsy 227
  pulmonary/mediastinal biopsy 134
  soft tissue biopsy 364
spina bifida 183
spindle cell hemangioma 438
splenectomy 294
splenic abscess 204, 207
splenic biopsy 223–4
splenic embolization 417
  partial 294–6, 417, 433, 436
    complications 296
    contraindications 294
    equipment 294
    indications 294
    patient preparation 295
    postprocedure and follow-up care 295–6
    technique 295
  total 294, 417
splenic rupture 280
splenic vein occlusion 414
splenomegaly 280
splenoportography 279–81
  complications 280–1
  contraindications 279
  equipment 279
  indications 279
  patient preparation 279
  postprocedure and follow-up care 280
  technical problems and pitfalls 280
  technique 280
spring-loaded biopsy device 216
staghorn calculus 330, 333
Staphylococcus spp. 112
  S. aureus 67, 99, 387
    methicillin-resistant see MRSA
  S. epidermidis 67, 295
StatSeal® powder 409

Steinman pin 390, 395
stents
  infection 343
  metallic 140–1
  migration 347–8
  occlusion 347
  silastic 343
  silicone 140
  tracheobronchial 140
  see also angioplasty and stenting; and specific types
stent insertion
  biliary stents 275
  tracheobronchial stents 140
  ureteral stents 2, 341–8
Steri-Strips® 408
sterile technique 66–7
Stevens–Johnson syndrome 234
stoma ulceration 175, 179
stomach see entries under gastric
Strecker stent 287
Streptococcus spp.
  S. pneumoniae 99
  S. pyogenes 99
streptodornase 109
streptokinase 72, 109, 465–72
subclavian vein catheters 28, 39, 41, 51–2
  equipment and patient preparation 51
  postprocedure and follow-up care 52
  technical variations 52
  technique 51–2
subcutaneous tunnel 49–50
  indwelling venous ports 77–80
Sublimaze® see fentanyl citrate
submandibular gland 369–70
subphrenic abscess 203, 205
suction drains 118
superior mesenteric vein occlusion 414
superior vena cava 26
supplies see equipment and supplies
supraventricular tachycardia 286
surgical anti-reflux procedures 157
surgical gastrostomy 153, 155
  complications 176
Surgicel® pads 409
synovial cell sarcoma 104
systemic pulmonary arterial supply 429, 431

T-lok® needle 388
Takayasu arteritis 458
talc 111, 208, 325
tamponade 318
tandem needle biopsy 134–6, 363
tape bridge 106
tears 39
Tegaderm® dressing 105, 167, 319, 408, 437

tenecteplase 469
tension pneumothorax 108
tetanus toxoid prophylaxis 367
tetracycline 111, 208, 325
Thal-Quick catheter 105–6
thermal ablation of bone tumors 397–9
  complications 399
  equipment 397
  indications 397–8
  patient preparation 397
  postprocedure and follow-up care 398
  technique 397, 399
thoracic aspiration and drainage 98–108
  complications 107–8
    chylothorax 108
    hemothorax 108
    pneumothorax 108
  empyema 99–100
  equipment 100–1
    access needles 102
    drainage catheters 103
  indications 100
  outcome measures 107
  patient preparation 101
    preprocedure imaging 101, 104
    preprocedure lab studies 101
  pleural effusion 98–9
  postprocedure and follow-up care 105–7
    catheters 105
    laboratory studies 107
  technique 101–5
thoracic interventions 97
  history 98
  interventional radiology 98
  marking lesions for resection 137–40
  see also specific interventions
thoracic transcatheter therapies
  chemical pleurodesis 109, 111
  chemotherapy 109
  complications 112
  equipment and patient preparation 110
  fibrinolysis 109–11
  indications 109–10
  postprocedure and follow-up care 111
  technique 110–11
  thrombolysis 109
thrombolysis 70–3, 465–72
  catheter design 72
  complications 471
  equipment 466–9
  indications 466–7
  intracavitary 109
  mechanical 71
  patient preparation 469–70
  postprocedure and follow-up care 471

technical problems and pitfalls 471
  technique 470–1
thrombophlebitis
  catheter-related 38
  septic 67
thrombosis
  catheter-related 73–4
    catheter position 74
    catheter stay duration 73
    mechanisms 73
  deep venous 26, 73–4, 472
thrombotic thrombocytopenic purpura 42
thrombus, tip occlusion 39–41
thyroglossal duct cysts 371
TIPS see transjugular intrahepatic portosystemic shunt
tissue adhesive 419
tissue plasminogen activator (tPA) 40, 99, 411, 465, 469
  catheter declotting 70, 72
topical anesthesia 17
Toradol® see ketorolac
total splenic embolization 294, 417
Towbin nephrostomy drain 315
tracheobronchial remnant 231–2
tracheobronchial stents 140
  complications 149–50
  equipment 144, 146
  indications 141–4
  issues and controversies 150
  metallic 140–1
  patient preparation 146
  postprocedure and follow-up care 149
  removal 141, 149
  silicone 140
  technique 146–9
    airway dilatation 146–9
    stent insertion 149
tracheobronchomalacia 141
tracheoesophageal fistula 232–3
tract seeding 228
transarterial intrahepatic chemoembolization (TACE) 291–3
  complications 293
  equipment 292
  indications 292
  patient preparation 292
  postprocedure and follow-up care 293
  technical variations 293
  technique 292–3
transbrachiocephalic access 54–5, 58
transcholecystic cholangiography (TCC) 258–9
  indications 258
  postprocedure and follow-up care 259
  technique 258–9

transcolonic puncture 174
transfemoral snare 39
transgluteal pelvic drainage 199
transhepatic access 58–9
  complications 65
  postprocedure and follow-up care 59
  ultrasound guidance 58
transhepatic biliary dilation, percutaneous (PTBD) 271–5
  complications 275
  equipment 272
  indications 271
  patient preparation 272
  postprocedure and follow-up care 274
  technical variations 273–5
    impassable strictures 273
  technique 272–3
transhepatic biliary drainage, percutaneous (PTD) 262–71
  complications 270–1
    bile leak 270
    catheter blockage 270
    hemorrhage 270–1
    pleural 270
  equipment 265, 267
  indications 263–4, 266
  postprocedure and follow-up care 270
  technical variations 269
  technique 265–9
    double-stick method 265–9
    single-stick method 265
transhepatic cholangiography, percutaneous (PTC) 252–8
  complications 258
  contraindications 253
  equipment 253–4
  indications 253
  patient preparation 253–4
  postprocedure and follow-up care 257
  technical variations 257
    carbon dioxide as contrast agent 257
    left lateral (subxiphoid) approach 257
  technique 254–7
    fluoroscopic guidance 255–7
    ultrasound guidance 255–6
transhepatic portal venography (TPV) 281–2
  complications 282
  contraindications 281
  equipment 281
  indications 281
  postprocedure and follow-up care 282
  technique 281–3

transjugular intrahepatic portosystemic shunt (TIPS) 286–91
  complications 290–1
  contraindications 287
  equipment 287
  indications 286–7
  patient preparation 287
  postprocedure and follow-up care 289
  technical problems and pitfalls 289
  technical variations 289
  technique 287–90
transjugular liver biopsy (TJLB) 276, 282–6
  complications 286
  equipment 284
  indications 284
  patient preparation 284
  postprocedure and follow-up care 286
  technical variations 285–6
    needle curvature 285
    ultrasound guidance 286
  technique 284–5
translumbar access 59–61
  ultrasound guidance 60
transplant vascular stenosis 456–8
  hepatic artery stenosis 456
  hepatic artery thrombosis 456, 466
  hepatic venous outflow obstruction 456–7, 459
transrectal drainage 199–200, 202
trapdoor catheter 187–8
Trellis™ thrombectomy system 469
trephine 389, 391
Treratola™ thrombectomy system 469
triamcinolone (Aristospan®) 383
trisomy-21 40
tumescent anesthesia 17
Tuoehy–Borst rotating hemostatic valve 60

ultrasonic Doppler flow detector 408
ultrasound 1, 5–7, 10
  abdominopelvic biopsy 216–17
  antegrade (pull) gastrostomy 160
  arthrography 379, 382
  aspiration and fluid drainage 195
  central venous catheters 26
    difficult access 58, 60
    internal jugular vein 45, 48
    PICCs 34–5
  hydronephrosis 301
  musculoskeletal interventions 358

nephrostomy 316
PTC 255–6
pulmonary/mediastinal biopsy 133
renal cyst aspiration 208
sclerotherapy of vascular malformations 442
soft tissue biopsy 363
thoracic interventions 98
transjugular liver biopsy 286
umbilical artery catheter-related aortic thrombosis 470
umbilical venous catheters 210
unicameral bone cysts 380
  see also bone cyst therapy
ureteral balloon dilation 336–41
  complications 339
  equipment 337
  indications 336–7
  patient preparation 337
  postprocedure and follow-up care 339
  technique 337–40
ureteral opening pressure 323
ureteral perforation 335
ureteral stent insertion 2, 341–8
  complications 347–9
  equipment 343, 345
  indications 341–4
  patient preparation 343

postprocedure and follow-up care 345–7
technique 343–6, 348
ureteroenteric anastomic strictures 330
ureteronephroscopy 336
ureteropelvic junction obstruction 299–304, 330, 350
  lower pole crossing vessels 301
  see also endopyelotomy
urine leakage 320
urinoma 320
urokinase 72, 99, 109, 465
uterine sound 49

VACTERL association 232, 300
van Andel catheter 338
vancomycin 12
varicocele sclerotherapy 447–9
vascular interventions 404–76
  angiography 405–13
  angioplasty and stenting 456–65
  arterial embolization 415–38
  hepatic arteriography 413–15
  pseudoaneurysm ablation 449–56

sclerotherapy 438–49
vena caval filters 472–6
vascular malformations
  embolization therapy 415, 419, 422
  high-flow 415, 419, 422, 438–9
  sclerotherapy 438–49
  slow-flow 438–9
VATS see video-assisted thoracoscopic surgery
vena caval filters 472–6
  complications 475–6
  contraindications 472
  equipment 472, 474
  indications 472–3
  patient preparation 474
  postprocedure and follow-up care 475–6
  technique 474–5
venography 33
venospasm 37
venous compression syndromes 460–4
venous recanalization 61–2
  equipment 61
  patient preparation 61
  postprocedure and follow-up care 62–5
  technique 61–4
venous thrombosis 73
Versed® see midazolam

Vicodin® see hydrocodone plus acetaminophen
video-assisted thoracoscopic surgery (VATS) 99
vitamin K 12, 254

Wallstent® 144, 287
warfarin 12
warming devices 10, 406
Whitaker (pressure–flow) perfusion test 2, 320–4
  complications 324
  equipment 321
  indications 321
  patient preparation 321
  postprocedure and follow-up care 323
  technical problems and pitfalls 324
  technical variations 323
  technique 321–3
    one-needle 322–3
    perfusion measurement 323
    two-needle 322
Williams syndrome 458
wires 10
wooden chest syndrome 19

Yueh sheathed needle 327

Z-stent 287